Ethics in Medicine

Ethics in Medicine

Historical Perspectives and Contemporary Concerns

edited by

Stanley Joel Reiser,
Arthur J. Dyck,
and
William J. Curran

The MIT Press
Cambridge, Massachusetts,
and London, England

Copyright © 1977 by
The Massachusetts Institute of
Technology

This book was set in VIP Optima by
DEKR Corporation and printed
and bound by Murray Printing Company
in the United States of America.

Second printing, 1977

Library of Congress Cataloging in
Publication Data
Main entry under title:

Ethics in medicine.

   Includes bibliographical references and
index.
   1. Medical ethics—Addresses, essays,
lectures. 2. Medical ethics—History—
Sources. I. Reiser, Stanley Joel. II. Dyck,
Arthur J., 1932–   . III. Curran, William J.
[DNLM: 1. Ethics, Medical. 2. Ethics,
Medical—History. 3. Physician-patient
relations. W50 E843]
R724.E823   174'.2   77–1876
ISBN 0-262-18081-2
ISBN 0-262-18081-2 (hardcover)
ISBN 0-262-68029-7 (paperback)

Contents

I. Ethical Dimensions of the Physician-Patient Relationship through History

VI. Procreative Decisions

VII. Suffering and Dying

Foreword

Eunice Kennedy Shriver and Sargent Shriver

Ethics is the oldest intellectual discipline in the Judeo-Christian tradition. The most distinguished thinkers of Western culture, such as Plato, Aristotle, and Aquinas, have devoted themselves to discovering the ethical principles of human behavior. It is gratifying that men and women of intelligence and insight are now bringing their minds to bear on the complex ethical problems of our own era. This book is a compilation of some of the most significant work that has been done in medical ethics. The Joseph P. Kennedy, Jr. Foundation is proud to give it its endorsement and support.

Cutting across the major disciplines of moral, legal, scientific, and religious thought, this book provides a universal context within which our individual human impulses can find their best expression. For some the vision of that context is humanistic; for others it is religious. For the humanistic vision, human life is intrinsically valuable. For the religious vision, human life is God's gift and receives its value from God. But those who locate their ethics within either vision can work together to discern and implement their fundamental ethical principles.

This book provides significant answers to troubling and difficult questions of human values. How should we distribute our national resources? How should we decide who receives medical care? Who is to be experimented on? How should severely handicapped infants be cared for? What are our duties to the powerless if we are to move beyond the boundaries of mere utility and declare ourselves a caring and just society?

The literature of medical ethics is not easily available to the student or the professional who is in need of wisdom, understanding, and intellectual support for his decisions. Even as medical ethics courses proliferate, the issues which demand ethical solutions grow more complex and far-reaching in their significance.

There is, for instance, the problem of human experimentation. Is there any ethical basis, as well as a legal or social basis, for experimentation on the retarded; on prisoners; on the fetus which will be aborted anyway? Those who measure human worth in terms of usefulness, or cost-effectiveness alone, see no conflict in treating the retarded, the poor, the imprisoned, and the aged, as objects, not as persons.

There is the problem of medical treatment. Should a kidney machine be available to a child with Down's syndrome (mongolism) as readily as to a businessman of 45? The utilitarian would say no, for the child with Down's syndrome cannot make a contribution to society that is equal to the businessman's contribution. But who will say yes? Which lawyer, which physician, which scientist, which theologian, which parent or child will say that the child with Down's syndrome is equally deserving? That that child, too, is a person, not an object; a human being equally worthy of our respect and our protection?

Science and technology have explored the atom, carried us to the stars, conquered the seas, and overcome famine and plague. Yet, without an acceptance of the ethical principles such as those examined in this book—dignity, respect for human life, equality, justice, sacrifice—science and technology alone will never give that affirmation without which the lives of all of us, at some time, will be in jeopardy.

At a time when the calculus of utility and cost-effectiveness dominates our value systems, it is refreshing to see the worth of every human being so strongly affirmed and so stoutly defended. For those of us who labor on behalf of the mentally retarded, the old, the sick, the helpless, this book articulates in many ways a rationale for doing so.

It is our hope that it may encourage many others, students and professionals alike, to recognize that, in the words of Jean Vanier, "A society which does not care for its weaker members is a society which lives in illusion. A society which rejects the weak is a society committing suicide."

Preface

We now are witnessing an unprecedented concern for human rights in the provision of medical care and the advancement of medical knowledge. This anthology of readings in medical ethics is one result of this concern. It explores the moral and ethical foundations of medical practice and medical science.

The readings are drawn from works in philosophical and religious ethics, history, political science, law, medicine, and biology. Most of the selections are republished in their entirety; several essays appear here for the first time. Illustrative cases that discuss moral problems raised in the readings follow most topically arranged sections. Most of the readings were first assembled for teaching medical ethics to undergraduate and graduate students at Harvard University whose academic focus ranged from the sciences to the humanities. This anthology, then, has been designed for people having diverse backgrounds and a broad range of interests in medical ethics.

No single criterion has been decisive in determining which selections have been included and which excluded from this anthology. Some selections were chosen because they have had or continue to have a significant place in the development of medical ethics and medical standards; some because they make a point in a concise and telling way; some because they both amuse and enlighten the reader; and some because they seemed to us to exhibit the best scholarship in a brief compass on the topic under discussion. These selections, though sometimes poised in opposition to one another, are designed to encourage and nourish, by way of reasoned discourse and investigation, our most humane impulses within the practice of medicine and medical ethics.

We acknowledge with gratitude the generous and continuing support since 1971 of the Joseph P. Kennedy, Jr. Foundation. Our thanks are given also to the National Endowment for the Humanities for its substantial assistance from 1972 to 1975.

Various persons have contributed in countless ways in bringing this anthology to fruition, some of whom we wish to identify for their particularly significant contributions. We owe more than we can say here to Eunice Kennedy Shriver, R. Sargent Shriver, Robert E. Cooke, and Robert Montague, all of the Kennedy Foundation, who have been a profound source of encouragement to us in all our work, in the preparation of this anthology, and in the development of the course out of which it grew. So often they shared with warmth and good humor their experiences and wisdom regarding the moral issues that are discussed in this book. Sissela Bok, while a Kennedy Fellow with the Interfaculty Program at Harvard, helped select readings and shared in the teaching of our first lecture course in medical ethics; she has continued to be a highly valued consultant. Larry Miller was a student assistant in gathering and assessing readings for that lecture course. Steven Anderson took the course as a student, and subsequently, as a research assistant, read and reread numerous selections with a view to their inclusion and exclusion. Barbara Goroll, Ilse Fersing, and Najla Salhaney provided indispensible assistance in helping to locate articles, typing, and preparing the manuscript. None of these people should be held responsible for our errors, but all of them have contributed to what we trust justifies this anthology and commends it to our readers.

Introduction

The term "medical ethics" is currently being used in a variety of ways. In one of its oldest but still current usages, medical ethics refers to a body of thinking and codes of conduct developed by the medical profession. Self-conscious reflection on standards of conduct is one of the defining characteristics of a profession. Therefore, it is not surprising that the development of medical ethics as a form of professional self-regulation has a history as long and venerable as the history of medicine itself. The Hippocratic Oath and modern codes of medical ethics, some of which are reproduced in this anthology, are visible evidence of the long span and continuity of medical ethics as an area of professional concern and activity.

Systematic intellectual reflection on what is right and wrong in the practice of medicine has also occurred within religious and philosophical ethics. From their very beginning the Jewish and Christian traditions in the West had a great deal to say about illness, healing, and the role of physicians and other health professionals, both in relation to patients and also to the larger society. During the medieval period, for example, Christianity rejected the Greek practice of reserving the best medical services for elites; the Christian tradition insisted on equal treatment for patients regardless of their ability to pay or their social status. In the writings of theologians and philosophers concerned with ethical issues, many of the contemporary moral dilemmas arising in the practice of medicine have been and are extensively discussed: special problems associated with the care of the dying; questions about the surgical removal of certain organs or the destruction of bodily functions—sterilization is a prime example; issues involving the taking of human life, which are raised by such practices as infanticide, abortion, and euthanasia; and the moral dilemmas that accompany the use of such medical innovations as organ transplantation, dialysis machines, and respirators.

Although the idea still persists that medical ethics is restricted to what is thought and practiced by health professionals, a critical reflection on moral issues in the practice of medicine is more lively today in fields outside medicine than at any other time in the modern period. New scientific, social, and legal developments have directed the attention of society to the values that inform medical decisions and have prompted health professionals to join with patients and experts in other disciplines to work toward resolving the moral problems of medical care. For example, the increasing use of sophisticated technology that maintains physiological existence in the midst of almost total cessation of brain function has led to a reexamination of euthanasia. Public debate over the controversial question of the right of women to have abortions has reemerged, a partial product of the human rights movements of the 1950s and 1960s. Concern about the rights of subjects in the conduct of human experimentation has become a matter of widespread discussion as a result of publicly aired abuses. And a belief in the right to a high standard of health care, which also became a powerful force in the United States in the 1960s, has prompted reflections and court decisions on the duties and obligations involved in the provision of health care.

As a result of these public concerns and the private reflections and discussions of physicians, medical ethics as understood by the medical profession has taken a new fork in the road from which it has not yet turned back, if it ever will. Medical journals now publish increasing numbers of articles in which physicians openly explore their thinking and practices concerning their ethical relationship to individual patients and to the general public, on issues such as abortion, euthanasia, eugenics, triage, and the cost-effectiveness of medical procedures. It is no wonder the ethicists, philosophers, lawyers, and other scholars, fortified by considerable access to the thinking and practices of medicine provided by more candid professionals, have stepped up their activities in the name of medical ethics. Indeed, there are invitations from the medical profession itself that bring their writings into the medical journals and, more recently, into the curriculum and ongoing intellectual dialogue of medical schools and teaching hospitals.

It is our position that medical ethics is fundamentally grounded in the moral principles and standards of reason that are a part of ethics generally, and in the cumulative wisdom and experience of medical knowledge and practice. The selections in this anthology cover all the topics and viewpoints presented in this introduction as well as many others arising in medicine. In keeping with the understanding of medical ethics that shapes this anthology, the writings of medical professionals, ethicists, philosophers, lawyers, sociologists, economists, and representatives from other disciplines are featured. The historical material provides a perspective regarding the persistence of certain themes, debates, and modes of argumentation.

I

Ethical Dimensions of the Physician-Patient Relationship through History

Introduction to Part I

The conduct resulting from a physician's sense of justice and morality and his responsiveness to fulfilling actions required by a promise or a contract have been periodically discussed in medical history—in oaths that tersely enumerate responsible and irresponsible medical acts and in monographs that discuss the general duties and obligations of physicians.

Many of the important works we possess on medicine that were products of the ancient world are found in the collection of documents known as the *Corpus Hippocraticum*. This material, largely written from the fifth to fourth century B.C., may represent the remains of the library of the Hippocratic school of medicine. Some of these works bear the stamp of a genius, Hippocrates, who was born on the Greek island of Cos in about 460 B.C. He belonged to a guild of physicians called the Asclepiadae. He traveled widely throughout Greece and was a well-known and widely sought healer during his life, which is reported variously to have spanned 85, 90, 104, or 109 years. Aristotle called him "the Great Hippocrates." Little more is known about the life of Hippocrates. Paradoxically, the oath that bears his name, which we reproduce along with other Hippocratic selections, probably was not written by him but more likely by the Pythagoreans, a philosophical sect started in the latter part of the fourth century B.C. Yet the approximation of the moral ideals expressed in the Hippocratic Oath with those of the early Christians perhaps accounts for the attention to and longevity of the oath in the Western world.

The archetype of a Christian version of the Hippocratic Oath was probably composed sometime during the first several centuries of the Christian era. The differences and similarities between the Greek and Christian Hippocratic oaths are interesting. The pagan version begins with an invocation to the deities Apollo, Asclepius, Health, and Panacea; the Christian oath begins by praising God the Father and Jesus Christ. It does not mention the pledge made by those who swore to the pagan version, to share their learning only with their own sons, the sons of their teachers, or those who had taken the oath. To Christians, who believed in brotherhood and universal benevolence, this statement probably seemed to stress elitism and trade-unionism. Still, both versions condemn abortion and euthanasia, emphasize decency and confidentiality as necessary qualifications for a medical practitioner, and promise fame to the healer who fulfills these obligations.

Three documents from the late Middle Ages are included in this section. Reproduced first is the law to regulate the practice of medicine, issued in the year 1240 or 1241 by Frederick II, Emperor of the Holy Roman Empire. It established stringent requirements for the learners and practitioners of medicine and sounds modern in tone and content. The high ideals that Frederick's law contains stand in contrast to the values expressed in the treatise *De Cautelis Medicorum* attributed to Arnald of Villanova (1235?–1311) and to the ethics of medical practice by the French surgeon Henri de Mondeville (1260–1320). A literary analysis of *De Cautelis Medicorum* suggests that it is a compendium of several texts by different hands. Probably these texts were materials assembled by Arnald for a treatise he never completed, but which was circulated by others under his name after he died. The treatise discusses the bedside manners of medieval physicians and patients, particularly the actions physicians might take against patients who tested the doctor's medical knowledge with the urine they brought him to examine. The evaluation of disease by inspecting the external character of a patient's urine, widely used in diagnosis at this time, often led to deceit by patient and doctor alike.

The moral conduct of surgeons, who were lower in social and professional standing than physicians, is discussed by Henri de Mondeville. His great concern about the doctor's fee in part demonstrates how difficult it was to collect in this period. But the emphasis that he and Arnald place on protecting the healer's self-interests contrasts sharply with the concern for the social image of medicine that preoccupied both Samuel Bard and Thomas Percival. Bard (1742–1821), a distinguished professor of medicine at the newly formed Kings College of Medicine in New York, and Percival (1740–1804), a well-known English physician to the Manchester Infirmary, both argued that good moral conduct benefited practitioner, profession, and patient. They called for high-principled behavior in dealing with the sick and disdained trickery.

Percival's treatise was a prototype for a number of codes of medical ethics. It particularly influenced the content of the code discussed by the American Medical Association at its founding meeting in 1846. The group of some one hundred doctors who convened in New York were particularly interested in reforming medical education in America and developing standards of conduct that would improve the practice of the "regular" medical profession. These changes, they hoped, would separate medicine from such rival healing sects as homeopaths, competition from whom increasingly distressed regular physicians. The code of ethics that emerged the following year announced a set of principles which promised good reputations for its subscribers. It could also indicate, the American physician Austin Flint wrote, "the proper course to those whose moral perceptions may be defective. It may prove a safeguard against the bias of personal interests. It thus contributes to the purity and dignity of the medical profession."[1] Although some physicians believed medical codes produced such harms as the stifling of individual initiative, an argument made by Lewis Pilcher in his 1883 essay, code writing continues into the modern period. This continuity is exemplified in the 1948 "Oath of Geneva" composed by the World Medical Association and the most recent (1957) version of the ethical code of the American Medical Association.

This section concludes with three historical and analytic essays on medical ethics by contemporary scholars. Ludwig Edelstein, a medical historian, examines the society of the ancient Greeks and the influential documents they produced on medical ethics. Jeffrey Berlant presents a sociological and economic analysis of medical ethics from the Renaissance to the modern period, in which he discusses how ethics have been used to organize physicians into social and professional groups. William May, who teaches religious studies, contrasts an approach to medical care as a gratuitous service to humanity with one that defines it as a responsive exchange of gifts and services. He explores the problems created for medicine by its emphasis on the first viewpoint.

Efforts to guide the moral behavior of physicians have a long and continuing history. The essays and primary source documents presented here constitute a representative and important part of it.

Note

1. Austin Flint, "Medical Ethics and Etiquette," *New York Medical Journal*, vol. 37, 1883, p. 286.

1

Selections from the Hippocratic Corpus: "Oath," "Precepts," "The Art," "Epidemics I," "The Physician," "Decorum," and "Law"

Hippocrates, trans. W. H. S. Jones, The Loeb Classical Library (Cambridge: Harvard University Press, 1923), vol. 1, pp. 164–165, 299–301, 317, 319, 321, 323, 325, 327; vol. 2, pp. 193, 203–205, 263–265, 293, 295, 297, 299, 301, 311, 313. By permission of the publishers.

Oath

I swear by Apollo Physician, by Asclepius, by Health, by Panacea and by all the gods and goddesses, making them my witnesses, that I will carry out, according to my ability and judgment, this oath and this indenture. To hold my teacher in this art equal to my own parents; to make him partner in my livelihood; when he is need of money to share mine with him; to consider his family as my own brothers, and to teach them this art, if they want to learn it, without fee or indenture; to impart precept,[1] oral instruction, and all other instruction[2] to my own sons, the sons of my teacher, and to indentured pupils who have taken the physician's oath, but to nobody else. I will use treatment to help the sick according to my ability and judgment, but never with a view to injury and wrong-doing. Neither will I administer a poison to anybody when asked to do so, nor will I suggest such a course. Similarly I will not give to a woman a pessary to cause abortion. But I will keep pure and holy both my life and my art. I will not use the knife, not even, verily, on sufferers from stone, but I will give place to such as are craftsmen therein. Into whatsoever houses I enter, I will enter to help the sick, and I will abstain from all intentional wrong-doing and harm, especially from abusing the bodies of man or woman, bond or free. And whatsoever I shall see or hear in the course of my profession, as well as outside my profession in my intercourse with men,[3] if it be what should not be published abroad, I will never divulge, holding such things to be holy secrets. Now if I carry out this oath, and break it not, may I gain for ever reputation among all men for my life and for my art; but if I transgress it and forswear myself, may the opposite befall me.

Precepts

III. Early determination of the patient's treatment—since only what has actually been administered will benefit; emphatic assertion is of no use—is beneficial but complicated. For it is through many turns and changes that all diseases settle into some sort of permanence.[4]

IV. This piece of advice also will need our consideration, as it contributes somewhat to the whole. For should you begin by discussing fees, you will suggest to the patient either that you will go away and leave him if no agreement be reached, or that you will neglect him and not prescribe any immediate treatment. So one must not be anxious about fixing a fee. For I consider such a worry to be harmful to a troubled patient, particularly if the disease be acute. For the quickness of the disease, offering no opportunity for turning back,[5] spurs on the good physician not to seek his profit but rather to lay hold on reputation. Therefore it is better to reproach a patient you have saved than to extort money from[6] those who are at death's door.

V. And yet some patients ask for what is out of the way and doubtful, through prejudice, deserving indeed to be disregarded, but not to be punished. Wherefore you must reasonably oppose them, as they are embarked upon a stormy sea of change. For, in heaven's name, who that is a brotherly[7] physician practises with such hardness of heart as not at the beginning to conduct a preliminary examination of every illness[8] and prescribe what will help towards a cure, to heal the patient and not to overlook the reward, to say nothing of the desire that makes a man ready to learn?

VI. I urge you not to be too unkind, but to consider carefully your patient's superabundance or means. Sometimes give your services for nothing, calling to mind a previous benefaction or present satisfaction.[9] And if there be an opportunity of serving one who is a stranger in financial straits, give full assistance to all such. For where there is love of man, there is also love of the art. For some patients, though conscious that their condition is perilous, recover their health simply through their contentment with the goodness of the physician. And it is well to superintend the sick to make them well, to care for the healthy to keep them well, but also to care for one's own self, so as to observe what is seemly.

VII. Now those who are buried in deep ignorance of the art cannot appreciate what has been said. In fact such men will be shown up as ignorant of medicine, suddenly exalted yet needing good luck. For should wealthy men gain some remission of their trouble, these quacks win reputation through a double good fortune, and if a relapse occurs they stand upon their dignity, having neglected the irreproachable methods of the art, wherewith a good physician, a "brother of the art" as he is called, would be at his best. But he who accomplishes his cures easily without making a mistake would transgress none of these methods through want of power;[10] for he is not distrusted on the ground of wickedness. For quacks do not attempt treatment when they see an alarming[11] condition, and avoid calling in other physicians, because they wickedly hate help. And the patients in their pain drift on a sea of twofold wretchedness for not having intrusted themselves to the end to the fuller treatment that is given by the art. For a remission of a disease affords a sick man much relief. Wherefore wanting a healthy condition they do not wish always to submit to the same treatment, therein being in accord with a physician's versatility.[12] For the patients are in need through heavy expenditure, worshipping incompetence and showing no gratitude when they meet it;[13] when they have the power to be well off, they exhaust themselves about fees, really wishing to be well for the sake of managing their investments or farms, yet without a thought in these matters to receive anything.[14]

VIII. So much for such recommendations. For remission and aggravation of a disease require respectively less or more medical assistance. A physician does not violate etiquette even if, being in difficulties on occasion over a patient and in the dark through inexperience, he should urge the calling in of others, in order to learn by consultation the truth about the case, and in order that there may be fellow-workers to afford abundant help. For when a diseased condition is stubborn and the evil grows, in the perplexity of the moment most things go wrong. So on such occasions one must be bold.[15] For never will I lay it down that the art has been condemned in this matter.[16] Physicians who meet in consultation must never quarrel, or jeer at one another. For I will assert upon oath, a physician's reasoning should never be jealous of another. To be so will be a sign of weakness. Those who act thus lightly are rather those connected with the business of the market-place. Yet it is no mistaken idea to call in a consultant. For in all abundance there is lack.[17]

IX. With all these things it will appear strong evidence for the reality of the art if a physician, while skilfully treating the patient, does not refrain from exhortations not to worry in mind in the eagerness to reach the hour of recovery. For we physicians take the lead in what is necessary for health. And if he be under orders the patient will not go far astray. For left to themselves patients sink through their painful condition, give up the struggle and depart this life. But he who has taken the sick man in hand, if he display the discoveries of the art, preserving nature, not trying to alter it, will sweep away the present depression or the distrust of the moment. For the healthy condition of a human being is a nature that has naturally attained a movement, not alien but perfectly adapted, having produced it by means of breath, warmth and coction of humours, in every way, by complete regimen and by everything combined, unless there be some congenital or early deficiency. Should there be such a thing in a patient who is wasting, try to assimilate to the fundamental nature.[18] For the wasting, even of long standing, is unnatural.

X. You must also avoid adopting, in order to gain a patient,[19] luxurious headgear and elaborate perfume. For excess of strangeness will win you illrepute, but a little will be considered in good taste, just as pain in one part is a trifle, while in every part it is serious. Yet I do not forbid your trying to please, for it is not unworthy of a physician's dignity.

XI. Bear in mind the employment of instruments and the pointing out of significant symptoms, and so forth.

XII. And if for the sake of a crowded audience you do wish to hold a lecture, your ambition is no laudable one, and at least avoid all citations from the poets, for to quote them argues feeble industry. For I forbid in medical practice an industry not pertinent to the art, and laboriously far-fetched,[20] and which therefore has in itself alone an attractive grace. For you will achieve the empty toil of a drone and a drone's spoils.

The Art

. . . I will define what I conceive medicine to be. In general terms, it is to do away with the sufferings of the sick, to lessen the violence of their diseases, and to refuse to treat those who are overmastered by their diseases, realizing that in such cases medicine is powerless. . . .

VIII. Some too there are who blame medicine because of those who refuse to undertake desperate cases, and say that while physicians undertake cases which would cure themselves, they do not touch those where great help is necessary; whereas, if the art existed, it ought to cure all alike. Now if those who make such statements charged physicians with neglecting them, the makers of the statements, on the ground that they are delirious, they would bring a more plausible charge than the one they do bring. For if a man demand from an art a power over what does not belong to the art, or from nature[21] a power over what does not belong to nature, his ignorance is more allied to madness than to lack of knowledge. For in cases where we may have the mastery through the means afforded by a natural constitution or by an art, there we may be craftsmen, but nowhere else. Whenever therefore a man suffers from an ill which is too strong for the means at the disposal of medicine, he surely must not even expect that it can be overcome by medicine. For example, of the caustics employed in medicine fire is the most powerful, though there are many others less powerful than it. Now affections that are too strong for the less powerful caustics plainly are not for this reason incurable; but those which are too strong for the most powerful plainly are incurable. For when fire operates, surely affections not overcome thereby show that they need another art, and not that wherein fire is the means. I apply the same argument to the other agents employed in medicine; when any one of them plays the physician false, the blame should be laid on the power of the affection, and not on the art. Now those who blame physicians who do not undertake desperate cases, urge them to take in hand unsuitable patients just as much as suitable ones. When they urge this, while they are admired by physicians in name, they are a laughing-stock of really scientific physicians. Those experienced in this craft have no need either of such foolish blame or of such foolish praise; they need praise only from those who have considered where the operations of craftsmen reach their end and are complete, and likewise where they fall short; and have considered moreover which of the failures should be attributed to the craftsmen, and which to the objects on which they practise their craft.

Epidemics

. . . In all dangerous cases you should be on the watch for all favourable coctions of the evacuations from all parts, or for fair and critical abscessions. Coctions signify nearness of crisis and sure recovery of health, but crude and unconcocted evacuations, which change into bad abscessions, denote absence of crisis, pain, prolonged illness, death, or a return of the same symptoms. But it is by a consideration of other signs that one must decide which of these results will be most likely. Declare the past, diagnose the present, foretell the future; practise these acts. As to diseases, make a habit of two things—to help, or at least to do no harm. The art has three factors, the disease, the patient, the physician. The physician is the servant of the art. The patient must co-operate with the physician in combating the disease.

The Physician

The dignity of a physician requires that he should look healthy, and as plump as nature intended him to be; for the common crowd consider those who are not of this[22] excellent bodily condition to be unable to take care of others. Then he must be clean in person, well dressed, and anointed with sweet-smelling unguents that are not in any way suspicious. This, in fact, is pleasing to patients. The prudent man must also be careful of certain moral considerations[23]—not only to be silent, but also of a great regularity of life,[24] since thereby his reputation will be greatly enhanced; he must be a gentleman in character, and being this he must be grave and kind to all. For an over-forward obtrusiveness is despised, even though it may be very useful. Let him look to the liberty of action that is his; for when the same things are rarely presented to the same persons there is content.[25] In appearance, let him be of a serious but not harsh countenance; for harshness is taken to mean arrogance and unkindness, while a man of uncontrolled laughter and excessive gaiety is considered vulgar, and vulgarity especially must be avoided. In every social relation he will be fair, for fairness must be of great service.[26] The intimacy also between physician and patient is close. Patients in fact put themselves into the hands of their physician, and at every moment he meets women, maidens and possessions very precious indeed. So towards all these self-control must be used. Such then should the physician be, both in body and in soul.

Decorum

VII. . . . The physician must have at his command a certain ready wit, as dourness is repulsive both to the healthy and to the sick. He must also keep a most careful watch over himself, and neither expose much of his person nor gossip to laymen, but say only what is absolutely necessary. For he realizes that gossip may cause criticism of his treatment. He will do none at all of these things in a way that savours of fuss or of show. Let all these things be thought out, so that they may be ready beforehand for use as required. Otherwise there must always be lack when need arises.

VIII. You must practise these things in medicine with all reserve, in the matter of palpation, anointing, washing, to ensure elegance in moving the hands, in the matter of lint, compresses, bandages, ventilation, purges, for wounds and eyetroubles, and with regard to the various kinds of these things, in order that you may have ready beforehand instruments, appliances, knives and so forth. For lack in these matters means helplessness and harm. See that you have a second physician's case, of simpler make, that you can carry in your hands when on a journey. The most convenient is one methodically arranged, for the physician cannot possibly go through everything.[27]

IX. Keep well in your memory drugs and their properties, both simple and compound,[28] seeing that after all it is in the mind that are also the cures of diseases,[29] remember their modes, and their number and variety in the several cases. This in medicine is beginning, middle and end.

X. You must have prepared in advance emollients classified according to their various uses, and get ready powerful[30] draughts prepared according to formula after their various kinds. You must make ready beforehand purgative medicines also,[31] taken from suitable localities, prepared in the proper manner, after their various kinds and sizes, some preserved so as to last a long time, others fresh to be used at the time, and similarly with the rest.

XI. When you enter a sick man's room, having made these arrangements, that you may not be at a loss, and having everything in order for what is to be done, know what you must do before going in. For many cases need, not reasoning, but practical help. So you must from your experience forecast what the issue will be. To do so adds to one's reputation, and the learning thereof is easy.

XII. On entering bear in mind your manner of sitting, reserve, arrangement of dress, decisive utterance, brevity of speech, composure, bedside manners, care, replies to objections, calm self-control to meet the troubles that occur, rebuke of disturbance, readiness to do what has to be done. In addition to these things be careful of your first preparation. Failing this, make no further mistake in the matters wherefrom instructions are given for readiness.[32]

XIII. Make frequent visits; be especially careful in your examinations, counteracting the things wherein you have been deceived at the changes.[33] Thus you will know the case more easily, and at the same time you will also be more at your ease.[34] For instability is characteristic of the humours, and so they may also be easily altered by nature and by chance. For failure to observe the proper season for help gives the disease a start and kills the patient, as there was nothing to relieve him. For when many things together produce a result there is difficulty. Sequences of single phenomena are more manageable, and are more easily learnt by experience.[35]

XIV. Keep a watch also on the faults of the patients, which often make them lie about the taking of things prescribed. For through not taking disagreeable drinks, purgative or other, they sometimes die. What they have done never results in a confession, but the blame is thrown upon the physician.

XV. The bed also must be considered. The season and the kind of illness[36] will make a difference. Some patients are put into breezy spots, others into covered places or underground. Consider also noises and smells, especially the smell of wine. This is distinctly bad, and you must shun it or change it.[37]

XVI. Perform all this calmly and adroitly, concealing most things from the patient while you are attending to him. Give necessary orders[38] with cheerfulness and serenity, turning his attention away from what is being done to him; sometimes reprove sharply and emphatically, and sometimes comfort with solicitude and attention, revealing nothing of the patient's future or present[39] condition. For many patients through this cause have taken a turn for the worse, I mean by the declaration I have mentioned of what is present,[40] or by a forecast of what is to come.

XVII. Let one of your pupils be left in charge, to carry out instructions without unpleasantness, and to administer the treatment. Choose out those who have been already admitted into the mysteries of the art, so as to add anything necessary, and to give treatment with safety. He is there also to prevent those things escaping notice that happen in the intervals between visits. Never put a layman in charge of anything, otherwise if a mischance occur the blame will fall on you.[41] Let there never be any doubt about the points which will secure the success of your plan,[42] and no blame will attach to you, but achievement will bring you pride.[43] So say beforehand all this at the time the things are done,[44] to those whose business it is to have fuller knowledge.[45]

XVIII. Such being the things that make for good reputation and decorum, in wisdom, in medicine, and in the arts generally, the physician must mark off the parts[46] about which I have spoken, wrap himself round always with the other,[47] watch it and keep it, perform it and pass it on. For things that are glorious are closely guarded among all men. And those who have made their way through them are held

in honour by parents and children; and if any of them do not know many things, they are brought to understanding by the facts of actual experience.

Law

I. Medicine is the most distinguished of all the arts, but through the ignorance of those who practise it, and of those who casually judge such practitioners, it is now of all the arts by far the *least esteemed*. The chief reason for this error seems to me to be this: medicine is the only art which our states have made subject to no penalty save that of dishonour, and dishonour does not wound those who are compacted of it. Such men in fact are very like the supernumeraries in tragedies. Just as these have the appearance, dress and mask of an actor without being actors, so too with physicians; many are physicians by repute, very few are such in reality.

II. He who is going truly to acquire an understanding of medicine must enjoy natural ability, teaching, a suitable place, instruction from childhood, diligence, and time. Now first of all natural ability is necessary, for if nature be in opposition everything is in vain. But when nature points the way to what is best, then comes the teaching of the art. This must be acquired intelligently by one who from a child has been instructed in a place naturally suitable for learning. Moreover he must apply diligence for a long period, in order that learning, becoming second nature, may reap a fine and abundant harvest.

III. The learning of medicine may be likened to the growth of plants. Our natural ability is the soil. The views of our teachers are as it were the seeds. Learning from childhood is analogous to the seeds' falling betimes upon the prepared ground. The place of instruction is as it were the nutriment that comes from the surrounding air to the things sown. Diligence is the working of the soil. Time strengthens all these things, so that their nurture is perfected.

IV. These are the conditions that we must allow the art of medicine, and we must acquire of it a real knowledge before we travel from city to city and win the reputation of being physicians not only in word but also in deed. Inexperience on the other hand is a cursed

treasure and store for those that have it, whether asleep or awake;[48] it is a stranger to confidence and joy, and a nurse of cowardice and of rashness. Cowardice indicates powerlessness; rashness indicates want of art. There are in fact two things, science and opinion; the former begets knowledge, the latter ignorance.

V. Things however that are holy are revealed only to men who are holy. The profane may not learn them until they have been initiated into the mysteries of science.

Notes

1. Apparently the written rules of the art, examples of which are to be found in several Hippocratic treatises. These books were not published in the strict sense of the word, but copies would be circulated among the members of the "physicians' union."

2. Probably, in modern English, "instruction, written, oral and practical."

3. This remarkable addition is worthy of a passing notice. The physician must not gossip, no matter how or where the subject-matter for gossip may have been acquired; whether it be in practice or in private life makes no difference.

4. Because changes and turns are common in the early stages, to fix the proper treatment early is a complicated matter.

5. I.e. from missed opportunities that have passed away while haggling over fees. It is possible that ἀναστροφή has here the sense of ἀναστρέφειν καρίδαν in Thucydides II. 49, "to upset." An acute disease is not the time to upset a patient with financial worries.

6. Or, if Coray's emendation be adopted, "to tease."

7. The word so translated is fairly common in the *Corpus* in the sense of "related." Here it evidently means "a loyal member of the family of physicians."

8. With Ermerins' reading, "all the illness."

9. Or, with εὐδοκιμίην, "your present reputation."

10. He is trusted, and so can do as he likes. Therefore want of power to influence a patient never compels him to transgress the medical code.

11. It is quite uncertain whether φλεβονώδεα is the correct reading, and equally uncertain what it means if it be correct. Erotian's note recognises two ancient readings, φλεδονώδεα, explained as τὰ μετὰ φλυαρίας καὶ πνευματώδους ταραχῆς ἐκκρινόμενα, and φλεβονώδεα, explained as τὰ μετ' ἀλγήματος οἰδήματα. But the general meaning must be "serious," "alarming."

12. The reader must suspect that in the words ἰητροῦ ποικιλίη is concealed an allusion to frequent changes of the medical attendant. "Changing their doctor every day."

The version in the text means that the patients frequently change their minds as do quacks, or as doctors must be ready to change their treatment at a moment's notice.

13. These patients ἀπορέουσιν, and so can scarcely be the same as the εὔποροι of the earlier part of the chapter. Perhaps οὐκ should be read before ἀχαριστέοντες, and the sense would then be, "they become poor by showing gratitude to quacks, when they might be well off by employing qualified men."

14. The greater part of this chapter is hopeless. There seems to be no connexion between the quack doctors of the first part and the wayward patients of the latter part. I suspect that an incongruous passage has been inserted here by some compiler, just as chapter fourteen was so inserted. Perhaps there are gaps in the text, the filling up of which would clear away the difficulty. Probably there is one after εἴνεκεν. If the latter part be not an interpolation, the general meaning seems to be that when patients grow worse under quack treatment, they change their doctor and hire another quack. So they both grow worse and lose money. They really want to get well to look after their business, but do not think of the right way to return to work again, i.e. of employing a qualified medical man.

15. Or (reading οὐ) "on such occasions one must not be self-confident."

16. I.e. that because a consultant is necessary the fault lies with the art of medicine.

17. No matter how much help you have you can never have enough.

18. I.e. try to bring the patient back to his normal condition.

19. Apparently, in order to increase your practice by fastidiousness in the matter of dress. But the expression is very strange, and should mean, "in order to effect a cure."

20. See p. 308.

21. The word φύσις (and φυσίων below) is difficult to translate. It refers to the natural powers of the human constitution, which may be too weak to resist the attack of a severe disease. Its ὄργανα are the means whereby we can influence the φύσις, the various bodily "organs" which can be affected by medicine and treatment generally. Gomperz translates φύσις by "Natur," and τοῖσι τῶν φυσίων ὀργάνοις by "durch die Kräfte der Körper."

22. The οὕτως of this sentence is not otiose: "those who are not well off in these respects" (i.e. of a healthy complexion and not too thin). Ermerins' emendation to αὐτοί is therefore not necessary, though it is ingenious.

23. Bensel's reading will mean "the following are important characteristics of a prudent soul."

24. It is easy to understand εἶναι with εὔτακτον from the εἶναι in the clause after the parenthesis. This understanding of a word or phrase in a first clause, which is actually used in a second clause, being unknown in modern English, is often a cause of obscurity.

25. So Littré. But it is more than doubtful if the Greek will bear this meaning. The reading of V (σκοπὸν) points to corruption of the text, as does the σπανίως ἔχουσιν of the MSS.

26. Bensel's emendation to the dative is very attractive, and is probably right: "for on many occasions one must come to the help of fairness."

27. I retain the reading of Littré without confidence, for διὰ μεθόδων is very curious Greek for "methodically," and M reads plainly περιέρχεσθαι. Hesychius has a gloss μεθόδιον = ἐφόδιον, and I suspect that we should read here διὰ μεθοδίων, and περιέρχεσθαι with M. The μεθόδια would be packets or compartments, filled with small quantities of the chief medical necessaries, with convenient instruments of a portable size, and so on, so that the physician, on arriving at his destination, would not be obliged "to go round everywhere" to get what he wanted. The article before λιτοτέρη is strange, and suggests that ἡ λιτοτέρη and perhaps ἡ διὰ χειρῶν are glosses.

28. Literally, "written down" because compounded according to a written formula.

29. Littré says, "si déjà sont dans l'esprit les notions sur le traitement." This is an impossible translation of εἴπερ ἄρα κ.τ.λ. Apparently Littré did not see that the εἴπερ clause is a parenthesis, and that καὶ οἱ τούτων continues the first clause. The general sense is, "carry your knowledge in your head, not on paper, seeing that it is with your mind that you must work a cure."

30. Littré takes τέμνειν δυνάμενα = "breuvages incisifs," whatever this may mean, adding that some critics suggest ἀνύειν for τέμνειν. It is more likely that τέμνειν is an imperatival infinitive, and that it has its usual meaning of "cutting simples." But δυνάμενα is strange, unless it means "having the appropriate δυνάμεις."...

31. Littré brackets ἐς τὰς καθάρσιας as a gloss, and he may be right. But Decorum is alternately over-concise and verbose, and ἐς τὰς καθάρσιας may have been added for the sake of clearness.

32. I agree with Littré that the text cannot be right, but I should hesitate to restore it confidently. I believe that here, too, we have the lecturer's rough, ungrammatical notes. The quaintness, the apparently purposed strangeness of the diction of this chapter makes me more than ever convinced that we have in Decorum the language of ritual and not of every-day life. In this particular case the sense is quite plain.

33. Apparently the "changes" shown by a disease in passing from one phase to another.

34. I can find no parallel for εὐμαρής in this sense, but the context makes it necessary to interpret it as I have done.

35. Such must be the meaning but the Greek is strange.

36. Littré takes γένεα to refer to different kinds of beds.

37. I suppose by eating something with a strong and pleasant odour.

38. Perhaps, "give encouragement to the patient to allow himself to be treated."

39. I am in doubt whether or not ἐνεστὼς in these two cases means "imminent." But ἐσομένων and ἐπεσομένων seem to suggest the meaning "present."

40. I make no attempt to correct the broken grammar, holding that the remarks are a lecturer's notes.

41. See note 40.

42. The meaning is very obscure.

43. The γένος of M points to the reading γάνος, "brightness," perhaps here "glory."

44. The meaning of ἐπὶ τῶν ποιεομένων is very uncertain.

45. Apparently ἐπιγιγνώσκω here means "to know in addition."

46. Probably a reference to Chapter I, ληφθείη δ' ἂν τούτων μέρεα.

47. What is τὴν ἑτέρην? I must once more revert to my suggestion that Decorum, with its stilted and often unnatural language, is full of the secret formulae of a medical fraternity, the most "holy" phrases being omitted or disguised. I think τὴν ἑτέρην is one of these phrases. Surely at the end of an address to "the brethren" (ἠδελφισμένος ἰητρός, Precepts V.) we should expect references to the mysteries of the craft. And this last chapter seems full of them. How else can we explain διατηρέοντα φυλάσσειν, παραδιδόντα (handing on the pass-words), εὐκλεᾶ διαφυλάσσεται, δι' αὐτῶν ὁδεύσαντες? The word σύνεσις, too, seems to be a word of this class.

48. A proverbial expression meaning "always."

2

W. H. S. Jones
From the Oath According to Hippocrates in So Far as a Christian May Swear It

Reprinted with permission of the publisher from W. H. S. Jones, *The Doctor's Oath: An Essay in the History of Medicine* (New York: Cambridge University Press, 1924), pp. 23, 25.

Blessed be God the Father of our Lord Jesus Christ, who is blessed for ever and ever; I lie not.

I will bring no stain upon the learning of the medical art. Neither will I give poison to anybody though asked to do so, nor will I suggest such a plan. Similarly I will not give treatment[1] to women to cause abortion, treatment neither from above nor from below[2]. But I will teach this art, to those who require to learn it[3], without grudging and without an indenture. I will use treatment to help the sick according to my ability and judgment. And in purity and in holiness I will guard my art[4]. Into whatsoever houses I enter, I will do so to help the sick, keeping myself free from all wrongdoing, intentional or unintentional, tending to death or to injury, and from fornication with bond or free, man or woman. Whatsoever in the course of practice I see or hear (or outside my practice in social intercourse) that ought not to be published abroad, I will not divulge, but consider such things to be holy secrets. Now if I keep this oath and break it not, may God be my helper in my life and art,[5] and may I be honoured among all men for all time. If I keep faith, well;[6] but if I forswear myself may the opposite befall me.[7]

Notes

1. φθόριον: *sc.* φάρμακον. The pagan oath has πεσσόν as the substantive.

2. Not in pagan oath. The phrase was apparently added to meet the case of those who thought that they could obey the Hippocratic oath if they used other means than a pessary to produce abortion.

3. The MSS vary here. I have translated Urb. 64, but Ambros. has "as is necessary, right and fitting for Christians to learn it," and Bonon. 3632 has "to those who wish to learn it."

4. Bonon. 3632 has (as in pagan oath) "my life and my art." Note that in the next sentence even unintentional (ἀκουσίης) harm is forbidden. The doctor must not be criminally negligent. The word ἀκουσίης is not in the pagan oath, but occurs in the strange manuscript Scorialensis Σ II 5.

5. Bonon. 3632 has "may God be my helper and guide in my life and art."

6. This sentence is not in Bonon. 3632, which has, however (as in the pagan oath), "but if I transgress and forswear myself."

7. I think the τέλους (or τέλος) of Urb. and Ambros. to be a mere blunder.

3

Frederick II
Medieval Law for the Regulation of the Practice of Medicine

Reprinted from James J. Walsh, *The Popes and Science: The History of the Papal Relations to Science During the Middle Ages and Down to Our Own Time* (New York: Fordham University Press, 1911), pp. 419–423.

It is usually presumed that the practice of medicine was on a very low plane during the Middle Ages, and that while only little was known about medical science, the methods of practicing the medical art were crude, as befitted an earlier time in evolution before modern advances had come. Any such impression is founded entirely on ignorance of the conditions which actually existed. In his studies in the history of anatomy in the Middle Ages, Von Töply[1] quotes the law for the regulation of the practice of medicine issued by the Emperor Frederick II in 1240 or 1241. The Law was binding on the two Sicilies, and shows exactly the state of medical practice in the southern part of Italy at this time. Everything that we think we have gained by magnificent advances in modern times is to be found in this law. A physician must have a diploma from a university and a license from the government; he must have studied three years before taking up medicine—then three years in a medical school, and then must have practiced with a physician for a year before he will be allowed to take up the practice of medicine on his own account. If he is to take up surgery, he must have made special studies in anatomy. The law is especially interesting because of its regulation of the purity of drugs, in which it anticipates by nearly seven centuries our Pure Drug Law. [Explanatory interpretations in this selection are those of James J. Walsh, author of the book from which the selection is excerpted.]

"While we are bent upon making regulations for the commonweal of our loyal subjects, we keep ever under our observation the health of the individual. In consideration of the serious damage and the irreparable suffering which may occur as a consequence of the inexperience of physicians, we decree that in future no one who claims the title of physician shall exercise the art of healing or dare to treat the ailing, except such as have beforehand, in our University of Salerno, passed a public examination under a regular teacher of medicine, and been given a certificate not only by the professor of medicine, but also by one of our civil officials, which declares his trustworthiness and sufficient knowledge. This document

must be presented to us, or in our absence from the kingdom to the person who remains behind in our stead, and must be followed by the obtaining of a license to practice medicine either from us or from our representative aforesaid. Violation of this law is to be punished by confiscation of goods and a year in prison for all those who in future dare to practice medicine without such permission from our authority.

"Since students cannot be expected to learn medical science unless they have previously been grounded in logic, we further decree that no one be permitted to take up the study of medical science without beforehand having devoted at least three full years to the study of logic." (Under logic at this time was included the study of practically all the subjects that are now taken up in the arts department of our universities. Huxley, in his address before the University of Aberdeen on the occasion of his inauguration as Rector of that University, said that "the scholars [of the early days of the universities] studied Grammar and Rhetoric; Arithmetic and Geometry; Astronomy, Theology and Music." He added: "Thus their work, however imperfect and faulty, judged by modern lights, it may have been, brought them face to face with all the leading aspects of the many-sided mind of man. For these studies did really contain, at any rate, in embryo—sometimes, it may be, in caricature—what we now call Philosophy, Mathematical and Physical Science, and Art. And I doubt if the curriculum of any modern university shows so clear and generous a comprehension of what is meant by culture as the old Trivium and Quadrivium does."[2])

"After three years devoted to these studies, he (the student) may, if he will, proceed to the study of medicine, provided always that during the prescribed time he devotes himself also to surgery, which is a part of medicine. After this, and not before, will he be given the license to practice, provided he has passed an examination in legal form as well as obtained a certificate from his teacher as to his studies in the preceding time. After having spent five years in study, he shall not practice medicine until he has during a full year devoted himself to medical practice with the advice and under the direction of an experienced physician. In the medical

schools the professors shall during these five years devote themselves to the recognized books, both those of Hippocrates as well as those of Galen, and shall teach not only theoretic, but also practical medicine.

"We also decree, as a measure intended for the furtherance of Public Health, that no surgeon shall be allowed to practice, unless he has a written certificate, which he must present to the professor in the medical faculty, stating that he has spent at least a year at that part of medicine which is necessary as a guide to the practice of surgery, and that, above all, he has learned the anatomy of the human body at the medical school, and is fully equipped in this department of medicine, without which neither operations of any kind can be undertaken with success nor fractures be properly treated.

"In every province of our Kingdom which is under our legal authority, we decree that two prudent and trustworthy men, whose names must be sent to our court, shall be appointed and bound by a formal oath, under whose inspection electuaries and syrups and other medicines be prepared according to law and only be sold after such inspection. In Salerno in particular, we decree that this inspectorship shall be limited to those who have taken their degrees as Masters in Physic.

"We also decree by the present law, that no one in the Kingdom, except in Salerno or in Naples (in which were the two universities of the Kingdom), shall undertake to give lectures on medicine or surgery, or presume to assume the name of teacher, unless he shall have been very thoroughly examined in the presence of a Government official and of a professor in the art of medicine.

"Every physician given a license to practice must take an oath that he shall faithfully fulfil all the requirements of the law, and in addition, whenever it comes to his knowledge that any apothecary has for sale drugs that are of less than normal strength, he shall report him to the court, and besides he shall give his advice to the poor without asking for any compensation. A physician shall visit his patient at least twice a day, and at the wish of his patient once also at night, and shall charge him, in case the visit does not require him to go out of the village or beyond the walls of the city, not more than one-half tarrene in gold for each day's service." (A tarrene in gold was equal to about thirty cents of our money. Money had at least twenty times the purchasing power at that time that it has now. At the end of the thirteenth century, according to an Act of the English Parliament, a workman received 4d [eight cents] a day for his labor, and according to the same Act of Parliament the following prices were charged for commodities: A pair of shoes cost eight cents, that is, a day's wages. A fat goose cost seven cents, less than a day's wages. A fat sheep unshorn cost thirty-five cents; shorn, about twenty-five cents. For four days' pay a man could get enough meat for himself and family to live on for a week, besides material out of which his wife could make excellent garments for the family. A fat hog cost twice as much as a fat sheep, and a bullock about six times as much.—J. J. W.) "From a patient whom he visits outside of the village or the wall of the town, the physician has a right to demand for a day's service not more than three tarrenes, to which may be added, however, his expenses, provided that he does not demand more than four tarrenes altogether.

"He (the regularly licensed physician) must not enter into any business relations with the apothecary, nor must he take any of them under his protection nor incur any money obligations in their regard." (Apparently many different ways of getting round this regulation had already been invented, and the idea of these expressions seemed to be to make it very clear in the law that any such business relationship, no matter what the excuse or method of it, is forbidden.—J. J. W.) "Nor must any licensed physician keep an apothecary's shop himself. Apothecaries must conduct their business with a certificate from a physician, according to the regulations and upon their own credit and responsibility, and they shall not be permitted to sell their products without having taken an oath that all their drugs have been prepared in the prescribed form, without any fraud. The apothecary may derive the following profits from his sales: Such extracts and simples as he need not keep in stock for more than a year before they may be employed may be charged for at the rate of three tarrenes an ounce." (90

cents an ounce seems very dear, but this is the maximum.) "Other medicines, however, which in consequence of the special conditions required for their preparation or for any other reason the apothecary has to have in stock for more than a year, he may charge for at the rate of six tarrenes an ounce. Stations for the preparation of medicines may not be located anywhere, but only in certain communities in the Kingdom, as we prescribe below.

"We decree also that the growers of plants meant for medical purpose shall be bound by a solemn oath that they shall prepare medicines conscientiously, according to the rules of their art, and as far as it is humanely possible that they shall prepare them in the presence of the inspectors. Violations of this law shall be punished by the confiscation of their movable goods. If the inspectors, however, to whose fidelity to duty the keeping of these regulations is committed, should allow any fraud in the matters that are entrusted to them, they shall be condemned to punishment by death."

Notes

1. Studien zur Geschichte der Anatomie im Mittelalter von Robert Ritter Von Töply (Leipzig, 1898).

2. Huxley, *Science and Education Essays* (New York: D. Appleton & Co., 1896), p. 197.

4

[Arnald of Villanova?]
From "On the Precautions That Physicians Must Observe"

Reprinted with permission of the publisher from "Bedside Manners in the Middle Ages: The Treatise De Cautelis Medicorum Attributed to Arnald of Villanova," trans. Henry E. Sigerist, *Quarterly Bulletin of Northwestern University Medical School*, vol. 20, 1946, pp. 139–142.

We must consider the precautions with regard to urines, by which we can protect ourselves against people who wish to deceive us. The very first shall consist in finding out whether the urine be of man or of another animal or another fluid; and if it is human urine it is diagnosed in four ways.

The second precaution is with regard to the individual who brings the urine. You must look at him sharply and keep your eyes straight on him or on his face; and if he wishes to deceive you he will start laughing or the color of his face will change, and then you must curse him forever and in all eternity.

The third precaution is also with regard to the individual who brings the urine, whether man or woman, for you must see whether he or she is pale, and after you have ascertained that this is the individual's urine, say to him: "Verily, this urine resembles you," and talk about the pallor, because immediately you will hear all about his illness. It commonly happens with poor people and those of moderate means that they go to the doctor when they are afflicted very seriously.

The fourth precaution is with regard to sex. An old woman wants to have your opinion. You inquire whose urine it is, and the old woman will say to you: "Don't you know it?" Then look at her in a certain way from the corner of your eye, and ask: "What relation is it of yours?" And if she is not too crooked, she will say that the patient is a male or female relation, or something from which you can distinguish the sex. Should she say: "We are not related," then ask what the patient used to do when he was in good health, and from the patient's doing you can recognize or deduce the sex.

The fifth precaution is that you must ask if the patient is old. If the messenger says yes, you must say that he greatly suffers from the stomach, and that he spits a lot, and in the morning more than at any other time, for old people have by nature a cold stomach.

The sixth precaution: whether this illness has lasted for a long time or not. If the messenger says that it has, you must say that the patient is altogether irritable and that one can help him, or some such talk. If he says no, you must say that the patient is altogether oppressed because in the beginnings of diseases there is much matter that oppresses the organ.

There is a seventh precaution, and it is a very general one; you may not find out anything about the case, then say that he has an obstruction in the liver. He may say: "No, sir, on the contrary he has pains in the head, or in the legs or in other organs." You must say that this comes from the liver or from the stomach; and particularly use the word, obstruction, because they do not understand what it means, and it helps greatly that a term is not understood by the people.

The eighth precaution is with regard to conception. An old woman consults you because the patient cannot become pregnant. Perhaps you do not know the cause but say that she cannot hold her husband's sperm which she could have done very well if she had been well disposed.

The ninth precaution is with regard to a woman, whether she is old or young; and this you shall find out from what is told you. Should she be very old, say that she has all the evils that old women have, and also that she has many superfluities in the womb. Should she, however, be young say that she suffers from the stomach, and whenever she has a pain further down, say that it comes from the womb or the kidneys; and whenever she has it in the anterior part of the head, then it comes from the stomach; and whenever on the left side, then it comes from the spleen; whenever to the right, then it comes from the liver; and when it is worse and almost impedes her eyesight, say that she has pains or feels a heaviness in the legs, particularly when she exerts herself.

The tenth precaution: you must keep yourself very busy spitting or blowing your nose and if the old woman pesters you with the urine say quite casually: "What concern is this of yours?" or "Why do you pester me so much?" If she says: "Yes, it concerns me," then you shall know the sex. If she says, no, ask as has been explained under the fourth precaution.

The eleventh precaution is taken with regard to white or yellow wine. If you have any doubts in this respect, be cautious and put the lid of the urinal down and pour out a little of the content in such a way that the wine in being poured out touches your finger. Then you must give her the urinal and act as if you were going to blow your nose whereby you put the finger that has been dipped in, on or next to your nose; then you will smell the odor of wine, whereupon you must take the urinal again and say to her: "Get away and be ashamed of yourself!"

The twelfth precaution is taken with respect to fluid made from figs and also nettles. Although you could recognize this under the first precaution, yet you will clearly see that the residue extends in the form of a circle touching the urinal and does not make a rotundity or pine cone like a true sediment.

The thirteenth precaution: whenever the old woman asks what disease the patient has, you must say: "You would not understand me if I told you, and it would be better for you to ask what he should do." And then she will see that you have judgment in the matter and will keep quiet. But perhaps she will say: "Sir, he is very hot; therefore he seems to have a fever."—"Thus it seems to you and other lay people who do not know how to distinguish between fever and other diseases."

The fourteenth precaution: When you have been called to a patient, feel the pulse before you examine the urine and make them [sic] talk so that the condition of the animal virtue becomes apparent to you. After having recognized these factors you will be able to evaluate the urine better and with more certainty and you may proceed thus.

The fifteenth precaution is: should the patient be in a bad condition so that you think that he may die the following day, do not go to him but send your servant to bring you the urine, or tell them to bring it to-morrow in the early morning because you wish that they prepare for the meal and that after you have seen the urine you will tell what they shall administer. And so from the report of the person who brings the urine you will be able to form an opinion about the patient, whether he is in good or bad condition.

The sixteenth precaution is that when you come to a patient you should always do something new lest they say that you cannot do anything without the books.

The seventeenth precaution is that if by hard luck you come to the home of the patient and find him dead and somebody perhaps says: "Sir, what have you come for?" You shall say that you have not come for that, and say that you well knew that he was going to die that night but that you wanted to know at what hour he had died.

The eighteenth precaution is that if you have a competitor whom you believe to be a shameless crook, be careful when you go to the house of the patient; perhaps he will stir up the urine for you and you will not be able to form a certain judgment from it.

The nineteenth precaution is the following: if two urines of the same patient are presented to you and you wish to know which was the first, ask at what time of the night he got up, for if he did at dawn or after digestion had taken place that urine which is more digested and red will be the first, if it has sediment. If, however, he got up before midnight or around that time, you may judge that the less digested and less red urine is the first.

No other deception can occur outside of these, but these points must be kept in mind, and you must be cautious because the physician is greatly honored if he knows how to be cautious, for he is asked questions many times.

II

Note that the physician must be learned in diagnosing, careful and accurate in prescribing, circumspect and cautious in answering questions, ambiguous in making a prognosis, just in making promises; and he should not promise health because in doing so he would assume a divine function and insult God. He should rather promise loyalty and attentiveness, should be discreet in making calls, and he must be careful in speech, modest in behavior and kind to the patient.

III

Physician! When you shall be called to a sick man, in the name of God seek the assistance of the Angel who has attended the action of the mind and from inside shall attend departures of the body.[1] You must know from the beginning how long the sick has been laboring, and in what way the illness has befallen him, and by inquiring about the symptoms, if it can be done, ascertain what the disease is. This is necessary because after having seen the

faeces and urine and the condition of the pulse you may not be able to diagnose the disease, but if you can announce the symptoms the patient will have confidence in you as in the author of his health and therefore one must devote greatest pains to knowing the symptoms.

Therefore, when you come to a house, inquire before you go to the sick whether he has confessed, and if he has not, he should confess immediately or promise[2] you that he will confess immediately, and this must not be neglected because many illnesses originate on account of sin and are cured by the Supreme Physician after having been purified from squalor by the tears of contrition, according to what is said in the Gospel: "Go, and sin no more, lest something worse happens to you."[3]

Entering the sickroom do not appear very haughty or over-zealous, and return, with the simple gesture, the greetings of those who rise to greet you. After they have seated themselves you finally sit down facing the sick; ask him how he feels and reach out for his arm, and all that we shall say is necessary so that through your entire behavior you obtain the favor of the people who are around the sick. And because the trip to the patient has sharpened your sensitivity, and the sick rejoices at your coming or because he has already become stingy and has various thoughts about the fee, therefore by your fault as well as his the pulse is affected, is different and impetuous from the motion of the spirits. When it has quieted down on both parts, you shall examine the pulse in the left arm because although the right side would be satisfactory, yet it is easier to diagnose the motion of the heart in the left arm on account of its vicinity to the heart. Be careful that the patient does not lie on the right side because the compression would hinder the sense motion, nor should he stretch the fingers or make a fist. While you apply the fingers of your right hand you shall support with the left the patient's arm, because from greater sensibility you will distinguish the different and various motions more easily, and also because the patient's arm being so to say weak requires your support. If the arm is very full and fleshy you must press your fingers hard so as to get into the depth; if it is weak and lean you can

feel the pulse sufficiently on the surface. You must examine the pulse to a hundred beats at the very least, so that you may form an opinion on the various kinds of pulses, and the patient's people should receive your words as the result of a long examination of the heart beat.

Finally you request to have the urine brought, and if the change in pulse indicates that the individual is sick, the kind of disease is still better indicated by the urine, but they will believe you to indicate and diagnose the disease not only from the urine but also from the pulse. While you look at the urine for a long time you pay attention to its color, substance and quantity and to its contents from the diversity of which you will diagnose the different kinds of diseases, as is taught in the Treatise on Urines, whereupon you promise health to the patient who is hanging on your lips. When you have left him say a few words to the members of the household, say that he is very sick, for if he recovers you will be praised more for your art; should he die his friends will testify that you had given him up.

Let me give you one more warning: do not look at a maid, or a daughter or a wife with an improper or covetous eye and do not let yourself be entangled in woman affairs—for there are medical operations that excite the helper's mind; otherwise your judgment is affected, you become harmful to the patient and people will expect less from you. And so, be pleasant in your speech, diligent and careful in your medical dealings, eager to help. And adhere to this without fallacy.

When you have been invited for dinner you should not throw yourself upon the party and at the table should not occupy the place of honor although it is customary to assign the place of honor to the priest and the physician. Then you should not disdain certain drinks, nor find fault with certain dishes, nor be disgusted perhaps because you are hardly accustomed to appease your hunger with millet bread in peasant fashion. If you act thus your mind will feel at ease. And while the attention is concentrated on the variety of dishes, inquire explicitly from some of the attendants about the patient or about his condition. If you do this the sick will have great confidence in you, because he sees that you cannot forget him in the midst of delicacies. When you leave the table and come to the sick, you must tell him that you have been served well, at which the patient greatly rejoices because he was very anxious to have you well served.

Notes

1. The text of the first sentence must be corrupt. Compare the text of de Renzi, "Codex Salernitanus of Breslau," in *Collectio Salernitana,* vol. 2 (Naples, 1853), pp. 72 ff., which is not too clear either.

2. The text should read *promittat* as de Renzi has, not *permittat.*

3. See Paul Diepgen. *Die Theologie und der arztliche Stand,* Berlin, 1922, p. 49 ff.

5

Henri de Mondeville on the Morals and Etiquette of Surgeons

Reprinted from D'Arcy Power, ed., *Treatises of Fistula in Ano,* by John Arderne (London: Kegan Paul, Trench, Trubner & Co., 1910), pp. xx–xxii.

. . . "A Surgeon ought to be fairly bold. He ought not to quarrel before the laity, and although he should operate wisely and prudently, he should never undertake any dangerous operation unless he is sure that it is the only way to avoid a greater danger. His limbs, and especially his hands, should be well-shaped with long, delicate and supple fingers which must not be tremulous. He ought to promise a cure to every patient, but he should tell the parents or the friends if there is any danger. He should refuse as far as possible all difficult cases, and he should never mix himself up with desperate ones. He may give advice to the poor for the love of God only, but the wealthy should be made to pay well. He should neither praise himself nor blame others, and he should not hate any of his colleagues. He ought to sympathise with his patients in their distress and fall in with their lawful requests so far as they do not interfere with the treatment. Patients, on the other hand, should obey their surgeons implicitly in everything appertaining to their cure. The surgeon's assistants must be loyal to their surgeon and friendly to his patients. They should not tell the patient what the surgeon said unless the news is pleasant, and they should always appear cheerful. They must agree amongst themselves as well as with the patients, and they must not be always grumbling, because this inspires fear and doubt in the patient."

De Mondeville then shows how an honest surgeon may be replaced and damaged by one who is less conscientious, for he says: "A rich man has the beginning of an inflammation. He calls in an upright surgeon, who says after examining him, 'Seigneur, there is no need for any operation here, because nature will relieve herself, etc.; but if the inflammation gets worse, send for me.' It then happens that the patient calls in another man who is a quack, and he is told, 'Seigneur, you have a great deal of inflammation, I can feel it inside, and if you are not treated at once you will certainly regret it.' This surgeon then sets to work and makes an inflammation, which he afterwards cures, so that the whole proceeding redounds to his credit and profit, for he discovered an inflammation which did not exist, whilst the first surgeon is damaged both in his reputation and his pocket because he did not find out what was not there."

"Then again, one of these second-rate surgeons will come to a sick man who is wealthy, and will say to him, with the voice of an archangel—taking care that no witnesses are present— 'Seigneur, you must remember that you are the one who is ill and in pain. It is not your son or your nephew. It is you who are kept awake by the pain whilst your friends and servants sleep. Others won't take care of you if you don't care of yourself. You are rich enough to get advice and to buy health and whatever else you want if you choose to do so. Riches are not more than health, nor is poverty worse than sickness. Have you not made the greater part of your money yourself and for yourself, so that if you are not a miser you can apply it to relieve your wants? Would to God that those who look after you so badly had your complaint. But all this is between ourselves, and what I tell you is only out of pity for you and for your good.' Then, in the absence of the patient, he speaks to the relatives and says, 'Seigneurs, this man has the greatest confidence in you, and, truly, if you lose him, you will lose an excellent friend. It is not to your credit either to let him go without advice, for if he died without advice you would be blamed everlastingly, even if it made him as poor as Job. He is really in great danger, and it is a serious case, but nature sometimes does better than we have any right to expect. He is sure to die if no one treats him, but if he is properly treated it is just possible that he will escape and not die. If he dies it won't be the result of the treatment, because he is nearly dead already, his only chance is to have a consultation, etc. I am speaking to you as a friend and not as a doctor.'

"But it is quite another matter when this same surgeon has to treat a poor man, for he says, 'I am really sorry for you, and I would gladly help you for the love of God only. But I am very busy just now with a lot of difficult cases, and, besides, the season is not a very favourable one for an operation. You can't afford to buy what is necessary for your case, such as drugs and dressings, so I would put it off until the summer. You will then be able to get the herbs and whatever else is wanted

and so save expense. The summer, too, is the best time for the poor.' When the same pauper comes back in the summer the surgeon says to him, 'I am very sorry that I put you off in the winter and told you to wait until the summer, because the winter is really the best time. Summer is too hot and there is a fear of stirring up the disease. I should advise you to wait until the hot weather is over.' And this goes on everlastingly, for this kind of surgeon never finds time to operate upon a pauper."

De Mondeville classifies his patients according to their ability to pay fees. "The first class are paupers who must be treated for nothing; the second class are a little better off, and may send presents of fowls and ducks; they pay in kind. The third class are friends and relations who pay no fixed fee, but send victuals or presents in token of gratitude, but no money. Our assistants ought to suggest the presents to this class, saying behind our backs, and as if we knew nothing about it, when anything is said about money, 'No, indeed, the Master would not like it, and you would do much better to make him a little present, though I am sure that he does not expect anything.' Indeed, a sharp assistant sometimes makes more by such suggestions than the Master does by his operation, and it is just like doubling the fee on account of the horse when the Master makes his visits on horseback. Then there is a class embracing those who are notoriously bad payers, such as our nobility and their households, government officials, judges, baillies and lawyers, whom we are obliged to treat because we dare not offend them. In fact, the longer we treat these people the more we lose. It is best to cure them as quickly as possible, and to give them the best medicines. Lastly, there is a class who pay in full and in advance, and they should be prevented from getting ill at all, because we are paid a salary to keep them in health."

The difficulty of obtaining payment for operations in the fourteenth century must have been very great, for De Mondeville still further emphasizes it and says, "The chief object of the patient, and the one idea which dominates all his actions, is to get cured, and when once he is cured he forgets his own obligation and omits to pay; the object of the surgeon, on the other hand, is to obtain his money, and he

should never be satisfied with a promise or a pledge, but he should either have the money in advance or take a bond for it. As the poet says, 'Sæpe fides data fallit, plegius plaidit, vadium valet—The promise is often broken, the security is worthless, the bond alone holds good.' "

Notes

1. "Chirurgie de Maître Henri de Mondeville, composée de 1306 à 1320," par Ed. Nicaise. Paris, 1893, pp. 91 et seqq.

2. "Soc. des Anciens Textes Français." Paris, 1897, tome i, p. 140.

6

Samuel Bard

From *A Discourse upon the Duties of a Physician*

Reprinted from Samuel Bard, *A Discourse upon the Duties of a Physician* . . . (New York: A. & J. Robertson, 1769), pp. 9–12.

. . . In your Intercourse with your Fellow Practitioners, let Integrity, Candour, and Delicacy be your Guides. There is a particular Sensibility of Disposition, which seems essential to delicate Honor, and which I believe is the best Counterpoise to Self-Interest. This I would by all Means advise you to cultivate, as you will meet with many Occasions where it only can direct your Conduct.

Never affect to despise a Man for the want of a regular Education, and treat even harmless Ignorance, with Delicacy and Compassion, but when you meet with it joined with foolhardiness and Presumption, you must give it no quarter.

On no Pretence whatever, practice those little Arts of Cunning and Dissimulation, which to the Scandal of the Profession, have been but too frequent amongst us. Nor ever attempt to raise your Fame on the Ruins of another's Reputation; and remember that you ought not only to be cautious of your Words, a Shrug or a Whisper, the stare of Surprise, or a piteous Exclamation of Sorrow, more effectually wound another's Reputation, and more clearly betray the Baseness of a Man's own Heart, than the loudest Expressions.

Do not pretend to Secrets, Panaceas, and Nostrums, they are illiberal, dishonest, and inconsistent with your Characters, as Gentlemen and Physicians, and with your Duty as Men— For if you are possessed of any valuable Remedy, it is undoubtedly your Duty to divulge it, that as many as possible may reap the Benefit of it; and if not, (which is generally the Case) you are propagating a Falsehood, and imposing upon Mankind.

In your Behaviour to the Sick, remember always that your Patient is the Object of the tenderest Affection, to some one, or perhaps to many about him; it is therefore your Duty, not only to endeavour to preserve his Life, but to avoid wounding the Sensibility of a tender Parent, a distressed Wife, or an affectionate Child. Let your Carriage be humane and attentive, be interested in his Welfare, and shew your Apprehension of his Danger, rather by your Assiduity to relieve, than by any harsh or brutal Expressions of it. On the other hand, never buoy up a dying Man with groundless Expectations of Recovery, this is at best a good natured and humane Deception, but too often it

arises from the baser Motives of Lucre and Avarice: besides, it is really cruel, as the stroke of Death is always most severely felt, when unexpected; and the grim Tyrant may in general be disarmed of his Terrors, and rendered familiar to the most timid, and apprehensive; either by frequent Meditation, by the Arguments of Philosophy, or by the Hopes and Promises of Religion. But even overlooking the important Concerns of Futurity; the Business of this Life may render such a Conduct highly dangerous and criminal; as those to whom the thoughts of Death are painful, are too apt when flattered with the Prospect of Recovery, to neglect the necessary Provision against a Disappointment, and by that Means involve their Families in Confusion and Distress.

Above all Things, avoid any ridiculous Expressions of Humour, at the bed-side of a sick Man; you cannot chuse a more unseasonable Opportunity for your Mirth; nor will you find a Person of a generous and benevolent Disposition, who can smile even at the Repetition of a Witticism, which carries with it the Appearance of so much Inhumanity.

Let your Prescriptions be simple, and as neat and agreeable as the Nature of the Remedy will permit— Nothing can be more absurd than the Farrago of some, nothing more disgustful than the Slovenliness of others; for it is impossible to learn the true Virtues of Medicines, from compound Prescriptions; and Inelegance frequently disappoints us of their Effects. —And as it is probable, from the Mode of Practice in this Country, that you will not only be the Prescribers, but likewise the Dispensers of your Medicines, let your Integrity be proof against the Temptation of unnecessarily multiplying Prescriptions, and trust rather to the Liberality of your Patient, than to the Quantity of your Physic, for your Reward. For altho' perhaps by this Method you may sometimes think your Services undervalued, yet you will always enjoy the superior Satisfaction of conscious Rectitude, which, by an honest Man, will ever be preferred to a trifling Emolument.

7

Thomas Percival
Of Professional Conduct

Reprinted from Thomas Percival, *Medical Ethics*, 3rd. ed. (Oxford: John Henry Parker, 1849), pp. 27–68.

Of Professional Conduct, Relative to Hospitals, or Other Medical Charities

1. *Hospital* Physicians and Surgeons should minister to the sick with due impressions of the importance of their office; reflecting that the ease, the health, and the lives of those committed to their charge depend on their skill, attention, and fidelity. They should study, also, in their deportment, so to unite tenderness with steadiness, and condescension with authority, as to inspire the minds of their patients with gratitude, respect, and confidence.

2. The choice of a Physician or Surgeon cannot be allowed to hospital patients, consistently with the regular and established succession of medical attendance. Yet personal confidence is not less important to the comfort and relief of the sick poor, than of the rich under similar circumstances; and it would be equally just and humane to enquire into and to indulge their partialities, by occasionally calling into consultation the favourite practitioner. The rectitude and wisdom of this conduct will be still more apparent, when it is recollected, that patients in hospitals not unfrequently request their discharge on a deceitful plea of having received relief, and afterwards procure another recommendation, that they may be admitted under the Physician or Surgeon of their choice. Such practices involve in them a degree of falsehood, produce unnecessary trouble, and may be the occasion of irreparable loss of time in the treatment of diseases.

3. The feelings and emotions of the patients, under critical circumstances, require to be known and to be attended to, no less than the symptoms of their diseases: thus, extreme timidity with respect to venesection contraindicates its use in certain cases and constitutions. Even the prejudices of the sick are not to be contemned, or opposed with harshness; for, though silenced by authority, they will operate secretly and forcibly on the mind, creating fear, anxiety, and watchfulness.

4. As misapprehension may magnify real evils, or create imaginary ones, no discussion concerning the nature of the case should be entered into before the patients, either with the House-Surgeon, the pupils of the hospital, or any medical visitor.

5. In the large wards of an infirmary the patients should be interrogated concerning their complaints in a tone of voice which cannot be overheard. Secrecy, also, when required by peculiar circumstances, should be strictly observed. And females should always be treated with the most scrupulous delicacy. To neglect or to sport with their feelings is cruelty; and every wound thus inflicted tends to produce a callousness of mind, a contempt of decorum, and an insensibility to modesty and virtue. Let these considerations be forcibly and repeatedly urged on the hospital pupils.

6. The moral and religious influence of sickness is so favourable to the best interests of men and of society, that it is justly regarded as an important object in the establishment of every hospital. The institutions for promoting it should therefore be encouraged by the Physicians and Surgeons, whenever seasonable opportunities occur; and, by pointing out these to the officiating clergyman, the sacred offices will be performed with propriety, discrimination, and greater certainty of success. The character of a Physician is usually remote either from superstition or enthusiasm; and the aid, which he is now exhorted to give, will tend to their exclusion from the sick wards of the hospital, where their effects have often been known to be not only baneful, but even fatal.

7. It is one of the circumstances which softens the lot of the poor, that they are exempt from the solicitudes attendant on the disposal of property. Yet there are exceptions to this observation; and it may be necessary that an hospital patient, on the bed of sickness and death, should be reminded by some friendly monitor of the importance of a last will and testament to his wife, children, or relatives, who otherwise might be deprived of his effects, of his expected prize-money, or of some future residuary legacy. This kind office will be best performed by the House-Surgeon, whose frequent attendance on the sick diminishes their reserve, and entitles him to their familiar confidence. And he will doubtless regard the performance of it as a duty; for whatever is right to be done, and cannot by another be so well done, has

the full force of moral and personal obligation.

8. The Physicians and Surgeons should not suffer themselves to be restrained by parsimonious considerations from prescribing wine, and drugs even of high price, when required in diseases of extraordinary malignity and danger. The efficacy of every medicine is proportionate to its purity and goodness; and on the degree of these properties, *caeteris paribus*, both the cure of the sick and the speediness of its accomplishment must depend. But, when drugs of inferior quality are employed, it is requisite to administer them in larger doses, and to continue the use of them a longer period of time; circumstances which probably more than counterbalance any savings in their original price. If the case, however, were far otherwise, no economy of a fatal tendency ought to be admitted into institutions, founded on principles of the purest beneficence, and which, in this age and country, when well conducted, can never want contributions adequate to their liberal support.

9. The Medical gentlemen of every charitable institution are in some degree responsible for, and the guardians of, the honour of each other. No Physician or Surgeon, therefore, should reveal occurrences in the hospital, which may injure the reputation of any one of his colleagues; except under the restriction contained in the succeeding article.

10. No professional charge should be made by a Physician or Surgeon, either publicly or privately, against any associate, without previously laying the complaint before the gentlemen of the Faculty belonging to the institution, that they may judge concerning the reasonableness of its grounds, and the measures to be adopted.

11. A proper discrimination being established in all hospitals between the Medical and Chirurgical cases, it should be faithfully adhered to by the Physicians and Surgeons on the admission of patients.

12. Whenever cases occur, attended with circumstances not heretofore observed, or in which the ordinary modes of practice have been attempted without success, it is for the public good, and in an especial degree advantageous to the poor, (who, being the most numerous class of society, are the greatest beneficiaries of the healing art) that new remedies and new methods of Chirurgical treatment should be devised. But in the accomplishment of this salutary purpose the gentlemen of the Faculty should be scrupulously and conscientiously governed by sound reason, just analogy, or well authenticated facts. And no such trials should be instituted without a previous consultation of the Physicians or Surgeons, according to the nature of the case.

13. To advance professional improvement, a friendly and unreserved intercourse should subsist between the gentlemen of the Faculty, with a free communication of whatever is extraordinary or interesting in the course of their hospital practice. And an account of every case or operation, which is rare, curious, or instructive, should be drawn up by the Physician or Surgeon to whose charge it devolves, and entered in a register kept for the purpose, but open only to the Physicians and Surgeons of the charity.

14. Hospital registers usually contain only a simple report of the number of patients admitted and discharged. By adopting a more comprehensive plan they might be rendered subservient to Medical science and beneficial to mankind. The following sketch is offered with deference to the gentlemen of the Faculty. Let the register consist of three tables: the first specifying the number of patients admitted, cured, relieved, discharged, or dead; the second, the several diseases of the patients, with their events; the third, the sexes, ages, and occupations of the patients. The ages should be reduced into classes; and the tables adapted to the four divisions of the year. By such an institution, the increase or decrease of sickness; the attack, progress, and cessation of epidemics; the comparative healthiness of different situations, climates, and seasons; the influence of particular trades and manufacturers on health and life; with many other curious circumstances, not more interesting to Physicians than to the community, would be ascertained with sufficient precision.

15. By the adoption of the register recommended in the foregoing article, Physicians and Surgeons would obtain a clearer insight into the comparative success of their hospital and private practice; and would be incited to a diligent investigation of the causes of such difference. In particular diseases it will be found to subsist in a very remarkable degree: and the discretionary power of the Physician or Surgeon in the admission of patients, could not be exerted with more justice or humanity, than in refusing to consign to lingering suffering and almost certain death a numerous class of patients, inadvertently recommended as objects of these charitable institutions. "In judging of diseases with regard to the propriety of their reception into hospitals," says an excellent writer, "the following general circumstances are to be considered:

"Whether they be capable of speedy relief; because, as it is the intention of charity to relieve as great a number as possible, a quick change of objects is to be wished; and also because the inbred disease of hospitals will almost inevitably creep in some degree upon one who continues a long time in them, but will rarely attack one whose stay is short.

"Whether they require in a particular manner the superintendence of skilful persons, either on account of their acute and dangerous nature, or any singularity or intricacy attending them, or erroneous opinions prevailing among the common people concerning their treatment. . . .

"Whether they be contagious, or subject in a peculiar degree to corrupt the air and generate pestilential diseases. . . .

"Whether a fresh and pure air be peculiarly requisite for their cure, and they be remarkably injured by any vitiation of it."[1]

16. But no precautions relative to the reception of patients who labour under maladies incapable of relief, contagious in their nature, or liable to be aggravated by confinement in an impure atmosphere, can obviate the evils arising from close wards, and the false economy of crowding a number of persons into the least possible space. There are inbred diseases which it is the duty of the Physician or Surgeon to prevent, as far as lies in his power, by a strict and persevering attention to the whole medical polity of the hospital. This comprehends the discrimination of cases admissible, air, diet, cleanliness, and drugs; each of which articles should be subjected to a rigid scrutiny at stated periods of time.

17. The establishment of a committee of the gentlemen of the Faculty, to be held monthly, would tend to facilitate this interesting investigation, and to accomplish the most important objects of it. By the free communication of remarks, various improvements would be suggested; by the regular discussion of them, they would be reduced to a definite and consistent form; and by the authority of united suffrages, they would have full influence over the governors of the charity. The exertions of individuals, however benevolent or judicious, often give rise to jealousy, are opposed by those who have not been consulted, and prove inefficient by wanting the collective energy of numbers.

18. The harmonious intercourse which has been recommended to the gentlemen of the Faculty will naturally produce frequent consultations, viz. of the Physicians on Medical cases, of the Surgeons on Chirurgical cases, and of both united in cases of a compound nature, which, falling under the department of each, may admit of elucidation by the reciprocal aid of the two professions.

19. In consultations on Medical cases the junior Physician present should deliver his opinion first, and the others in the progressive order of their seniority. The same order should be observed in Chirurgical cases; and a majority should be decisive in both: but if the numbers be equal, the decision should rest with the Physician or Surgeon under whose care the patient is placed. No decision, however, should restrain the acting practitioner from making such variations in the mode of treatment, as future contingences may require, or a farther insight into the nature of the disorder may shew to be expedient.

20. In consultations on mixed cases the junior Surgeon should deliver his opinion first, and his brethren afterwards in succession, according to progressive seniority. The junior Physician present should deliver his opinion after the senior Surgeon, and the other Physicians in the order above prescribed.

21. In every consultation the case to be considered should be concisely stated by the Physician or Surgeon who requests the aid of his brethren. The opinions relative to it should be delivered with brevity, agreeably to the preceding arrangement, and the decisions collected in the same order. The order of seniority among the Physicians and Surgeons may be regulated by the dates of their respective appointments in the hospital.

22. Due notice should be given of a consultation, and no person admitted to it except the Physicians and Surgeons of the hospital, and the House-Surgeon, without the unanimous consent of the gentlemen present. If an examination of the patient be previously necessary, the particular circumstances of danger or difficulty should be carefully concealed from him, and every just precaution used to guard him from anxiety or alarm.

23. No important operation should be determined upon, without a consultation of the Physicians and Surgeons, and the acquiescence of a majority of them. Twenty-four hours notice should be given of the proposed operation, except in dangerous accidents, or when peculiar circumstances occur which may render delay hazardous. The presence of a spectator should not be allowed during an operation, without the express permission of the operator. All extra-official interference in the management of it should be forbidden. A decorous silence ought to be observed. It may be humane and salutary, however, for one of the attending Physicians or Surgeons to speak occasionally to the patient, to comfort him under his sufferings, and to give him assurance (if consistent with truth,) that the operation goes on well, and promises a speedy and successful termination.[2]

As a hospital is the best school for practical Surgery, it would be liberal and beneficial to invite in rotation two Surgeons of the town, who do not belong to the institution, to be present at each operation.

24. Hospital consultations ought not to be held on Sundays, except in cases of urgent necessity; and on such occasions an hour should be appointed which does not interfere with attendance on public worship.

25. It is an established usage in some hospitals to have a stated day in the week for the performance of operations. But this may occasion improper delay, or equally unjustifiable anticipation. When several operations are to take place in succession, one patient should not have his mind agitated by the knowledge of the sufferings of another. The Surgeon should change his apron, when besmeared; and the table or instruments should be freed from all marks of blood, and every thing that may excite terror.

26. Dispensaries afford the widest sphere for the treatment of diseases, comprehending not only such as ordinarily occur, but those which are so infectious, malignant, and fatal, as to be excluded from admission into infirmaries. Happily also they neither tend to counteract that spirit of independence which should be sedulously fostered in the poor, nor to preclude the practical exercise of those relative duties, "the charities of father, son, and brother," which constitute the strongest moral bonds of society. Being institutions less splendid and expensive than hospitals, they are well adapted to towns of moderate size; and might even be established without difficulty in populous country districts. Physicians and Surgeons in such situations have generally great influence; and it would be truly honourable to exert it in a cause subservient to the interests of Medical science, of commerce, and of philanthropy.

The duties which devolve on gentlemen of the Faculty engaged in the conduct of Dispensaries, are so nearly similar to those of hospital Physicians and Surgeons, as to be comprehended under the same professional and moral rules. But greater authority and greater condescension will be found requisite in domestic attendance on the poor; and human nature must be intimately studied, to acquire that full ascendancy over the prejudices, the caprices, and the passions of the sick and of their relatives, which is essential to Medical success.

27. Hospitals appropriated to particular maladies are established in different places, and claim both the patronage and the aid of the gentlemen of the Faculty. To an asylum for female patients labouring under syphilis it is to be lamented that discouragements have been too often and successfully opposed. Yet whoever reflects on the variety of diseases to which the human body is incident, will find that a considerable part of them are derived from immoderate passions and vicious indulgences. Sloth, intemperance, and irregular desires are the great sources of

those evils which contract the duration and imbitter the enjoyment of life. But humanity, whilst she bewails the vices of mankind, incites us to alleviate the miseries which flow from them. And it may be proved that a Lock Hospital is an institution founded on the most benevolent principles, consonant to sound policy, and favourable to reformation and to virtue. It provides relief for a painful and loathsome distemper, which contaminates in its progress the innocent as well as the guilty, and extends its baneful influence to future generations. It restores to virtue and to religion those votaries whom pleasure has seduced or villany betrayed, and who now feel by sad experience that ruin, misery, and disgrace are the wages of sin. Over such objects pity sheds the generous tear, austerity softens into forgiveness, and benevolence expands at the united pleas of frailty, penitence, and wretchedness.[3]

No peculiar rules of conduct are requisite in the Medical attendance on Lock Hospitals: but, as these institutions must from the nature of their object be in a great measure shut from the inspection of the public, it will behove the Faculty to consider themselves as responsible in an extraordinary degree for their right government; that the moral, no less than the Medical purposes of such establishments may be fully answered. The strictest decorum should be observed in the conduct towards the female patients; no young pupils should be admitted into the house; every ministering office should be performed by nurses properly instructed; and books adapted to the moral improvement of the patients should be put into their hands, and given them on their discharge. To provide against the danger of urgent want, a small sum of money and decent clothes should at this time be dispensed to them; and, when practicable, some mode should be pointed out of obtaining a reputable livelihood.

28. Asylums for insanity possess accommodations and advantages, of which the poor must in all circumstances be destitute; and which no private family, however opulent, can provide. Of these schemes of benevolence all classes of men may have equal occasion to participate the benefits; for human nature itself becomes the mournful object of such institutions.

Other diseases leave man a rational and moral agent, and sometimes improve both the faculties of the head and the affections of the heart. But lunacy subverts the whole rational and moral character, extinguishes every tender charity, and excludes the degraded sufferer from all the enjoyments and advantages of social intercourse. Painful is the office of a Physician, when he is called upon to minister to such humiliating objects of distress; yet great must be his felicity, when he can render himself instrumental, under Providence, in the restoration of reason and in the renewal of the lost image of God. Let no one, however, promise himself this divine privilege, if he be not deeply skilled in the philosophy of human nature; for, though casual success may sometimes be the result of empirical practice, the *medicina mentis* can only be administered with steady efficacy by him, who, to a knowledge of the animal economy and of the physical causes which regulate or disturb its movements, unites an intimate acquaintance with the laws of association, the control of fancy over judgement, the force of habit, the direction and comparative strength of opposite passions, and the reciprocal dependences and relations of the moral and intellectual powers of man.

29. Even thus qualified with the prerequisite attainments, the Physician will find that he has a new region of Medical science to explore; for it is a circumstance to be regretted both by the Faculty and the public, that the various diseases which are classed under the title of insanity remain less understood than any others with which mankind are visited. Hospital institutions furnish the best means of acquiring more accurate knowledge of their causes, nature, and cure; but this information cannot be attained, to any satisfactory extent, by the ordinary attention to single and unconnected cases. The synthetic plan should be adopted; and a regular journal should be kept of every species of the malady which occurs, arranged under proper heads, with a full detail of its rise, progress, and termination; of the remedies administered, and of their effects in its several stages. The age, sex, occupation, mode of life, and (if possible,) hereditary constitution of each patient should be noted; and, when the event proves fatal, the brain and other organs affected should be

carefully examined, and the appearances on dissection minutely inserted in the journal. A register like this in the course of a few years would afford the most interesting and authentic documents, the want of which on a late melancholy occasion[4] was felt and regretted by the whole kingdom.

30. Lunatics are in a great measure secluded from the observation of those who are interested in their good treatment; and their complaints of ill-usage are so often false or fanciful, as to obtain little credit or attention, even when well founded. The Physician, therefore, must feel himself under the strictest obligation of honour, as well as of humanity, to secure to these unhappy sufferers all the tenderness and indulgence compatible with steady and effectual government.

31. Certain cases of mania seem to require a boldness of practice, which a young Physician of sensibility may feel a reluctance to adopt. On such occasions he must not yield to timidity, but fortify his mind by the councils of his more experienced brethren of the Faculty. Yet, with this aid, it is more consonant to probity to err on the side of caution than of temerity.

Hospitals for the small-pox, for inoculation, for cancers, etc., etc., are established in different places; but require no professional duties, which are not included under, or deducible from, the precepts already delivered.

Of Professional Conduct in Private or General Practice

1. The moral rules of conduct prescribed towards hospital patients should be fully adopted in private or general practice. Every case committed to the charge of a Physician or Surgeon should be treated with attention, steadiness, and humanity; reasonable indulgence should be granted to the mental imbecility and caprices of the sick; secrecy and delicacy, when required by peculiar circumstances, should be strictly observed; and the familiar and confidential intercourse, to which the Faculty are admitted in their professional visits, should be used with discretion, and with the most scrupulous regard to fidelity and honour.

2. The strictest temperance should be deemed incumbent on the Faculty; as the practice both of Physic and Surgery

at all times requires the exercise of a clear and vigorous understanding: and on emergencies, for which no professional man should be unprepared, a steady hand, an acute eye, and an unclouded head, may be essential to the well-being, and even to the life, of a fellow-creature. Philip of Macedon reposed with entire security on the vigilance and attention of his general Parmenio. In his hours of mirth and conviviality he was wont to say, "Let us drink, my friends; we may do it with safety, for Parmenio never drinks!" The moral of this story is sufficiently obvious when applied to the Faculty; but it should certainly be construed with great limitation by their patients.

3. A Physician should not be forward to make gloomy prognostications; because they savour of empiricism, by magnifying the importance of his services in the treatment or cure of the disease. But he should not fail on proper occasions to give to the friends of the patient timely notice of danger when it really occurs, and even to the patient himself, if absolutely necessary. This office, however, is so peculiarly alarming when executed by him, that it ought to be declined whenever it can be assigned to any other person of sufficient judgement and delicacy; for the Physician should be the minister of hope and comfort to the sick, that by such cordials to the drooping spirit he may smooth the bed of death, revive expiring life, and counteract the depressing influence of those maladies, which rob the philosopher of fortitude, and the Christian of consolation.

4. Officious interference in a case under the charge of another should be carefully avoided. No meddling enquiries should be made concerning the patient, no unnecessary hints given relative to the nature or treatment of his disorder, nor any selfish conduct pursued, that may directly or indirectly tend to diminish the trust reposed in the Physician or Surgeon employed. Yet, though the character of a professional busy-body, whether from thoughtlessness or craft, is highly reprehensible, there are occasions which not only justify, but require, a spirited interposition. When artful ignorance grossly imposes on credulity, when neglect puts to hazard an important life,

or rashness threatens it with still more imminent danger, a Medical neighbour, friend, or relative, apprized of such facts, will justly regard his interference as a duty. But he ought to be careful that the information on which he acts is well founded, that his motives are pure and honourable, and that his judgement of the measures pursued is built on experience and practical knowledge, not on speculative or theoretical differences of opinion. The particular circumstances of the case will suggest the most proper mode of conduct. In general, however, a personal and confidential application to the gentleman of the Faculty concerned, should be the first step taken, and afterwards, if necessary, the transaction may be communicated to the patient or to his family.

5. When a Physician or Surgeon is called to a patient who has been before under the care of another gentleman of the Faculty, a consultation with him should be proposed, even though he may have discontinued his visits. His practice also should be treated with candour, and justified, so far as probity and truth will permit: for the want of success in the primary treatment of a case is no impeachment of professional skill or knowledge; and it often serves to throw light on the nature of a disease, and to suggest to the subsequent practitioner more appropriate means of relief.

6. In large and opulent towns the distinction between the provinces of Physic and Surgery should be steadily maintained. This distinction is sanctioned both by reason and experience. It is founded on the nature and objects of the two professions; on the education and acquirements requisite for their most beneficial and honourable exercise; and tends to promote the complete cultivation and advancement of each. For the division of skill and labour is no less advantageous in the liberal than in the mechanic arts; and both Physic and Surgery are so comprehensive, and yet so far from perfection, as separately to give full scope to the industry and genius of their respective professors. Experience has fully evinced the benefits of the discrimination recommended, which is established in every well regulated hospital, and is thus expressly authorized by the Faculty themselves, and by those who have the best opportunities of judging

of the proper application of the healing art. No Physician or Surgeon, therefore, should adopt more than one denomination, or assume any rank or privileges different from those of his order.

7. Consultations should be promoted in difficult or protracted cases, as they give rise to confidence, energy, and more enlarged views in practice. On such occasions no rivalship or jealousy should be indulged: candour, probity, and all due respect should be exercised towards the Physician or Surgeon first engaged; and, as he may be presumed to be best acquainted with the patient and with his family, he should deliver all the medical directions agreed upon, though he may not have precedency in seniority or rank. It should be the province, however, of the senior Physician, first to propose the necessary questions to the sick, but without excluding his associate from the privilege of making farther enquiries, to satisfy himself, or to elucidate the case.

8. As circumstances sometimes occur to render a special consultation desirable, when the continued attendance of another Physician or Surgeon might be objectionable to the patient, the gentleman of the Faculty whose assistance is required, in such cases, should pay only two or three visits, and sedulously guard against all future unsolicited interference. For this consultation a double gratuity may reasonably be expected from the patient, as it will be found to require an extraordinary portion both of time and attention.

In Medical practice it is not an unfrequent occurrence, that a Physician is hastily summoned, through the anxiety of the family or the solicitation of friends, to visit a patient who is under the regular direction of another Physician, to whom notice of this call has not been given. Under such circumstances no change in the treatment of the sick person should be made, till a previous consultation with the stated Physician has taken place, unless the lateness of the hour precludes meeting, or the symptoms of the case are too pressing to admit of delay.

9. Theoretical discussions should be avoided in consultations, as occasioning perplexity and loss of time; for there may be much diversity of opinion concerning speculative points, with perfect agreement in those modes of

practice which are founded not on hypothesis, but on experience and observation.

10. The rules prescribed for hospital consultations may be adopted in private or general practice. And the seniority of a Physician may be determined by the period of his public and acknowledged practice as a Physician, and that of a Surgeon by the period of his practice as a Surgeon, in the place where each resides. This arrangement, being clear and obvious, is adapted to remove all grounds of dispute amongst Medical gentlemen; and it secures the regular continuance of the order of precedency established in every town, which might otherwise be liable to troublesome interruptions by new settlers, perhaps not long stationary.

11. A regular academical education furnishes the only presumptive evidence of professional ability, and is so honourable and beneficial, that it gives a just claim to pre-eminence among Physicians, in proportion to the degree in which it has been enjoyed and improved. Yet, as it is not indispensably necessary to the attainment of knowledge, skill, and experience, they who have really acquired in a competent measure such qualifications without its advantages, should not be fastidiously excluded from the privileges of fellowship. In consultations especially, as the good of the patient is the sole object in view, and is often dependent on personal confidence, the aid of an [any?] intelligent practitioner ought to be received with candour and politeness, and his advice adopted, if agreeable to sound judgement and truth.

12. Punctuality should be observed in the visits of the Faculty, when they are to hold consultation together; but, as this may not always be practicable, the Physician or Surgeon who first arrives at the place of appointment, should wait five minutes for his associate, before his introduction to the patient, that the unnecessary repetition of questions may be avoided. No visits should be made but in concert, or by mutual agreement; no statement or discussion of the case should take place before the patient or his friends, except in the presence of each of the attending gentlemen of the Faculty, and by common consent; and no prognostications should be delivered, which are not the result of previous deliberation and concurrence.

13. Visits to the sick should not be unseasonably repeated; because, when too frequent, they tend to diminish the authority of the Physician, to produce instability in his practice, and to give rise to such occasional indulgences, as are subversive of all Medical regimen.

Sir William Temple has asserted, that ''an honest Physician is excused for leaving his patient, when he finds the disease growing desperate, and can, by his attendance, expect only to receive his fees, without any hopes or appearance of deserving them.'' But this allegation is not well founded; for the offices of a Physician may continue to be highly useful to the patient and comforting to the relatives around him even in the last period of a fatal malady, by obviating despair, by alleviating pain, and by soothing mental anguish. To decline attendance under such circumstances would be sacrificing to fanciful delicacy and mistaken liberality that moral duty which is independent of, and far superior to, all pecuniary appreciation.

14. Whenever a Physician or Surgeon officiates for another who is sick or absent during any considerable length of time, he should receive the fees accruing from such additional practice; but, if this fraternal act be of short duration, it should be gratuitously performed, with an observance always of the utmost delicacy towards the interest and character of the professional gentleman previously connected with the family.

15. Some general rule should be adopted by the Faculty in every town relative to the pecuniary acknowledgements of their patients; and it should be deemed a point of honour to adhere to this rule with as much steadiness as varying circumstances will admit: for it is obvious that an average fee, as suited to the general rank of patients, must be an inadequate gratuity from the rich, who often require attendance not absolutely necessary, and yet too large to be expected from that class of citizens, who would feel a reluctance in calling for assistance without making some decent and satisfactory retribution.

But in the consideration of fees, let it ever be remembered, that, though mean ones from the affluent are both unjust and degrading, yet the characteristical beneficence of the Profession is inconsistent with sordid views and avaricious rapacity. To a young Physician it is of great importance to have clear and definite ideas of the ends of his Profession, of the means for their attainment, and of the comparative value and dignity of each. Wealth, rank, and independence, with all the benefits resulting from them, are the primary ends which he holds in view; and they are interesting, wise, and laudable: but knowledge, benevolence, and active virtue, the means to be adopted in their acquisition, are of still higher estimation; and he has the privilege and felicity of practising an art, even more intrinsically excellent in its mediate than in its ultimate objects. The former, therefore, have a claim to uniform pre-eminence.

16. All members of the Profession (including Apothecaries, as well as Physicians and Surgeons.) together with their wives and children, should be attended gratuitously by any one or more of the Faculty residing near them whose assistance may be required; for, as solicitude obscures the judgement, and is accompanied with timidity and irresolution, Medical men, under the pressure of sickness, either as affecting themselves or their families, are peculiarly dependent upon each other. But visits should not be obtruded officiously; as such unasked civility may give rise to embarrassment, or interfere with that choice on which confidence depends. Distant members of the Faculty, when they request attendance, should be expected to defray the charges of travelling; and, if their circumstances be affluent, a pecuniary acknowledgement should not be declined: for no obligation ought to be imposed, which the party would rather compensate than contract.

17. When a Physician attends the wife or child of a member of the Faculty, or any person very nearly connected with him, he should manifest peculiar attention to his opinions, and tenderness even to his prejudices. For the dear and important interests which the one has at stake, supersede every consideration of rank or seniority in the other; since the mind of a husband, a father, or a friend, may receive a deep and lasting wound, if the disease terminate fatally, from the adoption of means he could not approve, or the rejection of those he wished to be tried. Under such delicate circumstances,

however, a conscientious Physician will not lightly sacrifice his judgement; but will urge with proper confidence the measures he deems to be expedient, before he leaves the final decision concerning them to his more responsible coadjutor.

18. Clergymen who experience the "res angusta domi" should be visited gratuitously by the Faculty. And this exemption should be an acknowledged general rule, that the feeling of individual obligation may be rendered less oppressive. But such of the clergy as are qualified either from their stipends or fortunes to make a reasonable remuneration for Medical attendance, are not more privileged than any other order of patients. Military or naval subaltern officers in narrow circumstances are also proper objects of professional liberality.

19. As the first consultation by letter imposes much more trouble and attention than a personal visit, it is reasonable on such an occasion to expect a gratuity of double the usual amount: and this has long been the established practice of many respectable Physicians. But a subsequent epistolary correspondence on the further treatment of the same disorder may justly be regarded in the light of ordinary attendance, and may be compensated as such according to the circumstances of the case or of the patient.

20. Physicians and Surgeons are occasionally requested to furnish certificates, justifying the absence of persons who hold situations of honour and trust in the army, the navy, or the civil departments of government. These testimonials, unless under particular circumstances, should be considered as acts due to the public, and therefore not to be compensated by any gratuity. But they should never be given without an accurate and faithful scrutiny into the case; that truth and probity may not be violated, nor the good of the community injured, by the unjust pretences of its servants. The same conduct is to be observed by Medical practitioners when they are solicited to furnish apologies for non-attendance on juries, or to state the valetudinary incapacity of persons appointed to execute the business of constables, church-wardens, or overseers of the poor. No fear of giving umbrage, no view to present or future emolument, nor any motives of friendship, should

incite to a false, or even dubious declaration; for the general weal requires that every individual who is properly qualified should deem himself obliged to execute, when legally called upon, the juridical and municipal employments of the body politic; and to be accessory by untruth or prevarication to the evasion of this duty, is at once a high misdemeanour against social order, and a breach of moral and professional honour.

21. The use of quack medicines should be discouraged by the Faculty, as disgraceful to the Profession, injurious to health, and often destructive even of life. Patients, however, under lingering disorders, are sometimes obstinately bent on having recourse to such as they see advertised or hear recommended with a boldness and confidence which no intelligent Physician dares to adopt with respect to the means that he prescribes. In these cases, some indulgence seems to be required to a credulity that is insurmountable; and the patient should neither incur the displeasure of the Physician, nor be entirely deserted by him. He may be apprized of the fallacy of his expectations, whilst assured at the same time that diligent attention should be paid to the process of the experiment he is so unadvisedly making on himself, and the consequent mischiefs, if any, obviated as timely as possible. Certain active preparations, the nature, composition, and effects of which are well known, ought not to be proscribed as quack medicines.

22. No Physician or Surgeon should dispense a secret nostrum, whether it be his invention, or exclusive property; for, if it be of real efficacy, the concealment of it is inconsistent with beneficence and professional liberality; and if mystery alone give it value and importance, such craft implies either disgraceful ignorance or fraudulent avarice.

23. The *esprit du corps* is a principle of action founded in human nature, and, when duly regulated, is both rational and laudable. Every man who enters into a fraternity engages by a tacit compact not only to submit to the laws, but to promote the honour and interest, of the association, so far as they are consistent with morality and

the general good of mankind. A Physician, therefore, should cautiously guard against whatever may injure the general respectability of his Profession; and should avoid all contumelious representations of the Faculty at large, all general charges against their selfishness or improbity, and the indulgence of an affected or jocular scepticism concerning the efficacy and utility of the healing art.

24. As diversity of opinion and opposition of interest may in the Medical, as in other professions, sometimes occasion controversy and even contention; whenever such cases unfortunately occur, and cannot be immediately terminated, they should be referred to the arbitration of a sufficient number of Physicians or of Surgeons, according to the nature of the dispute; or to the two orders collectively, if belonging both to Medicine and Surgery. But neither the subject matter of such references, nor the adjudication, should be communicated to the public; as they may be personally injurious to the individuals concerned, and can hardly fail to hurt the general credit of the Faculty.

25. A wealthy Physician should not give advice gratis to the affluent, because it is an injury to his professional brethren. The office of Physician can never be supported but as a lucrative one, and it is defrauding in some degree the common funds for its support, when fees are dispensed with, which might justly be claimed.

26. It frequently happens that a Physician, in his incidental communications with the patients of other Physicians or with their friends, may have their cases stated to him in so direct a manner, as not to admit of his declining to pay attention to them. Under such circumstances his observations should be delivered with the most delicate propriety and reserve: he should not interfere in the curative plans pursued, and should even recommend a steady adherence to them, if they appear to merit approbation.

27. A Physician, when visiting a sick person in the country, may be desired to see a neighbouring patient who is under the regular direction of another Physician, in consequence of some sudden change or aggravation of symptoms. The conduct to be pursued on such an occasion is to give advice

adapted to present circumstances, to interfere no farther than is absolutely necessary with the general plan of treatment, to assume no future direction unless it be expressly desired, and, in this case, to request an immediate consultation with the practitioner antecedently employed.

28. At the close of every interesting and important case (especially when it hath terminated fatally,) a Physician should trace back in calm reflection all the steps which he had [has?] taken in the treatment of it. This review of the origin, progress, and conclusion of the malady, of the whole curative plan pursued, and of the particular operation of the several remedies employed, as well as of the doses and periods of time in which they were administered, will furnish the most authentic documents on which individual experience can be formed. But it is in a moral view that the practice is here recommended; and it should be performed with the most scrupulous impartiality. Let no self-deception be permitted in the retrospect; and, if errors either of omission or commission are discovered, it behoves that they should be brought fairly and fully to the mental view. Regrets may follow, but criminality will thus be obviated; for good intentions, and the imperfection of human skill which cannot anticipate the knowledge that events alone disclose, will sufficiently justify what is past, provided the failure be made conscientiously subservient to future wisdom and rectitude in professional conduct.

29. The opportunities which a Physician not unfrequently enjoys, of promoting and strengthening the good resolutions of his patients suffering under the consequences of vicious conduct, ought never to be neglected. And his counsels, or even remonstrances, will give satisfaction, not disgust, if they be conducted with politeness, and evince a genuine love of virtue, accompanied by a sincere interest in the welfare of the person to whom they are addressed.

30. The observance of the Sabbath is a duty to which Medical men are bound, so far as is compatible with the urgency of the cases under their charge. Visits may often be made with sufficient convenience and benefit, either before the hours of going to church, or during the intervals of public worship; and in many chronic ailments the sick, together with their attendants, are qualified to participate in the social offices of religion, and should not be induced to forego this important privilege by the expectation of a call from their Physician or Surgeon.

31. A Physician who is advancing in years, yet unconscious of any decay in his faculties, may occasionally experience some change in the wonted confidence of his friends. Patients, who before trusted solely to his care and skill, may now request that he will join in consultation, perhaps with a younger coadjutor. It behoves him to admit this change without dissatisfaction or fastidiousness, regarding it as no mark of disrespect, but as the exercise of a just and reasonable privilege in those by whom he is employed. The junior practitioner may well be supposed to have more ardour than *he* possesses in the treatment of diseases, to be bolder in the exhibition of new medicines, and disposed to administer old ones in doses of greater efficacy. And this union of enterprise with caution, and of fervour with coolness, may promote the successful management of a difficult and protracted case. Let the Medical parties, therefore, be studious to conduct themselves towards each other with candour and impartiality; co-operating by mutual concessions in the benevolent discharge of professional duty.

32. The commencement of that period of senescence, when it becomes incumbent on a Physician to decline the offices of his profession, it is not easy to ascertain; and the decision on so nice a point must be left to the moral discretion of the individual. For, one grown old in the useful and honourable exercise of the healing art, may continue to enjoy, and justly to enjoy, the unabated confidence of the public; and, whilst exempt in a considerable degree from the privations and infirmities of age, he is under indispensable obligations to apply his knowledge and experience in the most efficient way to the benefit of mankind: for the possession of powers is a clear indication of the will of our Creator concerning their practical direction. But in the ordinary course of nature the bodily and mental vigour must be expected to decay progressively, though perhaps slowly, after the meridian of life is past. As age advances, therefore, a Physician should from time to time scrutinize impartially the state of his faculties, that he may determine *bona fide* the precise degree in which he is qualified to execute the active and multifarious offices of his profession; and, whenever he becomes conscious that his memory presents to him with faintness those analogies on which Medical reasoning and the treatment of diseases are founded, that diffidence of the measures to be pursued perplexes his judgment, that, from a deficiency in the acuteness of his senses, he finds himself less able to distinguish signs or to prognosticate events, he should at once resolve (though others perceive not the changes which have taken place,) to sacrifice every consideration of fame or fortune, and to retire from the engagements of business. To the Surgeon under similar circumstances this rule of conduct is still more necessary; for the energy of the understanding often subsists much longer than the quickness of eye-sight, delicacy of touch, and steadiness of hand, which are essential to the skilful performance of operations. Let both the Physician and Surgeon never forget that their professions are public trusts, properly rendered lucrative whilst they fulfil them, but which they are bound by honour and probity to relinquish as soon as they find themselves unequal to their adequate and faithful execution. . . .

Notes

1. See Aikin's *Thoughts on Hospitals,* p. 21.

2. The substance of the five preceding articles (19–23) was suggested by Dr. Ferriar and Mr. Simmons, at the time when I was desired by them and my other colleagues to frame a code of rules for the Manchester Infirmary. The additions now made are intended to adapt them to general use.

3. See two Reports, intended to promote the establishment of a Lock Hospital at Manchester, in the year 1774, inserted in the Author's *Essays Medical, Philosophical, and Experimental,* vol. ii. p. 263. (*Works,* vol. iv. p. 203.)

4. [Alluding to the case of George III.]

8

American Medical Association

First Code of Medical Ethics

Reprinted from *Proceedings of the National Medical Convention 1846–1847*, pp. 83–106.

Introduction to the Code of Medical Ethics

Medical ethics, as a branch of general ethics, must rest on the basis of religion and morality. They comprise not only the duties, but, also, the rights of a physician: and, in this sense, they are identical with Medical Deontology—a term introduced by a late writer, who has taken the most comprehensive view of the subject.

In framing a code on this basis, we have the inestimable advantage of deducing its rules from the conduct of the many eminent physicians who have adorned the profession by their learning and their piety. From the age of Hippocrates to the present time, the annals of every civilized people contain abundant evidences of the devotedness of medical men to the relief of their fellow-creatures from pain and disease, regardless of the privation and danger, and not seldom obloquy, encountered in return; a sense of ethical obligations rising superior, in their minds, to considerations of personal advancement. Well and truly was it said by one of the most learned men of the last century: that the duties of a physician were never more beautifully exemplified than in the conduct of Hippocrates, nor more eloquently described than in his writings.

We may here remark, that, if a state of probation be intended for moral discipline, there is, assuredly, much in the daily life of a physician to impart this salutary training, and to insure continuance in a course of self-denial, and, at the same time, of zealous and methodical efforts for the relief of the suffering and unfortunate, irrespective of rank or fortune, or of fortuitous elevation of any kind.

A few considerations on the legitimate range of medical ethics will serve as an appropriate introduction to the requisite rules for our guidance in the complex relations of professional life.

Every duty or obligation implies, both in equity and for its successful discharge, a corresponding right. As it is the duty of a physician to advise, so has he a right to be attentively and respectfully listened to. Being required to expose his health and life for the benefit of the community, he has a just claim, in return, on all its members, collectively and individually, for aid to carry out his measures, and for all possible tenderness and regard to prevent needlessly harassing calls on his services and unnecessary exhaustion of his benevolent sympathies.

His zeal, talents, attainments and skill are qualities which he holds in trust for the general good, and which cannot be prodigally spent, either through his own negligence or the inconsiderateness of others, without wrong and detriment both to himself and to them.

The greater the importance of the subject and the more deeply interested all are in the issue, the more necessary is it that the physician—he who performs the chief part, and in whose judgment and discretion under Providence, life is secured and death turned aside—should be allowed the free use of his faculties, undisturbed by a querulous manner, and desponding, angry, or passionate interjections, under the plea of fear, or grief, or disappointment of cherished hopes, by the sick and their friends.

All persons privileged to enter the sick room, and the number ought to be very limited, are under equal obligations of reciprocal courtesy, kindness and respect; and, if any exception be admissible, it cannot be at the expense of the physician. His position, purposes and proper efforts eminently entitle him to, at least, the same respectful and considerate attentions that are paid, as a matter of course and apparently without constraint, to the clergyman, who is admitted to administer spiritual consolation, and to the lawyer, who comes to make the last will and testament.

Although professional duty requires of a physician, that he should have such a control over himself as not to betray strong emotion in the presence of his patient, nor to be thrown off his guard by the querulousness or even rudeness of the latter, or of his friends at the bedside, yet, and the fact ought to be generally known, many medical men, possessed of abundant attainments and resources, are so constitutionally timid and readily abashed as to lose much of their self possession and usefulness at the critical moment, if opposition be abruptly interposed to any part of the plan which they are about devising for the benefit of their patients.

Medical ethics cannot be so divided as that one part shall obtain the full and proper force of moral obligations on physicians universally, and, at the same time, the other be construed in such a way as to free society from all restrictions in its conduct to them; leaving it to the caprice of the hour to determine whether the truly learned shall be overlooked in favour of ignorant pretenders—persons destitute alike of original talent and acquired fitness.

The choice is not indifferent, in an ethical point of view, besides its important bearing on the fate of the sick themselves, between the directness and sincerity of purpose, the honest zeal, the learning and impartial observations, accumulated from age to age for thousands of years, of the regularly initiated members of the medical profession, and the crooked devices and low arts, for evidently selfish ends, the unsupported promises and reckless trials of interloping empirics, whose very announcements of the means by which they profess to perform their wonders are, for the most part, misleading and false, and, so far, fraudulent.

In thus deducing the rights of a physician from his duties, it is not meant to insist on such a correlative obligation, that the withholding of the right exonerates from the discharge of the duty. Short of the formal abandonment of the practice of his profession, no medical man can withhold his services from the requisition either of an individual or of the community, unless under circumstances, of rare occurrence, in which his compliance would be not only unjust but degrading to himself, or to a professional brother, and so far diminish his future usefulness.

In the discharge of their duties to Society, physicians must be ever ready and prompt to administer professional aid to all applicants, without prior stipulation of personal advantages to themselves.

On them devolves, in a peculiar manner, the task of noting all the circumstances affecting the public health, and of displaying skill and ingenuity in devising the best means for its protection.

With them rests, also, the solemn duty of furnishing accurate medical testimony in all cases of criminal accusation of violence, by which health is endangered and life destroyed, and in those other numerous ones involving the question of mental sanity and of moral and legal responsibility.

On these subjects—Public Hygiene and Medical Jurisprudence—every medical man must be supposed to have prepared himself by study, observation, and the exercise of a sound judgment. They cannot be regarded in the light of accomplishments merely: they are an integral part of the science and practice of medicine.

It is a delicate and noble task, by the judicious application of Public Hygiene, to prevent disease and to prolong life; and thus to increase the productive industry, and, without assuming the office of moral and religious teaching, to add to the civilization of an entire people.

In the performance of this part of their duty, physicians are enabled to exhibit the close connection between hygiene and morals; since all the causes contributing to the former are nearly equally auxiliary to the latter.

Physicians, as conservators of the public health, are bound to bear emphatic testimony against quackery in all its forms; whether it appears with its usual effrontery, or masks itself under the garb of philanthropy and sometimes of religion itself.

By an anomaly in legislation and penal enactments, the laws, so stringent for the repression and punishment of fraud in general, and against attempts to sell poisonous substances for food, are silent, and of course inoperative, in the cases of both fraud and poisoning so extensively carried on by the host of quacks who infest the land.

The newspaper press, powerful in the correction of many abuses, is too ready for the sake of lucre to aid and abet the enormities of quackery. Honourable exceptions to the once general practice in this respect are becoming, happily, more numerous, and they might be more rapidly increased, if physicians, when themselves free from all taint, were to direct the intention of the editors and proprietors of newspapers, and of periodical works in general, to the moral bearings of the subject.

To those who, like physicians, can best see the extent of the evil, it is still more mortifying than in the instances already mentioned, to find members of other professions, and especially ministers of the Gospel, so prone to give their countenance, and, at times, direct patronage, to medical empirics, both by their use of nostrums, and by their certificates in favour of the absurd pretensions of these impostors.

The credulous, on these occasions, place themselves in the dilemma of bearing testimony either to a miracle or to an imposture: to a miracle, if one particular agent, and it often of known inertness or slight power, can cure all diseases, or even any one disease in all its stages; to an imposture, if the alleged cures are not made, as experience shows that they are not.

But by no class are quack medicines and nostrums so largely sold and distributed as by apothecaries, whose position towards physicians, although it may not amount to actual affinity, is such that it ought, at least, to prevent them from entering into an actual, if not formally recognized, alliance with empirics of every grade and degree of pretention.

Too frequently we meet with physicians who deem it a venial error, in ethics, to permit, and even to recommend, the use of a quack medicine or secret compound by their patients and friends. They forget that their toleration implies sanction of a recourse by the people generally to unknown, doubtful and conjectural fashions of medication; and that the credulous in this way soon become the victims of an endless succession of empirics. It must have been generally noticed, also, that they, whose faith is strongest in the most absurd pretensions of quackery, entertain the greatest skepticism towards regular and philosophic medicine.

Adverse alike to ethical propriety and to medical logic, are the various popular delusions which, like so many epidemics, have, in successive ages, excited the imagination with extravagant expectations of the cure of all diseases and the prolongation of life beyond its customary limits, by means of a single substance. Although it is not in the power of physicians to prevent, or always to arrest, these delusions in their progress, yet it is incumbent on them, from their superior knowledge and better opportunities, as well as from their elevated vocation, steadily to refuse to extend to them the slightest countenance, still less support.

These delusions are sometimes manifested in the guise of a new and infallible system of medical practice,—the faith in which, among the excited believers, is usually in the inverse ratio of the amount of common sense evidence in its favour. Among the volunteer missionaries for its dissemination, it is painful to see members of the sacred profession, who, above all others, ought to keep aloof from vagaries of any description, and especially of those medical ones which are allied to empirical imposture.

The plea of good intention is not an adequate reason for the assumption of so grave a responsibility as the propagation of a theory and practice of medicine, of the real foundation and nature of which the mere medical amateur must necessarily, from his want of opportunities for study, observation, and careful comparison, be profoundly ignorant.

In their relations with the sick, physicians are bound, by every consideration of duty, to exercise the greatest kindness with the greatest circumspection; so that, whilst they make every allowance for impatience, irritation, and inconsistencies of manner and speech of the sufferers, and do their utmost to sooth and tranquilize, they shall, at the same time, elicit from them, and the persons in their confidence, a revelation of all the circumstances connected with the probable origin of the diseases which they are called upon to treat.

Owing either to the confusion and, at times, obliquity of mind produced by the disease, or to considerations of false delicacy and shame, the truth is not always directly reached on these occasions; and hence the necessity, on the part of the physician, of a careful and minute investigation into both the physical and moral state of his patient.

A physician in attendance on a case should avoid expensive complications and tedious ceremonials, as being beneath the dignity of true science and embarrassing to the patient and his family, whose troubles are already great.

In their intercourse with each other, physicians will best consult and secure their own self-respect and consideration from society in general, by a uniform courtesy and high-minded conduct towards their professional brethren. The confidence in his intellectual and moral worth, which each member of the profession is ambitious of obtaining for himself among his associates,

ought to make him willing to place the same confidence in the worth of others.

Veracity, so requisite in all the relations of life, is a jewel of inestimable value in medical description and narrative, the lustre of which ought never to be tainted for a moment, by even the breath of suspicion. Physicians are peculiarly enjoined, by every consideration of honour and of conscientious regard for the health and lives of their fellow beings, not to advance any statement unsupported by positive facts, nor to hazard an opinion or hypothesis that is not the result of deliberate inquiry into all the data and bearings of which the subject is capable.

Hasty generalization, paradox and fanciful conjectures, repudiated at all times by sound logic, are open to the severest reprehension on the still higher grounds of humanity and morals. Their tendency and practical operation cannot fail to be eminently mischievous.

Among medical men associated together for the performance of professional duties in public institutions, such as Medical Colleges, Hospitals and Dispensaries, there ought to exist, not only harmonious intercourse, but also a general harmony in doctrine and practice; so that neither students nor patients shall be perplexed, nor the medical community mortified by contradictory views of the theory of disease, if not the means of curing it.

The right of free inquiry, common to all, does not imply the utterance of crude hypotheses, the use of figurative language, a straining after novelty for novelty's sake, and the involution of old truths, for temporary effect and popularity, by medical writers and teachers. If, therefore, they who are engaged in a common cause, and for the furtherance of a common object, could make an offering of the extreme, the doubtful, and the redundant, at the shrine of philosophical truth, the general harmony in medical teaching, now desired, would be of easy attainment.

It is not enough, however, that the members of the medical profession be zealous, well informed and self-denying, unless the social principle be cultivated by their seeking frequent intercourse with each other, and cultivating, reciprocally, friendly habits of acting in common.

By union alone can medical men hope to sustain the dignity and extend the usefulness of their profession. Among the chief means to bring about this desirable end, are frequent social meetings and regularly organized Societies; a part of whose beneficial operation would be an agreement on a suitable standard of medical education, and a code of medical ethics.

Greatly increased influence, for the entire body of the profession, will be acquired by a union for the purposes of common benefit and the general good; while to its members, individually, will be insured a more pleasant and harmonious intercourse, one with another, and an avoidance of many heartburnings and jealousies, which originate in misconception, through misrepresentation on the part of individuals in general society, of each other's disposition, motives, and conduct.

In vain will physicians appeal to the intelligence and elevated feelings of the members of other professions, and of the better part of society in general, unless they be true to themselves, by a close adherence to their duties, and by firmly yet mildly insisting on their rights; and this not with a glimmering perception and faint avowal, but, rather with a full understanding and firm conviction.

Impressed with the nobleness of their vocation, as trustees of science and almoners of benevolence and charity, physicians should use unceasing vigilance to prevent the introduction into their body of those who have not been prepared by a suitably preparatory moral and intellectual training.

No youth ought to be allowed to study medicine, whose capacity, good conduct, and elementary knowledge are not equal, at least, to the common standard of academical requirements.

Human life and human happiness must not be endangered by the incompetency of presumptuous pretenders. The greater the inherent difficulties of medicine, as a science, and the more numerous the complications that embarrass in its practice, the more necessary is it that there should be minds of a high order and thorough cultivation, to unravel its mysteries and to deduce scientific order from apparently empirical confusion.

We are under the strongest ethical obligations to preserve the character which has been awarded, by the most learned men and best judges of human nature, to the members of the medical profession, for general and extensive knowledge, great liberality and dignity of sentiment, and prompt effusions of beneficence.

In order that we may continue to merit these praises, every physician, within the circle of his acquaintance, should impress both fathers and sons with the range and variety of medical study, and with the necessity of those who desire to engage in it, possessing, not only good preliminary knowledge, but, likewise, some habits of regular and systematic thinking.

If able teachers and writers, and profound inquirers, be still called for to expound medical science, and to extend its domain of practical application and usefulness, they cannot be procured by intuitive effort on their own part, nor by the exercise of the elective suffrage on the part of others. They must be the product of a regular and comprehensive system,—members of a large class, from the great body of which they only differ by the force of fortuitous circumstances, that gives them temporary vantage ground for the display of qualities and attainments common to their brethren.

John Bell, M. D.

Code of Medical Ethics

. . . The Committee appointed under the sixth resolution adopted by the Convention which assembled in New York, in May last, to prepare a Code of Medical Ethics for the government of the medical profession of the United States, respectfully submit the following Code.

Committee
John Bell,
Isaac Hays,
G. Emerson,
W. W. Morris,
T. C. Dunn,
A. Clark,
R. D. Arnold,

Philadelphia, June 5th, 1847.

Note.—Dr. Hays, on presenting this report, stated that justice required some explanatory remarks should accompany it. The members of the Convention, he observed, would not fail to recognize in parts of it, expressions with which they were familiar. On examining a great number of codes of ethics adopted by different societies in the United States, it was found that they

were all based on that by Dr. Percival, and that the phrases of this writer were preserved, to a considerable extent, in all of them. Believing that language which had been so often examined and adopted, must possess the greatest of merits for such a document as the present, clearness and precision, and having no ambition for the honours of authorship, the Committee which prepared this code have followed a similar course, and have carefully preserved the words of Percival wherever they convey the precepts it is wished to inculcate. A few of the sections are in the words of the late Dr. Rush, and one or two sentences are from other writers. But in all cases, wherever it was thought that the language could be made more explicit by changing a word, or even a part of a sentence, this has been unhesitatingly done; and thus there are but few sections which have not undergone some modification; while, for the language of many, and for the arrangement of the whole, the Committee must be held exclusively responsible.

Of the Duties of Physicians to Their Patients and of the Obligations of Patients to Their Physicians

Art. I—Duties of Physicians to Their Patients
1. A Physician should not only be ever ready to obey the calls of the sick, but his mind ought also to be imbued with the greatness of his mission, and the responsibility he habitually incurs in its discharge. Those obligations are the more deep and enduring, because there is no tribunal other than his own conscience, to adjudge penalties for carelessness or neglect. Physicians should, therefore, minister to the sick with due impressions of the importance of their office; reflecting that the ease, the health, and the lives of those committed to their charge, depend on their skill, attention and fidelity. They should study, also, in their deportment, so to unite *tenderness* with *firmness,* and *condescension* with *authority,* as to inspire the minds of their patients with gratitude, respect and confidence.

2. Every case committed to the charge of a physician should be treated with attention, steadiness and humanity. Reasonable indulgence should be granted to the mental imbecility and caprices of the sick. Secrecy and delicacy, when required by peculiar circumstances, should be strictly observed; and the familiar and confidential intercourse to which physicians are

admitted in their professional visits, should be used with discretion, and with the most scrupulous regard to fidelity and honor. The obligation of secrecy extends beyond the period of professional services;—none of the privacies of personal and domestic life, no infirmity of disposition or flaw of character observed during professional attendance, should ever be divulged by him except when he is imperatively required to do so. The force and necessity of this obligation are indeed so great, that professional men have, under certain circumstances, been protected in their observance of secrecy, by courts of justice.

3. Frequent visits to the sick are in general requisite, since they enable the physician to arrive at a more perfect knowledge of the disease,—to meet promptly every change which may occur, and also tend to preserve the confidence of the patient. But unnecessary visits are to be avoided, as they give useless anxiety to the patient, tend to diminish the authority of the physician, and render him liable to be suspected of interested motives.

4. A physician should not be forward to make gloomy prognostications, because they savour of empiricism, by magnifying the importance of his services in the treatment or cure of the disease. But he should not fail, on proper occasions, to give to the friends of the patient timely notice of danger, when it really occurs; and even to the patient himself, if absolutely necessary. This office, however, is so peculiarly alarming when executed by him, that it ought to be declined whenever it can be assigned to any other person of sufficient judgment and delicacy. For, the physician should be the minister of hope and comfort to the sick; that, by such cordials to the drooping spirit, he may smooth the bed of death, revive expiring life, and counteract the depressing influence of those maladies which often disturb the tranquillity of the most resigned, in their last moments. The life of a sick person can be shortened not only by the acts, but also by the words or the manner of a physician. It is, therefore, a sacred duty to guard himself carefully in this respect, and to avoid all things which have a tendency to discourage the patient and to depress his spirits.

5. A physician ought not to abandon a patient because the case is deemed

incurable; for his attendance may continue to be highly useful to the patient, and comforting to the relatives around him, even in the last period of a fatal malady, by alleviating pain and other symptoms, and by soothing mental anguish. To decline attendance, under such circumstances, would be sacrificing to fanciful delicacy and mistaken liberality, that moral duty, which is independent of, and far superior to all pecuniary consideration.

6. Consultations should be promoted in difficult or protracted cases, as they give rise to confidence, energy, and more enlarged views in practice.

7. The opportunity which a physician not unfrequently enjoys of promoting and strengthening the good resolutions of his patients, suffering under the consequences of vicious conduct, ought never to be neglected. His counsels, or even remonstrances, will give satisfaction, not offence, if they be proffered with politeness, and evince a genuine love of virtue, accompanied by a sincere interest in the welfare of the person to whom they are addressed.

Art. II—Obligations of Patients to Their Physicians 1. The members of the medical profession, upon whom are enjoined the performance of so many important and arduous duties towards the community, and who are required to make so many sacrifices of comfort, ease, and health, for the welfare of those who avail themselves of their services, certainly have a right to expect and require, that their patients should entertain a just sense of the duties which they owe to their medical attendants.

2. The first duty of a patient is, to select as his medical adviser one who has received a regular professional education. In no trade or occupation, do mankind rely on the skill of an untaught artist; and in medicine, confessedly the most difficult and intricate of the sciences, the world ought not to suppose that knowledge is intuitive.

3. Patients should prefer a physician, whose habits of life are regular, and who is not devoted to company, pleasure, or to any pursuit incompatible with his professional obligations. A patient should, also, confide the care of himself and family, as much as possible, to one physician, for a medical man who has become acquainted with the peculiarities of constitution, habits, and predispositions, of those he attends, is more likely to be successful in his treatment, than one who does not possess that knowledge.

A patient who has thus selected his physician, should always apply for advice in what may appear to him trivial cases, for the most fatal results often supervene on the slightest accidents. It is of still more importance that he should apply for assistance in the forming stage of violent diseases; it is to a neglect of this precept that medicine owes much of the uncertainty and imperfection with which it has been reproached.

4. Patients should faithfully and unreservedly communicate to their physician the supposed cause of their disease. This is the more important, as many diseases of a mental origin simulate those depending on external causes, and yet are only to be cured by ministering to the mind diseased. A patient should never be afraid of thus making his physician his friend and adviser; he should always bear in mind that a medical man is under the strongest obligations of secrecy. Even the female sex should never allow feelings of shame or delicacy to prevent their disclosing the seat, symptoms and causes of complaints peculiar to them. However commendable a modest reserve may be in the common occurrences of life, its strict observance in medicine is often attended with the most serious consequences, and a patient may sink under a painful and loathsome disease, which might have been readily prevented had timely intimation been given to the physician.

5. A patient should never weary his physician with a tedious detail of events or matters not appertaining to his disease. Even as relates to his actual symptoms, he will convey much more real information by giving clear answers to interrogatories, than by the most minute account of his own framing. Neither should he obtrude the details of his business nor the history of his family concerns.

6. The obedience of a patient to the prescriptions of his physician should be prompt and implicit. He should never permit his own crude opinions as to their fitness, to influence his attention to them. A failure in one particular may render an otherwise judicious treatment dangerous, and even fatal. This remark is equally applicable to diet, drink, and exercise. As patients become convalescent they are very apt to suppose that the rules prescribed for them may be disregarded, and the consequence but too often, is a relapse. Patients should never allow themselves to be persuaded to take any medicine whatever, that may be recommended to them by the self-constituted doctors and doctresses, who are so frequently met with, and who pretend to possess infallible remedies for the cure of every disease. However simple some of their prescriptions may appear to be, it often happens that they are productive of much mischief, and in all cases they are injurious, by contravening the plan of treatment adopted by the physician.

7. A patient should, if possible, avoid even the *friendly visits of a physician* who is not attending him,—and when he does receive them, he should never converse on the subject of his disease, as an observation may be made, without any intention of interference, which may destroy his confidence in the course he is pursuing, and induce him to neglect the directions prescribed to him. A patient should never send for a consulting physician without the express consent of his own medical attendant. It is of great importance that physicians should act in concert; for, although their modes of treatment may be attended with equal success when employed singly, yet conjointly they are very likely to be productive of disastrous results.

8. When a patient wishes to dismiss his physician, justice and common courtesy require that he should declare his reasons for so doing.

9. Patients should always, when practicable, send for their physician in the morning, before his usual hour of going out; for, by being early aware of the visits he has to pay during the day, the physician is able to apportion his time in such a manner as to prevent an interference of engagements. Patients should also avoid calling on their medical adviser unnecessarily during the hours devoted to meals or sleep. They should always be in readiness to receive the visits of their physician, as the detention of a few minutes is often of serious inconvenience to him.

10. A patient should, after his recovery, entertain a just and enduring sense

of the value of the services rendered him by his physician; for these are of such a character, that no mere pecuniary acknowledgment can repay or cancel them.

Of the Duties of Physicians to Each Other, and to the Profession at Large

Art. I—Duties for the Support of Professional Character 1. Every individual, on entering the profession, as he becomes thereby entitled to all its privileges and immunities, incurs an obligation to exert his best abilities to maintain its dignity and honour, to exalt its standing, and to extend the bounds of its usefulness. He should therefore observe strictly, such laws as are instituted for the government of its members;—should avoid all contumelious and sarcastic remarks relative to the faculty, as a body; and while, by unwearied diligence, he resorts to every honourable means of enriching the science, he should entertain a due respect for his seniors, who have, by their labours, brought it to the elevated condition in which he finds it.

2. There is no profession, from the members of which greater purity of character, and a higher standard of moral excellence are required, than the medical; and to attain such eminence, is a duty every physician owes alike to his profession, and to his patients. It is due to the latter, as without it he cannot command their respect and confidence, and to both, because no scientific attainments can compensate for the want of correct moral principles. It is also incumbent upon the faculty to be temperate in all things, for the practice of physic requires the unremitting exercise of a clear and vigorous understanding; and, on emergencies for which no professional man should be unprepared, a steady hand, an acute eye, and an unclouded head may be essential to the well-being, and even to the life, of a fellow creature.

3. It is derogatory to the dignity of the profession, to resort to public advertisements or private cards or handbills, inviting the attention of individuals affected with particular diseases—publicly offering advice and medicine to the poor gratis, or promising radical cures; or to publish cases and operations in the daily prints or suffer such publications to be made;—to invite laymen to be present at operations,—to boast of cures and remedies,—to adduce certificates of skill and success, or to perform any other similar acts. These are the ordinary practices of empirics, and are highly reprehensible in a regular physician.

4. Equally derogatory to professional character is it, for a physician to hold a patent for any surgical instrument, or medicine; or to dispense a secret *nostrum*, whether it be the composition or exclusive property of himself, or of others. For, if such nostrum be of real efficacy, any concealment regarding it is inconsistent with beneficence and professional liberality; and, if mystery alone give it value and importance, such craft implies either disgraceful ignorance, or fraudulent avarice. It is also reprehensible for physicians to give certificates attesting the efficacy of patent or secret medicines, or in any way to promote the use of them.

Art. II— Professional Services of Physicians to Each Other 1. All practitioners of medicine, their wives, and their children while under the paternal care, are entitled to the gratuitous services of any one or more of the faculty residing near them, whose assistance may be desired. A physician afflicted with disease is usually an incompetent judge of his own case; and the natural anxiety and solicitude which he experiences at the sickness of a wife, a child, or any one who by the ties of consanguinity is rendered peculiarly dear to him, tend to obscure his judgment, and produce timidity and irresolution in his practice. Under such circumstances, medical men are peculiarly dependent upon each other, and kind offices and professional aid should always be cheerfully and gratuitously afforded. Visits ought not, however, to be obtruded officiously; as such unasked civility may give rise to embarrassment, or interfere with that choice, on which confidence depends. But, if a distant member of the faculty, whose circumstances are affluent, request attendance, and an honorarium be offered, it should not be declined; for no pecuniary obligation ought to be imposed, which the party receiving it would wish not to incur.

Art. III—Of the Duties of Physicians as Respects Vicarious Offices 1. The affairs of life, the pursuit of health, and the various accidents and contingencies to which a medical man is peculiarly exposed, sometimes require him temporarily to withdraw from his duties to his patients, and to request some of his professional brethren to officiate for him. Compliance with this request is an act of courtesy, which should always be performed with the utmost consideration for the interest and character of the family physician, and when exercised for a short period, all the pecuniary obligations for such service should be awarded to him. But if a member of the profession neglect his business in quest of pleasure and amusement, he cannot be considered as entitled to the advantages of the frequent and long-continued exercise of this fraternal courtesy, without awarding to the physician who officiates the fees arising from the discharge of his professional duties.

In obstetrical and important surgical cases, which give rise to unusual fatigue, anxiety and responsibility, it is just that the fees accruing therefrom should be awarded to the physician who officiates.

Art. IV—Of the Duties of Physicians in Regard to Consultations 1. A regular medical education furnishes the only presumptive evidence of professional abilities and acquirements, and ought to be the only acknowledged right of an individual to the exercise and honours of his profession. Nevertheless, as in consultations the good of the patient is the sole object in view, and this is often dependent on personal confidence, no intelligent regular practitioner, who has a license to practice from some medical board of known and acknowledged respectability, recognized by this association, and who is in good moral and professional standing in the place in which he resides, should be fastidiously excluded from fellowship, or his aid refused in consultation when it is requested by the patient. But no one can be considered as a regular practitioner, or a fit associate in consultation, whose practice is based on an exclusive dogma, to the rejection of the accumulated experience of the profession, and of the aids actually furnished by anatomy, physiology, pathology, and organic chemistry.

2. In consultations no rivalship or jealousy should be indulged; candour, probity, and all due respect should be exercised towards the physician having charge of the case.

3. In consultations the attending physician should be the first to propose the necessary questions to the sick; after which the consulting physician should have the opportunity to make such farther inquiries of the patient as may be necessary to satisfy him of the true character of the case. Both physicians should then retire to a private place for deliberation; and the one first in attendance should communicate the directions agreed upon to the patient or his friends, as well as any opinions which it may be thought proper to express. But no statement or discussion of it should take place before the patient or his friends, except in the presence of all the faculty attending, and by their common consent; and no *opinions* or *prognostications* should be delivered, which are not the result of previous deliberation and concurrence.

4. In consultations, the physician in attendance should deliver his opinion first; and when there are several consulting, they should deliver their opinions in the order in which they have been called in. No decision, however, should restrain the attending physician from making such variations in the mode of treatment, as any subsequent unexpected change in the character of the case may demand. But such variation and the reasons for it ought to be carefully detailed at the next meeting in consultation. The same privilege belongs also to the consulting physician if he is sent for in an emergency, when the regular attendant is out of the way, and similar explanations must be made by him, at the next consultation.

5. The utmost punctuality should be observed in the visits of physicians when they are to hold consultation together, and this is generally practicable, for society has been considerate enough to allow the plea of a professional engagement to take precedence of all others, and to be an ample reason for the relinquishment of any present occupation. But as professional engagements may sometimes interfere, and delay one of the parties, the physician who first arrives should wait for his associate a reasonable period, after which the consultation should be considered as postponed to a new ap-

pointment. If it be the attending physician who is present, he will of course see the patient and prescribe; but if it be the consulting one, he should retire, except in case of emergency, or when he has been called from a considerable distance, in which latter case he may examine the patient, and give his opinion in *writing* and *under seal,* to be delivered to his associate.

6. In consultations, theoretical discussions should be avoided, as occasioning perplexity and loss of time. For there may be much diversity of opinion concerning speculative points, with perfect agreement in those modes of practice which are founded, not on hypothesis, but on experience and observation.

7. All discussions in consultation should be held as secret and confidential. Neither by words nor manner should any of the parties to a consultation assert or insinuate, that any part of the treatment pursued did not receive his assent. The responsibility must be equally divided between the medical attendants,—they must equally share the credit of success as well as the blame of failure.

8. Should an irreconcilable diversity of opinion occur when several physicians are called upon to consult together, the opinion of the majority should be considered as decisive, but if the numbers be equal on each side, then the decision should rest with the attending physician. It may, moreover, sometimes happen, that two physicians cannot agree in their views of the nature of a case, and the treatment to be pursued. This is a circumstance much to be deplored, and should always be avoided, if possible, by mutual concessions, as far as they can be justified by a conscientious regard for the dictates of judgment. But in the event of its occurrence, a third physician should, if practicable, be called to act as umpire, and if circumstances prevent the adoption of this course, it must be left to the patient to select the physician in whom he is most willing to confide. But as every physician relies upon the rectitude of his judgment, he should, when left in the minority, politely and consistently retire from any further deliberation in the consultation, or participation in the management of the case.

9. As circumstances sometimes occur to render a *special consultation* desirable, when the continued attendance of two physicians might be objectionable to the patient, the member of the faculty whose assistance is required in such cases, should sedulously guard against all future unsolicited attendance. As such consultations require an extraordinary portion both of time and attention, at least a double honorarium may be reasonably expected.

10. A physician who is called upon to consult, should observe the most honorable and scrupulous regard for the character and standing of the practitioner in attendance: the practice of the latter, if necessary, should be justified as far as it can be, consistently with a conscientious regard for truth, and no hint or insinuation should be thrown out, which could impair the confidence reposed in him, or affect his reputation. The consulting physician should also carefully refrain from any of those extraordinary attentions or assiduities, which are too often practiced by the dishonest for the base purpose of gaining applause, or ingratiating themselves into the favour of families and individuals.

Art. V—Duties of Physicians in Cases of Interference 1. Medicine is a liberal profession, and those admitted into its ranks should found their expectations of practice upon the extent of their qualifications, not on intrigue or artifice.

2. A physician, in his intercourse with a patient under the care of another practitioner, should observe the strictest caution and reserve. No meddling inquiries should be made; no disingenuous hints given relative to the nature and treatment of his disorder: nor any course of conduct pursued that may directly or indirectly tend to diminish the trust reposed in the physician employed.

3. The same circumspection and reserve should be observed, when, from motives of business or friendship, a physician is prompted to visit an individual who is under the direction of another practitioner. Indeed, such visits should be avoided, except under peculiar circumstances, and when they are made, no particular inquiries should be instituted relative to the nature of the disease, or the remedies employed, but

the topics of conversation should be as foreign to the case as circumstances will admit.

4. A physician ought not to take charge of, or prescribe for a patient who has recently been under the care of another member of the faculty in the same illness, except in cases of sudden emergency, or in consultation with the physician previously in attendance, or when the latter has relinquished the case or been regularly notified that his services are no longer desired. Under such circumstances no unjust and illiberal insinuations should be thrown out in relation to the conduct or practice previously pursued, which should be justified as far as candour, and regard for truth and probity will permit; for it often happens, that patients become dissatisfied when they do not experience immediate relief, and, as many diseases are naturally protracted, the want of success, in the first stage of treatment, affords no evidence of a lack of professional knowledge and skill.

5. When a physician is called to an urgent case, because the family attendant is not at hand, he ought, unless his assistance in consultation be desired, to resign the care of the patient to the latter immediately on his arrival.

6. It often happens, in cases of sudden illness, or of recent accidents and injuries, owing to the alarm and anxiety of friends, that a number of physicians are simultaneously sent for. Under these circumstances courtesy should assign the patient to the first who arrives, who should select from those present, any additional assistance that he may deem necessary. In all such cases, however, the practitioner who officiates, should request the family physician, if there be one, to be called, and, unless his further attendance be requested, should resign the case to the latter on his arrival.

7. When a physician is called to the patient of another practitioner, in consequence of the sickness or absence of the latter, he ought, on the return or recovery of the regular attendant, and with the consent of the patient, to surrender the case.

8. A physician, when visiting a sick person in the country, may be desired to see a neighbouring patient who is under the regular direction of another physician, in consequence of some sudden change or aggravation of symptoms. The conduct to be pursued on such an occasion is to give advice adapted to present circumstances; to interfere no farther than is absolutely necessary with the general plan of treatment; to assume no future direction, unless it be expressly desired; and, in this last case, to request an immediate consultation with the practitioner previously employed.

9. A wealthy physician should not give advice *gratis* to the affluent; because his doing so is an injury to his professional brethren. The office of a physician can never be supported as an exclusively beneficent one; and it is defrauding, in some degree, the common funds for its support, when fees are dispensed with, which might justly be claimed.

10. When a physician who has been engaged to attend a case of midwifery is absent, and another is sent for, if delivery is accomplished during the attendance of the latter, he is entitled to the fee, but should resign the patient to the practitioner first engaged.

Art. VI—Of Differences between Physicians 1. Diversity of opinion, and opposition of interest, may, in the medical, as in other professions, sometimes occasion controversy and even contention. Whenever such cases unfortunately occur, and cannot be immediately terminated, they should be referred to the arbitration of a sufficient number of physicians, or a *court-medical.*

As peculiar reserve must be maintained by physicians towards the public, in regard to professional matters, and as there exist numerous points in medical ethics and etiquette through which the feelings of medical men may be painfully assailed in their intercourse with each other, and which cannot be understood or appreciated by general society, neither the subject matter of such differences nor the adjudication of the arbitrators should be made public, as publicity in a case of this nature may be personally injurious to the individuals concerned, and can hardly fail to bring discredit on the faculty.

Art. VII—Of Pecuniary Acknowledgments 1. Some general rules should be adopted by the faculty, in every town or district, relative to *pecuniary*

acknowledgments from their patients; and it should be deemed a point of honour to adhere to these rules with as much uniformity as varying circumstances will admit.

Of the Duties of the Profession to the Public, and of the Obligations of the Public to the Profession

Art. I—Duties of the Profession to the Public 1. As good citizens, it is the duty of physicians to be ever vigilant for the welfare of the community, and to bear their part in sustaining its institutions and burdens: they should also be ever ready to give counsel to the public in relation to matters especially appertaining to their profession, as on subjects of medical police, public hygiene, and legal medicine. It is their province to enlighten the public in regard to quarantine regulations,—the location, arrangement, and dietaries of hospitals, asylums, schools, prisons, and similar institutions,—in relation to the medical police of towns, as drainage, ventilation, etc.,—and in regard to measures for the prevention of epidemic and contagious diseases; and when pestilence prevails, it is their duty to face the danger, and to continue their labours for the alleviation of the suffering, even at the jeopardy of their own lives.

2. Medical men should also be always ready, when called on by the legally constituted authorities, to enlighten coroners' inquests and courts of justice, on subjects strictly medical,— such as involve questions relating to sanity, legitimacy, murder by poisons or other violent means, and in regard to the various other subjects embraced in the science of Medical Jurisprudence. But in these cases, and especially where they are required to make a post-mortem examination, it is just, in consequence of the time, labour and skill required, and the responsibility and risk they incur, that the public should award them a proper honorarium.

3. There is no profession, by the members of which, eleemosynary services are more liberally dispensed, than the medical, but justice requires that some limits should be placed to the performance of such good offices. Poverty, professional brotherhood, and certain public duties referred to in section

1 of this chapter, should always be recognized as presenting valid claims for gratuitous services; but neither institutions endowed by the public or by rich individuals, societies for mutual benefit, for the insurance of lives or for analogous purposes, nor any profession or occupation, can be admitted to possess such privilege. Nor can it be justly expected of physicians to furnish certificates of inability to serve on juries, to perform militia duty, or to testify to the state of health of persons wishing to insure their lives, obtain pensions, or the like, without a pecuniary acknowledgment. But to individuals in indigent circumstances, such professional services should always be cheerfully and freely accorded.

4. It is the duty of physicians, who are frequent witnesses of the enormities committed by quackery, and the injury to health and even destruction of life caused by the use of quack medicines, to enlighten the public on these subjects, to expose the injuries sustained by the unwary from the devices and pretensions of artful empirics and impostors. Physicians ought to use all the influence which they may possess, as professors in Colleges of Pharmacy, and by exercising their option in regard to the shops to which their prescriptions shall be sent, to discourage druggists and apothecaries from vending quack or secret medicines, or from being in any way engaged in their manufacture and sale.

Art. II—Obligations of the Public to Physicians 1. The benefits accruing to the public directly and indirectly from the active and unwearied beneficence of the profession, are so numerous and important, that physicians are justly entitled to the utmost consideration and respect from the community. The public ought likewise to entertain a just appreciation of medical qualifications;—to make a proper discrimination between true science and the assumptions of ignorance and empiricism,—to afford every encouragement and facility for the acquisition of medical education,—and no longer to allow the statute books to exhibit the anomaly of exacting knowledge from physicians, under liability to heavy penalties, and of making them obnoxious to punishment for resorting to the only means of obtaining it.

9

Lewis S. Pilcher
Codes of Medical Ethics

Reprinted from *An Ethical Symposium: Being a Series of Papers Concerning Medical Ethics and Etiquette from the Liberal Standpoint* (New York: G. P. Putnam's Sons, 1883), pp. 42–55.

Ethical questions relate to the most delicate relations of life; they have to do with the hidden springs of action which prompt to any given course; they involve the instincts and impulses, as well as the reason and judgment of the individual; they constitute a domain in which every man is his own rightful sovereign, and an uninvited intrusion into which by others he has the right to regard and resent as an impertinence.

Every principle and instinct of manhood leads an individual to assert his right of independent judgment in matters that pertain to his feelings and conduct, and to admit of no restrictions by his fellows upon his practices, so long as the comfort and well-being of others is not trespassed upon.

The paternal government to which children are subjected is based on the truth that children are incapable of judging for themselves, and must be guided and corrected until they arrive at years of discretion. But even with children there may be such a thing as too much government. It certainly is the part of wisdom for a parent to realize when his parental solicitude may be relaxed, and to adapt himself to the changed circumstances. A parent may formulate a set of rules to which he may require the child to conform in his outward conduct as long as the child is dependent on him for support. An employer may establish similar rules, conformity to which he may require as a condition of remaining in his employment. In both instances such conformity is a mark of dependence, or a badge of servitude, and endured only by stress of necessity. A freeman rejoices in the right to regulate his own conduct, his manners, and morals, subject only to those limitations which the equal rights of other creatures impose upon him.

After this statement of general truths as to rules of ethics, it becomes of interest to inquire whether there is any thing in the peculiarities of membership in the medical profession which should make matters of medical ethics an exception to those principles which apply to ethics in general.

Any remarks upon the nobility of the profession of medicine would be trite; it claims for itself, and the willing tribute of others accords to it, the preëminence among the callings that men give themselves to, for the devotion to humanity, the high courage in the face of danger, the self-sacrifice for the relief of others, the public spirit, the liberality of views, and the general culture which the duties, the studies, and the influences of the profession tend to develop, and which its members, as a class, display.

A physician is not a member of a guild or corporation, the rules of which he must comply with in order to retain his membership therein, and to enjoy its benefits, but a member of a liberal profession, the rules of which are the unwritten law of humanity, and the special requirements of which must vary much according to the peculiarities of his environment. The approval of his own conscience, the respect and good-will of his colleagues, and the confidence of the people will always be the marks that will indicate the perfection with which he complies with the ethics of his profession,— while their loss is the worst of penalties that can follow his dereliction.

Of all classes of men, physicians are certainly least in the condition of children that need paternal watchguard and rules of conduct; and yet the singular spectacle is witnessed in the United States of America, at the present time, of a very large proportion of its physicians insisting upon the necessity of such provisions, either for their own guidance, or as a standard by which they may try the conduct of others. To one who has a high opinion of the dignity of his own manhood, as well as of the deference due his professional position, such a spectacle is a pitiful one, that might well excite his antipathy to the agents that have made it possible.

Even were it true that there were such difficult elements or complexities either in the relations of physicians to the public, or to each other, that it would be improbable that the average educated mind would be capable of deciding for himself his duty in the various junctures that might arise, there is no authority from whom the needed ethical laws could emanate. The physician is a freeman; he has ceased to recognize paternal interference with his judgment; he wears the livery of no employer; he acknowledges the restrictions of no trades-union. If, however, as an individual, he chooses to abdicate his dignity and put himself under a yoke, he has the right to do it, but he has no right to require that others shall follow his example.

Nevertheless, in defiance of this principle, certain associations of medical men in this country, have assumed the right to prescribe a fixed code of rules of conduct, not alone as the laws for their own guidance, but also as the standard by which they presume to fix the right to professional fellowship of all physicians.

However praiseworthy may be the desire to foster an elevated ideal of professional conduct among physicians, in which these codes have undoubtedly had their origin, the attempt to arbitrarily force them upon the acceptance of individuals, is a trespass upon individual rights that can be excused only either on the plea of great necessity, or on the promise of extreme benefit to be derived from such a course.

At the first annual meeting of the American Medical Association held in Baltimore in May, 1848, the president, in his opening address, made the statement, that the profession of medicine had become corrupt and degenerate, to the forfeiture of its social position, and of the homage which it had formerly spontaneously and universally received. That the truth of this averment was everywhere recognized and proclaimed, and that as an association they were imperatively instructed to purify its taints and abuses, and restore it to its former elevation and dignity, and that they were to seek a reform in medicine through a proper regard to its future glory and usefulness.

To remedy this state of things, to purify and elevate the profession of medicine in the United States, was to be the vocation of the association, and one of the earliest steps taken by it was the formulation and adoption of a code of ethics which, in the words of Austin Flint, should be indispensable for the sake of reference whenever differences of opinion should arise, an index to the proper course to those whose moral perceptions may be defective, and a safeguard against the bias of personal interest. (*N.Y. Medical Journal*, March 17, 1883, p. 286.)

No one can question the right, however much they may question the taste and dignity of the proceeding, of any association establishing specific rules of conduct for its members, if it chooses, and requiring conformity to these rules as a requisite to membership. So, in this case, this association had the right to establish its code, and to require that all its members, and all organizations which would be affiliated with it, should accept this code.

In addition to this, however, the adherents of this association, during the years that have passed since then, have claimed that this code was binding as well upon all members of the medical profession, and have proclaimed as unworthy of professional recognition those who refused allegiance to it.

Such claims have derived special force from the fact that this code contains sentiments that are marked by a spirit of propriety and dignity, and that it manifests an exalted ideal of the mission of the physician. Well might it be thus marked; for it is chiefly a copy of a code of ethics prepared, at the close of the last century, by a learned and pious physician of England, Dr. Percival, of Manchester, for the direction of his own son, who was about to engage in the practice of medicine. In the dedication, the father states that in its composition his thoughts were directed to his son "with the tenderest impulse of paternal love," and the body of rules which he framed form a proper legacy from a father to a son, while they reflect the greatest honor on the mind and heart of the author which they mirror.

It will not fail to suggest itself, however, that what may have been a very fitting and touching legacy from a father to his son, may become quite another thing when set up as the ultimatum of ethical law for the profession of a continent, and that ideas and directions, however noble the thought that animated them, which were timely in the days when Pitcairn was still carrying the "gold-headed cane," and when the voice of Dr. Brocklesby's barber, exclaiming, "Make way for Dr. Brocklesby's wig," had not yet died away from High Change, may demand to be differently stated in the latter part of the nineteenth century.

Waiving, for the present, the question of the right of any association of men to assume to dictate laws of conduct for a profession, it is to be acknowledged that it was done, and that other local associations, state, county, and town, accepted the code provided without question, until an organization was perfected that extended over the whole country, bound together by this code as its common bond. For a whole generation the great mass of the educated physicians of the country have been professedly dominated by it, and not until within the past three years has its rule been called in question.

During all these years, nevertheless, its enforcement, whenever attempted, has been a trespass on individual rights. The conditions which reigned in the medical profession in this country a generation ago, may or may not have been of a character to create the necessity of attempting its enactment; it is immaterial now to inquire into that. The living question to-day is whether the benefits derived from it in the past, and certain to be conferred by it in the future, are of that extreme character which alone could pardon an attempt to continue its existence.

It is claimed,[1] that the result of the promulgation of this code in the special manner described has been to cause medical men of the present day to feel it a duty to sustain the younger members of the profession, to treat them with courtesy and kindness, to save them from their errors, and to encourage them in all their good work; that it has put the seal of condemnation on all "isms," and developed an esprit de corps that has enlarged the boundaries of our science, and greatly increased the usefulness and social standing of the profession.

It may be claimed with some plausibility, on the other hand, that the period has been one in which there has been a general improvement in the material, mental, and moral tone of the country; that it has been a time of wonderful change and progress in every department of life; and that the medical profession has simply responded to the stimulus of its surroundings, the causes of whatever changes may really have taken place in its tone and bearing being extrinsic quite as much as intrinsic. It may be said—and much might be found to corroborate it—that it has not even kept pace with other learned callings in the advances which these years have produced, although the latter have not enjoyed the "invaluable blessings" (Atlee) of distinct codes of ethics. It may be said that equal, even greater, relative prog-

ress in elevating the standard of attainments among medical men, of advancing the science of medicine, and of securing for its practitioners the respect due them, has taken place during the same period of time in other countries where the safeguard and help of a formal ethical code, such as that of the American Medical Association, has not been provided.

There is room, then, for differences of opinion as to the real causes that have been most active in making the medical profession of this country what it is to-day.

As for myself, after a careful consideration of the pros and cons as to the benefits which the profession of the United States have thus far derived from the Code of Ethics of the American Medical Association, I am not able to see that they have been or are likely to be of such an extreme character as to reconcile me to accept it as the sole and authoritative guide by which my professional conduct must be fixed, nor to cause me to recognize in any man, or set of men, the right to bring me to bar for judgment.

Moreover, my own observation of medical men and manners during the twenty-one years that have passed since, as a medical student, I first felt myself identified with the medical profession, has caused me to feel, more and more strongly as the years have passed by, that the attitude of medical men in this country in matters of ethics, toward each other and toward the community, was radically wrong, and that it was working injury to the best interests of the profession as a whole.

The first injury, that I have believed discernible as flowing from the attempt to define in detail the methods by which the conduct of physicians in the various relations of life should be performed, is that it has tended to foster the creation of, and to give prominence to, a class of men who think much of the strict letter of the code, often to the forgetting of its spirit—medical Pharisees, who tithe the anise and cumin of medical etiquette, who make broad their ethical phylacteries, and thank God that they are not as other men are, but who nevertheless feel at liberty to coolly ride rough-shod over the rights of others when such rights

are not protected by any distinct provision of the code.

The second count in my indictment against the code is, that it has fostered and maintained a spirit of censoriousness in the profession. It tends to make every man a spy upon his neighbor, and has made persecutions of the most petty nature possible. It has placed in the hands of certain men a weapon to use against those that are weaker. It has created a multitude of star-chambers all over the land, in which men have assumed the right to sit in judgment upon and to exercise discipline over their peers as to the motives and methods of their professional conduct. The kinds and doses of medicines he uses, the theories of cure that he may indulge, his methods of commanding the confidence of his patients, the amounts he may charge for his services, the persons to whom he may give advice,—these and many like things physicians have claimed to be empowered to regulate for each other under the provisions of the code.

A third imputation upon the practical workings of the code is, that most of its provisions have, in general, been ignored, while attention has chiefly been centred upon a single part of its provisions, and that the least important, which has been so interpreted and enforced as to cause public attention to be continually attracted to a single form of medical error, in such a way as to create for it sympathy and to promote its growth in the esteem of the public.

A fourth evil has existed in the great unevenness which has prevailed in the manner in which infractions of the code have been subjected to discipline. It has often appeared that its provisions could be observed or disregarded at will by men who were prominent and influential, while the obscure and weak alone were expected to implicitly comply with it. Men who have been notorious for their infractions both of its spirit and letter have repeatedly received the honors of the association which created and maintained it; and in every city there are many who violate it without any attempt being made to subject them to discipline. Flagrant violations by powerful medical organizations have for years been the subject of general comment, but never of discipline.

It would be possible to still further elaborate statements of harmful tendencies, which thus far have accompanied the domination of this code of ethics in this country, but this must suffice. In conclusion, I have but to say that if my premises have been correct, there is but one logical outcome to my reasoning, viz.: the rejection of the present code of the American Medical Association, or of any like set of definite ethical rules, by whomsoever framed, as of any authority to control my professional acts.

I trust that even the most enthusiastic supporter of the code that I reject, will acknowledge that my conclusion is not necessarily dictated by a mercenary spirit, nor yet the result of a low standard of professional honor and dignity. I may, and do, welcome this code as a treatise on the moral aspects of medical life, as of value for reference and counsel, but for my decision as to what my action in any given case may be, I hold myself responsible to my own conscience alone.

Notes

1. The President's address before the American Medical Association, 1883, by John L. Atlee, M.D., LL.D.

10
World Medical Association Declaration of Geneva

Reprinted from *World Medical Association Bulletin*, vol. 1, 1949, pp. 109–111.

Declaration of Geneva

Adopted by the General Assembly of The World Medical Association at Geneva, Switzerland, September, 1948.

At the time of being admitted as Member of the Medical Profession.

I solemnly pledge myself to consecrate my life to the service of humanity.

I will give to my teachers the respect and gratitude which is their due;

I will practice my profession with conscience and dignity,

The health of my patient will be my first consideration:

I will respect the secrets which are confided in me;

I will maintain by all the means in my power, the honor and the noble traditions of the medical profession;

My colleagues will be my brothers;

I will not permit considerations of religion, nationality, race, party politics or social standing to intervene between my duty and my patient;

I will maintain the utmost respect for human life, from the time of conception; even under threat, I will not use my medical knowledge contrary to the laws of humanity.

I make these promises solemnly, freely and upon my honor.

In this very concise resume and of which the Medical Code will be for the most part only an amplification, a development or explanation, we wish to add the short introduction of the Code of Ethics of the Canadian Medical Association.

Our Canadian conferes have, in a few very high-sounding and dignified phrases, defined what a Code of Ethics should contain and what it should only contain.

Introductory

"As ye would that men should do to you, do ye even so to them," is a Golden Rule for all men. A Code of Ethics for physicians can only amplify or focus this and other golden rules and precepts to the special relations of practice. As a stream cannot rise above its source, so a code cannot change a low-grade man into a high-grade doctor, but it can help a good man to be a better man and a more enlightened doctor. It can quicken and inform a conscience, but not create one. Only in a few things can it decree "thou shalt" or "thou shalt not," but in many things it can urge "thou shouldst," or "thou shouldst not." While the highest service they can give to humanity is the only worthwhile aim for those of any profession, it is so in a special sense for physicians, since their services concern immediately and directly the health of the bodies and minds of men.''

The text adopted follows. It has been submitted to all national medical associations and will receive final consideration at the General Assembly in London.

Duties of Doctors in General

A doctor must always maintain the highest standards of professional conduct.

A doctor must not allow himself to be influenced merely by motives of profit.

The following practices are deemed unethical:

a. Any self-advertisement except such as is expressly authorized by the national code of medical ethics.

b. Taking part in any plan of medical care in which the doctor does not have complete professional independence.

c. To receive any money in connection with services rendered to a patient other than the acceptance of a proper professional fee, or to pay any money in the same circumstances without the knowledge of the patient.

Under no circumstances is a doctor permitted to do anything that would weaken the physical or mental resistance of a human being except from strictly professional reasons in the interest of his patient.

A doctor is advised to use great caution in publishing discoveries. The same applies to methods of treatment whose value is not recognized by the profession.

When a doctor is called upon to give evidence or a certificate he should only state that which he can verify.

Duties of Doctors to the Sick

A doctor must always bear in mind the importance of preserving human life from conception. Therapeutic abortion may only be performed if the conscience of the doctor and the national laws permit.

A doctor owes to his patient complete loyalty and all the resources of his science. Whenever an examination or treatment is beyond his capacity he should summon another doctor who has the necessary ability.

A doctor owes to his patient absolute secrecy on all which has been confided to him or which he knows because of the confidence entrusted to him.

A doctor must give the necessary treatment in emergency, unless he is assured that it can and will be given by others.

Duties of Doctors to Each Other

A doctor ought to behave to his colleagues as he would have them behave to him.

A doctor must not entice patients from his colleagues.

A doctor must observe the principles of ''The Declaration of Geneva'' approved by The World Medical Association.

11

American Medical Association

Principles of Medical Ethics (1957)

Reprinted with permission of the American Medical Association.

Preamble These principles are intended to aid physicians individually and collectively in maintaining a high level of ethical conduct. They are not laws but standards by which a physician may determine the propriety of his conduct in his relationship with patients, with colleagues, with members of allied professions, and with the public.

Section 1 The principal objective of the medical profession is to render service to humanity with full respect for the dignity of man. Physicians should merit the confidence of patients entrusted to their care, rendering to each a full measure of service and devotion.

Section 2 Physicians should strive continually to improve medical knowledge and skill, and should make available to their patients and colleagues the benefits of their professional attainments.

Section 3 A physician should practice a method of healing founded on a scientific basis; and he should not voluntarily associate professionally with anyone who violates this principle.

Section 4 The medical profession should safeguard the public and itself against physicians deficient in moral character or professional competence. Physicians should observe all laws, uphold the dignity and honor of the profession and accept its self-imposed disciplines. They should expose, without hesitation, illegal or unethical conduct of fellow members of the profession.

Section 5 A physician may choose whom he will serve. In an emergency, however, he should render service to the best of his ability. Having undertaken the care of a patient, he may not neglect him; and unless he has been discharged he may discontinue his services only after giving adequate notice. He should not solicit patients.

Section 6 A physician should not dispose of his services under terms or conditions that tend to interfere with or impair the free and complete exercise of his medical judgment and skill or tend to cause a deterioration of the quality of medical care.

Section 7 In the practice of medicine a physician should limit the source of his professional income to medical services actually rendered by him, or under his supervision, to his patients. His fee should be commensurate with the service rendered and the patient's ability to pay. He should neither pay nor receive commission for referral of patients. Drugs, remedies or appliances may be dispensed or supplied by the physician provided it is in the best interests of the patient.

Section 8 A physician should seek consultation upon request; in doubtful or difficult cases; or whenever it appears that the quality of medical service may be enhanced thereby.

Section 9 A physician may not reveal the confidences entrusted to him in the course of medical attendance, or the deficiencies he may observe in the character of patients, unless he is required to do so by law or unless it becomes necessary in order to protect the welfare of the individual or of the community.

Section 10 The honored ideals of the medical profession imply that the responsibility of the physician extend not only to the individual, but also to society, and these responsibilities deserve his interest and participation in activities that have the purpose of improving both the health and the well-being of the individual and the community.

12

Ludwig Edelstein

From "The Professional
Ethics of the Greek
Physician"

Reprinted with permission of the publisher from the *Bulletin of the History
of Medicine*, vol. 30, 1956, pp. 392–
418. Copyright © The Johns Hopkins
University Press.

. . . I wish to outline the various ethical positions taken by ancient physicians. In particular, it will be my aim to find out when and where the idea originated that medicine itself imposes certain obligations upon the physician, obligations summed up in the magic phrase "love of humanity." For, in my opinion, this lofty ideal was not the only one in antiquity that motivated the help proffered by medical men to those who suffer and are in distress. Over a long period of time other concepts of medicine and therefore other obligations and duties were held in high esteem. Rome was not built in one day.

Now at first glance it may seem as if such a contention were in fact quite unwarranted. For is it not in one of the Hippocratic writings, the essay called *Precepts*, that the statement occurs . . . : "Where there is love of man, there is also love of the art" (ch. 6)? Is it not said in another Hippocratic book, the treatise *On the Physician,* that the doctor must be a "lover of man" (ch. 1)? And does not Galen, no mean judge in these matters, expressly assert that Hippocrates, Empedocles, Diocles, and not a few of the other early physicians healed the sick because of their love of mankind (*De Placitis Hippocratis et Platonis*, ed. I. Müller, p. 765)? In the classical age of Greek civilization, then, the ethic of philanthropy seems already to have been securely established.

But if one scrutinizes carefully the context in which the word "philanthropy" appears in the so-called Hippocratic writings just mentioned, he realizes that it means no more than a certain friendliness of disposition, a kindliness, as opposed to any misanthropic attitude. A "philanthropic" doctor in the sense in which the term is used in the treatise *On the Physician* (ch. 1) will comport himself in a dignified manner; for aggressiveness and obtrusiveness are despicable; sour looks, harshness, arrogance, vulgarity, are disagreeable.[1] Likewise, the Hippocratic *Precepts* (ch. 6) understands by the doctor's "philanthropy" his kindheartedness and his willingness to accommodate his fees to the patient's circumstances. He should also treat strangers and paupers, even if they are unable to pay him. That is, he should be charitable, recalling some of the benefits which he may have received himself in the past, or thinking of the good name that his charitableness is likely to make for him in the future. If he acts thus, if such "philanthropy" is present on his part, then also "love of the (medical) art" will be kindled in his patients, a state of mind that greatly contributes to their speedy recovery, especially when they are dangerously sick. No more—and no less—is implied by the famous aphorism: "Where there is love of man, there is also love of the art."[2]

"Philanthropy," then, in the two Hippocratic treatises designates a proper behavior toward those with whom the physician comes in contact during treatment; it is viewed as a minor social virtue, so to say. And it was indeed in this way that the word, which later came to have such an exalted connotation, was commonly understood in the classical age and far down into the Hellenistic era.[3] Moreover, according to recent investigations, the book *On the Physician* was composed at the earliest between 350 and 300 B.C. *Precepts* cannot have been written before the first century B.C. or A.D. Neither the one nor the other treatise provides evidence for the ethics of the early Greek physician.[4] I trust that Osler, the scholar, would forgive me for dissenting from him in a question of interpretation and of chronology in which he followed the opinion of his time. I am sure he would not have wished me to put acceptance of authority before acceptance of the results of continued research.

As for Galen and his verdict, far be it from me to deny that even in the classical period there may have been men who dedicated themselves to medicine out of an instinctive compassion for the sufferings of their fellow men. But to assume that such a feeling, made conscious and, under whatever name, elevated to an ideal, could have extended to all mankind, would be the unhistorical projection of later concepts into an age entirely ignorant of them. To be sure, some of the Sophists taught that by nature all human beings—free, slave, and barbarian—are equal. The adherents of the rising enlightenment questioned existing conditions and extolled a natural or divine law of morality over the changing demands of the day. However, the time had not yet come to think in terms of obligations toward humanity.[5]

Most important, those treatises of the *Corpus Hippocraticum* which were written during the fifth and fourth centuries B.C. and reflect the situation then prevailing, show clearly, I suggest, that even the best among the physicians were not concerned at all with such considerations as Galen imputes to them. Their ethics was not one of the heart or of inner intention. It was shaped by rather different values.

For the early Hippocratic books are concerned exclusively with a body of rules prescribing a certain behavior during the physician's working hours, with medical etiquette, one might say. It is explained how the doctor's office —his *iatreion*—should be set up, how it should or should not be equipped. Bedside manners are discussed, the right way to enter a sick room, to converse with the patient; whether or not to give a prognosis of the outcome of the disease if there is danger of a fatal issue. The surgeon is admonished not to make a show of the application of bandages or of operations, since to do what is proper is preferable to indulging in the mere display of one's dexterity. It is urged that a treatment once started should be completed, and that the physician should not withdraw his help from the sick so as to avoid blame or other unwelcome consequences.[6]

Such injunctions, and many more that could be cited, are dictated by the wish to uphold a certain standard of performance and serve to distinguish the expert from the charlatan. From Homeric times the physician had been an itinerant craftsman; even in the classical age, few physicians stayed in the cities of their birth or took up permanent residence elsewhere. Living here today, there tomorrow, they were not subject to the ordinary social strictures and pressures which result from the integration of the crafts into a community, and which tend to insure the reliability of the workmen. Besides, no medical schools existed; training was not required, everybody was free to practice medicine, the state did not issue any license. Under these circumstances abuses abounded and went unpunished. They could be prevented only by the individual's decision to make himself responsible before the

bar of his own conscience, the conscience of a good craftsman, and this responsibility he assumed by the adoption of a strict etiquette. A great achievement indeed! For not only did the physician thus voluntarily establish a set of values governing sound treatment, he also gave, so to say, a personal pledge of safety to his patients, badly needed in a world that knew of no other protection for them.[7]

Yet at no point does the Hippocratic physician aim farther. Medicine to him is but the proper application of his knowledge to the treatment of diseases. "The medical art," it is maintained in one of the rare expositions of the character of medicine to be found in the *Corpus Hippocraticum*, "has to consider three factors, the disease, the patient, the physician. The physician is the servant of his art, and the patient must cooperate with the doctor in combatting the disease" (*Epidemics*, I, 11). In other words, it is the sole purpose of the good physician to achieve the objective of his art, to save his patient from the threat of death, if possible; to help him, or at least not to harm him, as the famous saying has it (*ibid.*). His ethic consists in doing his task well, in perfecting his skill; it is an ethic of outward achievement rather than of inner intention.[8]

As for the physician's motives in practicing medicine, he was engaged in it in order to make a living. Nor was there any conflict between his pecuniary interests and the exigencies of craftsmanship, as long as he remembered that love of money, of easy success, should not induce him to act without regard for the benefit of the patient, or, to speak with Ruskin, that the good workman rarely thinks first of his pay, and that the knack of getting well paid does not always go with the ability to do the work well. If he learned to forget personal advantage for the sake of doing the right thing, he had, in his opinion, done all that was necessary.[9]

And society fully approved of such an attitude, as follows with certainty from a memorable passage in the first book of Plato's *Republic* (340 C ff.). The question there debated is whether self-interest is at the root of all human endeavor and therefore also of political activity. Parallels from the various arts, and especially the comparison with medicine, are used in order to decide the issue. The physician in the precise

sense of the term is not a money maker or an earner of fees, Socrates holds, but a healer of the sick (341 C), just as it may be said of all the other arts that they were invented not for the sake of personal advantage, but rather for the purpose of performing a service, and most effectively at that. Medicine itself therefore has no concern for the advantage of medicine or of the physician, but only for that of the patient and his bodily welfare (342 C). Like every art, *qua* art, it looks out for the good of that which is its object. And when Socrates is asked rather mockingly: "Is this true of the shepherd also? Does he too have the good of his flock in mind?" (343 A ff.), he answers emphatically: "*qua* shepherd, yes." The fact that he sells the wool and makes money by so doing is not an intrinsic property of the art of shepherding; it belongs to another art, that of money making. For "if we are to consider it 'precisely' medicine produces health but the fee-earning art the pay, and architecture a house but the fee-earning art accompanying it the fee, and so with all the others, each performs its own task and benefits that over which it is set" (346 D). Yet the subsidiary art of fee earning cannot be entirely separated from the art producing health. "Unless pay is added to it," there would be no benefit for the craftsman, and consequently he would be unwilling to go to the trouble of taking care of the troubles of others. This is why everybody expects to make money with his craft, and why pay must be provided by those who benefit from the craft. Otherwise the self-interest of the craftsman would not be satisfied (346 E–347 A).

All the interlocutors in the dialogue agree on this conclusion—and I think none of their contemporaries would have gainsaid their admission: the artisan has fulfilled his duty if he is intent primarily upon the aim of his art—that is, in the case of medicine, upon restoring health to the body—and thinks of his income afterwards. No other obligations are incumbent upon him, no other personal qualities are demanded of him.[10] It is also clear that in the society of the fifth and fourth centuries, medicine is a craft like all the others and in no way differentiated from them. Completely free of any idealization of work as such, and considering it a dire necessity rather than an ennobling activity, the classical age judged all manual labor only by the standard of expertness and performance. What can, properly speaking, be called morality, it found realized in man's private life, and preeminently in his life as a citizen. Even medicine, therefore, remained impervious to moral considerations.[11]

But at this point your patience with my argument should be exhausted, and I must face the objection which no doubt will have been on your minds for some time: how does all this square with the content of the Hippocratic *Oath*? Certainly, the *Oath* prescribes a most refined personal ethics for the physician. It enjoins upon him a life pleasing to gods and men, a life almost saintly and bound by the strictest rules of purity and holiness. It makes him renounce all intentional injustice or mischief. Here a morality of the highest order is infused into medical practice. Have not centuries upon centuries seen in the Hippocratic *Oath* the prototype of all medical ethics?

I trust that I am second to none in my appreciation of this document. Yet its picture of the true physician is evidence not of the thought of the classical era which I have so far considered, but of a movement which started in the latter part of the fourth century B.C.— the time when the *Oath* was composed —and extended through the Hellenistic period down to the time of Galen. Through it, the ethics of the medical craftsman was reshaped in accordance with the various systems of philosophy. The new standards characteristic of the second stage in the development of ancient medical ethics originated in a revaluation of the arts and crafts and in the transformation of the medical craft into a scientific pursuit.

To speak first of the change in attitude toward the crafts, Aristotle already raised the problem "whether artisans too ought not to have goodness, seeing that they often fall short of their duties through intemperance." But he decided that unlike the slave who is subject to "unlimited servitude," the artisan is subject only to "limited servitude," namely the performance of his particular job, and therefore is obligated only to do his task; his moral goodness is his own affair (*Politics*, 1260 a 36–b2; cf. *Nic. Eth.* 1105 a 26

ff.). The so-called Pythagoreans of Aristotle's time, however, insisted on the moral implications of workmanship and considered it, if not a "noble toil" in the modern sense of the term, at least a matter of moral concern. They even claimed that "the good" could be achieved especially well through the crafts.[12] In Hellenistic philosophy such a belief became more widespread. Aristotle's successors distinguished the "happy life" and the "good life"—the one presupposing independent means, the other to be led by him who has to have an occupation. In both, man is asked to fulfill the moral law. Finally, the Stoa recognized the acquisition of money through any kind of work as compatible with the moral order and taught that in whatever station in life one may find oneself, one can and must live up to the rules of ethics.[13] Such an entirely new appraisal of the crafts surely was facilitated by the fact that virtue or morality was increasingly identified not with the objective content of human actions, but rather with the inner attitude of the human agent. The principal criterion of right or wrong came to be found almost exclusively in the proper use of things, good, bad, or indifferent, rather than in the things themselves.[14]

Now, once it was realized that the craftsman can partake in virtue, the narrow limitations of the old ethics of good craftsmanship were swept aside. The moral issues latent in the pursuit of medicine, which the classical age had either failed to see, or failed to emphasize, were brought out into the open. The so-called deontological writings of the *Corpus Hippocraticum*, the *Oath*, the treatise *On the Physician*, *Precepts*, and *On Decorum*—the three latter composed in Hellenistic times, if not at the beginning of the Christian era—take up the various questions concerning medical ethics and try to give an answer to them from different philosophical points of view.[15]

Does not the practice of medicine involve the physician in the most intimate contact with other human beings? Is he not sometimes called upon to make decisions that reach far beyond the mere application of technical knowledge and skill? In the Hippocratic *Oath* that responsibility which is peculiarly the doctor's is defined in agreement with the way of life instituted by Pythagoras.[16] And what about

the patient who is putting himself and "his all" into the hands of the physician? How can he be sure that he may have trust in the doctor, not only in his knowledge, but also in the man himself? Such confidence, according to the book *On the Physician*, can be aroused only if the physician asks himself what he should be like "in regard to his soul." Consequently the author of this treatise—perhaps the oldest known "introduction to medicine" which is posterior to the *Oath* by approximately two or three generations—prescribes for "the soul" of the physician self-control, regularity of habits, justness and fairness, a proper and good behavior, in short, all the virtues of the "gentleman." It is the doctrine of the Aristotelian school, I think, which is here adapted to medicine.[17]

Again, in the *Precepts* and in the book *On Decorum* it is the Stoic outlook which predominates. In the former treatise, gentleness and kindheartedness are commended. The physician ought to be charitable, especially toward him who is a stranger and in financial straits (ch. 6). In keeping with such a kindly and tolerant attitude the good physician—the "fellow workman," as he is called (ch. 7)—must also be ready at all times to call in another physician as a consultant, and he must not quarrel with his confrères either. Thus, aspects of medical practice neglected in the *Oath* and in the essay *On the Physician*, are elucidated in the light of general moral considerations.[18] The essay *On Decorum*, on the other hand, though abounding in detailed advice on moral situations as they may arise in the course of a treatment, mainly discusses the "wisdom" of the physician. For "between wisdom and medicine there is no gulf; in fact, medicine possesses all the qualities that make for wisdom" (ch. 5), that is, wisdom "applied to life," "directed toward seemliness and good repute" (ch. 1), which should be carefully distinguished from its opposite, from false or sham philosophy. A physician who has the right kind of philosophy is indeed "the equal of a god"; his are all the virtues one can think of (ch. 5). To put it in the technical language of the Stoic school, to which the author of the treatise owes allegiance, the true physician is the peer of the sage.[19]

Perhaps you are astonished at the fact that all these treatises which I have characterized briefly are so strongly imbued with philosophy. And thinking again of the Hippocratic *Oath* you may wonder why the ancient physician could not rest satisfied with the stipulation of his oath which seems to tell him all he has to know about his duties. But the Hippocratic *Oath* originally was a literary manifesto, a programme laid down by one who wished to set matters right in accordance with his own convictions. It was not an oath taken by all physicians, if indeed it was ever taken at all by any one before the end of antiquity.[20] Throughout Hellenistic times and in the first centuries of the Christian era no common agreement existed concerning an ethical code binding for the medical practitioner. As was the case with the medical etiquette of old, no moral stipulations were accepted voluntarily. The writers of whom I have spoken were individuals trying to find out for themselves how to conduct their business in the right way. Just like Osler, they believed they could see their own work in truer perspective by taking "the larger view." And in this endeavor where could they turn for instruction except to philosophy? Ancient religion had no moral or metaphysical message. In the vacuum that resulted from the disappearance of the city state, from the breakdown of the old ideal of civic virtue, philosophy alone could still provide guidance. It was, and it intended to be, not merely the domain of academics, but rather the inspiration of everybody who refused to get lost in doing his daily chores and was in search of standards on which to orientate himself. To be sure, adherence to whatever dogma seemed to the individual nearest to the truth did not yet make him a "philosopher-in-precept," and this holds also for the authors of the deontological writings. Philosophy gave them a *Weltanschauung* which enabled them to solve the task they had set for themselves.[21]

Yet I must turn now to a consideration of the other factor which, as I suggested before, was responsible for the acceptance of a philosophical ethic on the part of the physician: I mean the change of the medical art into medical science. Ever since the fifth and fourth centuries some physicians had interested themselves in the physiological and biological theories of the philosophers and had made use of them in their own work. Thereby they created scientific medicine, if I may use this term to designate the type of medicine that went beyond the practical application of traditional knowledge and demanded research into the nature of the body and of all the factors that may have a bearing upon it.[22] While throughout antiquity merely technical skill and empirical proficiency constituted the equipment of the average physician who as a craftsman was trained through apprenticeship with another physician-craftsman, the medical "scientists" studied philosophy. In the Hellenistic era they belonged to the various medical sects for which the unity of philosophy and medicine was axiomatic. And the new spirit in which medicine was thus approached soon made itself felt also in medical practice. The ethics of these physicians became identical with that of the philosophical school to which they professed allegiance as scientists.

The first testimony to this effect is perhaps the Hippocratic *Law* written at approximately the same time as the *Oath*. Many physicians, the author of the short and almost enigmatic treatise holds, are physicians "by repute"; very few are physicians "in reality." Rather have the majority, "like the supernumeraries in tragedies," merely "the appearance, dress, and mask of an actor without being actors" (ch. 1). He who wishes to win the reputation of being a physician "not only in name, but in deed," must go through a proper training, that is, a philosophical training. Its result will also be "cheerfulness" and "joyousness," instead of "cowardice" and "rashness," which betray "helplessness" and "want of knowledge" (ch. 4). This is the Democritean ideal of theoretical speculation, according to which the man of true insight is at the same time necessarily the man of truly good character.[23]

While here the ethics of the scientific physician still remains vague and shadowy, it manifests itself in its fully developed form in the doctrine of the Hellenistic Empiricists whose sect was of the sceptic persuasion. The empirical physician therefore, like all sceptic philosophers, accepts the established rules of life which, though by no means representing absolute truth, have the sanction of probability. In accordance with the common aim of men, he practices medicine for the sake of reputation or of money, of neither of which he desires to have too much or too little, but just as much as is adequate and guarantees peace of mind. In his character and behavior he evinces tranquillity and gentleness. In his work he is not given to unnecessary talk, but prefers action; talking much or talking big is the habit of those who, unlike the empiricist and sceptic, believe in speculative theories. In his writings and in his research he is truthful, not intent on winning an argument à *tout prix*, or on displaying his conceit. On the whole, then, he follows in the wake of the day, relying on indubitable data of sense perception and experience; living thus, he lives like Hippocrates himself who, in the opinion of the sceptics, had of course been a sceptic, and as a sceptic had equalled the fame of Asclepius.[24]

Evidence on the ethical teaching of the early dogmatic sects is almost entirely lacking. A happy chance has preserved at least one testimony which bears witness to the preoccupation of Erasistratus with medical ethics. "Most fortunate indeed," he says, "wherever it happens that the physician is both, perfect in his art and most excellent in his moral conduct. But if one of the two should have to be missing, then it is better to be a good man devoid of learning than to be a perfect practitioner of bad moral conduct, and an untrustworthy man—if indeed it is true that good morals compensate for what is missing in art, while bad morals can corrupt and confound even perfect art."[25] Further details of the deontology of the Herophilean and Erasistratean sects may be contained in the writings of Galen, the great systematizer of medicine. At any rate, his little essay *That the Best Physician also is a Philosopher* gives an exhaustive account of later dogmatic ethics. It can be summed up in the demand that the physician should be contemptuous of money, interested in his work, self–controlled and just. Once he is in possession of these basic virtues, he will have all the others at his command as well (ch. 3). And how is such moral eminence to be achieved? Like Galen, the true physician must become a philosopher himself, an adherent of Plato, or rather of the Platonism of Galen's time, which was fused with Aristotelianism and Stoicism.[26]

With this short description of Galen's views I have come to the end of my analysis of the various attitudes taken by the scientist-physicians and by the craftsmen-physicians during the second stage in the development of medical ethics. The important consequence of the movement which I have described hardly needs reemphasis. The morality of outward performance characteristic of the classical era was now supplemented by a morality of inner intention. The physician—whether as an amateur philosopher or as a philosopher in his own right—had learned to regard his patient not only as the object of his art, but also as a fellowman to whom he owed more than knowledge alone, however great, can provide. He had learned to face him not only as a master of techniques, but also as a virtuoso in moral conduct.

Can one then go one step further and claim that between the end of the fourth century B.C. and the second century A.D. medicine had been elevated to the rank of the most philanthropic art? Have I answered also the specific question raised at the very beginning of my discussion? Have I uncovered the origin of the humanism which Osler admired in Greek medicine? It may almost seem so. For surely, in Galen's opinion, the physician who accepts his philosophy will be led to practice medicine out of love of humanity, the motive which Galen is willing to attribute even to Hippocrates, as I mentioned before. And since nowhere else, neither in the deontological writings of the *Corpus Hippocraticum*, nor in the teaching of any of the other medical sects, philanthropy is mentioned as the inspiration of the doctor, one should conclude that it was dogmatic medicine, as formulated by Galen or maybe by one of his predecessors, which gave rise to medical humanism.[27]

But Galen's own appraisal of the possible motivations of medical practice, I am afraid, makes it impossible to rest satisfied as yet. For as he says (*De Placitis*, p. 763 f. ed. Müller) on the authority of the same passage in Plato's *Republic* to which I referred in my analysis of classical medicine, the physician's particular job is to take care of the health of the body, although it may be for a variety of reasons that he practices medicine. Some physicians engage in it for the sake of money, some for the sake of exemption from public duties—physicians in Galen's time were sometimes granted such privileges[28]—some few for love of mankind, just as still others for glory or honor. In so far as they are able to bring health to their patients, all of them are named physicians; in so far as they do what they do for different reasons, the one is called a "philanthropist," the other a lover of honor, the third a lover of glory, the fourth a lover of money. Therefore, Galen continues (p. 764 f.), the aim of the physician as physician is not glory or money, as the Empiricist Menodotus claimed; this may have been true of himself, but others in the past surely had different aims in mind. The motive of glory or money or of philanthropy is a matter of personal choice; it has no intrinsic connection with the pursuit of medicine.[29] For in regard to every craft it is necessary to distinguish between its common characteristics and those which belong to the individual practicing it. Failure to make this distinction is bad logic, irreconcilable with the tenets of Plato and Hippocrates alike.

This argumentation of Galen, so utterly devoid of ethical overtones or of any feeling of moral indignation, shows clearly that in his opinion philanthropy is not indissolubly joined with the practice of medicine. It is, so to say, a superfluity of riches on the part of the physician. What is expected of him is only that he should be an expert in medicine. However, no rules of behavior can be stated absolutely. For Galen as well as for the other moralizing physicians medical ethics remains relative to the respective philosophies to which they adhere at their own discretion. Whoever differs from their views is a bad philosopher, to be sure, but he is not necessarily a bad physician or a bad man. Various motivations of medical practice, therefore, are quite legitimate; no one single or definite virtue is enjoined upon the doctor by his task. From the point of view of medicine, his specific morality is incidental rather than essential.

Does this amount to the admission that the ancients never identified medicine with love of humanity? That they did not know of any strictly professional medical ethics dictated by the aim of medicine itself? By no means. Almost a hundred years before Galen there must have been a clear realization of a medical humanism inherent in the task of the physician. Scribonius Largus, a writer of the early first century A.D., speaks of it as something quite self-evident to himself and his readers. It still remains for me to elicit the full meaning of the doctrine in question from the few sentences in which Scribonius alludes to it, to determine its historical antecedents, and to sketch its later fate.[30]

Scribonius has embodied his views on the moral conduct of the physician in the preface to his book *On Remedies* in which he wishes to demonstrate the importance of treatment by drugs. Why is it, he asks (p. 2, 8 ed. Helmreich), that his colleagues refrain from the application of drugs? Are they unfamiliar with them? This would be just reason for accusing them of negligence. Or are they aware of the usefulness of drugs, yet deny their use to others? If so, they are even more culpable, "because they burn with envy, an evil that must be despised by all men, and especially by the physician who is himself despised by gods and men if his heart is not full of sympathy (*misericordiae*) and humaneness (*humanitatis*) in accordance with the will (*voluntatem*) of medicine itself" (p. 2, 15–19).

But the sympathy and humaneness "willed" by medicine imply more than that the physician should not withhold his knowledge from his patients. The true physician, Scribonius continues, "is not allowed to harm anybody, not even the enemies of the state (*hostibus*). He may fight against them with every means as a soldier (*miles*) or as a good citizen (*vir bonus*), should this be demanded of him. [As a physician, he cannot and must not fight or harm them], since medicine does not judge men by their circumstances in life (*fortuna*), nor by their character (*personis*). Rather does medicine promise (*pollicetur*) her succor in equal measure to all who implore her help, and she professes (*profitetur*) never to be injurious to anyone." (p. 2, 19–26). For, as Scribonius reiterates in conclusion, "medicine is the knowledge of healing, not of hurting. If she does not try in every way to help the sick with all means at her disposal, she fails to offer to men the sympathy she promises" (*hominibus quam pollicetur misericordiam*, p. 3, 5–8).

Obviously, according to Scribonius, the sympathy and humaneness required of the physician are due to everybody in equal measure. Humaneness (*humanitas*) for him is not merely a friendliness of behavior, it is a "proficiency and benevolence toward all men without distinction," it truly is "love of mankind," as *humanitas* was defined at that time in correspondence with the then prevailing meaning of the Greek word φιλανθρωπία.[31] Besides, sympathy and love of humanity constitute positive rules, and obedience to them supersedes all other allegiances that the doctor may have as a good citizen or as a soldier. They are the special obligation of the physician which he cannot violate under any circumstances. Most important, the one and only right standard of conduct is enforced upon him by medicine itself, just as is the standard of adequate knowledge. Unless he knows all that he ought to know and makes use of it for the benefit of the sick, he fails in his duty. He is as remiss, or even more so, if he does not fulfill his specific moral responsibility. Here, the ethics of inner intention and that of outward performance have become an inseparable unity; both are derived from the task to be achieved, from the "will" and "promise" of medicine itself, both are equally essential for medicine and the physician.

It is hardly by chance therefore that Scribonius calls medicine not merely an "art" or a "science," but a "profession" (*professio*, p. 2, 18; 27). This word, in the language of his time, was applied to workmanship in preference to the older and morally indefinite terms, in order to emphasize the ethical connotations of work, the idea of an obligation or a duty on the part of those engaged in the arts and crafts. It approximates most closely the Christian concept of "vocation" or "calling," except of course that for him who has been "called" to do a job his obligations are ordained by God, while for the member of an ancient profession

his duties result from his own understanding of the nature of his profession.[32] But this difference of the ancient ethos of work from that of later ages does not lessen the strict validity of the rules to be observed. The true physician, Scribonius says, like a soldier, is "bound in lawful obedience to medicine by his military oath" (p. 2, 20–21). On the other hand, he who acts in a way unbecoming to a physician is a deserter, as it were; he is "deservedly despised by gods and men" (*diis hominibusque invisus merito*, ch. 199; cf. p. 2, 19: *diis et hominibus invisi esse debent*); he has "against the law transgressed the proper boundaries of the profession" (ch. 199).[33] He is, one might say, disqualified as a physician, for it is no longer up to him how he should conduct himself.

That such an ideal of medical humanism is foreign to the spirit of Hippocratic ethics, Scribonius admits himself. Even in the *Oath* which in his opinion is the work of Hippocrates, the "founder of our profession" (p. 2, 27), he can find his views at best by implication. For, as he puts it, Hippocrates forbids the physician to give an abortive remedy to a woman, "and thereby has gone a long way toward preparing the mind of the learners for the love of humanity. For he who thinks it to be a crime to injure future life still in doubt, how much more criminal must he judge it to hurt a full grown human being" (p. 2, 30–3, 2)?[34] But if Scribonius' concept of medical ethics goes in fact beyond the demands of the classical period, if it is distinct from the teaching of all the deontological treatises and all the medical sects I have discussed, where and when did it originate?

That Scribonius himself formulated the code of behavior which he upholds, I cannot believe; for he does not argue about it, nor defend it, he simply presupposes it and takes it for granted, as I pointed out before. In addition, reading his account one cannot fail to be reminded of the doctrine concerning human life and human obligations which characterize the Stoic philosophy of humanism evolved in the second century B.C. by Panaetius and embedded in Cicero's book *On Duties*,

the manual of all later humanism, ancient and Christian, secular and religious alike. Here if anywhere in antiquity, a programme of a professional ethics was firmly established.[35]

For first of all, Panaetius, as Cicero represents him, accepted and even enhanced the more positive evaluation of the arts and crafts which earlier philosophers had made of them, granting that virtue has its place even among craftsmen. Medicine, next to architecture and education, is expressly mentioned and singled out by Cicero as socially acceptable, because it demands a high degree of insight and contributes something useful to life; it is therefore, he says, a "proper" (*honestae*) occupation for those for whose station in life it is fitting (*On Duties*, I, 42, 151).[36]

But Panaetius' positive appreciation of the various occupations implies much more than a general approval of the activities indispensable for man's welfare and for civilization. Although philosophically speaking virtue is one and the same, and it is impossible to have any one virtue without having all of them (II, 10, 35 [Panaetius]), different aspects of this one and indivisible virtue in which all men share come to the fore in the various pursuits of human life and have to be practiced without fail. To give an example, the judge must always adhere to the truth, while the lawyer may sometimes defend the probable, even if this may not quite coincide with the truth (II, 14, 51 [Panaetius]). Obviously, here man's particular task imposes upon him certain obligations; each one has its own morality, from which there is no exception. For the judge is not permitted to indulge in any bias or favoritism out of friendship; while sitting as a judge, he is not supposed to act as a friend (III, 10, 43).[37]

If one asks why this should be so, the answer is that the individual who practices any occupation is playing a certain role. It may be one derived from chance circumstances, the place in society to which he is born and by which his inclination toward a particular career and also his opportunities for it are conditioned; it may be one which he assumes through his own free decision, through a deliberate choice of an occupation (I, 32, 115 ff.) But whether the role be inherited or chosen, one must act one's part as the role demands it, just as in the two roles which nature, in addition, has assigned to everyone—as a human being who has the same duties as all other human beings, and as an individual endowed with specific intellectual and emotional gifts (I, 30, 107 ff.)—one must live up to "the lines one has to speak." It is therefore that the judge must always utter the truth, that he is not permitted to listen to the voice of friendship, "for he lays down the role (or mask) of the friend when putting on that of the judge" (III, 10, 43). What is fitting for the one, is not so for the other.[38]

Now is this not fundamentally the way in which Scribonius views medicine and the obligations imposed by it? The role which the physician plays in the tragedy, or comedy, of life demands of him the virtue of humaneness, sympathy, or commiseration. His lines are to be spoken in this spirit. Consequently as little as Cicero's judge in his professional activity can ever be in a situation justifying his failure to cling to the truth—though there are other professions in which this virtue may sometimes come second—so Scribonius' physician must never neglect love of humanity and all the duties it entails. Certainly, commiseration and humaneness are not demanded of him alone; but they are his professional virtues, just as truthfulness is the distinctive virtue of him who sits in court notwithstanding the fact that it is required of everybody. Only when he steps out of his role, so to say, is the member of a profession free to follow another code of morals. The physician may take on the role of a citizen or of a soldier, and in that case he may fight and kill the enemy. Yet as long as he acts his professional part, he has to stick to his cue. Otherwise, he would cease to be a physician, in the same manner in which the judge who indulges in favoritism ceases to be the representative of justice.

The similarity between Scribonius' concept of a profession and that of Cicero, in my opinion, is so striking that the former can hardly be thought to be independent of the latter.[39] Perhaps Scribonius consulted the same sources of which Cicero made use and found his inspiration there. Perhaps he drew from a lost treatise on medicine and its professional obligations influenced by Panaetius' Stoicism; treatises on other professions and their duties

are known to have been written at the turn of the first century B.C. to the first century A.D. In whichever way Scribonius learned of the views of his predecessors, the principal tenets of the creed which his book attests for the first time must have their roots in the Stoic humanism transmitted through Cicero.[40]

As for the later history of this strictly professional kind of ethics, few testimonies are extant. The novelist Apuleius refers to certain physicians who hold it unfitting for "the medical sect" to be guilty of anyone's death, because they have learned that "medicine is sought out not for the purpose of destroying men but rather for that of saving them" (Metamorphoses, X, 11). His contemporary, Soranus, the great rival of Galen, mentions some colleagues of his who regard it as their duty to banish abortives not only because Hippocrates said one should do so, but also "because it is the specific task of medicine to guard and preserve what has been engendered by nature" (Gynaecology, I, 60).[41] While these passing remarks do hardly more than rephrase Scribonius' formulations, a poem composed by an otherwise unknown Stoic philosopher, Sarapion—he too lived in the second century A.D.—shows, I think, a certain evolution of the original theory. For in this poem, entitled On the Eternal Duties of the Physician, and inscribed on stone in the Athenian temple of Asclepius, the god of medicine and of the physicians, the god who prided himself most of all on his virtue of philanthropy, the "eternal duties" of the doctor are said to be: "First to heal his mind and to give assistance to himself before giving it to anyone [else]" and to "cure with moral courage and with the proper moral attitude."[42] Then "he would be like god savior equally of slaves, of paupers, of rich men, of princes, and to all a brother, such help he would give. For we are all brothers. Therefore he would not hate anyone, nor would he harbor envy in his mind." Here, the thought of Scribonius, the philosophy advocated by Cicero, is restated in the language of late Stoicism, in its new terms of human brotherhood, which indeed foreshadow the categories of Christian medical ethics.[43]

Finally the quintessence of pagan medical humanism was expressed by Libanius in a moving speech which medicine addresses to the young physician starting out on his career: "You desired to be one of the healers (of sickness), you had the benefit of having (good) teachers. Now, practice your art faithfully. Be reliable; cultivate love of man; if you are called to your patient, hasten to go; when you enter the sickroom, apply all your mental ability to the case at hand; share in the pain of those who suffer; rejoice with those who have found relief; consider yourself a partner in the disease; muster all you know for the fight to be fought; consider yourself to be of your contemporaries the brother, of those who are your elders the son, of those who are younger the father. And if anyone of them neglects his own affairs, remember that this is not permissible for yourself, and that it is your duty to be to the sick what the Dioscuri are to the sailor (in distress)."[44]

Is it by chance that the evidence concerning the survival of the humanistic ideal does not seem to go beyond the second half of the fourth century A.D.? Since on the whole the material for the history of medical ethics is so fragmentary, one hesitates to hazard judgment. Yet one may say with assurance that from the third century, Stoic philosophy—of which the doctrine of professional ethos formed part and parcel—ceased to have influence. The Neo-Platonists established Galen as the unchallenged authority in medicine. Through him, the philosophical ethics of the scientist-physician, which had never quite lost its appeal, came to predominate among the learned. Among the general practitioners of late antiquity, the teaching of the deontological writings of the Corpus Hippocraticum seems to have prevailed.[45] As for the rising caste of especially privileged physicians—those who as city officials were granted immunity from public duties, and those who became court physicians—it is hard to believe that they should have been keen on following the precepts of brotherly love. As I mentioned before, Galen already noted that the city physicians accepted their position in order to be relieved from the staggering burden of "indirect taxation." The "courtly" ethics discernable even in his writings, according to which the physician will treat the emperor and his family, and all wealthy people for that matter, differently from what he proposes to do in the case of the poor, implies principles hardly compatible with Scribonius' love of mankind, or Sarapion's belief in the brotherhood of men.[46]

In the short span of time during which ancient medical humanism was current, once it had finally been formulated in opposition to the ideals of earlier generations, it most likely remained restricted to a small minority of physicians. Scribonius himself divined the slim chances for general acceptance of his belief and put the responsibility for this failure upon the patients. "Rarely," he says (p. 4, 9 ff.), "does anyone make an evaluation of the doctor before putting himself and his family under his care. And yet, if people have their portrait painted, they will first try to make sure of the artist's qualities on the basis of that which experience can tell, and then select and hire him." It is no wonder, therefore, he continues (p. 4, 15), that so many physicians rest content with little effort. Where no intelligent selection is made, where the good and the bad are held in equal esteem, "everybody will practice medicine as he sees fit" (p. 4, 24). The true reason for the relative ineffectualness of Scribonius' programme probably lies in a shortcoming which it shared with all the other ancient attempts to shape medical practice in accordance with moral concepts. None of them had the backing of institutions or organizations that had the power to enforce rules of conduct.[47] Yet, this very fact makes the achievement of the individuals who aspired to a medical ethics all the more impressive. It is praiseworthy indeed that under the given circumstances so many—some whose names history has recorded, and others whose identity has been obliterated—heeded Sarapion's appeal "to heal their own minds first" before giving help to their patients; that they were willing to forego material advantage for the law of their own conscience; that they took the initiative in raising and clarifying the moral issue, thereby laying the foundation for all later medical ethics.

It seems safe to add that among the ideals conceived by the ancients none was loftier than that which envisages love of humanity as the professional virtue of the physician. Even the Hippocratic *Oath* assumes full significance and dignity only if interpreted in the way in which it was understood by Scribonius and those who came after him. That this ideal of professional ethics also is the one most difficult to live up to, goes without saying. In fact, one cannot help wondering whether unending failure rather than even momentary success must not be the inevitable fate of those who commit themselves in earnest to such a seemingly utopian doctrine. For does it not essentially amount to the demand that the physician should be a citizen of two states, as it were, the one here and now, where he has obligations to his country, the other "laid up in heaven," where he is obligated to mankind alone? How can such a conflict of duties ever be fully resolved?

Notes

1. U. Fleischer, *Untersuchungen zu den pseudohippokratischen Schriften* Παραγγελίαι, Περὶ ἰητροῦ *und* Περὶ εὐσχημοσύνης (Neue Deutsche Forschungen, Abt. Klass. Philologie), 1939, pp. 1; 54, seems to take φιλάνθρωπος to refer to "love of mankind." Yet Jones is surely right in translating the word as "kind to all," and μισάνθρωπος, the term contrasted with it immediately afterwards, as "unkind" (*Hippocrates*, II, pp. 311; 313 [Loeb Classical Library; see p. 7, this volume]; cf. also E Littré, *Oeuvres complètes d'Hippocrate*, vol. 9, 1861, pp. 205–7: humain—dur).

2. The usual interpretation, "where there is love of man (on the part of the physician), there is also love of the art (on his part)," is refuted by the immediately following words: "For some patients, though conscious that their condition is perilous, recover their health simply through their contentment with the goodness of the physician." The previous sentence then must contain an assertion as to the patients' attitude, and it can only be "love of the art" felt by them in consequence of the doctor's philanthropy, contentment with the goodness of the physician, of which the author is speaking. In his opinion the question of fees discussed in ch. 6 has psychologically important consequences for the recovery of the sick. If the doctor is reasonable in his charges, or even willing to undertake the treatment without compensation, he creates an atmosphere of confidence that is helpful for the restoration of health. In the same spirit the writer, in an earlier chapter (4), has warned against discussing fees at the beginning of the cure because worry regarding fees is "harmful to a troubled patient, particularly if the disease is acute." Fleischer, *op. cit.*, p. 38, has clearly seen that the sequence of the statements made in chapter 6 points to the meaning:

"wenn der Arzt Menschenfreund ist, sind die Menschen Freunde seiner Kunst." Nevertheless he tries to save the common interpretation, believing that the term "love of the art" is more often predicated of the representative of the art and that the latter's "wish for knowledge" forms the starting point of the discussion. But the context is quite a different one, as I have tried to show in the text. Nor is it "love of mankind" that is here made "the motive of medical practice." In *Precepts* too the author speaks of "love of man," having warned at the beginning of the chapter against "disdain of man" (ἀπανθρωπίη, "not to be unkind," Jones, *op. cit.*, I, p. 319 [p. 5, this volume]; âpreté, Littré, *op. cit.*, vol. 9, p. 259). "Philanthropy" then appears here in exactly the same contrast as in the treatise *On the Physician*.

3. The word φιλάνθρωπος originally was used only of gods and kings to denote their benevolent attitude toward men, i.e., toward their inferiors (or of animals who are friendly toward men). From the second half of the fourth century B.C. it began to be applied more generally and to be interpreted as kindliness and friendliness of individuals in their social contacts (cf. S. Lorenz, *De progressu notionis* φιλανθρωπίας, Diss. Leipzig, 1914, pp. 8 ff.; 14 ff.; 19 ff.; also J. Heinemann, s.v. "Humanismus," *Realencyclopädie der classischen Altertumswissenschaft*, Supplementband 5, 1931, col. 298). The contrast φιλάνθρωπος—μισάνθρωπος is usual in the fourth century (Lorenz, p. 25 f.); for the Peripatetic and Stoic interpretations of the term φιλανθρωπία as kindness, which is reflected in the Hippocratic respective treatises, cf. below, notes 18 and 19.

4. For the late date of *On the Physician* and *Precepts* in general, cf. now Fleischer, *passim*, and below, notes 19, 20.

5. W. W. Tarn, "Alexander, Cynics and Stoics," *Amer. Journ. Philol.*, 60, 1939, p. 44, rightly says that even the cosmopolitanism of the fourth-century Cynics has nothing to do "with any belief in the unity of mankind or a human brotherhood." It is a negative rather than a positive creed (cf. also Heinemann, *loc. cit.*, col. 291). And the same holds true of the advocacy of the equality and kinship of men by Hippias and others (cf. Heinemann, *ibid.*, col. 287), or the "cosmopolitanism" to be found in Democritus and Euripides (cf. W. Nestle, *Vom Mythos zum Logos*, 1942, p. 380 f.). Lorenz' attempt to show that at least in the philosophical language of the fourth century philanthropy had the wider sense which it had later on (*op. cit.*, pp. 35 ff.), is refuted by the testimonies themselves. Still in Aristotle φιλανθρωπία is but an emotion, an instinctive feeling of friendliness and kinship that exists between men as members of the same species, just as animals of the same race feel akin to one another (cf. J. Burnet, *The Ethics of Aristotle*, 1900, ad 1155 a 16 ff.; also H. v. Arnim, *Arius Didymus' Abriss der peripatetischen Ethik*, Sitzb. Wien, philos. hist. Kl., 204, No. 3, 1926, p. 107).

6. For a more detailed picture of the rules of behavior, cf. L. Edelstein, Περὶ ἀέρων und

die Sammlung der Hippokratischen Schiften (Problemata, 4), 1931, pp. 93 ff. (this will be quoted as *Problemata*). Cf. also W. H. S. Jones, *Hippocrates*, II, Introductory Essay V.

7. The term used by the true physician in setting himself apart from the charlatan is that of "expertness," which is at the same time "goodness" (ἀνδραγαθικώτερον καὶ τεχνικώτερον); cf. e.g. *Hippocratis Opera*, ed. H. Kuehlewein, II, 1902, pp. 236, 18–237, 1; and in general, *Problemata*, pp. 95–98. For the lack of supervision of the medical art on the part of civil authorities, cf. *ibid.*, p. 89 f.

8. Here I am concerned only with the ideal of medical practice, as it emerges from the Hippocratic writings. How far reality could fall behind this ideal, how far the ancient physician could deviate from strictly medical considerations in order to attract patients, I have tried to show in *Problemata*, chs. 2 and 3.

9. That the competent Hippocratic physician was willing to forego momentary success and easy gain, follows e.g. from the surgical writings (cf. *Hippocratis Opera*, ed. Kuehlewein, II, pp. 168, 3 ff.; 175, 8 ff.; *Problemata*, pp. 97–99, where I should not have quoted however a passage from the later *Precepts*.) The Ruskin quotation I have borrowed from P. Shorey (*Plato, The Republic*, I, [Loeb], *ad* 346 A).

10. In the Platonic passage referred to Socrates argues according to the beliefs generally held; the passage therefore is especially illuminating for the common attitude towards the crafts. Aristotle too maintains that the function of medicine is that of causing health, not of producing wealth (*Politics*, 1258 a 10 ff.), though by some it is wrongly turned into mere money making, as if this were the aim of medicine (*ibid.*). From the point of view of economic theory, medicine belongs to that "art of acquisition" which deals with exchange, and is "labor for hire" (μισθαρνία 1258 b 25).

11. That the classical age did not know of the concept of "professions" but ranged the artist, the physician, and others with the common workmen or craftsmen (τεχνῖται) has been emphasized especially by A. E. Zimmern, *The Greek Commonwealth*, 1915, pp. 257 ff. For the contrast between the classical attitude toward work and the modern concept of the "nobility of toil," cf. H. Michell, *The Economics of Ancient Greece*, 1940, p. 14. It is because of the facts referred to that I cannot agree with W. Müri's statement that the Hippocratic physician is the "Vertreter des Standes" and as such "in seinem Auftreten nicht mehr ganz frei" (*Arzt und Patient bei Hippokrates*, Beilage z. Jahresber. über d. städt. Gymnasium in Bern, 1936, p. 35). W. A. Heidel's chapter on the medical profession (*Hippocratic Medicine*, 1941, pp. 26–39) also is vitiated by his failure to consider the particular social and moral values prevailing in the world in which the Hippocratic "doctor" practiced.

12. The attitude of the Pythagoreans of the late fourth century toward the crafts I have discussed in *The Hippocratic Oath*, 1943,

p. 60. Their views are the more significant since, generally speaking, the fifth and fourth centuries considered the workman not only déclassé, but evinced a definite prejudice against him, contrary to the preclassical generations, a prejudice to be found in aristocratic and democratic societies alike (cf. Michell, *op. cit.*, pp. 11 ff.; also M. Pohlenz, "Die Lebensformen, Arbeit und Erwerb" in *Der Hellenische Mensch*, ch. XIII, pp. 357 ff. That an exception was made in regard to the physician [*ibid.*, p. 359] is not attested). Among the few who at least maintained that for the poor it is shameful to remain idle rather than to work was the "historical" Socrates (cf. Pohlenz, *ibid.*, p. 358), whose teaching seems to have been important also for the development of a concept of professional ethics. Cf. below, note 37.

13. The Stoic philosophy of work, as it was formulated by Chrysippus, has been most adequately interpreted by A. Bonhöffer, *Die Ethik des Stoikers Epictet*, 1894, "Exkurs" IV, pp. 233 ff. For the importance of Stoic theories of the second and first centuries A.D. with regard to medical ethics, see later in this chapter. The Peripatetic doctrine concerning the life of the ordinary citizen and the act of acquisition is attested by Stobaeus (*Eclogae*, II, pp. 143, 24 ff.; 149, 21–23, ed. Wachsmuth, and Arnim, *op. cit.*, p. 90). I need not enter here into a discussion of the question whether the system outlined in Stobaeus can be traced altogether to Theophrastus (cf. Arnim, *op. cit.*, pp. 83 ff.), or whether it is influenced at least in part by Stoicism (R. Walzer, *Magna Moralia und Aristotelische Ethik* [Neue Philol. Unters., VII], 1929, p. 191 f.; also O. Regenbogen, *s.v.* "Theophrastos," *Realencycl.*, Suppl. VII, cols. 1492–94). However, it is important to note that the verdict of Aristotle's *Politics* according to which workmanship may be noble or ignoble depending on how much or how little virtue it requires as an accessory (1258 b 38 f.), must be considered an interpolation along the lines of later Peripatetic ethics. For it is in contradiction to Aristotle's general position. That the sentence in question is an addition has been suspected for other reasons by W. L. Newman, *The Politics of Aristotle*, II, 1887, p. 203; the whole chapter in which the statement occurs differs in many respects from the rest of the text, cf. E. Barker, *The Politics of Aristotle*, 1946, p. 29, note 3.

14. I should mention at least that at the turn of the fourth to the third century economic theory also began to consider the crafts in a new light. The Ps. Platonic dialogue *Eryxias* discussing the relation between wealth and virtue (393 A) entertains the notion that the crafts are not barter or "limited service," as Aristotle held (cf. above, note 12), but rather are to be classified under possession of wealth, and are thus more noble. The "expert pilot" and the "skilled physician" are the examples adduced (394 E); cf. M. L. W. Laistner, *Greek Economics*, 1923, p. xxviii f. The right, that is, the moral use of such "wealth" of practical skill forms the subject of a considerable part of the conversation

reported in this dialogue, the only extant Greek treatise which deals exclusively with economic problems.

15. The following analysis of the deontological writings which go into minute details of medical practice, is not intended to be exhaustive. I shall simply consider a number of salient features that within the context of my discussion seem to characterize the teaching of these essays.

16. For the Pythagorean origin of the *Oath* and its date, cf. Edelstein, *The Hippocratic Oath*, especially p. 59 f.

17. Fleischer's dating of the treatise *On the Physician* in the third century (*op. cit.*, p. 56 f.) seems convincing to me. (H. Diller, *Gnomon*, 17, 1941, p. 30, thinks it unlikely that the book was written after 300 B.C.). The short summary of ethics given by the "Hippocratic" author is usually related to the protreptic-paraenetic literature of the time (cf. J. F. Bensel, "De medico libellus ad codicum fidem recensitus," *Philologus*, 78, 1922, pp. 102–4; also Müri, *op. cit.*, p. 37), or is linked in addition with the content of introductory manuals on the crafts which became common in the Hellenistic era (Fleischer, *op. cit.*, p. 54 f.). Yet, the right behavior of the physician is defined at least once in the typically Aristotelian manner as "a mean between extremes." ("In appearance let him be of a serious, but not harsh countenance, for surliness is taken for arrogance and unkindness, while a man of uncontrolled laughter and excessive gaiety is considered vulgar"). Details of the precept also fall in line with Peripatetic terminology and doctrine. The concept of surliness (αὐθάδεια) is used here in the restricted and derogatory sense which it came to have in the Peripatetic school (*Magna Moralia*, 1192 b 31; Stobaeus, p. 146, 8, and Walzer, *op. cit.*, p. 161, n. 1). As Bensel already noted (p. 105), the word "vulgar" (φορτικός) is applied to him who indulges in excessive laughter, just as it is in *Nic. Eth.*, 1128 a 3 ff. Self-control (ἐγκράτεια) commended in the Hippocratic essay is treated as one of the main virtues in *Magna Moralia*, in contrast to the genuine Aristotelian ethics (Walzer, *op. cit.*, pp. 98; 106). The use of the term friendliness (φιλάνθρωπος, cf. above, note 3) agrees with that to be found in the Ps. Aristotelian treatise *On Virtues and Vices* (1251 b 35; cf. 1251 b 16; 1250 b 33; also Theophrastus *apud* Stobaeus, *Florilegium*, 3, 50). Finally, the ideal of the "gentleman" (τὸ δὲ ἦθος εἶναι καλὸν καὶ ἀγαθόν) remains valid throughout the history of Peripatetic ethics (Stobaeus, p. 147, 23). It is true, the ethics propounded in the book *On the Physician* is that of common morality, but as one has rightly said, the later Peripatos restored "bourgeois morality" (Walzer, *op. cit.*, p. 188). For the Peripatetic concern with the life of the ordinary citizen, cf. above, note 13. I should add that the Peripatetic flavor of the "Hippocratic" essay speaks for its being dated after 300 B.C.

18. *Precepts* is usually held to be Epicurean in origin, cf. now Fleischer, *op. cit.*, pp. 10 ff. However Bensel, *op. cit.*, pp. 96; 98, rightly doubted an influence of Epicurus on

any of the deontological writings because Epicurus (Fr. 196 ed. Usener) considers all forms of life which are not directed toward the happy life merely vulgar activities. Epicurean philosophy seems the only Hellenistic system that does not share in the rehabilitation of the crafts (cf. Philodemus, On Oeconomics, XXIII, 18 ff.). And indeed, the moral teaching of Precepts is Stoic rather than Epicurean. The term φιλανθρωπία, as it is used here (cf. above, note 3), corresponds to the meaning which the word has for the Chrysippean Stoa (φιλικὴ χρῆσις ἀνθρώπων [Stoicorum Veterum Fragmenta, III, 292 ed. Arnim]), and in its emphatically moral connotation differs significantly from the more utilitarian recommendation of φιλανθρωπία by the Epicureans (Philodemus, op. cit., XXIV, 29). The injunction on fees laid down in Precepts is paralleled by Chrysippus' statements on fees for teaching (St. V. Fr., 701). The definition of medicine as "habit" (ἕξις, ch. 2) is that of the Stoa (cf. e.g., St. V. Fr., II, 393; III, 111). That the epistemological theories, too, are Stoic rather than Epicurean, I hope to show elsewhere. The date of Precepts has been fixed by Fleischer (op. cit., p. 24) in the first or second century A.D. At any rate, the book must be late Hellenistic.

19. The Stoic influence on the treatise On Decorum is generally recognized (e.g. Jones, Hippocrates, II, p. 270 f.) and has been traced in detail by Fleischer (op. cit., especially pp. 78; 90: 101 ff.). The latter also dates the essay in the first-second century A.D. A reexamination of the background of the Stoic theories here adopted may perhaps lead to the assumption of a slightly earlier date. But this too I must leave for another investigation.

20. Scribonius Largus, perhaps the first to mention the Oath, maintains that Hippocrates began medical instruction by administering this vow (Compositiones, p. 2, 27 f. ed. Helmreich). This of course is mere conjecture. Such books as Ps. Soranus, Introductio ad medicinam (V. Rose, Anecdota Graeca et Graeco-Latina, II, 1870) speak of a medical oath and of the oath of Hippocrates (pp. 244, 27; 245, 16 f.). In the fourth century A.D. Libanius (Κατὰ ἰατροῦ φαρμακέως, 9) refers to "the oath taken by physicians when entering upon the practice of their profession" (cf. R. Pack, "Note on a 'Progymnasma' of Libanius," Amer. Jour. Philol., 69, 1948, p. 300), and many such oaths were in fact current (Pack, ibid.). That any of them were obligatory, cannot be proved. According to Ps. Oribasius, Comment. in Aphorismos Hippocratis, ed. Basileae, 1535, p. 7, the Oath was the first book to be read by the beginner, cf. K. Deichgräber, "Die ärztliche Standesethik des hippokratischen Eides," Quellen u. Stud. z. Gesch. d. Naturwiss. u. d. Medizin, III, 2, 1932, p. 93, n. 1, and the material there given on other oaths, p. 95, n. 33; p. 97, n. 42.

21. It is usual to designate the ethics of the Oath as "Berufsethos" (cf. e.g. Pohlenz, op. cit., p. 334); Müri uses this term in his analysis of the picture of the ideal physician, as it is given in the deontological writings (op. cit., p. 39). In a loose sense, such a characterization is surely not unjustified. But it is important to note that none of the "Hippocratic" treatises here discussed considers the obligations of the physician as inherent in his medical task. They rather adapt philosophical ethics to medicine.

22. For a more detailed interpretation of "scientific" medicine, cf. L. Edelstein, "The Relation of Ancient Philosophy to Medicine," Bull. Hist. Med., 26, 1952, pp. 301 ff.

23. In the interpretation of the Law I follow Wilamowitz, Hermes, 54, 1919, pp. 46 ff. F. Müller's attempt (Hermes, 75, 1940, pp. 39 ff.) to date the Law in the fifth century B.C. to me is unconvincing. As Fleischer says (op. cit., p. 46), it is perhaps impossible to date the essay exactly, because many of its concepts became common stock in the discussion of moral problems. Yet the book cannot be earlier than Democritus, some of whose central ethical concepts are here presupposed, as Wilamowitz has shown. Nor will it be much later than the end of the fourth century, since unalloyed Democritean teaching did not long survive. Jones (Hippocrates, II, p. 275) connects the Law with the doctrine of secret medical societies, which he thinks might have existed in Greece, since at the end of the Law it is proclaimed: "Holy things are shown to holy men; to the profane it is not lawful to show them until these have been initiated into the rites of knowledge." But the description of "knowledge" through the metaphor of the mysteries is not uncommon with Greek philosophers (cf. E. Frank, Knowledge, Will and Belief, 1955, pp. 63 f.; 67). Wilamowitz, op. cit., p. 49, already compared ἱερὰ πρήγματα in the Law with the ἱερὸν πνεῦμα that, according to Democritus, inspires the poet. Jones' translation of ἠδελφισμένος (Precepts, ch. 5) as "one made a brother" (of a secret society) involves an unnecessary change of the best manuscript tradition ἠδελφισμένως, for the meaning of which cf. Fleischer, op. cit., p. 36.

24. Cf. K. Deichgräber, Die griechische Empirikerschule, 1930, p. 322 f. Especially important is the statement, p. 82, 29 ff.: οἷος δ᾽ ἐστι καθ᾽ ὅλον τὸν βίον ὁ σκεπτικός, τοιοῦτός ἐστι περὶ τὴν ἰατρικὴν ὁ ἐμπειρικός. Ch. 11 of Galen's Subfiguratio Empirica treats "De moribus et dictis que debent esse in empericis." For the sceptics' conformance with the established laws, cf. e.g. M. M. Patrick, The Greek Sceptics, 1929, p. 51.

25. Cf. Ps. Soranus, Introductio ad medicinam (Rose, Anecdota Graeca et Graeco-Latina, II, p. 244, 16-23): "Disciplinarum autem ceterarum minime sit expers [sc. medicus], sed et circa mores habeat diligentiam. iuxta enim Erasistratum felicissimum quidem est ubi utraeque res fuerint, uti et in arte sit perfectus et moribus sit optimus. si autem unum de duobus defuerit, melius est virum esse bonum absque doctrina quam artificem perfectum mores habentem malos et improbum esse. modesti

si quidem mores quod in arte deest honestate repensare videntur, culpa autem morum artem perfectam corrumpere atque improbare potest." The Introductio which forms part of a collection of Quaestiones Medicinales (cf. Rose, op. cit., p. 169), though hardly by Soranus, is based on good ancient sources. There is no reason to doubt the authenticity of the quotation from Erasistratus.

26. E. Wenkebach, "Der hippokratische Arzt als das Ideal Galens," Quell. u. Stud. z. Gesch. d. Nat. u. d. Med., III, 1932-33, p. 372 f., stresses the influence of Hippocratic medicine on Galen's ideal as outlined in the treatise referred to. But although Galen identifies his philosophy with that of Hippocrates, one must remember that for him, Hippocrates and Plato agree in almost all points. Besides, he says expressly (ch. 3) that philosophy is indispensable for medical practice, just as it is for medical theory; in addition to logic and physics, the physician must take up the third part of philosophy, namely ethics.

27. On the evidence of Galen's claim that "Diocles practiced medicine out of love of mankind" (cf. above), K. Deichgräber, Professio medici, Zum Vorwort des Scribonius Largus, Abh. Akad. Mainz, Geistes- u. Sozialwiss. Klasse, 1950, No. 9), tentatively suggests that the association between medicine and philanthropy may be due to the influence of the Peripatos (p. 866, n. 1). Yet, for Aristotle, and even for Theophrastus, φιλανθρωπία is not "love of humanity" (cf. above, notes 5 and 17). As late as in Stobaeus' report on Peripatetic ethics the κοινὴ φιλανθρωπία, as it is called in contradistinction of the φιλία among friends (II, 121, 22; 120, 20), is not represented as one of the main virtues (cf. Heinemann, op. cit., col. 298); it rather is a natural sympathy that prompts men to help other men in dire need and not think of themselves only (p. 120, 20-121, 22). Much as the Peripatos contributed to the Hellenistic concept of the unity of men, it was the Stoa that stressed the rational duties inherent in the idea of humanity (M. Pohlenz, Die Stoa, I, 1948, pp. 136-39). And even in the Stoic school justice was at first the obligation stressed in connection with cosmopolitanism; love of mankind came to be fully recognized only in the first century A.D. (Pohlenz, ibid., p. 315; Bonhöffer, op. cit., p. 106). I should be inclined, therefore, to believe that philanthropy became integrated into the ethical teaching of the dogmatic physicians not long before Galen's time, if indeed it was not Galen himself who accepted the ideal of philanthropy in accordance with his Stoic leanings.

28. Cf. below.

29. In That the Best Physician also is a Philosopher Galen once speaks of medicine as a τέχνη οὕτω φιλάνθρωπος (ch. 2). The detailed refutation of Menodotus shows that by the term in question Galen can only mean that medicine is "philanthropic" because it removes the sufferings of men.

30. The fact that Scribonius upholds a humanistic ethics has often been noticed, of course; cf. *e.g.* J. Hirschberg, *Vorlesungen über hippokratische Heilkunde*, 1922, p. 35. A detailed analysis of Scribonius' views has recently been given by K. Deichgräber, *op. cit.* (cf. above, note 27).

31. I am quoting the definition of *humanitas* which Gellius gives (*Noctes Atticae*, XIII, 17) as the one commonly accepted. Hienemann, *Realencycl.*, col. 306, has shown that in the literature of the first century A.D. the words *humanitas* and *humanus* and their Greek equivalents are used in the sense attested by Gellius.

32. M. Weber, "Die protestantische Ethik und der Geist des Kapitalismus," *Ges. Aufsätze z. Religionssoziologie*, I. 1920, analyzing the meaning of the term *Beruf* or "calling" has pointed up its difference from the classical concept of work (p. 63). He has also noted, however, that in Latin, such words as *officium* (cf. also below, n. 40), *munus*, and *professio* (originally denoting, it seems, the duty of making a tax declaration) came to assume "eine unserem Wort 'Beruf' in jeder Hinsicht ziemlich ähnliche Gesamtbedeutung . . . natürlich durchaus diesseitig, ohne jede religiöse Färbung" (p. 63, n. 1).

33. The simile of fighting and military service used by Scribonius is quite common in Latin philosophy (cf. *e.g.* Pohlenz, *Die Stoa*, I, 1948, p. 314); it also occurs in the language of the mysteries so often applied to knowledge in general, cf. above, note 23, and *Amer. Journ. Philol.*, 72, 1951, p. 430, n. 6.

34. Scribonius concludes that Hippocrates apparently "thought it of great value for everyone to preserve the name and honor of medicine in purity and holiness, conducting himself after their design" (p. 3, 2–5). Thereby he translates into the language of his professional ethics the Pythagorean concepts of purity and holiness used in the *Oath* with reference to the art which the physician practices and to the life which he leads (ἁγνῶς δὲ καὶ ὁσίως διατηρήσω βίον ἐμὸν καὶ τέχνην ἐμήν). It is unwarranted, I think, to infer from this adaptation of the famous sentence in the *Oath* that Scribonius has a "religiös getönte Humanität" (Deichgräber, *op. cit.* [cf. above, note 27], p. 861).

35. R. Reitzenstein, *Werden und Wesen der Humanität im Altertum*, 1907, p. 15, already suggested that the philosophy of Panaetius gave rise to a "*Standesethik*"; cf. also Heinemann, *op. cit.*, col. 294.

36. In accordance with their own aristocratic prejudice and with the prejudice of the society in which they live, Panaetius and Cicero consider political and public activities the only ones proper for a gentleman (cf. M. Pohlenz, "Antikes Führertum," *Neue Wege z. Antike*, 2. Reihe, H. 3, 1934, p. 83 f.). The views of the older Stoics in this respect had been more liberal; cf. above, note 14.

37. Panaetius surely was not the first to discuss the particular virtues pertaining to an occupation. His teacher, Antipater (*St. V. Fr.*, III, 61 f.), had engaged in a famous dispute about "business ethics" with his predecessor, Diogenes (*St. V. Fr.*, III, 49). The casuistry of the old Stoa insists on the fact that for the physician it is permissible to lie (III, 513), that neither he, nor the judge is allowed to indulge in commiseration "with the suffering of his neighbors" (III, 451). The beginnings of such a "differenzierende Ethik" may be traced even to the Sophists, and especially to the Xenophontian Socrates (cf. E. Norden, in *Hermes*, 40, 1905, pp. 521 ff.; F. Wehrli, "Ethik und Medizin," *Mus. Helveticum*, 8, 1951, p. 45 f.). However, the recognition that virtuous action may differ with different people and different positions in life is still a far cry from the acknowledgement of professional virtues. At any rate, they seem not to have been appraised systematically before Panaetius.

38. The discussion summarized in the text makes it clear that, in Cicero's view, each "profession" or career has its own ethos. The example of the judge is obviously used as particularly appropriate to Roman conditions; cf. also above, note 37.

39. Deichgräber (*op. cit.*, pp. 865 ff.) assumes that the ethics outlined by Scribonius is original with him, though with reference to ch. 199 he admits that "die Frage der professio der Medizin hat [for Scribonius] allgemeineren Charakter" (p. 859). This in itself is an indication, it seems, that he is merely applying to medicine a general theory of professional behavior. The physician to the emperor Claudius must surely have been familiar with Stoicism. He was the freer to accept Panaetius' teaching which did not influence the established medical sects, because he himself apparently did not belong to any of the schools of his age (Deichgräber, p. 865 f.).

40. E. Norden has drawn attention to the specific literature "De officiis judicis" which starts to appear around the middle of the first century A.D. (*Hermes*, 40, 1905, p. 512 f.). It differs from the usual type of "Introductions" to any given art in that here only the moral obligations of the judge are considered. With Cicero and his contemporaries the word *officium* comes to mean not only the objective task of an art, but also, if not preeminently, the duties incumbent upon the artist (cf. E. Bernert, *De vi atque usu vocabuli officii*, Diss. Breslau, 1930, pp. 25 ff.; 29 ff.; and above, note 32). Gellius mentions books on the juridical "office" in both Latin and Greek (*Noctes Atticae*, XIV, 2, 1). Panaetius and his pupils, Posidonius and Hecaton, wrote Περὶ τοῦ καθήκοντος; other Stoic books "On Duties" are known from Seneca (cf. H. Gomoll, *Der stoische Philosoph Hekaton*, 1933, pp. 27 ff.); the work of the artisan is considered as an *officium*, as a moral obligation, by Cicero (*De officiis*, I, 7, 22) as well as by Seneca (*De beneficiis*, III, 18, 1; cf. Gomoll, p. 77 f.). In the Stoic treatises just referred to the obligations toward one's country and toward other groups to which the individual

may belong were set forth, or they were defined according to certain virtues. For the importance of philanthropy in late Stoic ethics, cf. above, note 27; below, note 43. The details of the general theory of professions as it was developed in the Middle Stoa I hope to discuss in an investigation of Stoic ethics. That the works on duties began to pay attention also to medicine is the more likely since physicians by this time were granted citizenship, and medicine was practiced even by free-born Romans (cf. K. H. Below, *Der Arzt im römischen Recht*, Münch. Beitr. z. Papyrusforschung u. antiken Rechtsgeschichte, 37, 1953, p. 20 f.).

41. I should mention that Galen's refutation of Menodotus (cf. above) may be an indirect reflection of the fight about the new professional ethics. Menodotus was a pupil of the Sceptic Antiochus (cf. Deichgräber, *Empirikerschule*, p. 212), who leaned toward Stoicism and deviated in many respects from his school. Possibly his assertion that the physician's aim is money or honor was intended as the antithesis of the ethos of philanthropy. Also, Seneca's contention that men owe more to the physician than financial remuneration (*De beneficiis*, VI, 16, 1) may be a reference to physicians of the type Scribonius depicts, although elsewhere he acknowledges the fact that medical knowledge and moral goodness do not always go together (*Ep.* 87, 17). Finally, could not Pliny's notorious diatribe against the physicians best be understood if his judgment was determined by the humanistic ideal? For Pliny is careful in mentioning that all the crimes committed by physicians should be attributed to the individuals and not to the medical art (XXIX, 21 f.).

42. Cf. P. L. Maas and James H. Oliver, "An Ancient Poem on the Duties of a Physician," *Bull. Hist. Med.*, 7, 1939, pp. 315 ff. The translation is Oliver's, whose emendation [αἰ]ώνια I also accept against Maas' [Παι]ώνια (cf. p. 320, n. 6).

43. Maas in his commentary (*loc. cit.*, p. 323) says, ad vv. 12 ff.: "color Epicteteus, ne dicam Christianus." It seems to me that the poem can be adequately understood within the confines of late Stoicism that so often approximates Christian ethics. For the brotherhood of men cf. *e.g.* Epictetus, I, 13, 3 f.; Seneca, *Ep.*, 95, 52: "natura nos cognatos edidit . . . haec nobis amorem indidit mutuum." Sarapion enumerating man's various stations in life spells out Scribonius' claim that medicine does not judge men by their circumstances in life or by their personality. Both proscribe envy (Sarapion: [ζᾶλος]; Scribonius: *invidentia*). While Sarapion derives from the brotherhood of men the duty not to hate anyone, Scribonius expresses the same thought positively through his concept of *humanitas*. (In the lines of the poem which I have omitted there are certain parallels with the deontological writings of the *Corpus Hippocraticum* noted by Oliver, p. 318, notes 2, 3; p. 320, note 4). Later Christian passages closely resembling the main drift of Sarapion's poem are to be found *e.g.* in L. C. MacKinney, "Medical Ethics and Etiquette

in the Early Middle Ages," *Bull. Hist. Med.,* *26,* 1952, pp. 6; 11 f.; 27. Only one feature sharply distinguishes pagan humanism from the Christian attitude and that of the nineteenth-century humanist reformers (for whom cf. I. Galdston, "Humanism and Public Health," *Bull. Hist. Med., 8,* 1940, pp. 1032 ff.): pagan ethics lacks any recognition of social responsibilities on the part of the physician. Although sickness was understood in rational terms, and some diseases were traced to social conditions, even the gospel of brotherly love took account only of the relationship between the individual doctor and the individual patient. Immediate help rather than long-range improvement remained the watchword. In general, cf. O. Temkin in *Social Medicine: Its Derivations and Objectives,* ed. I. Galdston, 1949, pp. 3 ff.

44. Κατὰ ἰατροῦ φαρμακέως, 6–7. Libanius writes in the vein of Cynic and Stoic popular philosophy, probably echoing older traditions. Already to Seneca and his generation, the physician had become "the friend" of the patient (*De beneficiis,* VI, 16, 1) sympathizing with him and loved in return as a friend (*ibid.,* 4–6); cf. above, note 41.

45. Cf. e.g. the *Introductio* of Ps. Soranus, *op. cit.,* p. 245, 17; 22; 33. Even the late deontological writings soon became integrated into some of the collections of the Hippocratic works compiled in the Christian era; cf. Fleischer, *op. cit.,* pp. 108 ff.

46. For Galen's rules concerning treatment of the imperial family and of the rich, cf. e.g. *Opera Omnia* (ed. Kühn), vol. 13, pp. 635–38; 14, p. 659; also 12, p. 435. Surely, the distinctions here made became even more marked when the hierarchic structure of the empire was consolidated. The importance of the class of city physicians has been pointed up through Herzog's interpretation of an edict of Vespasian in which their privileges are set forth (*Urkunden zur Hochschulpolitik der römischen Kaiser,* Sitzberichte Berlin, 1935, pp. 967 ff.; cf. also Below, *op. cit.,* pp. 23 ff.). Following perhaps the example of Augustus, Vespasian granted to all physicians exemption from taxes and from the burden of having soldiers billeted in their houses. Antoninus Pius revoked this edict and introduced a *numerus clausus* for the privileged physicians in each city (cf. Below, *op. cit.,* pp. 34 ff.); Galen's rather damning statement on those who practice medicine in order to be tax-exempt—to my knowledge never quoted in the pertinent literature—may throw some light on Antoninus' reasons for curtailing the benefits of Vespasian's edict. The imperial policy, in my opinion, was motivated by the recognition of the usefulness of medicine to the state, a topic widely discussed at that time (Quintilian, *Inst. Orat.,* VII, 1, 38; 4, 39; also Ps. Quintilian, *Declamationes,* 268). Herzog ascribes Vespasian's action to the recognition of medical philanthropy (*op. cit.,* p. 985), and restores the text accordingly (v. 6). Yet he himself concludes from the passages in Quintilian and from other statements that Vespasian invested physicians with the right to form corporations on account of "the usefulness of medicine" (p. 982 f.). It was not until Byzantine times that the privileges granted were made dependent on sufficient technical knowledge and on the morally unobjectionable character of the recipient (Below, *op. cit.,* p. 41).

47. Throughout antiquity, medicine remained free from supervision by civil authorities. Even Roman law dealt only with cases of death attributed to the physician's treatment.

13

Jeffrey L. Berlant
From "Medical Ethics and Monopolization"

Percivalean Ethics and Monopolization

Thomas Percival (1740–1804) is best remembered as the foremost spokesman for the conservative wing of the medical Enlightenment in England by virtue of his *Medical Ethics,* written in 1794 and published in 1803. Born in England, he entered the great medical school at Edinburgh and received his M.D. from Leyden in 1765. That year, he was also made a Fellow of the Royal Society and settled in Manchester to practice. Well known for his social and philosophical work, he corresponded regularly with Franklin, Voltaire, Diderot and D'Alembert. In 1791, he was asked by the medical staff of the Manchester Infirmary "to draw up a scheme of professional conduct relative to hospitals and other medical charities,"[1] following a dispute among house staff in 1789 that had led to resignations. Percival had close friends on both sides in the dispute, and his work apparently had some conciliatory effect. The code itself consisted of four sections: "Of Professional Conduct, Relative to Hospitals, or Other Medical Charities," "Of Professional Conduct in Private or General Practice," "Of the Conduct of Physicians Towards Apothecaries," and "Of Professional Duties, in Certain Cases which Require a Knowledge of Law." I will deal only with the section on private or general practice, for it was on the basis of this section that half a century later the newly founded American Medical Association constructed its own "Code of Medical Ethics" and claimed continuity with Percival's famous work.

Percival's section on general practice contains advice in six areas: trust building, consultations among physicians, taking over another physician's patient, economic policy, promoting the honor and interests of the profession, retrospection, and miscellany. His advice in each area will first be reviewed and then its role in the profession's institutionalization examined, particularly its role in monopolization.

The bulk of Percival's trust-building prescriptions are general moral rules of conduct: attention, steadiness, humanity, secrecy, delicacy, and confidence. Others pertain to the physician's quality of mind: temperance for the sake of clear thought, and retirement when senility sets in. Others have to do more specifically with handling the patient: reasonable numbers of visits to the sick, not abandoning doomed patients, admonitions to patients suffering from the wages of sin, observance of the Sabbath for both themselves and the patient except in emergencies, and abstention from gloomy prognostications to maintain hope and comfort in the sick except when the patient must make his own death arrangements.[2]

Such trust-inducing devices bear specific relationships to monopolization. In a general way, trust inducement increases the market value of medical services and helps convert them into commodities. Similarly, it flatters doctors and helps integrate them into a professional group, thereby furthering group formation. It also creates a paternalistic relationship toward the patient, which may undermine consumer organization for mutual self-protection, thereby maintaining consumer atomization. Essentially, it persuades the patient that he need not protect his own interests, either by himself or by organized action. Through atomization of the public into vulnerable patients, paternalism results in the profession's dealing with fragmented individuals instead of bargaining groups. Moreover, by appealing to patient salvation fantasies, trust inducement can stimulate interpatient competition by increasing each patient's desire to see that nothing stand between the doctor and himself. Much of the emotional power of the sentiment of the "doctor-patient relationship" resides in this wish of the patient to save himself at any cost to himself or others. When sick or dying, the patient is most likely to see any obstacle between himself and the doctor as a personal threat. Consequently, the patient becomes willing to accept the profession's desire not to deal with outside parties for the sake of privileged access to services—just in case. Yet another monopolistic consequence is the use of trust inducement to legitimize licensing privileges. Since legislators and other political figures cannot usually judge the quality of medical services, trust inducement plays a major role in political persuasion for obtaining legal privileges.

Consultations among physicians occupy a large part of Percival's work. The basic rule of conduct covering them is worth quoting in its entirety:

Consultations should be promoted in difficult or protracted cases, as they give rise to confidence, energy and more enlarged views in practice. On such occasions no rivalship or jealousy should be indulged. Candour, probity and all due respect should be exercised towards the physician or surgeon first engaged. And as he may be presumed to be best acquainted with the patient and with his family, he should deliver all the medical directions agreed upon, though he may not have precedency in seniority or rank.[3]

In other words the consulting physician should conduct the consultation in the presence of the doctor who called him into the case. Both physicians should try to arrive together, examine together "that the unnecessary repetition of questions may be avoided," and discuss the case together with the patient or his friends only after having agreed on what the patient should be told and what the prognosis should be. Protracted consultations with a doctor "objectionable to the patient" should be limited to two or three visits, and the consulted physician should be given "a double gratuity" for an "extraordinary portion of both time and attention," presumably to compensate him for having to deal with an unpleasant and unappreciative patient. Consultations should be preferred with physicians with "a regular academic education," but can be had with an uneducated "intelligent practitioner" for "the good of the Patient."[4]

These rules for consultations bear one major and one minor relationship to monopolization. Their manifest purpose, of course, is to prevent disputes so that doctors will share information and skill. The rule which maintains the attending physician's control, however, and the admonition against rivalry appear to be anticompetitive devices. Though encouraging consultation might be interpreted as encouraging group solidarity, it is probably equally important as a group integrative device for encouraging membership loyalty. Consultations distribute income among group members as well as information and skill, and such distribution can be important in times of oversupply of practitioners. And since consultations add another fee to a patient's case, they may bring a greater total income into the profession. So, anticompetition is the major purpose of these rules, and

group integration a minor one. The rule permitting consultations with uneducated practitioners is interesting in historical retrospect and does not seem to contribute to the group's monopolization or institutionalization. It is interesting because of a later movement in the United States to prevent exactly such consultations, a clearer example of monopolistic restrictionism. In this area, at least, Percival's ethics are not as monopolistic as they might have been. The rules discouraging competition, however, are still applicable in any oversupply situation, whether prior to the creation of modern restrictive systems of medical education or currently in certain overstaffed urban areas.

Percival also pays considerable attention to the problem of taking over another physician's patient. A physician called in by a patient on a case not helped by another physician should first consult with the previous physician, ostensibly to better understand the case. If the patient has already contacted the physician, perhaps during a visit with another patient of the physician, the previous physician's general plan of treatment should be followed, unless conditions warrant otherwise, in which case the previous physician should be consulted. An anxious patient who cannot wait for a consultation should be similarly handled. A physician should intervene on his own judgment only if consultation is precluded by "the lateness of the hour" or the urgency of the situation. No consultation is called for when taking over for a sick or absent physician. A physician who is questioned by a patient about treatment by another physician need not consult with the other physician but "should not interfere in the curative plans pursued; and should even recommend a steady adherence to them, if they appear to merit approbation."[5] In short, in such cases, a physician should continue the initiated therapy and, when possible, praise it if he can.

Essentially, these rules discourage criticism and thereby contribute to monopolization. They are in this respect more important for the institutionalization of the profession than are rules of consultation. Like rules of consultation, they discourage competition for patients by preventing patients

from comparing the advice of physicians and "shopping around." The noncompetitive, cooperative implications of consultations apply here as well. Self-silencing of criticism prevents the breakdown of patient and public trust in the profession and so plays an additional role in monopolization: inhibiting external controls on the profession. A breakdown of trust can lead to consumer protective organizations, as has been suggested; open criticism can undermine professional claims of keeping its own house clean and invite governmental controls. Insofar as monopolization includes policy-making authority, external controls narrow the range of legitimate professional policy making and thwart monopolization. That controls in one area of professional policy making, such as quality or costs, would lead to controls in others is probably not inevitable, yet one gets the impression that professional leaders see monopolistic powers as interdependently woven upon the same assumption: loss of one privilege might undermine all. So, these rules reduce both internal competition and external controls, protecting the group from dissolution into individualized practitioners.

Percival also offers rules for economic conduct, all of which are variants of the principle of the sliding scale (different fees for patients who meet certain criteria). The basic rule was set in honorific terms:

Some general rule should be adopted by the faculty in every town relative to the pecuniary acknowledgements of their patients, and it should be deemed a point of honour to adhere to this rule with as much steadiness as varying circumstances will admit. For it is obvious that an average fee, as suited to the general rank of patients, must be an inadequate gratuity from the rich, who often require attendance not absolutely necessary, and yet too large to be expected from that class of citizens who would feel a reluctance, in calling for assistance, without making some decent and satisfactory retribution.[6]

Payment, furthermore, should be based on the economic standing of the patient and not of the physician. Percival specifically warns of the danger in not always charging "the affluent, because it is an injury to his professional brethren. The office of physician can never be supported but as a lucrative one; and it is defrauding, in some degree, the common funds for its support, when fees are dispensed with, which might justly be claimed."[7] Consultations by letter should be charged doubly, because it "imposes much more trouble and attention than a personal visit." While the poor should pay less, some patients should pay nothing. Patients otherwise under the care of a sick or absent physician, mendicant clergymen, military and naval subaltern officers, and "persons who hold situations of honour and trust in the army, the navy, or the civil departments of government" who require sickness certificates all should be treated gratis as "acts due to the public and therefore not to be compensated by any gratuity."[8] Physicians, surgeons, and their immediate families are also to receive free care.[9]

While a sliding scale does not seem to be as monopolistic as uniform fees, there is little question that it is economically rational, at least when there is a shortage of patients. To accept whatever patients can afford is more profitable than to turn away those who cannot afford a fixed fee. At the same time, Percival opposed competing for patients when he opposed undercharging the affluent. He is at first confusing when he claims that wealthy physicians should maintain full fees in behalf of the profession's collective solvency, since the members of the profession do not share income. He implies, however, that a physician may collect all he can from a patient but should not collect less, for price competition might develop. The temptation is particularly great for wealthier physicians who can afford to charge less, perhaps for the sake of prestige, and divert solvent patients from poorer physicians. In this sense, Percival is correct that maintaining full fees helps the profession's collective solvency, but only because wealthier physicians forego a competitive advantage. It also furthers professional solidarity by encouraging physicians to think of their mutual interests.

The monopolistic effects of the provision of free care to certain groups may not be as clear as for other rules, yet they are present. It could be interpreted as the creation of political allies by morally indebting strategically placed officials and influential persons. Unfortunately, if these people were not

in positions where they could help the profession politically, winning a sense of obligation might have been useless. Nonetheless, discounting the cost of care for those with whom solidarity might be useful potentially contributes to monopolization. While a physician's emotional ties might indeed harm his technical judgment when treating his family, free care by an unrelated physician also builds professional solidarity by making treatment a less economic and more personal relationship. It helps the physician feel he is a special person, set off from the rest of society, tied through bonds of generosity and love to other members of the profession. Consequently, this quasi-fraternal device makes the physician more emotionally committed to protecting and furthering the interests of the profession and in general more disposed to accepting the cooperative attitudes which help form the profession into a unitary supply source. Similarly in this spirit of cooperation, doctors are expected to help one another out for a short time by taking over gratis the care of a patient when necessary. These devices are conducive to professional solidarity and help reduce nonmonopolistic competition. More important, however, by accepting responsibility for even the poor, Percival declares a monopoly for physicians over the care of all patients. This claim for authority over the medical market, as I shall later show, is not as economically rational or as effective a method of actual domination of the market as is the setting of fixed fees. But as part of the emergent ideology of the modern medical profession, it seems consistent with attempts to eliminate external competitors.

In other passages, Percival calls on physicians to defend the honor of the profession by withholding criticism:

The *Esprit de Corps* is a principle of action founded in human nature, and when duly regulated, is both rational and laudable. Every man who enters into a fraternity engages, by a tacit compact, not only to submit to the laws, but to promote the honour and interest of the association, so far as they are consistent with morality, and the general good of mankind. A physician, therefore, should cautiously guard against whatever may injure the general respectability of his profession; and should avoid all contumelious representations of the faculty at large; all

general charges against their selfishness or improbity; and the indulgence of an affected or jocular skepticism, concerning the efficacy and utility of the healing art.[10]

Physicians should refrain from criticizing individual practitioners as well as the profession as a whole. A physician should not publicly criticize another for incompetence uncovered during a consultation or during treatment of another's patients taken over for a while, or for incompetence discovered in any other way. Other means for influencing the course of treatment should be employed privately. He should also not make public the existence of controversies over the proper course of treatment; he should submit such controversies in private to an arbitration board of professionals, who may then make a public stand.[11]

Percival's comments on criticism fall into two broad categories: criticism of the profession as a whole and criticism of individual practitioners. As will be seen, they overlap in certain respects. Criticism of the profession as a whole is antimonopolistic in the sense that it opposes trust-inducement devices. This association to trust is contained in the functionalist argument as well, that is, that physicians should do nothing to make patients mistrust their physician, for care will be more difficult to perform. The monopolistic consequences of trust inducement, to repeat, are commodity creation, integration of physicians, consumer atomization, and inducement of legal privileges. And to the extent that criticism undermines trust, it also undermines these monopolistic consequences.

Criticism of individual practitioners undermines monopolization through three mechanisms. It can be a competitive device for winning over patients from other physicians, i.e., a market substitute for lower fees. Criticism can invite outsiders to apply self-protective controls on professional activities by implying that the profession cannot regulate itself or "keep its own house clean." Criticism of individual practitioners can also contribute to criticism of the profession as a whole, since failure to self-regulate implies misplacement of public trust in the profession. All criticism is antimonopolistic in another sense: it tends to counter the fraternalization of practitioners, even when made in private. It is a latent source of conflict which can divide the profession and lead to group dissolution. For criticism not to have such effects, it must be set off from normal interaction and defined as impersonal. Percival, however, does not touch on this problem of private criticism. On the basis of this analysis of Percival's work, I can say in summary that criticism in public is antimonopolistic, because it destroys trust, invites counter-monopolistic actions by outsiders, and can act as a competitive device.

Percival includes a section on the moral importance of looking back at cases to learn from them:

At the close of every interesting and important case, especially when it had terminated fatally, a physician should trace back, in calm reflection, all the steps which he had taken in the treatment of it. This review of the origin, progress, and conclusion of the malady; of the whole curative plan pursued; and of the particular operation of the several remedies employed, as well as of the doses and periods of time in which they were administered, will furnish the most authentic documents on which individual experience can be formed. But it is in a moral view that the practice is here recommended; and it should be performed with the most scrupulous impartiality. Let no self-deception be permitted in the retrospect; and if errors, either of omission or commission, are discovered, it behooves that they should be brought fairly and fully to the mental view. Regrets may follow, but criminality will thus be obviated. For good intentions, and the imperfections of human skill which cannot anticipate the knowledge that events alone disclose, will sufficiently justify what is past, provided the failure be made conscientiously subservient to future wisdom and rectitude in professional conduct.[12]

The retrospection clause is interesting from a monopolization perspective because of its expectations about the behavior of others. To the extent that it is interpretable as an injunction against criticism of individual practitioners, the clause shares the monopolistic consequences of all such injunctions. Since the retrospection clause excuses poor practice if the physician learns from his mistakes, however, it tends to favor leniency and carelessness. The relationship of this clause to trust-inducement, then, is ambiguous. It might undermine public trust by announcing that physicians make mistakes—recognizing human fallibility only reduces moral re-

sponsibility; it does not reassure the patient that errors will not occur—and by not calling for penalties for errors. [Sic.] So it might seem antimonopolistic. But allowing in a semipublic document such as a code of ethics that physicians err is more than compensated for by concealing errors in everyday practice. And leaving accountability for mistakes to individual conscience rather than collective professional action—a notable omission in Percival—amounts to a suppression of both public and private internal criticism.

The 1847 "Code of Ethics" of the American Medical Association states well the implications of Percival's individualistic statement about retrospection. Care for the sick, it held, constitutes an obligation "the more deep and enduring, because there is no tribunal, other than his own conscience to adjudge penalties for carelessness or neglect."[13] One would thus expect official actions against incompetence to be low in the profession. Some evidence bears this out. In America, incompetence has rarely been grounds for license revocation. In New York State, for instance, 230 complaints of unprofessional conduct and malpractice registered with the State Licensing Board between 1926 and 1939 resulted in only one disciplinary action and no suspension or revocation of license. In 1961, only five states disciplined physicians in any way for professional incompetence.[14]

A study of 938 "disciplinary actions" by state licensing boards between 1963 and 1967 suggested little change. Only seven actions were due to "gross malpractice" (0.7 percent); the type of action (revocation or reprimand) was not specified. These figures may not be complete, no uniform centralized statistical compilation exists, and the author of these recent studies had to compile his figures from the files of the Federation of State Medical Boards of the United States. His 1965 study found that only seven states had laws against both mental and physical incompetence; eighteen had provisions for physical or professional incompetence (defined as the inability to perform medicine), and twenty-seven covered mental incompetence specifically. Twelve states had no specific legal provisions for medical incompetence in any form. Indeed, "The constitutions and bylaws of 38 state medical

societies did not specify incompetence as a cause for action against their members. In the states which did have such provisions, members could be expelled for incompetence. But only seven societies had ever disciplined physicians because of incompetence."[15] These observations are consistent with a Percivalean reluctance to have professionals declared incompetent by the profession. Ethics could have exerted force as determinants of the profession's social organization, and so their latent monopolistic implications may well have had practical consequences.

Percival had some miscellaneous passages which bear varying degrees of relevance for monopolization. They are mentioned here only for the sake of thoroughness. Physicians called in to treat another physician's family should offer sincere advice but leave the final decision to the summoning physician regardless of rank, seniority, or other considerations. His rationale is that "the mind of a husband, a father, or a friend may receive a deep and lasting wound, if the disease terminated fatally, from the adoption of means he could not approve, or the rejection of those he wished to be tried."[16] The consequences for monopolization in this passage are minimal. Quack medicines are not to be used even if the patient wishes them; they would, one might think, be the methods of those outside the interest group and might be interpretable as an endorsement. Another passage calls for the rigid separation of "the provinces of physic and surgery" on the grounds that each has its special area of expertise. Though this sounds paternalistic through assuring competence, it is more precisely an acknowledgment of the status pretensions of the Royal College of Physicians of London, which had asserted its superiority over the surgeons for centuries.[17]. . .

One of the most conspicuous themes in Percival's medical ethics is his opposition to any form of competition. He opposes price competition and any claims which might distinguish one physician from another, i.e., quality competition. This is in marked contrast to the deep interest in competitive devices of one of Percival's contemporaries, the liberal Adam Smith. Since

Smith's *Wealth of Nations* was published in 1776, one would expect that an educated man such as Percival was familiar with the arguments of Smith. Even though Percival never mentions Smith, he appears to have responded to liberalism in his code of ethics. Unlike Smith, Percival also opposes individualizing tendencies in social organization. Seeing dangers such as unchecked exploitation by individual practitioners, Percival favors the idea of a principled honorable fraternity of self-denying practitioners. One of his arguments in behalf of professional silence, in fact, hits at the dangers of individualized medicine; he is troubled by Montaigne's complaint about physicians."That they perpetually direct variations in each other's prescriptions. 'Whoever saw,' says he, 'one physician approve of the prescription of another, without taking something away, or adding something to it? By which they sufficiently betray their act, and make it manifest to us, that they therein more consider their own reputation, and consequently their profit, than their patient's interest.' "[18]

Unlike Smith, Percival seriously questions the advantages of relying on economic motives for social organization. Instead of trying to arrange material rewards to maximize certain types of behavior—as would a modern social engineer—Percival wants physicians to transcend their personal motives. He believes in the possibility of virtuous men as the outcome of honorific appeals, and he wishes to solve the problem of power by having physicians be virtuous men. Toward this end, he apparently wants to create an internally consistent body of moral advice which an ideally moral man could follow. He finds consistency a difficult task, and he is clearly upset by this, for instance, when he discusses the dilemma between lying and gloomy prognosticating in fatal cases.[19]

Percival's social theory is two-pronged. He wants an intermediate social group between state and the individual with which physicians can identify; he wants an ethical code to integrate and guide members in their conduct. The purpose of the intermediate group is to provide a sense of status honor to buttress the ethical code, but the preservation and protection of the group is also one purpose of the code.

While one can easily see how the code can serve the group's interests, one has more difficulty with the role of the group in maintaining the code. When Percival declines to call for group sanctions, one wonders how he expects to have virtuous men follow the code without coercion or group controls on behavior. Apparently, he believes that virtuous men of spontaneous good conscience can exist without group regulation and without sanctions. This stand is consistent with his rejection of economic motivation for professional action. Percival evidently believes in the fundamental goodness of human nature and on this basis rejects the need for sanctions. To assert the need for professional criticism and regulation would impugn the good character of physicians. The ethics in this light are presented as a set of wise ideals which require no punishment for violations. All the group can do is provide a body of men with whom one would be proud to associate. Percival evidently believed in the power of revealed reason: physicians have a single most rational way to behave and, once shown the way, will follow. Percival's role is to be the voice of Reason.

As a social philosopher, Percival stands as a naively saintly man: he disdains conflict, bourgeois competitiveness, and group coercion; he envisions conscientious men, professional identification with a higher cause, and the superiority of ethical wisdom over social controls. Percival embraces the idea of a strong profession composed of strong members committed to the goodness of their cause; how this might be accomplished did not, as with many Enlightenment thinkers, seem problematic to him. Presumably the rationality of men once shown the way would be sufficient. . . .

The closest tradition to Percival's ethics was no doubt the statutes of the Royal College of Physicians of London (RCP). Indeed, documents with statutes listed as "penal" in 1543 and "ethical" in 1563 include many ideas later found in Percival's work. A consulting physician may not ethically dismiss the attending physician or change treatment without agreement; only the patient had the right to dismiss his attending physician. Physicians are expected to conduct consultations in private, outside the presence of the patient, and

are not to criticize one another in public. A 1601 statute prohibits the use of a remedy or treatment kept secret from the College's officers.

Other "ethical" statutes differ from Percival's ethics: consultation with unlicensed persons carries a fine, bargaining for fees except when previously underpaid is prohibited. Information and even the names of medicines are not to be given to the public, ostensibly to prevent misuse. Curiously, violation of these rules resulted only in fines, as determined by a scale. Expulsion from the College could occur only if the offender protested or resisted punishment; this act constituted a breach of oath.[20]

Most RCP statutes were set forth under the leadership of a Dr. Caius, who introduced a large body of ceremonial ornamentations to the College's affairs. These ceremonial additions in language, dress, organizational structure and meetings are suggestive of European secret societies.[21] The ethics of the period would seem consistent with this development, particularly those denying information about medicines, treatment, and the practice of medicine in general, and even about disputes over a specific patient's care. The reluctance to expel members and their easy reentry into the College is also consistent with a body more concerned with preserving its secret knowledge than with eliminating incompetents. The possession of collective secret knowledge is of course consistent with monopolistic action insofar as the knowledge is sought by buyers, that is, as scarcity creation. In this respect, the College differed from secret societies in that secret societies had little or nothing to sell.

When the Enlightenment began in England, the question of the rationality of the corporation system, typified by the RCP, arose. One major system of medical ethics, John Gregory's, specifically attacked the monopolistic medical corporations. John Gregory was a professor at the great medical school at Edinburgh, and presumably his independent position there influenced his conclusions about the problem with organized practitioners. His ethics found considerable following. They were written in 1770, circulated widely, found popularity on the Continent during the early nineteenth century, and were promoted in post-revolutionary America by Benjamin Rush.[22]

Gregory's writings on the obligations of the physician to the patient are similar to those Percival later wrote and will not be reviewed here. Unlike Percival, he suggests few regulations for intraprofessional relations, the so-called "medical etiquette," except for consultations even with nonregular physicians and no "arrangements with apothecaries," such as kickbacks and fee splitting.

Gregory's ethical code, however, stands in opposition to the monopolistic codes of the RCP and of the later Percivalean work. Percival saw the forces binding the profession into a group—esprit de corps, a common academic training, and support of each other's reputations—as the source of the best in medicine, as something to be encouraged. Without this group basis, medicine would lose its professionality and hence its excellence. Gregory challenged this central presumption and thereby also the medical profession's elitist autonomy as an independent institutional body. The domination of medical thought by men of the practicing profession, he explained, distorted the pursuit of medical knowledge and blocked the development and delivery of medical care. The profession offered a set of personal ends to physicians other than the furthering of knowledge:

Much wit has indeed, in all ages, been exerted upon our profession; but after all, we shall find that this ridicule has rather been employed against physicians than physick. There are some reasons for this sufficiently obvious. Physicians, considered as a body of men, who live by medicine as a profession, have an interest separate and distinct from the honour of the science. In pursuit of this interest, some have acted with candour, with honour, with the ingenuous and liberal manners of gentlemen. Conscious of their own worth, they disdained every artifice, and depended for success on their real merit. But such men are not the most numerous in any profession. Some impelled by necessity, some stimulated by vanity, and others anxious to conceal ignorance, have had recourse to various means and unworthy arts to raise their importance among the ignorant, who are always the most numerous of mankind. Some of these arts have been an affectation of mystery in all their writings and conversations relating to their profession; an affectation of knowledge, inscrutable to all, except the adepts in the science; an air of perfect confidence in their own skill and abilities; and a demeanor solemn, contemptuous, and highly expressive of self-sufficiency. These arts, however well they might succeed with the rest of mankind, could not escape the censure of the more judicious, nor elude the ridicule of men of wit and humor. The stage, in particular, has used freedom with the professors of the salutary art; but as is evident, that most of the satire is levelled against the particular notions, or manners of individuals, and not against the science itself.[23]

He criticizes two characteristics of the profession: formalism and restriction of knowledge. The formalities which the profession institutes to appear dignified can interfere with the primary purposes of the profession as a liberal discipline devoted to medical science and the care of humanity. Considerations such as the university where a physician obtains his degree or even the possession of a medical degree are to be overridden by the plight of the patient:

It is a physician's duty to do everything in his power that is not criminal, to save the life of his patient, and to search for remedies from every source and from every hand, however mean and contemptible. This, it may be said, is sacrificing the dignity and interests of the faculty. But I am not here speaking of the private police of a corporation, or the little arts of a craft. I am treating of the duties of a liberal profession, whose object is the life and health of the human species, a profession to be exercised by gentle men of honour and ingenuous manners; the dignity of which can never be supported by means that are inconsistent with its ultimate objects, and that only tend to increase the pride and fill the pockets of a few individuals.[24]

The attempts by physicians, surgeons, and apothecaries to separate each other's domains, while reasonable to the extent that men should preferably do what they can do best, should be complied with only if the patient's welfare is not sacrificed. In fact, separation into the three domains is prudent and imprudent for the same reason: meritorious skill and liberal knowledge best serve the patient. When the formality of separation comes before the judicious application of skill and knowledge, the patient is wronged:

As a doctor's degree can never confer sense, the title alone can never command regard; neither should the want of it deprive any man of the esteem and deference due to real merit. If a surgeon or apothecary has had the education, and acquired the knowledge of a physician, he is a physician to be respected and treated accordingly. There are certain limits, however, between the two professions, which ought to be attended to; as they are established by the customs of the country, and by the rules of their several societies. But a physician, of a candid and liberal spirit, will never take advantage of what a nominal distinction, and certain privileges, give him over men, who, in point of real merit, are his equals; and will feel no superiority, but what arises from superior learning, superior abilities, and more liberal manners. He will despise those distinctions founded in vanity, self-interest, or caprice; and will be careful, that the interests of science and mankind shall never be hurt by a punctilious adherence to formalities.[25]

Gregory's second criticism struck more directly at the type of professional organization Percival and other conservatives advocated: an autonomous, self-regulating body of elitist experts who made a living by treating patients and who sought to maximize the distance between medical man and patient, using secrecy and systematic ignorance to accentuate the disadvantageous position of the patient. Gregory believed, however, that confining practice "entirely to a class of men who live by it as a profession, is unfavorable to the progress of the art."[26] The love of and devotion to medicine as an art, differentially distributed among physicians, "is often checked by a necessary attention to private interest." In most arts compromise by private interest is acceptable because "all mankind are judges." But in the case of medicine and of medicine alone, the public is in no position to judge the merit of a practitioner; medical practice is too private and medical science kept too secret.[27] A physician with an acquaintance with "the outlines of practice," good presence, and good sense can persuade the public of his merit and become successful, for the public assumes that a physician clever in nonmedical matters will also be good in medicine. Gregory was taken aback, however, by the success of some incompetents who had little to recommend them even outside of medicine. The public could not seem to judge good physicians even by analogy. Like the conservative, then, Gregory concluded that the public could not judge accurately the technical merit of a physician.

Gregory posed for himself this problem: granted, the public cannot evaluate physicians accurately and so cannot direct itself to the best doctors; only the physician's own profession can judge his merit and direct patients to men of superior merit; *but* the collective interests of the practicing profession require that superior merit be concealed so that competition not occur.[28] Therefore, the private interests of the profession led to the concealment of information which might benefit the medical interests of patients.

Gregory also saw other disadvantages to leaving medical knowledge solely in the hands of practitioners. Thorough, careful research can best be done by a man whose practice does not take up his time or distract his attention. Freedom to question existing practices and knowledge is also more available to the gentleman who is not bound to adhere to a systematic body of professionally acceptable procedures and treatments. In fact, the quack has a scientific advantage over the legal practitioner in that he can depart with impunity from conventional methods to experiment with something new, whether a drug or a procedure. The quack does not often contribute to science, however, because his ignorance prevents him from carrying out useful experiments or recognizing important results when they occur.[29]

Gregory's solution was to encourage medical learning outside of the confines of the practicing profession. He thus advocated review of merit by men of liberal education (i.e., gentlemanly education) versed in medicine, who did not practice medicine for a living; they would be least likely to let personal economic interest interfere with a just judgment. Such gentlemen, moreover, would not be hurried by the pressures of their business to provide only a cursory examination and would "possess that tranquility of mind which is so requisite in every kind of investigation."[30] Gregory's comments were directed toward "gentlemen" who were by definition literate and liberally educated; yet they might as well have been applied to anyone with education. Gregory's position was that, for the layman, any knowledge of medicine is better than none. The task, then, was to educate nonpractitioners in medicine, a task he found plausible.

"Surely it is not a matter of such difficulty, for a gentleman of a liberal education, to learn so much of medicine as may enable him to understand the best books on the subject, and to judge of merit of those physicians to whom he commits the charge of his own health, and the health of those more immediately under his care and protection."[31] His criticism of the practicing profession, then, became an analysis of the causes of public inability to evaluate practitioners. As a consistent rationalist, he believed that if the public or even some among the public were sufficiently well educated, competent practitioners would not be placed at a disadvantage.

Knowledge of medicine could be put to many other uses. In an emergency when a physician cannot be reached, the knowledge could be helpful. Quacks would not flourish as widely or cause as much harm if they, as well as the public, were more knowledgable and less receptive to quasi-magical remedies. Finally, those who cannot afford medical care would suffer less harm by drawing more on science and less on the folklore of nature cures. "Patients are so far from being left to nature, when no physician is called, that they are commonly oppressed with a succession of infallible cures recommended by quacks or their weak and officious friends."[32] It would, in turn, effect a good influence on the medical profession to have a well educated public, for physicians would then be conduced to improve their technical skill rather than develop sales techniques for "the most ignorant, and consequently the most conceited part of mankind," the public with its prejudices and caprices born of ignorance.[33]

The division between Percival's conservative and Gregory's liberal versions of Enlightenment medicine is best captured in Gregory's concluding comments. For Percival, the Enlightenment and rationality were available only to elites paternalistically bound to assuming the burden of protecting the public. For him, the only conceivable authority in medical matters was the practicing medical profession as represented by the licensing bodies of the Royal Colleges. In his perspective, if physicians would only rise above the temptations

of personal interest, society would be well served. Gregory rejected much of this formulation, claiming that the public was capable of assuming more responsibility for its own medical welfare than Percival would allow, and that the medical practitioner compromised some of the goals of the profession. Put another way, Percival tended to identify the practitioner with the profession, while Gregory restricted practitioners to one limited sphere within the profession. Practitioners permit much harm by letting private interests intrude in the form of increasing the value of medical services through systematically ensuring that the public remain medically ignorant. By restricting knowledge to practitioners they could hinder scientific research, thereby subverting the fundamental commitment of the medical profession to the growth of medical knowledge.

For Percival, the strength of the profession lay in the corporate body of practicing professionals whose group identity encouraged the development of a personal ethical commitment to mankind. For Gregory, the strength of the profession lay in the individual mind's capacity to uncover medical knowledge and use it, despite the constraints of professional rituals and formalities, authoritarian orthodoxy, and economic inducements to play to the public's medically irrational and irrelevant demands. Above all, economic advantage from medical knowledge was not to be sought at the expense of humanity; professional organization that monopolized and exploited medical knowledge for economic ends was deplorable, not because it traded medical help for money, but because it impeded the spread and development of medical science.

Gregory was much troubled by the problem of creating an elite for the promotion of medical science in the presence of a dominant elite devoted to preserving its favorable position on the basis of demand for its services. The first elite is generated, in principle, by the ability of individuals to be selected on the basis of their meritorious development and dissemination of information. The second is created by the exclusion of practicing competitors by a professional group's monopolization and concealment of expert information, in the manner of a secret society. Gregory also recognized that these elites were not totally compatible: a well-educated public encourages the development of an elite of technically excellent practitioners, if the public is free to select its practitioners; but for this incompatibility to be minimized, information must be allowed and encouraged to spread to all sectors of society. The prime responsibility of the profession, then, is to produce and disseminate medical knowledge:

I hope I have advanced no opinions in these lectures that tend to lessen the dignity of a profession which has always been considered as most honourable and important. But, I apprehend, this dignity is not to be supported by a narrow, selfish, corporation-spirit; by self-importance; a formality in dress and manners, or by an affectation of mystery. The true dignity of physic is to be maintained by the superior learning and abilities of those who profess it, by the liberal manners of gentlemen, and by that openness and candour, which disdain all artifice, which invite to a free inquiry, and thus boldly bid defiance to all that illiberal ridicule and abuse to which medicine has been so much and so long exposed.[34]

Unlike Percivalean ethics, Gregory's ethics were antimonopolistic in the extreme, and they disapproved of arrangements which emphasized the profession's collective interests. According to him, the satisfaction of the personal interests of physicians should be turned to the advantage of the patient by spreading knowledge so that competitive meritorious service can be recognized and rewarded. Organizational devices that satisfy the personal interests of physicians without promoting superior care, using appeals to the honor of the profession and other mutually protective devices, should have no place in ethical medicine. . . .

The conservative Percival wrote his ethics at a time when the elitist medical corporations had come under democratic attack, particularly by economic liberals. As an apology for the corporations, Percival's work was superb; as a means for integrating the profession, it was unsurpassed. As an instrument for solidarity, it was particularly suitable for extending the monopolistic controls of the RCP to the newly professionalized surgeons and apothecaries. Therefore, on the basis of this comparative study, one can say that Percivalean ethics were probably an organizational tool for bolstering the system of licensing corporations through the encouragement of monopolistic traditions for

all professionals, an important device for suppressing competition between different types of professionals which might have been exacerbated by the appearance of increasing numbers of professional corporations.

The Vicissitudes of the AMA's Medical Ethics

Percival's ethics spread beyond Great Britain, particularly into the English-speaking countries. When the American Medical Association (AMA) was founded in Philadelphia in 1846, for example, it adopted a code of ethics supposedly based on Percival's medical ethics. Though the AMA's 1847 "Code of Ethics" was allegedly only a cleaning up of linguistic oddities, it substantially changed the meaning of a number of Percival's suggestions. The codes changed several times again, in 1903, 1912, 1949, and 1957. . . .

The most distinctive change in American medical ethics was the adoption of fee fixing instead of the sliding scale. While the 1847 "Code" retained the rule that wealthy physicians should charge for services, it omitted the sliding scale altogether. Percival, it may be recalled, had called for each physician to know the means of his patients: "Some general rule should be adopted by the faculty in every town relative to the pecuniary acknowledgements of their patients," but this general rule should be varied according to circumstances.[35] The AMA simply called for "some general rules" to be established in every town or district, relative to pecuniary acknowledgements from their patients, which should be adhered to as "uniformly" as possible.[36] The sliding scale was replaced by what today would be called the "usual, customary, prevailing rate": a uniform charge for everyone in a local area delimited by the local medical society. The 1903 "Principles" went a step further and suggested that "some general rules" be adopted "relative to the minimum pecuniary acknowledgement from their patients." The new code thus permitted a physician to price his services above the going rate, letting him risk pricing himself out of the medical market. The advantage of this permissive upper limit was that a physician could raise his fees for his established following, i.e., his "practice,"

and increase his income, even though he might not engage in competitive undercutting. In this way, ethical conduct could help maximize both the profession's collective interests and the individual practitioner's personal interests. The profession could price services above competitive market value; the practitioner could try for an income as high as he might command.

The principles of uniform fee setting (fee fixing) and a sliding scale (fee discrimination) are two types of economic conduct which can be found mixed in any concrete situation. Fee discrimination maximizes income per patient; fee fixing maximizes income per unit service, that is, within the total market. Their relative economic rationality varies according to the state of the market: a sliding scale is most rational in an oversupply market, where maximizing the number of patients is a problem; uniform fees are most rational in an undersupply market, where patients are plentiful, and selecting more affluent patients is a challenge. Their consequences for the distribution of care differ: a sliding scale tries to provide care for all patients; uniform fees tend to create two classes of patients—paying and charity patients. In either system, however, they may prevent some ill people from becoming patients. A sliding scale may lead to making care inaccessible to some, using various noneconomic mechanisms; uniform fees may also make care inaccessible by denying it to those who do not pay. Both also require a certain amount of noncompetition; they both assume that physicians will not undercut each other by embracing price competition. In short, price competition tends to minimize what patients must pay for services; a sliding scale maximizes what they must pay; and uniform fees select only patients who can pay a set minimum. Thus, both fee discrimination and fee fixing are consistent with monopolization, though in different ways, for they both require group cooperation to prevent price competition from making inroads. Since concrete situations are by and large only imperfectly monopolistic, price competition, price discrimination, and price fixing may all be present in any given instance.

Most remarkably, all recommendations for setting fees were omitted entirely in the 1912 "Principles of

Ethics'' of the AMA. Only a section prohibiting fee splitting and defending the right of physicians to charge for referrals appears:

Sec. 3. It is detrimental to the public good and degrading to the profession, and therefore unprofessional, to give or to receive a commission. It is also unprofessional, to divide a fee for medical advice or surgical treatment, unless the patient or his next friend is fully informed as to the terms of the transaction. The patient should be made to realize that a proper fee should be paid the family physician for the service he renders in determining the surgical and medical treatment suited to the condition and in advising concerning those best qualified to render any special service that may be required by the patient. [37]

Though the disappearance of rules for economic conduct (except for fee splitting) might be interpretable as an example of actual demonopolization, the profession's contemporary political setting suggests why these rules were omitted in 1912. Following the passage of the Sherman Act in 1890, antitrust prosecution of the profession became possible. As early as 1898, price fixing had been found by the courts to violate section one of the Sherman Act, inasmuch as it gave offenders "the power to charge unreasonable prices had they chosen to do so." Not until 1927, however, was price fixing illegal per se. [38] Antitrust legislation probably was not very threatening to the medical profession at first because of the infrequency of prosecution. But during Taft's administration, antitrust suits, instituted by Attorney General Wickersham from 1909 to 1913, rapidly increased in number and peaked in 1913, the year following the revised code of ethics of the AMA. [39] Presumably, an official document of the profession which called for uniform fees was an open invitation for prosecution at a time when the targets of prosecution were uncertain but increasing in number. So, this instance of apparent demonopolization may in fact have had profound and theoretically interesting monopolistic consequences. This theoretical issue will be addressed again later in this chapter.

The 1949 "Code of Ethics" also omitted references to setting fees, but they reappear in the 1957 "Code." By 1957, the physician's fee was supposed to be "commensurate with the services rendered and the patient's ability to pay. [40] This passage apparently tries to combine uniform fees with a sliding scale, without making clear that these are separate and somewhat contradictory philosophical positions. At best this passage represents a return to Percivalean fee discrimination. Why the issue of the patient's ability to pay reentered medical ethics in America at this late date also seems to require an explanation in terms of the profession's political setting, for nothing in the profession's internal organizational needs for structuring economic conduct accounts for the swing away from uniform fees. The question of which political developments were crucial will be addressed later.

The ethics of the AMA departed from Percivalean ethics on a number of other issues as well. Some of these changes were only marginally significant. American medical ethics, for instance, added one qualification after another to the ancient commandment of professional secrecy: the physician was at first required to divulge information when "imperatively required to do so" (1847), then when "imperatively required by the laws of the state" (1903), and then to prevent spread of a communicable disease (1912). Other changes were not as marginal. Percival had handled the question of public awareness of medical controversies by requiring that disputes be submitted to a professional board of arbitrators for a public stand. The 1847 ethics of the AMA demanded that "neither the subject matter of such differences nor the adjudication of the arbitrators should be made public, as publicity in a case of this nature may be personally injurious to the individuals concerned, and can hardly fail to bring discredit on the faculty. [41] This position is even more monopolistic than Percival's, in that it denies the public substantial knowledge of the existence of controversies and so reduces the probability of public criticism and consumer organization.

American medical ethics depart from Percivalean ethics in two other very important areas: permissible consultations and permissible settings for practice.

Percival had said that consultations with intelligent practitioners without academic training were permissible. Presumably such consultations worked both ways: the ethical physician might both send and receive referrals from marginal practitioners. The 1847 "Code of Ethics," however, prohibited consultations with anyone "whose practice is based on an exclusive dogma." [42] This blanket prohibition against all consultations with "irregular" practitioners was modified in 1903 to prohibit only referrals to irregulars. Many physicians had argued that closing off part of the medical market by denying eligibility for care to patients under the care of nonorthodox physicians made little sense. If nonorthodox physicians were going to recruit patients for orthodox physicians, the orthodox physicians could take advantage of this recruitment while simultaneously justifying it as the patient's finally receiving "proper" care. This position stood until 1949, when the "Principles of Ethics" forbade consultations with "cultists": "Such consultation lowers the honor and dignity of the profession in the same degree in which it elevates the honor and dignity of those who are irregular in training and practice." [43] Apparently, by 1949 the AMA had returned to a position similar to that of 1847. The 1957 "Ethics," for reasons to be discussed later, excluded mention of consultations with nonorthodox physicians. So, while Percivalean ethics had concentrated on eliminating internal competition among licensed physicians, American medical ethics also tried to eliminate external competition by controlling practitioner conduct. . . . ethical controls were a relatively ineffective means for doing so.

American medical ethics faced up to a different internal competition problem than did Percival and so added a new ethical concern to those of traditional Percivalean ethics. The 1903 "Principles" was the first to confront the problem: "Poverty, mutual professional obligations, and certain . . . public duties . . . should always be recognized as presenting valid claims for gratuitous services; but neither institutions endowed by the public or the rich, or by societies for mutual benefit, for life insurance, or for analogous purposes, nor any profession or occupation, can be admitted to possess such privilege." [44] This prohibition attacked what later was called "contract practice," in which doctors were salaried to provide unlimited services to all members of a voluntary organization. The conventional objection to contract practice was that doctors were made to carry too many patients for the performance of good medicine and that payments for treatment out of the doctor's own pocket tended to impoverish physicians. By demanding fees for services within these institutional arrangements, medical ethics could prevent such abuses of physicians and possibly of patient interests. The AMA disapproved of agencies offering medical services to patients and tried to establish the principle that only the medical profession may set the value of services. Institutional contract practice threatened the monopolistic interests of the profession in a number of ways: it created competition with independent physicians by offering medical services to patients at a low yearly membership charge; undermined the idea that medical services are discrete commodities that possess exchange value; provided patients with an organizational base for potentially opposing the medical profession; and placed in nonprofessional hands the right to make a number of policies about the number of patients doctors would see, the amount of services to be provided, the doctor's choice of patients, and other conditions of work. Not all contract practice plans contained these features, but as a type, they presented these threats. Later, the 1912 "Principles of Ethics" specifically attacked contract practice under Section 2: "It is unprofessional for a physician to dispose of his services under conditions that make it impossible to render adequate services to his patient or which interfere with reasonable competition among the physicians of a community. To do this is detrimental to the public and to the individual physician, and lowers the dignity of the profession."[45] This passage is interesting, for it ironically opposes one form of internal competition (between employed and independent practitioners) by appealing to the value of competition among independents, so that a patently nonmonopolistic structural feature—competition—acquires monopolistic consequences.

Between 1912 and 1949, the date of the next major ethical revision, the medical profession confronted the growth of a variety of institutions and arrangements that have come to be known as "third parties." Any intervening person or institution between the physician and the patient has usually been called a "third party," but governmental medical plans have usually been carefully separated from so-called "voluntary" medical institutions by the AMA. In the thirty-seven year period, the AMA had to come to terms with a variety of medical institutions that challenged the traditional means of monopolistic control: commercial health insurance plans, specialty clinics such as the Mayo Clinic, prepaid plans such as Kaiser-Permanente, and the Blue Cross and Blue Shield Plans (which were semi-autonomous). Some of these organizations grew with the support of the AMA, some were able to survive by coming to terms with local medical societies, and others had to bring suit against the AMA and its constituent societies.[46] Though the interests of the profession would have favored continued atomization of consumers and equal competition among professionals, these intermediate institutions became established and stimulated the AMA to create criteria to distinguish which third parties would henceforth be unacceptable.

The 1949 "Principles" contains four sections which introduce these criteria. First, institutions "should meet such costs as are covered by the contract under which the service is rendered," i.e., physicians should not have to pay out of their own pockets for services to subscribers.[47] Second, contract practice, defined as "an agreement between a physician or a group of physicians, as principals or agents, and a corporation, organization, political subdivision or individual, whereby partial or full medical services are provided for a group or class of individuals on the basis of a fee schedule, or for a salary or for a fixed rate per capita" was no longer unethical per se if it did not violate the ethical provisions of the "Principles of Medical Ethics" or cause "deterioration of the quality of the medical services rendered."[48] Third, restriction of choice of physician was not unethical per se in the event that a third party "by law or volition . . . assumes legal responsibility and provides for the cost of medical care and indemnity for occupational disability." This section apparently permitted the ethical operation of the health services of the Veterans Administration, a form of restricted choice of physician and the only health service in the United States that could have assumed the broad liabilities demanded by the 1949 "Principles." Fourth, "A physician should not dispose of his professional attainments or services to any hospital, lay body, organization, group or individual, by whatever name called, or however organized, under terms or conditions which permit exploitation of the services of the physician for the financial profit of the agency concerned."[49] But apparently commercial health insurance companies, profit-making organizations, were not considered exploiters of the services of the physician. This clause evidently served as a basis for the AMA to oppose organizational arrangements it did not favor, without making explicit its criteria for exploitation.

The criteria that the AMA enunciated should be restated: remuneration for all physician services and costs, maintenance of the quality of services, maintenance of ethical standards, free choice of physician except in the case of broad custodial institutional care, no "exploitation" of services for the profit of others. Aside from asserting the profession's commitment to quality service, the provisions created conditions for a one-way flow of resources into the profession by covering costs incurred in the course of delivering services and by forbidding "exploitation" by others for profit: if anyone should gain profits from medical services, it should be physicians. The Principles also discouraged competition between private and institution-based physicians by calling for free choice of physicians so that patients would not be drawn to low-cost or free sources of care. "Free choice" in this context meant that all physicians should be able to be reimbursed by third parties, regardless of patient preference.

The 1949 criteria were also no doubt a reaction to the European and British health organization experiences. General practitioners under the National Health Insurance system of 1911 and the National Health Service of 1948 in

Britain had elected to receive capitation fees, which provided a fixed payment by the government for each patient treated during the year and registered on a doctor's "panel." Whatever costs the physician incurred by treating his panel had to be paid out of the capitation money. Also, since the National Health Service provided free medical services for patients who belonged to the NHS, the market for private practice, while not eliminated, was greatly reduced. Doctors did not have to join the NHS; patients did not have to go to NHS doctors. Yet free choice, as defined by the AMA, was not a feature of the NHS, since the program did not pay for services to an NHS patient delivered by nonparticipant physicians. In Britain this distinction presented no problems, since reportedly nearly 100 percent of general practitioners were enrolled in the NHS.[50] The effect on the private medical market, however, was crushing in Britain, and the AMA's ethical opposition to arrangements that might have had similar effects in the United States is very understandable.

The *Journal of the American Medical Association* printed a remarkable speech that suggests the AMA's uneasiness about contemporary events in Britain. This speech, by Clem Whitaker of the public relations firm of Whitaker and Baxter, was the AMA's "Report of the Coordinating Committee," and appeared only three pages before the 1949 "Principles of Ethics." Its relevant part calls on American physicians to oppose developments at home similar to those in Britain for the sake of both patients and the moral fiber of America:

Britain began with compulsory health insurance on a supposedly moderate scale back in 1911. Since then the cancer of socialization has spread to almost every part of the British economy. It has eaten up the Bank of England, the cable and wireless services, civil aviation, the transportation industry, the coal industry, the electric industry and more recently the gas industry, and now it is about to spread to the steel industry.

There were those in Britain, when compulsory health insurance was first proposed, who thought it was a harmless experiment. And some of their cousins live here in America. But today Britain is plunging headlong toward a regimented society that will blot out every vestige of liberty for the British people, unless the tide is turned back.

This truth we know—and this truth we must some way make all America know: when medicine is socialized, the beginning of the end is in sight. It is one of the final, irrevocable steps toward complete state socialism. And at the end of that road is loss of everything that means most to free men.

This, without doubt, is the greatest emergency any of you ever has confronted in all your years of practice. Not just one life hangs in the balance, but the life of a nation is in your hands—a nation that has become the last hope of all the liberty-loving people in the world.

In all reverence, I want to say: Thank God that this House of Delegates and the American Medical Association have accepted the challenge. Thank God for the courage, the sound convictions and tireless energy of American doctors.

This isn't just a heavy obligation that has been laid upon you, and I am sure that you don't look at it that way. This is the greatest opportunity any of us ever will have to serve America, to champion our good way of life and to play a vital part in shaping the destiny of our country. The plague of socialization, with all its demoralizing consequences, has become epidemic throughout most of the world. It has impaired and crippled the productive capacity of great nations and stripped them of their political independence. It has undermined the character, the moral fiber and the individual initiative of untold millions who were once prideful, self-reliant, self-supporting people. It has made them serfs of their own governments, dependent on government for their very existence.[51]

Invoking such important values, Whitaker and Baxter called on the American medical profession to produce a highly mobilized response against a series of governmental plans, starting at that time with Truman's National Health Insurance plan. The preservation of a private medical market was transformed from a parochial medical problem to the level of a great international cause. In comparison, changes in medical ethics, while consistent with this reaction, were a mild response to the problem.

In a number of ways, American medical ethics favored monopolization more than Percivalean ethics did. The expanded concept of medical service which prohibited fee splitting, the call for uniform fees, the increased use of secrecy to maintain public trust, the attack on external competitors, and the attack on internal competition by physicians in organized practices were

all more monopolistic than Percival's simple plea for noncompetition and solidarity. Since the American medical ethics were written by the AMA rather than by any single person, they should be related to the role of the AMA in monopolization. One issue is the degree to which the AMA could claim control over the conduct of individual practitioners. The 1847 "Code" did not specifically require membership in the AMA for ethical standing but suggested a number of criteria for determining the boundaries of the legitimate profession: a regular medical education, nonadherence to an exclusive dogma, a license to practice from some medical board of known and acknowledged respectability recognized by the association, and "good moral and professional standing in the place in which he resides."[52] As such, the Association claimed the right to decide which practitioners were ethical. The 1903 "Principles," however, called on physicians to join "the organized body of the profession as represented in the community in which he resides." All of these county medical societies should affiliate with state medical societies, and those with the American Medical Association.[53] Even though the AMA had changed the title of ethics from a Code to Principles, and called the document only suggestive and advisory, the implication was still present: an ethical physician must belong to the American Medical Association and its constituent bodies. Those who did not belong could not be ethical physicians.

The 1903 "Principles," however, did not do away with all sanctions. There remained, of course, informal prestige sanctions; but even more important, since the advisory status of the ethics applied only to the AMA, state and local medical societies could still apply a variety of penalties for violations of the AMA's ethics. So, in effect, the AMA claimed the right to determine the conduct of physicians through enforced membership and control at a local level. The 1912 "Principles," however, do not mention any ethical responsibility on the part of physicians to join the AMA and local medical societies. This omission may well have been consistent with the political realities of impending antitrust prosecution. If the AMA had achieved virtually 100 percent control of the medical profession, it might have become subject to antitrust prosecution as a corporate organization which had eliminated competitors. By permitting physicians ethical status without joining the AMA, the AMA could avoid prosecution by dissociating the corporate entity of the Association from the body of licensed practitioners and by denying Association control of practitioners. The AMA has in fact taken the tack that physicians are independent men whose activities cannot be dictated by medical societies; medical societies cannot command where to work or what fees to charge. The medical societies can still declare specific activities unethical and refuse or terminate membership in the society, but constraining limits are not authoritative commands issued by the AMA. This absence of demonstrable organizational authority over the behavior of physicians, in the sense of issuing commands, may have helped prevent antitrust prosecution of the AMA and in any event helps explain why the role of the AMA, as spelled out in ethics, changed between 1903 and 1912.

The role of the AMA as an instrument for the cultivation of fellowship, for the exchange of professional experience, for the advancement of medical knowledge, for the maintenance of ethical standards, and for the promotion in general of the interests of the profession and the welfare of the public, in 1903 was later reduced to a "preferable" board of arbitrators to settle differences of opinion between disputing physicians.[54] In contrast to the 1903 document, the 1912 "Principles" provided the AMA with a comparatively passive manifest political role within the profession. By 1949, medical ethics again called for membership in the Association and prohibited association with marginal practitioners. This resurgence of manifest control probably reflects the profession's greater experience with the politics of antitrust prosecution and the discovery that certain types of control are more vulnerable than others.

The preceding examination of American medical ethics has raised certain theoretical problems. On a number of issues, certain codes have been more monopolistic than Percival's, while others at least at first seem less so. Even though interpreting the call for uniform fees as monopolistic is

straightforward, interpreting the removal of ethical regulations for setting fees is ambiguous. One might well say that the retraction of such passages represents actual demonopolization, that these ethics do not order the conduct of physicians in a monopolistic direction. Before so concluding, however, one should realize that a monopolization strategy has multiple components and that manifest demonopolization of this kind may constitute latent monopolization by solving certain requirements for monopolization.

To be sure, as one finds time and again, codes of ethics may contain nonmonopolistic or even antimonopolistic rules; therefore, I have not been trying to demonstrate that everything in the world of medical ethics is monopolistic. My study of ethics so far has attempted to elucidate the ways in which ethics can contribute to the capacity of a group to engage in monopolistic action. In other words, I have so far considered the requirements of economic monopolization, i.e., the organizational requirements for domination of the market, but I have paid insufficient attention to the problem of politically oriented monopolization: the exigencies imposed by constraints from the political community. What are now required are heuristic concepts for the analysis of the political aspects of monopolization. Two such concepts are offered for consideration: the constraints of audiences on ethics, and the divergence of public and private codes of ethics.

One approach to the profession's political setting is the investigation of audiences addressed by the code of ethics. Percival's ethics for the most part addressed only physicians and responded to the political setting simply by encouraging paternalistic attitudes and by currying favor with politically strategic people. The 1847 "Code" specifically addressed both physician and patient, even including long passages about the duties and obligations of the patient to his physician. These were dropped in 1903 because of their adverse effect on public opinion. One prominent theme in them, however, was that patients should be totally loyal to the physician or find another doctor, an alternative to consumer organization for dissatisfied patients.

By 1903, apparently, state legislatures were an important audience. The

fight for state licensing privileges had just been won in the few preceding decades, and the ethics tended to be concerned with justifying these newly won privileges. The compromising of professional secrecy by legal responsibility for testimony on the medical condition of patients, and the replacing of an attack on practitioners of exclusive dogma with a defense of Association practitioners as scientific, tended to affirm the profession's sense of civic duty and reaffirm the scientific basis of licensing restrictions. As I have suggested, by 1912 the United States Justice Department may well have been an audience. Noteworthy in this context is the appearance of the ideology that the profession exists to serve the public good—its "ideal of service to humanity"—an ideology absent in ethical systems prior to 1912. Apparently, appeals to science were insufficient for legitimizing licensing and other monopolistic privileges, and so appeals to public and human service were added. By 1949 the key new audience was probably federal legislators. A whole series of plans for nationalizing health care delivery were countered with a series of principles about what would constitute unethical practice for physicians. Presumably, the message to this audience was that laws should not be made which would violate professional ethics and which would incidentally put the independent practitioner at a competitive disadvantage.

The 1957 "Principles of Ethics," which has so far received minimal attention in this chapter, appears to be an ingenious solution to the problem of conflicting requirements for a monopolization strategy. While the previous AMA codes all bear a common resemblance, this code is much more general and idealistic. . . . [See Chapter 11, this book.]

The 1957 "Principles" eliminated virtually all regulations concerning consultations, the duty to affiliate with medical societies, restrictions on institutional arrangements, and any stated role of the AMA in medical affairs. Also important are the inclusion of conflicting demands for fees and services as if they were not contradictory: fees "commensurate with the services rendered" are presumably set according to some standard for the evaluation of services; fees set in accordance with "the patient's ability to pay" work against such standardization. Also, the service ideal of "improving both the health and the well-being of the individual and the community" admits that service to individuals may not constitute community service, but does not go very far toward reconciling the two. These ambiguities suggest that the 1957 "Principles" attempts to resolve internal differences by including everything in a sufficiently vague manner as to offend no one yet provide everyone with a sense of ethical conduct. Whatever the political and social functions of the 1957 "Principles," it is no longer a detailed code of regulations for professional behavior but a statement of professional ideals: service to humanity, medical skill, science, moral and legal correctness, free exercise of skills, fair fees, use of consultations, secrecy under most conditions, and responsibility to both individuals and the community. In one sense, no physician can live up to these ethical standards because they are so abstract and general that they result in practical conflicts. In another sense, all physicians could meet these standards because they are stated as ideals, and ideals are understood to be compromised by reality. Infractions cannot reasonably be punished in most cases because physicians can meet these ideals at least to some degree most of the time.

Vagueness does not, however, imply decline in control. The telling thing about the 1957 "Principles" is that they do not replace the 1949 "Principles of Medical Ethics"; both are in effect. One might argue that the 1957 ethics are but an abstraction of general principles from the 1949 work, but they seem to be quite different documents. The interpretation I offer is that the 1957 ethics and the 1949 ethics address different audiences. Presumably the 1957 ethics are a statement of ideals for public consumption, and the 1949 ethics are detailed private norms for conduct, for which members of the AMA can still be held accountable. By this means, the monopolistic consequences of medical ethics have been made even less public than before.

The comparative study of medical ethics in America has demonstrated that the codes have indeed departed in certain respects from Percival's ethics,

at times becoming more monopolistic but at other times losing certain key monopolistic features. I have attempted to maintain the view that medical ethics are an organizational tool for monopolization but have expanded this perspective to see ethics serving this end in different ways. There has probably been a shift in purpose for medical ethics from a Percivalean means for ordering the conduct of physicians to a means for legitimizing the monopolistic privileges of the profession to the powers-that-be and to the public, though this shift has by no means been total. Medical ethics have probably been strained in recent years to serve both functions, and the device of dual codes of ethics—public and private codes—may help ease this strain. The trend toward making monopolistic features of the profession less public suggests that American society may have become in certain respects less receptive to monopolization by social groups, and that relative submersion of monopolistic features of the profession's organization has been the general strategy for dealing with this change in receptivity. . . .

Notes

1. Chauncey D. Leake, ed., *Percival's Medical Ethics* (Baltimore: Williams & Wilkins, 1927), p. 31

2. *Ibid.*, sections I–III, XIII, XXIX–XXXII, pp. 90–91, 97–98, 107–111. [The passages under discussion are reprinted as part of Chapter 7 of this volume.]

3. *Ibid.*, p. 38.

4. *Ibid.*, sections VII, VIII, X–XII, pp. 94–97.

5. *Ibid.*, sections VI, VIII, XIV, XXVI, XXVII, pp. 93–97.

6. *Ibid.*, section XV, pp. 98–100.

7. *Ibid.*, p. 105.

8. *Ibid.*, p. 102.

9. *Ibid.*, sections XIV, XV, XVI, XVIII–XX, XXV, pp. 98–103, 105.

10. *Ibid.*, pp. 104–105.

11. *Ibid.*, sections IV, IX, XIV, XXIII, XXIV, pp. 92–93, 95–96, 98, 104–105.

12. *Ibid.*, pp. 106 ff.

13. *Ibid.*, p. 219.

14. Robert Feinbaum, "The Doctor and the Public: A Case Study of Professional Politics" (Doctoral dissertation, Department of Sociology, University of California, Berkeley, 1967), p. 32.

15. Robert C. Derbyshire, *Medical Licensure and Discipline in the United States* (Baltimore and London: Johns Hopkins Press, 1969), pp. 77, 79, 87.

16. Leake, *op. cit.* (n. 1, above), p. 101.

17. Joseph F. Kett, *The Formation of the American Medical Profession: The Role of Institutions, 1780–1860* (New Haven and London: Yale University Press, 1968), p. 2.

18. Leake, *op. cit.* (n. 1, above), p. 197.

19. *Ibid.*, pp. 194–195.

20. Sir George Clark, *A History of the Royal College of Physicians of London,* 2 vols. (Oxford: Clarendon Press for the Royal College of Physicians, 1964, 1966), pp. 96–97, 180–181.

21. Georg Simmel, "The Secret Society," in *The Sociology of Georg Simmel,* ed. Kurt H. Wolff (London: The Free Press of Glencoe, Collier-Macmillan, 1950), pp. 355–360.

22. E. H. Ackerknecht, "Zur Geschichte der Medizinischen Ethik," *Praxis* 176 (1964), p. 580.

23. John Gregory, *Lectures on the Duties and Qualifications of a Physician* (London: Strahan and T. Cadell, 1772), p. 60.

24. *Ibid.*, pp. 39–40.

25. *Ibid.*, p. 62.

26. *Ibid.*, p. 213.

27. *Ibid.*, p. 215.

28. *Ibid.*, p. 216.

29. *Ibid.*, pp. 219–223.

30. *Ibid.*, pp. 218–220.

31. *Ibid.*, p. 228.

32. *Ibid.*, p. 233.

33. *Ibid.*, pp. 234–235.

34. *Ibid.*, pp. 237–238.

35. Leake, *op. cit.* (n. 1, above), section XV.

36. *Ibid.*, p. 235.

37. *Ibid.*, p. 269.

38. A. D. Neale, *The Antitrust Laws of the United States of America: A Study of Competition Enforced by Law* (Cambridge: At the University Press, 1962), p. 35.

39. "During the 49 years from 1891 to 1939 it had instituted an average of less than nine cases a year and a maximum of 27 cases a year (in 1913) . . . several of the prosecutions instituted by Attorney General Wickersham (1909–1913) called for the dissolution of trusts." Fritz Machlup, *The Political Economy of Monopoly: Business, Labor, and Government Policies* (Baltimore: Johns Hopkins Press, 1952), p. 184, n. 4.

40. "Principles of Medical Ethics" (American Medical Association, 1957), pp. VI–VIII. [Reprinted as Chapter 11 of this volume.]

41. Leake, *op. cit.* (n. 1, above), p. 235.

42. *Ibid.*, p. 229.

43. "Principles of Medical Ethics," *J.A.M.A.* 140 (25 June 1949), p. 701.

44. Leake, *op. cit.* (n. 1, above), p. 253.

45. *Ibid.*, pp. 268–269.

46. Herman Miles Somers and Anne Ramsay Somers, *Doctors, Patients, and Health Insurance: The Organization and Financing of Medical Care* (Washington, D.C.: The Brookings Institution, 1961), pp. 292, 347–354.

47. "Principles," (1949), *op. cit.*, p. 703.

48. *Ibid.*

49. *Ibid.*

50. Rosemary Stevens, *Medical Practice in Modern England: The Impact of Specialization and State Medicine* (New Haven and London: Yale University Press, 1966,) p. 183.

51. "Report of Coordinating Committee," *J.A.M.A.* 140 (25 June 1949), p. 697.

52. Leake, *op. cit.* (n. 1, above), pp. 228–229.

53. *Ibid.*, pp. 243–244.

54. *Ibid.*, pp. 243, 268.

14

William F. May

Code and Covenant or Philanthropy and Contract?

Reprinted in expanded and revised form with permission of author and publisher from the *Hastings Center Report*, vol. 5, December 1975, pp. 29–38.

When it first broke in the news the Summer of 1975, the case of the Marcus twins (gynecologists at a teaching hospital in New York City) posed in vivid circumstances several difficult and illuminating problems in professional ethics; problems which worry both laymen and doctors. The usual analysis of such problems, which appeals to the language of Philanthropy and Contract, boggles at the Marcus case. The categories of Code and Covenant (which are related to Philanthropy and Contract as *genera* to *species*) offer at least the beginnings of solutions to the professional ethical problems embodied in the case.

The Marcus brothers were physicians who, although technically expert (they wrote one of the best current textbooks on gynecology) and professionally and sympathetically involved, allowed themselves to become addicted to barbiturates, to miss appointments, and to offer consultation, diagnosis, and treatment while under the observable influence of drugs. They retained skill and expertise enough, however, to refrain from killing any of their patients. Their colleagues and the institutions in which they worked were slow to blow the whistle on them.

The Marcus case poses ethical problems for the professional. At what point is a doctor who prescribes drugs for himself misusing his technical expertise? At what point does a professional's duty to laymen override his duties to his fellow professionals? At what point does professional courtesy become professional whitewash? Is there a duty to a profession, as distinct from a duty to those individuals who practice the profession and those who benefit from its practice? These problems tend to concern the layman more than the experts in moral philosophy. Professional moralists tend to apply their analytical skills to issues they find intellectually interesting. They tend to solve moral puzzles rather than outline the foundations for professional character. They have produced in recent years elegant work on abortion, euthanasia, organ transplants, scarce medical resources and other subjects tantalizing at a theoretical level. The layman meanwhile is concerned with more prosaic questions. He wonders whether the doctor's real loyalty is to the patient or to the guild. Are medical societies, hospitals, and other health agencies ready and willing to weed out incompetent or unscrupulous practitioners? Will the profession find ways of challenging those doctors who order unwarranted surgery, charge fees that always press against the ceiling, play Ping Pong with referrals, process patients through their office with the speed of salts, or commit the sick to the hospital with indecorous haste?

Such blatantly unethical behavior (perhaps its self-evident wrongness explains why the professional moralist seldom attends to it) stirs the layman's anger. The profession seems to belong to an elite, utterly beyond the reach of his criticism. Certainly the physician is beyond serious challenge from the nurse and the social worker. His professional hegemony is well-nigh total over other health professionals. As long as doctors are in scarce supply and badly distributed, they are also beyond the reach of consumer criticism—except through the melodramatic, spotty, random, and sometimes, in its own right, unjust resort to the malpractice suit. For the same reason to date, they have not been seriously limited—except for the demands of paperwork—by outside agencies—the government, Blue Shield, and insurance companies. Under current conditions, the maintenance of professional standards of conduct depends largely on the doctor's own internal sense of professional obligation and on the willingness of the profession to enforce standards of conduct on its members.

This essay on the basis of professional ethics will therefore divide into two questions: why, despite the existence of medical codes and enforcement procedures, is the medical profession reluctant to engage in serious self-criticism? How are the concepts of code and covenant useful in interpreting professional duties and in establishing their obligatory power?

When the *New York Times* first carried its story on the Marcus brothers, it seemed a potentially scandalous reminder that the profession is loath to accept responsibility for professional discipline. The death of the gynecologists exposed both the ineffectualness of the well-intentioned New York Medical Society and the possible lack of zeal of the teaching hospital in protecting patients from two derelict professionals.

As it turned out, the case was not quite so pure an instance of *noblesse néglige* as it first appeared. The New York Hospital did write a letter terminating the services of the gynecologists. (Unfortunately for the reputation of the hospital and the profession, the termination date set in the letter preceded their death only by seventeen days, and, at a stage so far along the road of addiction that the body weight of these six footers at death was 115 and 100 pounds each.) Officials also made the point that the work of professionals is always monitored by colleagues in the hospital but they conceded that such controls would not apply to the Marcus brothers' private practice. In this as in other cases of solo practice, the patient—certainly the unsophisticated patient—is unprotected by the profession from its incompetent or unscrupulous members.

Whatever the final disposition of the Marcus brothers' case, a fundamental problem remains—and grows—that deserves the attention of moralists; that is, the tension in medical ethics between obligations to patients and obligations to one's fellow professionals. The tendency in the profession is to take the latter duties more seriously than the former. Professional ethics has traditionally had two social vectors: one concerned with behavior toward patients or clients; the other, with conduct toward one's colleagues. When concern for colleagues prevails, professional ethics reduces itself to courtesy within a guild. Certain arguable responsibilities to patients (such as informing them about incompetent treatment) are not simply eclipsed, they are professionally denied, that is, they are viewed as a breach of the discretionary bonds that pertain within the guild. Thus an inversion occurs. A report on incompetent or unethical behavior to patients becomes a breach in "professional ethics," that is, a breach in courtesy.

There are many reasons both material and ideological for the reluctance of doctors to engage in professional self-criticism and regulation. First, like any professional group, doctors find themselves in a complex, interlocking network of relations with fellow professionals: they extend favors, incur debts;

exchange referrals; intertwine personal histories. The bond with fellow professionals grows, while ties with patients seem transient. Further, any society organized around certain ends tends to generate a sense of community among professional staff members serving those ends. This experience of collegiality becomes an end in its own right and subtly takes precedence over the needs of the population served. Hence criticism gets muted.

Second, professional self-regulation may be even more difficult to achieve in medicine because self-criticism seems somewhat more natural to lawyers and academicians whose work goes on in an adversarial or, at least, a disputatious setting. The doctor, however, has a special role in relation to his patients, quasi-priestly-parental, which seems more severely subverted by criticism. Trust is a very important ingredient in the relationship; criticism seems outside the boundaries of professional behavior.

Third, the doctor's authority, while great, is precarious. The analogy often drawn between the authority of the modern doctor and the traditional power of the parent and priest obscures an important difference between them in the security of their status. The modern doctor's position, while exalted, is inherently less stable. Apotheosized by many of his patients, he is resented bitterly if his hand slips publicly but once. The reason for this instability lies in differing sources to authority. Parents and priests in traditional society derived their authority from sacred powers perceived to be creative, nurturant, and beneficent. Given this positive derivation of power, human defect in the authority figure could be tolerated. The power of good would prevail despite human lapse. The modern doctor's authority, however, is reflexively derived from a grim negativity; that is, from the fear of death. This self-same power of death that exalts him and makes him the most highly paid, the most authoritative, professional in the modern world threatens to bring him low if through his own negligence, unscrupulousness or incompetence, he endangers the life of his patient. Thus while the modern physician enjoys much more prestige and authority than the contemporary teacher or lawyer, his position as a professional is, in one sense, more precarious than theirs. Resentment against him is potentially much greater. Professional self-criticism in academic life or in the law seems like child's play compared with medicine. The slothful teacher deprives me merely of the truth; the negligent lawyer forfeits my money, or, at worst, my freedom; but the incompetent doctor endangers my life. The stakes seem much higher in the case of medicine. The profession is tempted to draw its wagons around in a circle when any of its members are challenged.

Fourth, Americans of all walks of life have a morally healthy suspicion of officiousness. They are loath to press charges against their neighbors or colleagues. They are peculiarly sensitive to the injustice and hypocrisy of those who are zealous about the sliver in their neighbor's eye while unmindful of the beam in their own. Better, then, to comply with moral standards in one's own professional conduct, but, beyond that, to live and let live. It is difficult, after all, to tell the difference between an honest mistake and culpable negligence. Who can know enough about a particular medical case to second-guess the physician in charge? Is it not better to keep one's mouth shut? Must a person be his colleague's keeper?

This revulsion against officiousness deserves sympathy, but it fails to respect fully the special moral situation of the professional. Professionals are those who, on the basis of their special knowledge and competence, claim final right to pass judgment in professional matters) on colleagues or would-be colleagues. The state honors and supports this right when it establishes licensing procedures under the control of professionals and backs up these procedures by prosecuting imposters and pretenders. In effect, the state sanctions a monopoly (a limitation on the supply of professionals) from which, to be sure, patients profit, but also from which the professional profits—handsomely, financially. If the professional were in fact, a free-lance entrepreneur (as the myth would have it) without the protection of the monopoly, he would not fare nearly so well.

Professional accountability therefore cannot be restricted to the question of

one's own personal competence; it includes also the question of the competence of the guild. The right to pass judgment on colleagues carries with it the duty so to judge; otherwise doctors profit from a monopoly established by the state without enforcing those standards the need for which alone justified the monopoly. The license to practice is based on the prior license to license. If the license to practice carries with it the duty to practice well, the license to license carries with it the duty to judge and monitor well.

Ethical standards sag and falter when they are no longer accepted as universally binding. The usual test of whether an individual holds an ethical principle to be universally valid is whether he concedes its application not only to others but to himself. No one can make of himself an exception. The famous confrontation between King David and Nathan the prophet was devoted to that point. The king who makes judgments and enforces laws shall live by the law himself.

Today, however, in professional ethics, the test of moral seriousness may depend not simply upon personal compliance with ethical principles, but upon the courage to hold others accountable. Otherwise, the doctor's oath to his patients has yielded to the somewhat tarnished majesty of the guild.

A fifth and final cause for reserve in pressing for disciplinary action is neither exclusively modern nor American. It is prepared for in principle as far back as the Hippocratic Oath. The ancient oath made an important distinction between two sets of obligations: those that pertain to the doctor's treatment of his patients and those he accepts toward his teacher and his teacher's progeny. Obligations to one's fellow professionals flow from an original indebtedness of the student to his teacher; consequently, they acquire a gravity that makes them take precedence over obligations to patients.

To explore this distinction in obligations, we will need to press back into alternative ways of conceptualizing professional ethics and corresponding perceptions of its binding power. For this reason, in the second section of this essay, we will examine certain root

terms for interpreting professional obligation, specifically the concepts of code, covenant, philanthropy, and contract. This investigation will take us beyond the somewhat narrower issue of professional discipline with which we began, but it remains a topic to which, in closing, we will need to return.

The Hippocratic Oath is a useful place to begin not only because of its prominence in medicine, but because it forces reflection on the distinction between code and covenant. The oath itself includes three elements: first, codal duties to patients; second, covenantal obligations to colleagues; and, third, the setting of both within the context of an oath to the gods, specifically, the gods of healing.

The duties of a physician toward his patients, as elaborated in the oath, include a series of absolute prohibitions (against performing surgery, assisting patients in attempts at suicide or abortion, breaches in confidentiality, and acts of injustice or mischief toward the patient and his household, including sexual misconduct); more positively, the physician must act always for the benefit of the sick (the chief illustration of which is to apply dietetic measures according to the physician's best judgment and ability), and, more generally, to keep them from harm and injustice.

The second set of obligations, directed to the physician's teacher, his teacher's children and his own, require him to accept full filial responsibilities for his adopted father's personal and financial welfare, and to transmit without fee his art and knowledge to the teacher's progeny, his own, and to other pupils, but only those others who take the oath according to medical law.

In his monograph on the Hippocratic Oath, Ludwig Edelstein characterizes those obligations that a physician undertakes toward his patients as an ethical code and those assumed toward the professional guild and its perpetuation as a covenant. Just why this difference in terminology is appropriate, Edelstein does not say. In my judgment, the chief reason for resorting to the word covenant in describing the second set of obligations is the fact of indebtedness. The doctor may have duties to his patients, but he owes something to his teacher. He is the beneficiary of goods and services received to which his filial services are responsive. This is one of the hallmarks of covenant. Both the Hammurabi Code and the Mosaic Law detail those statutes that will give shape to a civilization; in this respect, they are alike. But the biblical covenant differs in that it places the moral duties of the people within the all-important context of a divine act of deliverance: "I am the Lord thy God who brought thee out of the land of Egypt, the house of bondage." Thus the promises which the people of Israel make at Mt. Sinai to obey the statutes of God are responsive to goods already received. Analogously, in the Hippocratic Oath, the physician undertakes obligations to his teacher and his progeny out of gratitude for services already rendered. It will be one of the contentions of this essay that the development of the practice of modern medicine, for understandable reasons, has tended to reinforce this particular and ancient distinction between code and covenant and opted for code as the ruling ideal in relations to patients, but not with altogether favorable consequences for the moral health of the profession.

The Hippocratic Oath, of course, includes a third element: the vow or religious oath proper, directed to the gods. "I swear by Apollo, the physician, and Aesculapius and health and all-heal and all the Gods and Godesses that, according to my ability and judgment, I will keep this oath and stipulation." A religious reference appears again in the statement of duties to patients: "In purity and holiness I will guard my life and art"; and the promise-maker finally petitions: "If I fulfill this oath and do not violate it, may it be granted to me to enjoy life and art . . . ; if I transgress it and swear falsely, may the opposite of all this be my lot."

This religious oath, in the literal sense, makes a "professional" out of the man who takes it. He professes or testifies thereby to the power of healing of which his duties to patients and his obligations to his teacher are a specification. Swearing by Apollo and Aesculapius is at the ontological root of his life. He professes those powers by which his own state of being is altered. Henceforth he is a professional, a professor of healing.

It is an intriguing, but not quite resolvable, question as to whether this oath is an ingredient of a covenant or simply a part of the full meaning of a code. In some respects, it is like a covenant. The physician makes a promise which has a reference to the gods from whom the profession of healing is ultimately derived. This religious promise becomes then the basis for that secondary promise or covenant which the physician makes to care for his teacher and for those duties which he undertakes toward his patients. His promise by the gods gives gravity and shape to the whole. Yet in two important respects the oath itself differs from a biblical covenant: it offers no prefatory statement about the actions of the divine to which the human promise is responsive; and, second, its form is such as to deemphasize the responsive nature of the physician's action, for he swears *by* the gods instead of promises *to* the gods to undertake his professional duties.

Similarly, the question can be raised as to whether this religious vow should be interpreted as part of the full meaning of a code, but, to argue this case, the concept of code needs to be expanded to include more than it means currently in the medical profession.

The word "code" in current professional ethics usually has two meanings—depending on the way in which professional duties are mediated. It can refer alternatively to those *unwritten* and habitual modes of behavior that are transmitted chiefly in a clinical setting from generation to generation of physicians or to those *written* codes, beginning with the Hippocratic Oath and concluding with the various AMA codes that have had wide currency in this country. Technical proficiency is the prized ideal in the informal codes of behavior passed on from doctor to doctor; the ideal of philanthropy (that is, the notion of gratuitous service to humankind) looms larger in the more official, engraved tablets of the profession.

Code, however, covers a third form of activity—above and beyond habitual modes of behavior and collections of written statutes—it refers also to special languages, coded messages, and solemn oaths within special groups. It is this third aspect of code which may be most ethically illuminating; for it implies a special initiation, a profession of allegiance, the possession of a key, and a mutual understanding available only to those who have undergone an alteration in their being which privileges them to use the codebook, the vocabulary, and the technical proficiency.

This third dimension of code prompted us to suggest that the religious vow in the Hippocratic Oath might be interpreted in codal as well as covenantal terms. The professional not only enters into a relationship with a patient, a colleague, or a guild, but also makes a *profession* in and through which his being is altered. He recognizes that his subsequent life for good or ill is derived from this profession. Whenever the medical guild fails to recognize this third aspect of code, it reduces itself to the ideal of technical proficiency alone or it tries to elevate itself to the compensatory and ultimately pretentious concept of philanthropy.

The Current Codal Ideal of Technical Proficiency

Both the ideal of technical proficiency and the skills that go with it are transmitted largely in a clinical setting. A code operating in this milieu shapes human behavior in a fashion somewhat similar to habits and rules. A habit, as Peter Winch has pointed out,[1] is a matter of doing the same thing on the same kind of occasion in the same way. A moral rule is distinct from a habit in that the agent in this instance *understands what is meant* by doing the same thing on the same kind of occasion in the same way. Both habits and rules are categorical, universal, and to this degree ahistorical, they do not receive their authority from particular events by which they are authorized or legitimated. They remain operative categorically on all similar occasions. *Never* assist patients in attempts to suicide or abortion or never break a confidence except under certain specified circumstances.

A code is usually categorical and universal in the aforementioned senses but not in the sense that it is binding on any and all groups. Hammurabi's code is obligatory only for particular peoples. Moreover, inner circles within certain societies—whether professional or social groups—develop their special codes of behavior. We think of code words or special codes of behavior among friends, workers in the same company, or professionals within a guild. These codes offer directives not only for the content of action, but also for its form. In its concern with appropriate form, a code, partly understood, moves in the direction of the aesthetic. It becomes less concerned with what is done or why it is done than with how it is done; so reduced, a code becomes preoccupied with matters of style and decorum. Thus medical codes include directives not only on the content of therapeutic action, but also on the fitting style for professional behavior including such matters as dress, discretion in the household, fitting behavior in the hospital, and prohibitions on self-advertisement.

Insofar as a code becomes more exclusively concerned with style, image, and decorum, it runs the danger of detaching itself from its ontological root. Style functions to protect the stylist from the assaults of life (and death) and to preserve him also from any alterations in his own being. This tendency to move ethics in the direction of aesthetics, rather than ontology, is conveniently illustrated in the work of the modern novelist who is most associated with the aesthetic ideal of a code—Ernest Hemingway. The ritual killing of a bull in the short stories and novels of Hemingway offers a paradigm for the professional; the bullfighter symbolizes an ethic in which stylish performance becomes everything.

. . . the bull charged and Villalta charged and just for a moment they became one. Villalta became one with the bull and then it was over. (*In Our Time,* Hemingway.)

For the Hemingway hero, there is no question of permanent commitments to particular persons, causes, or places. Robert Jordan of *For Whom the Bell Tolls* does not even remember the "cause," "power," or "profession" for which he came to Spain to fight. Once he is absorbed in the ordeal of war, the test of a man is not a cause to which he is committed but his conduct from moment to moment. Life is a matter of eating, drinking, loving, hunting, and dying well; Jordan can no longer "profess" a cause or sustain a long-term commitment; just like Catherine in *A Farewell to Arms,* he must die. Hemingway writes about lovers, briefly joined, but rarely about marriage or the family. Just for a moment, lovers become one and then it is over.

The bullfighter, the wartime lover, the doctor—all alike—must live by a code that eschews involvement; for each there comes a time when the thing is over; matters are terminated by death. At best, one can hope to escape from the pain of time; thus the aesthetic aspires to the timeless. Men must learn to live beautifully, stylishly, fittingly. Discipline is all, according to the aesthetic code. There is a right and a wrong way to do things. And the wrong way usually results from a deficiency in technique or from an excessive preoccupation with one's ego. The bad bullfighter either lacks technique or he lets his ego—through fear or vanity—get in the way of his performance. The conditions of beauty are technical proficiency and a style wholly purified of disruptive preoccupation with oneself. Literally, however, when the critical moment is consummated, it is over, it cannot shape the future. Partners must fall away; only the code remains.

For several reasons, the medical profession has been attracted to the aesthetic ideal of code for its interpretation of its ethics. First, such a code requires one to subordinate the ego to the more technical question of how a thing is done and done well. At its best, the discipline of a code cultivates the aesthetic. It encourages a proficiency that is quietly eloquent. It conjoins the good with the beautiful. Since the technical demands of medicine have become so great, the standards of the guild are largely transmitted by apprenticeship to those whose preeminent skills define the real meaning of the profession. All the rest is a question of disciplining the ego to the point that nervousness, fatigue, faintheartedness, and temptations to self-display (including gross efforts at self-advertisement) have been smoothed away.

A code is additionally attractive in that it does not, in and of itself, encourage personal involvement with the patient; and it helps free the physician of the destructive consequences of that personal involvement. Compassion, in the strictest sense of the term, "suffering with," has its disadvantages in the professional relationship. It will not do to pretend that one is the second person of the Trinity, prepared with every patient to make the sympathetic descent into his suffering, pain, particular form of crucifixion, and hell. It is

enough to offer whatever help one can through finely honed services. It is important to remain emotionally free so as to be able to withdraw the self when those services are no longer pertinent, when as Hemingway says, "it is over." Such is the attraction of the codal ideal of technical proficiency.

The Ideal of a Covenant

A covenant, as opposed to a code, has its roots in specific historical events. Like a code, it may give inclusive shape to behavior, but it always has reference to a specific historical exchange between partners leading to a promissory event. Edelstein was quite right in distinguishing code from covenant in the Hippocratic Oath. Rules governing behavior toward patients have a different ring to them from that fealty which a physician owes to his teacher. Loyalty to one's instructor is founded in a specific historical event—that original transaction in which the student received his knowledge and art. He receives, in effect, a specific gift from his teacher which deserves his life-long loyalty, a gift that he perpetuates in his own right and turn as he offers his art without fee to his teacher's children and his own progeny. Covenant ethics is responsive in character.

In its ancient and most influential form, a covenant usually included the following elements: first, an original experience of gift between the soon-to-be covenanted partners; and, second, a covenant promise based on this original or anticipated exchange of gifts, labors, or services. However, these temporal and contractual elements of a covenant were but two aspects of a tripartite concept: a covenant included not only an involvement with a partner in time, and a responsive contract, but the notion of a change of being; a covenanted people is a people changed utterly by the covenant. This third aspect of covenant is, like the third aspect of the concept code, ontological in nature. The aesthetic code attempts to remove style from time; a contract has a limited duration in time, but a covenant imposes a change on all moments. A mechanic can act under a contract, and then, when not fixing the piston, act without regard to the contract, but a covenanted people is covenanted while eating, sleeping, working, praying, stealing, cheating, healing, or blundering. Paul remarks, in effect, "When you eat, eat to the glory of God, and when you fast, fast to the glory of God, and when you marry, marry to the glory of God, and when you abstain, abstain to the glory of God."[2] When the professional is initiated, he is covenanted, and the physician is a healer when he is healing, and when he is sleeping, when he is practicing, and when he is malpracticing. A covenant changes the shape of the whole life of the covenanted. It changes the totality of the subsequent life of the covenanted in two ways: first, it contains very specific contractual obligations; the law of Moses, and the Talmudic code based on this law changed the life of the covenanted, by specifying not only the way in which God was to be worshipped, but in their methods of stewing kids; a physician contracts not only to do no harm, but specifically to educate free of charge other professionals' kids. However, the covenant changes are not restricted to the codified and specified changes. It alters the covenanted pervasively in his being; at the beginning of the oath, the physician seals himself, and his whole life, to the gods through his profession. This second change is ontological.

The scriptures of ancient Israel are littered with such covenants between men and controlled throughout by that singular covenant which embraces all others. The covenant between God and Israel includes the aforementioned elements: (1) a gift (the deliverance of the people from Egypt); (2) an exchange of promises (at Mt. Sinai); and (3) the shaping of all subsequent life by the promissory event. God "marks the forehead" of the Jews forever, as they respond by accepting an inclusive set of ritual and moral commandments by which they will live. These commands are both specific enough to make the future duties of Israel concrete (e.g., the dietary laws), yet summary enough (e.g., love the Lord thy God with all thy heart . . .) so as to require a fidelity that exceeds any specification.[3]

For some of the reasons already mentioned, the bond of covenant, in the classical period, tended to define and bind together medical colleagues to one another, but it did not figure large in interpreting the relations between the doctor and his patients. The

doctor receives his professional life from his teacher; this gift establishes a bond between them and prompts him to assume certain life-long duties not only toward the teacher (and his financial welfare), but toward his children. This symbolic bond with one's teacher acknowledged in the Hippocratic Oath is strengthened in modern professional life by all those exchanges between colleagues to which reference was made in the opening section of this essay—referrals, favors, personal confidences, and collaborative work on cases. Thus loyalty to colleagues is a responsive act for gifts already, and to be, received.

Duties to patients are not similarly interpreted in the medical codes as a responsive act for gifts or services received. This is the essential feature of covenant conspicuously missing in the interpretation of professional duties to patients from the Hippocratic Oath to the modern codes of the AMA. Compensatorily, the profession has tended to elaborate the codal ideal of philanthropy.

Philanthropy versus Covenantal Indebtedness

The medical profession includes in its written codes an ideal that Hemingway never shared and that seldom looms large in the ethic of any self-selected inner group—the ideal of philanthropy. The medical profession proclaims its dedication to the service of mankind. This ideal is implicitly at work in the Hippocratic Oath and the culture out of which it emerged;[4] it continues in the Code of Medical Ethics originally adopted by the American Medical Association at its national convention in 1847 and it is elaborated in contemporary statements of that code.

This ideal of service, in my judgment, succumbs to what might be called the conceit of philanthropy when it is assumed that the professional's commitment to his fellow man is a gratuitous, rather than a responsive or reciprocal, act flowing from his altered state of being. Statements of medical ethics that obscure the doctor's prior indebtedness to the community are tainted with the odor of condescension. The point is obvious if one contrasts the way in which the code of 1847 interprets the obligations of patients and

the public to the physician, as opposed to the obligations of the physician to the patient and the public. On this particular question, I see no fundamental change from 1847 to 1957.

Clearly the duties of the patient are founded on what he has received from the doctor:

The members of the medical profession, upon whom is enjoined the performance of so many important and arduous duties, toward the community, and who are required to make so many sacrifices of comfort, ease, and health, for the welfare of those who avail themselves of their services, certainly have a right to expect and require that their patients should entertain a just sense of the duties which they owe to their medical attendants. (Art. II, Sect. 1, "Obligations of Patients to Their Physicians," Code of Medical Ethics, American Medical Association, May 1847; Chicago: A.M.A. Press, 1897.)

In like manner, the section on the Obligations of the Public to Physicians (Art. II, Sect. 1) emphasizes those many gifts and services which the public has received from the medical profession and which are the basis for its indebtedness to the profession.

The benefits accruing to the public, directly and indirectly, from the active and unwearied beneficiaries of the profession, are so numerous and important that physicians are justly entitled to the utmost consideration and respect from the community.

But turning to the preamble for the physician's duties to the patient and the public, we find no corresponding section in the code of 1847 (or 1957) which founds the doctor's obligations on those gifts and services which he has received from the community. Thus we are presented with the picture of a relatively self-sufficient monad, who, out of the nobility and generosity of his disposition and the gratuitously accepted conscience of his profession, has taken upon himself the noble life of service. The false posture in all this blurts out in one of the opening sections of the 1847 code. Physicians "should study, also, in their deportment so as to unite tenderness with firmness, and condescension with authority, so as to inspire the minds of their patients with gratitude, respect and confidence."

I do not intend to demean the specific content of those duties which the codes set forth in their statement of the duties of physicians to their patients, but I am critical of the setting or context in which they are placed. Significantly the code refers to the *Duties* of Physicians to their Patients but to the *Obligations* of Patients to their Physicians. The shift from "Duties" to "Obligations" may seem slight, but, in fact, I believe it is a revealing adjustment in language. The AMA thought of the patient and public as *indebted* to the profession for its services but the profession has accepted its *duties* to the patient and public out of noble conscience rather than a reciprocal sense of indebtedness.

Put another way, the medical profession imitates God not so much because it exercises power of life and death over others, but because it does not really think itself beholden, even partially, to anyone for those duties to patients which it lays upon itself. Like God, the profession draws its life from itself alone. Its action is wholly gratuitous.

Now, in fact, the physician is in very considerable debt to the community. The first of these debts is already adumbrated in the original Hippocratic Oath. He is obliged to someone or some group for his education. In ancient times, this led to a special sense of covenant obligation to one's teacher. Under the conditions of modern medical education, this indebtedness is both substantial (far exceeding the social investment in the training of any other professional) and widely distributed (including not only one's teachers but those public monies on the basis of which the medical school, the teaching hospital, and research into disease, are funded).

In view of the fact that many more qualified candidates apply for medical school than can be admitted and many more doctors are needed than the schools can train, the doctor-to-be has a second order of indebtedness for privileges that have almost arbitrarily fallen his way. While the 1847 code refers to the "privileges" of being a doctor it does not specify the social origins of those privileges. Third, and not surprisingly, the codes do not make reference to that extraordinary social largesse that befalls the physician, in payment for services, in a society where need abounds and available personnel is limited. Further, the codes

do not concede the indebtedness of the physician to those patients who have offered themselves as subjects for experimentation or as teaching material (either in teaching hospitals or in the early years of practice). Early practice includes, after all, the element of increased risk for patients who lay their bodies on the line as the doctor "practices" on them. The pun in the word but reflects the inevitable social price of training. This indebtedness to the patient was most recently and eloquently acknowledged by Judah Folkman, M.D., of Harvard Medical School in a Class Day Address.

In the long run, it is better if we come to terms with the uncertainty of medical practice. Once we recognise that all our efforts to relieve suffering might on occasion cause suffering, we are in a position to learn from our mistakes and appreciate the debt we owe our patients for our education. It is a debt which we must repay—it is like tithing.

I doubt that the debt we accumulate can be repaid our patients by trying to reduce the practice of medicine to a forty-hour week or by dissolving the quality of our residency program just because certain groups of residents in the country have refused, through legal tactics, to be on duty more than every fourth or fifth night or any nights at all.

And, it can't be repaid by refusing to see Medicaid patients when the state can't afford to pay for them temporarily.

But we can repay the debt in many ways. We can attend postgraduate courses and seminars, be available to patients at all hours, teach, take recertification examinations; maybe in the future even volunteer for national service; or, most difficult of all, carry out investigation or research." [5]

The physician finally is indebted to his patients not only for a start in his career. He remains unceasingly in their debt in its full course. This continuing reciprocity of need is somewhat obscured for we think of the mature professional as powerful and authoritative rather than needy. He seems to be a self-sufficient virtuoso whose life is derived from his competence while others appear before him in their neediness, exposing their illness, their crimes, or their ignorance, for which the professional, as doctor, lawyer, or teacher, offers remedy.

In fact, however, a reciprocity of giving and receiving is at work in the professional relationship that needs to be acknowledged. In the profession of teaching, for example, the student

needs the teacher to assist him in learning, but so also the professor needs his students. They provide him with regular occasion and forum in which to work out what he has to say and to rediscover his subject afresh through the discipline of sharing it with others. Likewise, the doctors needs his patients. No one can watch a physician nervously approach retirement without realizing how much he has needed his patients to be himself.

A covenantal ethics helps acknowledge this full context of need and indebtedness in which professional duties are undertaken and discharged. It also relieves the professional of the temptation and pressure to pretend that he is a demigod exempt from human exigency.

Contract or Covenant

While criticizing the ideal of philanthropy, I have emphasized the elements of exchange, agreement, and reciprocity that mark the professional relationship. This leaves us with the question as to whether the element of the gratuitous should be suppressed altogether in professional ethics. Does the physician merely respond to the social investment in his training, the fees paid for his services, and the terms of an agreement drawn up between himself and his patients, or does some element of the gratuitous remain?

To put this question another way: is covenant simply another name for a contract in which two parties calculate their own best interests and agree upon some joint project in which both derive roughly equivalent benefits for goods contributed by each? If so, this essay would appear to move in the direction of those who would interpret the doctor-patient relationship as a legal agreement and who want, on the whole, to see medical ethics draw closer to medical law.

The notion of the physician as contractor has certain obvious attractions. First, it represents a deliberate break with more authoritarian models (such as priest or parent) for interpreting the role. At the heart of a contract is informed consent rather than blind trust; a contractual understanding of the therapeutic relationship encourages full respect for the dignity of the patient, who has not, because of illness, forfeited his sovereignty as a human being. The notion of a contract includes an exchange of information on the basis of which an agreement is reached and a subsequent exchange of goods (money for services); it also allows for a specification of rights, duties, conditions, and qualifications limiting the agreement. The net effect is to establish some symmetry and mutuality in the relationship between the doctor and patient.

Second, a contract provides for the legal enforcement of its terms—on both parties—and thus offers both parties some protection and recourse under the law for making the other accountable for the agreement.

Finally, a contract does not rely on the pose of philanthropy, the condescension of charity. It presupposes that people are primarily governed by self-interest. When two people enter into a contract, they do so because each sees it to his own advantage. This is true not only of private contracts but also of that primordial social contract in and through which the state came into being. So argued the theorists of the eighteenth century. The state was not established by some heroic act of sacrifice on the part of the gods or men. Rather men entered into the social contract because each found it to his individual advantage. It is better to surrender some liberty and property to the state than to suffer the evils that would beset men apart from its protection. Subsequent enthusiasts about the social instrument of contracts,[6] have tended to measure human progress by the degree to which a society is based on contracts rather than status. In the ancient world, the Romans made the most striking advances in extending the areas in which contract rather than custom determined commerce between people. In the modern world, the bourgeoisie extended the instrumentality of contracts farthest into the sphere of economics; the free churches, into the arena of religion. Some educationists today have extended the device into the classroom (as students are encouraged to contract units of work for levels of grade); more recently some women's liberationists would extend it into marriage; and still others would prefer to see it define the professional relationship. The movement, on the whole, has the intention of laicizing

authority, legalizing relationships, activating self-interest, and encouraging collaboration.

In my judgment, some of these aims of the contractualists are desirable, but it would be unfortunate if professional ethics were reduced to a commercial contract. First, the notion of contract suppresses the element of gift in human relationships. Earlier I verged on denying the importance of this ingredient in professional relations, when I criticized the medical profession for its conceit of philanthropy, for its self-interpretation as the great giver. In fact, this earlier criticism was not an objection to the notion of gift but to the moral pretension of a profession whenever it pretends to be the exclusive giver. Factually, the professional is also the beneficiary of gifts received. It is unbecoming to adopt the pose of spontaneous generosity when the profession has received so much from the community and from patients, past and present.

But the contractualist approach to professional behavior falls into the opposite error of minimalism. It reduces everything to tit for tat. Do no more for your patients than what the contract calls for. Perform specified services for certain fees and no more. The commercial contract is fitting instrument in the purchase of an appliance, a house, or certain services that can be specified fully in advance of delivery. The existence of a legally enforceable agreement in professional transactions may also be useful to protect the patient or client against the physician or lawyer whose services fall below a minimal standard. But it would be wrong to reduce professional obligation to the specifics of a contract alone.

Professional services in the so-called helping professions are directed to subjects whose needs are in the nature of the case rather unpredictable. The professional deals with the sickness, ills, crimes, needs, and tragedies of humankind. These needs cannot be exhaustively specified in advance for each patient or client. The professions therefore must be ready to cope with the contingent, the unexpected. Calls upon services may be required that exceed those anticipated in a contract or for which compensation may be available in a given case. These services moreover

are more likely to be effective in achieving the desired therapeutic result if they are delivered in the context of a fiduciary relationship that the patient or client can really trust.

Contract and covenant, materially considered, seem like first cousins; they both include an exchange and an agreement between parties. But, in spirit, contract and covenant are quite different. Contracts are external; covenants are internal to the parties involved. Contracts are signed to be expediently discharged. Covenants have a gratuitous, growing edge to them that spring from ontological change and are directed to the upbuilding of relationships.

There is a donative element in the upbuilding of covenant—whether it is the covenant of marriage, friendship, or professional relationship. Tit for tat characterizes a commercial transaction, but it does not exhaustively define the vitality of that relationship in which one must serve and draw upon the deeper reserves of another.

This donative element is important not only in the doctor's care of the patient but in other aspects of health care. In a fascinating study of *The Gift Relationship,* the late economist, Richard M. Titmuss, compares the British system of obtaining blood by donations with the American partial reliance on the commercial purchase and sale of blood. The British system obtains more and better blood, without the exploitation of the indigent, which the American system has condoned and which our courts have encouraged when they refused to exempt non-profit blood banks from the antitrust laws. By court definition, blood exchange becomes a commercial transaction in the United States. Titmuss expanded his theme from human blood to social policy by offering a sober criticism of the increased commercialism of American medicine and society at large. Recent court decisions have tended to shift more and more of what had previously been considered as services into the category of commodity transactions with negative consequences he believes for the health of health delivery systems.[7] Hans Jonas has had to reckon with the importance of voluntary sacrifice to the social order in a somewhat comparable essay on "Human Experimentation."[8] Others have done so on the subject of organ transplants.

The kind of minimalism that a contractualist understanding of the professional relationship encourages produces a professional too grudging, too calculating, too lacking in spontaneity, too quickly exhausted to go the second mile with his patients along the road of their distress.

Contract medicine encourages not only minimalism, it also provokes a peculiar kind of maximalism, the name for which is "defensive medicine." Especially under the pressure of malpractice suits, doctors are tempted to order too many examinations and procedures for self-protection. Paradoxically, contractualism simultaneously tempts the doctor to do too little and too much for the patient—too little in that one extends oneself only to the limits of what is specified in the contract, yet, at the same time, too much in that one orders procedures useful in protecting oneself as the contractor even though not fully indicated by the condition of the patient. The link between these apparently contradictory strategies of too little and too much is the emphasis in contractual decisions on self-interest.

Three concluding objections to contractualism can be stated summarily. Parties to a contract are better able to protect their self-interest to the degree that they are informed about the goods bought and sold. Insofar as contract medicine encourages increased knowledge on the part of the patient, well and good. Nevertheless the physician's knowledge so exceeds that of his patient that the patient's knowledgeability alone is not a satisfactory constraint on the physician's behavior. One must at least, in part, depend upon some internal fiduciary checks which the professional (and his guild) accept.

Another self–regulating mechanism in the traditional contractual relationship is the consumer's freedom to shop and choose among various vendors of services. Certainly this freedom of choice needs to be expanded for the patient by an increase in the number of physicians and paramedical personnel. However, the crisis circumstances under which medical services are often needed and delivered does not always provide the consumer with the kind of leisure or calm required for discretionary judgment. Thus normal marketplace controls cannot be relied upon fully to protect the consumer in dealings with the physician.

For a final reason, medical ethics should not be reduced to the contractual relationship alone. Normally conceived, ethics establishes certain rights and duties that transcend the particulars of a given agreement. The justice of any specific contract may then be measured by these standards. If, however, such rights and duties adhere only to the contract, then a patient might legitimately be persuaded to waive his rights. The contract would solely determine what is required and permissible. An ethical principle should not be waivable (except to give way to a higher ethical principle). Professional ethics should not be so defined as to permit a physician to persuade a patient to waive rights that transcend the particulars of their agreement.

The Donative mode seems to provide for a more satisfactory analysis than the philanthropic or the contractual, but it shares their flaws. Analysis based on Donative elements suggests that the professional fulfills his contract, lives up to his specified technical code, and then, gratuitously, throws in something extra to sweeten the pot. All of these tools of analysis allow the analyst to evade the uncomfortable and demanding ontological implications of Initiatory Code, Covenant as Chosen, and Profession as transformation. The ontological changes implied in Secret Code, Covenanted People, and Profession of a mystery are complete changes in substance which affect the total life of the professional. A carpenter who contracts to build a chair, when he eats an ice cream cone, does not eat it as a carpenter, nor, when he gets his union card, does he imply that his initiation has changed him utterly, relating him, before everything else, to the mystery of chair making or shellac. A profession of a mystery, in theological terms changes one from damned to saved; in professional terms, from a man who studies medicine, to a man who at all times embodies healing. Malpractice, then, is rather like the sin against the Holy Ghost, uncomfortable for those sinned against, but utterly negating the identity of the sinner. A professional eats to heal, drives to heal, reads to heal, comforts to heal, rebukes to heal, and rests to heal. The transformation is radical, and total. The Hippocratic Oath, under this ontological aspect, can be summarized: *aut medicus aut nihil;* from this moment, I am a healer or I am (literally) nothing. He takes his identity from that which he professes, and that which he professes, to which he is covenanted, whose code he will embody, transcends him and transcends his colleagues.

Transcendence and Covenant

Two characteristics of covenantal ethics have been developed in the course of contrasting it with the ideal of philanthropy and the legal instrument of contracts. As opposed to the ideal of philanthropy that pretends to wholly gratuitous altruism, covenantal ethics places the service of the professional within the full context of goods, gifts, and services received; thus covenantal ethics is responsive. As opposed to the instrument of contract that presupposes agreement reached on the basis of self-interest, covenantal ethics may require one to be available to the covenant partner above and beyond the measure of self-interest; thus covenantal ethics has an element of the gratuitous in it.

We have to reckon now with the potential conflict between these characteristics. Have we developed our notion of covenant too reactively to alternatives without paying attention to the inner consistency of the concept itself? On the one hand, we had cause for suspecting those idealists who founded professional duties on a philanthropic impulse, without so much as acknowledging the sacrifice of others by which their own lives have been nourished. Then we have reasons for drawing back from those legal realists and positivists who would circumscribe professional life entirely within the calculus of commodities bought and sold. But now, brought face to face, these characteristics conflict. Response to debt and gratuitous service seem opposed principles of action.

Perhaps our difficulty results from the fact that we have abstracted the concept of covenant from its original context within the transcendent. The indebtedness of a human being that make his life—however sacrificial—inescapably responsive cannot be fully appreciated by totaling up the varying sacrifices and investments made by others in his favor. Such sacrifices are there; and it is lacking in honesty not to acknowledge them. But the sense that one is inexhaustably the object of gift presupposes a more transcendent source of donative activity than the sum of gifts received from others. For the biblical tradition this transcendent was the secret root of every gift between human beings, of which the human order of giving and receiving could only be a sign. Thus the Jewish scriptures enjoin the covenanted people: when you harvest your crops, do not pick your fields too clean. Leave something for the sojourner for you were once sojourners in Egypt. Farmers obedient to this injunction were responsive, but not simply mathematically responsive to gifts received from the Egyptians or from strangers now drifting through their own land. At the same time, their actions could not be construed as wholly gratuitous. Their ethic of service to the needy flowed from Israel's original and continuing state of neediness and indebtedness before God. Thus action which, at a human level, appears gratuitous, in that it is not provoked by a specific gratuity from another human being, at its deepest level, is but gift answering to gift. This responsivity is theologically expressed in the New Testament as follows: "In this is love, not that we loved God, but that He loved us . . . if God so loved us, we also ought to love one another." (I John 4:10–11) In some such way, covenant ethics shies back from the idealist assumption that professional action is and ought to be wholly gratuitous and from the contractualist assumption that it be carefully governed by quotidian self-interest in every exchange.

A transcendent reference may also be important in laying out not only the proper context in which human service takes place but also the specific standards by which it is measured. Earlier we noted some dangers in reducing rights and duties to the terms of a particular contract. We observed the need for a transcendent norm by which contracts are measured (and limited). By the same token, rights and duties cannot be wholly derived from the particulars of a given covenant. What limits ought to be placed on the demands of an excessively dependent patient? At

what point does the keeping of one covenant do an injustice to obligations entailed in others? These are questions that warn against a covenantal ethics that sentimentalizes any and all involvements, without reference to a transcendent by which they are both justified and measured.

Further Reflections on Covenant

So far we have discussed those features of a covenant that affect the doctor's conduct toward his patient. The concept of covenant has further consequences for the patient's understanding of his role as patient, for the accountability of health institutions, for the placement of institutional priorities within other national commitments, and, finally, for such collateral problems as truth-telling.

Every model for the doctor-patient relationship establishes not only a certain image of the doctor, but also a specific concept of the patient. The image of the doctor as priest or parent encourages dependency in the patient. The image of the doctor as skillful technician encourages the patient to think of himself as passive host to a disease. The doctor and his technical procedures are the only serious agent in the relationship. The image of the doctor as covenanter or contractor bids the patient to become a more active participant both in the prevention and the healing of disease. He must bring a will-to-live and a will-to-health to the partnership.

Differing views of disease are involved in these differing patterns of relationship to the doctor. Disease today is usually interpreted by the layman as an extraordinary state, discrete and episodic, disjunctive from the ordinary condition of health. Illness is a special time when the doctor is in charge and the layman renounces authority over his life. This view, while psychologically understandable, ignores the build-up, during apparent periods of health, of those pathological conditions that invite the dramatic breakdown when the doctor "takes over."

The cardiovascular accident is a case in point. Horacio Fabrega[9] has urged an interpretation of disease and health that respects more fully the processive rather than the episodic character of

both disease and health. This interpretation, I assume, would encourage the doctor to monitor more continuously health and disease than ordinarily occurs today, to share with the patient more fully the information so obtained, and to engage the layperson in a more active collaboration with the doctor in health maintenance.

The concept of covenant has two further advantages for defining the professional relationship, not enjoyed by models such as parent, friend, or technician. First, covenant is not so restrictively personal a term as parent or friend. It reminds the professional community that it is not good enough for the individual doctor to be a good friend or parent to the patient, it is important also that whole institutions— the hospital, the clinic, the professional group—keep covenant with those who seek their assistance and sanctuary. Thus the concept permits a certain broadening of accountability beyond personal agency.

At the same time, however, the notion of covenant also permits one to set professional responsibility for this one human good (health) within social limits. The professional covenant concerning health should be situated within a larger set of covenant obligations that both the doctor and patient have to other institutions and priorities within the society at large. The traditional models for the doctor-patient relationship (parent, friend) tend to establish an exclusivity of relationship that obscures these larger responsibilities. At a time when health needs command $120 billion out of the national budget, one must think about the place that the obligation to the limited human good of health has amongst a whole range of social and personal goods for which men are compacted together as a society.

Although a covenantal ethic has implications for other collateral problems in biomedical ethics, I will restrict myself simply to one final issue that has not been viewed from the perspective of covenant: the question of truth-telling.

Key ingredients in the notion of covenant are promise and fidelity to promise. The philosopher J. I. Austin drew the distinction, now famous, between two kinds of speech: descriptive and performative utterances. In ordinary declarative or descriptive sentences, one describes a given item within the world. (It is raining. The tumor is malignant. The crisis is past.) In performative utterances, one does not merely describe a world; in effect, one alters the world by introducing an ingredient that would not be there apart from the utterance. Promises are such performative utterances. (I, John, take Thee, Mary. We will defend your country in case of attack. I will not abandon you.) To make or to go back on a promise is a very solemn matter precisely because a promise is world-altering.

In the field of medical ethics, the question of truth-telling has tended to be disposed of entirely as a question of descriptive speech. Should the doctor, as technician, tell the patient he has a malignancy or not? If not, may he lie or must he merely withhold the truth?

The distinction between descriptive and performative speech expands the question of the truth-telling in professional life. The doctor, after all, not only tells descriptive truths, he also makes or implies promises. (I will see you next Tuesday. Despite the fact that I cannot cure you, I will not abandon you.) In brief, the moral question for the doctor is not simply a question of telling truths, but of being true to his promises. Conversely, the total situation for the patient includes not only the disease he's got, but also whether others desert him or stand by him in his extremity. The fidelity of others will not eliminate the disease, but it affects mightily the human context in which the disease runs its course. What the doctor has to offer his patient is not simply proficiency but fidelity.

Perhaps more patients could accept the descriptive truth if they experienced the performative truth. Perhaps also they would be more inclined to believe in the doctor's performative utterances if they were not handed false diagnoses or false promises. That is why a cautiously wise medieval physician once advised his colleagues: "Promise only fidelity!"

The Problem of Discipline Revisited

The conclusion of this essay is not that covenantal ethics should be preferred to the exclusion of some of those values best symbolized by code and contract. If we return to the problem of discipline with which we began, we can see that both alternatives have resources for professional self-criticism.

Those who live by a code of technical proficiency have a standard on the basis of which to discipline their peers. The Hemingway novel, especially *The Sun Also Rises,* is quite clear about this. Those who live by a code know how to ostracize deficient peers. Indeed, any "in-group," professional or otherwise, can be quite ruthless about sorting out those who are "quality" and those who do not have the "goods." Medicine is no exception. Ostracism, in the form of discretely refusing to refer patients to a doctor whose competence is suspected, is probably the commonest and most effective form of discipline in the profession today.

Defendents of an ethic based on code might argue further that deficiencies in enforcement today result largely from too strongly developed a sense of covenantal obligations to colleagues and too weakly developed a sense of code. From this perspective, then, covenant is the source of the problem in the profession rather than the basis for its amendment. Covenantal obligation to colleagues inhibits the enforcement of code.

A code alone, however, will not in and of itself solve the problem of professional discipline. It provides only a basis for excluding from one's own inner circles an incompetent physician. But, as Eliot Freidson has pointed out in *Professional Dominance,* under the present system, the incompetent professional, when he is excluded from a given hospital, group practice, or informal circle of referrals, simply moves his practice and finds another circle of people of equal incompetence in which he can function. It will take a much stronger, more active and internal sense of covenant obligation to patients on the part of the profession to enforce standards within the guild beyond local informal patterns of ostracism. In a mobile society with a scarcity of doctors, local ostracism simply hands on problem physicians to other patients elsewhere. It does not address them.

Code patterns of discipline not only fall short of adequate protection for the patient, they also fail to be collegially responsible to the troubled physician. To ostracize may be the lazy way of handling a colleague when it fails altogether to make a first attempt at remedy and to address the physician himself in his difficulty.

At the same time, it would be unfortunate if the indispensable interest and pride of the medical profession in technical proficiency were allowed to lapse out of an expressed preference for a professional ethic based on covenant. Covenant fidelity to the patient remains unrealized if it does not include proficiency. A rather sentimental existentialism unfortunately assumes that it suffices morally for human beings to be "present" to one another. But in crisis, the ill person needs not simply presence but skill, not just personal concern but highly disciplined services targeted on specific needs. Code behavior, handed down from doctor to doctor, is largely concerned with the transmission of technical skills. Covenant ethics, then, must include rather than exclude the interests of the codes.

Neither does this essay conclude with a preference for covenant to the total exclusion of the interests of enforceable contract. While the reduction of medical ethics to contract alone incurs the danger of minimalism, patients ought to have recourse against those physicians who fail to meet minimal standards. They ought not to be dependent entirely upon disciplinary measures undertaken within the profession. There ought to be appeal to the law in cases of malpractice and for breach of contract explicit or implied.

On the other hand, a legal appeal cannot be sustained in the case of an injustice without assistance and testimony from physicians who take their obligations to patients and their profession seriously. If, in such cases, fellow physicians simply herd around and protect their colleague like a wounded elephant, the patient with just cause is not likely to get far. Thus the instrument of contract and other avenues of legal redress can be sustained only by physicians who have a sense of obligation to the patient and the profession. Needless to say, it would be better for all concerned if professional discipline and continuing education were so vigorously pursued within the profession as to cut down drastically on the number of cases that needed to reach the courts.

The author inclines to accept covenant as the most inclusive and satisfying model for framing questions of professional obligation. Covenant fidelity includes the code duty to become technically proficient; it includes the obligation to meet the minimal terms of contract, but it also requires much more. Moreover, this surplus of obligation may be to the final advantage not only of patients but also of colleagues. The Marcus case, or, if not that one, others like it, suggest a failure in covenant responsibilities not only to patients but to troubled colleagues.

Notes

1. *The Idea of a Social Science and its Relation to Philosphy* (New York: Humanities Press, 1958).

2. A paraphrase of Rom. 4:5–8 and I Cor. 10:31.

3. The most striking contemporary restatement of an ethic based on covenant is offered by Hemingway's great competitor and contemporary as a novelist—William Faulkner. See especially "Delta Autumn" and "The Bear" and *Intruder in the Dust.*

4. See P. Lain-Entralgo, *Doctor and Patient* (New York: McGraw-Hill, 1969), for his analysis of the classical fusion of *techne* with *philanthropia*, skill in the art of healing combined with a love of mankind defines the good physician.

5. *New York Times,* Op. Ed. Page, June 6, 1975.

6. Sir Henry Sumner Maine, *Ancient Law* (London: Oxford University Press, 1931).

7. Titmuss does not acknowledge that physicians in the United States have helped prepare for this commercialization of medicine by their substantial fees for services (as opposed to salaried professors in the teaching field or salaried health professionals in other countries).

8. Reprinted as Chapter 55 of this volume.

9. Horacio Fabrega, Jr., "Concepts of Disease: Logical Features and Social Implications," *Perspectives in Biology and Medicine,* Vol. 15, No. 4, Summer 1972.

Moral Bases of Medical Ethics

Introduction to Part II

Difficult decisions in contemporary medicine, whether arising out of new technologies such as respirators and kidney machines or from an increased emphasis on the rationality and autonomy of those who seek the professional services of medicine, are straining our courage and ability to make moral decisions that are satisfying and acceptable both to doctors and patients. In such a situation, it seems especially important to look at some of the best and representative thinking on principles of ethics as well as some of the contemporary efforts to apply and relate these to medicine.

From at least the time of Socrates, ethics has been engaged in a lively struggle against those who would undermine the usefulness of reasoned discourse about what is right or wrong. The struggle of Socrates against sophistry and cynicism about the possibility of articulating basic moral principles is as much with us today as it was twenty-five centuries ago. The attempt to identify moral principles is also a scientific effort to discover certain basic moral elements of our common life and to substitute as nearly as possible rational persuasion for sheer struggles of power and violent conflict.

Principles of Ethics

Major modes of moral reasoning and of thinking about the rationality of moral principles are considered in this subsection. The selections from the work of John Stuart Mill relate some of the clearest and most plausible statements of a utilitarian way of thinking about what makes actions right or wrong. Included in these excerpts from Mill is a concise statement of how utilitarians have tended to see the notion of justice. But in both our ordinary reasoning and in the discipline of ethics over the centuries, there is a constant debate over the extent to which it is reasonable or even moral to think in a utilitarian way about what is right or wrong. One of the most succinct and influential challenges to Mill and other utilitarian thinkers is the selection from Sir William David

Ross. Ross is not denying the moral significance of thinking about consequences. He is trying to show, among other things, that the morally significant relations in which we stand to various individuals, groups, and institutions are not exhaustively described by thinking about how we or they will be affected by the consequences of our behavior. Other morally significant relations derive from past and present interactions, such as the promises we have made and are making, or the debts we have incurred or are incurring.

It can be argued that justice is one of the most important moral principles, particularly where we are trying to assess the fairness of dealing with diverse interests and conflicts of interests, as one must in medicine. Because Ross does not have any extended discussion of justice, it is important to provide a significant challenge to Mill's utilitarian philosophy. The selection by John Rawls gives us the opportunity to determine which of these views seems more able to express our judgments of equity and fairness.

The selection from H. L. A. Hart is important for at least two reasons: as its title indicates, it delineates the way in which moral reasoning and moral principles relate to what a society puts into the form of laws and regulations it wishes in one way or another to enforce. On the other hand, this same essay, masterful in its conciseness and precision, offers some brief arguments for why it is rational for society to evolve and defend certain very basic moral rules or principles.

Ethics and Medicine

The major questions of ethics are outlined and discussed in the article by Arthur J. Dyck. Each of these major questions of ethics and of moral reasoning arise within the practice and thinking of the medical profession. Without denying some of the unique contributions that come from medical professionals themselves, the article illustrates some of the most practically vital ways in which moral reasoning occurs within and applies to medicine.

The essay by Paul Ramsey is another view of how ordinary moral reasoning and the reflection on it by ethicists intertwines with medical ethics as a professional enterprise. Ramsey's essay has the additional virtue of arguing for a certain way of conceptualizing moral bases of medical decision-making.

"Conceptual Foundations for an Ethics of Medical Care" is a collaborative effort by a religious ethicist, Albert R. Jonsen, and an ethically sensitive physician, Andre E. Hellegers. They argue that although rational conceptions of justice are essential to maintaining high ethical standards in medicine, they have not received as much attention as necessary.

In her intriguing essay, Sissela Bok analyzes various codes that have contributed to setting professional standards in medicine. From this analysis, she gleans valuable knowledge and insight into the way and the extent that medical standards as reflected in these codes have embodied some of the basic moral principles of ordinary moral discourse long pondered by philosophers and theologians. Like Jonsen and Hellegers, she notes a relative neglect of explicit attention to justice despite its obvious relevance to medicine. From this point of view, we have included selections on justice in this and other sections, particularly in Part VIII on rights and priorities in the provision of medical care.

Principles of Ethics

15

John Stuart Mill
From *Utilitarianism*

Reprinted from John Stuart Mill,
Utilitarianism, 4th ed. (London:
Longmans, Green, Reader, and Dyer,
1871), Chapter 2, pp. 8–31, Chapter 5,
pp. 88–96.

What Utilitarianism Is

A passing remark is all that needs be given to the ignorant blunder of supposing that those who stand up for utility as the test of right and wrong, use the term in that restricted and merely colloquial sense in which utility is opposed to pleasure. An apology is due to the philosophical opponents of utilitarianism, for even the momentary appearance of confounding them with any one capable of so absurd a misconception; which is the more extraordinary, inasmuch as the contrary accusation, of referring everything to pleasure, and that too in its grossest form, is another of the common charges against utilitarianism: and, as has been pointedly remarked by an able writer, the same sort of persons, and often the very same persons, denounce the theory "as impracticably dry when the word utility precedes the word pleasure, and as too practicably voluptuous when the word pleasure precedes the word utility." Those who know anything about the matter are aware that every writer, from Epicurus to Bentham, who maintained the theory of utility, meant by it, not something to be contradistinguished from pleasure, but pleasure itself, together with exemption from pain; and instead of opposing the useful to the agreeable or the ornamental, have always declared that the useful means these, among other things. Yet the common herd, including the herd of writers, not only in newspapers and periodicals, but in books of weight and pretension, are perpetually falling into this shallow mistake. Having caught up the word utilitarian, while knowing nothing whatever about it but its sound, they habitually express by it the rejection, or the neglect, of pleasure in some of its forms; of beauty, of ornament, or of amusement. Nor is the term thus ignorantly misapplied solely in disparagement, but occasionally in compliment; as though it implied superiority to frivolity and the mere pleasures of the moment. And this perverted use is the only one in which the word is popularly known, and the one from which the new generation are acquiring their sole notion of its meaning. Those who introduced the word, but who had for many years discontinued it as a distinctive appellation, may well feel themselves called upon to resume it, if by doing so they can hope to contribute anything towards rescuing it from this utter degradation.[1]

The creed which accepts as the foundation of morals, Utility, or the Greatest Happiness Principle, holds that actions are right in proportion as they tend to promote happiness, wrong as they tend to produce the reverse of happiness. By happiness is intended pleasure, and the absence of pain; by unhappiness, pain, and the privation of pleasure. To give a clear view of the moral standard set up by the theory, much more requires to be said; in particular, what things it includes in the ideas of pain and pleasure; and to what extent this is left an open question. But these supplementary explanations do not affect the theory of life on which this theory of morality is grounded—namely, that pleasure, and freedom from pain, are the only things desirable as ends; and that all desirable things (which are as numerous in the utilitarian as in any other scheme) are desirable either for the pleasure inherent in themselves, or as means to the promotion of pleasure and the prevention of pain.

Now, such a theory of life excites in many minds, and among them in some of the most estimable in feeling and purpose, inveterate dislike. To suppose that life has (as they express it) no higher end than pleasure—no better and nobler object of desire and pursuit—they designate as utterly mean and grovelling; as a doctrine worthy only of swine, to whom the followers of Epicurus were, at a very early period, contemptuously likened; and modern holders of the doctrine are occasionally made the subject of equally polite comparisons by its German, French, and English assailants.

When thus attacked, the Epicureans have always answered, that it is not they, but their accusers, who represent human nature in a degrading light; since the accusation supposes human beings to be capable of no pleasures except those of which swine are capable. If this supposition were true, the charge could not be gainsaid, but would then be no longer an imputation; for if the sources of pleasure were precisely the same to human beings and to swine, the rule of life which is good enough for the one would be good enough for the other. The comparison of the Epicurean life to that of beasts is felt as degrading, precisely because a beast's pleasures do not satisfy a human being's conceptions of happiness. Human beings have faculties more elevated than the animal appetites, and when once made conscious of them, do not regard anything as happiness which does not include their gratification. I do not, indeed, consider the Epicureans to have been by any means faultless in drawing out their scheme of consequences from the utilitarian principle. To do this in any sufficient manner, many Stoic, as well as Christian elements require to be included. But there is no known Epicurean theory of life which does not assign to the pleasures of the intellect, of the feelings and imagination, and of the moral sentiments, a much higher value as pleasures than to those of mere sensation. It must be admitted, however, that utilitarian writers in general have placed the superiority of mental over bodily pleasures chiefly in the greater permanency, safety, uncostliness, etc. of the former—that is, in their circumstantial advantages rather than in their intrinsic nature. And on all these points utilitarians have fully proved their case; but they might have taken the other, and, as it may be called, higher ground, with entire consistency. It is quite compatible with the principle of utility to recognise the fact, that some *kinds* of pleasure are more desirable and more valuable than others. It would be absurd that while, in estimating all other things, quality is considered as well as quantity, the estimation of pleasures should be supposed to depend on quantity alone.

If I am asked, what I mean by difference in quality in pleasures, or what makes one pleasure more valuable than another, merely as a pleasure, except its being greater in amount, there is but one possible answer. Of two pleasures, if there be one to which all or almost all who have experience of both give a decided preference, irrespective of any feeling of moral obligation to prefer it, that is the more desirable pleasure. If one of the two is, by those who are competently acquainted with both, placed so far above the other that they prefer it, even though knowing it to be attended with a greater amount of discontent, and would not resign it for any quantity of the other pleasure which their nature is capable of, we are justified in ascribing to the preferred enjoyment a superiority in quality, so far outweighing quantity as to render it, in comparison, of small account.

Now it is an unquestionable fact that those who are equally acquainted with, and equally capable of appreciating and enjoying, both, do give a most marked preference to the manner of existence which employs their higher faculties. Few human creatures would consent to be changed into any of the lower animals, for a promise of the fullest allowance of a beast's pleasures; no intelligent human being would consent to be a fool, no instructed person would be an ignoramus, no person of feeling and conscience would be selfish and base, even though they should be persuaded that the fool, the dunce, or the rascal is better satisfied with his lot than they are with theirs. They would not resign what they possess more than he, for the most complete satisfaction of all the desires which they have in common with him. If they ever fancy they would, it is only in cases of unhappiness so extreme, that to escape from it they would exchange their lot for almost any other, however undesirable in their own eyes. A being of higher faculties requires more to make him happy, is capable probably of more acute suffering, and is certainly accessible to it at more points, than one of an inferior type; but in spite of these liabilities, he can never really wish to sink into what he feels to be a lower grade of existence. We may give what explanation we please of this unwillingness; we may attribute it to pride, a name which is given indiscriminately to some of the most and to some of the least estimable feelings of which mankind are capable; we may refer it to the love of liberty and personal independence, an appeal to which was with the Stoics one of the most effective means for the inculcation of it; to the love of power, or to the love of excitement, both of which do really enter into and contribute to it: but its most appropriate appellation is a sense of dignity, which all human beings possess in one form or other, and in some, though by no means in exact, proportion to their higher faculties, and which is so essential a part of the happiness of those in whom it is strong, that nothing which conflicts with it could be, otherwise than momentarily, an object of desire to them. Whoever supposes that this preference takes place at a sacrifice of happiness—that the superior being, in anything like equal circumstances, is not happier than the inferior—confounds the two very different ideas, of happiness, and content. It is indisputable that the being whose capacities of enjoyment are low, has the greatest chance of having them fully satisfied; and a highly-endowed being will always feel that any happiness which he can look for, as the world is constituted, is imperfect. But he can learn to bear its imperfections, if they are at all bearable; and they will not make him envy the being who is indeed unconscious of the imperfections, but only because he feels not at all the good which those imperfections qualify. It is better to be a human being dissatisfied than a pig satisfied; better to be Socrates dissatisfied than a fool satisfied. And if the fool, or the pig, is of a different opinion, it is because they only know their own side of the question. The other party to the comparison knows both sides.

It may be objected, that many who are capable of the higher pleasures, occasionally, under the influence of temptation, postpone them to the lower. But this is quite compatible with a full appreciation of the intrinsic superiority of the higher. Men often, from infirmity of character, make their election for the nearer good, though they know it to be the less valuable; and this no less when the choice is between two bodily pleasures, than when it is between bodily and mental. They pursue sensual indulgences to the injury of health, though perfectly aware that health is the greater good. It may be further objected, that many who begin with youthful enthusiasm for everything noble, as they advance in years sink into indolence and selfishness. But I do not believe that those who undergo this very common change, voluntarily choose the lower description of pleasures in preference to the higher. I believe that before they devote themselves exclusively to the one, they have already become incapable of the other. Capacity for the nobler feelings is in most natures a very tender plant, easily killed, not only by hostile influences, but by mere want of sustenance; and in the majority of young persons it speedily dies away if the occupations to which their position in life has devoted them, and the society into which it has thrown them, are not favourable to keeping that higher capacity in exercise. Men lose their high aspirations as they lose their intellectual tastes, because they have not time or opportunity for indulging them; and they addict themselves to inferior pleasures, not because they deliberately prefer them, but because they are either the only ones to which they have access, or the only ones which they are any longer capable of enjoying. It may be questioned whether any one who has remained equally susceptible to both classes of pleasures, ever knowingly and calmly preferred the lower; though many, in all ages, have broken down in an ineffectual attempt to combine both.

From this verdict of the only competent judges, I apprehend there can be no appeal. On a question which is the best worth having of two pleasures, or which of two modes of existence is the most grateful to the feelings, apart from its moral attributes and from its consequences, the judgment of those who are qualified by knowledge of both, or, if they differ, that of the majority among them, must be admitted as final. And there needs be the less hesitation to accept this judgment respecting the quality of pleasures, since there is no other tribunal to be referred to even on the question of quantity. What means are there of determining which is the acutest of two pains, or the intensest of two pleasurable sensations, except the general suffrage of those who are familiar with both? Neither pains nor pleasures are homogeneous, and pain is always heterogeneous with pleasure. What is there to decide whether a particular pleasure is worth purchasing at the cost of a particular pain, except the feelings and judgment of the experienced? When, therefore, those feelings and judgment declare the pleasures derived from the higher faculties to be preferable *in kind*, apart from the question of intensity, to those of which the animal nature, disjoined from the higher faculties, is susceptible, they are entitled on this subject to the same regard.

I have dwelt on this point, as being a necessary part of a perfectly just conception of Utility or Happiness, considered as the directive rule of human conduct. But it is by no means an indispensable condition to the acceptance of the utilitarian standard; for that standard is not the agent's own greatest happiness, but the greatest amount of happiness altogether; and if it may possibly be doubted whether a noble character is always the happier for its nobleness, there can be no doubt that it makes other people happier, and that the world in general is immensely a gainer by it. Utilitarianism, therefore, could only attain its end by the general cultivation of nobleness of character, even if each individual were only benefited by the nobleness of others, and his own, so far as happiness is concerned, were a sheer deduction from the benefit. But the bare enunciation of such an absurdity as this last, renders refutation superfluous.

According to the Greatest Happiness Principle, as above explained, the ultimate end, with reference to and for the sake of which all other things are desirable (whether we are considering our own good or that of other people), is an existence exempt as far as possible from pain, and as rich as possible in enjoyments, both in point of quantity and quality; the test of quality, and the rule for measuring it against quantity, being the preference felt by those who, in their opportunities of experience, to which must be added their habits of self-consciousness and self-observation, are best furnished with the means of comparison. This, being, according to the utilitarian opinion, the end of human action, is necessarily also the standard of morality; which may accordingly be defined, the rules and precepts for human conduct, by the observance of which an existence such as has been described might be, to the greatest extent possible, secured to all mankind; and not to them only, but, so far as the nature of things admits, to the whole sentient creation.

Against this doctrine, however, arises another class of objectors, who say that happiness, in any form, cannot be the rational purpose of human life and action; because, in the first place, it is unattainable: and they contemptuously ask, What right hast thou to be happy? a question which Mr. Carlyle clenches by the addition, What right, a short time ago, hadst thou even *to be?* Next, they say, that men can do *without* happiness; that all noble human beings have felt this, and could not have become noble but by learning the lesson of Entsagen, or renunciation; which lesson, thoroughly learnt and submitted to, they affirm to be the beginning and necessary condition of all virtue.

The first of these objections would go to the root of the matter were it well founded; for if no happiness is to be had at all by human beings, the attainment of it cannot be the end of morality, or of any rational conduct. Though, even in that case, something might still be said for the utilitarian theory; since utility includes not solely the pursuit of happiness, but the prevention or mitigation of unhappiness; and if the former aim be chimerical, there will be all the greater scope and more imperative need for the latter, so long at least as mankind think fit to live, and do not take refuge in the simultaneous act of suicide recommended under certain conditions by Novalis. When, however, it is thus positively asserted to be impossible that human life should be happy, the assertion, if not something like a verbal quibble, is at least an exaggeration. If by happiness be meant a continuity of highly pleasurable excitement, it is evident enough that this is impossible. A state of exalted pleasure lasts only moments, or in some cases, and with some intermissions, hours or days, and is the occasional brilliant flash of enjoyment, not its permanent and steady flame. Of this the philosophers who have taught that happiness is the end of life were as fully aware as those who taunt them. The happiness which they meant was not a life of rapture; but moments of such, in an existence made up of few and transitory pains, many and various pleasures, with a decided predominance of the active over the passive, and having as the foundation of the whole, not to expect more from life than it is capable of bestowing. A life thus composed, to those who have been fortunate enough to obtain it, has always appeared worthy of the name of happiness. And such an existence is even now the lot of many, during some considerable portion of

their lives. The present wretched education, and wretched social arrangements, are the only real hindrance to its being attainable by almost all.

The objectors perhaps may doubt whether human beings, if taught to consider happiness as the end of life, would be satisfied with such a moderate share of it. But great numbers of mankind have been satisfied with much less. The main constituents of a satisfied life appear to be two, either of which by itself is often found sufficient for the purpose: tranquillity, and excitement. With much tranquillity, many find that they can be content with very little pleasure: with much excitement, many can reconcile themselves to a considerable quantity of pain. There is assuredly no inherent impossibility in enabling even the mass of mankind to unite both; since the two are so far from being incompatible that they are in natural alliance, the prolongation of either being a preparation for, and exciting a wish for, the other. It is only those in whom indolence amounts to a vice, that do not desire excitement after an interval of repose; it is only those in whom the need of excitement is a disease, that feel the tranquillity which follows excitement dull and insipid, instead of pleasurable in direct proportion to the excitement which preceded it. When people who are tolerably fortunate in their outward lot do not find in life sufficient enjoyment to make it valuable to them, the cause generally is, caring for nobody but themselves. To those who have neither public nor private affections, the excitements of life are much curtailed, and in any case dwindle in value as the time approaches when all selfish interests must be terminated by death: while those who leave after them objects of personal affection, and especially those who have also cultivated a fellow-feeling with the collective interests of mankind, retain as lively an interest in life on the eve of death as in the vigour of youth and health. Next to selfishness, the principal cause which makes life unsatisfactory, is want of mental cultivation. A cultivated mind—I do not mean that of a philosopher, but any mind to which the fountains of knowledge have been opened, and which has been taught, in any tolerable degree, to exercise its faculties—finds sources of inexhaustible interest in all

that surrounds it; in the objects of nature, the achievements of art, the imaginations of poetry, the incidents of history, the ways of mankind past and present, and their prospects in the future. It is possible, indeed, to become indifferent to all this, and that too without having exhausted a thousandth part of it; but only when one has had from the beginning no moral or human interest in these things, and has sought in them only the gratification of curiosity.

Now there is absolutely no reason in the nature of things why an amount of mental culture sufficient to give an intelligent interest in these objects of contemplation, should not be the inheritance of every one born in a civilized country. As little is there an inherent necessity that any human being should be a selfish egotist, devoid of every feeling or care but those which centre in his own miserable individuality. Something far superior to this is sufficiently common even now, to give ample earnest of what the human species may be made. Genuine private affections, and a sincere interest in the public good, are possible, though in unequal degrees, to every rightly brought up human being. In a world in which there is so much to interest, so much to enjoy, and so much also to correct and improve, every one who has this moderate amount of moral and intellectual requisites is capable of an existence which may be called enviable; and unless such a person, through bad laws, or subjection to the will of others, is denied the liberty to use the sources of happiness within his reach, he will not fail to find this enviable existence, if he escape the positive evils of life, the great sources of physical and mental suffering—such as indigence, disease, and the unkindness, worthlessness, or premature loss of objects of affection. The main stress of the problem lies, therefore, in the contest with these calamities, from which it is a rare good fortune entirely to escape; which, as things now are, cannot be obviated, and often cannot be in any material degree mitigated. Yet no one whose opinion deserves a moment's consideration can doubt that most of the great positive evils of the world are in themselves removable, and will, if human affairs continue to improve, be in the end reduced within narrow limits. Poverty, in any sense implying suffering, may be completely extinguished by the wisdom of society, combined with the good sense and providence of individuals. Even that most intractable of enemies, disease, may be indefinitely reduced in dimensions by good physical and moral education, and proper control of noxious influences; while the progress of science holds out a promise for the future of still more direct conquests over this detestable foe. And every advance in that direction relieves us from some, not only of the chances which cut short our own lives, but, what concerns us still more, which deprives us of those in whom our happiness is wrapt up. As for vicissitudes of fortune, and other disappointments connected with worldly circumstances, these are principally the effect either of gross imprudence, of ill-regulated desires, or of bad or imperfect social institutions. All the grand sources, in short, of human suffering are in a great degree, many of them almost entirely, conquerable by human care and effort; and though their removal is grievously slow—though a long succession of generations will perish in the breach before the conquest is completed, and this world becomes all that if will and knowledge were not wanting, it might easily be made—yet every mind sufficiently intelligent and generous to bear a part, however small and unconspicuous, in the endeavor, will draw a noble enjoyment from the contest itself, which he would not for any bribe in the form of selfish indulgence consent to be without.

And this leads to the true estimation of what is said by the objectors concerning the possibility, and the obligation, of learning to do without happiness. Unquestionably it is possible to do without happiness; it is done involuntarily by nineteen-twentieths of mankind, even in those parts of our present world which are least deep in barbarism; and it often has to be done voluntarily by the hero or the martyr, for the sake of something which he prizes more than his individual happiness. But this something, what is it, unless the happiness of others, or some of the requisites of happiness? It is noble to be capable of resigning entirely one's own portion of happiness, or

chances of it: but, after all, this self-sacrifice must be for some end; it is not its own end; and if we are told that its end is not happiness, but virtue, which is better than happiness, I ask, would the sacrifice be made if the hero or martyr did not believe that it would earn for others immunity from similar sacrifices? Would it be made, if he thought that his renunciation of happiness for himself would produce no fruit for any of his fellow creatures, but to make their lot like his, and place them also in the condition of persons who have renounced happiness? All honour to those who can abnegate for themselves the personal enjoyment of life, when by such renunciation they contribute worthily to increase the amount of happiness in the world; but he who does it, or professes to do it, for any other purpose, is no more deserving of admiration than the ascetic mounted on his pillar. He may be an inspiriting proof of what men *can* do, but assuredly not an example of what they *should*.

Though it is only in a very imperfect state of the world's arrangements that any one can best serve the happiness of others by the absolute sacrifice of his own, yet so long as the world is in that imperfect state, I fully acknowledge that the readiness to make such a sacrifice is the highest virtue which can be found in man. I will add, that in this condition of the world, paradoxical as the assertion may be, the conscious ability to do without happiness gives the best prospect of realizing such happiness as is attainable. For nothing except that consciousness can raise a person above the chances of life, by making him feel that, let fate and fortune do their worst, they have not power to subdue him: which, once felt, frees him from excess of anxiety concerning the evils of life, and enables him, like many a Stoic in the worst times of the Roman Empire, to cultivate in tranquillity the sources of satisfaction accessible to him, without concerning himself about the uncertainty of their duration, any more than about their inevitable end.

Meanwhile, let utilitarians never cease to claim the morality of self-devotion as a possession which belongs by as good a right to them, as either to the Stoic or to the Transcendentalist. The utilitarian morality does recognise in human beings the

power of sacrificing their own greatest good for the good of others. It only refuses to admit that the sacrifice is itself a good. A sacrifice which does not increase, or tend to increase, the sum total of happiness, it considers as wasted. The only self-renunciation which it applauds, is devotion to the happiness, or to some of the means of happiness, of others; either of mankind collectively, or of individuals within the limits imposed by the collective interests of mankind.

I must again repeat, what the assailants of utilitarianism seldom have the justice to acknowledge, that the happiness which forms the utilitarian standard of what is right in conduct, is not the agent's own happiness, but that of all concerned. As between his own happiness and that of others, utilitarianism requires him to be as strictly impartial as a disinterested and benevolent spectator. In the golden rule of Jesus of Nazareth, we read the complete spirit of the ethics of utility. To do as one would be done by, and to love one's neighbour as oneself, constitute the ideal perfection of utilitarian morality. As the means of making the nearest approach to this ideal, utility would enjoin, first, that laws and social arrangements should place the happiness, or (as speaking practically it may be called) the interest, of every individual, as nearly as possible in harmony with the interest of the whole; and secondly, that education and opinion, which have so vast a power over human character, should so use that power as to establish in the mind of every individual an indissoluble association between his own happiness and the good of the whole; especially between his own happiness and the practice of such modes of conduct, negative and positive, as regard for the universal happiness prescribes: so that not only he may be unable to conceive the possibility of happiness to himself, consistently with conduct opposed to the general good, but also that a direct impulse to promote the general good may be in every individual one of the habitual motives of action, and the sentiments connected therewith may fill a large and prominent place in every human being's sentient existence. If the impugners of the utilitarian morality represented it to their own minds in this its true character, I know not what recommendation possessed by any other morality they could possibly affirm to be wanting to it: what more beautiful or more exalted developments of human nature any other ethical system can be supposed to foster, or what springs of action, not accessible to the utilitarian, such systems rely on for giving effect to their mandates.

The objectors to utilitarianism cannot always be charged with representing it in a discreditable light. On the contrary, those among them who entertain anything like a just idea of its disinterested character, sometimes find fault with its standard as being too high for humanity. They say it is exacting too much to require that people shall always act from the inducement of promoting the general interests of society. But this is to mistake the very meaning of a standard of morals, and to confound the rule of action with the motive of it. It is the business of ethics to tell us what are our duties, or by what test we may know them; but no system of ethics requires that the sole motive of all we do shall be a feeling of duty; on the contrary, ninety-nine hundredths of all our actions are done from other motives, and rightly so done, if the rule of duty does not condemn them. It is the more unjust to utilitarianism that this particular misapprehension should be made a ground of objection to it, inasmuch as utilitarian moralists have gone beyond almost all others in affirming that the motive has nothing to do with the morality of the action, though much with the worth of the agent. He who saves a fellow creature from drowning does what is morally right, whether his motive be duty, or the hope of being paid for his trouble: he who betrays the friend that trusts him, is guilty of a crime, even if his object be to serve another friend to whom he is under greater obligations.[2] But to speak only of actions done from the motive of duty, and in direct obedience to principle: it is a misapprehension of the utilitarian mode of thought, to conceive it as implying that people should fix their minds upon so wide a generality as the world, or society at large. The great majority of good actions are intended, not for the benefit of the world, but for that of individuals, of which the good of the world is made up; and the thoughts of the most virtuous man need not on these occasions travel beyond the particular persons concerned, except so far as is necessary to assure himself that in benefiting them he is not violating the rights—that is, the legitimate and authorized expectations—of any one else. The multiplication of happiness is, according to the utilitarian ethics, the object of virtue: the occasions on which any person (except one in a thousand) has it in his power to do this on an extended scale, in other words, to be a public benefactor, are but exceptional; and on these occasions alone is he called on to consider public utility; in every other case, private utility, the interest or happiness of some few persons, is all he has to attend to. Those alone the influence of whose actions extends to society in general, need concern themselves habitually about so large an object. In the case of abstinences indeed—of things which people forbear to do, from moral considerations, though the consequences in the particular case might be beneficial—it would be unworthy of an intelligent agent not to be consciously aware that the action is of a class which, if practised generally, would be generally injurious, and that this is the ground of the obligation to abstain from it. The amount of regard for the public interest implied in this recognition, is no greater than is demanded by every system of morals; for they all enjoin to abstain from whatever is manifestly pernicious to society.

The same considerations dispose of another reproach against the doctrine of utility, founded on a still grosser misconception of the purpose of a standard of morality, and of the very meaning of the words right and wrong. It is often affirmed that utilitarianism renders men cold and unsympathizing; that it chills their moral feelings towards individuals; that it makes them regard only the dry and hard consideration of the consequences of actions, not taking into their moral estimate the qualities from which those actions emanate. If the assertion means that they do not allow their judgment respecting the rightness or wrongness of an action to be influenced by their opinion of the qualities of the person who does it, this is a complaint not against utilitarianism, but against having any standard of morality at all; for certainly no known ethical standard decides an action to be good or bad because it is done by a good or a bad man, still less because done by an amiable, a brave, or a benevolent man, or the contrary. These considerations are relevant, not to the estimation of actions, but of persons; and there is nothing in the utilitarian theory inconsistent with the fact that there are other things which interest us in persons besides the rightness and wrongness of their actions. The Stoics, indeed, with the paradoxical misuse of language which was part of their system, and by which they strove to raise themselves above all concern about anything but virtue, were fond of saying that he who has that has everything; that he, and only he, is rich, is beautiful, is a king. But no claim of this description is made for the virtuous man by the utilitarian doctrine. Utilitarians are quite aware that there are other desirable possessions and qualities besides virtue, and are perfectly willing to allow to all of them their full worth. They are also aware that a right action does not necessarily indicate a virtuous character, and that actions which are blameable often proceed from qualities entitled to praise. When this is apparent in any particular case, it modifies their estimation, not certainly of the act, but of the agent. I grant that they are, notwithstanding, of opinion, that in the long run the best proof of a good character is good actions; and resolutely refuse to consider any mental disposition as good, of which the predominant tendency is to produce bad conduct. This makes them unpopular with many people; but it is an unpopularity which they must share with every one who regards the distinction between right and wrong in a serious light; and the reproach is not one which a conscientious utilitarian need be anxious to repel.

If no more be meant by the objection than that many utilitarians look on the morality of actions, as measured by the utilitarian standard, with too exclusive a regard, and do not lay sufficient stress upon the other beauties of character which go towards making a human being loveable or admirable, this may be admitted. Utilitarians who have cultivated their moral feelings, but not their sympathies nor their artistic perceptions, do fall into this mistake;

and so do all other moralists under the same conditions. What can be said in excuse for other moralists is equally available for them, namely, that if there is to be any error, it is better that it should be on that side. As a matter of fact, we may affirm that among utilitarians as among adherents of other systems, there is every imaginable degree of rigidity and of laxity in the application of their standard: some are even puritanically rigorous, while others are as indulgent as can possibly be desired by sinner or by sentimentalist. But on the whole, a doctrine which brings prominently forward the interest that mankind have in the repression and prevention of conduct which violates the moral law, is likely to be inferior to no other in turning the sanctions of opinion against such violations. It is true, the question, What does violate the moral law? is one on which those who recognise different standards of morality are likely now and then to differ. But difference of opinion on moral questions was not first introduced into the world by utilitarianism, while that doctrine does supply, if not always an easy, at all events a tangible and intelligible mode of deciding such differences. . . .

Is, then, the difference between the Just and the Expedient a merely imaginary distinction? Have mankind been under a delusion in thinking that justice is a more sacred thing than policy, and that the latter ought only to be listened to after the former has been satisfied? By no means. The exposition we have given of the nature and origin of the sentiment, recognises a real distinction; and no one of those who profess the most sublime contempt for the consequences of actions as an element in their morality, attaches more importance to the distinction than I do. While I dispute the pretensions of any theory which sets up an imaginary standard of justice not grounded on utility, I account the justice which is grounded on utility to be the chief part, and incomparably the most sacred and binding part, of all morality. Justice is a name for certain classes of moral rules, which concern the essentials of human well-being more nearly, and are therefore of more absolute obligation, than any other rules for the guidance of life;

and the notion which we have found to be of the essence of the idea of justice, that of a right residing in an individual, implies and testifies to this more binding obligation.

The moral rules which forbid mankind to hurt one another (in which we must never forget to include wrongful interference with each other's freedom) are more vital to human well-being than any maxims, however important, which only point out the best mode of managing some department of human affairs. They have also the peculiarity, that they are the main element in determining the whole of the social feelings of mankind. It is their observance which alone preserves peace among human beings: if obedience to them were not the rule, and disobedience the exception, every one would see in every one else a probable enemy, against whom he must be perpetually guarding himself. What is hardly less important, these are the precepts which mankind have the strongest and the most direct inducements for impressing upon one another. By merely giving to each other prudential instruction or exhortation, they may gain, or think they gain, nothing: in inculcating on each other the duty of positive beneficence they have an unmistakeable interest, but far less in degree: a person may possibly not need the benefits of others; but he always needs that they should not do him hurt. Thus the moralities which protect every individual from being harmed by others, either directly or by being hindered in his freedom of pursuing his own good, are at once those which he himself has most at heart, and those which he has the strongest interest in publishing and enforcing by word and deed. It is by a person's observance of these, that his fitness to exist as one of the fellowship of human beings, is tested and decided; for on that depends his being a nuisance or not to those with whom he is in contact. Now it is these moralities primarily, which compose the obligations of justice. The most marked cases of injustice, and those which give the tone to the feeling of repugnance which characterizes the sentiment, are acts of wrongful aggression, or wrongful exercise of power over some one; the next are those which consist in wrongfully withholding from him something which is his due; in both cases, inflicting on him a positive hurt, either

in the form of direct suffering, or of the privation of some good which he had reasonable ground, either of a physical or of a social kind, for counting upon.

The same powerful motives which command the observance of these primary moralities, enjoin the punishment of those who violate them; and as the impulses of self-defence, of defence of others, and of vengeance, are all called forth against such persons, retribution, or evil for evil, becomes closely connected with the sentiment of justice, and is universally included in the idea. Good for good is also one of the dictates of justice; and this, though its social utility is evident, and though it carries with it a natural human feeling, has not at first sight that obvious connexion with hurt or injury, which, existing in the most elementary cases of just and unjust, is the source of the characteristic intensity of the sentiment. But the connexion, though less obvious, is not less real. He who accepts benefits, and denies a return of them when needed, inflicts a real hurt, by disappointing one of the most natural and reasonable of expectations, and one which he must at least tacitly have encouraged, otherwise the benefits would seldom have been conferred. The important rank, among human evils and wrongs, of the disappointment of expectation, is shown in the fact that it constitutes the principal criminality of two such highly immoral acts as a breach of friendship and a breach of promise. Few hurts which human beings can sustain are greater, and none wound more, than when that on which they habitually and with full assurance relied, fails them in the hour of need; and few wrongs are greater than this mere withholding of good; none excite more resentment, either in the person suffering, or in a sympathizing spectator. The principle, therefore, of giving to each what they deserve, that is, good for good as well as evil for evil, is not only included within the idea of Justice as we have defined it, but is a proper object of that intensity of sentiment, which places the Just, in human estimation, above the simply Expedient.

Most of the maxims of justice current in the world, and commonly appealed to in its transactions, are simply instrumental to carrying into effect the principles of justice which we have now spoken of. That a person is only responsible for what he has done voluntarily, or could voluntarily have avoided; that it is unjust to condemn any person unheard; that the punishment ought to be proportioned to the offence, and the like, are maxims intended to prevent the just principle of evil for evil from being perverted to the infliction of evil without that justification. The greater part of these common maxims have come into use from the practice of courts of justice, which have been naturally led to a more complete recognition and elaboration than was likely to suggest itself to others, of the rules necessary to enable them to fulfil their double function, of inflicting punishment when due, and of awarding to each person his right.

That first of judicial virtues, impartiality, is an obligation of justice, partly for the reason last mentioned; as being a necessary condition of the fulfilment of the other obligations of justice. But this is not the only source of the exalted rank, among human obligations, of those maxims of equality and impartiality, which, both in popular estimation and in that of the most enlightened, are included among the precepts of justice. In one point of view, they may be considered as corollaries from the principles already laid down. If it is a duty to do to each according to his deserts, returning good for good as well as repressing evil by evil, it necessarily follows that we should treat all equally well (when no higher duty forbids) who have deserved equally well of us, and that society should treat all equally well who have deserved equally well of it, that is, who have deserved equally well absolutely. This is the highest abstract standard of social and distributive justice; towards which all institutions, and the efforts of all virtuous citizens, should be made in the utmost possible degree to converge. But this great moral duty rests upon a still deeper foundation, being a direct emanation from the first principle of morals, and not a mere logical corollary from secondary or derivative doctrines. It is involved in the very meaning of Utility, or the Greatest-Happiness Principle. That principle is a mere form of words without rational signification, unless one person's happiness, supposed equal in degree (with the proper allowance made for kind), is counted for exactly as much as

another's. Those conditions being supplied, Bentham's dictum, "everybody to count for one, nobody for more than one," might be written under the principle of utility as an explanatory commentary.[3] The equal claim of everybody to happiness in the estimation of the moralist and the legislator, involves an equal claim to all the means of happiness, except in so far as the inevitable conditions of human life, and the general interest, in which that of every individual is included, set limits to the maxim; and those limits ought to be strictly construed. As every other maxim of justice, so this is by no means applied or held applicable universally; on the contrary, as I have already remarked, it bends to every person's ideas of social expediency. But in whatever case it is deemed applicable at all, it is held to be the dictate of justice. All persons are deemed to have a *right* to equality of treatment, except when some recognised social expediency requires the reverse. And hence all social inequalities which have ceased to be considered expedient, assume the character not of simple inexpediency, but of injustice, and appear so tyrannical, that people are apt to wonder how they ever could have been tolerated; forgetful that they themselves perhaps tolerate other inequalities under an equally mistaken notion of expediency, the correction of which would make that which they approve seem quite as monstrous as what they have at last learnt to condemn. The entire history of social improvement has been a series of transitions, by which one custom or institution after another, from being a supposed primary necessity of social existence, has passed into the rank of an universally stigmatized injustice and tyranny. So it has been with the distinctions of slaves and freemen, nobles and serfs, patricians and plebeians; and so it will be, and in part already is, with the aristocracies of colour, race, and sex.

It appears from what has been said, that justice is a name for certain moral requirements, which, regarded collectively, stand higher in the scale of social utility, and are therefore of more paramount obligation, than any others; though particular cases may occur in

which some other social duty is so important, as to overrule any one of the general maxims of justice. Thus, to save a life, it may not only be allowable, but a duty, to steal, or take by force, the necessary food or medicine, or to kidnap, and compel to officiate, the only qualified medical practitioner. In such cases, as we do not call anything justice which is not a virtue, we usually say, not that justice must give way to some other moral principle, but that what is just in ordinary cases is, by reason of that other principle, not just in the particular case. By this useful accommodation of language, the character of indefeasibility attributed to justice is kept up, and we are saved from the necessity of maintaining that there can be laudable injustice.

The considerations which have now been adduced resolve, I conceive, the only real difficulty in the utilitarian theory of morals. It has always been evident that all cases of justice are also cases of expediency: the difference is in the peculiar sentiment which attaches to the former, as contradistinguished from the latter. If this characteristic sentiment has been sufficiently accounted for; if there is no necessity to assume for it any peculiarity of origin; if it is simply the natural feeling of resentment, moralized by being made coextensive with the demands of social good; and if this feeling not only does but ought to exist in all the classes of cases to which the idea of justice corresponds; that idea no longer presents itself as a stumbling-block to the utilitarian ethics. Justice remains the appropriate name for certain social utilities which are vastly more important, and therefore more absolute and imperative, than any others are as a class (though not more so than others may be in particular cases); and which, therefore, ought to be, as well as naturally are, guarded by a sentiment not only different in degree, but also in kind; distinguished from the milder feeling which attaches to the mere idea of promoting human pleasure or convenience, at once by the more definite nature of its commands, and by the sterner character of its sanctions.

Notes

1. The author of this essay has reason for believing himself to be the first person who brought the word utilitarian into use. He did

not invent it, but adopted it from a passing expression in Mr. Galt's *Annals of the Parish*. After using it as a designation for several years, he and others abandoned it from a growing dislike to anything resembling a badge or watchword of sectarian distinction. But as a name for one single opinion, not a set of opinions—to denote the recognition of utility as a standard, not any particular way of applying it—the term supplies a want in the language, and offers, in many cases, a convenient mode of avoiding tiresome circumlocution.

2. An opponent, whose intellectual and moral fairness it is a pleasure to acknowledge (the Rev. J. Llewellyn Davies), has objected to this passage, saying, "Surely the rightness or wrongness of saving a man from drowning does depend very much upon the motive with which it is done. Suppose that a tyrant, when his enemy jumped into the sea to escape from him, saved him from drowning simply in order that he might inflict upon him more exquisite tortures, would it tend to clearness to speak of that rescue as 'a morally right action'? Or suppose again, according to one of the stock illustrations of ethical inquiries, that a man betrayed a trust received from a friend, because the discharge of it would fatally injure that friend himself or some one belonging to him, would utilitarianism compel one to call the betrayal 'a crime' as much as if it had been done from the meanest motive?"

I submit, that he who saves another from drowning in order to kill him by torture afterwards, does not differ only in motive from him who does the same thing from duty or benevolence; the act itself is different. The rescue of the man is, in the case supposed, only the necessary first step of an act far more atrocious than leaving him to drown would have been. Had Mr. Davies said, "The rightness or wrongness of saving a man from drowning does depend very much"—not upon the motive, but—"upon the *intention*," no utilitarian would have differed from him. Mr. Davies, by an oversight too common not to be quite venial, has in this case confounded the very different ideas of Motive and Intention. There is no point which utilitarian thinkers (and Bentham pre-eminently) have taken more pains to illustrate than this. The morality of the action depends entirely upon the intention—that is, upon what the agent *wills to do*. But the motive, that is, the feeling which makes him will so to do, when it makes no difference in the act, makes none in the morality: though it makes a great difference in our moral estimation of the agent, especially if it indicates a good or a bad habitual *disposition*—a bent of character from which useful, or from which hurtful actions are likely to arise.

3. This implication, in the first principle of the utilitarian scheme, of perfect impartiality between persons, is regarded by Mr. Herbert Spencer (in his "Social Statics") as a disproof of the pretensions of utility to be a sufficient guide to right; since (he says) the principle of utility presupposes the anterior principle, that everybody has an equal right to happiness. It may be more correctly described as supposing that equal amounts of happiness are equally desirable, whether felt by the same or by different persons. This, however, is not a presupposition; not a premise needful to support the principle of utility, but the very principle itself; for what is the principle of utility, if it be not that "happiness" and "desirable" are synonymous terms? If there is any anterior principle implied, it can be no other than this, that the truths of arithmetic are applicable to the valuation of happiness, as of all other measurable quantities.

16

W. D. Ross
From "What Makes Right Acts Right?"

Reprinted by permission of the publisher from W. D. Ross, *The Right and the Good* (Oxford: Clarendon Press 1930), pp. 16–29.

The real point at issue between hedonism and utilitarianism on the one hand and their opponents on the other is not whether "right" means "productive of so and so"; for it cannot with any plausibility be maintained that it does. The point at issue is that to which we now pass, viz. whether there is any general character which makes right acts right, and if so, what it is. Among the main historical attempts to state a single characteristic of all right actions which is the foundation of their rightness are those made by egoism and utilitarianism. But I do not propose to discuss these, not because the subject is unimportant, but because it has been dealt with so often and so well already, and because there has come to be so much agreement among moral philosophers that neither of these theories is satisfactory. A much more attractive theory has been put forward by Professor Moore: that what makes actions right is that they are productive of more *good* than could have been produced by any other action open to the agent.[1]

This theory is in fact the culmination of all the attempts to base rightness on productivity of some sort of result. The first form this attempt takes is the attempt to base rightness on conduciveness to the advantage or pleasure of the agent. This theory comes to grief over the fact, which stares us in the face, that a great part of duty consists in an observance of the rights and a furtherance of the interests of others, whatever the cost to ourselves may be. Plato and others may be right in holding that a regard for the rights of others never in the long run involves a loss of happiness for the agent, that "the just life profits a man." But this, even if true, is irrelevant to the rightness of the act. As soon as a man does an action *because* he thinks he will promote his own interests thereby, he is acting not from a sense of its rightness but from self-interest.

To the egoistic theory hedonistic utilitarianism supplies a much-needed amendment. It points out correctly that the fact that a certain pleasure will be enjoyed by the agent is no reason why he *ought* to bring it into being rather than an equal or greater pleasure to be enjoyed by another, though, human nature being what it is, it makes it not unlikely that he *will* try to bring it into being. But hedonistic utilitarianism in its turn needs a correction. On reflection it seems clear that pleasure is not the only thing in life that we think good in itself, that for instance we think the possession of a good character, or an intelligent understanding of the world, as good or better. A great advance is made by the substitution of "productive of the greatest good" for "productive of the greatest pleasure."

Not only is this theory more attractive than hedonistic utilitarianism, but its logical relation to that theory is such that the latter could not be true unless *it* were true, while it might be true though hedonistic utilitarianism were not. It is in fact one of the logical bases of hedonistic utilitarianism. For the view that what produces the maximum pleasure is right has for its bases the views (1) that what produces the maximum good is right, and (2) that pleasure is the only thing good in itself. If they were not assuming that what produces the maximum *good* is right, the utilitarian's attempt to show that pleasure is the only thing good in itself, which is in fact the point they take most pains to establish, would have been quite irrelevant to their attempt to prove that only what produces the maximum *pleasure* is right. If, therefore, it can be shown that productivity of the maximum good is not what makes all right actions right, we shall a *fortiori* have refuted hedonistic utilitarianism.

When a plain man fulfils a promise because he thinks he ought to do so, it seems clear that he does so with no thought of its total consequences, still less with any opinion that these are likely to be the best possible. He thinks in fact much more of the past than of the future. What makes him think it right to act in a certain way is the fact that he has promised to do so—that and, usually, nothing more. That his act will produce the best possible consequences is not his reason for calling it right. What lends colour to the theory we are examining, then, is not the actions (which form probably a great majority of our actions) in which some such reflection as "I have promised" is the only reason we give ourselves for thinking a certain action right, but the exceptional cases in which the consequences of fulfilling a promise (for instance) would be so disastrous to others that we judge it right not to do so. It must of course be admitted that such cases exist. If I have promised to meet a friend at a particular time for some trivial purpose, I should certainly think myself justified in breaking my engagement if by doing so I could prevent a serious accident or bring relief to the victims of one. And the supporters of the view we are examining hold that my thinking so is due to my thinking that I shall bring more good into existence by the one action than by the other. A different account may, however, be given of the matter, an account which will, I believe, show itself to be the true one. It may be said that besides the duty of fulfilling promises I have and recognize a duty of relieving distress,[2] and that when I think it right to do the latter at the cost of not doing the former, it is not because I think I shall produce more good thereby but because I think it the duty which is in the circumstances more of a duty. This account surely corresponds much more closely with what we really think in such a situation. If, so far as I can see, I could bring equal amounts of good into being by fulfilling my promise and by helping some one to whom I had made no promise, I should not hesitate to regard the former as my duty. Yet on the view that what is right is right because it is productive of the most good I should not so regard it.

There are two theories, each in its way simple, that offer a solution of such cases of conscience. One is the view of Kant, that there are certain duties of perfect obligation, such as those of fulfilling promises, of paying debts, of telling the truth, which admit of no exception whatever in favour of duties of imperfect obligation, such as that of relieving distress. The other is the view of, for instance, Professor Moore and Dr. Rashdall, that there is only the duty of producing good, and that all "conflicts of duties" should be resolved by asking "by which action will most good be produced?" But it is more important that our theory fit the facts than that it be simple, and the account we have given above corresponds (it seems to me) better than either of the simpler theories with what we really think, viz. that normally promise-keeping, for example, should come before benevolence, but that

when and only when the good to be produced by the benevolent act is very great and the promise comparatively trivial, the act of benevolence becomes our duty.

In fact the theory of "ideal utilitarianism," if I may for brevity refer so to the theory of Professor Moore, seems to simplify unduly our relations to our fellows. It says, in effect, that the only morally significant relation in which my neighbours stand to me is that of being possible beneficiaries by my action.[3] They do stand in this relation to me, and this relation is morally significant. But they may also stand to me in the relation of promisee to promiser, of creditor to debtor, of wife to husband, of child to parent, of friend to friend, of fellow countryman to fellow countryman, and the like; and each of these relations is the foundation of a *prima facie* duty, which is more or less incumbent on me according to the circumstances of the case. When I am in a situation, as perhaps I always am, in which more than one of these *prima facie* duties is incumbent on me, what I have to do is to study the situation as fully as I can until I form the considered opinion (it is never more) that in the circumstances one of them is more incumbent than any other; then I am bound to think that to do this *prima facie* duty is my duty *sans phrase* in the situation.

I suggest "*prima facie* duty" or "conditional duty" as a brief way of referring to the characteristic (quite distinct from that of being a duty proper) which an act has, in virtue of being of a certain kind (e.g. the keeping of a promise), of being an act which would be a duty proper if it were not at the same time of another kind which is morally significant. Whether an act is a duty proper or actual duty depends on *all* the morally significant kinds it is an instance of. The phrase "*prima facie* duty" must be apologized for, since (1) it suggests that what we are speaking of is a certain kind of duty, whereas it is in fact not a duty, but something related in a special way to duty. Strictly speaking, we want not a phrase in which duty is qualified by an adjective, but a separate noun. (2) "*Prima*" facie suggests that one is speaking only of an appearance which a moral situation

presents at first sight, and which may turn out to be illusory; whereas what I am speaking of is an objective fact involved in the nature of the situation, or more strictly in an element of its nature, though not, as duty proper does, arising from its *whole* nature. I can, however, think of no term which fully meets the case. "Claim" has been suggested by Professor Prichard. The word "claim" has the advantage of being quite a familiar one in this connexion, and it seems to cover much of the ground. It would be quite natural to say, "a person to whom I have made a promise has a claim on me," and also, "a person whose distress I could relieve (at the cost of breaking the promise) has a claim on me." But (1) while "claim" is appropriate from *their* point of view, we want a word to express the corresponding fact from the agent's point of view—the fact of his being subject to claims that can be made against him; and ordinary language provides us with no such correlative to "claim." And (2) (what is more important) "claim" seems inevitably to suggest two persons, one of whom might make a claim on the other; and while this covers the ground of social duty, it is inappropriate in the case of that important part of duty which is the duty of cultivating a certain kind of character in oneself. It would be artificial, I think, and at any rate metaphorical, to say that one's character has a claim on oneself.

There is nothing arbitrary about these *prima facie* duties. Each rests on a definite circumstance which cannot seriously be held to be without moral significance. Of *prima facie* duties I suggest, without claiming completeness or finality for it, the following division.[4]

(1) Some duties rest on previous acts of my own. These duties seem to include two kinds, (a) those resting on a promise or what may fairly be called an implicit promise, such as the implicit undertaking not to tell lies which seems to be implied in the act of entering into conversation (at any rate by civilized men), or of writing books that purport to be history and not fiction. These may be called the duties of fidelity. (b) Those resting on a previous wrongful act. These may be called the duties of reparation. (2) Some rest on previous acts of other men, i.e. services done by them to me. These may be

loosely described as the duties of gratitude.[5] (3) Some rest on the fact or possibility of a distribution of pleasure or happiness (or of the means thereto) which is not in accordance with the merit of the persons concerned; in such cases there arises a duty to upset or prevent such a distribution. These are the duties of justice. (4) Some rest on the mere fact that there are other beings in the world whose condition we can make better in respect of virtue, or of intelligence, or of pleasure. These are the duties of beneficence. (5) Some rest on the fact that we can improve our own condition in respect of virtue or of intelligence. These are the duties of self-improvement. (6) I think that we should distinguish from (4) the duties that may be summed up under the title of "not injuring others." No doubt to injure others is incidentally to fail to do them good; but it seems to me clear that non-maleficence is apprehended as a duty distinct from that of beneficence, and as a duty of a more stringent character. It will be noticed that this alone among the types of duty has been stated in a negative way. An attempt might no doubt be made to state this duty, like the others, in a positive way. It might be said that it is really the duty to prevent ourselves from acting either from an inclination to harm others or from an inclination to seek our own pleasure, in doing which we should incidentally harm them. But on reflection it seems clear that the primary duty here is the duty not to harm others, this being a duty whether or not we have an inclination that if followed would lead to our harming them; and that when we have such an inclination the primary duty not to harm others gives rise to a consequential duty to resist the inclination. The recognition of this duty of non-maleficence is the first step on the way to the recognition of the duty of beneficence; and that accounts for the prominence of the commands "thou shalt not kill," "thou shalt not commit adultery," "thou shalt not steal," "thou shalt not bear false witness," in so early a code as the Decalogue. But even when we have come to recognize the duty of beneficence, it appears to me that the duty of non-maleficence is recognized as a distinct one, and as *prima facie* more binding. We should

not in general consider it justifiable to kill one person in order to keep another alive, or to steal from one in order to give alms to another.

The essential defect of the "ideal utilitarian" theory is that it ignores, or at least does not do full justice to, the highly personal character of duty. If the only duty is to produce the maximum of good, the question who is to have the good—whether it is myself, or my benefactor, or a person to whom I have made a promise to confer that good on him, or a mere fellow man to whom I stand in no such special relation—should make no difference to my having a duty to produce that good. But we are all in fact sure that it makes a vast difference.

One or two other comments must be made on this provisional list of the divisions of duty. (1) The nomenclature is not strictly correct. For by "fidelity" or "gratitude" we mean, strictly, certain states of motivation; and, as I have urged, it is not our duty to have certain motives, but to do certain acts. By "fidelity," for instance, is meant, strictly, the disposition to fulfil promises and implicit promises *because we have made them*. We have no general word to cover the actual fulfilment of promises and implicit promises *irrespective of motive;* and I use "fidelity," loosely but perhaps conveniently, to fill this gap. So too I use "gratitude" for the returning of services, irrespective of motive. The term "justice" is not so much confined, in ordinary usage, to a certain state of motivation, for we should often talk of a man as acting justly even when we did not think his motive was the wish to do what was just simply for the sake of doing so. Less apology is therefore needed for our use of "justice" in this sense. And I have used the word "beneficence" rather than "benevolence," in order to emphasize the fact that it is our duty to do certain things, and not to do them from certain motives.

(2) If the objection be made, that this catalogue of the main types of duty is an unsystematic one resting on no logical principle, it may be replied, first, that it makes no claim to being ultimate. It is a *prima facie* classification of the duties which reflection on our moral convictions seems actually to reveal. And if these convictions are, as I would claim that they are, of the nature of knowledge, and if I have not

misstated them, the list will be a list of authentic conditional duties, correct as far as it goes though not necessarily complete. The list of *goods* put forward by the rival theory is reached by exactly the same method—the only sound one in the circumstances—viz. that of direct reflection on what we really think. Loyalty to the fact is worth more than a symmetrical architectonic or a hastily reached simplicity. If further reflection discovers a perfect logical basis for this or for a better classification, so much the better.

(3) It may, again, be objected that our theory that there are these various and often conflicting types of *prima facie* duty leaves us with no principle upon which to discern what is our actual duty in particular circumstances. But this objection is not one which the rival theory is in a position to bring forward. For when we have to choose between the production of two heterogeneous goods, say knowledge and pleasure, the "ideal utilitarian" theory can only fall back on an opinion, for which no logical basis can be offered, that one of the goods is the greater; and this is no better than a similar opinion that one of two duties is the more urgent. And again, when we consider the infinite variety of the effects of our actions in the way of pleasure, it must surely be admitted that the claim which *hedonism* sometimes makes, that it offers a readily applicable criterion of right conduct, is quite illusory.

I am unwilling, however, to content myself with an *argumentum ad hominem*, and I would contend that in principle there is no reason to anticipate that every act that is our duty is so for one and the same reason. Why should two sets of circumstances, or one set of circumstances, *not* possess different characteristics, any one of which makes a certain act our *prima facie* duty? When I ask what it is that makes me in certain cases sure that I have a *prima facie* duty to do so and so, I find that it lies in the fact that I have made a promise; when I ask the same question in another case, I find the answer lies in the fact that I have done a wrong. And if on reflection I find (as I think I do) that neither of these reasons is reducible to the other,

I must not on any *a priori* ground assume that such a reduction is possible.

An attempt may be made to arrange in a more systematic way the main types of duty which we have indicated. In the first place it seems self-evident that if there are things that are intrinsically good, it is *prima facie* a duty to bring them into existence rather than not to do so, and to bring as much of them into existence as possible. It will be argued in our fifth chapter that there are three main things that are intrinsically good—virtue, knowledge, and, with certain limitations, pleasure. And since a given virtuous disposition, for instance, is equally good whether it is realized in myself or in another, it seems to be my duty to bring it into existence whether in myself or in another. So too with a given piece of knowledge.

The case of pleasure is difficult; for while we clearly recognize a duty to produce pleasure for others, it is by no means so clear that we recognize a duty to produce pleasure for ourselves. This appears to arise from the following facts. The thought of an act as our duty is one that presupposes a certain amount of reflection about the act; and for that reason does not normally arise in connexion with acts towards which we are already impelled by another strong impulse. So far, the cause of our not thinking of the promotion of our own pleasure as a duty is analogous to the cause which usually prevents a highly sympathetic person from thinking of the promotion of the pleasure of others as a duty. He is impelled so strongly by direct interest in the well-being of others towards promoting their pleasure that he does not stop to ask whether it is his duty to promote it; and we are all impelled so strongly towards the promotion of our own pleasure that we do not stop to ask whether it is a duty or not. But there is a further reason why even when we stop to think about the matter it does not usually present itself as a duty: viz. that, since the performance of most of our duties involves the giving up of some pleasure that we desire, the doing of duty and the getting of pleasure for ourselves comes by a natural association of ideas to be thought of as incompatible things. This association of ideas is in the main salutary in its operation, since it puts a check on what

but for it would be much too strong, the tendency to pursue one's own pleasure without thought of other considerations. Yet if pleasure is good, it seems in the long run clear that it is right to get it for ourselves as well as to produce it for others, when this does not involve the failure to discharge some more stringent *prima facie* duty. The question is a very difficult one, but it seems that this conclusion can be denied only on one or other of three grounds: (1) that pleasure is not *prima facie* good (i.e. good when it is neither the actualization of a bad disposition nor undeserved), (2) that there is no *prima facie* duty to produce as much that is good as we can, or (3) that though there is a *prima facie* duty to produce other things that are good, there is no *prima facie* duty to produce pleasure which will be enjoyed by ourselves. I give reasons later for not accepting the first contention. The second hardly admits of argument but seems to me plainly false. The third seems plausible only if we hold that an act that is pleasant or brings pleasure to ourselves must for that reason not be a duty; and this would lead to paradoxical consequences, such as that if a man enjoys giving pleasure to others or working for their moral improvement, it cannot be his duty to do so. Yet it seems to be a very stubborn fact, that in our ordinary consciousness we are not aware of a duty to get pleasure for ourselves; and by way of partial explanation of this I may add that though, as I think, one's own pleasure is a good and there is a duty to produce it, it is only if we *think* of our own pleasure not as simply our own pleasure, but as an objective good, something that an impartial spectator would approve, that we can think of the getting it as a duty; and we do not habitually think of it in this way.

If these contentions are right, what we have called the duty of beneficence and the duty of self-improvement rest on the same ground. No different principles of duty are involved in the two cases. If we feel a special responsibility for improving our own character rather than that of others, it is not because a special principle is involved, but because we are aware that the one is more under our control than the other.

It was on this ground that Kant expressed the practical law of duty in the form "seek to make yourself good and other people happy." He was so persuaded of the internality of virtue that he regarded any attempt by one person to produce virtue in another as bound to produce, at most, only a counterfeit of virtue, the doing of externally right acts not from the true principle of virtuous action but out of regard to another person. It must be admitted that one man cannot compel another to be virtuous; compulsory virtue would just not be virtue. But experience clearly shows that Kant overshoots the mark when he contends that one man cannot do anything to *promote* virtue in another, to bring such influences to bear upon him that his own response to them is more likely to be virtuous than his response to other influences would have been. And our duty to do this is not different in kind from our duty to improve our own characters.

It is equally clear, and clear at an earlier stage of moral development, that if there are things that are bad in themselves we ought, *prima facie*, not to bring them upon others; and on this fact rests the duty of non-maleficence.

The duty of justice is particularly complicated, and the word is used to cover things which are really very different—things such as the payment of debts, the reparation of injuries done by oneself to another, and the bringing about of a distribution of happiness between other people in proportion to merit. I use the word to denote only the last of these three. In the fifth chapter I shall try to show that besides the three (comparatively) simple goods, virtue, knowledge, and pleasure, there is a more complex good, not reducible to these, consisting in the proportionment of happiness to virtue. The bringing of this about is a duty which we owe to all men alike, though it may be reinforced by special responsibilities that we have undertaken to particular men. This, therefore, with beneficence and self-improvement, comes under the general principle that we should produce as much good as possible, though the good here involved is different in kind from any other.

But besides this general obligation, there are special obligations. These may arise, in the first place, incidentally, from acts which were not essentially meant to create such an obligation, but which nevertheless create it. From the nature of the case such acts may be of two kinds—the infliction of injuries on others, and the acceptance of benefits from them. It seems clear that these put us under a special obligation to other men, and that only these acts can do so incidentally. From these arise the twin duties of reparation and gratitude.

And finally there are special obligations arising from acts the very intention of which, when they were done, was to put us under such an obligation. The name for such acts is "promises"; the name is wide enough if we are willing to include under it implicit promises, i.e. modes of behaviour in which without explicit verbal promise we intentionally create an expectation that we can be counted on to behave in a certain way in the interest of another person.

These seem to be, in principle, all the ways in which *prima facie* duties arise. In actual experience they are compounded together in highly complex ways. Thus, for example, the duty of obeying the laws of one's country arises partly (as Socrates contends in the *Crito*) from the duty of gratitude for the benefits one has received from it; partly from the implicit promise to obey which seems to be involved in permanent residence in a country whose laws we know we are *expected* to obey, and still more clearly involved when we ourselves invoke the protection of its laws (this is the truth underlying the doctrine of the social contract); and partly (if we are fortunate in our country) from the fact that its laws are potent instruments for the general good.

Or again, the sense of a general obligation to bring about (so far as we can) a just apportionment of happiness to merit is often greatly reinforced by the fact that many of the existing injustices are due to a social and economic system which we have, not indeed created, but taken part in and assented to; the duty of justice is then reinforced by the duty of reparation.

It is necessary to say something by way of clearing up the relation between *prima facie* duties and the actual or absolute duty to do one particular act in particular circumstances. If, as almost all moralists except Kant are agreed, and as most plain men think, it is sometimes right to tell a lie or to break a promise, it must be maintained that there is a difference between *prima facie* duty and actual or absolute duty. When we think ourselves justified in breaking, and indeed morally obliged to break, a promise in order to relieve some one's distress, we do not for a moment cease to recognize a *prima facie* duty to keep our promise, and this leads us to feel, not indeed shame or repentance, but certainly compunction, for behaving as we do; we recognize, further, that it is our duty to make up somehow to the promisee for the breaking of the promise. We have to distinguish from the characteristic of being our duty that of tending to be our duty. Any act that we do contains various elements in virtue of which it falls under various categories. In virtue of being the breaking of a promise, for instance, it tends to be wrong; in virtue of being an instance of relieving distress it tends to be right. Tendency to be one's duty may be called a parti-resultant attribute, i.e. one which belongs to an act in virtue of some one component in its nature. *Being* one's duty is a toti-resultant attribute, one which belongs to an act in virtue of its whole nature and of nothing less than this. This distinction between parti-resultant and toti-resultant attributes is one which we shall meet in another context also.

Another instance of the same distinction may be found in the operation of natural laws. *Qua* subject to the force of gravitation towards some other body, each body tends to move in a particular direction with a particular velocity; but its actual movement depends on *all* the forces to which it is subject. It is only by recognizing this distinction that we can preserve the absoluteness of laws of nature, and only by recognizing a corresponding distinction that we can preserve the absoluteness of the general principles of morality. But an important difference between the two cases must be pointed out. When we say that in virtue of gravitation a body tends to move in a certain way, we are referring to a causal influence actually exercised on it by another body or other bodies. When we say that in virtue of being deliberately untrue a certain remark tends to be wrong, we are referring to no causal relation, to no relation that involves succession in time, but to such a relation as connects the various attributes of a mathematical figure. And if the word 'tendency' is thought to suggest too much a causal relation, it is better to talk of certain types of act as being *prima facie* right or wrong (or of different persons as having different and possibly conflicting claims upon us), than of their tending to be right or wrong.

Notes

1. I take the theory which, as I have tried to show, seems to be put forward in *Ethics* rather than the earlier and less plausible theory put forward in *Principia Ethica*. . . .

2. These are not strictly speaking duties, but things that tend to be our duty, or *prima facie* duties.

3. Some will think it, apart from other considerations, a sufficient refutation of this view to point out that I also stand in that relation to myself, so that for this view the distinction of oneself from others is morally insignificant.

4. I should make it plain at this stage that I am *assuming* the correctness of some of our main convictions as to *prima facie* duties, or, more strictly, am claiming that we *know* them to be true. To me it seems as self-evident as anything could be, that to make a promise, for instance, is to create a moral claim on us in someone else. Many readers will perhaps say that they do *not* know this to be true. If so, I certainly cannot prove it to them; I can only ask them to reflect again, in the hope that they will ultimately agree that they also know it to be true. The main moral convictions of the plain man seem to me to be, not opinions which it is for philosophy to prove or disprove, but knowledge from the start; and in my own case I seem to find little difficulty in distinguishing these essential convictions from other moral convictions which I also have, which are merely fallible opinions based on an imperfect study of the working for good or evil of certain institutions or types of action.

5. For a needed correction of this statement, cf. next section.

17

John Rawls
Justice as Fairness

Reprinted with permission of the author and publisher from *Philosophical Review*, vol. 67, 1958, pp. 164–194.

1. It might seem at first sight that the concepts of justice and fairness are the same, and that there is no reason to distinguish them, or to say that one is more fundamental than the other. I think that this impression is mistaken. In this paper I wish to show that the fundamental idea in the concept of justice is fairness; and I wish to offer an analysis of the concept of justice from this point of view. To bring out the force of this claim, and the analysis based upon it, I shall then argue that it is this aspect of justice for which utilitarianism, in its classical form, is unable to account, but which is expressed, even if misleadingly, by the idea of the social contract.

To start with I shall develop a particular conception of justice by stating and commenting upon two principles which specify it, and by considering the circumstances and conditions under which they may be thought to arise. The principles defining this conception, and the conception itself, are, of course, familiar. It may be possible, however, by using the notion of fairness as a framework, to assemble and to look at them in a new way. Before stating this conception, however, the following preliminary matters should be kept in mind.

Throughout I consider justice only as a virtue of social institutions, or what I shall call practices.[1] The principles of justice are regarded as formulating restrictions as to how practices may define positions and offices, and assign thereto powers and liabilities, rights and duties. Justice as a virtue of particular actions or of persons I do not take up at all. It is important to distinguish these various subjects of justice, since the meaning of the concept varies according to whether it is applied to practices, particular actions, or persons. These meanings are, indeed, connected, but they are not identical. I shall confine my discussion to the sense of justice as applied to practices, since this sense is the basic one. Once it is understood, the other senses should go quite easily.

Justice is to be understood in its customary sense as representing but *one* of the many virtues of social institutions, for these may be antiquated, inefficient, degrading, or any number of other things, without being unjust. Justice is not to be confused with an all-inclusive vision of a good society; it is only one part of any such conception. It is important, for example, to distinguish that sense of equality which is an aspect of the concept of justice from that sense of equality which belongs to a more comprehensive social ideal. There may well be inequalities which one concedes are just, or at least not unjust, but which, nevertheless, one wishes, on other grounds, to do away with. I shall focus attention, then, on the usual sense of justice in which it is essentially the elimination of arbitrary distinctions and the establishment, within the structure of a practice, of a proper balance between competing claims.

Finally, there is no need to consider the principles discussed below as *the* principles of justice. For the moment it is sufficient that they are typical of a family of principles normally associated with the concept of justice. The way in which the principles of this family resemble one another, as shown by the background against which they may be thought to arise, will be made clear by the whole of the subsequent argument.

2. The conception of justice which I want to develop may be stated in the form of two principles as follows: first, each person participating in a practice, or affected by it, has an equal right to the most extensive liberty compatible with a like liberty for all; and second, inequalities are arbitrary unless it is reasonable to expect that they will work out for everyone's advantage, and provided the positions and offices to which they attach, or from which they may be gained, are open to all. These principles express justice as a complex of three ideas: liberty, equality, and reward for services contributing to the common good.[2]

The term "person" is to be construed variously depending on the circumstances. On some occasions it will mean human individuals, but in others it may refer to nations, provinces, business firms, churches, teams, and so on. The principles of justice apply in all these instances, although there is a certain logical priority to the case of human individuals. As I shall use the term "person," it will be ambiguous in the manner indicated.

The first principle holds, of course, only if other things are equal: that is, while there must always be a justification for departing from the initial position of equal liberty (which is defined by the pattern of rights and duties, powers and liabilities, established by a practice), and the burden of proof is placed on him who would depart from it, nevertheless, there can be, and often there is, a justification for doing so. Now, that similar particular cases, as defined by a practice, should be treated similarly as they arise, is part of the very concept of a practice; it is involved in the notion of an activity in accordance with rules.[3] The first principle expresses an analogous conception, but as applied to the structure of practices themselves. It holds, for example, that there is a presumption against the distinctions and classifications made by legal systems and other practices to the extent that they infringe on the original and equal liberty of the persons participating in them. The second principle defines how this presumption may be rebutted.

It might be argued at this point that justice requires only an equal liberty. If, however, a greater liberty were possible for all without loss or conflict, then it would be irrational to settle on a lesser liberty. There is no reason for circumscribing rights unless their exercise would be incompatible, or would render the practice defining them less effective. Therefore no serious distortion of the concept of justice is likely to follow from including within it the concept of the greatest equal liberty.

The second principle defines what sorts of inequalities are permissible; it specifies how the presumption laid down by the first principle may be put aside. Now by inequalities it is best to understand not *any* differences between offices and positions, but differences in the benefits and burdens attached to them either directly or indirectly, such as prestige and wealth, or liability to taxation and compulsory services. Players in a game do not protest against there being different positions, such as batter, pitcher, catcher, and the like, nor to there being various privileges and powers as specified by the rules; nor do the citizens of a country object to there being the different offices of government such as president, senator, governor, judge, and so on, each with their special rights and

duties. It is not differences of this kind that are normally thought of as inequalities, but differences in the resulting distribution established by a practice, or made possible by it, of the things men strive to attain or avoid. Thus they may complain about the pattern of honors and rewards set up by a practice (e.g., the privileges and salaries of government officials) or they may object to the distribution of power and wealth which results from the various ways in which men avail themselves of the opportunities allowed by it (e.g., the concentration of wealth which may develop in a free price system allowing large entrepreneurial or speculative gains).

It should be noted that the second principle holds that an inequality is allowed only if there is reason to believe that the practice with the inequality, or resulting in it, will work for the advantage of *every* party engaging in it. Here it is important to stress that *every* party must gain from the inequality. Since the principle applies to practices, it implies that the representative man in every office or position defined by a practice, when he views it as a going concern, must find it reasonable to prefer his condition and prospects with the inequality to what they would be under the practice without it. The principle excludes, therefore, the justification of inequalities on the grounds that the disadvantages of those in one position are outweighed by the greater advantages of those in another position. This rather simple restriction is the main modification I wish to make in the utilitarian principle as usually understood. When coupled with the notion of a practice, it is a restriction of consequence,[4] and one which some utilitarians, e.g., Hume and Mill, have used in their discussions of justice without realizing apparently its significance, or at least without calling attention to it.[5] Why it is a significant modification of principle, changing one's conception of justice entirely, the whole of my argument will show.

Further, it is also necessary that the various offices to which special benefits or burdens attach are open to all. It may be, for example, to the common advantage, as just defined, to attach special benefits to certain offices. Perhaps by doing so the requisite talent can be attracted to them and encouraged to give its best efforts. But any

offices having special benefits must be won in a fair competition in which contestants are judged on their merits. If some offices were not open, those excluded would normally be justified in feeling unjustly treated, even if they benefited from the greater efforts of those who were allowed to compete for them. Now if one can assume that offices are open, it is necessary only to consider the design of practices themselves and how they jointly, as a system, work together. It will be a mistake to focus attention on the varying relative positions of particular persons, who may be known to us by their proper names, and to require that each such change, as a once for all transaction viewed in isolation, must be in itself just. It is the system of practices which is to be judged, and judged from a general point of view: unless one is prepared to criticize it from the standpoint of a representative man holding some particular office, one has no complaint against it.

3. Given these principles one might try to derive them from a priori principles of reason, or claim that they were known by intuition. These are familiar enough steps and, at least in the case of the first principle, might be made with some success. Usually, however, such arguments, made at this point, are unconvincing. They are not likely to lead to an understanding of the basis of the principles of justice, not at least as principles of justice. I wish, therefore, to look at the principles in a different way.

Imagine a society of persons amongst whom a certain system of practices is *already* well established. Now suppose that by and large they are mutually self-interested; their allegiance to their established practices is normally founded on the prospect of self-advantage. One need not assume that, in all senses of the term "person," the persons in this society are mutually self-interested. If the characterization as mutually self-interested applies when the line of division is the family, it may still be true that members of families are bound by ties of sentiment and affection and willingly acknowledge duties in contradiction to self-interest. Mutual self-interestedness in the relations between families, nations, churches, and the like, is commonly associated with intense loyalty and devotion on the part of individual members. Therefore, one can form a more realistic conception of this society if one thinks of it as consisting of mutually self-interested families, or some other association. Further, it is not necessary to suppose that these persons are mutually self-interested under all circumstances, but only in the usual situations in which they participate in their common practices.

Now suppose also that these persons are rational: they know their own interests more or less accurately; they are capable of tracing out the likely consequences of adopting one practice rather than another; they are capable of adhering to a course of action once they have decided upon it; they can resist present temptations and the enticements of immediate gain; and the bare knowledge or perception of the difference between their condition and that of others is not, within certain limits and in itself, a source of great dissatisfaction. Only the last point adds anything to the usual definition of rationality. This definition should allow, I think, for the idea that a rational man would not be greatly downcast from knowing, or seeing, that others are in a better position than himself, unless he thought their being so was the result of injustice, or the consequence of letting chance work itself out for no useful common purpose, and so on. So if these persons strike us as unpleasantly egoistic, they are at least free in some degree from the fault of envy.[6]

Finally, assume that these persons have roughly similar needs and interests, or needs and interests in various ways complementary, so that fruitful cooperation amongst them is possible; and suppose that they are sufficiently equal in power and ability to guarantee that in normal circumstances none is able to dominate the others. This condition (as well as the others) may seem excessively vague; but in view of the conception of justice to which the argument leads, there seems no reason for making it more exact here.

Since these persons are conceived as engaging in their common practices, which are already established, there is no question of our supposing them to come together to deliberate as to how

they will set these practices up for the first time. Yet we can imagine that from time to time they discuss with one another whether any of them has a legitimate complaint against their established institutions. Such discussions are perfectly natural in any normal society. Now suppose that they have settled on doing this in the following way. They first try to arrive at the principles by which complaints, and so practices themselves, are to be judged. Their procedure for this is to let each person propose the principles upon which he wishes his complaints to be tried with the understanding that, if acknowledged, the complaints of others will be similarly tried, and that no complaints will be heard at all until everyone is roughly of one mind as to how complaints are to be judged. They each understand further that the principles proposed and acknowledged on this occasion are binding on future occasions. Thus each will be wary of proposing a principle which would give him a peculiar advantage, in his present circumstances, supposing it to be accepted. Each person knows that he will be bound by it in future circumstances the peculiarities of which cannot be known, and which might well be such that the principle is then to his disadvantage. The idea is that everyone should be required to make *in advance* a firm commitment, which others also may reasonably be expected to make, and that no one be given the opportunity to tailor the canons of a legitimate complaint to fit his own special condition, and then to discard them when they no longer suit his purpose. Hence each person will propose principles of a general kind which will, to a large degree, gain their sense from the various applications to be made of them, the particular circumstances of which being as yet unknown. These principles will express the conditions in accordance with which each is the least unwilling to have his interests limited in the design of practices, given the competing interests of the others, on the supposition that the interests of others will be limited likewise. The restrictions which would so arise might be thought of as those a person would keep in mind if he were designing a practice in which his enemy were to assign him his place.

The two main parts of this conjectural account have a definite significance. The character and respective situations of the parties reflect the typical circumstances in which questions of justice arise. The procedure whereby principles are proposed and acknowledged represents constraints, analogous to those of having a morality, whereby rational and mutually self-interested persons are brought to act reasonably. Thus the first part reflects the fact that questions of justice arise when conflicting claims are made upon the design of a practice and where it is taken for granted that each person will insist, as far as possible, on what he considers his rights. It is typical of cases of justice to involve persons who are pressing on one another their claims, between which a fair balance or equilibrium must be found. On the other hand, as expressed by the second part, having a morality must at least imply the acknowledgment of principles as impartially applying to one's own conduct as well as to another's, and moreover principles which may constitute a constraint, or limitation, upon the pursuit of one's own interests. There are, of course, other aspects of having a morality: the acknowledgment of moral principles must show itself in accepting a reference to them as reasons for limiting one's claims, in acknowledging the burden of providing a special explanation, or excuse, when one acts contrary to them, or else in showing shame and remorse and a desire to make amends, and so on. It is sufficient to remark here that having a morality is analogous to having made a firm commitment in advance; for one must acknowledge the principles of morality even when to one's disadvantage.[7] A man whose moral judgments always coincided with his interests could be suspected of having no morality at all.

Thus the two parts of the foregoing account are intended to mirror the kinds of circumstances in which questions of justice arise and the constraints which having a morality would impose upon persons so situated. In this way one can see how the acceptance of the principles of justice might come about, for given all these conditions as described, it would be natural if the two principles of justice were to be acknowledged. Since there is no way for anyone to win special advantages for himself, each might consider it reasonable to acknowledge equality as an initial principle. There is, however, no reason why they should regard this position as final; for if there are inequalities which satisfy the second principle, the immediate gain which equality would allow can be considered as intelligently invested in view of its future return. If, as is quite likely, these inequalities work as incentives to draw out better efforts, the members of this society may look upon them as concessions to human nature: they, like us, may think that people ideally should want to serve one another. But as they are mutually self-interested, their acceptance of these inequalities is merely the acceptance of the relations in which they actually stand, and a recognition of the motives which lead them to engage in their common practices. *They* have no title to complain of one another. And so provided that the conditions of the principle are met, there is no reason why they should not allow such inequalities. Indeed, it would be short-sighted of them to do so, and could result, in most cases, only from their being dejected by the bare knowledge, or perception, that others are better situated. Each person will, however, insist on an advantage to himself, and so on a common advantage, for none is willing to sacrifice anything for the others.

These remarks are not offered as a proof that persons so conceived and circumstanced would settle on the two principles, but only to show that these principles could have such a background, and so can be viewed as those principles which mutually self-interested and rational persons, when similarly situated and required to make in advance a firm commitment, could acknowledge as restrictions governing the assignment of rights and duties in their common practices, and thereby accept as limiting their rights against one another. The principles of justice may, then, be regarded as those principles which arise when the constraints of having a morality are imposed upon parties in the typical circumstances of justice.

4. These ideas are, of course, connected with a familiar way of thinking about justice which goes back at least to the Greek Sophists, and which regards the acceptance of the principles of justice as a compromise between persons of roughly equal power who would enforce their will on each other if they could, but who, in view of the equality of forces amongst them and for the sake of their own peace and security, acknowledge certain forms of conduct insofar as prudence seems to require. Justice is thought of as a pact between rational egoists the stability of which is dependent on a balance of power and a similarity of circumstances.[8] While the previous account is connected with this tradition, and with its most recent variant, the theory of games,[9] it differs from it in several important respects which, to forestall misinterpretations, I will set out here.

First, I wish to use the previous conjectural account of the background of justice as a way of analyzing the concept. I do not want, therefore, to be interpreted as assuming a general theory of human motivation: when I suppose that the parties are mutually self-interested, and are not willing to have their (substantial) interests sacrificed to others, I am referring to their conduct and motives as they are taken for granted in cases where questions of justice ordinarily arise. Justice is the virtue of practices where there are assumed to be competing interests and conflicting claims, and where it is supposed that persons will press their rights on each other. That persons are mutually self-interested in certain situations and for certain purposes is what gives rise to the question of justice in practices covering those circumstances. Amongst an association of saints, if such a community could really exist, the disputes about justice could hardly occur; for they would all work selflessly together for one end, the glory of God as defined by their common religion, and reference to this end would settle every question of right. The justice of practices does not come up until there are several different parties (whether we think of these as individuals, associations, or nations and so on, is irrelevant) who do press their claims on one another, and who do regard themselves as representatives of interests which deserve to be considered. Thus the previous account involves no general theory of human motivation. Its intent is simply to incorporate into the conception of justice the relations of men to one another which set the stage for questions of justice. It makes no difference how wide or general these relations are, as this matter does not bear on the analysis of the concept.

Again, in contrast to the various conceptions of the social contract, the several parties do not establish any particular society or practice; they do not covenant to obey a particular sovereign body or to accept a given constitution.[10] Nor do they, as in the theory of games (in certain respects a marvelously sophisticated development of this tradition), decide on individual strategies adjusted to their respective circumstances in the game. What the parties do is to *jointly* acknowledge certain *principles* of appraisal relating to their common *practices* either as already established or merely proposed. They accede to standards of judgment, not to a given practice; they do not make any specific agreement, or bargain, or adopt a particular strategy. The subject of their acknowledgment is, therefore, very general indeed; it is simply the acknowledgment of certain principles of judgment, fulfilling certain general conditions, to be used in criticizing the arrangement of their common affairs. The relations of mutual self-interest between the parties who are similarly circumstanced mirror the conditions under which questions of justice arise, and the procedure by which the principles of judgment are proposed and acknowledged reflects the constraints of having a morality. Each aspect, then, of the preceding hypothetical account serves the purpose of bringing out a feature of the notion of justice. One could, if one liked, view the principles of justice as the "solution" of this highest order "game" of adopting, subject to the procedure described, principles of argument for all coming particular "games" whose peculiarities one can in no way foresee. But this comparison, while no doubt helpful, must not obscure the fact that this highest order "game" is of a special sort.[11] Its significance is that its various pieces represent aspects of the concept of justice.

Finally, I do not, of course, conceive the several parties as necessarily coming together to establish their common practices for the first time. Some institutions may, indeed, be set up *de novo*;

but I have framed the preceding account so that it will apply when the full complement of social institutions already exists and represents the result of a long period of development. Nor is the account in any way fictitious. In any society where people reflect on their institutions they will have an idea of what principles of justice would be acknowledged under the conditions described, and there will be occasions when questions of justice are actually discussed in this way. Therefore if their practices do not accord with these principles, this will affect the quality of their social relations. For in this case there will be some recognized situations wherein the parties are mutually aware that one of them is being forced to accept what the other would concede is unjust. The foregoing analysis may then be thought of as representing the actual quality of relations between persons as defined by practices accepted as just. In such practices the parties will acknowledge the principles on which it is constructed, and the general recognition of this fact shows itself in the absence of resentment and in the sense of being justly treated. Thus one common objection to the theory of the social contract, its apparently historical and fictitious character, is avoided.

5. That the principles of justice may be regarded as arising in the manner described illustrates an important fact about them. Not only does it bring out the idea that justice is a primitive moral notion in that it arises once the concept of morality is imposed on mutually self-interested agents similarly circumstanced, but it emphasizes that, fundamental to justice, is the concept of fairness which relates to right dealing between persons who are cooperating with or competing against one another, as when one speaks of fair games, fair competition, and fair bargains. The question of fairness arises when free persons, who have no authority over one another, are engaging in a joint activity and amongst themselves settling or acknowledging the rules which define it and which determine the respective shares in its benefits and burdens. A practice will strike the parties as fair if none feels that, by participating in it, they or any of the others are taken advantage of, or

forced to give in to claims which they do not regard as legitimate. This implies that each has a conception of legitimate claims which he thinks it reasonable for others as well as himself to acknowledge. If one thinks of the principles of justice as arising in the manner described, then they do define this sort of conception. A practice is just or fair, then, when it satisfies the principles which those who participate in it could propose to one another for mutual acceptance under the aforementioned circumstances. Persons engaged in a just, or fair, practice can face one another openly and support their respective positions, should they appear questionable, by reference to principles which it is reasonable to expect each to accept.

It is this notion of the possibility of mutual acknowledgment of principles by free persons who have no authority over one another which makes the concept of fairness fundamental to justice. Only if such acknowledgment is possible can there be true community between persons in their common practices; otherwise their relations will appear to them as founded to some extent on force. If, in ordinary speech, fairness applies more particularly to practices in which there is a choice whether to engage or not (e.g., in games, business competition), and justice to practices in which there is no choice (e.g., in slavery), the element of necessity does not render the conception of mutual acknowledgment inapplicable, although it may make it much more urgent to change unjust than unfair institutions. For one activity in which one can always engage is that of proposing and acknowledging principles to one another supposing each to be similarly circumstanced; and to judge practices by the principles so arrived at is to apply the standard of fairness to them.

Now if the participants in a practice accept its rules as fair, and so have no complaint to lodge against it, there arises a prima facie duty (and a corresponding prima facie right) of the parties to each other to act in accordance with the practice when it falls upon them to comply. When any number of persons engage in a practice, or conduct a joint undertaking according to rules, and thus restrict their liberty, those who have submitted to these restrictions when required have the right

to a similar acquiescence on the part of those who have benefited by their submission. These conditions will obtain if a practice is correctly acknowledged to be fair, for in this case all who participate in it will benefit from it. The rights and duties so arising are special rights and duties in that they depend on previous actions voluntarily undertaken, in this case on the parties having engaged in a common practice and knowingly accepted its benefits.[12] It is not, however, an obligation which presupposes a deliberate performative act in the sense of a promise, or contract, and the like.[13] An unfortunate mistake of proponents of the idea of the social contract was to suppose that political obligation does require some such act, or at least to use language which suggests it. It is sufficient that one has knowingly participated in and accepted the benefits of a practice acknowledged to be fair. This prima facie obligation may, of course, be overridden: it may happen, when it comes one's turn to follow a rule, that other considerations will justify not doing so. But one cannot, in general, be released from this obligation by denying the justice of the practice only when it falls on one to obey. If a person rejects a practice, he should, so far as possible, declare his intention in advance, and avoid participating in it or enjoying its benefits.

This duty I have called that of fair play, but it should be admitted that to refer to it in this way is, perhaps, to extend the ordinary notion of fairness. Usually acting unfairly is not so much the breaking of any particular rule, even if the infraction is difficult to detect (cheating), but taking advantage of loop-holes or ambiguities in rules, availing oneself of unexpected or special circumstances which make it impossible to enforce them, insisting that rules be enforced to one's advantage when they should be suspended, and more generally, acting contrary to the intention of a practice. It is for this reason that one speaks of the sense of fair play: acting fairly requires more than simply being able to follow rules; what is fair must often be felt, or perceived, one wants to say. It is not, however, an unnatural extension of the duty of fair play to have it include the obligation which participants who have knowingly accepted the benefits of their common practice owe to each other to act in accordance with it when their performance falls due; for it is usually considered unfair if someone accepts the benefits of a practice but refuses to do his part in maintaining it. Thus one might say of the tax-dodger that he violates the duty of fair play: he accepts the benefits of government but will not do his part in releasing resources to it; and members of labor unions often say that fellow workers who refuse to join are being unfair: they refer to them as "free riders," as persons who enjoy what are the supposed benefits of unionism, higher wages, shorter hours, job security, and the like, but who refuse to share in its burdens in the form of paying dues, and so on.

The duty of fair play stands beside other prima facie duties such as fidelity and gratitude as a basic moral notion; yet it is not to be confused with them.[14] These duties are all clearly distinct, as would be obvious from their definitions. As with any moral duty, that of fair play implies a constraint on self-interest in particular cases; on occasion it enjoins conduct which a rational egoist strictly defined would not decide upon. So while justice does not require of anyone that he sacrifice his interests in that *general position* and procedure whereby the principles of justice are proposed and acknowledged, it may happen that in particular situations, arising in the context of engaging in a practice, the duty of fair play will often cross his interests in the sense that he will be required to forego particular advantages which the peculiarities of his circumstances might permit him to take. There is, of course, nothing surprising in this. It is simply the consequence of the firm commitment which the parties may be supposed to have made, or which they would make, in the general position, together with the fact that they have participated in and accepted the benefits of a practice which they regard as fair.

Now the acknowledgment of this constraint in particular cases, which is manifested in acting fairly or wishing to make amends, feeling ashamed, and the like, when one has evaded it, is one of the forms of conduct by which participants in a common practice exhibit their recognition of each other as

persons with similar interests and capacities. In the same way that, failing a special explanation, the criterion for the recognition of suffering is helping one who suffers, acknowledging the duty of fair play is a necessary part of the criterion for recognizing another as a person with similar interests and feelings as oneself.[15] A person who never under any circumstances showed a wish to help others in pain would show, at the same time, that he did not recognize that they were in pain; nor could he have any feelings of affection or friendship for anyone; for having these feelings implies, failing special circumstances, that he comes to their aid when they are suffering. Recognition that another is a person in pain shows itself in sympathetic action; this primitive natural response of compassion is one of those responses upon which the various forms of moral conduct are built.

Similarly, the acceptance of the duty of fair play by participants in a common practice is a reflection in each person of the recognition of the aspirations and interests of the others to be realized by their joint activity. Failing a special explanation, their acceptance of it is a necessary part of the criterion for their recognizing one another as persons with similar interests and capacities, as the conception of their relations in the general position supposes them to be. Otherwise they would show no recognition of one another as persons with similar capacities and interests, and indeed, in some cases perhaps hypothetical, they would not recognize one another as persons at all, but as complicated objects involved in a complicated activity. To recognize another as a person one must respond to him and act towards him in certain ways; and these ways are intimately connected with the various prima facie duties. Acknowledging these duties in *some* degree, and so having the elements of morality, is not a matter of choice, or of intuiting moral qualities, or a matter of the expression of feelings or attitudes (the three interpretations between which philosophical opinion frequently oscillates); it is simply the possession of one of the forms of conduct in which the recognition of others as persons is manifested.

These remarks are unhappily obscure. Their main purpose here, however, is to forestall, together with the remarks in Section 4, the misinterpretation that, on the view presented, the acceptance of justice and the acknowledgment of the duty of fair play depends in every day life solely on there being a *de facto* balance of forces between the parties. It would indeed be foolish to underestimate the importance of such a balance in securing justice; but it is not the only basis thereof. The recognition of one another as persons with similar interests and capacities engaged in a common practice must, failing a special explanation, show itself in the acceptance of the principles of justice and the acknowledgment of the duty of fair play.

The conception at which we have arrived, then, is that the principles of justice may be thought of as arising once the constraints of having a morality are imposed upon rational and mutually self-interested parties who are related and situated in a special way. A practice is just if it is in accordance with the principles which all who participate in it might reasonably be expected to propose or to acknowledge before one another when they are similarly circumstanced and required to make a firm commitment in advance without knowledge of what will be their peculiar condition, and thus when it meets standards which the parties could accept as fair should occasion arise for them to debate its merits. Regarding the participants themselves, once persons knowingly engage in a practice which they acknowledge to be fair and accept the benefits of doing so, they are bound by the duty of fair play to follow the rules when it comes their turn to do so, and this implies a limitation on their pursuit of self-interest in particular cases.

Now one consequence of this conception is that, where it applies, there is no moral value in the satisfaction of a claim incompatible with it. Such a claim violates the conditions of reciprocity and community amongst persons, and he who presses it, not being willing to acknowledge it when pressed by another, has no grounds for complaint when it is denied; whereas he against whom it is pressed can complain. As it cannot be mutually acknowledged it is a resort to coercion; granting the claim is possible only if one party can compel acceptance of what the other will not admit. But it makes no sense to concede claims the denial of which cannot be complained of in preference to claims the denial of which can be objected to. Thus in deciding on the justice of a practice it is not enough to ascertain that it answers to wants and interests in the fullest and most effective manner. For if any of these conflict with justice, they should not be counted, as their satisfaction is no reason at all for having a practice. It would be irrelevant to say, even if true, that it resulted in the greatest satisfaction of desire. In tallying up the merits of a practice one must toss out the satisfaction of interests the claims of which are incompatible with the principles of justice.

6. The discussion so far has been excessively abstract. While this is perhaps unavoidable, I should now like to bring out some of the features of the conception of justice as fairness by comparing it with the conception of justice in classical utilitarianism as represented by Bentham and Sidgwick, and its counterpart in welfare economics. This conception assimilates justice to benevolence and the latter in turn to the most efficient design of institutions to promote the general welfare. Justice is a kind of efficiency.[16]

Now it is said occasionally that this form of utilitarianism puts no restrictions on what might be a just assignment of rights and duties in that there might be circumstances which, on utilitarian grounds, would justify institutions highly offensive to our ordinary sense of justice. But the classical utilitarian conception is not totally unprepared for this objection. Beginning with the notion that the general happiness can be represented by a social utility function consisting of a sum of individual utility functions with identical weights (this being the meaning of the maxim that each counts for one and no more than one),[17] it is commonly assumed that the utility functions of individuals are similar in all essential respects. Differences between individuals are ascribed to accidents of education and upbringing, and they should not be taken into account. This assumption, coupled with that of diminishing marginal utility, results in a

prima facie case for equality, e.g., of equality in the distribution of income during any given period of time, laying aside indirect effects on the future. But even if utilitarianism is interpreted as having such restrictions built into the utility function, and even if it is supposed that these restrictions have in practice much the same result as the application of the principles of justice (and appear, perhaps, to be ways of expressing these principles in the language of mathematics and psychology), the fundamental idea is very different from the conception of justice as fairness. For one thing, that the principles of justice should be accepted is interpreted as the contingent result of a higher order administrative decision. The form of this decision is regarded as being similar to that of an entrepreneur deciding how much to produce of this or that commodity in view of its marginal revenue, or to that of someone distributing goods to needy persons according to the relative urgency of their wants. The choice between practices is thought of as being made on the basis of the allocation of benefits and burdens to individuals (these being measured by the present capitalized value of their utility over the full period of the practice's existence), which results from the distribution of rights and duties established by a practice.

Moreover, the individuals receiving these benefits are not conceived as being related in any way: they represent so many different directions in which limited resources may be allocated. The value of assigning resources to one direction rather than another depends solely on the preferences and interests of individuals as individuals. The satisfaction of desire has its value irrespective of the moral relations between persons, say as members of a joint undertaking, and of the claims which, in the name of these interests, they are prepared to make on one another;[18] and it is this value which is to be taken into account by the (ideal) legislator who is conceived as adjusting the rules of the system from the center so as to maximize the value of the social utility function.

It is thought that the principles of justice will not be violated by a legal system so conceived provided these executive decisions are correctly made.

In this fact the principles of justice are said to have their derivation and explanation; they simply express the most important general features of social institutions in which the administrative problem is solved in the best way. These principles have, indeed, a special urgency because, given the facts of human nature, so much depends on them; and this explains the peculiar quality of the moral feelings associated with justice.[19] This assimilation of justice to a higher order executive decision, certainly a striking conception, is central to classical utilitarianism; and it also brings out its profound individualism, in one sense of this ambiguous word. It regards persons as so many *separate* directions in which benefits and burdens may be assigned; and the value of the satisfaction or dissatisfaction of desire is not thought to depend in any way on the moral relations in which individuals stand, or on the kinds of claims which they are willing, in the pursuit of their interests, to press on each other.

7. Many social decisions are, of course, of an administrative nature. Certainly this is so when it is a matter of social utility in what one may call its ordinary sense; that is, when it is a question of the efficient design of social institutions for the use of common means to achieve common ends. In this case either the benefits and burdens may be assumed to be impartially distributed, or the question of distribution is misplaced, as in the instance of maintaining public order and security or national defense. But as an interpretation of the basis of the principles of justice, classical utilitarianism is mistaken. It *permits* one to argue, for example, that slavery is unjust on the grounds that the advantages to the slaveholder as slaveholder do not counterbalance the disadvantages to the slave and to society at large burdened by a comparatively inefficient system of labor. Now the conception of justice as fairness, when applied to the practice of slavery with its offices of slaveholder and slave, would not allow one to consider the advantages of the slaveholder in the first place. As that office is not in accordance with principles which could be mutually acknowledged, the gains accruing to the slaveholder, assuming them to exist, cannot be counted as in *any* way mitigating the injustice of the practice.

The question whether these gains outweigh the disadvantages to the slave and to society cannot arise, since in considering the justice of slavery these gains have no weight at all which requires that they be overridden. Where the conception of justice as fairness applies, slavery is *always* unjust.

I am not, of course, suggesting the absurdity that the classical utilitarians approved of slavery. I am only rejecting a type of argument which their view allows them to use in support of their disapproval of it. The conception of justice as derivative from efficiency implies that judging the justice of a practice is always, in principle at least, a matter of weighing up advantages and disadvantages, each having an intrinsic value or disvalue as the satisfaction of interests, irrespective of whether or not these interests necessarily involve acquiescence in principles which could not be mutually acknowledged. Utilitarianism cannot account for the fact that slavery is always unjust, nor for the fact that it would be recognized as irrelevant in defeating the accusation of injustice for one person to say to another, engaged with him in a common practice and debating its merits, that nevertheless it allowed of the greatest satisfaction of desire. The charge of injustice cannot be rebutted in this way. If justice were derivative from a higher order executive efficiency, this would not be so.

But now, even if it is taken as established that, so far as the ordinary conception of justice goes, slavery is always unjust (that is, slavery by definition violates commonly recognized principles of justice), the classical utilitarian would surely reply that these principles, as other moral principles subordinate to that of utility, are only generally correct. It is simply for the most part true that slavery is less efficient than other institutions; and while common sense may define the concept of justice so that slavery is unjust, nevertheless, where slavery would lead to the greatest satisfaction of desire, it is not wrong. Indeed, it is then right, and for the very same reason that justice, as ordinarily understood, is usually right. If, as ordinarily understood, slavery is always unjust, to this extent the utilitarian conception of justice might be admitted to differ from that of common moral opinion. Still the

utilitarian would want to hold that, as a matter of moral principle, his view is correct in giving no special weight to considerations of justice beyond that allowed for by the general presumption of effectiveness. And this, he claims, is as it should be. The every day opinion is morally in error, although, indeed, it is a useful error, since it protects rules of generally high utility.

The question, then, relates not simply to the analysis of the concept of justice as common sense defines it, but the analysis of it in the wider sense as to how much weight considerations of justice, as defined, are to have when laid against other kinds of moral considerations. Here again I wish to argue that reasons of justice have a *special* weight for which only the conception of justice as fairness can account. Moreover, it belongs to the concept of justice that they do have this special weight. While Mill recognized that this was so, he thought that it could be accounted for by the special urgency of the moral feelings which naturally support principles of such high utility. But it is a mistake to resort to the urgency of feeling; as with the appeal to intuition, it manifests a failure to pursue the question far enough. The special weight of considerations of justice can be explained from the conception of justice as fairness. It is only necessary to elaborate a bit what has already been said as follows.

If one examines the circumstances in which a certain tolerance of slavery is justified, or perhaps better, excused, it turns out that these are of a rather special sort. Perhaps slavery exists as an inheritance from the past and it proves necessary to dismantle it piece by piece; at times slavery may conceivably be an advance on previous institutions. Now while there may be some excuse for slavery in special conditions, it is never an excuse for it that it is sufficiently advantageous to the slaveholder to outweigh the disadvantages to the slave and to society. A person who argues in this way is not perhaps making a wildly irrelevant remark; but he is guilty of a moral fallacy. There is disorder in his conception of the ranking of moral principles. For the slaveholder, by his own admission, has no moral title to the advantages which he receives as a slaveholder. He is no more prepared than the slave to acknowledge the principle

upon which is founded the respective positions in which they both stand. Since slavery does not accord with principles which they could mutually acknowledge, they each may be supposed to agree that it is unjust: it grants claims which it ought not to grant and in doing so denies claims which it ought not to deny. Amongst persons in a general position who are debating the form of their common practices, it cannot, therefore, be offered as a reason for a practice that, in conceding these very claims that ought to be denied, it nevertheless meets existing interests more effectively. By their very nature the satisfaction of these claims is without weight and cannot enter into any tabulation of advantages and disadvantages.

Furthermore, it follows from the concept of morality that, to the extent that the slaveholder recognizes his position vis-à-vis the slave to be unjust, he would not choose to press his claims. His not wanting to receive his special advantages is one of the ways in which he shows that he thinks slavery is unjust. It would be fallacious for the legislator to suppose, then, that it is a ground for having a practice that it brings advantages greater than disadvantages, if those for whom the practice is designed, and to whom the advantages flow, acknowledge that they have no moral title to them and do not wish to receive them.

For these reasons the principles of justice have a special weight; and with respect to the principle of the greatest satisfaction of desire, as cited in the general position amongst those discussing the merits of their common practices, the principles of justice have an absolute weight. In this sense they are not contingent; and this is why their force is greater than can be accounted for by the general presumption (assuming that there is one) of the effectiveness, in the utilitarian sense, of practices which in fact satisfy them.

If one wants to continue using the concepts of classical utilitarianism, one will have to say, to meet this criticism, that at least the individual or social utility functions must be so defined that no value is given to the satisfaction of interests the representative claims of which violate the principles of justice. In this way it is no doubt possible to include these principles within the form of the utilitarian conception; but to do so is, of course, to change its inspiration altogether as a moral conception. For it is to incorporate within it principles which cannot be understood on the basis of a higher order executive decision aiming at the greatest satisfaction of desire.

It is worth remarking, perhaps, that this criticism of utilitarianism does not depend on whether or not the two assumptions, that of individuals having similar utility functions and that of diminishing marginal utility, are interpreted as psychological propositions to be supported or refuted by experience, or as moral and political principles expressed in a somewhat technical language. There are, certainly, several advantages in taking them in the latter fashion.[20] For one thing, one might say that this is what Bentham and others really meant by them, as least as shown by how they were used in arguments for social reform. More importantly, one could hold that the best way to defend the classical utilitarian view is to interpret these assumptions as moral and political principles. It is doubtful whether, taken as psychological propositions, they are true of men in general as we know them under normal conditions. On the other hand, utilitarians would not have wanted to propose them merely as practical working principles of legislation, or as expedient maxims to guide reform, given the egalitarian sentiments of modern society.[21] When pressed they might well have invoked the idea of a more or less equal capacity of men in relevant respects if given an equal chance in a just society. But if the argument above regarding slavery is correct, then granting these assumptions as moral and political principles makes no difference. To view individuals as equally fruitful lines for the allocation of benefits, even as a matter of moral principle, still leaves the mistaken notion that the satisfaction of desire has value in itself irrespective of the relations between persons as members of a common practice, and irrespective of the claims upon one another which the satisfaction of interests represents. To see the error of this idea one must give up the conception of justice as an executive decision altogether and refer to the notion of justice as fairness: that participants in a common practice be

regarded as having an original and equal liberty and that their common practices be considered unjust unless they accord with principles which persons so circumstanced and related could freely acknowledge before one another, and so could accept as fair. Once the emphasis is put upon the concept of the mutual recognition of principles by participants in a common practice the rules of which are to define their several relations and give form to their claims on one another, then it is clear that the granting of a claim the principle of which could not be acknowledged by each in the general position (that is, in the position in which the parties propose and acknowledge principles before one another) is not a reason for adopting a practice. Viewed in this way, the background of the claim is seen to exclude it from consideration; that it can represent a value in itself arises from the conception of individuals as separate lines for the assignment of benefits, as isolated persons who stand as claimants on an administrative or benevolent largesse. Occasionally persons do so stand to one another; but this is not the general case, nor, more importantly, is it the case when it is a matter of the justice of practices themselves in which participants stand in various relations to be appraised in accordance with standards which they may be expected to acknowledge before one another. Thus however mistaken the notion of the social contract may be as history, and however far it may overreach itself as a general theory of social and political obligation, it does express, suitably interpreted, an essential part of the concept of justice.[22]

8. By way of conclusion I should like to make two remarks: first, the original modification of the utilitarian principle (that it require of practices that the offices and positions defined by them be equal unless it is reasonable to suppose that the representative man in *every* office would find the inequality to his advantage), slight as it may appear at first sight, actually has a different conception of justice standing behind it. I have tried to show how this is so by developing the concept of justice as fairness and by indicating how this notion involves the mutual acceptance, from a general position, of the principles on which a practice is founded,

and how this in turn requires the exclusion from consideration of claims violating the principles of justice. Thus the slight alteration of principle reveals another family of notions, another way of looking at the concept of justice.

Second, I should like to remark also that I have been dealing with the *concept* of justice. I have tried to set out the kinds of principles upon which judgments concerning the justice of practices may be said to stand. The analysis will be successful to the degree that it expresses the principles involved in these judgments when made by competent persons upon deliberation and reflection.[23] Now every people may be supposed to have the concept of justice, since in the life of every society there must be at least some relations in which the parties consider themselves to be circumstanced and related as the concept of justice as fairness requires. Societies will differ from one another not in having or in failing to have this notion but in the range of cases to which they apply it and in the emphasis which they give to it as compared with other moral concepts.

A firm grasp of the concept of justice itself is necessary if these variations, and the reasons for them, are to be understood. No study of the development of moral ideas and of the differences between them is more sound than the analysis of the fundamental moral concepts upon which it must depend. I have tried, therefore, to give an analysis of the concept of justice which should apply generally, however large a part the concept may have in a given morality, and which can be used in explaining the course of men's thoughts about justice and its relations to other moral concepts. How it is to be used for this purpose is a large topic which I cannot, of course, take up here. I mention it only to emphasize that I have been dealing with the concept of justice itself and to indicate what use I consider such an analysis to have.

Notes

1. I use the word "practice" throughout as a sort of technical term meaning any form of activity specified by a system of rules which defines offices, roles, moves, penalties, defenses, and so on, and which gives the activity its structure. As examples one may think of games and rituals, trials and

parliaments, markets and systems of property. I have attempted a partial analysis of the notion of a practice in a paper "Two Concepts of Rules," *Philosophical Review*, LXIV (1955), 3–32.

2. These principles are, of course, well known in one form or another and appear in many analyses of justice even where the writers differ widely on other matters. Thus if the principle of equal liberty is commonly associated with Kant (see *The Philosophy of Law*, tr. by W. Hastie, Edinburgh, 1887, pp. 56 f.), it may be claimed that it can also be found in J. S. Mill's *On Liberty* and elsewhere, and in many other liberal writers. Recently H. L. A. Hart has argued for something like it in his paper "Are There Any Natural Rights?," *Philosophical Review*, LXIV (1955), 175–191. The injustice of inequalities which are not won in return for a contribution to the common advantage is, of course, widespread in political writings of all sorts. The conception of justice here discussed is distinctive, if at all, only in selecting these two principles in this form; but for another similar analysis, see the discussion by W. D. Lamont, *The Principles of Moral Judgment* (Oxford, 1946), ch. v.

3. This point was made by Sidgwick, *Methods of Ethics*, 6th ed. (London, 1901), Bk. III, ch. v., sec. 1. It has recently been emphasized by Sir Isaiah Berlin in a symposium, "Equality," *Proceedings of the Aristotelian Society*, n.s. LVI (1955–56), 305 f.

4. In the paper referred to in note 1, I have tried to show the importance of taking practices as the proper subject of the utilitarian principle. The criticisms of so-called "restricted utilitarianism" by J. J. C. Smart, "Extreme and Restricted Utilitarianism," *Philosophical Quarterly*, VI (1956), 344–354, and by H. J. McCloskey, "An Examination of Restricted Utilitarianism," *Philosophical Review*, LXVI (1957), 466–485, do not affect my argument. These papers are concerned with the very general proposition, which is attributed (with what justice I shall not consider) to S. E. Toulmin and P. H. Nowell-Smith (and in the case of the latter paper, also, apparently, to me); namely, the proposition that particular moral actions are justified by appealing to moral rules, and moral rules in turn by reference to utility. But clearly I meant to defend no such view. My discussion of the concept of rules as maxims is an explicit rejection of it. What I did argue was that, in the *logically special* case of practices (although actually quite a common case) where the rules have special features and are not moral rules at all but legal rules or rules of games and the like (except, perhaps, in the case of promises), there is a peculiar force to the distinction between justifying particular actions and justifying the system of rules themselves. Even then I claimed only that restricting the utilitarian principle to practices as defined strengthened it. I did not argue for the position that this amendment alone is sufficient for a complete defense of utilitarianism as a general theory of morals.

In this paper I take up the question as to how the utilitarian principle itself must be modified, but here, too, the subject of inquiry is not all of morality at once, but a limited topic, the concept of justice.

5. It might seem as if J. S. Mill, in paragraph 36 of Chapter v of *Utilitarianism*, expressed the utilitarian principle in this modified form, but in the remaining two paragraphs of the chapter, and elsewhere, he would appear not to grasp the significance of the change. Hume often emphasizes that *every* man must benefit. For example, in discussing the utility of general rules, he holds that they are requisite to the "well-being of every individual"; from a stable system of property "every individual person must find himself a gainer in balancing the account. . . ." "Every member of society is sensible of this interest; everyone expresses this sense to his fellows along with the resolution he has taken of squaring his actions by it, on the conditions that others will do the same." *A Treatise of Human Nature*, Bk. III, Pt. II, Section II, paragraph 22.

6. It is not possible to discuss here this addition to the usual conception of rationality. If it seems peculiar, it may be worth remarking that it is analogous to the modification of the utilitarian principle which the argument as a whole is designed to explain and justify. In the same way that the satisfaction of interests, the representative claims of which violate the principles of justice, is not a reason for having a practice (see sec. 7), unfounded envy, within limits, need not be taken into account.

7. The idea that accepting a principle as a moral principle implies that one generally acts on it, failing a special explanation, has been stressed by R. M. Hare, *The Language of Morals* (Oxford, 1952). His formulation of it needs to be modified, however, along the lines suggested by P. L. Gardiner, "On Assenting to a Moral Principle," *Proceedings of the Aristotelian Society*, n.s. LV (1955), 23–44. See also C. K. Grant, "Akrasia and the Criteria of Assent to Practical Principles," *Mind*, LXV (1956), 400–407, where the complexity of the criteria for assent is discussed.

8. Perhaps the best known statement of this conception is that given by Glaucon at the beginning of Book II of Plato's *Republic*. Presumably it was, in various forms, a common view among the Sophists; but that Plato gives a fair representation of it is doubtful. See K. R. Popper, *The Open Society and Its Enemies*, rev. ed. (Princeton, 1950), pp. 112–118. Certainly Plato usually attributes to it a quality of manic egoism which one feels must be an exaggeration; on the other hand, see the Melian Debate in Thucydides, *The Peloponnesian War*, Book V, ch. vii, although it is impossible to say to what extent the views expressed there reveal any current philosophical opinion. Also in this tradition are the remarks of Epicurus on justice in *Principal Doctrines*, XXXI–XXXVIII. In modern times elements of the conception appear in a more sophisticated form in

Hobbes *The Leviathan* and in Hume *A Treatise of Human Nature*, Book III, Pt. II, as well as in the writings of the school of natural law such as Pufendorf's *De jure naturae et gentium*. Hobbes and Hume are especially instructive. For Hobbes's argument see Howard Warrender's *The Political Philosophy of Hobbes* (Oxford, 1957). W. J. Baumol's *Welfare Economics and the Theory of the State* (London, 1952), is valuable in showing the wide applicability of Hobbes's fundamental idea (interpreting his natural law as principles of prudence), although in this book it is traced back only to Hume's *Treatise*.

9. See J. von Neumann and O. Morgenstern, *The Theory of Games and Economic Behavior*, 2nd ed. (Princeton, 1947). For a comprehensive and not too technical discussion of the developments since, see R. Duncan Luce and Howard Raiffa, *Games and Decisions: Introduction and Critical Survey* (New York, 1957). Chs. VI and XIV discuss the developments most obviously related to the analysis of justice.

10. For a general survey see J. W. Gough, *The Social Contract*, 2nd ed. (Oxford, 1957), and Otto von Gierke, *The Development of Political Theory*, tr. by B. Freyd (London, 1939), Pt. II, ch. ii.

11. The difficulty one gets into by a mechanical application of the theory of games to moral philosophy can be brought out by considering among several possible examples, R. B. Braithwaite's study, *Theory of Games as a Tool for the Moral Philosopher* (Cambridge, 1955). On the analysis there given, it turns out that the fair division of playing time between Matthew and Luke depends on their preferences, and these in turn are connected with the instruments they wish to play. Since Matthew has a threat advantage over Luke, arising purely from the fact that Matthew, the trumpeter, prefers both of them playing at once to neither of them playing, whereas Luke, the pianist, prefers silence to cacophony, Matthew is alloted 26 evenings of play to Luke's 17. If the situation were reversed, the threat advantage would be with Luke. See pp. 36 f. But now we have only to suppose that Matthew is a jazz enthusiast who plays the drums, and Luke a violinist who plays sonatas, in which case it will be fair, on this analysis, for Matthew to play whenever and as often as he likes, assuming, of course, as it is plausible to assume, that he does not care whether Luke plays or not. Certainly something has gone wrong. To each according to his threat advantage is hardly the principle of fairness. What is lacking is the concept of morality, and it must be brought into the conjectural account in some way or other. In the text this is done by the form of the procedure whereby principles are proposed and acknowledged (Section 3). If one starts directly with the particular case as known, and if one accepts as given and definitive the preferences and relative positions of the parties, whatever they are, it is impossible to give an analysis of the moral concept of fairness. Braithwaite's use of the theory of

games, insofar as it is intended to analyze the concept of fairness, is, I think, mistaken. This is not, of course, to criticize in any way the theory of games as a mathematical theory, to which Braithwaite's book certainly contributes, nor as an analysis of how rational (and amoral) egoists might behave (and so as an analysis of how people sometimes actually do behave). But it is to say that if the theory of games is to be used to analyze moral concepts, its formal structure must be interpreted in a special and general manner as indicated in the text. Once we do this, though, we are in touch again with a much older tradition.

12. For the definition of this prima facie duty, and the idea that it is a special duty, I am indebted to H. L. A. Hart. See his paper "Are There Any Natural Rights?," *Philosophical Review*, LXIV (1955), 185 f.

13. The sense of "performative" here is to be derived from J. L. Austin's paper in the symposium, "Other Minds," *Proceedings of the Aristotelian Society*, Supplementary Volume (1946), pp. 170–174.

14. This, however, commonly happens. Hobbes, for example, when invoking the notion of a "tacit covenant," appeals not to the natural law that promises should be kept but to his fourth law of nature, that of gratitude. On Hobbes's shift from fidelity to gratitude, see Warrender, *op. cit.*, pp. 51–52, 233–237. While it is not a serious criticism of Hobbes, it would have improved his argument had he appealed to the duty of fair play. On his premises he is perfectly entitled to do so. Similarly Sidgwick thought that a principle of justice, such as every man ought to receive adequate requital for his labor, is like gratitude universalized. See *Methods of Ethics*, Bk. III, ch. v, Sec. 5. There is a gap in the stock of moral concepts used by philosophers into which the concept of the duty of fair play fits quite naturally.

15. I am using the concept of criterion here in what I take to be Wittgenstein's sense. See *Philosophical Investigations* (Oxford, 1953); and Norman Malcolm's review, "Wittgenstein's *Philosophical Investigations*," *Philosophical Review*, LXIII (1954), 543–547. That the response of compassion, under appropriate circumstances, is part of the criterion for whether or not a person understands what "pain" means, is, I think, in the *Philosophical Investigations*. The view in the text is simply an extension of this idea. I cannot, however, attempt to justify it here. Similar thoughts are to be found, I think, in Max Scheler, *The Nature of Sympathy*, tr. by Peter Heath (New Haven, 1954). His way of writing is often so obscure that I cannot be certain.

16. While this assimilation is implicit in Bentham's and Sidgwick's moral theory, explicit statements of it as applied to justice are relatively rare. One clear instance in *The Principles of Morals and Legislation* occurs in ch. x, footnote 2 to section XL: ". . . justice, in the only sense in which it has a meaning, is an imaginary personage,

feigned for the convenience of discourse, whose dictates are the dictates of utility, applied to certain particular cases. Justice, then, is nothing more than an imaginary instrument, employed to forward on certain occasions, and by certain means, the purposes of benevolence. The dictates of justice are nothing more than a part of the dictates of benevolence, which, on certain occasions, are applied to certain subjects. . . ." Likewise in *The Limits of Jurisprudence Defined*, ed. by C. W. Everett (New York, 1945), pp. 117 f., Bentham criticizes Grotius for denying that justice derives from utility; and in *The Theory of Legislation*, ed. by C. K. Ogden (London, 1931), p. 3, he says that he uses the words "just" and "unjust" along with other words "simply as collective terms including the ideas of certain pains or pleasures." That Sidgwick's conception of justice is similar to Bentham's is admittedly not evident from his discussion of justice in Book III, ch. v of *Methods of Ethics*. But it follows, I think, from the moral theory he accepts. Hence C. D. Broad's criticisms of Sidgwick in the matter of distributive justice in *Five Types of Ethical Theory* (London, 1930), pp. 249–253, do not rest on a misinterpretation.

17. This maxim is attributed to Bentham by J. S. Mill in *Utilitarianism*, ch. v, paragraph 36. I have not found it in Bentham's writings, nor seen such a reference. Similarly James Bonar, *Philosophy and Political Economy* (London, 1893), p. 234 n. But it accords perfectly with Bentham's ideas. See the hitherto unpublished manuscript in David Baumgardt, *Bentham and the Ethics of Today* (Princeton, 1952), Appendix IV. For example, "the total value of the stock of pleasure belonging to the whole community is to be obtained by multiplying the number expressing the value of it as respecting any one person, by the number expressing the multitude of such individuals" (p. 556).

18. An idea essential to the classical utilitarian conception of justice. Bentham is firm in his statement of it: "It is only upon that principle [the principle of asceticism], and not from the principle of utility, that the most abominable pleasure which the vilest of malefactors ever reaped from his crime would be reprobated, if it stood alone. The case is, that it never does stand alone; but is necessarily followed by such a quantity of pain (or, what comes to the same thing, such a chance for a certain quantity of pain) that the pleasure in comparison of it, is as nothing: and this is the true and sole, but perfectly sufficient, reason for making it a ground for punishment" (*The Principles of Morals and Legislation*, ch. ii, sec. iv. See also ch. x, sec. x, footnote i). The same point is made in *The Limits of Jurisprudence Defined*, pp. 115 f. Although much recent welfare economics, as found in such important works as I. M. D. Little, *A Critique of Welfare Economics*, 2nd ed. (Oxford, 1957) and K. J. Arrow, *Social Choice and Individual Values* (New York, 1951), dispenses with the idea of cardinal utility, and use instead the theory of ordinal utility as stated by J. R. Hicks, *Value and Capital*, 2nd ed. (Oxford, 1946), Pt. I, it assumes with

utilitarianism that individual preferences have value as such, and so accepts the idea being criticized here. I hasten to add, however, that this is no objection to it as a means of analyzing economic policy, and for that purpose it may, indeed, be a necessary simplifying assumption. Nevertheless it is an assumption which cannot be made in so far as one is trying to analyze moral concepts, especially the concept of justice, as economists would, I think, agree. Justice is usually regarded as a separate and distinct part of any comprehensive criterion of economic policy. See, for example, Tibor Scitovsky, *Welfare and Competition* (London, 1952), pp. 59–69, and Little, *op. cit.*, ch. VII.

19. See J. S. Mill's argument in *Utilitarianism*, ch. v, pars. 16–25.

20. See D. G. Ritchie, *Natural Rights* (London, 1894), pp. 95 ff., 249 ff. Lionel Robbins has insisted on this point on several occasions. See *An Essay on the Nature and Significance of Economic Science*, 2nd ed. (London, 1935), pp. 134–143, "Interpersonal Comparisons of Utility: A Comment," *Economic Journal*, XLVIII (1938), 635–41, and more recently, "Robertson on Utility and Scope," *Economica*, n.s. XX (1953), 108 f.

21. As Sir Henry Maine suggested Bentham may have regarded them. See *The Early History of Institutions* (London, 1875), pp. 398 ff.

22. Thus Kant was not far wrong when he interpreted the original contract merely as an "Idea of Reason"; yet he still thought of it as a *general* criterion of right and as providing a general theory of political obligation. See the second part of the essay, "On the Saying 'That may be right in theory but has no value in practice'" (1793), in *Kant's Principles of Politics*, tr. by W. Hastie (Edinburgh, 1891). I have drawn on the contractarian tradition not for a general theory of political obligation but to clarify the concept of justice.

23. For a further discussion of the idea expressed here, see my paper, "Outline of a Decision Procedure for Ethics," in the *Philosophical Review*, LX (1951), 177–197. For an analysis, similar in many respects but using the notion of the ideal observer instead of that of the considered judgment of a competent person, see Roderick Firth, "Ethical Absolutism and the Ideal Observer," *Philosophy and Phenomenological Research*, XII (1952), 317–345. While the similarities between these two discussions are more important than the differences, an analysis based on the notion of a considered judgment of a competent person, as it is based on a kind of judgment, may prove more helpful in understanding the features of moral judgment than an analysis based on the notion of an ideal observer, although this remains to be shown. A man who rejects the conditions imposed on a considered judgment of a competent person could no longer profess to *judge* at all. This seems more fundamental than his rejecting the conditions of observation, for these do not seem to apply, in an ordinary sense, to making a moral judgment.

18

H. L. A. Hart
Laws and Morals

Reprinted by permission of The
Clarendon Press, Oxford, from H. L. A.
Hart, *The Concept of Law*. Copyright
© 1965 by the Oxford University
Press, pp. 181–207.

Natural Law and Legal Positivism

There are many different types of relation between law and morals and there is nothing which can be profitably singled out for study as *the* relation between them. Instead it is important to distinguish some of the many different things which may be meant by the assertion or denial that law and morals are related. Sometimes what is asserted is a kind of connexion which few if any have ever denied; but its indisputable existence may be wrongly accepted as a sign of some more doubtful connexion, or even mistaken for it. Thus, it cannot seriously be disputed that the development of law, at all times and places, has in fact been profoundly influenced both by the conventional morality and ideals of particular social groups, and also by forms of enlightened moral criticism urged by individuals, whose moral horizon has transcended the morality currently accepted. But it is possible to take this truth illicitly, as a warrant for a different proposition: namely that a legal system *must* exhibit some specific conformity with morality or justice, or *must* rest on a widely diffused conviction that there is a moral obligation to obey it. Again, though this proposition may, in some sense, be true, it does not follow from it that the criteria of legal validity of particular laws used in a legal system must include, tacitly if not explicitly, a reference to morality or justice.

Many other questions besides these may be said to concern the relations between law and morals. In this chapter we shall discuss only two of them, though both will involve some consideration of many others. The first is a question which may still be illuminatingly described as the issue between Natural Law and Legal Positivism, though each of these titles has come to be used for a range of different theses about law and morals. Here we shall take Legal Positivism to mean the simple contention that it is in no sense a necessary truth that laws reproduce or satisfy certain demands of morality, though in fact they have often done so. But just because those who have taken this view have either been silent or differed very much concerning the nature of morality, it is necessary to consider two very different forms in which Legal Positivism has been rejected. One of

these is expressed most clearly in the classical theories of Natural Law: that there are certain principles of human conduct, awaiting discovery by human reason, with which man-made law must conform if it is to be valid. The other takes a different, less rationalist view of morality, and offers a different account of the ways in which legal validity is connected with moral value. We shall consider the first of these in this section and the next.

In the vast literature from Plato to the present day which is dedicated to the assertion, and also to the denial, of the proposition that the ways in which men ought to behave may be discovered by human reason, the disputants on one side seem to say to those on the other, "You are blind if you cannot see this" only to receive in reply, "You have been dreaming." This is so, because the claim that there are true principles of right conduct, rationally discoverable, has not usually been advanced as a separate doctrine but was originally presented, and for long defended, as part of a general conception of nature, inanimate and living. This outlook is, in many ways, antithetic to the general conception of nature which constitutes the framework of modern secular thought. Hence it is that, to its critics, Natural Law theory has seemed to spring from deep and old confusions from which modern thought has triumphantly freed itself; while to its advocates, the critics appear merely to insist on surface trivialities, ignoring profounder truths.

Thus many modern critics have thought that the claim that laws of proper conduct may be discovered by human reason rested on a simple ambiguity of the word "law," and that when this ambiguity was exposed Natural Law received its deathblow. It is in this way that John Stuart Mill dealt with Montesquieu, who in the first chapter of the *Esprit des Lois* naïvely inquires why it is that, while inanimate things such as the stars and also animals obey "the law of their nature," man does not do so but falls into sin. This, Mill thought, revealed the perennial confusion between laws which formulate the course or regularities of nature, and laws which require men to behave in certain ways. The former, which can be discovered by observation and reasoning, may be called "descriptive" and it is for the scientist thus to discover them; the latter cannot be so established, for they are not statements or descriptions of facts, but are "prescriptions" or demands that men shall behave in certain ways. The answer therefore to Montesquieu's question is simple: prescriptive laws may be broken and yet remain laws, because that merely means that human beings do not do what they are told to do; but it is meaningless to say of the laws of nature, discovered by science, either that they can or cannot be broken. If the stars behave in ways contrary to the scientific laws which purport to describe their regular movements, these are not broken but they lose their title to be called "laws" and must be reformulated. To these differences in the sense of "law," there correspond systematic differences in the associated vocabulary of words like "must," "bound to," "ought," and "should." So, on this view, belief in Natural Law is reducible to a very simple fallacy: a failure to perceive the very different senses which those law-impregnated words can bear. It is as if the believer had failed to perceive the very different meaning of such words in "You are bound to report for military service" and "It is bound to freeze if the wind goes round to the north."

Critics like Bentham and Mill, who most fiercely attacked Natural Law, often attributed their opponents' confusion between these distinct senses of law, to the survival of the belief that the observed regularities of nature were prescribed or decreed by a Divine Governor of the Universe. On such a theocratic view, the only difference between the law of gravity and the Ten Commandments—God's law for Man—was, as Blackstone asserted, the relatively minor one that men, alone of created things, were endowed with reason and free will; and so unlike things, could discover and disobey the divine prescriptions. Natural Law has, however, not always been associated with belief in a Divine Governor or Lawgiver of the universe, and even where it has been, its characteristic tenets have not been logically dependent on that belief. Both the relevant sense of the word "natural," which enters into Natural Law, and its general outlook minimizing the difference, so

obvious and so important to modern minds, between prescriptive and descriptive laws, have their roots in Greek thought which was, for this purpose, quite secular. Indeed, the continued reassertion of some form of Natural Law doctrine is due in part to the fact that its appeal is independent of both divine and human authority, and to the fact that despite a terminology, and much metaphysics, which few could now accept, it contains certain elementary truths of importance for the understanding of both morality and law. These we shall endeavour to disentangle from their metaphysical setting and restate here in simpler terms.

For modern secular thought the world of inanimate and living things, animals, and men is a scene of recurrent kinds of events and changes which exemplify certain regular connexions. Some at least of these, human beings have discovered and formulated as laws of nature. To understand nature is, in this modern view, to bring to bear on some part of it, knowledge of these regularities. The structure of great scientific theories does not of course mirror in any simple way observable fact, events, or changes; often, indeed, a great part of such theories consists of abstract mathematical formulations with no direct counterpart in observable fact. Their connexion with observable events and changes lies in the fact that, from these abstract formulations, generalizations may be deduced which do refer to, and may be confirmed or falsified by, observable events. A scientific theory's claim to forward our understanding of nature is therefore, in the last resort, dependent on its power to predict what will occur, which is based on generalizations of what regularly occurs. The law of gravity and the second law of thermodynamics are, for modern thought, laws of nature and more than mere mathematical constructions in virtue of the information they yield concerning the regularities of observable phenomena.

The doctrine of Natural Law is part of an older conception of nature in which the observable world is not merely a scene of such regularities, and knowledge of nature is not merely a knowledge of them. Instead, on this older outlook every nameable kind of existing thing, human, animate, and inanimate, is conceived not only as tending to maintain itself in existence but

as proceeding towards a definite optimum state which is the specific good—or the end (τέλος, finis) appropriate for it.

This is the teleological conception of nature as containing in itself levels of excellence which things realize. The stages by which a thing of any given kind progresses to its specific or proper end are regular, and may be formulated in generalizations describing the thing's characteristic mode of change, or action, or development; to that extent the teleological view of nature overlaps with modern thought. The difference is that on the teleological view, the events regularly befalling things are not thought of *merely* as occurring regularly, and the questions whether they *do* occur regularly and whether they *should* occur or whether it is *good* that they occur are not regarded as separate questions. On the contrary (except for some rare monstrosities ascribed to "chance") what generally occurs can both be explained and evaluated as good or what ought to occur, by exhibiting it as a step towards the proper end or goal of the thing concerned. The laws of a thing's development therefore should show both how it should and how it does regularly behave or change.

This mode of thinking about nature seems strange when stated abstractly. It may appear less fantastic if we recall some of the ways in which even now we refer at least to living things, for a teleological view is still reflected in common ways of describing their development. Thus in the case of an acorn, growth into an oak is something which is not only regularly achieved by acorns, but is distinguished unlike its decay (which is also regular) as an optimum state of maturity in the light of which the intermediate stages are both explained and judged as good or bad, and the "functions" of its various parts and structural changes identified. The normal growth of leaves is required if it is to obtain the moisture necessary for "full" or "proper" development, and it is the "function" of leaves to supply this. Hence we think and speak of this growth as what "ought naturally to occur." In the case of the action or movements of inanimate things, such ways of talking seem much less plausible unless they are artifacts designed by human beings for a purpose. The notion that a stone on falling to the ground is realizing some appropriate "end" or returning to its "proper place," like a horse galloping home to a stable, is now somewhat comic.

Indeed, one of the difficulties in understanding a teleological view of nature is that just as it minimized the differences between statements of what regularly happens and statements of what ought to happen, so too it minimizes the difference, so important in modern thought, between human beings *with* a purpose of their own which they consciously strive to realize and other living or inanimate things. For in the teleological view of the world, man, like other things, is thought of as tending towards a specific optimum state or end which is set for him and the fact, that he, unlike other things, may do this consciously, is not conceived as a radical difference between him and the rest of nature. This specific human end or good is in part, like that of other living things, a condition of biological maturity and developed physical powers; but it also includes, as its distinctively human element, a development and excellence of mind and character manifested in thought and conduct. Unlike other things, man is able by reasoning and reflection to discover what the attainment of this excellence of mind and character involves and to desire it. Yet even so, on this teleological view, this optimum state is not man's good or end because he desires it; rather he desires it because it is already his natural end.

Again, much of this teleological point of view survives in some of the ways in which we think and speak of human beings. It is latent in our identification of certain things as human *needs* which it is *good* to satisfy and of certain things done to or suffered *by* human beings as *harm* or *injury*. Thus, though it is true that some men may refuse to eat or rest because they wish to die, we think of eating and resting as something more than things which men regularly do or just happen to desire. Food and rest are human needs, even if some refuse them when they are needed. Hence we say not only that it is natural for all men to eat and sleep, but that all men ought to eat and rest sometimes, or that it is naturally good

to do these things. The force of the word "naturally," in such judgments of human conduct, is to differentiate them both from judgments which reflect mere conventions or human prescriptions ("You ought to take off your hat"), the content of which cannot be discovered by thought or reflection, and also from judgments which merely indicate what is required for achieving some particular objective, which at a given time one man may happen to have and another may not. The same outlook is present in our conception of the *functions* of bodily organs and the line we draw between these and mere causal properties. We say it is the function of the heart to circulate the blood, but not that it is the function of a cancerous growth to cause death.

These crude examples designed to illustrate teleological elements still alive in ordinary thought about human action, are drawn from the lowly sphere of biological fact which man shares with other animals. It will be rightly observed that what makes sense of this mode of thought and expression is something entirely obvious: it is the tacit assumption that the proper end of human activity is survival, and this rests on the simple contingent fact that most men most of the time wish to continue in existence. The actions which we speak of as those which are naturally good to do, are those which are required for survival; the notions of a human need, of harm, and of the *function* of bodily organs or changes rests on the same simple fact. Certainly if we stop here, we shall have only a very attenuated version of Natural Law: for the classical exponents of this outlook conceived of survival (*perseverare in esse suo*) as merely the lowest stratum in a much more complex and far more debatable concept of the human end or good for man. Aristotle included in it the disinterested cultivation of the human intellect, and Aquinas the knowledge of God, and both these represent values which may be and have been challenged. Yet other thinkers, Hobbes and Hume among them, have been willing to lower their sights: they have seen in the modest aim of survival the central indisputable element which gives empirical good sense to the terminology

of Natural Law. "Human nature cannot by any means subsist without the association of individuals: and that association never could have place were no regard paid to the laws of equity and justice."[1]

This simple thought has in fact very much to do with the characteristics of both law and morals, and it can be disentangled from more disputable parts of the general teleological outlook in which the end or good for man appears as a specific way of life about which, in fact, men may profoundly disagree. Moreover, we can, in referring to survival, discard, as too metaphysical for modern minds, the notion that this is something antecedently fixed which men necessarily desire because it is their proper goal or end. Instead we may hold it to be a mere contingent fact which could be otherwise, that in general men do desire to live, and that we may mean nothing more by calling survival a human goal or end than that men do desire it. Yet even if we think of it in this common-sense way, survival has still a special status in relation to human conduct and in our thought about it, which parallels the prominence and the necessity ascribed to it in the orthodox formulations of Natural Law. For it is not merely that an overwhelming majority of men do wish to live, even at the cost of hideous misery, but that this is reflected in whole structures of our thought and language, in terms of which we describe the world and each other. We could not subtract the general wish to live and leave intact concepts like danger and safety, harm and benefit, need and function, disease and cure; for these are ways of simultaneously describing and appraising things by reference to the contribution they make to survival which is accepted as an aim.

There are, however, simpler, less philosophical, considerations than these which show acceptance of survival as an aim to be necessary, in a sense more directly relevant to the discussion of human law and morals. We are committed to it as something presupposed by the terms of the discussion; for our concern is with social arrangements for continued existence, not with those of a suicide club. We wish to know whether, among these social arrangements, there are some which may illuminatingly be ranked as natural laws discoverable by reason, and what their relation is to human law and morality. To raise this or any other question concerning *how* men should live together, we must assume that their aim, generally speaking, is to live. From this point the argument is a simple one. Reflection on some very obvious generalizations—indeed truisms—concerning human nature and the world in which men live, show that as long as these hold good, there are certain rules of conduct which any social organization must contain if it is to be viable. Such rules do in fact constitute a common element in the law and conventional morality of all societies which have progressed to the point where these are distinguished as different forms of social control. With them are found, both in law and morals, much that is peculiar to a particular society and much that may seem arbitrary or a mere matter of choice. Such universally recognized principles of conduct which have a basis in elementary truths concerning human beings, their natural environment, and aims, may be considered the *minimum content* of Natural Law, in contrast with the more grandiose and more challengeable constructions which have often been proffered under that name. In the next section we shall consider, in the form of five truisms, the salient characteristics of human nature upon which this modest but important minimum rests.

The Minimum Content of Natural Law

In considering the simple truisms which we set forth here, and their connexion with law and morals, it is important to observe that in each case the facts mentioned afford a *reason* why, given survival as an aim, law and morals should include a specific content. The general form of the argument is simply that without such a content laws and morals could not forward the minimum purpose of survival which men have in associating with each other. In the absence of this content men, as they are, would have no reason for obeying voluntarily any rules; and without a minimum of co-operation given voluntarily by those who find that it is in their interest to

submit to and maintain the rules, coercion of others who would not voluntarily conform would be impossible. It is important to stress the distinctively rational connexion between natural facts and the content of legal and moral rules in this approach, because it is both possible and important to inquire into quite different forms of connexion between natural facts and legal or moral rules. Thus, the still young sciences of psychology and sociology may discover or may even have discovered that, unless certain physical, psychological, or economic conditions are satisfied, e.g. unless young children are fed and nurtured in certain ways within the family, no system of laws or code of morals can be established, or that only those laws can function successfully which conform to a certain type. Connexions of this sort between natural conditions and systems of rules are not mediated by *reasons*; for they do not relate the existence of certain rules to the conscious aims or purpose of those whose rules they are. Being fed in infancy in a certain way may well be shown to be a necessary condition or even a *cause* of a population developing or maintaining a moral or legal code, but it is not a *reason* for their doing so. Such causal connexions do not of course conflict with the connexions which rest on purposes or conscious aims; they may indeed be considered more important or fundamental than the latter, since they may actually explain why human beings have those conscious aims or purposes which Natural Law takes as its starting points. Causal explanations of this type do not rest on truisms nor are they mediated by conscious aims or purposes: they are for sociology or psychology like other sciences to establish by the methods of generalization and theory, resting on observation and, where possible, on experiment. Such connexions therefore are of a different kind from those which relate the content of certain legal and moral rules to the facts stated in the following truisms.

Human Vulnerability

The common requirements of law and morality consist for the most part not of active services to be rendered but of forbearances, which are usually formulated in negative form as prohibitions.

Of these the most important for social life are those that restrict the use of violence in killing or inflicting bodily harm. The basic character of such rules may be brought out in a question: If there were not these rules what point could there be for beings such as ourselves in having rules of *any* other kind? The force of this rhetorical question rests on the fact that men are both occasionally prone to, and normally vulnerable to, bodily attack. Yet though this is a truism it is not a necessary truth; for things might have been, and might one day be, otherwise. There are species of animals whose physical structure (including exoskeletons or a carapace) renders them virtually immune from attack by other members of their species and animals who have no organs enabling them to attack. If men were to lose their vulnerability to each other there would vanish one obvious reason for the most characteristic provision of law and morals: *Thou shalt not kill.*

Approximate Equality

Men differ from each other in physical strength, agility, and even more in intellectual capacity. Nonetheless it is a fact of quite major importance for the understanding of different forms of law and morality, that no individual is so much more powerful than others, that he is able, without co-operation, to dominate or subdue them for more than a short period. Even the strongest must sleep at times and, when asleep, loses temporarily his superiority. This fact of approximate equality, more than any other, makes obvious the necessity for a system of mutual forbearance and compromise which is the base of both legal and moral obligation. Social life with its rules requiring such forbearances is irksome at times; but it is at any rate less nasty, less brutish, and less short than unrestrained aggression for beings thus approximately equal. It is, of course, entirely consistent with this and an equal truism that when such a system of forbearance is established there will always be some who will wish to exploit it, by simultaneously living within its shelter and breaking its restrictions. This, indeed is, as we later show, one of the natural facts which makes the step from merely moral to organized, legal forms of control a necessary one. Again, things might have been otherwise. Instead of being approximately equal there might have been some men immensely stronger than others and better able to dispense with rest, either because some were in these ways far above the present average, or because most were far below it. Such exceptional men might have much to gain by aggression and little to gain from mutual forbearance or compromise with others. But we need not have recourse to the fantasy of giants among pygmies to see the cardinal importance of the fact of approximate equality: for it is illustrated better by the facts of international life, where there are (or were) vast disparities in strength and vulnerability between the states. This inequality, as we shall later see, between the units of international law is one of the things that has imparted to it a character so different from municipal law and limited the extent to which it is capable of operating as an organized coercive system.

Limited Altruism

Men are not devils dominated by a wish to exterminate each other, and the demonstration that, given only the modest aim of survival, the basic rules of law and morals are necessities, must not be identified with the false view that men are predominantly selfish and have no disinterested interest in the survival and welfare of their fellows. But if men are not devils, neither are they angels; and the fact that they are a mean between these two extremes is something which makes a system of mutual forbearances both necessary and possible. With angels, never tempted to harm others, rules requiring forbearances would not be necessary. With devils prepared to destroy, reckless of the cost to themselves, they would be impossible. As things are, human altruism is limited in range and intermittent, and the tendencies to aggression are frequent enough to be fatal to social life if not controlled.

Limited Resources

It is a merely contingent fact that human beings need food, clothes, and shelter; that these do not exist at hand in limitless abundance; but are scarce, have to be grown or won from nature, or have to be constructed by human toil. These facts alone make indispensable some minimal form of the institution of property (though not necessarily individual property), and the distinctive kind of rule which requires respect for it. The simplest forms of property are to be seen in rules excluding persons generally other than the "owner" from entry on, or the use of land, or from taking or using material things. If crops are to grow, land must be secure from indiscriminate entry, and food must, in the intervals between its growth or capture and consumption, be secure from being taken by others. At all times and places life itself depends on these minimal forbearances. Again, in this respect, things might have been otherwise than they are. The human organism might have been constructed like plants, capable of extracting food from air, or what it needs might have grown without cultivation in limitless abundance.

The rules which we have so far discussed are *static* rules, in the sense that the obligations they impose and the incidence of these obligations are not variable by individuals. But the division of labour, which all but the smallest groups must develop to obtain adequate supplies, brings with it the need for rules which are *dynamic* in the sense that they enable individuals to create obligations and to vary their incidence. Among these are rules enabling men to transfer, exchange, or sell their products; for these transactions involve the capacity to alter the incidence of those initial rights and obligations which define the simplest form of property. The same inescapable division of labour, and perennial need for co-operation, are also factors which make other forms of dynamic or obligation-creating rule necessary in social life. These secure the recognition of promises as a source of obligation. By this device individuals are enabled by words, spoken or written, to make themselves liable to blame or punishment for failure to act in certain stipulated ways. Where altruism is not unlimited, a standing procedure providing for such self-binding operations is required in order to create a minimum form of confidence in the future behaviour of others, and to ensure the predictability necessary for co-operation. This is most obviously needed where what is to be exchanged or jointly planned are mutual services, or wherever goods which are to be exchanged or sold are not simultaneously or immediately available.

Limited Understanding and Strength of Will

The facts that make rules respecting persons, property, and promises necessary in social life are simple and their mutual benefits are obvious. Most men are capable of seeing them and of sacrificing the immediate short-term interests which conformity to such rules demands. They may indeed obey, from a variety of motives: some from prudential calculation that the sacrifices are worth the gains, some from a disinterested interest in the welfare of others, and some because they look upon the rules as worthy of respect in themselves and find their ideals in devotion to them. On the other hand, neither understanding of long-term interest, nor the strength or goodness of will, upon which the efficacy of these different motives towards obedience depends, are shared by all men alike. All are tempted at times to prefer their own immediate interests and, in the absence of a special organization for their detection and punishment, many would succumb to the temptation. No doubt the advantages of mutual forbearance are so palpable that the number and strength of those who would co-operate voluntarily in a coercive system will normally be greater than any likely combination of malefactors. Yet, except in very small closely knit societies, submission to the system of restraints would be folly if there were no organization for the coercion of those who would then try to obtain the advantages of the system without submitting to its obligations. "Sanctions" are therefore required not as the normal motive for obedience, but as a *guarantee* that those who would voluntarily obey shall not be sacrificed to those who would not. To obey, without this, would be to risk going to the wall. Given this standing danger, what reason demands is *voluntary* co-operation in a *coercive* system.

It is to be observed that the same natural fact of approximate equality between men is of crucial importance in the efficacy of organized sanctions. If some men were vastly more powerful than others, and so not dependent on their forbearance, the strength of the malefactors might exceed that of the supporters of law and order. Given such inequalities, the use of sanctions could not be successful and would involve dangers at least as great as those which were designed to suppress. In these circumstances instead of social life being based on a system of mutual forbearances, with force used only intermittently against a minority of malefactors, the only viable system would be one in which the weak submitted to the strong on the best terms they could make and lived under their "protection." This, because of the scarcity of resources, would lead to a number of conflicting power centres, each grouped round its "strong man": these might intermittently war with each other, though the natural sanction, never negligible, of the risk of defeat might ensure an uneasy peace. Rules of a sort might then be accepted for the regulation of issues over which the "powers" were unwilling to fight. Again we need not think in fanciful terms of pygmies and giants in order to understand the simple logistics of approximate equality and its importance for law. The international scene, where the units concerned have differed vastly in strength, affords illustration enough. For centuries the disparities between states have resulted in a system where organized sanctions have been impossible, and law has been confined to matters which did not affect "vital" issues. How far atomic weapons, when available at all, will redress the balance of unequal power, and bring forms of control more closely resembling municipal criminal law, remains to be seen.

The simple truisms we have discussed not only disclose the core of good sense in the doctrine of Natural Law. They are of vital importance for the understanding of law and morals, and they explain why the definition of the basic forms of these in purely formal terms, without reference to any specific content or social needs, has proved so inadequate. Perhaps the major benefit to jurisprudence from this outlook is the escape it affords from certain misleading dichotomies which often obscure the discussion of the characteristics of law. Thus, for example, the traditional question whether

every legal system *must* provide for sanctions can be presented in a fresh and clearer light, when we command the view of things presented by this simple version of Natural Law. We shall no longer have to choose between two unsuitable alternatives which are often taken as exhaustive: on the one hand that of saying that this is required by "the" meaning of the words "law" or "legal system," and on the other that of saying that it is "just a fact" that most legal systems do provide for sanctions. Neither of these alternatives is satisfactory. There are no settled principles forbidding the use of the word "law" of systems where there are no centrally organized sanctions, and there is good reason (though no compulsion) for using the expression "international law" of a system, which has none. On the other hand we do need to distinguish the place that sanctions must have within a municipal system, if it is to serve the minimum purposes of beings constituted as men are. We can say, given the setting of natural facts and aims, which make sanctions both possible and necessary in a municipal system, that this is a *natural necessity*; and some such phrase is needed also to convey the status of the minimum forms of protection for persons, property, and promises which are similarly indispensable features of municipal law. It is in this form that we should reply to the positivist thesis that "law may have any content." For it is a truth of some importance that for the adequate description not only of law but of many other social institutions, a place must be reserved, besides definitions and ordinary statements of fact, for a third category of statements: those the truth of which is contingent on human beings and the world they live in retaining the salient characteristics which they have.

Legal Validity and Moral Value

The protections and benefits provided by the system of mutual forbearances which underlies both law and morals may, in different societies, be extended to very different ranges of persons. It is true that the denial of these elementary protections to any class of human beings, willing to accept the corresponding restrictions, would offend the principles of morality and justice to which all modern states pay, at any rate, lip

service. Their professed moral outlook is, in general, permeated by the conception that in these fundamentals at least, human beings are entitled to be treated alike and that differences of treatment require more to justify them than just an appeal to the interests of others.

Yet it is plain that neither the law nor the accepted morality of societies need extend their minimal protections and benefits to all within their scope, and often they have not done so. In slave-owning societies the sense that the slaves are human beings, not mere objects to be used, may be lost by the dominant group, who may yet remain morally most sensitive to each other's claims and interests. Huckleberry Finn, when asked if the explosion of a steamboat boiler had hurt anyone, replied, "No'm: killed a nigger." Aunt Sally's comment "Well it's lucky because sometimes people do get hurt" sums up a whole morality which has often prevailed among men. Where it does prevail, as Huck found to his cost, to extend to slaves the concern for others which is natural between members of the dominant group may well be looked on as a grave moral offence, bringing with it all the sequelae of moral guilt. Nazi Germany and South Africa offered parallels unpleasantly near to us in time.

Though the law of some societies has occasionally been in advance of the accepted morality, normally law follows morality and even the homicide of a slave may be regarded only as a waste of public resources or as an offence against the master whose property he is. Even where slavery is not officially recognized, discriminations on grounds of race, colour, or creed may produce a legal system and a social morality which does not recognize that all men are entitled to a minimum of protection from others.

These painful facts of human history are enough to show that, though a society to be viable must offer *some* of its members a system of mutual forbearances, it need not, unfortunately, offer them to all. It is true, as we have already emphasized in discussing the need for and the possibility of sanctions, that if a system of rules is to be imposed by force on any, there must be a sufficient number who accept it voluntarily. Without their voluntary co-operation, thus creating *authority*, the coercive power of law and government cannot be established. But coercive power, thus established on its basis of authority, may be used in two principal ways. It may be exerted only against malefactors who, though they are afforded the protection of the rules, yet selfishly break them. On the other hand, it may be used to subdue and maintain, in a position of permanent inferiority, a subject group whose size, relatively to the master group, may be large or small, depending on the means of coercion, solidarity, and discipline available to the latter, and the helplessness or inability to organize of the former. For those thus oppressed there may be nothing in the system to command their loyalty but only things to fear. They are its victims, not its beneficiaries.

In the earlier chapters of this book we stressed the fact that the existence of a legal system is a social phenomenon which always presents two aspects, to both of which we must attend if our view of it is to be realistic. It involves the attitudes and behaviour involved in the voluntary acceptance of rules and also the simpler attitudes and behaviour involved in mere obedience or acquiescence.

Hence a society with law contains those who look upon its rules from the internal point of view as accepted standards of behaviour, and not merely as reliable predictions of what will befall them, at the hands of officials, if they disobey. But it also comprises those upon whom, either because they are malefactors or mere helpless victims of the system, these legal standards have to be imposed by force or threat of force; they are concerned with the rules merely as a source of possible punishment. The balance between these two components will be determined by many different factors. If the system is fair and caters genuinely for the vital interests of all those from whom it demands obedience, it may gain and retain the allegiance of most for most of the time, and will accordingly be stable. On the other hand it may be a narrow and exclusive system run in the interests of the dominant group, and it may be made continually more repressive and unstable with the latent threat of upheaval. Between

these two extremes various combinations of these attitudes to law are to be found, often in the same individual.

Reflection on this aspect of things reveals a sobering truth: the step from the simple form of society, where primary rules of obligation are the only means of social control, into the legal world with its centrally organized legislature, courts, officials, and sanctions brings its solid gains at a certain cost. The gains are those of adaptability to change, certainty, and efficiency, and these are immense; the cost is the risk that the centrally organized power may well be used for the oppression of numbers with whose support it can dispense, in a way that the simpler régime of primary rules could not. Because this risk has materialized and may do so again, the claim that there is some further way in which law *must* conform to morals beyond that which we have exhibited as the minimun content of Natural Law, needs very careful scrutiny. Many such assertions either fail to make clear the sense in which the connexion between law and morals is alleged to be necessary; or upon examination they turn out to mean something which is both true and important, but which it is most confusing to present as a necessary connexion between law and morals. We shall end this chapter by examining six forms of this claim.

Power and Authority
It is often said that a legal system must rest on a sense of moral obligation or on the conviction of the moral value of the system, since it does not and cannot rest on mere power of man over man. We have ourselves stressed, in the earlier chapters of this book, the inadequacy of orders backed by threats and habits of obedience for the understanding of the foundations of a legal system and the idea of legal validity. Not only do these require for their elucidation the notion of an accepted rule of recognition . . . but, as we have seen in this chapter, a necessary condition of the existence of coercive power is that some at least must voluntarily co-operate in the system and accept its rules. In this sense it is true that the coercive power of law presupposes its accepted authority. But the dichotomy of "law based merely on power" and "law which is accepted as morally

binding" is not exhaustive. Not only may vast numbers be coerced by laws which they do not regard as morally binding, but it is not even true that those who do accept the system voluntarily, must conceive of themselves as morally bound to do so, though the system will be most stable when they do so. In fact, their allegiance to the system may be based on many different considerations: calculations of long-term interest; disinterested interest in others; an unreflecting inherited or traditional attitude; or the mere wish to do as others do. There is indeed no reason why those who accept the authority of the system should not examine their conscience and decide that, morally, they ought not to accept it, yet for a variety of reasons continue to do so.

These commonplaces may have become obscured by the general use of the same vocabulary to express both the legal and the moral obligations which men acknowledge. Those who accept the authority of a legal system look upon it from the internal point of view, and express their sense of its requirements in internal statements couched in the normative language which is common to both law and morals: "I (You) ought," "I (he) must," "I (they) have an obligation." Yet they are not thereby committed to a *moral* judgment that it is morally right to do what the law requires. No doubt if nothing else is said, there is a presumption that any one who speaks in these ways of his or others' legal obligations, does not think that there is any moral or other reason against fulfilling them. This, however, does not show that nothing can be acknowledged as legally obligatory unless it is accepted as morally obligatory. The presumption which we have mentioned rests on the fact that it will often be pointless to acknowledge or point out a legal obligation, if the speaker has conclusive reasons, moral or otherwise, to urge against fulfilling it.

The Influence of Morality on Law
The law of every modern state shows at a thousand points the influence of both the accepted social morality and wider moral ideals. These influences enter into law either abruptly and

avowedly through legislation, or silently and piecemeal through the judicial process. In some systems, as in the United States, the ultimate criteria of legal validity explicitly incorporate principles of justice or substantive moral values; in other systems, as in England, where there are no formal restrictions on the competence of the supreme legislature, its legislation may yet no less scrupulously conform to justice or morality. The further ways in which law mirrors morality are myriad, and still insufficiently studied: statutes may be a mere legal shell and demand by their express terms to be filled out with the aid of moral principles; the range of enforceable contracts may be limited by reference to conceptions of morality and fairness; liability for both civil and criminal wrongs may be adjusted to prevailing views of moral responsibility. No "positivist" could deny that these are facts, or that the stability of legal systems depends in part upon such types of correspondence with morals. If this is what is meant by the necessary connexion of law and morals, its existence should be conceded.

Interpretation
Laws require interpretation if they are to be applied to concrete cases, and once the myths which obscure the nature of the judicial processes are dispelled by realistic study, it is patent . . . that the open texture of law leaves a vast field for a creative activity which some call legislative. Neither in interpreting statutes nor precedents are judges confined to the alternatives of blind, arbitrary choice, or "mechanical" deduction from rules with predetermined meaning. Very often their choice is guided by an assumption that the purpose of the rules which they are interpreting is a reasonable one, so that the rules are not intended to work injustice or offend settled moral principles. Judicial decision, especially on matters of high constitutional import, often involves a choice between moral values, and not merely the application of some single outstanding moral principle; for it is folly to believe that where the meaning of the law is in doubt, morality always has a clear answer to offer. At this point judges may again make a choice which is neither

arbitrary nor mechanical; and here often display characteristic judicial virtues, the special appropriateness of which to legal decision explains why some feel reluctant to call such judicial activity "legislative." These virtues are: impartiality and neutrality in surveying the alternatives; consideration for the interest of all who will be affected; and a concern to deploy some acceptable general principle as a reasoned basis for decision. No doubt because a plurality of such principles is always possible it cannot be *demonstrated* that a decision is uniquely correct: but it may be made acceptable as the reasoned product of informed impartial choice. In all this we have the "weighing" and "balancing" characteristic of the effort to do justice between competing interests.

Few would deny the importance of these elements, which may well be called "moral" in rendering decisions acceptable; and the loose and changing tradition or canons of interpretation, which in most systems govern interpretation, often vaguely incorporate them. Yet if these facts are tendered as evidence of the *necessary* connexion of law and morals, we need to remember that the same principles have been honoured nearly as much in the breach as in the observance. For, from Austin to the present day, reminders that such elements *should* guide decision have come, in the main, from critics who have found that judicial law-making has often been blind to social values, "automatic," or inadequately reasoned.

The Criticism of Law
Sometimes the claim that there is a necessary connexion between law and morality comes to no more than the assertion that a *good* legal system must conform at certain points, such as those already mentioned in the last paragraph, to the requirements of justice and morality. Some may regard this as an obvious truism; but it is not a tautology, and in fact, in the criticism of law, there may be disagreement both as to the appropriate moral standards and as to the required points of conformity. Does the morality, with which law must conform if it is to be good, mean the accepted morality of the group whose law it is, even though this may rest on superstition or may withhold its benefits and protection from slaves or subject classes? Or does

morality mean standards which are enlightened in the sense that they rest on rational beliefs as to matters of fact, and accept all human beings as entitled to equal consideration and respect?

No doubt the contention that a legal system must treat all human beings within its scope as entitled to certain basic protections and freedoms, is now generally accepted as a statement of an ideal of obvious relevance in the criticism of law. Even where practice departs from it, lip service to this ideal is usually forthcoming. It may even be the case that a morality which does not take this view of the right of all men to equal consideration, can be shown by philosophy to be involved in some inner contradiction, dogmatism, or irrationality. If so, the enlightened morality which recognizes these rights has special credentials as the true morality, and is not just one among many possible moralities. These are claims which cannot be investigated here, but even if they are conceded, they cannot alter, and should not obscure, the fact that municipal legal systems, with their characteristic structure of primary and secondary rules, have long endured though they have flouted these principles of justice. What, if anything, is to be gained from denying that iniquitous rules are law, we consider below.

Principles of Legality and Justice
It may be said that the distinction between a good legal system which conforms at certain points to morality and justice, and a legal system which does not, is a fallacious one, because a minimum of justice is necessarily realized whenever human behaviour is controlled by general rules publicly announced and judicially applied. Indeed we have already pointed out, in analysing the idea of justice, that its simplest form (justice in the application of the law) consists in no more than taking seriously the notion that what is to be applied to a multiplicity of different persons is the same general rule, undeflected by prejudice, interest, or caprice. This impartiality is what the procedural standards known to English and American lawyers as principles of "Natural Justice" are designed to secure. Hence, though the most odious laws may be justly applied, we have,

in the bare notion of applying a general rule of law, the germ at least of justice.

Further aspects of this minimum form of justice which might well be called "natural" emerge if we study what is in fact involved in any method of social control—rules of games as well as law—which consists primarily of general standards of conduct communicated to classes of persons, who are then expected to understand and conform to the rules without further official direction. If social control of this sort is to function, the rules must satisfy certain conditions: they must be intelligible and within the capacity of most to obey, and in general they must not be retrospective, though exceptionally they may be. This means that, for the most part, those who are eventually punished for breach of the rules will have had the ability and opportunity to obey. Plainly these features of control by rule are closely related to the requirements of justice which lawyers term principles of legality. Indeed one critic of positivism has seen in these aspects of control by rules, something amounting to a necessary connexion between law and morality, and suggested that they be called "the inner morality of law." Again, if this is what the necessary connexion of law and morality means, we may accept it. It is unfortunately compatible with very great iniquity.

Legal Validity and Resistance to Law
However incautiously they may have formulated their general outlook, few legal theorists classed as positivists would have been concerned to deny the forms of connexion between law and morals discussed under the last five headings. What then was the concern of the great battle-cries of legal positivism: "The existence of law is one thing; its merit or demerit another,"[2] "The law of a State is not an ideal but something which actually exists . . . it is not that which ought to be, but that which is,"[3] "Legal norms may have any kind of content"?[4]

What these thinkers were, in the main, concerned to promote was clarity and honesty in the formulation of the theoretical and moral issues raised by the existence of particular laws which were morally iniquitous but were enacted in proper form, clear in

meaning, and satisfied all the acknowledged criteria of validity of a system. Their view was that, in thinking about such laws, both the theorist and the unfortunate official or private citizen who was called on to apply or obey them, could only be confused by an invitation to refuse the title of "law" or "valid" to them. They thought that, to confront these problems, simpler, more candid resources were available, which would bring into focus far better, every relevant intellectual and moral consideration: we should say, "This is law; but it is too iniquitous to be applied or obeyed."

The opposed point of view is one which appears attractive when, after revolution or major upheavals, the Courts of a system have to consider their attitude to the moral iniquities committed in legal form by private citizens or officials under an earlier régime. Their punishment may be felt socially desirable, and yet, to procure it by frankly retrospective legislation, making criminal what was permitted or even required by the law of the earlier régime, may be difficult, itself morally odious, or perhaps not possible. In these circumstances it may seem natural to exploit the moral implications latent in the vocabulary of the law and especially in words like *ius, recht, diritto, droit* which are laden with the theory of Natural Law. It may then appear tempting to say that enactments which enjoined or permitted iniquity should not be recognized as valid, or have the quality of law, even if the system in which they were enacted acknowledged no restriction upon the legislative competence of its legislature. It is in this form that Natural Law arguments were revived in Germany after the last war in response to the acute social problems left by the iniquities of Nazi rule and its defeat. Should informers who, for selfish ends, procured the imprisonment of others for offences against monstrous statutes passed during the Nazi régime, be punished? Was it possible to convict them in the courts of post-war Germany on the footing that such statutes violated the Natural Law and were therefore void so that the victims' imprisonment for breach of such statutes was in fact unlawful, and procuring it was itself an offence?[5] Simple as the

issue looks between those who would accept and those who would repudiate the view that morally iniquitous rules cannot be law, the disputants seem often very unclear as to its general character. It is true that we are here concerned with alternative ways of formulating a moral decision not to apply, obey, or allow others to plead in their defence morally iniquitous rules: yet the issue is ill presented as a verbal one. Neither side to the dispute would be content if they were told, "Yes: you are right, the correct way in English (or in German) of putting that sort of point is to say what you have said." So, though the positivist might point to a weight of English usage, showing that there is no contradiction in asserting that a rule of law is too iniquitous to be obeyed, and that it does not follow from the proposition that a rule is too iniquitous to obey that it is not a valid rule of law, their opponents would hardly regard this as disposing of the case.

Plainly we cannot grapple adequately with this issue if we see it as one concerning the proprieties of linguistic usage. For what really is at stake is the comparative merit of a wider and a narrower concept or way of classifying rules, which belong to a system of rules generally effective in social life. If we are to make a reasoned choice between these concepts, it must be because one is superior to the other in the way in which it will assist our theoretical inquiries, or advance and clarify our moral deliberations, or both.

The wider of these two rival concepts of law includes the narrower. If we adopt the wider concept, this will lead us in theoretical inquiries to group and consider together as "law" all rules which are valid by the formal tests of a system of primary and secondary rules, even though some of them offend against a society's own morality or against what we may hold to be an enlightened or true morality. If we adopt the narrower concept we shall exclude from "law" such morally offensive rules. It seems clear that nothing is to be gained in the theoretical or scientific study of law as a social phenomenon by adopting the narrower concept: it would lead us to exclude certain rules even though they exhibit all the other complex characteristics of law. Nothing, surely, but confusion could follow from a proposal to leave the study of such rules to another discipline, and certainly no history or other form of legal study has found it profitable to do this. If we adopt the wider concept of law, we can accommodate within it the study of whatever special features morally iniquitous laws have, and the reaction of society to them. Hence the use of the narrower concept here must inevitably split, in a confusing way, our effort to understand both the development and potentialities of the specific method of social control to be seen in a system of primary and secondary rules. Study of its use involves study of its abuse.

What then of the practical merits of the narrower concept of law in moral deliberation? In what way is it better, when faced with morally iniquitous demands, to think "This is in no sense law" rather than "This is a law but too iniquitous to obey or apply"? Would this make men more clear-headed or readier to disobey when morality demands it? Would it lead to better ways of disposing of the problems such as the Nazi régime left behind? No doubt ideas have their influence; but it scarcely seems that an effort to train and educate men in the use of a narrower concept of legal validity, in which there is no place for valid but morally iniquitous laws, is likely to lead to a stiffening of resistance to evil, in the face of threats of organized power, or a clearer realization of what is morally at stake when obedience is demanded. So long as human beings can gain sufficient co-operation from some to enable them to dominate others, they will use the forms of law as one of their instruments. Wicked men will enact wicked rules which others will enforce. What surely is most needed in order to make men clear sighted in confronting the official abuse of power, is that they should preserve the sense that the certification of something as legally valid is not conclusive of the question of obedience, and that, however great the aura of majesty or authority which the official system may have, its demands must in the end be submitted to a moral scrutiny. This sense, that there is something outside the official system, by reference to which in the last resort the individual must solve his problems of obedience, is surely more likely to be kept alive among those who are accustomed to think that rules of law may be iniquitous, than among those who think that nothing iniquitous can anywhere have the status of law.

But perhaps a stronger reason for preferring the wider concept of law, which will enable us to think and say, "This is law but iniquitous," is that to withhold legal recognition from iniquitous rules may grossly oversimplify the variety of moral issues to which they give rise. Older writers who, like Bentham and Austin, insisted on the distinction between what law is and what it ought to be, did so partly because they thought that unless men kept these separate they might, without counting the cost to society, make hasty judgments that laws were invalid and ought not to be obeyed. But besides this danger of anarchy, which they may well have overrated, there is another form of oversimplification. If we narrow our point of view and think only of the person who is called upon to *obey* evil rules, we may regard it as a matter of indifference whether or not he thinks that he is faced with a valid rule of "law" so long as he sees its moral iniquity and does what morality requires. But besides the moral question of obedience (Am I to do this evil thing?) there is Socrates' question of submission: Am I to submit to punishment for disobedience or make my escape? There is also the question which confronted the post-war German courts, "Are we to punish those who did evil things when they were permitted by evil rules then in force?" These questions raise very different problems of morality and justice, which we need to consider independently of each other: they cannot be solved by a refusal, made once and for all, to recognize evil laws as valid for any purpose. This is too crude a way with delicate and complex moral issues.

A concept of law which allows the invalidity of law to be distinguished from its immorality, enables us to see the complexity and variety of these separate issues; whereas a narrow concept of law which denies legal validity to iniquitous rules may blind us to them. It may be conceded that the German informers, who for selfish ends procured the punishment of others under monstrous laws, did what morality forbad; yet morality may also demand that the state should punish only those who, in doing evil, did what the state at the time forbad. This is the principle of *nulla poena sine lege*. If inroads have to be made on this principle in order to avert something held to be a greater evil than its sacrifice, it is vital that the issues at stake be clearly identified. A case of retroactive punishment should not be made to look like an ordinary case of punishment for an act illegal at the time. At least it can be claimed for the simple positivist doctrine that morally iniquitous rules may still be law, that this offers no disguise for the choice between evils which, in extreme circumstances, may have to be made.

Notes

1. Hume, *Treatise of Human Nature*, III. ii, "Of Justice and Injustice."

2. Austin, *The Province of Jurisprudence Defined*, Lecture V, pp. 184–5.

3. Gray, *The Nature and Sources of the Law*, S. 213.

4. Kelsen, *General Theory of Law and State*, p. 113.

5. See the judgment of 27 July 1940, Oberlandsgericht Bamberg, 5 *Süddeutsche Juristen-Zeitung*, 207: discussed at length in H. L. A Hart, "Legal Positivism and the Separation of Law and Morals," in *Harvard L. Rev. lxxi* (1958), 598, and in L. Fuller, "Positivism and Fidelity to Law," ibid., p. 630. But note corrected account of this judgment *infra*, pp. 254–5.

Ethics and Medicine

19

Arthur J. Dyck
Ethics and Medicine

Reprinted by permission of author and publisher from *Linacre Quarterly*, August 1973, pp. 182–200.

The voluntary consent of the human subject is absolutely essential. This means that the person involved should have legal capacity to give consent; should be so situated as to be able to exercise free power of choice, without the intervention of any element of force, fraud, deceit, duress, over-reaching, or other ulterior form of constraint or coercion; and should have sufficient knowledge and comprehension of the elements of the subject matter involved as to enable him to make an understanding and enlightened decision. This latter element requires that before the acceptance of an affirmative decision by the experimental subject there should be made known to him the nature, duration, and purpose of the experiment; the methods and means by which it is to be conducted; all inconveniences and hazards reasonably to be expected; and the effects upon his health of person which may possibly come from his participation in the experiment.

Articles of the Nuremberg Tribunal [1]

The declarations of Nuremberg symbolize and express two significant characteristics of the contemporary situation of medicine: a heightened responsiveness to the needs, wants and rights of patients; a heightened awareness of the increasing difficulty of knowing what is right, and hence of knowing how best to benefit the patient and prevent harm. These concerns have arisen within the medical profession itself, but they are shared by the public at large.

Technological advances that make it possible to transplant organs and keep the heart and lungs going when the brain is no longer functioning, the ability to diagnose genetic defects while the developing child is still in the womb, the experimentation with techniques that would make it possible to grow babies outside the womb, the rising costs and complexity of delivering health care with its adverse effects on the poor, and the existence of medical experiments that are of no immediate benefit to patients who are subjects, are all facts of modern life known and reflected upon not only by physicians but also by the public, and by the media that conveys so much of this information to the public.

The past decade has given rise to a flurry of literature that documents and agonizes over moral dilemmas within contemporary medicine. Some of this literature is designed to shock and alarm us. Thus, for example, Pappworth writes a book entitled

Human Guinea Pigs in which a number of cases are cited as clear deviations from the morality of traditional medical practice.[2] Within the profession, Henry Beecher, in a widely read essay, discussed cases that he judged to be violations of existing medical codes, and hence unethical.[3] One cause for alarm, then, among those who are reflecting upon contemporary medical practice arises from perceived departures from traditional values, including those already embodied in medical codes.

Quite another kind of alarm is being expressed, this by people who tend to assume that technological innovations in medicine and medical science are generally good and ought to be vigorously pursued. Such writers express the concern that traditional values—often the focus is on religious values—continue to stand in the way of medical innovation and progress.[4] Whereas people used to oppose surgery, blood transfusions, inoculations, etc., now they oppose new definitions of death, transplants, in-vitro fertilization, etc. Some of these writers, therefore, are inclined to call for nothing less than a new ethic that will clarify the benefits of medical innovation and the necessity of assuming various risks in order to get these benefits.[5]

Decision-Making

Sharp differences of opinion evoke still another kind of reaction to the morally problematic character of contemporary medical decision-making. We see this, for example, in the area of employing a technique like amniocentesis.[6] To justify the risks of this diagnostic technique to discover whether the child developing in the womb has certain defects, physicians often leave the decision in the hands of the pregnant woman. She is the one who will decide whether she will have an abortion should her developing child be diagnosed as defective. This approach to medical decision-making is one of individualizing those decisions because individuals differ as to whether or when abortion for defective fetuses is morally justifiable.

Sharply contrasting with the tendency to individualize medical decisions is a call for much more stringent regulation of the medical profession, whether by the legislatures, government agencies, and/or the courts.[7] The desire for more stringent regulation comes from those who wish to see time-honored formulations of moral values enforced. It comes also from those who want to see new values enshrined in medicine: some physicians, for example, seek to have euthanasia, mercy killing, legalized.

Whatever their merit, these responses to contemporary moral dilemmas in medicine are inadequate. They are made without explicitly offering the framework for understanding the relationship between ethical standards and medical practice implied by the policies they advocate. The purpose of this essay is to seek some clarity about the way in which ethical questions arise within medical practice and to suggest a framework for formulating moral policy. Obviously this brief essay will only make a beginning of this dual enterprise.

In characterizing the nature and scope of ethics, it is possible to outline the concerns of this discipline by specifying its three major questions. The major questions of ethics are normative, metaethical, and strategic.[8] Normative questions are raised in an effort to discover the most generally and universally recognizable values that specify the right- and wrong-making characteristics of actions, and the goodness and badness of persons and various states of being. Questions of metaethics have as their concern the understanding of the nature of moral discourse and the processes by which moral judgments and debates are decided, argued, and justified or criticized. Questions of strategy are focused upon the way in which moral decisions are implemented and social policy is formulated and carried out. What we wish to do in this essay is use these three types of questions, that serve to define the nature and scope of ethics, to clarify the nature and scope of ethical debates concerning contemporary medical practices. Indeed, we wish to indicate how these three types of questions elucidate the nature and scope of medical ethics, both as a subspecialty within ethics generally and as a set of practical moral issues that arise for both physicians and patients in the pursuit of health and health care.

Normative Questions for Medicine

In her fascinating study of the more universally and generally held human values, Tamara Dembo found that health was high on the list.[9] Indeed, one of the effects of improvements in medicine has been to increase the expectations both physicians and the public have regarding the possibility of achieving health and maintaining it. The most startling achievements of medicine, and particularly of public health measures, has come in the form of greatly reduced death rates from infectious and communicable diseases. The decreases in infant mortality that result greatly raise the prospects of longevity.

With longevity, however, come increases in diseases that affect aging adults, such as cancer and heart disease, diseases which may also be related to our contemporary style of life. It is precisely the increased ability to prolong life that poses what appears to be the most fundamental question of values for the practitioners and recipients of modern medical care. Someone dying from cancer, for example, can be kept alive much longer than ever before. Even patients whose brains are severely damaged can be fed and have their hearts and lungs maintained, sometimes for periods of more than two years. Also at the beginning of life, where the ability to perform abortions is coupled with an increasing ability to diagnose various types of fetal deformities, questions about the support of nascent life in the womb also arise. Situations, therefore, exist within contemporary medicine where the increased expectation for health is not always compatible with the very strong desire for maintaining life as long as possible. For as we have noted, there are circumstances under which it is possible to sustain bodily functions under conditions of extremely poor health. At the same time, it is possible to choose to have only healthy infants.

But should health and a certain quality of life be considered a more important value than life itself? Or to put the question another way, is quality of life—a certain state of health and well-being—the dominant value by which we should judge what to do as physicians and what we wish as patients or should life itself be the dominant value? This it seems to me poses one of the most critical and far-reaching issues in the history of ethics and medicine.

A rather startlingly candid editorial in *California Medicine* compares two ethical systems with regard to their understanding of the value of life.[10] One is the Judeo-Christian ethic. This ethic, so the editorial claims, sees life as an absolute value and causes physicians to prolong and repair life regardless of the cost and circumstances. Alternatively, there is a new ethic that rejects the Judeo-Christian formulation of absolute devotion to life. In the view of the editorial, the adoption of this new ethic is beginning in the practice of abortion where quality of life arguments are used to give the moral justification for abortions, and will extend to various forms of euthanasia. The editorial does not give us a very clear indication as to the range of cases in which killing could be justified by this new quality of life ethic.

Stoicism

This editorial exhibits a very penetrating grasp of one of the most significant moral debates in contemporary medicine. However, it has oversimplified the alternatives considerably. For one thing, it is not true as the editorial alleges, that the quality of life ethic would be a new ethic. Ironically, Christianity had its beginning at a time when the high value it put on individual life distinguished it sharply from other more dominant religious and ethical systems. One such powerful philosphy was Stoicism. The Stoic could definitely justify suicide in circumstances where a person no longer felt life to be worthwhile. For the Stoic, the freedom to exercise rational control over one's own destiny was such a weighty value that it always provided an option to the continuation of one's own life.[11]

Christianity also found itself in opposition to the widespread practices of infanticide and abortion that prevailed at the time of its inception. Where Christianity came to dominate, infanticide and abortion came to be seen as evils. Laws to curb such evils came to be enacted.[12] The editorial claims that this legacy of Judaism and Christianity is waning, and an outlook, which as we have noted is more akin to traditional Stoicism, is beginning to take its place. There is no clear evidence to support this assessment of trends.

It's unfair to contrast the Judeo-Christian ethic with the new ethic by arguing that the former is absolutistic and the latter relativistic. This obscures the issue of the difference between an ethic in which life itself is a significant value, and an ethic in which questions of life and death are always questions of the quality of life, so that quality of life and not life itself is the value to be weighed in relation to other values.

Judaism and Christianity have never, except for certain of their sects which espouse absolute pacifism, taken the view that it is never morally justifiable to kill. Capital punishment and self-defense have always had their defenders within these traditions. The just war tradition has developed a whole set of sophisticated criteria designed to constrain rulers and armed forces from killing, but which at the same time state the conditions under which a war waged in self-defense may be just.[13] In these traditions, therefore, life is looked upon as a good in itself to which each individual has a right. At the same time, however, this right may be forfeited by those individuals who threaten or rob others of their right to life. The value placed upon life is so weighty that it is not at all easy to justify capital punishment and war. These traditions have especially strong constraints against killing any innocent party, that is, any individual who could in no sense be construed as being an intentional threat or danger to the life of anyone else. Hence the prohibition against infanticide did take an absolute form.

A quality of life ethic does not treat life as a good in itself. Life as a value is always life of a certain kind and the right to life is always subject to question: it cannot be assumed.

To see how this ethic functions, consider the following case of a Mongoloid (Downs Syndrome) child who was deliberately allowed to die.[14] Soon after birth it was discovered that a child, diagnosed as Mongoloid, required surgery. This surgery does involve some risks but is usually successful and permits a child to realize its physical potential. Obviously it does nothing for whatever degree of mental retardation the child would experience from Down's Syndrome. Although mentally retarded, such individuals are usually happy and may sometimes manage a degree of independence that includes earning one's own living and setting up an independent household. In this particular case, the parents did not give permission for surgery and their physician acceded to the parents' wishes. He ordered nothing by mouth and fifteen days later the infant was dead.

What kind of argument led the participants to justify infanticide? On the side of the parents there was a strong desire to have a normal child, coupled with a very negative view of mental retardation on the part of the mother who had had some exposure to such children. Both parents did not want the suffering and anguish either of trying to rear such a child or of institutionalizing it. Presumably they also did not wish a life of mental retardation for their child. Whatever other assumptions were made by their physician, there was a strong feeling that institutionalization of an undesirable quality was the only prospect for this child and, given the attitudes of the parents, this was seen quite literally as a fate worse than death. (As it turned out, it was learned later that there are couples in that area who would gladly adopt mentally retarded children. This fact, however, is not essential to understanding quality of life arguments.)

Quality of Life

The essential feature of all quality of life arguments is the proposition that there is such a thing as a life not worth living. Life itself is not what is good: only life of a certain kind, life with a certain degree of intelligence, potential for development, or whatever, is considered valuable. Those who argue in this way will disagree with respect to what it is that gives life value, how much of it one has to possess in order to have a right to life, and who it is that has the authority to specify that certain individuals will not, for whatever reason, be granted a right to life. Some would restrict the decision as to what qualities bestow value upon life to the individual whose life it is. This view is very hard to maintain, however, because it cannot apply to the very young, the senile, the severely mentally ill or those who have lost their capacity for conscious life. If mercy killing is to be applied in such instances, it cannot be considered voluntary at the time in which people find themselves to be in one of those conditions.[15]

Someone may argue that there is really no alternative to a quality of life view. There are occasions when it seems necessary to sacrifice life. One could cite here the declaration of one highly revered partriot when he exclaims "Give me liberty or give me death!" However, this affirmation need not be made from the standpoint of a quality of life ethic. One can take the view that life is a significant good in itself to which every individual has a right and, at the same time, claim that there are other values of great significance to which individuals have a right, such as liberty and justice.

There are situations in which the deprivation of liberty or the perpetuation of injustices are so severe that one might well morally justify risk to one's life and limb in order to increase liberty or decrease injustice. In a situation of enslavement, for example, there may be a point at which the sacrifice of some lives may bring about the kind of freedom and justice that will greatly reduce suffering and death among the enslaved. Civil disobedience, rebellion, or even revolution may, under certain circumstances, satisfy the criteria involved for waging a just war. Using the just war criteria, the respect for life is never lost. One can never kill in order to improve one's material welfare or happiness. But one may wage war to rectify grave injustices and overcome oppression. The injustices and oppression of slavery can be so great that those who are slaves experience a great deal of premature death, whether as infants or adults deprived of proper care, or as young people or adults so poorly fed and worked so hard that the usual chances for a normal life expectancy are severely reduced.

The right to life, therefore, is fundamentally linked to maintaining and respecting rights to liberty and justice. In the case of the Mongoloid child, the complete deprivation of liberty—the child is not allowed to grow up and decide for itself whether life is worth living—means in that case the complete loss of the right to live. Similarly, where abnormalities such as mental retardation are used to decide the merit of a life, a merit view of justice is brought into play. The merit view of justice does not presume that each individual has an equal right to life, liberty, and the goods of this world, including due process, the cornerstone of any system of justice. Rather these rights have to be earned in some way.

Ethical or political systems that entertain a merit view of justice are at fundamental odds with the principle of equity. In John Rawls' recent monumental work on justice, he recognizes that certain kinds of inequities, for example differences in income, may be justifiable but only if all persons, including those with less income, stand to benefit.[16] From the standpoint of those who see life as a good in itself, life is one of those benefits. From the standpoint of certain quality of life arguments, however, life under certain circumstances is not considered a benefit.

Utilitarian

This brings us to another important normative question. Not only does one's system of ethics hinge on the particular values such as life, liberty, and justice, affirmed by it, but also on the mode of moral reasoning employed. One common method of moral reasoning is what is called in ethics utilitarian. A system of ethics that employs only utilitarian reasoning is one in which the rightness and wrongness of actions, and the goodness of persons and of social ends, are all judged by some standard of utility. The rights of individuals to life, liberty, and justice are not presumed. Such rights must be established by their utility.

One of the narrower forms of contemporary utilitarian reasoning is that of judging policies by computing their cost effectiveness. If the utility of a project exceeds its disutility, it can be justified. Thus in medical literature one finds arguments for aborting deformed fetuses on the grounds that the costs of aborting are so much less than the costs of sustaining the children who would be born.[17] Similarly there are those who argue that the costs of certain kinds of treatment, where the chances of recovery are statistically highly improbable or involve people who are poor risks, may justify withholding treatment from such individuals.

Formalistic modes of normative reasoning are to be distinguished from utilitarian modes in that formalists allege that the rightness or wrongness of actions or practices does not depend solely upon their consequences. Formalists need not, therefore, reject all utilitarian reasoning but see utility as at most one right-making characteristic of actions and practices among others such as justice, truth-telling, gratitude, reparation, etc. One of the most widely respected and regnant formalist systems is that of W. D. Ross.[18]

The question no doubt arises in the minds of our readers at this point just how it is that one decides that certain characteristics of actions are right- or wrong-making characteristics, and certain characteristics of things or social ends are good or evil. Closely related to this is the further question as to what individuals and groups speak with authority on moral issues in medicine and what it is that confers such authority. These are questions of metaethics to which we now turn.

Metaethical Questions for Medicine

There has been, and there continues to be a strong presumption within the profession of medicine that the profession itself provides the best basis for deciding what is right and wrong in questions of medical research and care. Medical ethics in this view is defined, understood, and practiced by medical professionals. Among medical professionals, those with a doctor's degree in medicine carry the most weight. The proposition that a particular group is best qualified to make and to criticize moral judgments pertaining to their own interests and work is not self-evidently true or false. Whether one believes it to be true or false depends in large measure on one's view of the nature of moral judgments and moral decision-making processes.

Books on medical ethics by specialists in ethics do not uniformly presuppose the special expertise of the medical profession to make moral judgments about medical cases. Joseph Fletcher in *Morals and Medicine* does not presume to be doing medical ethics.[19] Fletcher claims that he is dealing with the ethics of medical care and that in so doing he is not dealing with medical ethics, a term usually used for the rules governing the social conduct and graces of the medical profession: "Medical ethics is the business of the medical profession, although certainly it has to fall somewhat within the limits of social obligation."[20] Fletcher recognizes that some professionals would give medical ethics as a professional concern a loftier definition. He cites Dr. George Jacoby as saying that medical ethics deals with "the question of the general attitude of the physician toward the patient: to what extent his duty obligates him to intervene in the patient's interest, and what demands the physician has a right and duty to make upon the patient's relatives in regard to obedience and subordination for the purposes of treatment."[21] Fletcher notes that Dr. Jacoby nowhere says anything about the demands the patient has a right and duty to make upon physicians. Fletcher then claims that it is this other perspective, namely the patient's point of view, that he tries to take in examining the morals, principles and values that are at stake in medical care.

Despite Fletcher's distinction between an ethics of medical care and medical ethics as professional ethics, his own book is virtually always referred to as a book in medical ethics. When physicians speak of the book in this way, I think it is because they presume that the issues raised by Fletcher are issues for them as professionals: nothing about medical care is outside the expertise of the physician; certainly nothing about medical care is outside the concern of the physician. When ethicists refer to Fletcher's book as a book in medical ethics, they share the assumption that medical ethics is part of ethics generally and that what distinguishes medical ethics from ethics generally is its concern with the moral questions that arise in and from the practice of medicine.

Thus when Paul Ramsey set out to write a book on patient care entitled *The Patient as Person,* the subtitle is "Explorations in Medical Ethics."[22] In the preface to his book, he makes his

view of the relation between medical ethics and ethics generally very explicit:

problems of medical ethics . . . are by no means technical problems on which only the expert (in this case, the physician) can have an opinion. They are rather the problems of human beings in situations in which medical care is needed. Birth and death, illness and injury, are not simply events the doctor attends. They are moments in every human life.

. . . The question, What ought the doctor to do? is only a particular form of the question, What should be done?

. . . I hold that medical ethics is consonant with the ethics of a wider human community. The former is (however special) only a particular case of the latter. The moral requirements governing the relations of physician to patients and researcher to subjects are only a special case of the moral requirements governing any relations between man and man. Canons of loyalty to patients or to joint adventurers in medical research are simply particular manifestations of canons of loyalty of person to person generally.[23]

Ramsey has the utmost respect for the moral sensitivity of physicians. Nevertheless, he is not sanguine that the medical profession and its codes will suffice to guide contemporary medicine through its ethical dilemmas:

In the medical literature there are many articles on ethics which are greatly to be admired. Yet I know that these are not part of the daily fare of medical students, or of members of the profession when they gather together as professionals or even for purposes of conviviality. I do not believe that either the codes of medical ethics or the physicians who have undertaken to comment on them and to give fresh analysis of the physician's moral decisions will suffice to withstand the omnivorous appetite of scientific research or of a therapeutic technology that has a momentum and a life of its own.

The Nuremberg Code, the Declaration of Helsinki, various "guidelines" of the American Medical Association, and other "codes" governing medical practice constitute a sort of "catechism" in the ethics of the medical profession. These codes exhibit a professional ethics which ministers and theologians and members of other professions can only profoundly respect and admire. Still, a catechism never sufficed. Unless these principles are constantly pondered and enlivened in their application they become dead letters. There is also need that these principles be deepened and sensitized and opened to further humane revision in face of all the ordinary and the newly emerging situations which a doctor

confronts—as do we all—in the present day. In this task none of the sources of moral insight, no understanding of the humanity of man or for answering questions of life and death, can rightfully be neglected.[24]

This does not mean that medical ethics is best left to those trained in ethics only. Ramsey argues that physicians can do medical ethics but not without some training in ethics; similarly ethicists need exposure to the fields of medicine to which their ethical reflections are directed. Above all, Ramsey argues that the medical profession should no longer believe that the personal integrity of physicians alone is enough "to deal with the contemporary quandaries of medical ethics."[25]

Whereas Ramsey does not become explicit about the metaethical presuppositions that inform his view, a recent essay by Robert Veatch does.[26] This essay argues on theoretical grounds that medical ethics should not be the province of medical practitioners only and that medical decisions cannot be morally justified if they are construed as matters of personal opinion. The fact that these decisions of medical care are made by physicians does not by itself suffice to raise them above the level of personal opinion.

In discussing the relationship between medical ethics and ethics generally, Veatch describes a common debate that occurs between those trained in medicine and those who are not. Veatch cites a case where a woman was diagnosed to be dying from cancer. The medical student who presents the case considers it appropriate to tell the women gently and diplomatically that although the medical staff will do all that it can to treat her condition, it cannot give her assurances that she will recover. The physician who is the student's supervisor and the other physicians participating in the discussion to which Veatch alludes claimed that as physicians they have a unique ethical duty to do no harm to the patient. The physicians were in agreement that telling the patient she has cancer will harm her and therefore it is wrong to tell her this. Nonphysicians discussing this case disagreed with the physicians regarding the factual question of whether the bad news about cancer would adversely affect the patient and also as to whether the decision ought finally to be based on the principle of not harming or on the principle of truth-telling. What raises the metaethical question here is the claim of the physicians that their understanding of moral norms or principles is unique to the medical profession and should be given priority in medical cases over the judgments of nonprofessionals.

Veatch argues that these physicians were actually claiming that there are specific moral rules applicable in medicine which are valid for physicians qua physicians, and that the general rules and expectations of the larger society may, in specific cases, be justifiably abrogated by them. As Veatch notes, this is an implicit acceptance of a particular metaethical position, namely that of social relativism which argues that to say of an action that it is right or wrong is to say that it is in accord with the mores of one's group. Veatch is quite right in asserting that this metaethical position is not one that ethicists would defend.[27] It is a meaningful question to ask whether anything considered right or wrong by one's group is in fact right or wrong. Indeed, it is a growing consensus in contemporary ethical theory that the peculiarity of moral assertions is precisely that they are assertions that claim to be universalizable.[28] In other words, the decision not to tell the truth to a dying patient is one that one would expect any right-thinking person to make if one in fact claims that this is the right decision in cases of this sort.

Personal Relativism

The difficulties of relativistic theories of ethics cannot be thoroughly discussed here but have been elsewhere.[29] There is, however, another point at issue that deserves some elaboration. There are those among physicians, and this view seems to be quite common, who assume that moral decisions are personal decisions and that physicians can do no more than other human beings when faced with moral dilemmas, which is to search diligently their own consciences. This presumption is also a metaethical position for which the medical literature gives no justification. With respect to this form of relativism, ethical theory is more divided, but at the same time strong objections to it and plausible alternatives are not hard to find.[30] It is enough for our purposes

here simply to indicate that one of the working assumptions of some physicians is not one for which they have offered rational and cogent arguments. Where one stands with respect to such an issue makes a lot of difference for one's conception of the nature of medicine as a science and as an art. It goes without saying that those who implicitly or explicitly adhere to doctrines of social or personal relativism in ethics can more easily justify the private and/or professional nature of medical ethics, feeling no intellectual or moral obligation to know what is discovered by professional ethicists or even what is thought to be right or wrong by the general public except insofar as opinions of the public may represent political and/or legal power to influence decisions by medical practitioners.

There is another important implication of metaethical theories like social and personal relativism. If one is a social relativist, there is no way to decide who among differing groups should have the say regarding questions of right or wrong. Personal relativism is also ultimately without a basis for adjudicating disputes among groups or persons. In practice, relativists tend to give the nod in moral decisions to the persons who have the most expertise regarding the factual data relevant to the decisions being made. This means that where the doctors of medicine are considered the experts par excellence in matters of health, they are granted the ultimate power of moral decision-making in medical cases. Veatch refers to this as the fallacy of generalization of expertise. It is a fallacy because, as Veatch and other ethicists generally hold, moral decisions are not based only upon factual matters narrowly defined. Furthermore, the same facts are seen differently from the perspective of various disciplines.

The value of truth for a dying patient may quite justifiably be perceived quite differently by someone like a minister who may well consider it a great benefit for all concerned if dying persons face the question of their own dying. This kind of benefit may or may not be accepted on purely medical grounds depending upon one's conception of health and of medicine as well as one's conception of the relation between

bodily and psychic functions. In any event, the judgment as to whether one ought to reflect upon one's dying is not self-evidently a strictly medical decision, even if the term health is stretched to cover every aspect of a person's well-being. Health so defined becomes the concern of everyone, including a great variety of professionals in addition to those trained in medicine.

Albeit in a very preliminary way, our discussion of metaethical assumptions illustrates some of the ways in which metaethical theories, whether held implicitly or explicitly, influence very practical or strategic questions of moral policy, such as who will be accorded the authority and power to decide moral issues in medical care and how the decisions made will be implemented. In short, metaethical theories have great practical import for moral strategy or policy. This is so because metaethical theory is a theory about the nature of the processes of moral decision-making, particularly of the kind of justification that one offers for one's moral judgments. Metaethics seeks to assess the extent to which such justifications are rational or irrational, subjective or objective, and private or universalizable. Let us look at some of the practical moral problems of medical decision-making and raise some questions about these in the light of certain metaethical criteria.

Questions of Moral Policy for Medicine

Moral policy refers to that portion of the total ethical enterprise in which whatever is known or believed to be true in normative theory as well as metaethical theory is applied to specific moral issues and the methods used to cope with them. Decisions about what is right or wrong, good or bad, are not solely decided, nor ought they to be, on the basis of ethical theory per se. Ethical theory provides one of the essential components of any adequate moral decision, namely a method of moral reasoning.

Moral reasoning about specific moral issues, such as whether to do or to have an abortion, a sterilization, a kidney transplant, etc. has two components: reasoning about general principles as illustrated by our discussion of the difference between formalists and utilitarians; reasoning as to the best processes by which to arrive at a decision. Policy debates, however, hinge not only on the nature of one's moral reasoning but on the perception one has of relevant facts, the kinds of loyalties one has, such as loyalties to one's family, one's ethnic group, one's profession, one's religion, one's nation, etc., and also one's more theological or quasi-theological assumptions about the nature of reality, particularly the nature of persons.[31] An example of a quasi-theological assumption that greatly influences policy would be that persons are very prone to evil, and hence laws and sanctions are very important for preventing evil, as compared with an assumption that people are prone to do what is good and interference in their freedom tends to be more harmful than beneficial. Some of the disputes among physicians about the regulation of research often reflect a difference of opinion as to whether individuals doing research are more prone to be influenced by desires for money, advancement, and fame or by the desire to know the truth and benefit humanity. Obviously the direction of one's thinking about policy can be tipped in one direction or another by such considerations.

Wielding power in decision-making depends a great deal upon who has the facts that are relevant to what is being decided. Physicians have a great deal of power in medical cases by reason of their express certification to make diagnoses and engage in intervention where assistance in matters of health is being sought and by reason of the general respect accorded this certification by the public and by other professionals concerned with health and illness, such as ministers, lawyers, judges, politicians, etc. It is also important to note that there are a whole range of occupational roles other than that of the physician involved in medical care. These persons, such as nurses, physiotherapists, counselors, voluntary aides, etc., tend to have a definitely subordinate role in medical decision-making wherever these persons lack an M.D.

There are two strategies, therefore, that serve to secure the power of the licensed physician to have the final say in matters of medical care: one is to perpetuate the notion that the proper knowledge of medicine is conferred by those institutions accredited to grant the M.D. degree; the other is to keep the precious knowledge possessed by the holder of the M.D. within the confines of that profession and to share it as little as possible with any other professional or with the patient.

Sharing of Power

Now we are not arguing that the power and role of expert knowledge per se be diminished or denigrated. The question before us is rather the extent to which the power that comes from possessing such knowledge should be shared and to what extent.

Consider the following case: a man is seriously ill, so ill that there is a high probability that he may die.[32] The physician does not convey this to the patient nor does he inform the man's minister of this diagnosis. A nurse, however, connected with the case takes it upon herself to tell the man's minister before he sees the patient of precisely how serious the man's illness is judged to be. The minister, with some trepidation, but with firm resolve, decides to share this information with the patient.

When this incident was reported to a class of graduate students in religion, some of whom were training for the ministry and some of whom were obtaining higher degrees specializing in ethics, there was considerable criticism of the minister's action. Many felt that the minister should not have taken this upon himself without consulting with the doctor. Indeed some felt strongly that the minister must have the attending physician's consent to talk to the patient about dying. The minister in this instance disagreed sharply. He viewed the man who was in danger of dying as one who was not only paying the physician to carry out whatever duties were incumbent upon him as a physician, but as one who was also paying the minister to carry out his duties. The question as to whether a person who may be dying should reflect upon this possibility or actuality as the case may be is as much a question of the welfare of the patient as the question as to whether discussions of dying will have an adverse physical effect upon a patient. The difficult question as to whether in fact a particular patient will have adverse physical reactions to the topic of death—it appears that this is much less often the case than is supposed—is not the critical question if one's concern about the patient is for that patient's total welfare. A lawyer or a friend or a relative concerned about whether a proper will has been made out, a minister concerned about whether persons have achieved a proper attitude toward their own limited powers as human beings, a nurse concerned with the anxieties of patients who want to know, all raise important considerations about what is beneficial for patients. If physicians are the only ones who know that a given person is dying, the power of what is best for the patient in the light of that fact resides totally with him or with her. Is this the way it ought to be?

One immediate reaction to this question is that it depends upon the particular case that one has in mind. But that response misses the point of the question, which is the question as to whether it is best for attending physicians to make the decision that they indeed will be the only ones who know the prognosis of patients. It is of course the case that many physicians, whether for moral reasons or for others, will share their knowledge of the prognosis of a patient, sometimes only with persons responsible for the care of that patient, sometimes with those persons as well as with relatives and friends of patients, and sometimes with all of these and patients as well. The question is what persons should be involved in the decision about who shares in this knowledge?

Information Controlled

The principle that some knowledge must be shared with patients is well established. We are not therefore talking about totally withholding information from patients or from other persons concerned with patients' care and well-being. Patients, or those who are spokesmen for patients, sign consent forms that include some details about medical interventions that are being contemplated. Surgical interference, for example, requires consent and the necessity for consent is only waived in extreme emergency to save lives where it is not possible to obtain consent in the time required. Furthermore, as indicated in the articles of the Nuremberg tribunal, any procedure considered to be experimental is acknowledged as requiring informed and voluntary consent of the patient or subject. Although this requirement is sometimes violated in spirit or quite literally, nevertheless these violations are considered deviations from accepted norms of medical practice and are subject to censure and negative sanctions. Nevertheless, it is still the case that physicians largely control, on an individual and collective basis, what information is conveyed to patients. They also control, for the most part, what information is conveyed to all others concerned with the welfare of patients.

Now this situation may be seen to be less than optimum in at least two major ways. First of all, the knowledge possessed by physicians by reason of their training is important to know if the patient's welfare is to be served, but it is not the only knowledge that is relevant to the welfare of patients. Secondly, moral decision-making involves a process that includes knowledge of factual information as one of its important components, but not as its only component. The first point involves many interesting questions that we do not have space to discuss here: questions about conceptions of health and disease, and conceptions of what various kinds of expertise contribute to the enhancement of health, the diminution of disease, and the increase in individual and community well-being. The role and scope of contemporary medicine in enhancing human well-being is not self-evident. Some of its benefits to those whose lives have been saved and lengthened are fairly indisputable, but contemporary medicine with its armament of powerful drugs, its quest for new knowledge through research using humans, does not always engage in practices that are non-controversially beneficial.

The second point is one that requires some comment. As we noted earlier, the components of moral decision-making and the nature of this process is what a metaethical theory is designed to elucidate. Despite certain variations among theorists in detail, there is a growing consensus in contemporary metaethical theory that moral judgments are rational to the degree that they are factually informed, relatively disinterested, relatively dispassionate, and made in the light of a vivid imagination as to how others are affected by the action or practice being decided.[33] The power and role of factual information we have already illustrated. These other components of moral decision-making merit some clarification. The best examples of disinterestedness and dispassionateness are found in the procedures used to govern judicial processes in the courtroom. Thus judges would not be seen as fit to try their own children or loved ones, nor if they owned stock in a company, to judge an alleged wrong-doing of that company. We have come, albeit belatedly, to recognize some of the subtleties of racial interest, if not prejudice, and we act accordingly to see that black jurors are involved in the trials of blacks. In a perfect world this would not in principle be necessary but that is not the kind of world that we live in, certainly not with respect to the way our judgments are influenced by our interests and our passions.[34]

Experiments

The physician-patient relationship is greatly simplified if the relationship is purely between physicians who are committed to constraint from doing any harm to patients and to employing only those therapeutic interventions that can reasonably be expected to improve the conditions of patients. However, many physicians are part of the ceaseless quest of modern medicine for knowledge so that patients can also become subjects in experiments and as such may find themselves at the receiving end of risk-filled interventions that have a low, or even no, probability of benefiting them.

Physicians who also see themselves as scientists cannot be viewed as disinterested parties in the care and welfare of their patients. Because of the great power that physicians have by reason of their knowledge, the requirement of informed consent where the knowledge of the procedures are conveyed by the scientist-physician hardly guarantees that disinterested judgments as to what are justified risks will be made.

This is one of the reasons why procedures for achieving more disinterestedness in decisions involving experimentation have been set up by agencies such as the FDA and NIH.[35] Increasingly these agencies are also recognizing that the committees that are to review research before it will be funded by government money should include nonscientists and nonphysicians who will help to represent interests that are not primarily those of a medical scientist or even a physician. Such persons may take a harder look at the scientific merit of proposed experiments, but equally if not more important is their role in articulating the point of view and interests of those who are potential subjects in any experiment.

Increasing the representation of interests that are nonmedical and nonresearch oriented not only serves to protect individuals but also serves to determine whether or not certain kinds of medical interventions will create desirable or undesirable social policies. To take one extreme example, decisions to undertake experiments to perfect the technique of in-vitro fertilization, that is of creating and sustaining human life outside the womb, may well be motivated by the physicians' desire to provide children for couples who would otherwise be childless. However, these experiments and their results, while hypothetically beneficial on an individual basis, may not represent a sound social policy. The question of regulation is not one that physicians can be expected to be disinterested or dispassionate about. By the same token, physicians can rightly claim that uninformed lay persons may have their views of this distorted by their passions and interests. The whole purpose of democratic processes from a moral point of view is to achieve a higher measure of disinterestedness, dispassionateness, and vivid imagination of how various parties are affected by one policy or another. To accomplish this, democratic processes seek to maximize participation of diverse interests, or at least to achieve representation of those diverse interests and to establish procedures by which persons and groups are guaranteed due process.

Here we touch on one of the critical strategic moral issues in contemporary medicine. The relations between physicians and patients are not governed purely by the moral conscientiousness of physicians and the sophistication of patients. Groups like the poor and blacks suffer ill health in part because, for various reasons, they either do not avail themselves of existing medical care for which they are eligible, or when they do so, they encounter difficulties intentionally or unintentionally perpetrated by persons and modes of care that are not well understood or appreciated, and which may or may not be best for them. Again, this situation is only partially rectified by injecting into the delivery of medical care persons from ethnic and/or minority groups that are not now well represented. There are also larger policy questions having to do with health education, with alleviation of poverty, with the location and nature of health facilities, and also with the locus and nature of the administrative control of these facilities.

Clearly, our brief essay could only encompass a framework for discussion. There are so many questions that require substantive analysis. Our failure to take up some of these questions in greater detail is not due to a lack of desire but rather to a self-confessed choice that it was important to put some of these questions into a larger framework, a framework suggested by the nature and scope of the ethical enterprise itself. There is no question that the assumption throughout has been that the concerns of the medical profession and of medical ethics as an enterprise are very much the concern of everyone but particularly of ethicists who reflect on the most general nature of ethics and moral decision-making. In no way do we wish to minimize thereby the significance and the benefits of the expertise that comes to us from medicine. We have only suggested ways of thinking and of formulating policy that may increase these benefits for all concerned.

Notes

1. Paul Ramsey, *The Patient as Person,* New Haven: Yale University Press, 1970, p. 1.

2. London: Routledge & Kegan Paul, 1967; reprinted in paperback; Boston: Beacon Press, 1968; and Harmondsworth: Penguin Books, 1969.

3. "Ethics and Clinical Research," *New England Journal of Medicine,* June 16, 1966, Vol. 274, pp. 1354–1360. [Reprinted as Chapter 51 of this volume.]

4. Joseph Fletcher is one of the most outspoken representatives of this view; see, for example, "Our Shameful Waste of Human Tissue: An Ethical Problem for the Living and the Dead," in D. R. Cutler (ed.), *Updating Life and Death,* Boston: Beacon Press, 1968.

5. Editorial: "A New Ethic for Medicine and Society," *California Medicine,* 113:67–68, 1970.

6. See the essay by Karen Lebacqz in the May, 1973, issue of the *Linacre Quarterly.* [Reprinted as Chapter 64 of this volume.]

7. For a discussion of regulation by government agencies, see William J. Curran, "Governmental Regulation of the Use of Human Subjects in Medical Research: The Approach of Two Federal Agencies," in P. A. Freund (ed.), *Experimentation with Human Subjects,* New York: Braziller, 1969.

8. See Arthur J. Dyck, "Questions of Ethics," *Harvard Theological Review,* Oct., 1972.

9. "A Theoretical and Experimental Inquiry into Concrete Values and Value Systems," in B. Kaplan and S. Wapner (eds.), *Perspectives in Psychological Theory,* New York: International Universities Press, 1960.

10. *Op. cit.*

11. Stoicism as a euthanasia ethic is discussed in more detail in Arthur J. Dyck, "An Alternative to the Ethic of Euthanasia," in R. H. Williams (ed.), *To Live and To Die: When, Why and How?,* New York: Springer-Verlag, 1973. [The essay is reprinted as Chapter 85 of this volume.]

12. John T. Noonan, Jr., "An Almost Absolute Value in History," in J. T. Noonan, Jr. (ed.), *The Morality of Abortion,* Cambridge: Harvard University Press, 1970; and George H. Williams, "Religious Residues and Presuppositions in the American Debate on Abortion," *Theological Studies* 31:1, March, 1970, pp. 10–75.

13. Ralph B. Potter, Jr., *War and Moral Discourse,* Richmond: John Knox Press, 1969, pp. 43–46.

14. This case is depicted in a film "Who Shall Survive?" made and distributed by the Joseph P. Kennedy, Jr. Foundation.

15. For a discussion of these issues, see Arthur J. Dyck, "An Alternative to the Ethic of Euthanasia," *op. cit.*

16. *A Theory of Justice,* Cambridge: Harvard University Press, 1971.

17. See Karen Lebacqz, *op. cit.,* for a discussion of such views.

18. *The Right and the Good,* Oxford, 1930, Chapter 2. [Chapter 16, this volume.]

19. Boston: Beacon Press, 1960.

20. *Ibid.,* p. 5.

21. *Ibid.,* p. 6.

22. New Haven: Yale University Press, 1970.

23. *Ibid.,* pp. xi–xii.

24. *Ibid.,* pp. xv–xvi.

25. *Ibid.,* p. xviii.

26. "Medical Ethics: Professional or Universal?," *Harvard Theological Review,* Oct., 1972.

27. W. K. Frankena, *Ethics,* Englewood Cliffs: Prentice-Hall, 1963, pp. 92–94, and Bernard Williams, *Morality: An Introduction to Ethics,* New York: Harper and Row, 1972, pp. 20–26.

28. W. K. Frankena, *ibid.,* pp. 94–96.

29. W. K. Frankena, *ibid.,* pp. 92–94, and Bernard Williams, *op. cit.,* pp. 20–26.

30. *Ibid.* See also the discussions of relativism by R. B. Brandt, *Ethical Theory,* Englewood Cliffs: Prentice-Hall, 1959.

31. Ralph B. Potter, Jr., *War and Moral Discourse, op. cit.,* pp. 23–29.

32. This is an actual case but somewhat changed to hide the identity of persons involved.

33. The clearest formulation of this kind of theory is by Roderick Firth, "Ethical Absolutism and the Ideal Observer Theory," *Philosophy and Phenomenological Research* 12 (1952), pp. 317–345. See also W. K. Frankena, *op. cit.,* pp. 94–96.

34. As we noted earlier, policy judgments hinge in part on the loyalties of those who make them. Loyalties are "interests" and "passions." If moral policy is to be rational, the loyalties must take on the universal perspective that is implied in disinterestedness and dispassionateness.

35. William J. Curran, *op. cit.*

20

Paul Ramsey
The Nature of Medical Ethics

Reprinted with permission of author and publisher from Robert Veatch, Willard Gaylin, and Councilman Morgan, eds., *The Teaching of Medical Ethics* (Hastings-on-Hudson, New York: Institute of Society, Ethics and the Life Sciences [Hastings Center], 1971), pp. 14–28.

We have first a language problem. The word "ethics" can be used to point to the *ethos* of a given culture or period; "morality," to refer to *mores*, the actual behavior of people, the decisions they make or are likely to make; and "normative" can be associated with the normal, or average. The roots of all three words mean almost the same thing: patterns of behavior. If this is all ethics means, "medical ethics" could appeal to the "customary practice" of the profession as its only standard.

We need—even simply by agreement—some differentiation in the use of these terms. I shall mean by "ethics" the science of right or wrong conduct, praise—or blameworthy behavior. Thus, to engage in normative medical ethics means to reflect upon what should be done, whether this is actually the case or an ideal or action-guide to be espoused. Similarly, aesthetics means an inquiry into the nature of beauty, whether of an actual vase or score, or one yet to be composed. Ethics means making rationally defendable judgments about "morality." For our purposes, the word "normative" simply adds force to this meaning of the ethical. Normative medical ethics, then, means the application of evaluative norms of some sort in appraisal of practices in medicine. In terms of "is-ought," we would be trying, as the outcome of ethical discourse, to tell what ought not to be that may now be done, or what ought to be that is now not done.

This conference is a sign of hope that we can prepare ourselves, and the young men and women who are our students, to face the many new moral dilemmas (or old dilemmas in new form) which we face because of the triumphs of medical research and the promise of medical technology. The conference is also a sign of crisis—a moral crisis in the ethics of the medical profession because of the moral crisis in modern culture generally. I think it can no longer be assumed that we are agreed on moral action-guides, the practice of virtue, the premises and principles of the highest, most humane, most bracing ethics, or what a moral agent owes to anyone who bears a human countenance. If not, then medical ethics can no longer consist of etiquette and a few codes, or following the example of our teachers in moral matters also.

In fact, ethical inquiry and discourse begin only when we discover we are in disagreement about what we ought to do. Then we are forced back upon our premises, and we must seek together in the human community and in the medical profession to find agreement at a deeper level. We must ask about what makes anything right. We need to find out if we can agree upon the right-making or wrong-making features of moral attitudes, actions, roles or relations, before returning to the specific case where we first disagreed over what ought to be done. That is ethics proper. It is also why in any age every moral agent is an ethicist if he will only let himself go, and be one; and why in a period in which there is a moral consensus, ethics mainly gives backing to the consensus and few are needed for that important function. In an age, however, when ancient landmarks have been removed, and we are trying to do the unthinkable, namely, build a civilization without an agreed civil tradition and upon the absence of a moral consensus, everyone needs to be an ethicist to the extent of his capacity for reflection and his desire to be and to know that he is a responsible person. (Under conditions of moral disagreement, the impulse to be responsible and the task of knowing more fully the meaning of responsibility lead in the same direction.)

The conclusion, it seems to me, is that normative medical ethics is impossible unless medical education and the profession generally becomes in a significant measure more literate. How to introduce medical ethics into a curriculum that in first year must be largely memorization and for the remaining years must be the acquirement of the manual skills and art of medicine, I do not practically know. But unless we mean to make medical education more literate, indeed more literary, ethics can find no proper place in it, except in some defaced form; and lest we foster in ourselves illusions, I suggest we adjourn. We should rather leave ethics as a sediment from the liberal arts years, to be socialized away by medical education as it now is. In no case is medical ethics as a discipline fostered by discussing cases in the absence of a framework of analysis, nor is it accomplished by "Gee Whiz!"

social concerns on the part of first and second year students. Ethics is not a matter of concerns or passion (praiseworthy as these may be in moral agents); it is rather an intellectual inquiry. Therefore, education in medical ethics must necessarily be primarily literate.

Two things, additionally, medical ethics is not. It is not the same as *law* (or medical jurisprudence) and it is not a matter of deciding the *procedures* (Who shall decide?, for example) for making moral or professional decisions.

What I mean by distinguishing ethics from law can be explained by a single illustration. When the Director of a program of amniocentesis followed by the abortion of fetuses discovered to be afflicted with a serious degenerative, soon fatal and presently untreatable genetic disease said, "It would be *wrong* to offer the procedure of intrauterine screening to· a woman pregnant beyond x-weeks, even though both she and her husband were screened and found to be carriers," the reason given in support of this seeming moral judgment was: "Because we cannot offer her any medical *good,* namely, the certainty of avoiding the birth of an irreversibly dying baby, with the opportunity to try again for a normal one." Further discussion revealed that the physician meant to say that since the law of his state prohibited abortions after x-weeks, he had no medical benefit to offer, etc. His words, "It would be *wrong* to offer the procedure of interuterine screening, etc." meant simply "Abortions are against the law after x-weeks."

At most, he may have meant to say, It would be wrong for me to do a useless procedure, or to deceive her about my willingness to grant her the same outcome as to others in the screening. But those lesser moral judgments trace home and depend upon what was legal or illegal. Can we not say that the physician's original statement (which when delivered had the force of a fundamental medical ethical verdict) rested upon a considerable confusion of law with ethics? He did not cite any degree of greater danger to the mother from late abortion, which anyway could hardly have failed to be overridden by the benefit to her of avoidng the birth of an infant afflicted so fatally.

Moreover, if his original verdict had been a medico-moral judgment it would have been an entirely irrational one—like seriously claiming that something that is right on one side of the Pyrenees can be wrong on the other. The physician did not cite any morally relevant features justifying the procedure with genetic abortion *before* x-weeks that are not still present *after* x-weeks. The features he believed to be right-making were simply illegal after that.

This is not to say that disobedience to law is not an ethical matter. If the physician said, It would be *wrong* for me to break the law that good may come, the question at issue would have been the morality of civil disobedience. Instead, he ascribed wrongfulness to offering a medical procedure to the woman, etc. That was a confusion of legality with medical morality, or an attempt to derive the latter from the former.

Nor am I saying that there are no interconnections between ethics and law, or denying the law's function as moral influence and teacher. Many people, in fact, take their judgments of right and wrong from what the law allows or forbids. Whether they should do so is an ethical question.

Nor do I mean to deny—I mean rather now to affirm—that in the fabric of the law we have a depository of ethical decision-making, a civil tradition from the past until now, in which we can see morality "writ large," a continuity of moral judgments developed over time and honed in the prism of case after case. (Ethics is, among other things, the critical study of the grounds and validity of those decisions.) No judge ever says, "I discern in this case justice to be x." Instead, his judgment is framed by conceptualized precedents in past similar sorts of cases. He brings the present case under the appropriate past judgments; or else, noting dissimilarities in the instant case, he creatively expands the ethical and legal concepts available from past cases.

For this reason, the law touching medical-ethical cases could be extraordinarily instructive in medical ethics. All the particularities of a case are brought up, but in the framework of precedental concepts of right action.

At the same time, this points to a difference between the case-method in legal education and the case method in teaching medical ethics. In the former, theoretical notions are built into the cases. The latter needs radical supplement by ethical analytical material that is not to be found by staring at the bare case, unless we are to deem the pouring of the contents of one empty mind into another to be the discussion of a medical ethical problem. A law student using the case method is never without precedental concepts of justice or fairness. Indeed, he has the same set of action-guides for similar sorts of cases. Must not the medical student be provided like resources?

There are, of course, the various codes or lists of principles drawn up by various medical societies since the Nuremberg Code, together with the commentaries on them written by many wise physicians and discussion of various cases in the light of these principles, with arguments pro and con for revisions. A remarkable professional ethics, I would say. Perhaps we may look forward to graduates of medical schools who can discuss these matters with the subtlety and agility that a law student must know of the law embedded in the cases to which he must appeal.

However, there would be real analogy between the case method in medical ethics teaching and the case method in legal instruction if, but only if, peer committees in medical centers did more than reject or accept research protocols, if they wrote opinions saying why, if there were majority and dissenting opinions each advancing an argument, if future decisions appealed to the articulation of principles governing in past cases or subscribed to by other peer committees in like cases. Otherwise, we still have a laissez-faire decisional system in which proposals are voted up or down, but without the deciding group having to draw upon a larger community of professional ethical decisions and without being put on its mettle by knowing it is contributing to a living body of medical ethics, its growth or erosion.

A second thing medical ethics is *not:* it is not a matter of settling the *procedures* for deciding difficult medico-moral issues. The error of thinking in terms of decision-making models is the special temptation of a professional ethics in a relativistic age and in a pluralistic culture. So, in the absence of a moral consensus, it becomes of first importance to decide who shall decide. In abortion, the woman exclusively? Or both parents? Or the woman with her physician? Or is there a public policy interest in the question? We light upon peer committees as a way to insure surveillance of a researcher's moral practices as well as scientific aspects of his design. And then there is discussion of whether there should be representatives of "the public" on peer committees. Who shall tell the dying patient—the physician or a member of his family? Finally, there are elaborate proposals for a rank-order of family members in decisions to allow a patient to die.

These procedural questions are not unimportant. Yet it must be said that ethics is concerned with *what* should be decided—the right and wrong of it—not primarily with *who* shall decide, or *how*. Indeed we would not be able to determine the appropriate decision-maker if we had no notion of the appropriate decision to be made. We cannot appraise procedures except in terms of greater or less likelihood that worthy choices will be forthcoming. Absent any normative ethics on the urgent moral questions we face, however, and inevitably deciding-who-shall-decide becomes a substitute for ethical inquiry and discourse about what ought to be done (whoever does it).

Robert M. Veatch is also extraordinarily concerned to perfect decisional procedures, but from a different base—that of a universal ethics. The words in the Hippocratic Oath by which a physician promises to "abstain from whatever harm or injustice" require that "a medical ethics should be an integral component of a universal ethic, one which neither dichotomizes the ethical and the scientific nor makes ethical rightness dependent upon membership in a particular professional group." Veatch wants no more ethical expertise ascribed to medical professionals than to the Defense Department. ". . . technical competence does not an ethical expert make."

We may agree with Veatch that professional ethics is only a special case of the ethics of a wider human community. We may also agree with him that

there is no ethics without some universal warrants or principles. Still that should not lead us simply in the direction of setting up decision-making procedures based mainly in that wider community. For even if we are not relativists we must still acknowledge that there are plural "views of the universal." Each of us worships the Lord under his own vine and fig tree (in a sense Scripture did not mean) and none can persuade another that he has "a universal view."

In the absence of a moral consensus nourishing the roots of a professional medical ethics without much thoughtful reflection on the part of physicians and medical students, the medical profession could and should contribute as well as any other to the renewal of moral discourse in a pluralistic age. For all the moral crisis in medical practice and in our civilization generally, I myself would still trust "the ethical physician" to discern the issues we face as well or better than some overawed, excessively scientifically minded member of "the public." To say that is not "the fallacy of generalization of expertise." It is simply to say that to whom more is given of facing birth and death and pain and suffering in between, of him more is required in moral discernment in an age when that no longer flows from the decencies of one moral universe or the religious faiths in which men formerly lived.

The trick is to turn our attention decisively away from decisional procedures, supported for whatever reason, if we mean to engage in ethical inquiry, from the *who* or *how* to the *what*, to the features of attitude and actions that make them right, and to principles of ethical appraisal. So far as I can see physicians today can contribute as well as anyone, and medical education as well as any other, to the moral history of mankind. But, for the reasons already given, medical ethics must become more literate, if any light upon our pathway is to come from that source.

I shall conclude by sketching the broad outlines of a normative medical ethics, a model of ethical decision-making—with, as illustrations, a few of the sorts of verdicts, principles or action-guides which, I believe, are the upshot of proper ethical reasoning in the context of medical practice. Not

surprising, these are some of the principles of our existing medical ethics.

Our first move must be to agree on a term to express the ultimate requirement or standard or warrant binding in all cases upon the helping and healing professions. I suggest the word "care" (or "respect") for human life)—not "care" in the sense of specific kinds of medical care, but "care" as a strong, ethical expression, the source of particular moral obligations and our court of final appeal for deciding the features of actions and practices that make what we do right or wrong.

"Care" has the advantage of locating medical ethics within the ethics of a wider human community. It also locates our model for medical decision-making alongside other models: Jewish ethics whose ultimate norm is *hesed* or steadfast fidelity to the covenant of life with life and Christian ethics whose final appeal and criteria of judgment is Christian love and compassion. Religious ethics would be inclined to ascribe "sanctity" to human life and call for more than "care" and "respect" for life. We need not go into that, since "care" can be understood in a strong sense and may blend in one degree or another with those other sources of judgment. Medical ethics, we can minimally say with an editorial in *California Medicine*, has "had the blessing of the Judeo-Christian tradition"; but we need not be concerned with the interconnections between medical ethics and other models of normative decision-making.

Our next move must be to ask, What does care require?

That question takes two forms. It breaks down into two sorts of questions productive of two sorts of answers, which are important to keep clear as we proceed to unfold proper ethical reasoning toward applications.

One can say, first, that we are to tell what we should do in a particular dilemma by making sure we know the facts of that situation and the options it affords and then asking which specific action takes most care of human life—present lives and (in the case of research) future lives. In more or less discrete decisions in the face of more or less unique problematic cases we are to ask, What singular deed or design of ours is most likely to embody or convey care or respect for human life?

We ask, Will this or that procedure care for the patient more? Or we ask, Will this or that research design be productive of the more significant benefit for the ongoing community of medical care?

This first form of our question is productive of balancing decisions to operate or not to operate in particular cases. It is also productive of the second Article of the Nuremberg Medical Code which states the requirement that an experiment on human subjects "should be such as to yield fruitful results for the good of society, unprocurable by any other method or means of study, and not random and unnecessary in nature." These are essentially prudential decisions concerning what care requires, which only the physician or researchers are competent to make and which they make case after case, from protocol to protocol, in extending medical care.

The second form of the question, however, leads to answers of a different order. One can say, secondly, in medical ethics that we are to tell what we ought to do, not only by asking which particular action or research design is most caring, but also by asking which *rules of practice,* what *principles* of action, what moral institutions or "covenants of loyalty" (as I prefer to call them) would, if maintained or established in the ethics of the medical profession, prove generally most caring for the dignity of man in patients or research subjects? Some contemporary philosophers call answers to this question "rules of the game"; and I suggest that there are universal rules of the game called caring.

This sort of ethical reasoning from an ultimate norm is productive, for example, of the first Article of the Nuremberg Medical Code, which requires a free and informed consent in human experimentation. Now, the physician must make prudential judgments in applying that principle in medical care and research. For this reason some physicians are under the impression that they are engaged in the same sort of activity when they judge a patient's or subject's consent to be an understanding, voluntary one as they are

when they make balancing judgments to operate or not or in perfecting protocols.

In this they are mistaken. In the latter case, the physician tries to respond aptly to a particular situation. In the former, he is asking the applicable meaning of a principle of medical ethics, a rule of professional practice. He is exploring the requirements of a governing moral notion. He asks what he should do in order to abide by a "covenant of loyalty" between persons who are physician/researchers and persons who are patients or subjects.

To repeat: the two forms of our original question are: What should we do in particular actions or designs in order, case by case, to extend the greatest care? and, What rules of practice render the medical profession most careful and respectful of the dignity of all concerned?

Next we come to the question of priority of one over the other of these two sorts of ethical reasoning. I suggest that there are sound grounds for saying that rules of practice or covenants of loyalty should be accorded priority over an ethics of doing the most good on the whole, if there are cases of irresolvable conflict between them.

To illustrate from another realm: the practice of promise-making and promise-keeping. If you promise a dying friend, no one else knowing, to take care of his two retarded children, why should you keep that promise if you come upon two other children who are very bright, equally destitute, your funds are limited, and there is no other recourse? Without here saying that promise-keeping is absolutely without exception binding upon us, I would suggest the promise to one's dying friend ought to be kept even in face of the fact that one can do far more good on the whole by, instead, taking care of those other two children.

Dr. Henry K. Beecher made the same sort of priority-judgment between the first and second Articles of the Nuremberg Medical Code. If an experiment is moral it is moral in its inception; it does not become moral because it produces valuable data (or is wisely calculated to do so). Beecher goes on to criticize the language of the second provision because it opens the

door to violations of the first, and much else besides. "The words 'for the good of society' must be viewed with distaste, even alarm. Undoubtedly all sound work has this as its ultimate aim, but such high-flown expressions are not necessary and have been used within recent memory as cover for outrageous ends" (Beecher, 1959). That verdict he repeats in his recent book: ". . . The *bonum communum* was precisely the rationalization claimed by the Nazis"; "In Rule 2, the phrase 'for the good of society' is unsavory" (Beecher, 1970).

That may go too far in downgrading the second Article as also a manifestation of an ethics of care. Still, it needs to be acknowledged that there is a possible collision between these two requirements. One of the Articles places an independent limit upon the use of the other; and fidelity to the being and well-being, and to the humanity, of everyone now engaged in helping to make medical progress takes priority. A major task in the ethical practice of medicine is to harmonize these requirements and to stay within the boundaries of permissible practice fixed by both together.

As an illustration of what goes on in normative medical ethics, it is most important for us to see that care leads to these two provisions through different modes of ethical reasoning. In the one case we are led to a *benefits*-requirement by asking which particular actions or designs are productive of greater care for human life. In the other case, we are led to the *consent*-requirement by asking which practice-rule or principle of loyalty includes and exhibits care for all presently concerned.

Note also that if we assign priority to a benefits-requirement (the second Article), that takes us all the way to Utilitarianism. Concerning that I will simply say that that would be to try to resurrect a dead horse. If that seems too extreme a statement, let me simply report that among the majority of philosophers doing ethics today, Utilitarianism has been dead for decades. So, I can revise my remark and say that if a crisis of medical ethics today is the threat it will go overboard for Utilitarianism, then such an eventuality would mean a most remarkable breakdown of communication between two leading professions in our society: physicians and ethicists, without parallel in periods past. In the present day, when nonutilitarian requirements in morality are being eroded in society generally and can no longer be counted on silently to inform the physician's conscience, I have to conclude, again, that in future ethical physicians and medical ethics generally must become more literate and establish explicit communication with the writings and reflections of ethicists. The conclusion I regret, since medical ethics worked better when moral consensus was intact and there was less need for ethical reflection and analysis.

Let us now replay our model of an ethics of care in other illustrations. Here we come to some disputed conclusions, but ones that still show the crux to be our same two questions: What does care require in this particular situation? and What does care require as a general practice, in all like situations?

In hemodialysis, or like instances of placing a patient on a sparse medical resource whose absence would be fatal, decision must be made as to who shall live, who die. If medical care asks only, what helps most in this particular situation? it unavoidably gets into judging competitively the comparative social worthiness of two patients who both need the only available kidney machine. However, if we ask, as we should also ask, What does care require as a rule of practice, expressive of loyalty and respect for all lives concerned in the issue? Sound moral reasoning would, I suggest, incline us to adopt the controls of some form of lottery, or of a "first come, first served" arrangement, upon the vagaries of our private judgments about who most deserves to live. That alone would insure that, within the limits of possibility, care will be distributed equally to all who are in need, that we respect everyone who bears a human countenance. In the minimal form of equality of opportunity to live or to die when tragically all cannot be saved, such a practice-rule insures that everyone counts, and no one counts for more than one (as would be the case if we applied criteria of comparative social worthiness).

Another illustration of a basic rule of medical practice is: Never directly take the life of a terminal patient, or intervene to hasten his death. Medical care as a moral institution can never mean that. This is a prohibition constitutive of the game of medical care, to be compared with rules of the game in football defining "offside" or forbidding more than eleven men in play: these proscriptions are without exception; they tell us the game we are playing, and lay down the basic roles of the players in relation to one another.

But in football there are other rules that are only advice to the players as to how most of the time they should play the game—like, punt on fourth down. Everyone knows there are exceptions to that rule. One should be prepared to violate it in appropriate situations. So also there are summary directives to physicians within the institution of medical care which tell them how most of the time to play that game, but not always—like, Try and try again to cure your patient; struggle with him to save his life. Still everyone should know that doctors ought not always do that. There comes a time when medical care no longer means continuing exquisite efforts to cure and to save life. To be sure, medical care always means to cherish and respect life, and that can never mean killing patients. But there comes a time when to cherish and respect life means to care but *only* to care for the dying, no longer to oppose death, to accept its coming, to comfort and to keep company with the dying, not to prolong their dying but to make a human presence in that solitude, never to desert them, to insure as much dignity as possible to the dying in their passage. In the words of the old revival hymn, medical care need not always mean trying to "rescue the perishing," but it does always mean to "care for the dying." So unlike the prohibition of killing the innocent, the injunction to cure and save life is not a universal requirement of medical practice. How could it be, since cure is not always possible, and will finally become impossible in all cases? Care never ceases; yet care, never ceasing, has no duty to do the impossible or the useless.

Thus, I would argue that an ethics of care prolongs itself into a professional ethics consisting of several sorts of things: (1) rules constitutive of medical care, like the consent-requirement, the prohibition of killing, and randomizing life and death decisions, which are always binding, (2) directives to cure and save life which true care sometimes suspends and replaces by comfort and dignity for the dying, and (3) balancing situational decisions, such as to operate or not to operate, or to use this research protocol or that.

Objection will be forthcoming to the more strenuous of these conclusions, to the view that professional medical ethics, like any other ethics, consists also of universally binding obligations. The objection will be that there are always "exceptions." I shall contend that this is only seemingly so, and that "exceptions" to rules of practice are themselves implied by the fidelity-principle in question and are themselves "universals," only more specifically defined. To show this, let us consider again the consent-requirement and its supposed "exceptions."

No man is good enough, or for that matter wise enough, to treat another without his understanding consent. Besides, medical care is a joint venture in which patient and physician ideally should both say, I cure. Therefore, the consent-requirement is a universal rule of medical practice. Yet there is an evident sort of "exception" where this seems not required as in the case of highway accident victims. We might say that if a physician stops on the road to Jericho, instead of passing by on his way to read a research paper before a scientific gathering or to visit his regular paying patients, he is self-selected as good enough to practice medicine without the needy man's expressed consent. But the point is not whether that was subjectively an ethical physician or not. The question is rather what makes us objectively certain that was right to do. We could say that in these instances a physician practices medicine without consent— an exception to the rule. Instead we say, correctly I believe, that the unconscious man "constructively" consented to procedures from which he may have suffered harm if the physician bungles. Why do we imply that he did? The answer is by an application of the *reversibility*-test, which shows that in the case of highway accident victims the requirement of consent is only being extended and applied. The physician exchanges places with the man by the side of the road, and thus sustains in himself the claims of the absolutely universalizable principle that human need calls for rescue, that a man in need "consents" to be helped.

Notice that the consent-requirement is in no way weakened; its meaning might rather be said to be extended, explained and applied.

In any case, the "exception" indicates a *class* or *sort* of case having relevant moral features in common. These are as universalizable as was the original rule before the exception was added. The exception to the need for consent—if such it is—still tells us, as a guide to action, that similar agents should do likewise in similar situations. *One* who is a physician, not just *I* who am, nor just because that is a socially worthy individual over there by the side of the road, should stop to help in emergencies even if he had no covenant or contract with me to be his physician. The moral judgment remains intact, even if all personal pronouns are removed (who I am or who he is—except for the relation of care). Even if suddenly there were no more crushed bodies along the highways, that would still be the right thing to do. Even if never repeated again, what was done is essentially repeatable. In stopping to help without prior patient consent, the physician wills what he does to be a universal moral law governing medical practice. He prescribes for himself and all men a moral institution.

To obtain another so-called "exception" to universal rules of medical practice, let us say—as I would argue—that one entailment of the consent-requirement is that no one should give proxy consent for children or other incompetents to hazardous trials unless those are at least remotely in their behalf medically. (That "unless" is already an "exception" which again shows that exceptions to moral rules always define a *class* of actions, never unique situations.) Suppose we say, then, that a rule of medical practice is "Never subject children to the unknown possible hazards of medical investigations having no possible relation to their own treatment." To that we must promptly add, "except in epidemic conditions." That exception

simply explains, extends and applies the rule. It takes account of the fact that the dangers from which the child needs protection need not be already resident beneath his own skin. He is already subject to predictable risks from exposure to crippling epidemic, for example, of Polio. He can therefore be treated as one of a population, and those risks be weighed against the risks, which are not negligible, of entering him into field-trials of a vaccine. To do this *is* in his behalf medically, and therefore to put parental consent in place of the consent he cannot maturely give is quite valid. We only do what anyone, any parent should do. This, again, illustrates the reversibility-test and the universalizability-test in deciding the ethical thing to do. The personal pronouns are removed, any idiosyncratic or situationally unique features are removed, and the moral judgment remains intact. Such decisions are clearly not like deciding to operate or not to operate. In the latter case, one decides what care requires in a particular situation. In the former, one decides what actions fall under a rule of care and loyalty to the dignity of persons who are patients.

One cannot even do violence to the consent of another except within the consent-requirement as a canon of medical practice (as but an instance of a wider ethics of respect for persons), no more than one can commit an "error" or draw a "walk" unless he is playing the game of baseball, which has some exceptionless rules. In the practice of medicine, too, there are constitutive principles. Otherwise, there are no infractions; and physicians are only technicians going about doing the most good, on the whole, in ways that can only be mistaken, never in any meaningful sense moral violations.

Finally, mention should be made of the role of ethical reflection in perhaps helping to solve the difficult problem of setting medical priorities. To date, I have been convinced that there is no rational way to determine medical and social priorities, beyond every man's and every group's sense of justice entering into contention in our annual struggle over the Federal budget (plus the incidence of Senatorial and Presidential illnesses). However, Professor

John Rawls of Harvard University has recently published a volume entitled *A Theory of Justice*. This book bids to become the outstanding work on ethics published in this century. In Professor Rawls' concept of "justice as fairness," he is especially concerned with "distributive justice," with the priority-problem and with establishing principles by which inequities in a society might be justified as compatible with fairness to everyone concerned. How, without an actual egalitarianism and without a dynamic society contingently fixing priorities unequally, can there be a well-ordered society founded on an equal liberty?

Rawls' proposal for the critical appraisal of political and social institutions (including, I suggest, medical institutions, practices and inequities) is that "the higher expectations of those better situated are just if and only if they work as part of a scheme which improves the expectations of the least advantaged members of the society." He requires, even in a less than perfectly just world, that "the expectation of all those better off at least contribute to the welfare of the more unfortunate. That is, if their expectations were decreased, the prospects of the least advantaged would likewise fall." Inequities, to be justified, must "make a difference" to the representative least advantaged man: "an inequality of opportunity must enhance the opportunity of those with the lesser opportunity."

Is it not correct to say that today the medical profession has largely adopted a Utilitarian calculus of the greatest sum of good as the only overarching social philosophy by means of which to deal with the problem of medical priorities? Then the fact that Rawls' book is a superdreadnought sent out to do battle with the last remnants of Utilitarianism throws into striking relief the breakdown of communication between sectors in the intellectual leadership of our society. I suggest that *A Theory of Justice*—justice as fairness—provides a worthy framework for mutual discussion if in medical ethics we mean to become more self-conscious and critically reflective about our task. That is, if we mean to do ethics.

References

Beecher, Henry K. "Experiment in Man," *Journal of the American Medical Association* 169, No. 5 (January 31, 1959), p. 468.

Beecher, Henry K. *Research and the Individual.* Boston, Mass.: Little, Brown and Co., 1970, pp. 77, 232.

Ramsey, Paul. *The Patient as Person.* New Haven, Conn.: Yale University Press, 1970, pp. 266–275.

Rawls, John. *A Theory of Justice.* Cambridge, Mass.: Harvard University Press, 1971, pp. 75, 78, 303.

Veatch, Robert M. *Medical Ethics: Professional or Universal?* A Working Paper of the Institute of Society, Ethics and the Life Sciences, pp. 1, 2, 4, 5.

21

Albert R. Jonsen and Andre E. Hellegers

Conceptual Foundations for an Ethics of Medical Care

Reproduced with permission of the National Academy of Sciences from Laurence R. Tancredi, ed., *Ethics of Health Care* (Washington: National Academy of Sciences, 1974), pp. 3–20.

I

Medical ethics is currently in a muddle. Many questions are asked, but few answers are offered. Many anxieties are aired, but few are assuaged. Worst of all, the diversity of subjects discussed and the variety of arguments propounded makes one wonder whether there is any proper subject matter or proper methodology deserving the name, "medical ethics."

During July 1973, when this essay was first conceived, the newspapers carried three major, and many minor, stories about "medical ethics." In New York, a respected physician was accused of injecting potassium chloride into his dying cancer patient. In Chicago, the American Medical Association commented on the standards governing the ownership of stock in pharmaceutical companies by individual physicians and by the Association itself. In Aiken, South Carolina, three obstetricians refused, for what they called "social reasons," to deliver the babies of welfare mothers unless the mothers submitted to sterilization. All three stories were headlined "medical ethics." Euthanasia, financial investments, sterilization for social reasons: all three concern behavior by physicians, all three pertain, immediately or remotely, to the practice of medicine. This may justify use of "medical," but what justifies the "ethics"?

The title of this essay, while rather grandiose, refers to the modest task of stating the propriety of denominating certain sorts of considerations as medical "ethics" or the "ethics" of medical care. This essay is designed as a road map for this conference on Health Care and Changing Values. It will, hopefully, provide to its participants the main features of the topography of that ancient realm of the mind called ethics, through which modern medicine must travel.

Popularly, ethics seems to mean any body of prescriptions and prohibitions, do's and don'ts, that people consider to carry uncommon weight in their lives. When their lives are deeply involved in certain activities, ethics can refer to the rules that guide those activities. The *Lexicon* of the Sydenham Society[1] defined "ethics, medical" as "the laws of the duties of medical men to the public, to each other and to themselves with regard to the exercise of their profession. In this purview, euthanasia, financial investments in drugs, and sterilization for social reasons obviously belong to the family of ethics.

However, ethics, at least for most ethicians, means much more than a body of prescriptions and prohibitions. Ethics means the critical assessment and reconstruction of such bodies in the context of a comprehensive theory of human morality. By "morality" the present authors mean the actual behavior of human beings, involving judgments, actions, and attitudes, constructed around rationally conceived and effectively based norms whereby that behavior can be judged right or wrong and around values whereby states effected by that behavior are judged good or bad. By "ethics" the authors mean an academic discipline, a systematic set of propositions that constitute the intellectual instruments for the analysis of morality.

This discipline seeks to elucidate how the norms and values are established and perceived and how the actions are justified. It inquires how one argues and should argue from norms and facts to decisions. It tries to show how values and norms are related to purposes and results. To accomplish such analyses, a theory must be elaborated, within which these elements are comprehensively described and coherently articulated. It provides, when rightly done, not only a descriptive discipline of morality, but a normative one as well, for its analysis purports to reveal the roots of obligation and value appreciation, thereby exposing not how men do *in fact* behave, but how *in principle* they should behave. Ethics, then, is the normative discipline of morality.[2]

An adequate ethics would be a theoretical system capable of suggesting some answers to the sorts of questions arising about morality. The authors believe that since there are at least three sorts of questions, an adequate ethics would consist of at least three principal theories, which we call, in reverence to the traditions of the discipline, the theory of virtue, the theory of duties, and the theory of the common good.

In response to questions like, "What sort of person can rightly be called a morally good man?," the theory of virtue will expatiate on the character of

moral agents, like attitudes, habits, affections, and motives. In response to questions like, "What ought I to do in this situation?," the theory of action will discuss the nature of action, its objectives, goals, intentions, consequences, and conditions for freedom, and voluntariness. In response to questions like, "What is the best form of human society?," the theory of common good seeks to understand not the good man alone nor his right actions but the social institutions that make and are made by good men acting rightly.

Medical ethics is, we believe, a species of the genus *Ethics*. It should, then, be constructed out of the three essential theories of ethics. In this essay we contend that, traditionally, medical ethics has dwelt mostly within two of those three theories, namely, the theories of virtue and of duty. Both of these theories, while in need of refurbishing and modernization, remain indispensable to medical ethics. But the nature of contemporary medicine demands that they be complemented by the third essential theory—the common good. We shall review two traditional forms of medical ethics, indicating their relationship to the classical ethical theories. We shall then state the condition of modern medicine that calls for the theory of the common good. We suggest that this does not merely add an appendix to medical ethics but that it can be the source of a new concept of the discipline that can profoundly affect the more traditional theories of virtue and duty.

II

The term "medical ethics" is frequently applied to those statements of professional standards that are set forth in "codes." There are many such codes, but we shall select the *Ethical Principles of the American Medical Association* as a paradigm. We believe that our analysis applies generally to what is sometimes called "code ethics."[3]

The AMA code, adopted in 1847 and revised four times (1903, 1912, 1947, 1955), now consists of ten sections in which such subjects as consultations and precedence, scientific competence, professional courtesy, cooperation with nonphysician health personnel, solicitation of patients, fees, conditions of practice, and confidentiality

are treated. Some of these subjects are discussed at length but, for the most part, the principles are succinctly expressed. For example, "It is unethical . . . for a physician to provide or prescribe unnecessary services or unnecessary ancillary facilities" (Section 4). "The acceptance of rebates on appliances and prescriptions or of commissions from those who aid in the care of patients is unethical" (Section 7). The preamble states that "these principles . . . are not immutable laws to govern the physician, for the ethical practitioner needs no such laws; rather they are standards by which he may determine the propriety of his own conduct." The substance of the code, which comes to 67 pages in its latest edition, consists of these standards that serve to "standardize" the more common transactions, social and economic, between physicians, between physicians and patients, and between physicians and third parties, such as legal authorities, insurance providers, and the press. We call these standards "pragmatic directions."[4]

Interspersed among these pragmatic directions are occasional exhortations to cultivate certain virtues considered proper to the physician. A citation from the Hippocratic literature opens Section 1: The physician "should be modest, sober, patient, prompt to do his whole duty without anxiety; pious without going so far as superstition, conducting himself with propriety in his profession and in all the actions of his life." Physicians are expected, notes Section 2, "in their relationship with patients, with colleagues and with the public, to maintain under God, as they have down the ages, the most inflexible standards of personal honor." At various points, the virtues of fearlessness, benevolence, patience, and delicacy are recommended. The Preamble notes that, while "interpretation of these principles by an appropriate authority will be required at times . . . as a rule . . . the physician who is capable, honest, decent, courteous, vigilant, and an observer of the Golden Rule, and who conducts his affairs in the light of his own conscientious interpretation of these principles will find no difficulty in the discharge of his professional obligations."[5]

Pragmatic standards for common transactions predominate; exhortations to virtue are sparse and, one might cynically say, perfunctory. The predominance of the pragmatic directions has prompted many to refer to the codes as an "etiquette" rather than an "ethic." One of the first codes is *Decorum*, more literally the *Etiquette*, found in the Hippocratic corpus; during the nineteenth century medical codes were frequently called "etiquettes." Dr. Chauncey Leake[6] writes in the preface to his edition of *Percival's Medical Ethics*, which served as exemplar for the early AMA codes:

The term "medical ethics" introduced by Percival is a misnomer. Based on Greek traditions of good taste . . . it refers chiefly to the rules of etiquette developed in the profession to regulate the professional contacts of its members with each other . . . medical etiquette is concerned with the conduct of physicians toward each other and embodies the tenets of professional courtesy. Medical ethics should be concerned with the ultimate consequences of the conduct of physicians toward their individual patients, and toward society as a whole, and it should include consideration of the will and motive behind this conduct.

The concept of etiquette is enticing because it sidesteps the pitfalls of having to define morality. An etiquette is a set of conventional rules, usually quite arbitrary, that reflect behavior in polite society. With obvious repugnance, but impeccable *noblesse oblige*, Lord Chesterfield admonished his son, "Without hesitation, kiss the Pope's slipper or whatever else the etiquette of that court requires." An etiquette is hardly susceptible to ethical analysis, for it is seldom possible or profitable to attempt to justify its precepts, which are either simply "just done" or devised with a clear view to avoiding arguments about precedence, confusion over procedures, etc.

Etiquette is then a set of rules for external behavior that may be presumed to come from an internally virtuous man. Obviously, the external behavior may not reflect the internal man. Yet this is not sufficient to become cynical about the rules of etiquette. At best, they will truly reflect virtue. At worst, they are likely to keep the individual on his *qui vive*.

However, the word "etiquette" is a misleading description of the codes.

They do consist predominantly of pragmatic and arbitrary standards of behavior. But the sparse, almost perfunctory, exhortations to virtue in the modern codes are the faded tokens of their ancestry as ethics. The immediate progenitor of the American codes, Percival's *Medical Ethics,* is a treatise on the "Gentleman Physician." In the eighteenth century, "gentleman" denoted much more than a polite, gracious, considerate man with *savoir faire*. It was a synonym for the virtuous man. A century earlier, Izaak Walton[7] had written, "I would rather prove myself a Gentleman, by being learned and humble, valiant and inoffensive, virtuous and communicable than by a fond ostentation of riches." The long tradition of medicine, from the Hippocratic corpus through the Admonita and Epistulae of the Middle Ages, the *Medicus Politicus* of the Renaissance and the eighteenth century treatises on *Duties* and *Character of the Physician* is replete with exhortations to virtues proper to those who would practice medicine. This whole tradition mingles these exhortations with pragmatic directions about bedside manners, consultations, and fees; but the vision of the "upright man instructed in the art of healing" predominates.

These exhortations to virtue tend to dwindle, almost disappear, in more recent codes. Apparently, they seem to some superfluous, for they belabor the obvious. To others, they seem futile, for they cannot be enforced. Again, they seem vacuous, for they offer no practical guidance for action. Finally, they might seem embarrassing, for they smack of posturing for public consumption.

However, we suggest that these exhortations to virtue constitute the heart of code ethics. Indeed, they are the justification for calling the codes "ethics" at all. They give to the pragmatic directions a moral substance without which they are, indeed, merely etiquettes. Their disappearance in current codes is not merely a mildly deplorable withering of a charming, but rather quaint, affirmation of the good, the true, and the beautiful. It reflects fundamental uncertainty about the character desired in the person who would practice medicine.

The theory of virtue is a treatise about moral character. It has always been recognized that moral judgments

bear not only on the rightness or wrongness of discrete actions but also upon the goodness or badness of rather fixed states of persons who perform actions. Although "virtue" and "vice" are words with Victorian tone, great ethicists from Aristotle through Kant to Hartmann have used them to describe rationally intended, effectively rooted attitudes whereby persons consistently seem to incline toward certain sorts of behavior. Terms such as benevolence, honesty, trustworthiness, and sobriety described particular modes of these states of character.[8]

The great ethicists have always noted that while a spectrum of virtues should adorn the good man, particular dispositions were proper to certain roles: courage to the soldier, fairness to the judge, discretion to the ruler. A theory of virtue in medical ethics must explore that disposition most proper to the relationship between physician and patient—trust.

The patient approaching the physician suffers from more than his illness; he suffers from significant social disadvantages. He enters a mysterious domain, where arcane knowledge and rare skills rule. He is nervous, fearful, and perhaps even terrified. He places himself in the hands of a fallible human being. The novelist Kurt Vonnegut writes sardonically in *Goodbye, Mr. Rosewater*, "The most exquisite pleasure in the practice of medicine comes from nudging a layman in the direction of terror, then bringing him back to safety again." The potential for such sadism, which does lie within any physician's power, must be countered by the bond of trust. This bond—or as Paul Ramsey aptly titles it, covenant—arises from more than a contract; it is nourished by the evident trustworthiness of the physician.[9]

Codes do not create virtue. Their pragmatic directions establish certain regularities of procedure that elicit public confidence. But confidence elicited is fulfilled and confirmed only in the personal relationship that Pedro Lain Entralgo[10] calls "the medical friendship," a delicate alliance that must simultaneously encourage confidence and discourage dependency. The apparent fading of this friendship, under the cold exigencies of scientific skill, technical expertise, harried services, and, frankly, cupidity, has been blamed by many as the major cause of the "dehumanization" of care.

In sum, code ethics, as they now exist, might be called the archeological ruins of a doctrine of medical virtue. The codes are, in their present form, collections of pragmatic directions that mark the outer walls of the physician-patient covenant. Their inspiration and the inner confirmation of this covenant require the virtue of trustworthiness. Restoration of exhortations to virtue in the codes would not, of course, ensure the actual existence of virtue in physicians. This comes from the manner in which the profession selects and socializes its members, from exemplarity, and from exercise. Nonetheless, the theory of virtue in medical ethics requires serious reflection on the virtues proper to the physician and on the obstacles to their realization in contemporary settings and in contemporary men. Multiplication of codes, regulations, statutes, and standards, particularly if they are expected to be self-enforcing, as are most professional codes, is futile unless those to whom they are addressed comprehend and possess the virtues of the physician.

III

Virtue is the inner spirit of morality; action is its outer manifestation. The virtuous physician without skill may be comfort, but cold comfort, to one seeking cure. Medicine is a practical science: theory and experience evoked in clinical decision and action. Medical ethics, then, must be as concerned about the rightness of acts as about the goodness of the agent. A theory of virtue is a necessary, but not sufficient, part of medical ethics.

Ethics provides a second complementary theory, often called theory of duty, that defines the criteria whereby actions are judged right or wrong. It analyzes the relationship between intentions and consequences, motivations and circumstances. It studies the conditions of freedom and responsibility underlying imputation of guilt and innocence.

The need for an ethical analysis of actions comprising clinical practice is demonstrated in daily news articles on euthanasia, transplantation, and experimental trials. Serious efforts have been made to provide such an analysis. Jewish medical ethics is predominantly a doctrine of duties. Joseph Fletcher's pioneer work in medical ethics applies utilitarian theory of action to clinical acts. The present authors wish to use as an example the natural law theory of duties as it is found in Roman Catholic medical ethics. A volume on medical ethics in the Catholic tradition contains lengthy discussions of specific clinical actions such as euthanasia, abortion, transplantation, obstetrical techniques, and cosmetic surgery. Pope Pius XII had intense interest in questions of medical ethics and his frequent statements, delivered before distinguished medical societies, lent authoritative tone to the theologians' efforts.[11]

The medical ethics of this tradition is, in a very proper sense, a doctrine of duties. Medical interventions and procedures are analyzed in light of an explicitly formulated ethical system of principles and argumentation that can be broadly described as natural law.

The first affirmation of the system is that God has dominion over his creation, the human body, while man is granted a derived dominion over his body that he must exercise in view of the divinely appointed finality of his body and its functions. Because he is ultimately not his own, man has an obligation to preserve his life and health. Any mutilation of his body is an abuse of the derived dominion, unless that mutilation contributes to the good of the whole body. This affirmation, entitled the principle of totality, is the proximate governing principle of Catholic medical ethics.[12]

Other carefully defined principles allow the Catholic moral theologian to thread a precise path through the complexities of medical procedures. The principle of double effect can be invoked when an intervention involves the problem of finding moral justification for both the physical evil of mutilation and some other evil such as the death of a fetus removed in a salpingectomy done for ectopic pregnancy. The distinction between ordinary and extraordinary means of sustaining life, elaborated within the context of the principles of divine dominion and totality, provide to physician and patient thoughtfully defined ethical grounds for making painful ultimate decision about life and death.[13]

The theory of duty elaborated in Roman Catholic ethics describes an act in terms of (1) the *object*, that is, the objective design of the act and its immediate consequences; (2) the *end*, that is, the intention of the agent; and (3) the *circumstances*, that is, time, place, office, and other relevant concrete conditions of the act. In this approach, all three elements of an act must be right before the act is considered objectively moral. Criteria for evaluating the rightness of the action and its elements are such principles as divine and derived dominion and, more directly, the principle of totality.

In this scheme, a surgical intervention in the case of an ectopic pregnancy, described in terms of its objective, might be called a salpingectomy. The circumstances are advanced erosion of the fallopian tube, the presence of a fetus, and the absence of any therapeutic possibilities other than radical resection. The surgeon intends the removal of the eroding tube and tolerates the inevitable death of the developing fetus. The act would be judged morally right, for in its object, in the intention of the surgeon, and in the given circumstances, it effects the restoration of the integrity of the patient. The abortion is neither intended nor is it the principal objective of the act. It is, in the technical language of this school, an "indirect" abortion.

The purpose of this description and evaluation of actions is to enable the agent to discern actions that are morally right from those that are morally wrong. Morally right actions must or may be performed. Morally wrong action must be avoided. Thus, this doctrine of duties contains a doctrine of obligation, grounded in the principle of divine and derived dominion, which distinguishes between obligatory, permissible, and forbidden actions. There is an absolute moral obligation to refrain from morally wrong acts and a conditional moral obligation to perform right acts. The purpose of the theory of duties is to guarantee the moral rectitude of medical intervention. Almost every medical procedure of diagnosis and therapy requires an invasion of the sphere of the patient's physical and psychological independence.

Two points are particularly notewor-thy about this example of a theory of duties. First, the principle of totality is defined in terms of the integrity of the *physical* organism of an individual per-son. Efforts have been made, from time to time, to extend its range to *social* or *interpersonal* totality, but these have never been enthusiastically adopted. Thus, early discussions of homografts, such as renal transplants, tended to disapproval because of the nonbene-ficial mutilation of the donor. The suggestion that the bond of charity could thereby be strengthened between donor and recipient won little favor and the transplantation was finally jus-tified on grounds more consonant with traditional doctrine of totality, namely that donation of one of paired organs did not absolutely impair functional in-tegrity. Similarly, attempts to defend contraception by means other than periodic abstinence on the basis that hormonal alteration or tubal ligation would, ultimately, improve the psychological and physical well-being of a woman or benefit the total family situation were met with disfavor. The principle of totality remains tightly linked to physical integrity of single persons, rather than their psychological or social integrity.[14]

This problem has been framed in terms of the traditional Roman Catholic use of the principle of totality. How-ever, it is not a problem unique to that particular form of the theory of duties. Most efforts to formulate a theory of duties, in particular, those influenced by Kantian ethics, have a tendency to thrust the single act or the isolated agent onto center stage and leave the interrelationships of acts and agents in the shadows.

Second, any theory of duties issues prescriptions, prohibitions, and permis-sions. The physician committed to this moral reasoning must refrain from pro-hibited interventions. Even though cer-tain concessions are made for unwill-ing and compelled cooperation in im-moral acts, the physician's moral duty is quite clear. Direct abortion, direct sterilization, positive euthanasia are clearly forbidden. Refusal to perform these actions assures the moral integrity of the physician's conscience. How-ever, from the point of view of those who do not share the physician's con-science, his refusal to perform an act is perceived as denial of a benefit to the

petitioner. While any single petitioner might seek that benefit elsewhere, could it be that the conscientiously act-ing physician, by accumulation of his decisions and by his efforts to effect public policy in favor of his con-science, might impede some public good? And what if all physicians were of identical mind on the issue and all patients of opposite mind?[15]

Both of these problems, the restric-tion of the principle of totality to the *physical* integrity of single persons and the possibility of disagreement between adherents of this theory of duty and the possible demands of a broader public, suggest that a theory of duties, while necessary, may not be sufficient for adequate ethics. To the extent that such theories concentrate on discreet acts and individual intentions, they ne-glect the ethical issues arising from the intersection of multiple actions in institutions and society. Thus, an adequate ethics calls for an explicit reflection on the morality of institutions and on the relationship, and possible clash, between social values and indi-vidual values. Classical ethics has made such a reflection. It can be con-veniently called a theory of the com-mon good.

IV

The ethical theories of virtue and of duty are complemented by a theory of the common good. A theory of the common good seeks to elucidate the nature of human communities. These are the institutional forms that human actions create and human virtues sus-tain and, in their turn, should become the objective conditions nurturing virtue and sustaining action. This theory should treat two principal ques-tions: First, what is the "common" good or goods? Second, how should they be distributed? The first question inquires about the goods and values that are necessary for individuals and for the society. In the present context, "health and health care" might be discussed as common goods. This is a crucial dis-cussion for ethics of medical care. However, the second question, prop-erly called the problem of social jus-tice, will be the problem to which we shall attend in the remainder of this paper.[16]

Before considering this problem, it is important to realize that the theory of

the common good is not merely a separate third chapter of ethical con-cepts that should be glanced at from time to time whenever a "social ques-tion" arises. Properly conceived, the theory of the common good is a third dimension in which virtues and actions take on a depth and tone that they do not have in isolation. The very mean-ing of a virtue or an action depends on its social or institutional setting. For example, lying and deception can be viewed and analyzed as a private in-teraction between two individuals, as in the recent drama *Sleuth*. But when they are considered within the struc-tures of public trust, authority and re-sponsibility that constitute an institu-tion, for example government, quite different issues arise. In what sense, for example, does the problem of National Defense Security morally qualify an act of deception? And, analogously, would a National Health Security be sufficient warrant to deceive patients, or experi-mental subjects, about the nature of what was being done to them?

It must be clear that considerations of the common good do not *ipso facto* override considerations of individual rectitude of action. Rather, the purpose of the doctrine of the common good is to consider how conflicts may be avoided, reconciled or, more impor-tantly, how the institutional structure can be designed so as to avoid conflict, how to reconcile discord, and how to compensate unjust harm.

There is little or nothing that can be identified as a doctrine of the common good in contemporary ethics of medi-cal care. There is, of course, a convic-tion on the part of most professionals that they do serve the common good in a significant way. Yet there is, further, a contention on the part of many pro-fessionals that the practice of medicine involves significant social injustices. The authors do not intend to argue either conviction or contention. Neither of them, however valid, constitutes a theory of the common good. Such a theory must consist of a comprehensive description of the exigencies of medi-cal care and the institutional forms that serve these exigencies at present. It must propose criteria whereby these in-stitutional forms can be analyzed and criticized, not only in terms of the exigencies of care, but in light of certain exigencies of human moral existence. These latter exigencies, when seen in the light of social institutions, have been most clearly expressed by the great ethicists in terms of a doctrine of justice.

Justice, while a virtue, or personal characteristic, of individuals, is above all the "virtue" of institutions.[17] An institution may be judged ethically "good" if it exhibits in its organizational structure and in its procedures the characteristics of justice. The establishment of a just society, for the great ethicists, required not merely the assembling of many just men but the design of social institutions, laws, policies, and economics in which the habits, inclinations, and intentions of just men could be realized in public policy and practice. It is curious that while we often speak of just laws, just courts, just taxes, just contracts, we do not often speak of just medicine.

If, however, justice is pre-eminently the virtue of institutions, our failure to apply the criteria of justice to medicine may result from our failure to recognize that medicine has become, in fact, an institution. Medicine has, in recent years, evolved from a practice, a private technical interaction between two parties, through a profession, a socially coherent, publicly recognized group that defines the conditions under which those private transactions take place, to an institution.[18]

By an institution, we mean a complex interaction of professionals, paraprofessionals, and the public, on informational, economic, and occupational levels, in identifiable physical environments, whose coordinated decisions and actions have magnified public impact and is recognized culturally and legally as affecting the public welfare in a significant way. Law enforcement, the free market, religion, higher education are institutions in this broad sense.

Just as the free market once consisted of a solo producer exchanging his product for consideration by a single buyer (and still, in essence, consists of that) so the medical transaction once was, and still essentially is, a solo physician diagnosing and treating a single patient. But that essential transaction has gradually been surrounded by the indispensable cooperation of

other people, by accessory producers, by physical environments, by customary and legal prescriptions. The face-to-face decisions made in the private transaction have magnified public impact since they now engage the attention of multiple other parties, nurses, druggists, insurance carriers, etc. The coordinated decisions and actions of the institutions have magnified public impact because accepted forms of diagnosis and treatment, research, and prevention engage the manufacture of products, the construction of buildings, and the enactment of laws.

Modern medicine, then, is an institution that incorporates a profession that practices a technique and an art. The practice remains, indeed, at the heart of the institution, but it cannot be adequately performed or understood outside of it. Doctrines of virtue and action supply ideals and norms and pragmatic directions for the profession and for the practitioner; a doctrine of the common good must be added to provide an ethics for the institution.

It must be emphasized again that a doctrine of the common good does not supplant the other two modes of ethical analysis. All three doctrines are required for an adequate ethics. The practice of medicine, once conceived as the relief of the suffering of one person by another properly qualified person, was adequately analyzed in ethical terms by the two doctrines of virtue and of duty. Today, however, the institutionalization of practice and profession calls for an institutional ethic. On the other hand, the possibility that misjudgments about the ethical exigencies of virtue and duty might be propagated throughout the institution, still demands a careful ethical scrutiny of quality of individual character and rectitude of single actions.

Institutions are vehicles for the distribution of the benefits and burdens of social life, and it is the function of the principles of justice to determine fair and equitable assignment of rights and duties and fair and equitable distribution of benefits and burdens.[19]

An institution possesses an identity, an organization, and resources that enable activities performed by its members to have an extensivity and perpetuity that they otherwise could not have. By extensivity, we mean that activities can have effects on a broad

contemporary population. By perpetuity, we mean that they can be prolonged in time by affecting future populations. It may be argued that medical actions always factually had effects that fulfilled these definitions of extensivity and perpetuity. However, the development of epidemiology and biostatistics has made the dimensions of this extensivity and perpetuity vividly evident in contemporary medicine.

Only the institutional form provides the exchange of information, the continuity and cooperation, the designation of qualified participants and the utilization of physical and financial resources to support extensivity and perpetuity. A profession may have an identity based on possession of similar knowledge and techniques and may cooperate to share and assure possession of them, but a professional, as such, did not deliberately utilize information and resources to effect extensivity and perpetuity. Medicine has, in the last 100 years, by virtue of certain scientific and technical accomplishments, evolved from a profession with knowledge of limited effects in time and space to an institution with knowledge of extensive and perpetuated effects.

The most pressing ethical issues of modern medicine arise from the potential for extensivity and perpetuity inherent in its new institutional status. At one time a medical intervention was perceived as a transaction between a physician and a patient. The benefits and the costs were, for the most part, thought to be quite strictly limited to that transaction. Today, benefits and costs are known to be distributed broadly in many ways. Financial costs of medical research and education are borne by an extensive public. Costs of care are borne by insurance purchasers and tax payments. Resource allocation distributes benefits of research to certain afflicted populations at a cost to others. Certain treatment modalities impose burdens on those other than the treated. The effects of certain medical interventions can be perpetuated into future generations, for example, the burden of heredity of certain genetic diseases such as diabetes and hemophilia. Formerly, these patients often did not live long enough to reproduce and hence the defective gene was eliminated from the pool. Techniques for genetic diagnosis and control are directed toward modification of inheritable characteristics.

Where benefits and burdens can be so distributed, the problem of justice arises. Some who will benefit will not bear costs; some who will bear costs will not benefit. When this situation depends not on chance or accident but on planned and conscious decisions about the structure of the institution, it is necessary to ask, "What justifies the imposition of a burden, a cost, a risk, on any single individual?" Why should one individual benefit at the apparent cost of another? These are the questions at the heart of each of the serious ethical issues of medicine as they are of justice.

The problem of access to medical care is the most obvious field for the application of the concept of justice. This appears to be, on its face, a problem of distributive justice. A subset of this problem is the allocation of scarce resources, such as renal dialysis. However, many other problems that are not usually considered in terms of justice involve deliberate distribution of costs and benefits. Randomized clinical trials, particularly when one of the alternatives is a proven therapeutic agent, involves costs without compensating benefit to certain individuals. An increasing number of therapeutic modalities lay burdens of risk on others than the beneficiaries such as drugs administered to pregnant mothers. In the near future, nuclear-powered artificial hearts—and, perhaps in the further, but real future, DNA therapy through viral agents—will have this effect. The entire realm of genetic control, whether it utilizes elimination of births or elimination of defective genomes, raises the question of justice to future generations. Psychosurgery and psychoactive drug therapy, while they may be conceived as interventions beneficial to the individual, have the potential to impose stringent limitations on that individual's freedom from which others may benefit socially, politically, and economically. The classical problem of euthanasia is aggravated by the institutionally supported potential for prolonging dying at great cost, emotional and financial, to survivors.

Finally, the nagging, but ill-defined, problem of dehumanization of medical care may obtain clarity within the concepts of justice. The great jurisprudent, Georgio del Vecchio, wrote, "The ideal criteria of justice . . . demand the equal and perfect recognition . . . of the quality or personality in oneself as in all others for all possible interactions among several subjects."[20] Dehumanization is, at bottom, unequal and imperfect recognition of the quality of personality, an entity most difficult to quantitate under the criteria required for a just theory of the common good.

Many of the moral problems of medicine appear to be problems of justice. Many of the old problems of medicine, placed in the modern setting, seem to have been transmuted from problems of virtue or duty, into problems of justice. Yet, the theories of justice long familiar to ethics have not been fully mined for their relevance to the moral problems of medicine. The authors are not so naïve as to suppose that the ancient conflicts of individual versus institution and personal duty versus social good will be resolved by yet another invocation of the doctrine of justice. Still, to the extent that considerations of justice contribute to the design of institutions of medicine and to policies governing its practice, many moral problems may be either avoided or ameliorated.

The traditional definition of justice is "giving to each his due." The problem of justice is defining what is "due" to each. This is done, first, by recognizing that the "each" of the definition is both everyman (with a basic humanness shared by all), and the single person, different in ability, merit, and need from all others. Justice thus requires an impartiality resting on the fundamental similarity of all persons and an equity that allows for different treatment justified by different conditions of ability and merit. Effecting justice becomes the continual process of critical scrutiny of the reasons proposed for different treatment of persons. This scrutiny must measure particular considerations against universal characteristics, the claims of ability, merit, and need against the claims of equality of liberty, consideration, and treatment. So stated, the conundrum is not vastly different than the problem of reconciling the age-old precept to give to each

according to his need with that of giving to each according to his merit.[21]

The requirements of a theory of justice are not satisfied by the proposition that an act or institution is ethically justified when it produces the "greater good for the greater number." This thesis, called Utilitarianism, has been much disputed by ethicists and its inherent defects revealed. Nonetheless, it appears to be the dominant ethic for many policymakers in scientific medicine.[22] The problem of the lesser number, disadvantaged for the sake of the greater, remains unsolved.

In medicine, this problem can be particularly pressing, for traditionally medicine has favored the good of individuals, while the law has favored the common good. Today, the realization of extensivity and perpetuity of modern medicine place many medical interventions directly within the sphere of the common good. Whether the problems thus raised can be "justly" solved depends on how deeply modern medical practitioners and policymakers reflect on the profound moral dilemmas and theses of the theory of justice. They must refuse to relax those dilemmas either by a facile appeal to the "inestimable social benefits of medicine," on the one hand, or to the "inviolable individual rights of patient or practitioner," on the other. Neither assertion can stand alone; both must be comprehended within an adequate theory of justice. Above all, public policy relative to the shape of institutions, the flow of money and people through them, the regulation of their powers, and vigilance over their performance must be devised with the requirements of justice foremost in mind.

Several final points should be made about "just" medicine. First, the cynical often say, "Ethics is no more than the simulation of good intentions." Doctrines of virtue, because virtue can be so easily simulated by scoundrels, are most susceptible to this pessimistic criticism. Doctrines of duty can take refuge in excuses and protestations of ignorance. But doctrines of justice rest on different ground. Their concern is the fair and equitable structure and function of institutions. In this theory of ethics, we are concerned about the institutional forms that set up problems in certain ways and restrict or expand the alternatives for their solution. We do not limit our attention to good intentions alone or to the outcome of single actions. We are concerned about the assignment of rights and duties, the design of offices and tasks, the currents of resources, and support that can best eliminate problems of unfair distribution of burdens and benefits and can best enable virtuous character and right action.

Second, the advent of institutions heralds the appearance of laws. Medicine has always been governed, to a greater or lesser degree, by civil law. Medicine has seldom been happy under that governance. "Just" medicine raises the menacing threat of medical practice cribbed, cabined, and confined by statute and regulation. This need not necessarily be the case. Justice and law are not synonymous. A theory of justice is concerned basically with the design of institutions. Institutional design can be created and effected by innumerable agencies other than the state. The profession, related professions and industries, interested and impartial groups, organized and unorganized consumers can, if allowed and enabled, assist in institutional design. However, to the extent that civil law and regulations are advisable, a doctrine of justice is indispensable. It alone can provide the vision of just and equitable distribution that the enacted law should, imperfectly, piecemeal, but steadily, seek to realize. Without a doctrine of just medicine, laws and regulations will be haphazard, aimless, and for this reason frustrating to professional and consumer alike.

In conclusion, then, the thesis of this essay might be restated in terms of an ancient Roman definition of the entire field of ethics: *Honeste vivere, nemini laedere, suum cuique tribuere*—live uprightly, hurt no one, give to each his due. The authors have attempted to state the conceptual foundations for an ethics of medical care under similar titles. It must consist, they maintain, of three essential theories of ethics applied to the unique enterprise of medicine and health care. The theory of virtue concerns those dispositions and qualities that define uprightness of life for those who practice medicine

and engage in care. The theory of duties concerns criteria that enable the practitioner to recognize acts that ultimately harm those who seek his help. The theory of justice concerns the establishment of fair and equitable institutions for the practice of medicine and the provision of care. It is the authors' impression that in discussions of medical ethics these questions are often jumbled, that their theoretical bases are unrecognized, and that their intellectual history is unknown. They contend that fruitful progress might be made if future discussions acknowledge the distinction and the interrelation of these three theories of ethics and undertake their careful application to the difficult moral problems of modern medicine. This will make, they hope, for better medicine, for better ethics, and for a better ethics for medical care.

References and Notes

1. *Lexicon of Medicine and Applied Sciences.* London, The Sydenham Society, 1881–1889.

2. Frankena, W., *Ethics,* Englewood Cliffs, Prentice-Hall, 1963, pp. 1–10. Wallace, G., and Walker, A. (ed.), *The Definition of Morality.* London, Methuen, 1970.

3. *Opinions and Reports of the Judicial Council.* Chicago, American Medical Association, 1969. On the ethical nature of codes, see Veatch, R., Medical ethics: professional or universal? *Harvard Theolog. Rev.,* 65:531–559, 1972. On the history of the AMA code, see Konold, D., *A History of American Medical Ethics.* Madison, University of Wisconsin, 1962.

4. Our intention is to give an *ethical* analysis of codes. A sociological analysis can be found in Freidson, E., *The Profession of Medicine.* New York, Dodd-Mead, 1970.

5. This echoes an early critique of the AMA code: "Were the great rule of Christian ethics present to the mind of the physician, 'do unto others as ye would that they would should do unto you,' there would be but little necessity for societal codes." Duglison, R., On the present state of medicine in the United States. *Br. Foreign Med. Rev.* 3:227, 1837.

6. Leake, C., *Percival's Medical Ethics.* Baltimore, Williams & Wilkins, 1927, pp. 1–2; Leake, C., Theories of ethics and medical practice. *J. Am. Med. Assoc.* 208:842–847, 1969. On the term "etiquette," see Jones, W. H. S., *The Doctor's Oath.* Cambridge, University Press, 1924; and *Ancient medical etiquette, Hippocrates II.* Cambridge, University Press, 1923.

7. *Compleat Angler* 1:13, 1653. See King, L. S. *The Medical World of the Eighteenth Century.* Chicago, University of Chicago Press, 1958, p. 256.

8. Klubertanz, G., *Habits and Virtues.* New York, Appleton, Century, Crofts, 1965.

9. Ramsey, P., *Patient as Person.* New Haven, Yale University Press, 1970, preface.

10. Lain Entralgo, P., *Doctor and Patient.* New York, McGraw-Hill, 1969.

11. Pius XII, *The Human Body,* Boston, St. Paul Press, 1960. See Healy, E., *Medical Ethics.* Chicago, Loyola Press, 1959; Kelly, G., *Medico-Moral Problems.* St. Louis, Catholic Hospital Association, 1958; Paquin, J., *Morale et Médecine.* Montreal, L'Immaculee-Conception, 1960.

12. Aquinas T., *Summa Theologica* II–II, q. 65, a.l.

13. Kelly, G., On the duty of using artificial means to preserve life, *Theolog. Stud.* 11:203–220, 1950; 12:550–556, 1951.

14. Nolan, M., Principle of totality in moral theology, *Absolutes in Moral Theology.* Edited by C. Curran. Washington, Corpus, 1968; Curran, C., *Medicine and Morals.* Washington, Corpus, 1970.

15. This problem is reflected in the debate over the Code of the Catholic Hospital Association. See Catholic hospital ethics: report of the Commission on Ethical Directions for Catholic Hospitals. *Linacre Q.* 39, Nov. 1972; Brennan J., Quicksands of compromise. Reich, W., Policy vs. ethics. McCormick, R., Not what the Catholic hospitals ordered. *Linacre Q.* 39, Feb. 1972.

16. Our use of the terms "common good" and "social justice" may be elucidated by the following: "Social justice [is] the equal treatment of all persons except as inequality is required by relevant, that is, just-making, considerations . . . it takes equality of treatment to be a *prima facie* requirement of justice, but allows that it may on occasion be overruled by other principles of justice . . . the differences in treatment are not justified simply by arguing that they are conducive to the general good life, but by arguing that they are required for the good lives of the individuals concerned. It is not as if one must first look to see how the general good is best subserved and only then can tell what treatment of individuals is just. Justice entails the presence of equal *prima facie* rights prior to any consideration of utility." Frankena, W., The concept of social justice, *Social Justice.* Edited by R. Brandt, Englewood Cliffs, Prentice-Hall, 1962, pp. 13, 15.

17. Rawls, J., *Theory of Justice.* Cambridge, Harvard University Press, 1971, Ch. 2.

18. Mechanic, D., *Medical Sociology.* Glencoe, Free Press, 1968, Ch. 10–11.

19. Rawls, *op. cit.,* p. 55.

20. del Vecchio, G., *Justice.* Edinburgh, University Press, 1952, p. 116.

21. del Vecchio, G., *op. cit.;* Perelman, C., *Justice.* New York, Random House, 1967; Friedrick, C., Chapman, J. (ed.), *Nomos VI: Justice.* New York, Atherton Press, 1963.

22. ". . . the dicta of that school [Utilitarianism] . . . are still used as part of the language of men of science." Singer, G., Underwood, E. A., *A Short History of Medicine*. New York, Oxford Press, 1962, p. 208. For critique of Utilitarianism, see, among others, Lyons, D., *Forms and Limits of Utilitarianism*. Oxford, Clarendon Press, 1965.

22

Sissela Bok
The Tools of Bioethics

This essay is excerpted from an address delivered at the Eastern Sociological Society meeting in Boston, March 26, 1976. Its subject is more fully explored in a forthcoming book. Copyright by Sissela Bok.

I would like to consider, first, some fundamental principles of bioethics and, second, whether bioethics as a discipline possesses workable and rigorous methods whereby these principles can be brought to bear on real and complex human conflicts. Since bioethics is one form of applied ethics, any such questioning of its methodology must also question that of applied ethics in general.

It is especially important to ask these questions now, for today philosophers and social theorists are asked to participate in social choice as they have not been asked since antiquity. At that time, their assistance, while sought by some, was often feared or thought outright disastrous by many. The Roman Senate impatiently decreed in 161 B.C., for example, that all philosophers should be banished from the city, along with all teachers of rhetoric. This thought has surely occurred to many policy-makers since.

In part, this impatience is due to the trivialization which philosophers can bestow upon human predicaments; in part, it is also due to the carelessness of some intellectuals pronouncing on human conflicts from a distance. To a considerable extent, however, the response results from a sense of *threat*—a feeling now experienced by those affected by the social choices in bioethics.

For philosophers, theologians, and social theorists now participate in such choices as what national policy should govern biomedical research on prisoners, or kidney dialysis programs, or fetal research; and their participation cannot help being a threat to those whose scientific and medical activities are at stake. The most natural and immediate response to such a threat is to question the criteria used in the policy choices, the assumptions underlying them, and the methods of arriving at conclusions.

Such questioning is legitimate and crucial. What is *not* legitimate is to hold as many do that outsiders need not worry about the ethics of science and medicine; that these enterprises are somehow value-free; or that any ethical problems which do come up are adequately taken care of within the professions without meddling from the outside.

One of the simplest and best definitions of ethics was put down by

Diogenes Laertius in the 3rd century A.D.[1] He reported that, for Epicurus,

Ethics deals with things to be sought and things to be avoided, with ways of life and with the "telos." (Telos is the chief good or the end of action.)

Ethics, according to such a view, must be taken into account whenever human choice is at stake. Using such a definition, it is clear that there are no more fundamental ethical choices than those which are made in medicine and in science. What *should* we seek through these fields? And what ought we to try to avoid? What ways of life should we encourage? What can doctors choose to do or to avoid to affect our health? And how do their own life-styles affect the care that they provide for others? These questions are at least as central to us all as what happens to our property, our schooling, or our right to vote.

To be blind to moral dimensions of what human beings do to one another is as much of a handicap as to be visually blind or unable to have memories. But it is a more insidious handicap since it is often not recognized as one. Those who are thus deprived stumble through the world of humans unaware that their perception is flawed—and do untold harm to those whose lives they affect. It is in this category that we must place those who insist that there are no ethical considerations in science or in medicine.

The *need* for ethical inquiry, therefore, is great. And the choices made—individually and socially—in the biomedical areas are moral choices at bottom. But the recognition that this is so only sharpens the question of what tools exist for making such choices wisely.

Principles

The principles of bioethics flow together from the health professions and from moral philosophy. They have been expressed through the centuries in codes and oaths and writings by physicians. There are no principles of ethics in medicine which have not also been expressed in moral philosophy. But some general principles of moral philosophy have found more frequent echoes in medicine than others—and some have been almost entirely neglected.

The two fundamental principles of doing good and of not doing harm—of beneficence and of nonmaleficence—are the most immediately relevant to medical practitioners. To preserve life and good health; to ward off illness, pain, and death—these are the perennial tasks of physicians. Their published prayers and oaths[2] express their awareness of needing a very special sense of responsibility in caring for the sick. These principles of helping others and, above all, of not harming them, have found powerful expression at all times in the history of medicine:

Day and night, thou shalt endeavor for the relief of patients with all thy heart and soul. Thou shalt not desert or injure thy patient even for the sake of thy living.[3]

And the ranking of these two principles—the fact that, regardless of what help one brings, one must at the very least not affect patients for the worse—is expressed by Hippocrates in the *Epidemics*:

As to diseases, make a habit of two things—to help, or at least to do no harm.[4]

Because doctors have access to the most intimate concerns of patients, two kinds of harm they might bring to patients have been prohibited in the codes with special urgency: sexual exploitation and breach of confidentiality.[5] Other more general statements have also warned doctors to keep their patients from injustice and from the attention of quacks.

The documents stress the trust and the guild-dictated behavior which should prevail among physicians. They should treat family members of doctors free of charge, regard students as sons, not interfere with one another's practice, and not compete in unseemly ways. Percival's *Medical Ethics*,[6] first published in 1803, is especially vocal on these matters. Percival goes so far as to explain that even a wealthy physician should avoid giving free advice to his affluent patients, because to do so would be an injury to his "professional brethren."

These professional courtesies operate to smooth the relationships between physicians. Insofar as they help subdue the inclination to profit from human misery, they serve patients as well as the profession. But insofar as they prevent a physician from interfering with

the incompetent or malicious practice of fellow physicians, they obviously do a disservice to patients, by concealing from them what could affect their life and health most profoundly.

The two principles of beneficence and nonmaleficence have nevertheless traditionally been thought to apply mostly to the physician's conduct toward his own patients. But major new conflicts have sprung up recently with the advent of human experimentation and transplantation. For in experiments on human beings, subjects are often placed at some risk of harm or maleficence in order that society or future sufferers from the disease may be benefitted. And in transplantation, as of kidneys, one person is being harmed in order to save the life of another. As a result of these developments, the weighing of benefits and harms has taken on a new complexity. How *can* one weigh harm done to some against benefits to others? No matter how hard or how simple, such a process of weighing has been thought by many to constitute the essence of medical decision making. But the simple statement by Amatus,[7] that he had "never brought about sickness," could no longer be made by most physicians.

Other principles have also been stated in the medical literature—strongly at times, feebly at times; they have even been suppressed or forgotten altogether at times. The principle of equality is most interesting in this respect. Some oaths in antiquity were eloquent on the subject. An inscription on the Sanctuary of Asclepius, for instance, on the south slope of the Acropolis, reads:

he [physician] would be like God: saviour equally of slave, of paupers, of rich men, of princes, and to all a brother.[8]

And a Canon of Medicine, China, Han Dynasty, 200 B.C.–200 A.D., holds that:

He should have bowels of mercy on the sick and pledge himself to relieve suffering among all classes. Aristocrat or commoner, poor or rich, aged or young, beautiful or ugly, enemy or friend, native or foreigner, and educated or uneducated, all are to be treated equally. He should look upon the misery of the patient as if it were his own.

And the oath long thought to have been written by Maimonides[9] states:

Preserve the strength of my body and of my soul that they ever be ready to cheerfully help and support rich and poor, good and bad, enemy as well as friend. In the sufferer let me see only the human being.

By comparison, the *absence* of any thought that the physician should care equally for all is very striking in the Hippocratic Oath,[10] the most widely disseminated oath even today. Nor do the Principles of Ethics of the American Medical Association venture such a notion. The principle of equality, therefore, is only asserted at times, and is absent in today's most commonly used codes in the United States.

The vaster questions of social justice have not, on the whole, been discussed at all in these historical documents. In the past, as now, principles of medical ethics have been primarily principles for *individual* behavior—between health professionals and patients, or between one health professional and another.[11] The increased pressure to consider moral principles governing institutions and societies is beginning to force attention towards questions of medical justice. What is a just allocation of medical resources—among citizens of a community, a state, or even the world? And what roles do equality, beneficence, and nonmaleficence play in such schemes of allocation? These most important of all ethical inquiries are not addressed at all in traditional codes of medical ethics.

Another principle of ethics which is absent in virtually all documents of medical ethics is that of *veracity*—of informing patients truthfully about their condition and prognosis.[12] One of the few who claimed such a principle was Amatus:

If I lie, may I incur the eternal wrath of God and of His angel Raphael, and may nothing in the medical art succeed for me according to my desires.[13]

Other writings either veil this subject in silence, or assume, as Plato stated in the *Republic*,[14] that lies are acceptable from a physician since they are told to us for our own good—as a form of medicine. It is only recently, with the loss in trust and with our awareness of the risks we can run from a false diagnosis, a deceptive prognosis, or treatment we are duped into believing that we need, that the principle of veracity is coming to the forefront.[15] And it is only with the working out of all that informed consent implies and what kind of information it presupposes, that

truth-telling and deception are coming to be discussed in a serious way in the health professions.

The absence of concern with veracity reflects in turn the absence of another and more general principle of ethics which is only now being pressed into medical contexts. This is the principle of patient *autonomy*. For while the codes are vocal on the *physician's* liberty, or autonomy in certain respects, they have long been silent on that of the patient. Yet when ethics is defined as an inquiry into human choice and goals, the question of *who chooses* is obviously crucial. This is especially true of choices having to do with illness and health, and, most of all, with what should be done to one's own body.

There are two ways to interfere with legitimate autonomous choices by patients: through overt coercion, and through manipulating the information reaching patients so that they accept what they would not have chosen had they been correctly informed. Both of these forms of assault on autonomy— direct coercion and deception—are especially controversial in medicine because they are undertaken in the name of the *patient's best interest,* and cannot therefore always be discounted. Yet Professor Talcott Parsons has rightly stated that:

The sick person is peculiarly vulnerable to exploitation and at the same time peculiarly handicapped in arriving at a rationally objective appraisal of his situation.[16]

The principle of autonomy, if respected, would lessen this exploitation while increasing the chances for personal appraisal of their predicament by patients.

The major moral principles in medical ethics, of nonmaleficence, beneficence, justice, equality, veracity, and autonomy, therefore, are no different from those debated in ethics more generally. In both domains, the same disagreements come up as to whether one or two of these principles in reality account for all the rest.[17] The same disagreements arise in both about what rights we have with respect to, for example, not being lied to or not being harmed, or about what is a justifiable distribution of resources.

Different theories answer these questions in different ways. Some even claim that ethics can give no answers of this kind. But most theories recognize that ethical principles must at least possess certain formal characteristics. Recently, Baier and Rawls have discussed these characteristics.[18] Three which are crucial are *generality, universality,* and *publicity* (or universal teachability).[19]

To be *general*, a principle should be capable of formulation without recourse to proper names. Thus a principle holding that all that which Mussolini desires is right or good fails to be general in this sense.

A principle which is *universal in application* is one which holds for everyone. Most moral principles are of this kind, but some are not. A form of egoism holding that rules apply to others only, not to oneself, or one's social group, is incapable of living up to this criterion.

Principles which fail on these two grounds usually also fail to comply with the criterion of *publicity*. A principle should be capable of public statement and expression. The same is true, in my opinion, of any application of a moral principle to a concrete situation. Those who argue for and against the extension of the principle of informed consent to experimentation on children ought to be able to do so openly and in advance. Of course, this does not mean that one must always go through such a process. But it should be *possible* to do so.

Such principles of ethics as emerge from a reading of the medical literature do satisfy these criteria. And they provide inspiration and guidance with respect to the humane treatment of patients, the avoidance of harm and unnecessary suffering, and the safeguarding of confidentiality and dignity.

But three major circumstances prevent them from providing the protection for patients which they should ideally inspire. In the first place, as we have seen, certain principles of ethics are nearly nonexistent in writings on *medical* ethics. Secondly, many clear principles of medical ethics are disregarded by a number of practitioners. And thirdly, these principles often conflict in such a way that even those who wish to uphold them are uncertain as to what action to choose.

Complex Moral Problems

Sometimes there is no disagreement whatsoever, in theory. Every tradition of applied ethics and of medical ethics would condemn those surgeons who deceive patients into thinking they must have operations which they do not need. Similarly, all traditions would condemn those physicians who, employed by industries, examine workers without letting them know that they suffer from illnesses acquired at work. Yet it is well known that innumerable acts of these and other similarly unethical kinds are performed. What is at fault here is not moral reasoning nor the appeal to moral principles. Rather, blame must go to individual callousness and weaknesses in the social structure which permit the pursuit of these practices.

But there are a great many ethical conflicts in medicine where there is no such agreement even in principle, let alone in practice. These are complex conflicts, causing health professionals to divide sharply about what ethical dimensions are at stake. Some of these conflicts arise out of marginal or uncertain aspects of the clear abuses mentioned above. Some have caused bitter disagreement since the beginnings of medicine—how best to care for dying patients, for instance, or whether to allow abortion, or how to distribute scarce medical resources.

Other divisive conflicts confront us now with increasing urgency as a result of modern developments in medical technology and knowledge. Problems posed by the possibility of cloning, or by organ transplantation, or by fetal research or by psychosurgery—these problems all produce genuine disagreement about what *is* best, most beneficial, least harmful, or most conducive to equality.

The moral dilemmas which produce these disagreements share one or more elements of complexity. The information on which choice must be based in these dilemmas is often inadequate, biased, and not of uniform relevance. The individuals involved have divergent, often clashing, interests. And several moral principles are in sharp conflict. Finally, more than one person often claim to be decision makers.

In dilemmas with some or all of these characteristics of complexity, intelligent, well-informed, and well-intentioned persons can sincerely disagree about what should be done. And the disagreement does not spring up in neat categories between holders of different faiths or traditions. It is rather *within* each tradition that suicide or abortion or distribution of health care cause disputes over and over again. . . .

We need, therefore, two different strategies for dealing with moral problems in medicine and science. In the clear cases where all theories agree, what is needed is not so much moral reasoning as the mobilization of public opinion and social change to increase accountability and combat abuse. So long as these are not successful, individuals need also to consider efforts at self-defense, so that they will not be hurt by the abuses in question. But for the more complex problems, we need methods and clarity before we can even reach the point of evaluating social policy, incentives and disincentives, and self-protection. And it is with respect to these complex problems that theologians and philosophers and social theorists have been asked for help with the greatest urgency.

Notes

1. Diogenes Laertius, *Lives of Eminent Philosophers* (Cambridge: Harvard University Press, 1925), vol. 2, pp. 559–560.

2. See Donald E. Konold, "History of the Codes of Medical Ethics," forthcoming, in the *Encyclopedia of Bioethics,* and M. B. Etziony, *The Physician's Creed: An Anthology of Medical Prayers, Oaths and Codes of Ethics* (Springfield, Ill.: Charles C. Thomas, 1973).

3. From a Hindu oath of initiation, reproduced in Etziony, *The Physician's Creed.*

4. Hippocrates, *Epidemics,* tr. W. H. S. Jones, in *Hippocrates* Vol. I. (Note: a more faithful translation would read: "to help or not to harm." It may be the interpretation of Hippocrates rather than his own words which has done the ranking.)

5. Every professional relationship gives rise to special kinds of benefits and harms. As a result, some have imagined that medical ethics and legal ethics and other professional ethics are somehow separable from more general principles of morality. There is no need, however, to postulate such separateness. The special harms and benefits can be understood in terms of beneficence, nonmaleficence and other general principles in combination with the specific contracts undertaken in the professional relationship.

6. Thomas Percival, *Medical Ethics* (Oxford: John Henry Parker, 1849).

7. A celebrated Jewish physician who died in 1568 from the plague.

8. The thought that the physician should feel a sense of brotherhood, or kinship, with the patient recurs often in antiquity, in medical and religious texts. It expresses the ideal of *fraternity,* which is an extension, or qualification, of that of equality. The physician can either act as a brother in giving of his expertise to a patient or, more rarely, see himself as brother to all those who suffer, feeling their pain, sharing their lot. To whatever extent this sense of fellow-feeling exists, it stands in sharp contrast to the distant "professional" manner which is another response to suffering and represents another way of trying to cope. (For a brief discussion of "fraternity," see J. Rawls, *A Theory of Justice* [Cambridge: Harvard University Press, 1971], pp. 105–106.)

9. Now attributed to Marcus Herz, and thought to have been published in 1783. See Etziony, *The Physician's Creed.*

10. The Hippocratic Oath makes use of equality only in the limited sense that the physician foreswears sexual advances to those in the household of the sick, be they female or male, free or slave.

11. Much interest has also been accorded questions of medical *etiquette*—governing questions of the appearance of physicians, of grooming and courtesy. See A. R. Jonsen and A. Hellegers, "Conceptual Foundations for an Ethics of Medical Care," in *Ethics of Health Care,* for an excellent discussion of medical ethics and etiquette in the codes and oaths. [The essay is reprinted as Chapter 21 of this volume.]

12. Lying *between* health professionals, on the other hand, has always been thought unprincipled. For a thoughtful discussion of the differences between duties that doctors think they owe each other and duties owed to their patients, see William F. May, "Code, Covenant, Contract, or Philanthropy," *Hastings Center Report* 5, 29–38. [Reprinted as Chapter 14 of this volume.]

13. Reproduced in "The Ethics of the Practice of Medicine from the Jewish Point of View," Harry Friedenwald, *Johns Hopkins Hospital Bulletin,* August 1917, 256–261.

14. Plato, *Republic* (Cambridge, Harvard University Press, 1930), 389b–d.

15. As literature attests (see, for example, Molière's *Le Médecin Malgré Lui*), patients have always been suspicious of physicians and quacks. But not until this century have these concerns been so consistently voiced and supported by law.

16. Talcott Parsons, *The Social System* (New York: The Free Press, 1951). See pp. 436–465 for an analysis of "the sick role."

17. Thus W. K. Frankena, in *Ethics* (Englewood Cliffs: Prentice-Hall, 1973), holds that beneficence and justice (interpreted as equal treatment) are the only principles we

need to recognize. G. J. Warnock, in *The Object of Morality* (London: Methuen, 1971), sees beneficence, nonmaleficence, fairness, and nondeception.

18. K. Baier, *The Moral Point of View* (New York: Random House, 1965), Ch. VIII; and J. Rawls, *A Theory of Justice*, pp. 130–136.

19. Rawls and Baier add a fourth—ordering—and a fifth—finality—which will not be stressed in these pages. *Ordering* requires that the principles adopted make possible an ordering of conflicting claims. This criterion cannot be accepted in empirical dilemmas without a methodology as yet lacking in all theories of ethics. See pages which follow. *Finality* requires that reasoning from the principles be conclusive. This, again, is more an ideal than a possible achievement in applied ethics.

III

Regulation, Compulsion, and Consumer Protection in Clinical Medicine and Public Health

Introduction to Part III

The two earlier sections analyzed the ethical foundations of medical practice from the point of view of the relationship between physician and patient and the moral structure of that relationship. The enforcement of ethical standards in medicine was assumed by most authors to come through sanctions, either professional or legal or both, directed against the physician. Thus most of the ethical and ethical-legal codes in the field are addressed almost exclusively to physicians. The patient tends to play a passive role with neither rights nor responsibilities—except to benefit by the treatment he receives.

This situation is changing. Through more universal public education and heavy exposure to medical coverage in the mass media, the average patient is much more knowledgeable about his or her body, its pathology, and, very important, about the dangers as well as the potential benefits of prescribed modes of medical treatment. Some aspects of the emerging ethical issues involved in the changing role of the patient are explored in this section. We examine the patient's right to refuse treatment as well as to accept it. We see the moral, ethical, and legal dilemmas for physicians and other health-care personnel in caring for patients who refuse even lifesaving treatment.

This section begins with Joseph Healey's examination of the role of law in overseeing the actions of patients and physicians as they negotiate the terms under which medical care will be dispensed. The statement of the American Hospital Association on the rights of hospitalized patients that follows is a useful summary of the human rights currently recognized as inherently possessed by all patients. This statement asserts that the duty to respect patient's rights rests on the health-care institution as well as upon the physician, which is a significant departure from the earlier positions of the hospitals and the medical profession under which the institution carried no such ethical or legal responsibility. Each of the principles begins with the phrase: "The

patient has the right . . ." No granting of a benefit or privilege comes from the physician or hospital to the patient. The right exists for the patient *as a patient,* independent of the provider. This phrase is even used for the last two principles, which seem more related to obligations of the patient to pay his hospital bill and to obey the hospital's rules and regulations than to any rights of the patient as such. Is this evidence of the continued reluctance of the medical community to place responsibility directly on the patients? Or is it a reflection of the "public relations" overtones of the statement?

Robert Cooke next explores the interactions between law and ethics in the restrictions placed on the liberties of mentally retarded people. His concern with the inherent rights of individuals is also reflected in the statement by the President's Committee on Mental Retardation. It enumerates the rights and needs of the mentally disabled person and recommends procedures to give him equality under the law.

The articles on lifesaving medical treatment, organ transplantation, and sickle cell anemia also focus on the individual rather than on the physician or other health-care professionals. In his exploration of the legal and ethical protections of bodily integrity, Norman Cantor argues the case for respecting the decision of an independent and rational adult to refuse lifesaving therapy. In discussing organ transplantation, Paul Freund is mainly concerned with the justifications for allowing a person to donate a vital part of his body to someone else in desperate need of it. In the examination of sickle cell anemia Philip Reilly raises questions about the legal authority being exercised in regard to public screening for the existence of a disease or the inherited potential for a disease. He points out the weaknesses as well as the strengths of the legislation in the field and presents some second thoughts about the wisdom of such public programs. What are the elements of compulsion in these programs, which were supposedly intended for individual as well as public good? What are the dangers?

What is the role for medical ethics in this field? When is compulsion justified in medical care?

Part III concludes with more general philosophical materials on individual freedom and paternalism. As modern society concentrates more and more power in the state, individuals look to the governments not only for protection of their common welfare, but for securing their freedoms as well. When these interests clash, which is the higher value? The issues of compulsion and freedom will recur in nearly every section in this collection. We have only made a start in our analysis here.

23

Joseph M. Healey, Jr.
Legal Regulation of Medicine: An Overview

This chapter has not been previously published.

The relationship between law and medicine in twentieth century America has been characterized by a dramatic increase in the forms and extent of legal regulation of the medical care process. Many practitioners of the healing arts have regarded this increasing regulation with a great deal of anger, suspicion, and frustration. They have joined Franz Ingelfinger, editor of the *New England Journal of Medicine*, in protesting the contemporary ''legal hegemony in medicine'' which seems so widespread:

Examples of the lawyer's pervasiveness in medical decision making abound. Who needs to be reminded of his role in the current malpractice mania? If medical care is costly, the doctor defensive and the patients suspicious, the referee must share part of the blame. By the means of actual or threatened court action, lawyers determine not only the particulars of treatment, but also who will get treatment, where and under what conditions. Courts decide on who will get blood transfusions, and whether or not treatment will be meted out in a given case. Courts decide on who will get medical education. Even when doctors try to clean their own house, courts may order reinstatement of a suspended staff member. Courts may also decide on the overall administrative practices of medicine, on who may or may not practice, on the payment of the physician, on the conversation permitted and required between the doctor and patient, and on the kinds of records kept.[1]

Though Dr. Ingelfinger's examples may be overstated,[2] they constitute an important reminder of what is a critical question for every society: the appropriate role of the legal system in regulating the medical care process. This is by no means a new question, nor one whose importance is confined to contemporary America.[3] But the strong demand in our society for more regulation, greater accountability and increased responsibility in the practice of medicine makes our need to confront this question of particular significance. What are legitimate goals to be sought in legal regulation of the medical care process? How have these goals been pursued? To what extent does the law play a role in formulating the physician's mandate from society? We find these questions raised in a variety of settings from one end of the life cycle to the other, from the case of Kenneth

Edelin, in which a Boston obstetrician was convicted of manslaughter for failing to preserve fetal life during an abortion,[4] to the case of Karen Quinlan, a young woman living for months in a coma whose parents sued to have her respirator disconnected.[5] Not everyone who exercises the increased power is comfortable with it. Judge Muir wrote in his opinion dealing with the plight of Karen Quinlan: ''The onus of the judicial process for me, in this instance, is unparalleled.''[6] Yet these considerations only remind us how important it is to appreciate the law's role in regulating health care so that we might begin to address the vast agenda of unfinished societal policies in which law and medicine must play an important role.

For a variety of reasons—some rooted in our Anglo-American legal history, others rooted in the concept of law itself—the law in its relationship with medicine has functioned in three chief ways:
1. as an influence on the quality of medical care;
2. as a source of human values to be reflected in the physician-patient relationship;
3. as a boundary of medical decision making.
Each has played an important role in regulating the medical care process, and will now be discussed.

When a person is sick, there are limits to what he can do to regain health. These limits involve a restriction of who can provide him with health care in our society. This regulatory scheme begins with a medical practice act which establishes a limitation on who may practice medicine. The Iowa Code contains a series of regulations typical of those existing throughout the United States. Its provisions declare, in part, that a license shall be required for practitioners of those healing arts which are recognized by the government of Iowa: medicine and surgery, podiatry, osteopathy, nursing, and so forth.[7] The Code defines actions that constitute the practice of medicine, such as a public declaration of one's availability to patients; treating people by means of drugs or surgery.[8] It also provides for the establishment of boards to conduct examinations for medical licenses, most of whose members must be licensed to practice the specialty for which the license is granted.[9] The Code specifies other licensing requirements such as a diploma from a medical school approved by the medical examiners, and a year of internship at an approved hospital.[10] Offenses which can lead to revocation or suspension of one's license are enumerated: fraud in procuring the license, incompetency, misleading or deceptive representations to patients, engaging in "unethical conduct or practice harmful to the public," habitual intoxication or drug addiction, conviction of a felony.[11]

The goal of licensure is to protect the health and safety of the patient by controlling those who may practice medicine or provide other forms of health care in society.

The concept of licensure has been criticized as failing to be an effective quality control, especially after a license is initially granted. Such criticisms have resulted in the alteration of some state medical examining boards to include consumer representatives and the granting of additional authority to them to supervise professional conduct. Some sentiment exists for a restructuring of the licensing mechanism to require relicensing every five or ten years. This concept has not yet received widespread acceptance.

A second, and equally important attempt to influence the quality of medical care is represented by medical malpractice. The medical malpractice system has been the subject of much criticism and many misconceptions during the recent "malpractice crisis." Malpractice is not a relatively recent development. It is a regular part of the law of torts whose roots extend back through the Anglo-American common law system to a time preceding the invasion of William the Conqueror. It is not a system which applies only to physicians. It is the same system which is applied to the conduct of persons in society (to determine the existence of negligence) and to the conduct of persons who belong to a profession specifically. It is the same system which applies to the conduct of lawyers, dentists, architects, barbers, and other professionals.

There are five elements to a malpractice case. For malpractice to exist and for liability to be assigned, each of these five elements must be present:
1. Duty:
this element has two parts: (a) did the accused (the defendant) owe the injured person (the plaintiff) a duty? (b) what was the nature of the duty owed (the standard of care)?

The accused person must have owed a duty to the injured party. This duty may arise from a relationship between the two persons. In medicine, such a duty arises from the beginning of the physician-patient relationship.

The duty owed is generally stated in terms of reasonableness (what would a reasonable practitioner of ordinary skill and training have done in the same or similar circumstances?). In most cases, this is a question of medical judgment, determined by the testimony of medical experts.[12]
2. Breach of the Duty:
for this element to be present, the conduct of the defendant must have been of such a nature as to violate the duty owed to the injured party. This determination is generally a question of fact to be made by the jury.
3. Causation: Direct:
for this element to be present, there must be a direct, causal relation between the action committed by the defendant and the injuries suffered by the plaintiff.
4. Causation: Proximate:
for this element to be present, there must be sufficient closeness between the action of the defendant and the injuries suffered by the plaintiff so that it is not superseded by the actions of another subsequent party.
5. Damages:
for this element to be present, the plaintiff must have suffered actual harm. The negligence system is not designed to compensate for theoretical or potential harms. For recovery, it is necessary to prove that actual damages were suffered.

The medical malpractice system applies to both the actions of an individual and the actions of an institution.[13] It is a system that has several goals. It is designed to influence the quality of medical care by encouraging responsibility in medicine and discouraging negligent treatment of patients. It is a compensation mechanism through which injured parties can claim damages resulting from negligent medical care. It is interesting to note that in medical malpractice, as in the licensure system, the medical profession plays a key role. The malpractice "crisis" is complex. But the roots of the problem seem to be found in such things as the depersonalization of the modern doctor-patient relationship, the excessive expectations of the modern patient, the disregard of the patient's right to consent to treatment, and the uncertainties faced by insurance companies in judging the risks of writing a policy for a given physician. In any event, the malpractice system is the primary form of redress for an injured patient and remains an important influence on the quality of medical care.

In its development over the past 900 years, certain human values have been incorporated into the Anglo-American system of justice. They include the value of human life, the principle of self-determination, the right to privacy, and many others. The law reflects these values in its relations with other institutions in society including medicine. One can define, from a legal perspective, three aspects of the physician-patient relationship which reflect some of these values:
1. The contractual aspect:
the physician-patient relationship is a voluntary one in which the assent of each party is necessary before obligations flow from the relationship.[14]
2. The consensual aspect:
the physician-patient relationship is based on the exercise of self-determination by the patient through consent to treatment.[15]
3. The quality assurance aspect:
the physician-patient relationship involves the quality of compliance with the standards of medical practice in accordance with the medical malpractice system.

Each of these three characteristics has been the source of major controversies during the past ten years. Does a hospital have an obligation to provide emergency medical care to everyone who comes seeking it?[16] What must be disclosed to a patient about to undergo a life-threatening operation? Questions like these reflect the substantial tension which exists currently between the clinical judgment of a physician, the expectation, demand, need and right of the patient consumer, and the best interests of society.

The law has also functioned as a boundary of medical decision making.

In this sense, the law joins science, economics, philosophy, and theology in helping the physician to face the questions: what can I do and what should I do? There are two important sources of legal obligations to keep in mind. The first is composed of those obligations which all citizens of society share. The prohibition against homicide is a good example. A person who is a physician does not have any less an obligation to avoid the unjust taking of life than does any citizen. The second involves those obligations which have special application because a person is a physician. The obligations deriving from the physician-patient relationship are a good example of these.

It is important also to keep in mind that the perspectives of law, science, economics, philosophy, and theology complement each other, and are not substitutes for each other. Thus, the failure of the law to forbid an activity is not necessarily an indication of its endorsement of the activity. Often this represents an indication by legal authorities that moral persuasion is more appropriate than outright legal prohibition. The contemporary controversy over the legality of abortion is an example of this problem.[17]

Two explicit goals of legal regulation of medical care can be discerned in the various law-medicine interactions:
1. the promotion and protection of the public health, safety, and welfare;
2. the protection of human rights and civil liberties.

The power of the state to enact laws to encourage and assure the public well-being is called the "police power." It is an inherent power of a sovereign government. Thus each of the fifty states possesses the power to regulate in this manner while the national government (a government of delegated power) does not.[18] The police power has been employed in a wide variety of circumstances from compulsory health care procedures[19] to the medical licensure system. While the goal of promoting and protecting societal well-being is a widely accepted goal, application of the general principles to specific circumstances has been the source of much litigation.[20]

The protection of human rights and civil liberties is likewise an important goal of the regulation of the health care process. We have witnessed during the past fifteen years the increasing recognition that the patient possesses rights as a citizen which are not surrendered by becoming sick. It is easy to overlook, however, the fact that the physician is likewise a citizen whose values and rights deserve consideration. The solution to the imbalance of power which has traditionally existed between physician and patient is not to consider one as superior to the other, but to understand the important role each plays in health care, and the need to involve law, medicine, philosophy, and theology in the ongoing process of reflection on the many problems which exist. The central issue considered in such reflection should be the nature of the physician's mandate from society. What do we as citizens expect from medical providers? What rights do we want to see respected in the physician-patient relationship?

Law, philosophy, and theology raise questions about the ends of medicine, the nature of man, the goals of society, and the values and systems which shape the context in which medicine is practiced. But lawyers, philosophers, and theologians are not competent to practice medicine. It is the physician and the patient who are the center of the medical decision-making process. By stimulating public discussion and by clarifying for the physician the importance of legal regulation, we begin to address the ultimate goal of legal regulation: the best health care possible, delivered in a manner consistent with the rights of patient and provider.

Appendix

Iowa Medical Practice Act

147.2 License Required No person shall engage in the practice of medicine and surgery, podiatry, osteopathy, osteopathic medicine and surgery, chiropractic, physical therapy, nursing, dentistry, dental hygiene, optometry, pharmacy, cosmetology, barbering, funeral directing or embalming as defined in the following chapters of this title, unless he shall have obtained from the state department of health a license for that purpose.

148.1 Persons Engaged in Practice For the purpose of this title the following classes of persons shall be termed to be engaged in the practice of medicine and surgery:

1. Persons who publicly profess to be physicians or surgeons or who publicly profess to assume the duties incident to the practice of medicine or surgery.

2. Persons who prescribe, or prescribe and furnish medicine for human ailments or treat the same by surgery.

3. Persons who act as representatives of any person in doing any of the things mentioned in this section.

147.15 Professional Qualifications Every dental, podiatry, chiropractic, nurse, optometry, pharmacy, cosmetology, barbering, and funeral director and embalmer examiner shall be a person licensed to practice the profession for which the board, of which he is a member, conducts examinations for licenses to practice such profession. The medical examiners shall consist of eight persons, six of whom shall be licensed to practice medicine and surgery and two of whom shall be licensed to practice osteopathic medicine and surgery. Three of the physical therapy examiners shall be licensed to practice physical therapy and one of the physical therapy examiners shall be licensed to practice medicine and surgery.

148.3 Requirements for License

Each applicant for a license to practice medicine shall:

1. Present a diploma issued by a medical college approved by the medical examiners. The medical examiners may accept, in lieu of a diploma from a medical college approved by them, all of the following.
a. A diploma issued by a medical college which has been neither approved nor disapproved by the medical examiners; and
b. The completion of three years of training as a resident physician, which training has been approved by or is acceptable to the medical examiners; and
c. The recommendation of the educational council for foreign medical graduates, incorporated or similar accrediting agency.

2. Pass an examination prescribed by the medical examiners in the subjects of anatomy, chemistry, physiology,

materia medica and therapeutics, obstetrics, pathology, theory and practice, and surgery; but in the subjects of materia medica and therapeutics, and theory and practice, each applicant shall be examined in accordance with the teachings of the school of medicine which he desires to practice. The board of medical examiners may require written, oral, and practical examinations of the applicant.

3. Present to the state department of health satisfactory evidence that applicant has completed one year of internship in a hospital approved by the state board of medical examiners. No hospital shall be approved which does not provide the internship without expense to the intern.

4. Be a citizen of the United States or have legally declared his intention of becoming a citizen.

148.4 Certificates of a National Board

The state department of health may with the approval of the medical examiners, accept in lieu of the examination prescribed in section 148.3 a certificate of examination issued by the national board of medical examiners of the United States of America, but every applicant for a license upon the basis of such certificate shall be required to pay the fee prescribed for licenses issued under reciprocal agreements.

Revocation of Licenses

147.55 Grounds A license to practice a profession shall be revoked or suspended when the licensee is guilty of any of the following acts or offenses:

1. Fraud in procuring his license.

2. Incompetency in the practice of his profession.

3. Knowingly making misleading, deceptive, untrue, or fraudulent, representations in the practice of his profession or engaging in unethical conduct or practice harmful to the public. Proof of actual injury need not be established.

4. Habitual intoxication or addiction to the use of drugs.

5. Conviction of a felony. A copy of the record of conviction or plea of guilty shall be conclusive evidence.

Notes

1. Ingelfinger, F., Legal hegemony in medicine, *N. Eng. J. Med.*, 293: 825–826, 1975.

2. Cf. Chayet, N., Hegemony in medicine revisited, *N. Eng. J. Med.*, 294: 547–548, 1976.

3. Cf. Camps, F. (ed.), *Gradwohl's Legal Medicine*. (Bristol: John Wright and Sons Ltd., 1968) pp. 1–13, 18–22.

4. *Commonwealth* v. *Kenneth Edelin* (Docket Number 81823, Superior Court of Massachusetts, Suffolk County, 1975).

5. *In the Matter of Karen Quinlan* (Docket No. C-201-75, Superior Court of New Jersey, Chancery Division, Morris County, 1975).

6. *Ibid.*, p. 22A.

7. Iowa Code 147.2 (see Appendix for licensure sections of Iowa Code discussed here).

8. Iowa Code 148.1.

9. Iowa Code 147.15.

10. Iowa Code 148.3–4.

11. Iowa Code 147.55.

12. For an exception to this general principle, cf. *Canterbery* v. *Spence*, 464 F.2d. 772 (D.C. cir. 1972): informed consent.

13. Curran, W. J., and Shapiro, E., *Law, Medicine and Forensic Science* (2nd ed.) (Boston: Little, Brown, 1970) pp. 529–599, 610–621.

14. For an exception to this general rule, cf. Curren and Shapiro, op. cit., pp. 639–645.

15. Cf. note 12.

16. Cf. note 14.

17. *Roe* v. *Wade*, 410 U.S. 116 (1973) United States Supreme Court. For text of opinion see Chapter VI, pp. 116–178.

18. For a more complete discussion of the police power, cf. Grad, F., *Public Health Law Manual* (Washington, D.C.: American Public Health Association, 1973) pp. 5–8.

19. Cf. Curran and Shapiro, op. cit., pp. 668–687.

20. Ibid.

24

American Hospital Association Statement on a Patient's Bill of Rights

Reprinted with the permission of the American Hospital Association from *Hospitals,* vol. 47, February 1973, p. 41.

The American Hospital Association presents a Patient's Bill of Rights with the expectation that observance of these rights will contribute to more effective patient care and greater satisfaction for the patient, his physician, and the hospital organization. Further, the Association presents these rights in the expectation that they will be supported by the hospital on behalf of its patients, as an integral part of the healing process. It is recognized that a personal relationship between the physician and the patient is essential for the provision of proper medical care. The traditional physician-patient relationship takes on a new dimension when care is rendered within an organizational structure. Legal precedent has established that the institution itself also has a responsibility to the patient. It is in recognition of these factors that these rights are affirmed.

1. The patient has the right to considerate and respectful care.

2. The patient has the right to obtain from his physician complete current information concerning his diagnosis, treatment, and prognosis in terms the patient can be reasonably expected to understand. When it is not medically advisable to give such information to the patient, the information should be made available to an appropriate person in his behalf. He has the right to know, by name, the physician responsible for coordinating his care.

3. The patient has the right to receive from his physician information necessary to give informed consent prior to the start of any procedure and/or treatment. Except in emergencies, such information for informed consent should include but not necessarily be limited to the specific procedure and/or treatment, the medically significant risks involved, and the probable duration of incapacitation. Where medically significant alternatives for care or treatment exist, or when the patient requests information concerning medical alternatives, the patient has the right to such information. The patient also has the right to know the name of the person responsible for the procedures and/or treatment.

4. The patient has the right to refuse treatment to the extent permitted by law and to be informed of the medical consequences of his action.

5. The patient has the right to every consideration of his privacy concerning his own medical care program. Case discussion, consultation, examination, and treatment are confidential and should be conducted discreetly. Those not directly involved in his care must have the permission of the patient to be present.

6. The patient has the right to expect that all communications and records pertaining to his care should be treated as confidential.

7. The patient has the right to expect that within its capacity a hospital must make reasonable response to the request of a patient for services. The hospital must provide evaluation, service, and/or referral as indicated by the urgency of the case. When medically permissible, a patient may be transferred to another facility only after he has received complete information and explanation concerning the needs for and alternatives to such a transfer. The institution to which the patient is to be transferred must first have accepted the patient for transfer.

8. The patient has the right to obtain information as to any relationship of his hospital to other health care and educational institutions insofar as his care is concerned. The patient has the right to obtain information as to the existence of any professional relationships among individuals, by name, who are treating him.

9. The patient has the right to be advised if the hospital proposes to engage in or perform human experimentation affecting his care or treatment. The patient has the right to refuse to participate in such research projects.

10. The patient has the right to expect reasonable continuity of care. He has the right to know in advance what appointment times and physicians are available and where. The patient has the right to expect that the hospital will provide a mechanism whereby he is informed by his physician or a delegate of the physician of the patient's continuing health care requirements following discharge.

11. The patient has the right to examine and receive an explanation of his bill regardless of source of payment.

12. The patient has the right to know what hospital rules and regulations apply to his conduct as a patient.

No catalog of rights can guarantee for the patient the kind of treatment he has a right to expect. A hospital has many functions to perform, including the prevention and treatment of disease, the education of both health professionals and patients, and the conduct of clinical research. All these activities must be conducted with an overriding concern for the patient, and, above all, the recognition of his dignity as a human being. Success in achieving this recognition assures success in the defense of the rights of the patient.

25

Robert E. Cooke

Ethics and Law on Behalf of the Mentally Retarded

Reprinted with permission of the author and publisher from *Pediatric Clinics of North America,* vol. 20, No. 1, February 1973, pp. 259–268.

Nearly five and a half million American citizens "are significantly impaired in their ability to learn and adapt to the demands of society," according to the *Report of the President's Panel on Mental Retardation* published in 1962. The figure today is probably closer to six million. While less than 10 per cent of these impaired persons are so severely limited in their intellectual development as to require constant care or supervision, all of them are affected in one way or another by the myriad of laws and administrative practices that control admission to institutions; establish criteria for guardianship; determine the validity of marriages and the grounds for annulment and divorce; assign custody of children; provide for *ad hoc* "incompetency" (to sue or be sued, to hold a driver's license, to vote, to make a contract, or a conveyance, or a will, etc.); govern the determinations in the criminal law under which one may be held incompetent to stand trial, be adjudicated a "defective delinquent," or be acquitted "by reason of insanity," or declared a sexual psychopath; and fix the conditions under which retardates may be confined, tranquilized, sterilized, placed in "seclusion," and their property managed by others.

Richard C. Allen
The Retarded Citizen: Victim of Mental and Legal Deficiency[2]

Traditionally, the pediatrician has remained uninvolved, unconcerned, and uninformed regarding the ethical and legal problems of the mentally retarded. Psychiatrists in general are somewhat familiar with the law, by virtue of their involvement with the processes of institutional commitment. However, more and more, the pediatrician is expected to provide expert guidance and advice to parents and to societal institutions regarding the retarded. Many are now advisors to local chapters of the Association for Retarded Children, and they often serve on state and city commissions.

Previous societies have rather episodically reviled or revered, deified or destroyed the handicapped. It has become acceptable to abort the retarded before birth; yet the attitude toward them after birth is inconsistent. In some circumstances, we do all we can to preserve life; in others, such as mongolism with complications requiring surgical correction, we deny it. Even when life is preserved, the retarded are generally relegated to second class citizenship, devoid of opportunities or even basic liberties.

As our society becomes more technologically sophisticated and demands more and more freedom from discomfort, the productivity of each individual and the benefit-to-cost ratio of each expenditure becomes increasingly important. On this scale, the mentally retarded cannot compete, at least in short-term gains. Special classes for the mentally retarded are in direct competition for personnel and funds, for example, with reading disability programs, programs for the superior child, the normal child, etc. Although no detailed analysis has yet been carried out, it is likely that better education for the normal child would be the most "profitable," simply because of the impact of much larger numbers.

Therefore, why should people care? Is there another yardstick by which worth of persons or programs may be judged? Is there a reason for caring, when there is relatively little material benefit to society? Is there an advantage to society for selflessness—for caring without immediate gain?

Since law represents to a substantial degree a somewhat delayed codification of the ethics of society, it is essential to discuss not only the legal provisions pertaining to mental retardation, but also to consider the social and ethical factors involved in the protection of the dependent and, especially, the mentally retarded. Additionally, because of the limited reversibility of their disability, the mentally retarded represent a model of societal concern for all handicapped groups—the aged, the mentally ill, the alcoholic, even the impoverished.

Toleration of Difference

Philosophers, sociologists, and psychologists have long described man as a social animal. His behavior and his biology must be described in terms of his relationships with other men. Cooperative rather than mutually destructive behavior permits evolutionary progress of the species. Therein, cultural heritage plays an enormous role in transmitting the practices most likely to produce satisfactory social adjustment.

Rules of conduct—politeness, for example—have undoubtedly evolved, not as God-given prescriptions, but as practices that have led most efficiently to social harmony and productivity. If all the participants at a meeting shout at once, all transactions cease immediately. In all such situations, the easier that man can interact with other men, the greater the opportunity for accomplishment.

How is the problem of mental retardation related to this process? The mentally retarded to a large extent represent nonthreatening examples of difference, and a basic requirement of all social intercourse is tolerance of difference. No two individuals (even monozygotic twins) are identical; hence, "different from me" must be acceptable.

The profoundly retarded, as well as the severely maimed, the aged, and certainly the severely ill and dying, are psychologically threatening. As Jean Vanier has pointed out, the fear of death forces even well motivated people to avoid responsibility to the injured, the dying, and the unsightly.[12]

The mentally retarded are often noticeably different, but their acceptance is generally less threatening, since their behavior is frequently childlike—happy, rather than depressing. Even the mongoloid with a severe degree of mental retardation is a delightful child when accepted by a family.

The Balance of Rights and Responsibility

It is not surprising that society has worked out adjustments which prevent serious social imbalance. In a totalitarian state, primitive or sophisticated, the aggregation of power and self-generating social benefits are kept in check. Maoism, for example, demands periodic return to the earth of the educated and advantaged. In a free society, such coercive direction is considered undesirable and the advantaged—biologically, behaviorally, and culturally—are free to achieve and accumulate more and more. Only through personal restraint, respect of the rights of the less fortunate, and the assumption of responsibility can social balance be achieved. Modern genetics and developmental biology have proven that no two individuals are the same—that there are biological advantages of a greater or lesser degree throughout society.

Thus, social balance—the assurance of rights to all, not just the favored—demands that as the individual achieves more, he must assume greater responsibility for the rights of others and be less concerned for his own rights.

How such an ethic is taught or transmitted as part of our cultural heritage is not clear, but certainly the acceptance of the handicapped and the retarded, as an integral part of every aspect of our society—school, recreation, family life—can assist in this process of tolerance and responsibility.

Legal Rights

Although in theory, society has guaranteed the rights of the dependent through protective statutes and institutions, in actual day-to-day operation, many of these protective aspects are misused to protect the rights of the normal and to disenfranchise the mentally retarded. Nowhere is the abuse more flagrant than in the care of the institutionalized retarded.

Only within the last few years has a reform movement been initiated through a series of class action suits. This development—the use of litigation as a means of achieving reform—must become familiar to all pediatricians, for they will be called upon sooner or later to assist on behalf of one side or the other. The civil rights movement initiated such an approach, and its application seems limitless.

The laws and statutes regarding the mentally retarded can be looked upon in three broad classes, based upon their inherent purposes: (1) prevention of mental retardation, (2) protection of the community, and (3) civil rights and protection of the mentally retarded person.

Laws and Statutes Directed at Prevention

Although there are substantial differences in regulations from one state to another, most states require premarital or prenatal blood tests to prevent congenital syphilis. Likewise, testing of the newborn for phenylketonuria is mandatory in most states. Physical abuse of the child is also prohibited, though frequently ineffectively. Mental abuse or intellectual deprivation can occur with little chance for legal action.

As a consequence of the misapplied or misunderstood genetics of the 1920's . . . many states retain statutes prohibiting marriage of the retarded. For the mentally retarded in the community, this usually presents no problem, because tests of intelligence are almost never carried out before marriage licenses are issued. The institutionalized retarded person, however, must obtain permission from the superintendent of the institution, almost always without the protection of due process. This permission is rarely given, and then usually only after sterilization of the prospective wife.

The sterilization of the retarded also represents an effort to prevent the birth of mentally retarded offspring. It, too, represents a misconception that intelligence is determined by a single gene or at most a few, and that the spread of mental retardation can be prevented by sterilization of all retarded. In ruling in favor of compulsory sterilization, Chief Justice Holmes in 1927 (Buck vs. Bell) declared . . . that "three generations of imbeciles are enough." According to Kittrie, "the state's interest in the maintenance of the quality of the species, Holmes held, was superior to any individual's power of procreation."[9]

The fact that mild mental retardation is possibly a multifactorial result of environmental forces interacting with many genes has been appreciated only in recent years, and the related concept that each of us carries deleterious mutant genes is as yet understood by only a small part of the general population.

Surgical sterilization of the mentally retarded is permitted by statute in 26 states.[2] In 23 of these states, it can be performed without consent. Even where permission is required, institutions frequently utilize coercive measures, such as offering discharge from the institution or the opportunity for marriage, greater freedom, and the like, in exchange for agreement to be sterilized. Truly informed consent without coercion is unlikely in most cases under these circumstances.[10]

Surgical sterilization of the mentally retarded is still a relatively common practice on demand of the parents, and less frequently on demand of a social agency. In general, such requests are aimed at preventing pregnancy and are usually on behalf of a female child, although occasionally a male is sterilized to "protect the community." Physicians have at times unwittingly been used to carry out a sort of sterilization by isolation. The institutionalization of mildly retarded attractive girls to protect against pregnancy is fairly frequent. Such action is generally motivated by the comfort and pride of the family, rather than the benefit of the child.

If there is a real, not imagined, high risk of pregnancy, and if serious restriction of social freedom is the alternative, then temporary, not permanent, contraceptive measures should be employed. Unfortunately, if promiscuity is a concern, sterilization simply offers a license to the family for neglect of the retarded child or young adult.

According to the rich experience of Doctor George Tarjan at Pacific State Hospital in California, the retarded are in general more responsible, more puritanical in conduct, and more sensitive to rules of proper conduct in sex matters than normal individuals. Without recourse to sterilization by surgery or isolation, "the extramarital conception rate of our women patients would have given pride to any college president or high school principal."[11] In one state's statutes, the effort to prevent reproduction by isolation is euphemistically referred to: "The Division of Mental Retardation shall provide the number of residencies as can be used advantageously, giving preference first to *women of child-bearing age.*"

Anecdotal evidence does exist for the successful marital adjustment with child-bearing among the retarded.[7] Various studies have been done on groups of previously institutionalized retarded individuals who married. These studies showed widely diverse outcomes— from excellent to poor adjustment. Failures to adapt were more related to personality problems than to low IQ's. Successful adjustment required, as would be expected, considerable continuing guidance. The value of special guidance in education and employment for the mentally retarded is now appreciated, but specialized counselling for and during marriage is not yet common, even in such highly socialized states as Denmark, Sweden, or the Netherlands.

A statute still extant in several states prohibits first cousin marriages. Modern genetics has clearly shown that the children of such parents have an increased but still low frequency of abnormality (less than 1 in 100). Such laws should be repealed before they lead to the enactment of laws designed to prohibit marriage of carriers of mutant genes with a far higher risk of abnormal offspring (1 in 4).

Protection of the Community

Although the majority of commitments to institutions are alleged to be for the benefit of the retarded person, the argument being that services needed by the mentally retarded are only available there, few institutions provide active habilitation for the majority of their occupants. Institutionalization of the profoundly and severely retarded may assist a sorely pressed family and prevent major social dislocation of parents or siblings. But such action should not be automatic, and should occur only after the family is advised and grants their well considered consent.

The moderately retarded, especially the young, fare far better in the community. Institutionalization in such instances represents a failure of the community to provide adequate educational and vocational activities. Commitment, voluntary or involuntary, of the mildly retarded is totally unjustified, and leads to a serious loss of the common civil and human rights that can be fully appreciated by the mildly retarded. By such action, usually without due process (trial by judge or jury), the rights to vote, to drive, to inherit, and to make a will or contract are lost. For example, if the retarded inherits property, the institution acquires that property to defray the costs of care.[3]

Commitment in a sense is always involuntary; the retarded person does not decide his own fate. Parents, social workers, judges, and physicians decide a course of action in "the retarded's best interests." Indeed, many times children are institutionalized less for their own benefit than for the convenience or comfort of others. Rarely does a court inquire into the possibility of using community resources or foster care instead of institutionalization. Indeed, rarely is the judge even aware of them.

The retarded individual is almost never represented by counsel, has no appeal mechanism, and may be institutionalized without review for a lifetime. It is, therefore, essential that no one be committed without a careful hearing and/or jury trial, which will include all the constitutional protections present in other types of civil proceedings.

While institutionalized, the retarded individual can be the victim of administrative whimsy directed at what is interpreted as his "best interests."[4] For example, where feeding is difficult, one institution frequently performs gastrostomy. Parents at times may be poor advocates under such circumstances, in part because of lack of information, in part because of many unconscious or conscious biases, and in part because of implied or explicit threats of retribution against their child if complaints are lodged.

These inadequacies, which occur in every state, may well be corrected in the coming decade by a series of class action suits that have established in the Federal Courts the right of the mentally retarded to receive adequate treatment. A final order and opinion, setting standards for minimum constitutionally and medically adequate treatment and establishing a detailed procedure for implementation, was handed down on April 13, 1972 (Wyatt vs. Stickney— Alabama, 1971). The judge also appointed a 7 member "human rights committee" for Partlow State School and Hospital, a public institution for the mentally retarded in Tuscaloosa, Alabama, and included a patient on this committee. Similar class action suits have been filed in New York, Massachusetts, Georgia, Tennessee, and Missouri.[8]

These rulings have included a detailed prescription for personnel requirements and a habilitation program for each and every resident, as well as periodic reassessment. The general principle endorsed is that each child or adult is entitled to the least restrictive treatment possible to fulfill his or her potential. The operation of the institution should copy the developmental model of Wolfensberger, rather than the traditional medical model which resembles the operation of a psychiatric institution.[13]

Civil Rights

In the process of "protecting the community," legislatures have in general preempted the rights of the mentally retarded to vote, to drive, to enter into contracts, and to assign property by will or covenant.[1] Fortunately, in the actual granting of such licenses or rights, rarely are measurements made of adaptive capacity.

When the retarded is involved in or suspected of involvement in crime, no statutes exist that deny him rights accorded to every citizen. Yet, in practical operation of the courts, the retarded offender is frequently deprived of these rights. Bertram Brown has clearly shown that the mentally retarded are three times more common in the population of federal prisons than in the general population.[5] Such data have sometimes been erroneously interpreted to mean that retardation is characterized by criminal tendencies.

In fact, however, such statistics show that the retarded individual is less able than others to protect his legal rights. In a study of the legal process for suspected mentally retarded offenders, Allen et al. have shown that the mentally retarded, at the time of arrest, have far more frequently waived their constitutional rights against making self-incriminating statements.[3] (Two thirds so acted, and in over one half of such cases, self-incriminating statements were used as evidence.) The retarded are easily cajoled into confession; 59 per cent pleaded guilty, compared with less than 10 per cent of the nonretarded. They have waived right to counsel and to jury trial far more than the criminal with average intelligence. Likewise, reduction of charge is far less frequent with the retarded, suggesting that when counsel is provided, the lawyer or judge does not communicate as readily with the mentally retarded offender. In 88 per cent of the convictions, no appeal of judgment or sentence was made.

Competence to stand trial and to understand right and wrong are difficult determinations. The courts must come to act on behalf of the retarded, and articulate the responsibility of society toward them. The use of flexible criteria that are dependent upon the situation would seem desirable, since each retarded individual and each situation varies enormously. The doctrine of "diminished responsibility" in the retarded would seem more appropriate than the so-called M'Naghten rule (ability to distinguish right from wrong),

the Durham test (irresistible impulse as consequence of mental disease), or the American Law Institute criterion (inability to appreciate criminality of conduct).[5] This doctrine of diminished responsibility states that the defendant is neither wholly responsible nor wholly irresponsible; it calls for recognition of and allowance for varying degrees of mental impairment.

Laws Protecting the Individual and His Rights

From the strictly legalistic point of view, the mentally retarded do not differ whatsoever in rights from the normal; they are entitled to education, care, and protection under the law. However, class action suits, as mentioned above, have clearly established that, in practice, many of these rights are not guaranteed. In Pennsylvania, the courts (Civil Action No. 71–42) have now ruled that every child is entitled to education commensurate with his abilities, regardless of intelligence.[8] Such an action will lead shortly to the development and implementation of public programs for the moderately, severely, and profoundly retarded, in addition to the mildly retarded in every state. Similar class action suits regarding the right to education have been filed in the District of Columbia and California.

Although every hospital or physician usually feels it necessary and desirable to intercede with the courts on behalf of minor patients requiring life-saving treatment for which parents will not give permission, it has been routine in many hospitals (and even intimated by textbooks) that pressure on parents or the court for permission to operate on a child with Down's syndrome and duodenal atresia should not be exerted. Enough interest has recently been generated nationally by a case from Johns Hopkins to indicate that legal advice should be obtained in all similar cases in the future if parental permission is not given. Several families have volunteered their services as foster parents if successful surgery is performed, so that institutionalization or care by the natural parents does not represent the only possibilities for care.

Just as society or parents cannot violate the right of the mentally retarded to live, neither should it be possible for parents or administrators to

volunteer the retarded for experimentation or for donation of organs for transplantation. Unless the medical experimentation has a reasonable chance of benefit to the retarded person himself, no volunteering of another person's well being should be tolerated— ethically or legally.

The rights of an individual to life, to education, and to freedom from harassment will require the establishment of advocacy or guardian measures which do not exist in most areas at the present time. Guardianship may be conceived of as a legal form of social guidance, but fiscal guidance, advice in use of property, and law, are needed as well. It should be as limited as possible in scope, minimally restrictive of the retarded individual, and should be reexamined regularly.

Wolfensberger has urged the development of citizen advocacy for the handicapped.[13] The advocate may be a unit, such as the local Association for Retarded Children or, more informally, a mature person who represents the interests of another as if they were his own. Such citizen advocacy must extend into the institutions, as well as the community, to assure full respect for the institutionalized as a member of our society, since administrative practices often fall far short of what is desirable.

Although families are not prevented by statute from bearing children when risks of retardation exist, prospective parents may have great difficulty in adopting retarded children. Social agencies, in the past at least, have been inappropriately anxious to spare knowledgeable parents some discomforts, even to the detriment of the infant. If parents unwittingly adopt a child who within a 5-year-period is discovered to be mentally retarded, annulment of the adoption is possible in many states. Such statutes seem discriminatory toward adopted children, since families do not have the legal right to discard their natural children if they prove to be defective. If adoption is to be a complete substitute for child bearing, as it can be from all points of view including emotional commitment, parents should expect risks, hardships, and imperfections, just as with natural children.

Free Choice Principle

In concluding this review of the ethical and legal considerations of the mentally retarded, mention should be made of a recommended change in the financing of the care of the mentally retarded. At the present time, most institutional programs and some community programs are direct operations of state or local public agencies. Parents have almost no options except for home care, or care by the state, with or without formal commitment. Such a monopolistic system was originally developed as a public service comparable to public schools. But in contrast to students in public schools, retarded individuals and their families are often either unwilling or unable to make their needs known to the bureaucracy responsible for providing this care.

In our society, individual needs have traditionally been met by the free enterprise system, with competition leading to improved products (or the belief that they are), and adaptation to the needs of most citizens. If parents were given, through a voucher system, purchasing power equivalent to the billions being expended from general tax revenues by federal, state, and local bureaucracies, smaller, more responsive facilities would arise in response to the market. Some concern has been expressed that such a free choice system would lead to exploitation of families and of the adult retarded without a family. In general, however, parents remain the most interested advocates for the child, and every adult retarded should have a surrogate parent as his personal advocate. It is to be hoped that some enlightened states or the Social Security System itself may respond to this need in years to come.[6]

References

1. Allen R. C., Legal rights of the institutionalized retardate: Equal justice for the unequal. *Ment. Retard.*, 7: (no. 6): 2, 1969.

2. Allen, R. C., The retarded citizen: Victim of mental and legal deficiency. *Maryland Law Forum*, 2:4, 1971.

3. Allen, R. C., Ferster, E. Z., and Weihofen, H., *Mental Impairment and Legal Incompetency*. Englewood Cliffs, New Jersey, Prentice-Hall, 1968.

4. Blatt, B., *Exodus from Pandemonium*. Boston, Massachusetts, Allyn and Bacon, 1970.

5. Brown, B. S., and Courtless, T. F., *The Mentally Retarded Offender*. The President's Commission on Law Enforcement and Administration of Justice.

6. Cooke, R. E., The free choice principle in the care of the mentally retarded. In Kugel, R. B., and Wolfensberger, W. (eds.): *Changing Patterns in Residential Services for the Mentally Retarded*. A President's Committee on Mental Retardation Monograph, Washington, D.C. 1969, pp. 359-365.

7. Edgerton, R. B., *The Cloak of Competence: Stigma in the Lives of the Mentally Retarded*. Berkeley and Los Angeles, University of California Press, 1967.

8. Friedman, P., *Mental Retardation and the Law: A Report on Status of Current Court Cases*. Publication of the Center for Law and Social Policy, Washington, D.C., June 9, 1972.

9. Kittrie. N., *The Right to be Different*. Baltimore, Maryland, Johns Hopkins Press, 1971.

10. *Report of the Task Force on Law*. President's Panel on Mental Retardation, Washington, D.C., 1963.

11. Tarjan, G., Sex: A tri-polar conflict in mental retardation. Presented at The Joseph P. Kennedy, Jr. Foundation International Symposium on Human Rights, Retardation and Research, Washington, D.C., October 16, 1971.

12. Vanier, J., Remarks made at Fifth Annual International Post-Graduate Symposium on Mental Retardation, Paris, France, March 18-28, 1972.

13. Wolfensberger, W., A new approach to decision-making in human management services. In Kugel, R. B., and Wolfensberger, W. (eds.): *Changing Patterns in Residential Services for the Mentally Retarded*. A President's Committee on Mental Retardation Monograph, Washington, D.C., 1969, pp. 367-381.

26

Full Citizenship and Legal Rights of the Retarded Person

Reprinted from U.S. Department of Health, Education and Welfare, *Report to the President, Mental Retardation: Century of Decision* (Washington, D.C.: Government Printing Office, 1976), pp. 58-60.

Mentally retarded people have in the past suffered extensive discrimination in the exercise of constitutional rights. During the past 10 years, significant advancements have geen made in defining the legal status of the mentally disabled person, in clarifying and establishing procedures of due process, and in implementing the retarded person's equality under the law. This represents only a beginning, however. The retarded person still suffers from the persistence of past inequities and the discriminatory restriction of rights.

The basic premises on which the following discussion and recommendations rest are these:

Retarded people have the same rights, legal and constitutional, as every other United States citizen, including the rights of due process and equal protection of the laws.

Retarded people can be more independent and can function more competently and responsibly than is commonly believed—mental retardation and incompetency are not synonymous.

Full citizenship exercised by a retarded person in a community setting is possible and is in the public interest.

On the basis of these assumptions, which have been increasingly recognized during the last decade in the legislatures, the courts and in society in general, a number of specific rights deserve special attention in order to remedy the effects of past discrimination. These include, but are not limited to the following:

The right of equal access to quality health care, both medical and dental, and social services adapted to need;

The right to residential programs and other supportive services in settings most conducive to development and independence;

The right to equal educational opportunity adapted to need;

The right to equal employment opportunity and economic security;

The right to marry and bear children;

The right of due process and equal protection of the law in the criminal justice system;

The right to vote.

Prior to discussion of these rights, two key terms need to be clarified: *competence and consent.*

Every mentally retarded person, as every other citizen, is presumed to be competent. Only where there has been a full due process hearing can anyone's rights be restricted on the basis of incompetence. This restriction of rights should be limited to the specific problems which the individual has been shown to be unable to handle and which involve possible harm to himself or others. There should be a recognition of gradations and separability of competences, e.g., the individual who is unable to make a formal contract involving sums of money should not be deprived of all right to make money transactions, nor lose all civil rights because of this inability. The idea that, because a person is incompetent to do one thing, he is therefore incompetent to do all things is absurd, and contrary to the facts of everyday life. Legal incompetency, which is generally taken to mean an inability of the person to manage his own affairs, should be based on facts to be determined for a specifiable set of circumstances, at an appropriately conducted hearing, and established in a specific legal judgment. Incompetency, once a judgment has been made, should be subject to automatic periodic review and rights restored when evidence of the previous impediment is no longer found to exist.

The concept of consent directly relates to the presumption of competence of each mentally retarded individual in the absence of a legal finding to the contrary. Consent requires an informed decision by an individual. A mentally retarded person should be presumed able to make informed decisions when presented with pertinent facts and in language he understands. However, the more serious the decision and the more there is a question of an individual's ability to understand and weigh the facts, and thus give informed consent, the more there is a need for review of the decision by a personal representative or advocate recognized as competent to consult with the retarded person and to speak in his behalf.

The concepts of competence and consent are not static. The movement to protect the legal rights of the mentally retarded citizen is based on a challenge to the traditional view of the retarded person as an individual with little or no ability to learn, to develop or to function within the framework of citizenship. As scientific knowledge and direct experience with the accomplishments of retarded people have increased, so our perception of the limitations of ability has been altered. The potential for growth and development of the retarded citizen, given appropriate opportunities to learn and to use his learning under supportive conditions, has become an emerging concept. The conditions of consent must not be locked into inflexible definitions, but must allow for future modification in the light of expanding knowledge and educational skill.

The following statements represent the President's Committee's views on rights of retarded persons and the conditions governing their possible limitation.

The Right to Equal Access to Quality Health and Social Services Adapted to Need

The right to be free from the arbitrary denial of lifesaving medical services. This right is premised on a recognition of the universal value of human life and the recognition that mentally retarded persons must be allowed equal access to medical services to preserve their lives. Such a right rules out any practice which would "allow" a retarded person to die based upon a judgment that the quality of life of a retarded person is less than that of other citizens, or any routine policies or guidelines predetermining the withdrawal of life support from impaired newborn babies based on predicted development potential.

The right to medical and medically related services on an equal basis with other citizens. This right includes all medical, dental, and surgical treatments available, as well as occupational and physical therapy, speech and language services, etc., as they may be indicated.

The right to be protected from unnecessary and experimental research procedures. Such a right prevents mentally retarded individuals from being subjects of medical or behavioral experimentation, unless the individual or his legal representative has given an informed consent, consistent with regulations promulgated under law governing the use of human subjects in research.

The right to health services necessary to prevent or control mental retardation. The right includes access to nutritional and dietary programs, maternal care, and beneficial medication. It includes also the right to be free of unnecessary and debilitating drugs employed solely for behavioral restraint.

The right to have access to all available social services which facilitate the retarded person's adjustment to society or which facilitate his development. This right precludes an agency from denying services solely on the basis of mental retardation.

27

Norman L. Cantor

A Patient's Decision to Decline Lifesaving Medical Treatment: Bodily Integrity versus the Preservation of Life

Reprinted with permission of author and editors from *Rutgers Law Review*, vol. 26, 1973, pp. 228–264.

The scene is a local community hospital. The patient is a 25-year-old man or woman suffering from a perforated ulcer, potentially fatal but curable by a simple operation. The patient is unmarried, childless, and fully coherent. With the threat of death looming, physicians request that the patient consent to surgery and an accompanying blood transfusion. The patient refuses because: (a) religious convictions forbid either the surgery[1] or the blood transfusion,[2] (b) the patient wants to die because of shame and anxiety over recent financial or romantic setbacks; (c) the patient wants to die because he or she is also the victim of a terminal illness which will inevitably entail considerable pain and gradual bodily degeneration; or (d) the patient is refusing treatment as a symbolic protest against a governmental policy, such as Viet Nam, and will only submit to surgery when that policy is officially changed. The hospital administrator, acting on the principle that a hospital's paramount mission is to preserve life, seeks a judicial order appointing himself temporary guardian for purposes of consenting to the necessary lifesaving medical treatment.

Can or should a judge grant the relief requested? Does refusal to intervene entail acceptance of a "right to die" in the context of suicide and euthanasia? Does it matter whether the patient is motivated by reasons of conscience or simply by the will to die? Does it matter that the patient has dependents who will be disadvantaged by his or her death? The strong temptation is to respond positively to the opportunity to preserve life. Judges have been anguished by the knowledge that failure to order treatment would likely mean the patient's death, particularly where the patient did not really wish to die but was only following religious dictates.[3] Religious freedom, bodily integrity, or individual self-determination appear as evanescent or ephemeral principles in the face of an immediate threat to life. Yet, both religious freedom and control of one's body are cherished values in our society, and both are of constitutional dimension when threatened by governmental invasion.[4]

The above questions should not be resolved by visceral reaction. Careful analysis of legal protections for bodily integrity, constitutional standards, and governmental interests asserted as justifications for judicial intervention is necessary. While the reported cases are relatively few,[5] there has been no dearth of legal commentary on judicial compulsion of lifesaving medical treatment.[6] Previous treatments of this topic, however, have largely failed to examine all the potential interests, or to assess the degree of harm posed to these interests by refusal of medical care.[7] This article is intended to avert that weakness. Hopefully, it will contribute to resolution of a public policy issue—judicially compelled lifesaving treatment[8]—which undoubtedly arises with considerably more frequency than the number of reported cases would indicate.[9] Additionally, fixing the delicate constitutional balance between bodily integrity and the preservation of life in this context may have significant ramifications for such issues as abortion, contraception, sterilization, and population control.

Background—Cases and Commentators

Judicial intervention to secure lifesaving medical treatment most commonly involves minors whose parents voice religious objections to blood transfusions or operations. In these situations, the cases have uniformly upheld state interference with parents' control in order to safeguard the children.[10] Religious objections have been overridden by resort to the state's traditional parens patriae authority—its right and duty to protect the disabled, meaning those unable to care for themselves. Normally, this parens patriae doctrine is embodied in "neglect" statutes authorizing state intervention for parental failure to provide necessary medical care.[11] But there have been indications that such intervention would be forthcoming even in the absence of specific legislation.[12] In short, protection of child welfare has been viewed as a paramount state interest and courts have consistently ordered lifesaving medical treatment for minors.

No similar "neglect" statutes authorize judicial interference when competent adults fail to secure necessary medical treatment, nor does the common law parens patriae doctrine extend beyond protection of the disabled. Moreover, adults' cases have usually entailed religious or other principled objections to treatment raised by the patient whose own bodily integrity is threatened. The cases involving adults' refusal of treatment are, therefore, considerably more complex than those involving minors and the judicial results have varied accordingly.

Where the patient declining care was a parent of a minor child, the courts have been prone to appoint a guardian to authorize treatment.[13] The most famous example is Application of the President and Directors of Georgetown College.[14] There, a 25-year-old female Jehovah's Witness had refused a blood transfusion despite mortal danger posed by a ruptured ulcer. The patient was the mother of a seven month old child but both the patient and her husband refused to authorize the transfusion.[15] After a United States district court judge had rejected the hospital's request for judicial intervention, Circuit Judge J. Skelly Wright authorized the transfusion, citing a number of considerations to support his decision. Primarily, he viewed the case as embodying an extension of the traditional parens patriae doctrine. Since the state could generally guard a child's well being, and prevent the child's abandonment, it could also act to prevent this "ultimate abandonment" of a child by its parent.[16] He failed, however, to clearly indicate whether the state's precise interest lay in avoiding a fiscal burden[17] or in preserving the emotional well being of a minor. Presumably, the latter was the predominant factor, since a spouse remained to provide economic security for the surviving child. Judge Wright also noted the interests of the hospital and physicians who had assumed responsibility for treatment and cure and wanted to pursue their professional skills. To let the patient die without a transfusion would run counter to their professional judgments and might expose them to civil or criminal liability.[18] This dilemma could be obviated by judicial authorization of treatment. Judge Wright also contended that court authorization would entail only minor infringement upon the patient's religious beliefs. According to

the court, the religious prohibition attached to consenting to a blood transfusion; thus, submission to a court-ordered transfusion would not contravene the patient's religious scruples.[19] Finally, in an effort to glean further support for judicial intervention, Judge Wright analogized a refusal of medical treatment to suicide and pointed toward criminal penalties for attempted suicide as proof of legitimate legislative opposition to suicide.[20] He could not rely heavily on the suicide analogy only because the legal status of attempted suicide in his jurisdiction was unclear.

The District of Columbia Circuit Court en banc refused to address the merits of the Georgetown College case, so it cannot be considered strong precedent in that jurisdiction.[21] Nonetheless, the case has had a considerable persuasive impact. It has been followed where minor dependents were involved,[22] where only a spouse would have survived the patient,[23] and where no dependents were present.[24]

The recent decision of the New Jersey Supreme Court in John F. Kennedy Memorial Hospital v. Heston[25] represents a major appellate call for judicial intervention even in the absence of minor children. The case dealt with a 22-year-old, unmarried woman who had been severely injured in an automobile accident. Although there was considerable dispute over the woman's competency at the time of hospital admission,[26] it was clear that she had been for some time a Jehovah's Witness opposed to blood transfusions, and her mother, also a Jehovah's Witness, refused to authorize a necessary blood transfusion. Upon petition of the hospital, a lower court judge appointed a temporary guardian and the transfusion was given. On appeal, New Jersey's highest court unanimously upheld the judicial action. The opinion by Chief Justice Weintraub cited two interests sufficient to justify judicial intervention—the state's interest in preserving life and the hospital's interest in pursuing its functions without the threat of liability.[27] The interest in "life" was recited without much elaboration as to the precise governmental concerns involved, whether economic, political, or simply paternalistic. As evidence of the state's legitimate concern with sustaining life, the opinion pointed to the legislative proscription of attempted suicide.[28] Chief Justice Weintraub observed that through the police, the state commonly intervenes to prevent suicide. He concluded that whatever interests justify such intervention also support the overriding of an individual's refusal of lifesaving attention. According to the court, "if the State may interrupt one mode of self-destruction, it may with equal authority interfere with the other."[29]

The court next considered the position of the hospital and staff in the controversy. Not to pursue lifesaving treatment would violate professional creeds. Moreover, civil liability might flow from failure to render treatment, unless a valid release was available. The court preferred to authorize treatment over the patient's objections rather than subject the professional staff to the task of assessing the patient's competency or a release's validity.[30]

The preceding discussion notwithstanding, judicial sentiment is by no means unanimous in favor of court-ordered treatment. The most articulate statement for the position opposing interference with a patient's decision is In re Brooks' Estate. [31] There, the patient, a female Jehovah's Witness, refused a transfusion necessary to the treatment of a peptic ulcer.[32] The patient had a spouse and adult children, but they did not oppose her refusal. In a unanimous decision, the Supreme Court of Illinois upheld the patient's right to determine her own fate. Although the hospital's representative asserted an overriding societal interest in protecting the lives of citizens, the court perceived no immediate threat to the public health, safety, or welfare sufficient to outweigh the patient's interest in religious freedom. The court commented:

Even though we may consider [Mrs. Brooks'] beliefs unwise, foolish or ridiculous, in the absence of an overriding danger to society we may not permit interference therewith . . . for the sole purpose of compelling her to accept medical treatment forbidden by her religious principles, and previously refused by her with full knowledge of the probable consequences.[33]

In dictum, the opinion conceded that the result might be different if Mrs. Brooks had minor children, since the state would then have an interest in preventing the children from becoming wards of the state.[34]

Judicial refusal to override a patient's rejection of medical treatment has been reached in several other cases. In Erickson v. Dilgard, [35] the court supported the patient's refusal of a blood transfusion despite a "very great chance" that the consequence would be death from internal bleeding. No reason for the refusal, religious or otherwise, was articulated in the opinion. The court nonetheless ruled in favor of individual self-determination, commenting:

[I]t is the individual who is the subject of a medical decision who has the final say and . . . this must necessarily be so in a system of government which gives the greatest possible protection to the individual in the furtherance of his own desires.[36]

In an unreported 1972 case,[37] a Milwaukee judge declined to appoint a temporary guardian for a 77-year-old woman who had refused to permit amputation of a gangrenous leg. Although the patient was physically weak, the court noted her clear determination to avoid the surgical procedure and ruled that competent adults have the prerogative of making life and death medical decisions about their own bodies. The court's opinion observed: "I believe we should leave [the patient] depart in God's own peace."[38] The patient died several weeks after the decision.[39]

Commentators upon patients' refusal of lifesaving treatment have expressed views almost as varied as those of the courts.[40] There is widespread support for judicial intervention where the patient has a minor child,[41] grounded on the public interest both in avoiding an economic burden and in protecting the emotional well being of a youngster. Beyond this point, attitudes toward compelled treatment diverge. Some sources regard the state's interest in preserving life as too chimerical to justify interference with an adult's private decision on how to control his body.[42] They perceive no real threat to public safety or welfare, or to the welfare of any third parties from a patient's refusal of treatment and, therefore, find no basis to override an individual's convictions. They note that although the law generally compels adults to care

for their dependents, it does not compel self-care.[43] Other sources concede governmental power to intercede and render lifesaving treatment but counsel against exercise of such authority.[44] According to this view, preservation of life promotes a healthy and thriving population and therefore constitutes an important societal interest. However, respect for individual self-determination and recognition that refusals of lifesaving treatment do not pose a substantial threat to societal well being dictate against judicial intervention. There is some sentiment that judicial compulsion of lifesaving treatment is not only permissible, but desirable.[45] According to this view, the state's interest in preserving life—even by overriding individual choice—is real and compelling. Not only is society preserved and strengthened by the sustenance of the patient, but general respect for the sanctity of life is reinforced. The traditional negative attitude of the law toward suicide and euthanasia is cited as support for interference with individual decisions consenting to death. These sources consider compelled treatment to be only a minor infringement upon religious liberty since the individual may follow all his religious dictates except in the life and death situation. Submission to court-ordered treatment would not violate the patient's religious convictions.

These divergent viewpoints, both judicial and scholarly, reflect the complexity of the issues involved in refusal of lifesaving medical assistance. Before attempting resolution of these delicate issues, however, it is important to consider the legal framework in which judges contemplating intervention must operate.

Constitutional and Common Law Standards

The "right" of an individual to determine when bodily invasions will occur is by no means a novel jurisprudential concept. Bodily integrity has often been recognized by the judiciary as an important value and has enjoyed protection under both the common law and the Constitution. In an 1891 decision repudiating attempts to compel a personal injury plaintiff to undergo pretrial medical examination, the United States Supreme Court commented:

No right is held more sacred, or is more carefully guarded, by the common law, than the right of every individual to the possession and control of his own person, free from all restraint or interference by others, unless by clear and unquestionable authority of law.[46]

More recently, the medical patient's right to bodily control has been embodied in the tort doctrine of informed consent. Under this doctrine, no medical procedure may be performed without a patient's consent, obtained after explanation of the nature of the treatment, substantial risks, and alternative therapies.[47] The theory is variously expressed as assault, battery, negligence, malpractice, or even trespass, but the underlying concept of protection of bodily integrity remains the crux of informed consent. The doctrine recognizes that the consequence of a physician's explanation and consultation may be a patient's refusal of treatment and assumption of the risk of harm.[48] Indeed, it has been acknowledged that the exercise of self-determination by the patient may mean the spurning of lifesaving assistance. As expressed by one court:

Anglo American law starts with the premise of thorough-going self determination. It follows that each man is considered to be master of his own body, and he may, if he be of sound mind, expressly prohibit the performance of lifesaving surgery, or other medical treatment. A doctor might well believe that an operation or form of treatment is desirable or necessary, but the law does not permit him to substitute his own judgment for that of the patient by any form of artifice or deception.[49]

There is an exception to the informed consent requirement in "emergency" situations, grounded not on the imminence of death, but on the patient's incapacity and the presumption that the patient would, if physically able, authorize medical treatment.[50] The emergency exception does not, therefore, affect the case of a competent adult or that of an adult whose convictions are asserted by a valid representative.

It is not suggested that the doctrine of informed consent precludes judicial intervention to compel lifesaving treatment. The doctrine is a judicial construct which can either be narrowly interpreted to bar only non-judicially authorized treatment or can be modified. Moreover, the threat of civil

liability for lifesaving treatment cannot be a very effective deterrent for physicians since the value of the benefit conferred—preservation of life—must be set off against any damages from the technical trespass.[51] But the doctrine of informed consent does demonstrate profound legal concern for bodily integrity and individual self-determination. These latter interests are directly at stake in resolving the issue of compelled lifesaving treatment.

The Constitution also bears directly upon resolution of the issue. Many, if not most, of the reported cases involve religiously motivated rejection of treatment, usually a Jehovah's Witness' refusal of a blood transfusion. In such instances, the free exercise clause of the first amendment (as applied to the states through the fourteenth amendment) is inevitably raised as the guarantor of individual choice. Since religious liberty is not absolute,[52] the issue is how to appraise compelled treatment in light of the first amendment. The applicable constitutional standard has been articulated as requiring a finding of "grave abuses" endangering "paramount state interests" to justify infringement of religious liberty.[53] The search for a paramount state interest is, therefore, an integral part of any free exercise case. The basic approach, however, requires balancing the state interests involved against the constitutional liberties at stake, keeping in mind that society, as well as the individual, benefits from the maintenance of basic liberties.

Last term, in *Wisconsin v. Yoder,*[54] the Supreme Court made eminently clear that balancing is the appropriate approach in a free exercise case. The Court addressed a Wisconsin statute requiring school attendance until age 16. The law was alleged to infringe upon free exercise of the Amish religion, which demanded devotion to nature and the soil and avoidance of worldly influence. The Amish contended that continued exposure to secular education beyond age 14 would undermine their youngsters' beliefs and eventually destroy the religion. In a six-to-one decision the Court upheld the Amish claim, finding that the threats to the Amish religion posed by the compulsory attendance law outweighed state interests in promoting an

effective political system (educated electorate) and a self-reliant population. Chief Justice Burger's majority opinion clearly articulated a balancing test.[55]

Yoder also demonstrates that use of a balancing test entails much more than the abstract weighing of "state interests" and "individual freedom." Assessment of the extent of harm threatened by enforcement or nonenforcement of the disputed statute or policy is required. For example, the *Yoder* opinion considered the magnitude of harm posed to the Amish religion by two additional years of education and the societal benefits derived from the two years.[56] The Court could not perceive significant benefits to the quality of citizenship or to the self-reliance of the population stemming from two more years of education. In short, the Court looked to the actual impact of the law upon both the state interests and religious freedoms invoked.[57]

This intricate balancing technique has important implications for the issue of court-ordered medical treatment. It suggests that abstract weighing of bodily integrity against the preservation of life is too simplistic. The underlying state interests must be determined and the harm to those interests from allowing patients to die must be assessed. For example, if the social harm lies in a diminished populace, the number of people likely to reject lifesaving medical treatment must be appraised. Similarly, the degree of interference with religious or philosophical tenets must be gauged. This type of analysis will be applied in succeeding pages.

Of course, the free exercise clause does not provide the only constitutional bulwark for bodily integrity. The emerging concept of privacy[58] undoubtedly gives constitutional dimension to the individual's asserted right to control his body. A "right to be let alone" has long been discussed in the context of the fourth amendment.[59] In *Schmerber v. California,*[60] concerning a police ordered blood test to procure proof of drunken driving, the Supreme Court applied fourth amendment limitations to a bodily invasion to obtain evidence of crime. While upholding the governmental intrusion in the context of that case, the Court acknowledged that "the integrity of an individual's person is a cherished value in our society," and that the human dignity and privacy at stake are "fundamental human interests."[61] Moreover, it is clear that personal privacy is protected by constitutional provisions other than the fourth amendment.[62] *Griswold v. Connecticut*[63] indicated that the constitutional source of personal privacy lies in the first, fourth, fifth, ninth, and fourteenth amendments.[64] While *Griswold* only dealt with marital privacy, there can be little doubt that the right to personal privacy extends well beyond a married couple's use of contraceptives. Last term, in *Eisenstadt v. Baird,*[65] a case involving the regulation of contraceptive dissemination, four Justices observed: "If the right of privacy means anything, it is the right of the *individual,* married or single, to be free from unwarranted governmental intrusion into matters so fundamentally affecting a person as the decision whether to bear or beget a child."[66] Nor can the concept of personal privacy be limited to matters of sexual privacy. In the context of challenges to abortion laws, several federal courts have spoken broadly of a woman's right to control her own body.[67] Indeed, this broad approach is necessary, for if only the decision of whether to beget children is constitutionally protected, it could be argued in abortion cases that the availability of contraceptives satisfies that interest. *Stanley v. Georgia*[68] also reinforces the notion that personal privacy extends well beyond matters of procreation. In ruling that a person could not be punished for private possession of obscene material, the Court acknowledged the "fundamental . . . right to be free, except in very limited circumstances, from unwarranted governmental intrusions into one's privacy."[69] These cases, taken together, indicate that basic physical privacy is entitled to constitutional protection from governmental invasion.

It would not be accurate to talk about an undifferentiated "right to privacy." There are many different facets of personal privacy including personal appearance, sexual conduct, confidentiality of personal information, a physical zone of privacy, privacy of belief and thought, and freedom from bodily intrusion. Not all of these interests may be regarded as fundamental. Moreover,

different constitutional provisions may protect different aspects of privacy. For example, governmental intrusions to obtain evidence of crime are governed by the fourth amendment, while personal belief is guarded by the first amendment and nonevidentiary bodily invasions are protected by a penumbral right of personal privacy. The point remains, however, that no more basic aspect of personal privacy can be found than bodily integrity, and this interest is entitled to concomitant constitutional protection.

In many instances, including refusal of medical treatment, a matter relating to bodily control also entails significant ramifications for a person's future lifestyle or condition. Refusal of treatment determines not just whether a bodily invasion will take place, but whether the patient will live. Abortion determines not just whether an operation takes place or a birth proceeds, but whether the mother will have an offspring to nurture, support, and raise. Because of such long range implications, I have referred to the refusal of lifesaving treatment as involving a right to self-determination, meaning liberty to choose a lifestyle or course of conduct. This interest has a constitutional dimension and is covered by the fourteenth amendment guarantee of liberty, that is, substantive due process. However, bodily control or integrity involves not just liberty to act, but preservation of a domain of personal privacy. Protection of the immediate person and surroundings of an individual is explicitly provided in the first, fourth, and fifth amendments, and by a broader right of privacy deriving from these explicit provisions.[70] My thesis is that this broader right of privacy will be viewed as a fundamental aspect of personal liberty, a prerequisite or predicate to the exercise of all other liberties. A strict scrutiny approach, including a search for a compelling state interest, should, therefore, be employed where governmental invasions of bodily privacy occur.[71] Although refusal of treatment involves both self-determination (liberty) and bodily control, it must be judged according to the stricter protections surrounding personal privacy.

This constitutional protection has import for consideration of compelled treatment. The person who declines medical assistance for philosophical or

personal reasons, as opposed to religious commands, can also invoke the Constitution. Of course, bodily control is no more an absolute prerogative than religious freedom,[72] but the constitutional standard used to test the validity of judicially compelled treatment will remain substantially the same whether the patient relies upon the free exercise clause or penumbral guarantees of privacy. That is, to justify an invasion of bodily integrity the state will have to demonstrate that a compelling state interest exists, and that it outweighs countervailing interests in individual rights.[73] As previously noted, this entails careful assessment of the asserted state interests and the extent of harm posed to them by upholding the individual's privacy and self-determination. With this standard in mind, consideration of the specific interests at stake in the issue of lifesaving treatment can be undertaken.

Analysis of Interests

A variety of public interests have been arrayed both by courts and commentators in support of judicial intervention to order lifesaving medical treatment for a reluctant patient. These interests run the gamut from a noble reference to the sanctity of life to a banal concern for the economic burden left by a patient who dies after refusing treatment. Most of these interests have been described briefly in the prior discussion of case law on point.[74] A few have not. All deserve careful scrutiny.

Preservation of Society

One writer has argued that the "importance of the individual's life to the welfare of society" precludes allowing a patient to spurn lifesaving treatment.[75] This is an appealing notion, but it cannot withstand critical examination. Certainly, a society and its duly constituted institutions have a strong and legitimate interest in their own preservation.[76] Any significant diminution in population might be a matter of real concern, but no one has ever suggested that the volume of persons declining medical treatment constitutes a threat to the maintenance of population levels. Nor is the refusal of treatment an act likely to be widely imitated or duplicated if openly allowed;[77] it is unlike narcotics addiction in that respect.[78] In short, society's existence is by no means threatened by patients' refusals of treatment.

The state also has a legitimate interest in promoting a thriving and productive population. Compulsory education laws are one manifestation of such an interest, yielding both economic and political benefits to society as a whole. In this context, the state might assert an interest in the productivity of an individual—talents, skills, taxpaying potential, military service potential—justifying compelled treatment to keep the individual alive. It is submitted, however, that this concern with productivity cannot override the competing interests in bodily integrity or religious liberty. In the first place, the marginal social utility involved is generally outweighed by the direct and immediate invasion of the patient's personal privacy,[79] both because of the small numbers involved and the attenuated impact on the economy. Secondly, in each instance of refusal, the societal interest would vary according to the individual patient's attributes. In terms of productivity, for example, an industrialist or nuclear physicist has more "social worth" than a vagrant. The problem here is obvious. It is both unseemly and unrealistic to measure the social worth of each patient who declines medical treatment.[80] One solution would be to assume the high value of every patient.[81] But this approach exalts the interest of government, the state, or society over individual self-determination.[82] It is also a fictive approach since in reality the vast majority of us do not contribute so much to the social fabric as to enable the state to claim a paramount interest in our preservation.

Sanctity of Life

The state has an indisputable interest in the preservation of life. The criminal law and police power are focused on the protection of public safety. But this use of governmental authority is grounded on the assumption that citizens invariably want to enjoy bodily safety and uninterrupted life. Where a competent individual chooses to decline lifesaving treatment, the normal congruity of interest between individual welfare and state protection against

death is disrupted. Entirely new interests, self-determination and privacy from state intrusions, are asserted. The assumption that the citizen demands self-preservation can no longer be operative.

Some writers have nonetheless argued that preservation of a resisting patient's life is relevant to the lives and safety of the general public. The theory is that by denying the patient an opportunity to choose death, a court promotes general respect for life. If a court acquiesced in a patient's rejection of treatment and consequent death, the value of life would be degraded since "any exception to the sanctity of life cannot but cheapen it."[83]

This argument cannot be taken lightly. Sanctity of life is not just a vague theological precept. It is the foundation of a free society. Indeed, libertarians recently campaigned against capital punishment on a similar theory that destruction of life (even the life of a convicted malefactor) degrades the value of life and undermines a society's regard for its sanctity. The countervailing consideration, of course, is the dignity tied up with bodily control and self-determination.

Control by men over their circumstances of action is, along with knowledge of their circumstances, an indispensable part of their personal integrity. Knowledge and control are what make the difference between puppets and people.[84]

It is true that non-interference in an individual's decision to refuse treatment may mean that the patient dies for a reason which may appear silly or inconsequential to most observers. But the rejection of lifesaving medical treatment normally represents a principled invocation of personal or religious convictions, not a deprecation of life. Restraint by courts would be impelled by profound respect for the individual's bodily integrity and religious freedom, not by disregard or disdain for the sanctity of life.[85] Human dignity is enhanced by permitting the individual to determine for himself what beliefs are worth dying for. Through the ages, a multitude of noble causes, religious and secular, have been regarded as worthy of self-sacrifice.[86] Certainly, most governments and societies, our own included, do not consider the sanctity of life to be the supreme value.

Nations still insist on the prerogative to engage in mass killing for furtherance of the "national interest," "wars of liberation," or the "defense of democracy."[87] Bodily control, self-determination, and religious freedom are beneficial both to the individual and to the society whose atmosphere and tone are determined by the human values which it respects.

Public Morals

As the debate over so-called victimless crimes[88] illustrates, the use of law to reinforce a dominant morality without tangible benefit to public health, safety, and welfare is fraught with difficulties. This is particularly true where the moral underpinnings of laws no longer enjoy a wide community consensus. Many laws aimed primarily at morality nonetheless have been enacted and we must acknowledge that all law is infused with some moral view.

These factors are relevant here because the rejection of lifesaving treatment is a form of suicide—in that it is a voluntary act undertaken with knowledge that death will likely result.[89] Suicide, in turn, has traditionally been anathema in a Judaeo-Christian culture. In the religious sphere, the revulsion toward suicide is grounded primarily on the sixth commandment and the belief that only a divinity can control the withdrawal of life.[90] Antipathy toward suicide, however, extends well beyond the theological realm and public attitudes have sometimes mirrored religious ones. The English common law attached both criminal and civil penalties to suicide or attempted suicide.[91] Suicide was viewed as an offense against nature, violating instincts of self-preservation, as well as an offense against God, the society, and the king. The common revulsion of western culture toward self-imposed death has, then, an ethical or moral base as well as a religious one. Self-destruction is considered to be contrary to man's natural inclinations, a deprivation of a person's productive capacity, an evil example to others and even a rude expression of contempt for society.[92] "Public morals," specifically the "immorality" of self-destruction, cannot provide a legitimate basis for intervention in the patient's decision however. Contemporary condemnation of suicide as "immoral" is largely clerical in nature and public attitudes toward suicide have markedly changed. While embarrassment about the subject persists, the individual is no longer generally regarded as a sinner or crazed demon.[93] Changes in law have accompanied changes in public opinion. In the vast majority of states, attempted suicide is no longer covered by the criminal law.[94] To the extent that anti-suicide laws remain on the books, they are directed toward authorizing officials to take temporary custody of the individual to prevent the immediate infliction of harm and to render psychological assistance.[95] Suicide is no longer considered, either legally or popularly, as inherently immoral. A morality grounded on an individual's service to the state would be threatened by a patient's conduct in refusing treatment. However, that moral scheme is not widely accepted within a democratic society which stresses maximum individual liberty compatible with the comfort and welfare of others.

Protection of the Individual against Himself

Normally, the state's police power is exercised for the general public's health, safety, or welfare. This is so even in the case of certain ostensibly individual invasions, such as compulsory immunizations or blood tests. There are a few areas of law, however, where the state apparently undertakes to protect the individual against his own imprudence.

The "snake cases," involving statutory prohibition of the public handling of snakes, provide one commonly cited example of government paternalism. A number of courts have sustained the validity of such statutes against claims by fundamentalist religious sects that the prohibitions interfere with their expression of religious faith.[96] These cases do not, however, stand for the proposition that government can readily interfere with an individual's course of conduct in order to prevent the individual from harming himself. For these statutes undoubtedly protect observers and peripheral participants, as well as the snake handlers themselves. No court has addressed the issue of whether a legislature could protect the handler alone.[97]

The motorcycle helmet cases are more apposite. Scores of state cases have considered challenges to statutes requiring motorcyclists to wear protective helmets.[98] Motorcyclists claim that their individual liberty and privacy are infringed without a corresponding protection of legitimate public interests. The majority of courts have avoided the basic issue of whether state concern for the welfare of the cyclist can justify such requirements; they have made strained findings that all highway travelers are protected because cyclists struck by stones or limbs might lose control of their vehicles and injure others.[99] Thus, the public health, safety, and welfare is being promoted. A number of courts have proceeded beyond this fictive argument to address whether the state may protect an individual from himself.[100] The results are inconclusive. Several cases have urged that the police power encompasses authority to protect individuals despite their reluctance to be safeguarded.[101] A few cases have rules that the helmet statutes constitute unconstitutional infringements of liberty, since they have only a tenuous relation to public safety or welfare.[102] It is submitted that without a clearer judicial consensus, and without Supreme Court guidance, the motorcycle helmet cases provide no resolution of whether the state can generally protect individuals against themselves. Certainly, they do not determine the outcome where a patient resists compelled treatment and invokes religious freedom or a right to bodily integrity as his protection. Indeed, constitutional standards may differ where liberty (substantive due process) is invoked as opposed to religious freedom or bodily privacy.

There is, however, an area of paternalistic state conduct which has universally been upheld despite its ostensible interference with individual freedom of choice. A plethora of pure food and drug laws, licensure schemes, and regulations controlling noxious substances exists which incidentally prevents consumers from injuring themselves.[103] Even where the restrictions apply to sellers or distributors, the objective is to prevent the buyer from subjecting himself to risks which the government deems unadvisable.[104]

Some observers have articulated concern about the legal implications of this interference with individual self-determination,[105] but these protective health measures nonetheless proliferate. They are generally salutary and are seldom challenged. Yet they may occasionally prevent consumer access to an enjoyable food (for example, swordfish, cyclamate-containing beverages) or to an experimental drug which might be highly beneficial.[106] The individual is effectively precluded from selecting his own risks. Because such protective laws remain judicially inviolate,[107] the question arises whether they provide an effective precedent for governmental prevention of individual risk-taking which might be extended to the life-saving medical treatment problem.

Most protective legislation is clearly warranted because it guards against abuses which individual consumers are generally helpless to detect or control. For example, most consumers cannot determine the minimum competency of a physician, the iodine content of a food, or the spoilage of meat without regulatory controls. Furthermore consumers alone may be impotent to eliminate the dangerous products of an entire industry (for example, flammable fabrics or unsafe cars). The regulated items also have such wide potential distribution that the public safety and welfare is actually promoted by the protective legislation. These observations about regulatory schemes, however, in no way apply to refusal of medical treatment, since judicial intervention to compel treatment is a very different matter than common regulatory controls. Although both forms of governmental action interfere with individual choice, the regulatory schemes are generally impelled by conditions which preclude real individual choice.[108] The elimination of dangerous products also constitutes, in most instances, a lesser deprivation than interference with religious liberty or bodily integrity.[109] Thus, while precedents may be cited for government efforts to preclude individual risk-taking, none sanction judicial intervention to protect a patient against his own decision to decline treatment. Clearly, there are limitations on attempts to guarantee the individual's safety, for otherwise an individual's personal habits, including eating and sleeping, would be potentially subject to governmental dictates.

The rights to freedom of religion and personal privacy circumscribe paternalistic impulses in the context of compelled medical treatment.

Protection of Third Parties

The patient's important interests in religious freedom or bodily integrity could be overridden if refusal of medical treatment were shown to inflict legally cognizable harm on persons other than the patient. Various third party injuries have been suggested by courts and commentators discussing compelled treatment. They all warrant consideration.

Surviving Adults The death of a relative or close friend may provoke grief, despair, or other emotional harm in the surviving person. This phenomenon will undoubtedly be present in cases of compelled treatment, and may be urged as a ground for judicial intervention.[110] It is submitted, however, that this factor cannot justify a court in overriding a patient's determination.[111] A variety of conduct by an individual may inflict emotional harm upon his loved ones. The dissolution of a marriage by separation or divorce, or simply abusive conduct toward loved ones can cause emotional wounds, yet no court would contemplate a judicial order to force an adult to be considerate or kind to adult relatives. A similar independence of conduct must be accorded to the patient who may be asserting religious or personal principles in his refusal of treatment. The emotional consequences to survivors will likely be temporary, should be tempered by respect for the patient's principled decision, and, in any event, do not outweigh the patient's interests at stake.

Fellow Patients One source has argued that a patient's rejection of lifesaving treatment will distract physicians, provoke turmoil in the hospital staff, and generally disrupt hospital procedure to the detriment of other patients.[112] This argument is speculative and seems rather farfetched. If the patient's choice is honored, precisely the converse of the predicted result should follow. That is, by declining treatment, medical care may well be reduced to the administration of analgesics, freeing staff to attend to other functions. Once a policy of

judicial nonintervention is established and publicized, the hospital staff will not expend futile effort in seeking court orders. Although there may be occasions when the rejection of therapy engenders medical complications which necessitate diverting hospital staff to the patient, this situation is more likely to be the exception than the rule and cannot operate as a general justification for judicial interference with patients' decisions.

Physicians Several courts have noted the interests of physicians in compelling lifesaving treatment.[113] One concern is that the physician, if required to respect the patient's choice to decline treatment, must act against his best professional judgment. It is difficult for a physician, trained and dedicated to preservation of life, to allow a salvageable patient to die. In addition, by withholding therapy, the physician may theoretically risk subsequent civil or criminal liability,[114] particularly if the physician were found to have honored an incompetent patient's choice.

While a physician's interest in proper practice of medicine is both valid and legally cognizable, the above concerns do not justify judicial intervention to compel lifesaving treatment. Unfettered exercise of medical judgment has never been a sacrosanct value. The doctrine of informed consent[115] is grounded on the premise that a physician's judgment is subservient to the patient's right to self-determination. Further, other situations exist where a physician's professional judgment is legally restricted or precluded. Laws governing contraception, narcotics, experimental drugs, and compulsory reporting[116] demonstrate that professional judgment is not always a paramount consideration. The assertion of constitutional interests in bodily integrity and free exercise of religion in the context of refusal of care deserve no less deference, even in derogation of a physician's best judgment. While it may be harrowing for a physician to determine whether a patient is voluntarily and competently declining lifesaving treatment,[117] difficult medical decisions must inevitably be made. This is so, for example, whenever a patient is certified as mentally ill for purposes of civil commitment or when a patient ostensibly consents to medical operations which entail substantial risks.

Surviving Minors As previously noted, both courts and commentators have supported judicial intervention to compel medical treatment where the patient is the parent of a minor child,[118] based on an extension of the parens patriae doctrine. Since the state can generally act to safeguard a child's welfare, it can act to prevent "ultimate abandonment" of a child by the parent's self-destruction. By keeping the parent alive, the child presumably benefits emotionally, by continued love and reassurance from the parent, and economically, by continued financial support.

The argument that a court should act to preserve the emotional well-being of children is an appealing one. The legitimacy of the state's interest can be sustained on either of two grounds: there may be altruistic concern with providing each child with a healthful environment, or, development of stable children may be viewed as promoting the political and social well-being of the country.[119] Of course, the loss of a parent will not always produce emotional harm in a child. Not all parents are loving and supportive of their children. It is conceivable that in some instances the surviving child would benefit emotionally from a court's acquiescence in the parent's decision to decline lifesaving treatment.[120] But judicial inquiry, on a case by case basis, into the complex emotional relationships among parents and children might well be too time-consuming and unpleasant to be undertaken. Assuming that the death of a parent will likely provoke some emotional harm to a surviving child, the question becomes whether that harm justifies exercise of the state's parens patriae authority to compel a patient to undergo unwanted treatment.

There are numerous situations where a child may be left alone by a parent with consequent emotional upheaval in the child. Death of a parent from natural causes, service in the armed forces, divorce, or even extended travel might cause some emotional wounds. Yet these unintended inflictions of emotional harm are never the source of state intervention; to suggest such intervention would undoubtedly provoke indignant cries of interference with personal liberty. Indeed, an infinite variety of parental conduct could be regulated if prevention of the infliction of emotional harm upon children were accepted as an unlimited basis for interference with parental conduct not intended to harm the child. The state could, under such a theory, compel medical checkups or dictate diets in order to preserve the health of parents.

Some interference with parental conduct is not only justified, but necessary, as the existence of "neglect" statutes demonstrates. Nevertheless, the loss of one of two parents because of the parent's adherence to religious or personal convictions in declining treatment is, arguably, too remote from the state's interest in a child's emotional well being to support judicial intervention.[121] Perhaps a legislature could make a contrary judgment and dictate intervention, but a court operating without such authorization must hesitate to intervene on the basis of protecting children's psychic well being.[122]

A second, less speculative basis exists for judicial intervention to preserve parents' lives—the economic interest of the state in avoiding the burden of supporting surviving children.[123] In many contexts, protection of the public fisc has served as a justification for state conduct or regulations which otherwise would be considered to infringe upon fundamental personal rights. This has been the case with compulsory sterilization laws,[124] motorcycle helmet laws,[125] and certain welfare regulations having an indirect impact on parents' behavior.[126] In *Wisconsin v. Yoder*,[127] the Supreme Court treated avoidance of "public wards" as a legitimate state interest to be balanced against competing individual rights. It must be conceded, then, that some judicial concern with the financial plight of a patient's survivors is both understandable and proper.

The economic issue is placed in even sharper perspective if the refusal of medical treatment threatens permanent disability but not death; for example, where rejection of a blood transfusion results in insufficient oxygen to the brain and consequent neurological damage. The ensuing permanent disability could result in the patient, as well as the surviving family, becoming public economic burdens. In such an instance, the economic impact would

be direct and probably substantial. Judicial intervention to avoid that impact would likely be sustained even in the face of constitutional challenges bottomed on privacy and religious freedom. Similar considerations would probably support judicial intervention where the patient by declining treatment would die and leave an impecunious family to be sustained by the public.[128]

Despite this concession, an important caveat should be considered before a court intervenes to compel treatment on an "avoidance of public wards" theory. The economic factors justifying intervention are not present in every case of a parent's refusal of treatment. The surviving spouse, accumulated savings, or other sources may be available to avoid penury even if the patient dies. Thus, the problem would have to be approached on a case by case basis and the economic circumstances sifted in each instance.[129] This type of judicial inquiry is neither difficult nor unseemly; courts commonly examine financial status with regard to support payments, bankruptcy, and enforcement of judgments, to cite a few examples. However, tying the question of judicial intervention to financial circumstances of the patient may prove distasteful to the judiciary. The effect is to tell the patient that his convictions will not be respected because he does not have enough money. It is at least arguable that this de facto wealth discrimination would violate the equal protection clause.[130] In any event, it appears rather mercenary to hinge exercise of rights of privacy and free exercise upon wealth. Perhaps the public should be expected to absorb the economic burden when the refusal of medical treatment leaves indigent survivors. Courts might well take this approach. In light of the relatively small number of people who can be expected to spurn medical treatment when they know their family will be left impecunious, the overall economic burden shifted to the public can be expected to be slight. Judges who rely on the public ward theory to compel lifesaving medical treatment will likely be impelled not by real concern for the public coffers, but by their personal distaste for the patient's decision.[131]

Implications For Other Areas of Law

Suicide

I have argued that a patient should normally have the prerogative of declining lifesaving medical treatment, both because of the constitutional principles involved and the lack of a sufficiently strong basis for judicial intervention. This raises important questions with regard to the legal status of suicide. Does a right to decline treatment imply a broader right to die? Or can judicial acquiescence in refusal of treatment be reconciled with traditional efforts of the legal system to prevent suicide? What of the patient whose rejection of treatment is tantamount to suicide because the patient wishes to die?

Several sources have contended that there is a close analogy between refusal of treatment and suicide, even where the refusal is not accompanied by a wish to die.[132] They argue that if an individual has a right to dictate his own death, the form—non-feasance in refusal of treatment as opposed to misfeasance in suicide—should not matter.[133] They point to the apparent legitimacy of governmental efforts to preclude suicide,[134] and assert that the same interests which justify such efforts also justify intervention to preclude refusal of treatment.[135] According to this view, it would be anomalous to permit refusal of treatment but to prevent suicide,[136] since the person who wishes to die is then obstructed but the person who wishes to live is permitted to die.

The meaning of "suicide," as contained in criminal statutes, may well exclude the case of a principled decision to refuse lifesaving medical treatment because such criminal enactments probably require a finding of specific intent to die,[137] a factor lacking in the religiously or philosophically motivated rejection of treatment. Although an actor is ordinarily presumed to intend the natural consequences of his act, this presumption would probably not be applied in this context; to do so would label the person who jumps in front of a car to save another a suicide. Similarly, refusal of treatment should not be considered to fall within the term "suicide" as contained in the criminal law. It is also true that attempted suicide has been eliminated from criminal codes in the vast majority of states.[138] Legislatures have recognized that deterrence is not accomplished by criminal sanctions of attempted suicide, and that intervention to secure treatment or assistance for the victim can be accomplished without need of the criminal law.[139] Yet, neither of these factors—narrowness of the technical definition of suicide or elimination of attempted suicide from the criminal law—negates the arguments of those who assert that the same interests supporting governmental intervention to block suicide also support judicial intervention to compel medical treatment. The issues of whether refusal of treatment is legally tantamount to suicide, or whether attempted suicide is a criminal offense, are therefore not determinative of whether a state can validly compel a reluctant patient to undergo treatment. If government efforts to prevent suicide are valid, and if the same interests supporting such efforts are applicable to the refusal of treatment, then the proponents of compelled treatment would appear to have a strong case. Their first premise, that efforts to prevent suicide by direct state intervention are valid, seems correct. One case raising a constitutional challenge to an attempted suicide statute was dismissed for want of a substantial federal question.[140] The question remains, however, whether the interests involved in suicide and refusal of treatment are sufficiently distinct to justify divergent legal treatment of the two phenomena.

The principal objective of governmental intervention in the area of suicide is to secure assistance for the individual. Such assistance is appropriate because many suicide attempts are the product of rash, unbalanced, or confused judgments. Admittedly, there is no simple explanation for the phenomenon of suicide. "A profound ambiguity of motives" characterizes both suicide in general and the actions of any particular individual.[141] For this reason, it is impossible to accurately categorize or quantify types of suicide. However, there seems to be a consensus that many suicide attempts are the products of mental disorder.[142] Some attempts are also acknowledged to be either conscious or subconscious cries for help, rather than determined efforts to die.[143] No criticism can be directed toward governmental efforts to reach

and assist persons who do not wish to die or whose action is the product of a temporary derangement. While it is true that the laws or practices aimed at preventing suicide do not differentiate according to the individual victim's motives, it is equally true that those factors cannot readily be determined without some initial intervention. "The natural and human thing to do with a person who is suddenly discovered attempting suicide is to interpose to prevent it."[144] Moreover, if the individual has made a deliberate choice to die, the state's intervention constitutes more a temporary postponement than a permanent proscription. A determined individual can likely find alternative times, places, and means to consummate his intended act. In the interim, intervention will only have ensured that the self-destruction is the product of a fixed and unalterable desire.[145]

Other elements differentiate the problem of suicide from refusal of medical treatment. The sheer magnitude of the suicide phenomenon makes it a cause for societal alarm. Over 20,000 people per year successfully commit suicide in the United States.[146] This accounts for 1% of annual deaths and places suicide among the 12 leading causes of death.[147] Even these figures do not expose the true magnitude of the problem; suicide is grossly underreported and many attempts at suicide are unsuccessful. In addition, there is some evidence that suicide produces an imitative effect, sometimes causing "epidemics" of self-destruction.[148] Even without this last speculative factor, the magnitude of the suicide phenomenon warrants serious governmental concern.

In sum, both the magnitude of the problem and certain attributes of the suicide phenomenon provide a solid basis for government intervention to prevent suicide. These factors are not, for the most part, present in refusal of lifesaving medical treatment. The volume of such refusals must be miniscule in comparison to attempted suicide. Most instances of refusal represent careful decisions to abide by religious or philosophical principles, and not rash attempts at self-destruction. There is normally an opportunity to test the sincerity, firmness, and rationality of a patient's decision to decline treatment without mooting the issue by medical

intervention. By insisting on his position, the patient directly invokes important constitutional principles of either religious freedom or personal privacy. Thus, there is ample basis for espousing governmental intervention in suicide cases while eschewing similar intervention to compel lifesaving medical treatment.

This leaves the problem of the patient who rejects medical treatment with the intent and wish to die, the patient who really is committing suicide by refusing treatment. This may be a small percentage of refusals of treatment; virtually every case which has come to my attention has involved a religiously motivated decision. But the suicidal refusal, particularly when the patient is suffering from serious illness and is threatened with loss of faculties, is not entirely implausible.[149] At the outset of this article I hypothesized several situations where the patient refusing treatment might be seeking death—the despondent patient who has lost the will to live, the terminally ill patient who wishes to avoid a painful deterioration and loss of dignity, and the protesting patient who hopes to become a political martyr. Even though these patients might not be making "principled" decisions in the sense of open reliance upon religious or philosophical scruples, serious considerations of bodily integrity and self-determination are still involved.

The important state interest in preventing rash or unbalanced self-destruction must be honored in this situation. Medical inquiry (or judicial inquiry if a court has been petitioned for intervention) into the patient's state of mind is appropriate. The patient must be competent and his decision to reject treatment must be deliberate and firm.[150] Otherwise, temporary intervention to provide psychological assistance (and medical treatment if the patient would die in the interim) is warranted, even if the patient's suicide wish is temporarily frustrated. If there is a genuine emergency, with no opportunity to assess the patient's state of mind, medical intervention should proceed.[151] If the patient demonstrates the requisite state of mind, however, and persists in refusal of treatment, that decision should be respected though tantamount to suicide. The distinction between principled and unprincipled action is not strong enough to warrant a different approach toward the suicide-patient than that taken toward the religiously motivated patient when both in reality are asserting rights to bodily integrity, personal privacy, and self-determination.[152] This position, that the patient wishing to die should be permitted to decline treatment, has distinct implications for legal approaches to suicide generally. In effect, it means that the "serious suicide," the person whose decision to die is clearly competent, deliberate, and firm, should be permitted to die. The form of self-destruction, refusal of treatment versus slashing of wrists or whatever, should not matter.[153]

Euthanasia

Euthanasia, or mercy killing, is generally defined as the deliberate killing by a physician or other party of a person suffering from a painful and terminal illness.[154] Although an affirmative act by the physician (for example, an injection) is normally thought to be a component of euthanasia, the withholding of medical treatment or therapy may be considered to be a form of euthanasia. I have argued that withholding of medical treatment at the request of a competent adult patient is not only legally defensible, but that a court cannot constitutionally intervene to authorize treatment. This raises several issues. Does my position conflict with established legal postures toward euthanasia? Does my position mean that euthanasia in the form of affirmative killing must also be countenanced?

It is well established in criminal law that an affirmative act of euthanasia constitutes homicide.[155] A person is not legally permitted to consent to the infliction of death upon himself by another. While judges and juries appear to show extreme solicitude toward persons accused of euthanasia, the act is clearly illegal under contemporary doctrine. The legal status of the physician who merely withholds treatment at the request of the patient is in great dispute. Most commentators merely state that the legality of such an act of omission is uncertain.[156] The precise issue is whether the special physician-patient relationship imposes upon the physician an automatic duty to take every step to preserve the patient's life. Glanville Williams asserts that a physician's inaction at the patient's behest is

probably lawful.[157] Yale Kamisar argues that the physician who withholds life-preserving treatment "commits criminal homicide by omission."[158] All sources agree that no physician has ever been indicted or convicted for any such crime.

The legal relationship between the physician and the dying patient is murky. Physicians commonly administer analgesics which shorten a patient's life.[159] No one apparently regards this as illegal. Even though death may be accelerated, the countervailing necessity to relieve suffering prevails. Also, a point is inevitably reached in the demise of a terminally ill patient when medical treatment no longer preserves life, but rather prolongs the act of dying.[160] It seems inconceivable that the patient's competent exercise of a right to decline further treatment could be denied at that point. Some authorities meet this last situation by acknowledging that "extraordinary" medical techniques need not be employed to keep a patient alive. Presumably, this would permit disconnecting extraordinary equipment. Yet no one has defined the term "extraordinary" with precision; blood transfusions and intravenous feeding are probably considered "ordinary," while heart-lung machines and artificial respirators are not.

In light of this general confusion regarding the physician's responsibility toward the dying patient, I have little difficulty extending my basic position—that a physician must legally respect a patient's decision to reject treatment—to the terminally ill patient. The same considerations of bodily integrity and self-determination apply. They assume added importance where the patient faces a loss of faculties and dignity before inevitably succumbing. I stop short, however, of espousing euthanasia in the form of affirmative physicians' acts to kill a patient.

The arguments in favor of affirmative acts of euthanasia are appealing; indeed, they rely on some of the same values which support the patient's refusal of treatment. The basic contention is that voluntary euthanasia supports human dignity. The suffering patient in the throes of terminal illness is relieved of the indignity of a life endured without faculties or self-control.[161] A host of objections have, however, been raised

against legalization. Some of them are spurious,[162] but others are substantial. For example, Professor Kamisar discusses at length the problem of assessing the "voluntariness" of a consent by a patient who, by definition, is a victim of terminal illness and is either experiencing considerable pain or is drugged.[163] Several sources also contend that legal acceptance of an act of killing where a life is "not worth living" would undermine respect for life and lay a foundation for acceptance of involuntary euthanasia.[164] Proponents of euthanasia have advanced a variety of protective procedural schemes to forestall some of these criticisms. Mandatory time intervals to allow a patient to contemplate or reconsider and intervention of neutral third parties or referees to confirm the diagnosis and verify the patient's consent have been proposed.[165]

The most serious argument against voluntary euthanasia—that it would eventually lead to involuntary euthanasia—is not convincing. So long as careful attention is paid to the capacity of a person to request euthanasia, there is a large gap between voluntary euthanasia and involuntary elimination of societal misfits. One does not necessarily flow from the other. I am bothered, however, by authorizing an affirmative act which would destroy another human being. A patient's request to terminate further therapy should be honored, but affirmative acts (injections, etc.) to terminate patients' lives should not be condoned.[166] If affirmative medical conduct to end the patient's life[167] is prohibited, the patient is allowed maximum opportunity to change his mind and demand treatment. The patient declining treatment normally remains alive for a period and thereby receives some opportunity to articulate or demonstrate any change of mind or to eliminate any mistake on the physician's part in comprehending the patient's wishes. Authorization of affirmative acts of mercy killing would necessitate changes in state criminal law which might arguably constitute official recognition of the "worthlessness" of some life. A physician's deference to a patient's decision to refuse medical treatment is not currently criminal, and no statutory changes are needed to sustain refusals of treatment. The physician who respects the patient's choice, as required by the doctrine of informed consent, is not concurring in the dying patient's possible evaluation of his life as "worthless," as might be the case if the physician voluntarily administered fatal drugs.

The line between withholding treatment at the patient's request and active administration of death may be difficult to draw and may seem somewhat arbitrary. This is particularly so where the "affirmative acts" are the disconnection of life-sustaining equipment or placement of a poison capsule within reach of the patient. Both acts fall somewhere in the spectrum between passive withholding of treatment and active administration of a fatal injection. While a determination can eventually be made as to whether disconnection of life-sustaining equipment is an "affirmative act," that determination will probably be based on a subjective characterization of the physician's action.[168] More importantly, it is not clear that active administration of death at the patient's request is morally very different from withholding treatment. Nonetheless, the considerations mentioned in the preceding paragraph lead me to the position that affirmative acts of euthanasia should continue to be proscribed while the patient's decision to decline lifesaving treatment must be respected. In any event, it is clear that acceptance of a right to decline treatment does not compel broad acceptance of euthanasia in all forms.

State Regulation of Human Reproduction

There are a number of other legal areas where bodily integrity and control are threatened by governmental interference. Interference with personal decisions concerning human reproduction—including abortion,[169] sterilization,[170] contraception,[171] and population control[172]—is one of these areas which has already become and will continue to be a constitutional battleground. The prior discussion of refusal of lifesaving medical treatment has direct implications for resolution of these controversies. Certainly, it affirms the constitutional status of bodily integrity and articulates the approach to be employed in testing the validity of governmental policies affecting procrea-

tion. In some instances, the conflicting interests involved are analogous to those interests involved in the issue of compelled medical treatment. For example, the abortion controversy arrays bodily control and self-determination against interests in the prospective life of the foetus[173] and in reinforcement of conventional morality.[174] Challenges to involuntary sterilization pit bodily integrity and self-determination against asserted state interests in promotion of a healthy population, protection of children's well-being, and state avoidance of economic burdens. The precise interests and degrees of harm to those interests vary as to each area of law. Detailed analysis of these topics has not been attempted here. It should be noted, however, that resolution of the issue of compelled medical treatment in favor of respecting the patient's decision and preserving bodily integrity does not necessarily mean that personal privacy should prevail on all of the above issues concerning human reproduction. The balancing process in each instance will be complex, defying easy prediction of constitutional results.[175]

Conclusion

As to an independent adult who genuinely objects to treatment, the patient's decision to refuse lifesaving treatment must be respected by the judiciary no matter what the reason for refusal. Respect for bodily integrity, as dictated by constitutional rights of personal privacy,[176] mandates this result in light of the inadequacy or inapplicability of asserted governmental interests in compelling treatment. Even where familial circumstances would constitutionally permit judicial intervention, a judge should normally respect the patient's decision. Intervention to protect survivors' emotional or economic interests, with concomitant government avoidance of fiscal burdens, would too often reflect judicial distaste for a decision to accept death rather than recognition of compelling state interests sufficient to override a patient's decision.

Acceptance of a patient's right to decline lifesaving treatment will mean emotional strain for both physicians and judges. On occasion, it will even be difficult to determine whether the

patient's decision is the product of a sound mind. Yet deference to the patient's refusal of treatment[177] reflects sensitivity toward personal interests in bodily integrity and self-determination, not callousness toward life.

Notes

1. Several religious sects treat disease solely by prayer and regard recourse to medical science as a gross act of non-faith. Cawley, *The Right to Live* 25–26 (1969) [hereinafter cited as Cawley].

2. Jehovah's Witnesses, while not objecting to medical treatment generally, believe that blood transfusions violate biblical injunctions against "eating blood." The biblical sources of these injunctions are Acts 15:28–29, Deuteronomy 12:33, Genesis 9:3–4, and Leviticus 17:10–14. The application of the biblical language to blood transfusions has sometimes been criticized as defective theological reasoning. See Ford, Refusal of Blood Transfusions by Jehovah's Witnesses, 10 *Cath. Law.* 212, 213 (1964) [hereinafter cited as Ford], but many Jehovah's Witnesses would rather die than receive a transfusion. They consider it to be "a serious violation of the law of God for which transgressors will be called upon by God to account for and be punished for their sins." Note, An Adult's Right to Resist Blood Transfusions: A View Through John F. Kennedy Memorial Hospital v. Heston, 47 *Notre Dame Law.* 571 (1972) [hereinafter cited as An Adult's Right to Resist]. See Jehovah's Witnesses v. King County Hosp., 278 F. Supp. 488, 502 (W.D. Wash. 1967), *aff'd.,* 390 U.S. 598 (1968).

3. *See* Application of President and Directors of Georgetown College, 331 F.2d 1000 (D.C. Cir.), *cert. denied* 377 U.S. 978 (1964); Powell v. Columbia Presbyterian Medical Center, 49 Misc. 2d 215, 216, 267 N.Y.S.2d 450, 452 (Sup. Ct. 1965) ("This woman wanted to live. I could not let her die!").

4. No constitutional issue arises if a private physician acts in his own professional capacity and renders treatment despite the patient's conscientious objections, but hospitals have commonly been the moving forces in cases involving adult patients who decline treatment. In such cases, state action is probably present either because of the public aspects of all hospitals or because of the judicial mandate commonly sought. *See* Eaton v. Grubbs, 329 F.2d 710 (4th Cir. 1964); Meyer v. Massachusetts Eye & Ear Infirmary, 330 F. Supp. 1328 (D. Mass. 1971). *Cf.* Shelley v. Kraemer, 334 U.S. 1 (1948). But see Mulvihill v. Julian Butterfield Memorial Hospital, 329 F. Supp. 1020 (S.D.N.Y. 1971). The cases favoring mandated treatment primarily assert state interests to justify judicial interference. *See* cases cited in nn. 21 & 22 *infra.* The professional interests of physicians or hospitals in rendering care would not, in themselves, warrant judicial intervention. See 250–51 *infra.*

5. Application of President and Directors of Georgetown College, 331 F.2d 1000 (D.C. Cir.), *cert. denied*, 377 U.S. 978 (1964); United States v. George, 239 F. Supp. 752 (D. Conn. 1965); In re Osborne, 294 A.2d 372 (D.C. Ct. App. 1972); In re Brooks Estate, 32 Ill. 2d 361, 205 N.E.2d 435 (1965); John F. Kennedy Hosp. v. Heston, 51 N.J. 576, 279 A.2d 670 (1971); Powell v. Columbia Presbyterian Medical Center, 49 Misc. 2d 215, 267 N.Y.S.2d 450 (Sup. Ct. 1965); Collins v. Davis, 44 Misc. 2d 622, 254 N.Y.S.2d 666 (Sup. Ct. 1964); Erickson v. Dilgard, 44 Misc. 2d 27, 252 N.Y.S.2d 705 (Sup. Ct. 1962). *Cf.* Winters v. Miller, 306 F. Supp. 1158 (E.D.N.Y. 1969), *rev'd on other grounds*, 446 F.2d 65 (2d Cir. 1971), *cert. denied*, 404 U.S. 985 (1971).

6. Ford, *supra* note 2; Robitscher, The Right to Die, 2 *Hastings Center Rep.*, Sept. 1972, at 11 (Inst. of Society, Ethics and Life Sci.); Sharpe & Hargest, Lifesaving Treatment for Unwilling Patients, 36 *Ford. L. Rev.* 695 (1968) [hereinafter cited as Sharpe & Hargest]; Note, Unauthorized Rendition of Lifesaving Medical Treatment, 53 *Calif. L. Rev.* 860 (1965) [hereinafter cited as Unauthorized Rendition]; Note, The Right to Die, 7 *Hous. L. Rev.* 654 (1970) [hereinafter cited as The Right to Die]; Note, Compulsory Medical Treatment and the Free Exercise of Religion, 42 *Ind. L.J.* 386 (1967) [hereinafter cited as Free Exercise]; Note, The Dying Patient: A Qualified Right to Refuse Medical Treatment, 7 *J. Fam. L.* 644 (1968) [hereinafter cited as The Dying Patient]; Note, Compulsory Medical Treatment: The State's Interest Re-evaluated, 51 *Minn. L. Rev.* 293 (1966) [hereinafter cited as State's Interest]; Note, The Refused Blood Transfusion: An Ultimate Challenge for Law and Morals, 10 *Nat. L.F.* 202 (1965) [hereinafter cited as The Refused Blood Transfusion]; Note, The Right to Die, 18 *U. Fla. L. Rev.* 591 (1966) [hereinafter cited as *U. Fla. L. Rev.*]; An Adult's Right to Resist, *supra* note 2; Note, Compulsory Medical Treatment and Constitutional Guarantees: A Conflict?, 33 *U. Pitt. L. Rev.* 628 (1972) [hereinafter cited as Compulsory Medical Treatment]; 64 *Mich. L. Rev.* 554 (1966); 60 *Nw. U. L. Rev.* 399 (1965); 39 *N.Y.U. L. Rev.* 706 (1964); 25 *Sw. L.J.* 745 (1971); 44 *Tex. L. Rev.* 190 (1965); 113 *U. Pa. L. Rev.* 290 (1964); 9 *Utah L. Rev.* 161 (1964). The foregoing list is not exhaustive.

7. One exception is an excellent student note which represents the most articulate statement supporting judicial intervention which I have read. See, Unauthorized Rendition, *supra* note 6.

8. This article deals with the problem of patients who are conscious and competent to articulate their opposition to treatment or who are represented by persons expressing the patient's previously articulated opposition. See note 15 *infra*.

9. There is no way of knowing how many people avoid a confrontation on the issue by refusing hospitalization. Many other cases undoubtedly go unreported when patients do not pursue an appeal after medical treatment has been ordered and rendered.

See Jehovah's Witness v. King County Hosp., 278 F. Supp. 488, 496 n.5 (W.D. Wash. 1967), *aff'd* 390 U.S. 598 (1968). See *N.Y. Times*, Jan. 28, 1972 at 42, col. 3; *Newark Star Ledger*, May 2, 1972, at E-3-L, cols. 7–8.

10. *See, e.g.*, People ex rel. Wallace v. Labrenz, 411 Ill. 618, 104 N.E.2d 769, *cert. denied*, 344 U.S. 824 (1952); State v. Perricone, 37 N.J. 463, 181 A.2d 751, *cert. denied*, 371 U.S. 890 (1962); Larsen, Child Neglect in the Exercise of Religious Freedom, 32 *Chi.-Kent L. Rev.* 283 (1954).

The results may be different where the treatment required is non-emergency in nature. See In re Green, 448 Pa. 338, 292 A.2d 387 (1972) (deference to parents' religious beliefs where child's life not immediately threatened).

11. *See* Morrison v. State, 252 S.W.2d 97 (K.C. Ct. App. 1952); People v. Pierson, 176 N.Y. 201, 68 N.E. 243 (1903); Cawley, *supra* note 1, at 158–59, 275.

12. State v. Perricone, 37 N.J. 463, 475, 181 A.2d 751, 759 (1962); In re Clark, 21 Ohio Op.2d 86, 87, 185 N.E.2d 128, 129 (Ohio Comm. Pleas 1962); 64 *Mich. L. Rev.* 554, 556 n.7 (1966). But see In re Frank, 41 Wash. 2d 294, 248 P.2d 553 (1952).

13. See An Adult's Right to Resist, *supra* note 2, at 572; The Right to Die, *supra* note 6, at 667; The Dying Patient, *supra* note 6, at 648.

14. 331 F.2d 1000 (D.C. Cir.), *cert. denied*, 377 U.S. 978 (1964).

15. I choose to treat this case as one involving interference with an adult's bodily control even though the patient was considered legally incompetent at the time judicial intervention was sought, since a spouse was present who, as a representative of the patient, asserted the patient's own scruples and objections in declining treatment. Some authorities argue that if the adult patient is incompetent, the court should treat the patient as it would a minor or disabled person and appoint a guardian. See *id.* at 1008; Compulsory Medical Treatment, *supra* note 6, at 629 n.7. *Cf.* Westing v. Commonwealth, 123 Ky. 95, 93 S.W. 646 (1906). This argument assumes that the representative spouse is under a special obligation to look out for the patient's well being and cannot properly refuse to authorize treatment. See, e.g., Comment, 39 *N.Y.U. L. Rev.* 706, 709–10 (1964). This argument ignores the fact that the spouse or other representative is asserting the patient's own beliefs as previously articulated. To reject the legitimacy of these asserted beliefs would be to deprive the patient of all conscientious scruples once his condition has deteriorated to the point of legal incompetency. The situation is different where the guardian or representative is attempting to impose his own convictions, either because the patient is a minor or because the patient has not previously expressed personal objections to treatment. Where the adult becomes incompetent without having previously articulated

his personal beliefs, and where loss of life or serious injury is threatened by the spouse's refusal to authorize treatment, judicial intervention is appropriate and the patient's interests in self-determination are not overridden. See In re Nemser, 51 Misc. 616, 273 N.Y.S.2d 624 (Sup. Ct. 1964); *N.Y. Times*, Jan. 28, 1972, at 42, col. 3 (wife opposes operation upon 79-year-old husband who has lost virtually all faculties). Similarly, if there is an emergency situation and the physicians are not clear that the "representative" is reflecting the patient's own position, treatment should be rendered.

16. 331 F.2d at 1008: "The patient had a responsibility to the community to care for her infant. Thus the people had an interest in preserving the life of this mother."

17. *Cf.* Winters v. Miller, 306 F. Supp. 1158, 1170 (E.D.N.Y. 1969), *rev'd on other grounds*, 446 F.2d 65 (2d Cir.), *cert. denied*, 404 U.S. 985 (1971).

18. Judge Wright was aware that a waiver might obviate the risk of civil liability, but apparently felt that a similar waiver could not eliminate the risk of a manslaughter prosecution. 331 F.2d at 1009.

19. 331 F.2d at 1009. A similar interpretation of Jehovah's Witnesses' religious precepts was rendered in United States v. George, 239 F. Supp. 752, 753 (D. Conn. 1965) and Powell v. Columbia Presbyterian Medical Center, 49 Misc. 2d 215, 216, 267 N.Y.S.2d 450, 451 (Sup. Ct. 1965). Both cases argued that the patients objected to authorizing their own transfusions, but did not have serious religious scruples against undergoing a court-ordered transfusion. If this position were accurate, the minor nature of the religious infringement would strengthen the case for judicial intervention. But the position simply does not comport with the adamant opposition expressed by many Jehovah's Witnesses to any blood transfusion, whether authorized by the patient or the court. See Jehovah's Witnesses v. King County Hosp., 278 F. Supp. 488 (W.D. Wash. 1967), *aff'd*, 390 U.S. 598, *rehearing denied*, 391 U.S. 961 (1968). This article will proceed on the basis that a blood transfusion, even if court-ordered, represents a serious breach of Jehovah's Witnesses' religious tenets and a serious violation of the individual patient's beliefs. *See also* The Refused Blood Transfusion, *supra* note 6, at 204.

20. [W]here attempted suicide is illegal by the common law or by statute, a person may not be allowed to refuse necessary medical assistance when death is likely to ensue without it. Only quibbles about the distinction between misfeasance and non-feasance, or the specific intent necessary to be guilty of attempted suicide, could be raised against this latter conclusion. 331 F.2d at 1008–09.

21. While the circuit court as a whole avoided the merits by declaring the matter moot, several judges, including (now Chief Justice) Burger, indicated misgivings about Judge Wright's decision. 331 F.2d at 1017–18.

22. Powell v. Columbia Presbyterian Medical Center, 49 Misc. 2d 215, 267 N.Y.S.2d 450. (Sup. Ct. 1965) (mother of 6 children given blood transfusion).

23. United States v. George, 239 F. Supp. 752 (D. Conn. 1965); Collins v. Davis, 44 Misc. 2d 622, 254 N.Y.S.2d 666 (Sup. Ct. 1964).

24. John F. Kennedy Memorial Hosp. v. Heston, 58 N.J. 576, 279 A.2d 670 (1971). *See also Newark Star Ledger*, May 2, 1972, at E-3-L, cols 7–8.

25. 58 N.J. 576, 279 A.2d 670 (1970).

26. *Id.* at 578, 279 A.2d at 671. The court eventually found that the patient had become disoriented and incoherent either upon admission or soon thereafter. In light of the patient's clear prior beliefs and the mother's assertion of religious scruples on her daughter's behalf, the court considered the case as if the patient's own beliefs were at stake. This approach is entirely appropriate where, as here, the representative is asserting the patient's own religious tenets. See note 15 *supra*.

27. 58 N.J. at 582–83, 279 A.2d at 673.

28. At the time of the *Heston* case, attempted suicide was a disorderly persons offense. See Law of May 9, 1957, ch. 34 [1957] Laws of N.J. 63 (repealed 1971). Since that date, all legislative prohibitions of attempted suicide have been repealed in New Jersey. See *N.J. Stat. Ann.* § 2A:85–5.1 (Supp. 1972).

29. 58 N.J. at 581, 279 A.2d at 673.

30. In United States v. George, 239 F. Supp. 752 (D. Conn. 1965), the court, ordering a blood transfusion for a Jehovah's Witness, also relied heavily on physicians' interests. The opinion there stressed the need to respect the physician's professional conscience, at least where the patient himself had initially sought medical treatment. *Id.* at 754.

31. 32 Ill. 2d 361, 205 N.E.2d 435 (1965).

32. Although the patient may have been incompetent at the time of the application for a court order, she had expressed her religious scruples to her physician over a period of 2 years. Her husband and adult children concurred in her beliefs. The court therefore regarded any potential intervention as a direct infringement upon her religious beliefs. See also note 15 *supra*.

33. 32 Ill. 2d at 373, 205 N.E.2d at 442.

34. *Id.* at 373, 205 N.E.2d at 440.

35. 44 Misc. 2d 27, 252 N.Y.S.2d 705 (Sup. Ct. 1962). Although the patient in *Erickson* had a son, there is no indication in the opinion that he was minor.

36. *Id.* at 28, 252 N.Y.S.2d at 706. See also *In re* Osborne, 294 A.2d 372 (D.C. Ct. App. 1972); People v. Pierson, 176 N.Y. 201, 211, 68 N.E. 243, 247 (1903) (dictum).

37. *In re* Raasch, No. 455–996 (Prob. Div., Milwaukee County Ct. Jan. 21, 1972). See also *Newark Star Ledger*, Jan. 26, 1972, at 21, cols. 1–8.

38. *In re* Raasch, No. 455–996 at 2, (Prob. Div., Milwaukee County Ct., supp. proceeding, Jan. 25, 1972). See *In re* Osborne, 294 A.2d 372 (D.C. Ct. App. 1972).

39. Letter from George James, court reporter, branch number 2, Probate Division, Milwaukee County Court to Norman L. Cantor, July 5, 1972.

40. For a summary listing of the literature, see note 6 *supra*.

41. *See, e.g., U. Fla. L. Rev., supra* note 6, at 603; State's Interest, *supra* note 6, at 305.

42. See, e.g., Compulsory Medical Treatment, *supra* note 6, at 635; An Adult's Right to Resist, *supra* note 2, at 577–78.

43. Cawley, *supra* note 1, at 278.

44. Sharpe & Hargest, *supra* note 6, at 704; The Dying Patient, *supra* note 6, at 656.

45. Unauthorized Rendition, *supra* note 6, at 872–73; Free Exercise, *supra* note 6, at 401.

46. Union Pacific Ry. v. Botsford, 141 U.S. 250, 251 (1891). See *also* note 56 *infra* and accompanying text.

47. See generally Comment, Failure to Inform as Medical Malpractice, 23 *Vand. L. Rev.* 754 (1970); Note, Informed Consent as a Theory of Medical Liability, 1970 *Wis. L. Rev.* 879 [hereinafter cited as Informed Consent]; Note, Restructuring Informed Consent: Legal Therapy for the Doctor-Patient Relationship, 79 *Yale L.J.* 1533 (1970). Judge Cardozo articulated the doctrine as follows: "Every human being of adult years and sound mind has a right to determine what shall be done with his own body; and a surgeon who performs an operation without his patient's consent commits an assault, for which he is liable in damages." Schloendorff v. Society of New York Hosp., 211 N.Y. 125, 129–30, 105 N.E. 92, 93 (1914).

48. See Informed Consent, *supra* note 47, at 883, 891.

49. Natanson v. Kline, 186 Kan. 393, 406–07, 350 P.2d 1093, 1104 (1960). *See also* Woods v. Brumlop, 71 N.M. 221, 226–27, 377 P.2d 520, 524 (1962).

50. See Unauthorized Rendition, *supra* note 6, at 863; The Right to Die, *supra* note 6, at 668–69.

51. See Curran & Shapiro, *Law, Medicine and Forensic Science* 813 (2d ed. 1970); Sharpe & Hargest, *supra* note 6, at 706.

52. *See, e.g.,* Zucht v. King, 260 U.S. 174 (1922) (vaccination); Reynolds v. United States, 98 U.S. 145 (1879) (polygamy).

53. Sherbert v. Verner, 374 U.S. 398, 406 (1963). See Free Exercise, *supra* note 6, at 393; An Adult's Right to Resist, *supra* note 2, at 576.

54. 406 U.S. 205 (1972).

55. *Id.* at 213.

56. *Id.* at 219–28.

57. But *cf.* State v. Armstrong, 39 Wash. 2d 860, 239 P.2d 545 (1952); Mountain Lakes Bd. of Educ. v. Maas, 56 N.J. Super. 245, 152 A.2d 394 (App. Div. 1959), aff'd, 31 N.J. 537, 158 A.2d 330 (1960).

58. See generally Fried, Privacy, 77 *Yale L.J.* 475 (1968); Griswold, The Right to be Let Alone, 55 *Nw. U.L. Rev.* 216 (1960); Gross, The Concept of Privacy, 42 *N.Y.U. L. Rev.* 34 (1967).

59. See Stanley v. Georgia, 394 U.S. 557 (1969); Olmstead v. United States, 277 U.S. 438, 478 (1928). "The overriding function of the Fourth Amendment is to protect personal privacy and dignity against unwarranted intrusion by the State." Schmerber v. California, 384 U.S. 757, 767 (1966).

60. 384 U.S. 757 (1966).

61. *Id.* at 772, 770.

62. See Katz v. United States, 389 U.S. 347, 350 (1967).

63. 381 U.S. 479 (1965).

64. See generally Lister, The Right to Control of the Use of One's Body, in *The Rights of Americans* 348–49 (Dorsen ed. 1970); Note, Legal Analysis and Population Control: The Problem of Coercion, 84 *Harv. L. Rev.* 1856, 1875–79 (1971).

65. 405 U.S. 438 (1972).

66. 405 U.S. at 453 (emphasis in original).

67. See e.g., Doe v. Scott, 321 F. Supp. 1385, 1390 (N.D. Ill.), *motion to shorten time to docket appeal denied*, 401 U.S. 969 (1971); Roe v. Wade, 314 F. Supp. 1217 (N.D. Tex. 1970), *prob. juris. postponed*, 402 U.S. 941 (1971), *reargued* 41 U.S.L.W. 3201 (U.S. Oct. 11, 1972); Doe v. Bolton, 319 F. Supp. 1048 (N.D. Ga. 1970), *prob. juris. postponed*, 402 U.S. 941 (1971), *reargued* 41 U.S.L.W. 3201 (U.S. Oct. 11, 1972); Babbitz v. McCann, 310 F. Supp. 219 (E.D. Wis. 1970) *appeal dismissed*, 400 U.S. 1 (1970), 320 F. Supp. 219 (E.D. Wis. 1970) *vacated and remanded* 402 U.S. 903 (1970). However, when the Supreme Court rules on pending challenges to state abortion laws, it is likely to acknowledge that governmental interference with bodily control is circumscribed by constitutional guarantees of privacy.

68. 394 U.S. 557 (1969).

69. *Id.* at 564.

70. See Stanley v. Georgia, 394 U.S. 557 (1969); Griswold v. Connecticut, 381 U.S. 479 (1965).

71. But *cf.* Wyman v. James, 400 U.S. 309 (1971).

72. See, e.g., Schmerber v. California, 384 U.S. 757 (1966); Jacobson v. Massachusetts, 197 U.S. 11 (1905).

73. *Cf.* Stanley v. Georgia, 394 U.S. 557, 568 n.11 (1969); Legal Analysis and Population Control, *supra* note 64, at 1880–82.

74. *See* notes 5 and 6 *supra* and accompanying text.

75. Unauthorized Rendition, *supra* note 6, at 862. See also *Free Exercise, supra* note 6, at 400.

76. See Dennis v. United States, 341 U.S. 494 (1951); Morrison v. State, 252 S.W.2d 97, 102 (Mo. Ct. App. 1952); Peterson v. Widule, 157 Wis. 641, 147 N.W. 966 (1914).

77. There have been historic instances when "epidemics" of suicide took place. See Alvarez, *The Savage God* 58, 109 (1970) [hereinafter cited as Alvarez]. But it is unlikely that someone who desires death would employ refusal of treatment as the means to die. There are a variety of poisons, gases, and weapons which are quicker and relatively painless. A person declining treatment might provide encouragement to others, but natural instincts of self-preservation are likely to prevail within the population.

78. See Kaplan, The Role of the Law in Drug Control, 1971 *Duke L.J.* 1065, 1067.

79. See note 54 *supra* and accompanying text.

80. 64 *Mich. L. Rev.* 554, 561 (1966). Imagine a situation where a court refused to intervene to order an amputation because, though the patient's life would be saved, the patient would be a "useless" cripple.

81. This is the approach urged in Unauthorized Rendition, *supra* note 6, at 872. But see The Dying Patient, *supra* note 6, at 652; *U. Fla. L. Rev., supra* note 6, at 600 n.28.

82. *In re* Osborne, 294 A.2d 372, 375 n. 5 (D.C. Ct. App. 1972); *U. Fla. L. Rev., supra* note 6, at 604.

83. Unauthorized Rendition, *supra* note 6, at 867.

84. Fletcher, *Morals and Medicine* 66 (1954).

85. Any contention that self-destruction by refusal of treatment would undermine popular respect for life is purely speculative. It is true that in ancient Roman society, where suicide was habitual and honored, there was an incredible indifference to life. Mass murder of Christians, slaves, and gladiators was not only tolerated, but encouraged at various times. Yet it is difficult to establish any causal relation between attitudes toward suicide and general respect for life. There have been other societies where suicide was accepted in limited contexts, but where life was generally revered. See Alvarez, *supra* note 77, at 52–53, 64–65.

86. Fletcher, *supra* note 84, at 194–95.

87. *See* Friedmann, Interference with Human Life: Some Jurisprudential Reflections, 70 *Colum. L. Rev.* 1058, 1066 (1970). Numerous instances have also occurred in which authorities have enlisted prisoners to undergo hazardous medical experiments. In one recently publicized horror story, the Public Health Service studied syphilitic males without rendering treatment. See *N.Y. Times*, Aug. 8, 1972, at 16, col. 4. It is arguable that significant numbers of lives could be saved by rigid enforcement of automobile and highway safety standards, or by governmental elimination of hand guns.

88. These include homosexuality among consenting adults, prostitution, alcoholism, drug abuse and the like. See generally Hart, *Law, Liberty and Morality* (1963); *Morality and the Law* (Wasserstrom ed. 1971); Sartorious, The Enforcement of Morality, 81 *Yale L.J.* 891 (1972).

89. This is not to say that it falls within the legal definition of suicide. See note 137 *infra* and accompanying text. Indeed, refusal of treatment is not suicide since the patient, unlike the genuine suicide, does not normally wish to die.

90. St. John-Stevas, *Life, Death and the Law* 248–50 (1961). There are other, less important religious objections to suicide which need not be elaborated here. *Id.*

91. *Id.* at 234–35; Williams, *The Sanctity of Life and the Criminal Law* 261–64 (1956) [hereinafter cited as Williams].

92. Williams, *supra* note 91, at 264, 267.

93. See generally Alvarez, *supra* note 77, at 74–75, 79. Interestingly, historical attitudes toward suicide have not always been negative. Both the Romans and Greeks esteemed suicide in some situations as a noble act. The early Christians accepted their martyrdom as a chance to obtain salvation. *Id.* at 43–76.

94. Williams, *supra* note 90, at 248.

95. Curran & Shapiro. *Law, Medicine and Forensic Science* 832 (1970). No serious pretense of punishment or deterrence can be retained.

96. See, e.g., State v. Massey, 229 N.C. 734, 51 S.E.2d 179 (1949), *appeal dismissed*, 336 U.S. 942 (1949); Harden v. State, 188 Tenn. 17, 216 S.W.2d 708 (1948); Hill v. State, 38 Ala. App. 623, 88 So.2d 880 (1956).

97. But see Lawson v. Commonwealth, 164 S.W.2d 972, 974 (Ky. 1942).

98. See generally Annot., 32 ALR 3d 1270 (1970); Note, Motorcycle Helmets and the Constitutionality of Self-Protective Legislation, 30 *Ohio St. L.J.* 355 (1969); 82 *Harv. L. Rev.* 469 (1969).

99. See, e.g., Everhardt v. City of New Orleans, 217 So.2d 400 (La. Sup. Ct. 1968); State v. Anderson, 3 N.C. App. 124, 164 S.E.2d 48 (1968).

100. A number of courts have accepted the argument that motorcycle helmet statutes are adequately supported by a state interest in averting an economic burden—costs of treatment and hospitalization for head injuries. See, e.g., State v. Laitinen, 77 Wash. 2d 130, 459 P.2d 789 (1969), *cert. denied*, 397 U.S. 1055 (1970). *Cf.* Winters v. Miller, 306 F. Supp. 1158, 1170 (E.D.N.Y. 1969) *rev'd on other grounds*, 446 F.2d 65 (2d Cir.), *cert. denied*, 404 U.S. 985 (1971). These courts have largely ignored the fact that the statutes are not narrowly drawn to apply only where insurance is not present.

A similar economic burden argument can be applied to the issue of refusal of medical treatment since the death of a patient may, in some instances, make the patient's survivors public wards. The issue is addressed at pp. 252–54 *infra*.

In State v. Congdon, 76 N.J. Super. 493, 185 A.2d 21 (Law Div. 1963), the court ruled that the state could compel an individual to take cover during an air raid drill. The opinion stated that pursuant to the police power the state could protect its citizens regardless of whether the individual wished to be protected. *Id.* at 506, 185 A.2d at 29. But it has been suggested that the result might better be rationalized by reliance on the state's interest in avoiding the economic burden of an injured person. See The Dying Patient, *supra* note 6, at 653.

101. See, e.g., People v. Carmichael, 56 Misc. 2d 388, 288 N.Y.S.2d 931 (Genesee County Ct. 1968); State v. Lee, 51 Hawaii 516, 465 P.2d 573 (Hawaii 1970).

102. See, e.g., American Motorcycle Ass'n v. Davids, 11 Mich. App. 351, 158 N.W.2d 72 (1968); State v. Betts, 21 Ohio Misc. 175, 182, 252 N.E.2d 866, 872 (Munic. Ct. 1969) ("Included in man's liberty is the freedom to be as foolish, foolhardy, or reckless as he may wish, so long as others are not endangered thereby.").

103. See generally Kaplan, *supra* note 78; Note, Health Regulation of Naturally Hazardous Foods: The FDA Ban on Swordfish, 85 *Harv. L. Rev.* 1025 (1972) [hereinafter cited as Health Regulation].

104. Kaplan, *supra* note 78, at 1079.

105. See Wilcox, Public Protection, Private Choices and Scientific Freedom: Food, Drugs and Environmental Hazards, 18 *Food Drug Cosm. L.J.* 321, 326 (1963); Health Regulation, *supra* note 103, at 1045–47.

106. One extension of paternalistic regulations may come if current proposals to force automobile drivers to wear seatbelts by interlocking seatbelts with ignitions are adopted. See 36 Fed. Reg. 12858–59 (1971).

107. United States v. Walsh, 331 U.S. 432 (1947); Purity Extract & Tonic Co. v. C.C. Lynch, 226 U.S. 192 (1912).

108. Sometimes, labeling or warning requirements are insufficient to protect the general public. For example, warnings may go unnoticed because too inconspicuous, or unheeded because the substance is addictive (e.g., narcotics, cigarettes) and individuals, once addicted, cannot exercise full self-control. Of course, there may be instances where warnings are inadequate only because people foolishly choose to ignore them. In those cases, regulatory bans constitute purely paternalistic efforts to preclude risk-taking by individuals. The FDA's swordfish ban is one recent example. See 36 Fed. Reg. 11, 514 (1971); Health Regulation, *supra* note 103.

109. *Cf.* People v. Woody, 61 Cal. 2d 716, 394 P.2d 813, 40 *Cal. Rptr.* 69 (1964).

110. Not all deaths because of refused treatment will have a harmful emotional impact. If the patient has a terminal illness and faces gradual deterioration, premature death because of refused treatment may be considered by the family to be a blessing. Because of the delicacy of the inquiry into family members' attitudes toward the patient's death, however, courts cannot be expected to address the matter on a case by case basis. The death must be presumed to constitute a source of grief to the surviving family.

111. See Free Exercise, *supra* note 6, at 400 for a contrary viewpoint.

112. Unauthorized Rendition, *supra* note 6, at 868.

113. See, *e.g.*, Application of President and Directors of Georgetown College, 331 F.2d 1000 (D.C. Cir.), *cert. denied*, 377 U.S. 978 (1964); United States v. George, 239 F. Supp. 752 (D. Conn. 1965); John F. Kennedy Memorial Hosp. v. Heston, 58 N.J. 576, 279 A.2d 670 (1971).

114. But see Ford, *supra* note 6, at 221.

115. See note 44 *supra* and accompanying text.

116. Compulsory reporting of child abuse, venereal disease and a variety of other contagious diseases is required by most states. See Rosenberg, Compulsory Disclosure Statutes, 280 *N. Eng. J. Med.* 1287 (1969).

117. Problems undoubtedly occur in evaluating the competency or capacity of any patient who declines lifesaving treatment. See Robitscher, *supra* note 6, at 13. Since the patient's condition is, by definition, potentially fatal, he will inevitably become confused or debilitated and unable to exercise rational judgment. Physicians and hospital staff must, in good conscience, resist the temptation to wait until the patient has lost competency before seeking judicial intervention. See State's Interest, *supra* note 6, at 300–01. Once the patient has made a clear decision while competent, it must be respected unless altered. Of course, if the patient suffering pain and anxiety renounces his "competent" decision to reject treatment, treatment should be rendered since no patient should be permitted to die against his apparent will. If the patient vacillates, treatment should be rendered unless in all moments of lucidity the patient rejects treatment.
   This means that care cannot be terminated if the person is afflicted with sudden incapacity or becomes incompetent before expressing his opposition to treatment. The consequence is to relegate some people to a painful and perhaps unwanted existence, for no one can reject treatment on behalf of the patient unless representing the patient's previously competently expressed position. See *N.Y. Times*, Jan. 28, 1972, at 42, col. 4 (judicial repudiation of a wife's efforts to prevent continued treatment of her husband, who had deteriorated to the point of having lost all faculties). This principle, authorizing only voluntary refusal of care, ultimately protects mongoloid children, idiots and the senile from manipulation.

118. See note 10 *supra* and accompanying text.

119. *Cf.* Wisconsin v. Yoder, 406 U.S. 205, 229–34 (1972); Prince v. Massachusetts, 321 U.S. 158, 168 (1944); Morrison v. State, 252 S.W.2d 97, 103 (Mo. Ct. App. 1952).

120. One source has suggested that judicial interference, resulting in a parent being kept alive, might produce permanent resentment on the part of the frustrated parent against the child whose existence forced the court to intervene. See *U. Fla. L. Rev.*, *supra* note 6, at 600. This seems rather farfetched since it would be the court and not the child which actually forced the violation of the parent's religious or philosophical precepts. It would be more plausible to argue that a parent's steadfast devotion to religious principle will be a source of pride and respect, and not hurt, for the surviving child. See State's Interest, *supra* note 6, at 301.

121. See Sharpe & Hargest, *supra* note 6, at 697. Note that practically all states provide for the voluntary surrender of a child by natural parents via adoption. This may, of course, cause emotional scars in the children.

122. *Cf. In re* Frank, 41 Wash. 2d 294, 248 P.2d 553 (1952).

123. See 64 *Mich. L. Rev.* 554, 560 (1966).

124. See, *e.g.*, *In re* Cavitt, 182 Neb. 712, 157 N.W.2d 171 (1968), *prob. juris. noted*, 393 U.S. 1078 (1969), *appeal dismissed*, 396 U.S. 996 (1970); *In re* Main, 162 Okla. 65, 19 P.2d 153, 156 (1933).

125. See, *e.g.*, State v. Odegaard, 165 N.W.2d 677, 679 (N.D. 1969); State v. Laitinen, 77 Wash. 2d. 130, 459 P.2d 789 (1969).

126. See, *e.g.*, Dandridge v. Williams, 397 U.S. 471 (1970).

127. 406 U.S. 205 (1972); see note 54 *supra* and accompanying text.

128. Savings to the public fisc cannot be used as an automatic or unlimited justification for infringement of individual liberty. Welfare residency requirements have not been sustained, even though they saved money for the state. Shapiro v. Thompson, 394 U.S. 618 (1969). A state may have to support religious practices of prison inmates despite the public burden. See Cruz v. Beto, 405 U.S. 319 (1972). Counsel must be provided to indigent criminal defendants despite the economic burden entailed. Argersinger v. Hamlin, 407 U.S. 25 (1972).
   Undoubtedly, a balancing test must be utilized to determine the validity of money saving measures which incidentally infringe upon personal liberties. A welfare mother could not be criminally punished for having additional children. But, apparently, benefits can be cut back for additional children, despite the impact on the mother's decision whether to bear children, in order to exact savings to the state. See Dandridge v. Williams, 397 U.S. 471 (1970).

129. See *In re* Osborne, 294 A.2d 372, 374 (D.C. Ct. App. 1972). *Cf.* Kaplan, *supra* note 78, at 1073.

130. *Cf.* Klein v. Nassau County Medical Center, 347 F. Supp. 496 (E.D.N.Y. 1972); Cantor, The Law and Poor People's Access to Health Care, 35 *Law & Contemp. Prob.* 901, 903–07 (1970). It is also arguable, of course, that the state's economic interests simply do not outweigh the patient's interests in religious freedom and bodily integrity. *See* note 128 *supra*.

131. *Cf.* Kaplan, *supra* note 78 at 1071.

132. See Unauthorized Rendition, *supra* note 6, at 867–69; John F. Kennedy Memorial Hosp. v. Heston, 58 N.J. 576, 279 A.2d 670 (1971).

133. Efforts to distinguish suicide from refusal of treatment on the basis of misfeasance versus non-feasance or the immorality of affirmative actions as opposed to passive refusal are unconvincing. See An Adult's Right to Resist, *supra* note 2, at 574; Ford, *supra* note 6, at 225. A person might passively commit suicide by refusing medical treatment with the desire to die.

134. See, *e.g.*, Penney v. Municipal Ct., 312 F. Supp. 938 (D.N.J. 1970).

135. See Compulsory Medical Treatment, *supra* note 6, at 634.

136. Unauthorized Rendition, *supra* note 6, at 871.

137. The Dying Patient, *supra* note 6, at 651 (1967). *E.g.*, Okla. Stat. Ann. tit. 21, § 812 (1958):
   Any person who, with intent to take his own life, commits upon himself any act dangerous to human life, or which if committed upon or toward another person and followed by death as a consequence would render the perpetrator chargeable with homicide, is guilty of attempting suicide.

138. See Williams, *supra* note 99, at 289.

139. *Id.* at 287–90; St. John-Stevas, *supra* note 90, at 256–58.

140. Penney v. Municipal Ct., 312 F. Supp. 938 (D.N.J. 1970).

141. Alvarez, *supra* note 77, at 111–20. See generally Durkheim, *Suicide* (1951); *The Cry for Help* (Ferberon & Schneidman, eds. 1961).

142. Estimates of the percentage of attempts where the actor was actually psychotic range from 20 to 30 percent. See generally *Suicidal Behavior, Diagnosis and Management* (Resnik ed. 1968). The estimate of cases where psychiatric illness or mental disorder was a factor range as high as 94 percent. See Robins, Murphy, Wilkenson, Gassner, & Kayes, Some Clinical Considerations in the Prevention of Suicide Based on a Study of 134 Successful Suicides, 49 *Am. J. Pub. Health* 888 (1959).

143. Alvarez, *supra* note 77, at 81; Williams, *supra* note 91, at 285.

144. Williams, *supra* note 91, at 292.

145. See *id.* at 293.

146. National Center for Health Statistics, *Suicide in the United States 1950–1964* (1967). See *Self-Destructive Behavior 5* (Hafen and Faux eds. 1972).

147. *Id.*

148. Alvarez, *supra* note 77, at 58, 109.

149. It is possible that the elderly patient in the *Raasch* case, *supra* note 37, spurned treatment because she wished to die. The opinion does not clarify whether the rejection of treatment was motivated by a wish to die or by distaste for the serious medical procedure (amputation of a leg) proposed.

150. Not all suicide is totally irrational. In some situations, a person makes a deliberate, "balanced" assessment that his life is no longer worth living. Alvarez, *supra* note 77, at 56–61. The decision may be the product of "perverted logic," but it is not the product of derangement. Of course, certain practical problems will undoubtedly occur in evaluating the competency or capacity of a patient who declines treatment. See note 117 *supra*.

151. The attempted suicide who is rushed to the hospital and who attempts to reject emergency assistance should nonetheless be treated.

152. As a practical matter, it might be possible to distinguish between the "principled patient" and the "suicide-patient." Even if the suicide attempted to assert religious scruples against receiving treatment, his subterfuge could probably be detected if there had been no prior articulation of such scruples. But suppose the patient were asserting a philosophical belief that each person should be able to determine his own time and way of dying. Philosophical principles and suicide would, in that instance, be intermingled.

153. Under my approach to suicide, even the Hindu "suttee"—the ritual in which the wife throws herself on the funeral pyre of her husband—would have to be tolerated if the wife's act were shown to be the product of deliberate consideration. *Contra,* Reynolds v. United States, 98 U.S. 145, 161–62 (1878) (dictum). It could be argued that suicidal refusal of treatment might be differentiated from suicides generally, on the basis of volume of cases involved, but this seems to be an artificial distinction.

154. See generally Fletcher, *Morals and Medicine,* 172–210 (1954); Meyers, *The Human Body and the Law,* 139–54 (1970); St. John-Stevas, *supra* note 90, at 262–80; Williams, *supra* note 91, at 311–49. All references herein are to voluntary euthanasia, killing at the request of the patient, unless otherwise noted.

155. Curran & Shapiro, *Law, Medicine and Forensic Science,* 130 (1970); Williams, *supra* note 91, at 318–19.

156. See The Right to Die, *supra* note 6, at 659; Meyers, *supra* note 154 at 147; Elkinton, The Dying Patient, The Doctor and the Law, 13 *Vill. L. Rev.* 740, 744 (1968).

157. Williams, *supra* note 91, at 326.

158. Kamisar, Some Non-Religious Views Against Proposed Mercy Killing Legislation, 42 *Minn. L. Rev.* 969, 982 n.41 (1958) [hereinafter cited as Kamisar].

159. See The Right to Die, *supra* note 6, at 661; Williams, *supra* note 91, at 324.

160. Meyers, *supra* note 154, at 159.

161. "To prolong life uselessly, while the personal qualities of freedom, knowledge, self-possession and control, and responsibility are sacrificed, is to attack the moral status of a person." Fletcher, *supra* note 154, at 191. See also *id.* at 176–86; Meyers, *supra* note 154, at 142–43; Williams, *supra* note 91, at 316.

162. The notion that the diagnosis of terminal illness might be erroneous, or that a miraculous cure *might* materialize, do not impress me as persuasive reasons for denying the patient a chance to avoid further misery and indignity. But see Kamisar, *supra* note 158, at 998.

163. *Id.* at 977–84, 986–90. See *supra* note 117 for similar problems in refusal of lifesaving treatment.

164. "[O]nce a concession about the disposability of innocent life is made in one sphere, it will inevitably spread to others. The recognition of voluntary euthanasia by the law would at once be followed by pressure to extend its scope to deformed persons and imbeciles, and eventually to the old and any one who could be shown to be 'burdens' to society." St. John-Stevas, *supra* note 90, at 272–73. See Kamisar, *supra* note 158, at 994, 1029–32.

165. See St. John Stevas, *supra* note 90, at 267; Williams, *supra* note 91, at 333.

166. In the case of the patient suffering pain, this course should only be followed after considerable care to evaluate the capacity of the patient.

167. The disconnection of supportive medical equipment is a perplexing problem. In one sense, this is an affirmative act by the physician. In another, it is merely a discontinuance of treatment which the patient had an initial right to reject. Wherever the line between valid and invalid conduct is drawn in this context, the result will be somewhat arbitrary. The patient receiving "extraordinary" medical assistance will likely be debilitated, and it will be difficult to determine competency to authorize discontinuance of equipment. See note 117 *supra*. On the other hand, classifying the disconnection of extraordinary medical equipment as a proscribed affirmative act will condemn some patients to an existence which is agonizing both for them and their families. My own feeling is that the discontinuance of special mechanical assistance is basically no different from cessation of chemotherapy and therefore ought to be accepted as a legitimate form of refusal of medical treatment.

168. *Id.*

169. See cases cited in note 67 *supra*.

170. See *In re* Cavitt, 182 Neb. 712, 157 N.W.2d 171 (1968), *prob. juris. noted,* 393 U.S. 1078 (1969), *appeal dismissed,* 396 U.S. 996 (1970).

171. Eisenstadt v. Baird, 405 U.S. 438 (1972).

172. *See* Friedmann, *supra* note 87, at 1069.

173. The "humanity" of a foetus appears to be more a metaphysical than a biological question. But there can be no doubt that a foetus, at whatever stage of development, represents a prospective human being and is at least a valid subject of state concern—even if this concern is held to be outweighed by countervailing interests in bodily control.

174. *But cf.* Eisenstadt v. Baird, 405 U.S. 432, 452–54 (1972).

175. For example, resolution of the question of population control might well depend upon the demographic situation at the time governmental controls are instituted, or upon the precise nature of the controls employed. See generally Legal Analysis and Population Control, supra note 64.

176. Where a patient articulates religious objections to treatment, freedom of religion offers a second constitutional basis for protection against judicial intervention. The constitutional standard for assessing the validity of intervention should be the same, however, whether religious freedom or privacy is the basis for the patient's resistance. Perhaps the assertion of two constitutional interests would strengthen the patient's case in the balancing process which ensues when compelling state interests are arrayed against constitutionally protected patient interests.

The religiously motivated patient resisting bodily invasion is inevitably invoking both privacy and religious freedom even though religious scruples form the immediate basis for resistance. If this were not so, if the patient were considered to be waiving constitutional rights to bodily integrity (personal privacy), a substantial difference in judicial result might be dictated. In some instances, courts might determine that a patient's religious scruples do not really mandate objection to court-ordered treatment. See note 19 *supra*. Alternatively, a patient's religious objections to treatment might be found to constitute such a small part of his religion's dogma that the degree of infringement upon religious freedom would be considered to be outweighed by countervailing governmental interests. See note 55 *supra* and accompanying text. Of course, this last situation is unlikely to arise, for if a patient is willing to die for the religious principles at stake they must be regarded as substantial religious precepts.

177. This deference does not mean that a state is precluded from intervening in most cases of attempted suicide, or that the state must authorize affirmative acts of "mercy killing." The "right" is to decline lifesaving treatment. See notes 153 and 167 *supra* and accompanying text.

28

Paul A. Freund

Organ Transplants: Ethical and Legal Problems

Reprinted with permission of the author and publisher from *Proceedings of the American Philosophical Society,* vol. 115, no. 4, 1971, pp. 276–281.

Until we secure an adequate supply of organs—natural or artificial—to meet the needs, there will be problems of allocation of these resources: from whom they should come and to whom they should be transferred. By what criteria should these decisions be made? The question implicates moral, legal, and medical considerations, which differ in the cases of removal after death and removal during life.

The moral and legal problems attending the taking of an organ from a cadaver appear to be well on the way to resolution. Although objection to the mutilation of a corpse has been traditional in Orthodox Judaism, as the life-saving potential of transplants has become clearer the resistance on religious grounds has weakened.[1] Legal obstacles have been more widespread. Under the principles of the common law a person could not in his lifetime determine by will or agreement how his bodily organs should be treated after death; and the authority of the next of kin was essentially limited to providing a decent burial. While more recent legal precedents could be construed to authorize the next of kin to donate organs, the authority was not beyond peradventure clear, and since the next of kin might be unknown, or unavailable, or hostile, the procedure for securing approval was at best unsatisfactory, especially in situations where the utmost promptness in removal was essential for the viability of the organ.[2]

The problem of obtaining the necessary consent has now been resolved from another direction. The Uniform Anatomical Gift Act, which has been adopted in forty-eight states, authorizes an individual to donate his body, or certain organs or tissues, for purpose of transplantation or other scientific use, by means of a relatively simple witnessed document, and there is a growing practice of using a card to signify his authorization.[3] Many persons are now card-carrying potential donors of organs. Alternatively, the Act authorizes the next of kin (in order of priority, beginning with a surviving spouse) to grant authorization. The most serious problems that remain in the field of transplants from cadavers are thus the biological ones: the medical requirement that certain organs,

notably the heart, be utilized in an oxygenated condition, precluding storage or even appreciable delay, and so necessitating early typing and matching of tissues.

Turning from the donation of organs after death to their donation for live transplants, we have to differentiate between paired and unpaired organs.

In the case of paired organs, like kidneys, the law is permissive, where the loss and the risk of further injury to the donor are moderate in relation to the anticipated benefit to the recipient. Indeed, a renal transplant has been authorized by a Massachusetts court even between minors who were twins, despite the rule that a child may not be made the subject of harm unless for his own benefit; the court reasoned, after interviewing the healthy twin, that he would suffer lasting psychic trauma if he were not allowed to contribute an organ to his brother so that they could continue to enjoy the blessings of life together.[4]

From the ground of permitting the donation of a paired organ to save a life, should the law move to the position of requiring such contributions, through a process of random selection? In Kantian terms, would we will a universal rule imposing an obligation on others to save us, and in return accept an obligation to save others in the same way? Compulsory vaccination is of course a different matter, since an unvaccinated person may be a positive menace. The law has hesitated to equate a duty to come to the aid of another with a duty to refrain from doing harm. Why should this reluctance persist? Three possible reasons can be suggested. First, there is a practical calculus. Compulsory giving may range along a spectrum from taxation to enforced martyrdom. There is an intuitively felt difference between the taking of one's substance and of one's selfhood. In a situation of catastrophe one can imagine a conscription of blood, which is self-replenishing, more readily than a conscription of organs. The disproportion between risk to the donor and expected benefit to the donee would have to be greater and surer to warrant compulsion than to support a voluntary sacrifice; otherwise we might be in the position of the traveler in the desert, carrying a canister of water sufficient for one person, who is obliged to share it with another and thereby causes two deaths. Secondly, there would be practical problems of selection among all possible donors, since randomness is not a self-defining concept. And finally, enforced giving would diminish the moral quality of the act, though this consideration would be less relevant if scope were also left for voluntary donations.

Coming now to the transplanting of an unpaired organ like the heart or liver, we confront the medical-moral-legal problem of how to obtain the organ early enough to make it viable and yet not secure it by performing a lethal operation on a living person. For a lethal operation, regardless of the consent of the subject, would be in violation of the criminal law. Why should this be so? Why should the law not recognize a right to dispose of one's life as one pleases? It is a question that has engaged philosophers from Socrates to Camus. There are, of course, many limitations in law and morals on an individual's freedom to do with himself as he will even though his action causes no particular harm to others. He may, for example, sell his services but may not sell himself into slavery. A secular explanation might take this form: since freedom of the will is the ground asserted for the legal privilege, an act that would irretrievably destroy this freedom forfeits the claim to immunity within its own terms. A similar rationale can be advanced for the law's protective intervention against self-destruction. But it would be disingenuous not to take account of the religious background of the law's concern.[5]

Although the Old Testament does not specifically denounce suicide, the Talmudists, building on the Sixth Commandment and other more remote Biblical texts, condemned the act. Plato, in the Laws (Book IX), justifies self-destruction when (as in Socrates' case) it is visibly ordained by an authoritative judgment, and he would bow also to the direction of Destiny, but in other cases it would be improper to take one's life without the approval of divine authority. The Christian disapproval derives from Augustine, who, it has been suggested, was disturbed by the excesses of a sect whose members, intent on the life hereafter, destroyed

themselves in hordes when they believed themselves to be in a state of grace. Aquinas reasoned that suicide was an act contrary to man's nature, that it diminished society, and that it usurped the divine function. Again an exception was recognized for divine direction, apprehended mainly by saints.

English law, reflecting this religious heritage doubtless reinforced by the king's interest in conserving the manpower of the realm, dishonored the body of a suicide and visited forfeiture of property upon his heirs. (Roman law, with impeccable logic, had decreed forfeiture only in cases where the suicide was committed in order to avoid conviction of an offense that itself would have entailed such forfeiture.) The practice of burying a suicide at a crossroads, with a stake driven into the ground (to prevent the evil spirits from rising and doing mischief) was formally abolished in England in 1823, and forfeiture continued until as late as 1870. There were, to be sure, escape valves in the law. A finding that the act was committed while the mind was unbalanced was one; and there might be a question whether the event was due to a positive self-destructive act or to a passive exposure to deadly forces (did the water come to Ophelia, or did she go to the water, in the quibble of the gravedigger?)

In America, the states have taken different positions on the criminality of an act of suicide—a question not wholly academic, since it determines whether an unsuccessful attempt is punishable and since it affects the question whether one who aids and abets a suicide is himself guilty of a crime. In a substantial but decreasing number of states, suicide is still classified as a crime. And even if it were not a crime, it would not follow inevitably that inducing or aiding and abetting would likewise be innocent. Innocence would logically follow if the reason for immunity of the suicide itself were a policy to encourage it; but if the policy is simply to tolerate it, or to recognize that a potential suicide is not deterred by a legal rule, there is no logical entailment that an accessory must likewise be granted a privilege. The bearing of this point on the performance by a surgeon of a consented-to lethal operation is evident.

There have been, to be sure, powerful dissenting voices amid the chorus of condemnation. The Stoics and Epicureans admired a rational decision to end one's life. When Horatio reaches for the poisoned cup in Hamlet's hands he exclaims, "I am more an antique Roman than a Dane" (that is, than an Englishman, as is generally to be understood in Shakespeare). In England, John Donne wryly ascribed the official rejection of suicide to a desire to conserve the supply of members of a depressed working class, and David Hume could see nothing more "unnatural" in hastening one's death than in averting it by dodging a dangerous falling stone. But these were voices of nonconformity.

Should there be a special rule in any event, however, for altruistic suicide? Certainly the sentiment of society does not condemn, but in fact extols, certain forms, at least, of self-willed death in the service of fellow men. The soldier who falls on a grenade to save the lives of his comrades, the firefighter who exposes himself to the flames to rescue another, the man who throws himself in front of a train to toss out of danger a fallen child—these are heroic figures, to be celebrated, not dishonored.

In comparing these examples of self-sacrifice with the willing of one's death for purposes of transplant, one should notice certain features of those instances. In each of them one or more of the following characteristics is present: the diversion of a deadly force; a vocation calling for disregard of self, upon which others may be relying; a sudden impulse, an almost reflexive act, that would not in any event be amenable to the encouragement or deterrence of law.

These may be distinctions without a difference. Perhaps the time has come to face straightforwardly the question whether a dying patient should not be allowed to consent to surgical intervention for the sake of saving another's life. Such an approach would at least have the merit of focusing on the ethical and social issues involved. Considerations of this kind would then be adduced and weighed in opposition. It would be argued that to confer this discretion on a patient would put him in a psychologically intolerable position: he would be under great pressure to follow the noble course; if he did not a stigma might attach to his name, and if he did he would, by setting an example, make the decision even more intolerable for others in a similar position.[6] That the question cannot arise because of legal constraints may be a salutary shield for those who wish to take leave of life in peace and gentleness. But the most telling argument is that which concerns the physician. To take on the role of an active intervenor to end a life—an executioner, as it might be made to appear—would introduce a confusion of functions that could be unsettling to a practitioner of medicine and could erode the absolute trust that ought to prevail on the part of patients toward their physician. The judgment whether to use extraordinary supportive measures to prolong the life of a hopelessly ill patient, and whether to withdraw such measures in order not to prolong the process of dying, is agonizing enough. At least in making those decisions the physician can reflect that he is allowing natural forces to prevail and is not becoming an active destroyer. Even this discretion, which received the approval of Pope Pius XII in 1957, has not unfailingly seemed manifestly right. We quote today the lines of Arthur Hugh Clough as if they were a forthright prescription of the moral course:

Thou shalt not kill, yet need not strive
Officiously to keep alive.

Actually the lines were highly ironic, part of a satirical poem called "The Latest Decalogue," containing such companion couplets as

Thou shalt not covet; but tradition
Approves all forms of competition.

It is a striking example of the ethical heresy of one generation becoming the moral dogma of another.

Perhaps, despite the cogent objections that have been offered, we shall one day reach a consensus that will accept the self-sacrifice of a living person through the intervention of a surgeon. But at present the approach has taken a different turn—a redefinition of death that will in fact, if not in primary purpose, facilitate the removal of viable organs for transplantation. The problem, in short, is defined as a scientific one. It is pointed out that death is a process, in which various organs cease to function at various times. Traditionally the crucial time has been taken to be the cessation of the natural

heartbeat. But, aside from the convenience of the test and the figurative view of the heart as the vital center, there is no compelling reason for making that organ the decisive one in determining death. The proposed new definition focuses on brain death, evidenced by an irreversible coma, which in turn is identified by absence of reflexes, lack of response to intense stimuli, cessation of natural breathing, and a flat electroencephalogram, recorded over a period of twenty-four hours. All of these signs can be consistent with a continuing natural heartbeat, reinforced by artificial respiration. A finding of death according to these criteria would justify both the withdrawal of supportive measures and the availability of the heart and other organs for transplant. As explained by Dr. Henry K. Beecher, the chairman of the group at Harvard which has proposed the new definition. "Death is to be declared and *then* the respirator turned off."[7]

A number of practical questions are raised by this proposal.[8] How infallible is it as a prognosticator that neural activity in the brain will not revive? The sponsors are confident of its reliability provided the patient has not been in a state of hypothermia or of narcotic toxicity. Should it be adopted in some quarters even though in others the traditional definition is retained, and if so may there not be awkward problems of determining priority of death among the victims of a common disaster, where priority may determine succession to property?[9] How will the new definition affect the physician's discretion regarding the use or continuance of extraordinary measures? Must the physician in all cases wait for a finding of brain death before the respirator is turned off, and if so may not the new definition produce the paradoxical result in some cases of actually extending the period of dying? What will be the logistical and legal problems of transporting a person declared dead but with a heartbeat supported by artificial respiration, who is moved to another state as a source of material for a transplant? Since, under the new definition, the body is a cadaver, what obstacles are presented by state laws that require special permission and embalming as a condition of transporting a body out of the state?

Beyond these practical problems there are deeper philosophical issues. Is the new definition a scientific tactic that obscures and diverts attention from the moral and social issues presented by extraordinary supportive measures and by the procedures for organ transplantation? Is it a convenient and plausible fiction—the tribute that change pays to continuity—which enables us to achieve new results without altering but merely by redefining the words of the old rules? Is it in effect an effort to answer some vexing, specific diverse questions by a definitional generality, as if the way to consider the problems of abortion were to work out a definition of "life"? One is reminded of the cautionary words of I. A. Richards:

The temptation to introduce premature ultimates—Beauty in Aesthetics, the Mind and its faculties in psychology, Life in physiology, are representative examples—is especially great for believers in Abstract Entities. The objection to such Ultimates is that they bring an investigation to a dead end too suddenly.[10]

It is not essential that these questions be answered; it is only important, perhaps, that they shall have been asked—important lest the scientists be taken to have resolved through their special competence what are searching moral questions—lest, in short, the complex inquiry be brought to an end too suddenly.

There is one further question that ought to be raised in connection with the selection of donors: should a person be encouraged or permitted to sell his organs for purposes of transplant? In the case of donations of blood, where the risk to the donor is negligible, the question is relatively unimportant. We would not object on moral grounds to paying someone to stand in line for us at a ticket counter, though we would have the most serious moral qualms about paying for someone to take our place in a conscript army.[11] To save oneself by putting another in mortal danger through trading on his poverty strikes one as an immoral bargain. Is the case different if the bargain is struck not by the more affluent beneficiary but more impersonally by the state or a philanthropic institution? The question is analogous to that raised by a so-called volunteer army, using the inducement of higher pay for service, and the answer is equally debatable.

The Uniform Anatomical Gift Act takes no position on the issue, leaving it to state law, although it can be said that the acceptability of compensation is strongest where the donation is to be made after death. In the case of an *inter vivos* transplant of serious nature, the allowance of a pecuniary motive is repugnant, as if society had a vested interest in maintaining an impoverished class of citizens to serve as risk-takers for others. If the need for organs is felt to be crucial, and if both payment and conscription are ruled out, a possibility remains of liberalizing the law concerning bodies at death, by enacting that post-mortem removal of organs may be effected unless the decedent or next of kin have affirmatively interposed an objection.[12] This is a step whose consideration ought to await evidence on the adequacy of the Uniform Act.

It is time to turn from the selection of donors to that of donees. Few decisions can be as harrowing as the choice of who shall live and who shall die, as any judge or governor can attest; and yet in those cases the law is dealing with persons whose guilt, at least in a legal sense, has been found, and where there is no constraint on sparing the lives of all. In our problem we are dealing with the constraints of scarcity and the consequent necessity of preferences for secular salvation and doom of innocent persons.

In 1943, when penicillin was in short supply for our forces in North Africa, two groups of soldiers could have benefited from its use: those who had contracted venereal disease, and those who suffered from infected battle wounds. The consulting surgeon advised, on moral grounds, that the wounded be given priority, but the medical officer in charge ruled that preference be given to the other group. The latter, he reasoned, could be restored to active duty more quickly, and immediate manpower was needed; moreover, if untreated they could be a threat to others. For good or ill, life's values are seldom so one-dimensional as they are on the front lines in wartime. Nevertheless efforts have been made to assess the comparative worth of patients to society in the rationing of scarce medical resources, notably renal dialysis equipment. At the center in Seattle, after a medical and psychiatric

screening to identify those patients who could benefit substantially from the treatment, they are evaluated by an anonymous but predominantly lay committee, operating under no more definite criteria than social worth, which in practice has been judged by such factors as the number and need of dependents and civic service performed, such as scout leadership, religious-social teaching, and Red Cross activities.[13] One less confident that one's middle-class values represent eternal verities or even the clear hope of the future might well find it impossible to serve on such a committee. More pointedly, where the facilities are operated by a public agency there is a real question whether some more articulated and warrantable standards must be formulated to satisfy the demands of the constitutional guarantees of due process of law and equal protection of the laws.[14] When mortals are called on to make ultimate choice for life or death among their innocent fellows, the only tolerable criterion may be equality of worth as a human being. Translated into practical terms this means a procedure for selection based on randomness within a group, or on objective factors like age or priority of application.

Scarcity of resources presents not only a problem of selection of donors and donees but of allocation of medical facilities and personnel between transplant and other undertakings. At a large teaching hospital in Boston the decision was made not to engage in heart transplant surgery at the present time. To have done so would have required a material inroad on the program of open-heart surgery, where the operative results have been favorable in eighty to ninety per cent of the cases. Meanwhile basic work on the biological aspects of transplantation continued. Not every institution that has undertaken heart transplants, it can be said, was ideally suited for the mission. Should the decision to engage or not to engage in this form of surgery be left to the individual institution, or should not an effort be made to ration this enterprise in order to achieve a minimum of dislocation and a maximum of scientific progress in the experimental stage of a promising therapeutic procedure?

The upshot of our whole discussion is that the choices enforced by a scarcity of resources, and the awesome moral questions raised by deliberate programs to increase the number of donors of viable organs, point to a search for a solution that would bypass these issues, so uncomfortable for human decision. It may not be thought an evasion, one hopes, to suggest that what is urgently needed is a program for the development of artificial organs, like teeth and limbs, to supersede the transplant of natural organs. The physical obstacles are admittedly formidable: how, for example, to provide a lasting and safe power supply for an implanted mechanical heart, and how to overcome the problem of clotting presented by a large foreign surface at the site of the heart. Yet the eventuality of biologists and engineers supplanting moralists and lawyers in the collaborative quest for bodily renewal is a consummation devoutly to be wished.

Notes

1. D. Daube, "Limitations on Self-Sacrifice in Jewish Law and Tradition," *Theology* 72 (1969): pp. 291, 299; Carroll, "The Ethics of Transplantation," *Amer. Bar Assn. Jour.* 56 (1970): pp. 137, 138. (The Chief Rabbi of Israel hailed the first heart transplant in that country; the rabbinate, at the same time, asserted that postmortem operations are prohibited by the Torah.)

2. ". . . in the light of current medical advances . . . existing 'anatomical' statutes, such as [the law providing for surrender of unclaimed bodies for the advance of medical science] are inadequate, and the need for appropriate statutory provision to implement the desires of the dying to aid the living is increasingly urgent." *Holland v. Metalious,* 105 N.H. 290, 293, 198 Atl.2d 654, 656 (1964).

3. The Uniform Act is set forth and analyzed in A. M. Sadler and B. M. Sadler, "Transplantation and the Law: The Need for Organized Sensitivity," *Georgetown Law Jour.* 57 (1968): p. 5.

4. W. J. Curran, "A Problem of Consent: Kidney Transplantation," *N.Y.U. Law Rev.* 34 (1959): p. 891.

5. The religious and historical background is described in Glanville Williams, *The Sanctity of Life and the Criminal Law* (Farber, London, 1958), c. 7, and N. St. John-Stevas, *Life, Death and the Law* (Indiana, Bloomington, 1961), c. 6, on which the following paragraphs draw.

6. Daube, *supra* note 1.

7. H. K. Beecher, "Scarce Resources and Medical Advancement," in *Experimentation with Human Subjects* (P. A. Freund, ed., Braziller, N.Y., 1970), pp. 67, 84.

8. See D. Rutstein, "The Ethical Design of Human Experiments," *op. cit. supra* note 7: pp. 383, 386–387. See also Paul Ramsey, *The Patient as Person* (Yale, New Haven, 1970), c. 2. This book, which came to my attention after this paper was prepared, is of great value for the whole discussion. Similarly valuable on the entire subject of transplants is the recent volume, David W. Meyers, *The Human Body and the Law* (Aldine, Chicago, 1970).

9. See e.g., *Smith v. Smith,* 229 Ark. 579, 317 S.W. 2d 275 (1958), pointing out that the Uniform Simultaneous Death Act, prescribing a rule of succession where deaths occur in a common disaster, applies only where there is no sufficient evidence to determine which party died first. The court rejected the "unusual and unique allegation" that a victim who remained unconscious for seventeen days had in fact, according to "modern medical science," died at the time of the accident.

10. I. A. Richards, *Principles of Literary Criticism* (Harcourt, Brace, New York, 1948), p. 40.

11. Nevertheless it is to be recalled that in our early history it was customary to condition the exemption of conscientious objectors from military service on their providing a substitute or the money necessary to engage one. See J. Cardozo, in *Hamilton v. Regents,* 293 U.S. 245, 266–277 (1934).

12. D. Sanders and J. Dukeminier, "Medical Advance and Legal Lag: Hemodialysis and Kidney Transplantation," *U.C.L.A. Law Rev.* 15 (1968): pp. 357, 410–413. [Reprinted as Chapter 97 of this volume.]

13. *Idem* at pp. 366–380.

14. See Note, "Patient Selection for Artificial and Transplant Organs," *Harv. Law Rev.* 82 (1969): pp. 1322, 1331–1337.

29

Philip Reilly
Sickle Cell Anemia Legislation

Reprinted without illustrations by permission of *The Journal of Legal Medicine,* September/October, November/December, 1973, pp. 39–48, 36–40.

Much confusion surrounds the meaning of the phrase, sickle cell anemia. The term has been used to include the homozygous state for the sickle gene (genotype aaB^{s}B^s) as well as the heterozygous states for the sickle cell gene combined with genes for either structural hemoglobin variants or various types of thalassemia. As of 1969, there were at least 14 identified sickling disorders.[1]

In this article, sickle cell disease shall mean the homozygous condition for the gene; sickle cell trait shall mean the heterozygous condition. Sickle cell anemia shall encompass both conditions.

Sickle cell anemia is an inherited abnormal hemoglobinopathy that predominantly afflicts blacks.[2] Persons with sickle cell trait are called carriers. About 35 per cent of their hemoglobin has a sickling potential.[3] With the exception of greater risk such persons run from sudden oxygen deprivation (for example, in a depressurized aircraft),[4] they lead normal lives.[5] Persons with sickle cell disease (who inherited a pair of the sickling genes) are burdened with an incurable and painful condition that manifests itself in infancy and continues throughout an attenuated life span.

Sickle cell hemoglobin differs from the normal by the substitution of glutamic acid by valine in the sixth position of the B chain of the molecule.[6] In a manner not perfectly understood, the substitution error causes a spatial alteration of the hemoglobin molecules that during deoxygenation permits them to stack.[7] In the person with the disease, sickling and unsickling are ongoing phenomena. At some point when the blood flow rate is sufficiently reduced, sickling becomes established. Capillary occlusion results. This causes anoxia; thus, more cells sickle. At some point, a "crisis" is reached.[8] Infarction of soft tissue and bone causes great pain for the patient.[9]

Sickle cell disease usually manifests itself in infancy.[10] A number of clinical features now are associated with the condition: massive enlargement of the spleen, unusual liability to salmonella organism infection, bone destruction, cardiopulmonary complications, and some liver and renal malfunction.[11] One or more of these complications may cause death, with infection being the leading cause.

Table 29-1
Status of State Sickle Cell Legislation

| State | Date Effective | Testing Situation | | | | | Mandatory | Target Population | Confiden- tiality | Counsel- ing | Education | Funding |
		Pregnancy	Neonatal	Public School	Premarital	Other						
Arizona	August 1972	X		X	X		No	No	No	No	No	No
California	July 1973			X	X		Yes^a	No	No	No	No	No
Georgia	April 1973		X		X		Yes^b	No	No	Yes	No	Yes
Illinois	December 1971			X	X		Yes^c	No	No	No	No	No
Indiana	1971			X	X		Yes^{a,c}	No	No	No	No	No
Louisiana			X				No	No	No	No	No	No
Maryland	July 1972	X			X		No	No	Yes	Yes	Yes	Yes
Massachusetts	July 1971			X			Yes^c	No	No	No	No	No
Mississippi	April 1972			X			Yes	No	No	No	Yes	No
Kentucky	January 1973		X		X		Yes	Yes^d	No	Yes	No	No
New York	September 1972			X	X		Yes	Yes^{e,f}	No	No	No	No
Virginia	April 1972			X	X	X^g	Yes	Yes^h	No	No	Yes	Yes
District of Columbia	September 1973			X			Yes	No	No	No	No	No

a. Permits religious objection to screening.
b. Premarital testing is not compulsory.
c. Screening is discretionary with the attending physician.
d. "Negroes" are specified by the law.
e. The law provides for testing those not of the "Causasian, Indian, or Oriental races" prior to obtaining a marriage license.
f. The law compels testing of pupils in "city school districts."
g. The law mandates testing of incarcerated persons.
h. A child is subject to testing upon reaching the age of six.

Perhaps the most unusual aspect of sickle cell anemia is its frequency. Numerous studies indicate that 7–9 per cent of the American black population carry the sickle cell trait; about 0.3 per cent suffer from the disease.[12] The abnormal hemoglobin is not strictly limited to blacks. It has been found in high frequency in Greeks, Sicilians, Arabs, southern Iranians, Asiatic Indians, some American Indians, and some Mexican populations.[13] A recent inconclusive screening of a white population in upstate New York uncovered an incidence of 0.5 per cent sickle cell trait.[14]

If it is assumed that one in 11 black persons carries the sickle cell trait, a simple calculation leads to a fairly accurate estimate of the number of persons in that group suffering from sickle cell disease. Because the disease is homozygous, a diseased child can only be the progeny of a mating between two trait parents.[15] If each parent carries a single normal gene and an abnormal gene, there is one chance in four that they will produce a normal child, one chance in four that they will have a child with disease, and two chances in four that they will produce a trait child like themselves. The odds are, therefore, that one out of every 484 blacks suffers from sickle cell disease.[16] Assuming approximately 22 million black persons in America, it is cautious to guess that 55,000 are suffering from sickle cell disease. Although not the most commonly inherited disorder, sickle cell disease is the hereditary illness most frequently fatal.[17]

If persons with sickle cell trait did not mate, obviously there would be a significant, rapid reduction of the disease. The methodology for effecting such a reduction provokes difficult ethical/legal questions.[18]

By 1970, an inexpensive, simple, relatively reliable test for sickle cell hemoglobin was available.[19] A few drops of a person's blood was all that was needed to determine if he or she had trait.[20] Today the testing methodology is quite refined.[21]

Some controversy surrounds the appropriate methods to be used in a screening program.[22] Generally, the problem is one of balancing the most economical procedure against a small but significant number of false test results. Further, some sickle cell testing methods miss a number of related hemoglobinopathies that other methods could uncover.[23]

Today it is economically feasible to test the entire population for sickle cell trait.[24] Testing programs involving only a few thousand people have proven to require an expenditure of less than a dollar per person.[25] Economies of scale would reduce the unit cost further. These figures do not, however, include costs of education and genetic counseling that Dr. James Bowman, professor of pathology at the Pritzker School of

Medicine and the Division of Biological Science, University of Chicago, and other articulate critics argue are necessary elements of any testing program.

As a rule, legislation mandating sickle cell anemia screening programs has failed to consider that the cost of actually administering the tissue test may be a small fraction of the total expenditure for a program that adequately provides for education and counseling of subjects tested. Many state laws, as a matter of fact, do not include a counseling provision.

In 1971, Massachusetts became the first state to enact a sickle cell anemia testing law.[26] Today at least 12 states and the District of Columbia have adopted sickle cell anemia screening laws.[27] Legislation has been considered in a number of other states.[28] The rapidity with which these laws have been created recalls the phenylketonuria[29] legislative craze several years ago. Recent passage of the National Sickle Cell Anemia Control Act, with a hefty budget of $115 million for diagnosis, control, treatment, and research,[30] seems likely to stimulate further state legislation.

The desire to see the millions spent on medical research pay public dividends certainly must have motivated some legislators. Yet, the ethnicity of the disease, the political mileage screening legislation seemed to provide, and a growing concern for health care in a society pressured by population problems were probably influential factors. The legislation has raised some novel legal problems.

A careful scrutiny of the laws currently in force suggests the haste with which they were passed. One is forced to conclude that the laws, as written, indicate a nearly complete failure of communication between the biomedical and legal professions. As will be demonstrated, state legislation often reflects a lack of understanding of the simple Mendelian laws of genetics or of the pathology of the sickle cell disease. A critique of the legislation suggests some appropriate areas for amendment or repeal.

In an era when privacy seems threatened, in a time of severe racial tensions, and amidst increased promise for a technology of eugenics,[31] sickle

cell anemia legislation provides an excellent forum to ponder germane ethical issues. It is hoped that a critical analysis of the current laws will stimulate more sophisticated biomedical legislation in the future.

Early sickle cell anemia legislation was usually considered and passed without objection.[32] The law, until recently, proved the concern of the state for health problems in the black community.[33] Often proposed by black legislators and rarely hampered by funding provisions, the law was politically expedient and, so it seemed, unimpeachable.

The legislative picture is changing. States continue to implement such laws. There is, however, a growing trend, particularly within the black community, to criticize laws that foster or compel mass screening of blacks.[34]

New York and New Jersey have in recent months been the sites for conferences on the sickle cell laws.[35] At these conferences an interdisciplinary panel of black citizens led by Dr. Bowman sharply criticized sickle cell anemia screening laws as harbingers of socioeconomic discrimination. In New York, there seemed to be immediate repercussions. State Senator Joseph Galiber held hearings to reconsider the New York law on March 6, 1973.

It appears that protests from the black community that sickle cell screening results in a new discrimination are not unjustified. Research by the New York State Department of Public Health indicates a significant number of life insurance companies charge a higher premium rate for the policy holder who is a known sickle cell trait carrier.[36] Yet, there does not appear to be evidence suggesting a documented reduction in life expectancy of trait individuals.

James Europe, a panelist at the sickle cell conferences, stated that his research indicated a growing number of employers required a sickle cell trait screening test for their employment physicals.[37] The spectrum of employers that request an applicant to undergo a test for sickle cell trait may soon include the U.S. armed forces,[38] the New York Metropolitan Transit Authority,[39] and major airlines.[40] It appears that certain job categories will be foreclosed to an individual with trait.[41] If this practice were adopted by the armed forces

alone, thousands of blacks would be precluded from possible careers in the service just as that option becomes more attractive. This can only exacerbate current unemployment problems of blacks.[42]

As of March 1973, 12 states and the District of Columbia have sickle cell anemia testing laws. Legislative action has been initiated in a number of states. Any compilation of state legislative activity in the area of sickle cell anemia screening could be inaccurate in a matter of weeks. Amendments to some of the laws are under consideration.[43] According to a recent survey, Massachusetts, the District of Columbia, Illinois, Virginia, and New York are contemplating changes to conform to the recent federal legislation.[44] Many of these changes are to repeal or amend mandatory laws.

The key issue in each of these laws is the manner in which screening shall be conducted. Nine states provide for screening prior to application for a marriage license, three for neonatal screening, two for screening of all pregnant women. Eight states and the District of Columbia provide for screening of public school children. One state, Virginia, mandates screening of incarcerated individuals. Obviously, several states have legislated multiple screening situations.

The issue of compulsion is the crucial factor in understanding the controversy that surrounds these laws. Only three states can easily be classified as having completely voluntary screening laws. Under Arizona law, a test must be premised upon consent of the individual or guardian. Louisiana has modeled its sickle cell law on the phenylketonuria statute. It also provides for neonatal screening, subject to parental objection. Maryland is the only state currently embracing voluntariness as a value in its screening legislation. It has been unique in its response to criticisms offered by the black community and concerned persons in the medical profession.

Nine states and the District of Columbia have sickle cell laws that are either explicitly compulsory or suggest compulsion. Few of the laws, however, are coupled with a clear enforcement mechanism. The District of Columbia, Georgia, Illinois, Massachusetts, New

York, and Virginia require a record of a sickle cell anemia test on a child's public school health certificate. (In Georgia, testing is specified for neonates but seems to be a prerequisite for public schooling.) In effect, public school could be closed to a child who did not subject himself to the test. The Mississippi screening law, also modeled along testing public school children, does not suggest that such a test be a prerequisite for attendance. Such an inference could, however, reasonably be made. Kentucky requires compulsory testing of Negro applicants for marriage licenses and of newborn Negroes. Failure to comply can result in a fine of "not less than $100 nor more than $300."[45]

Before attempting an analysis of the sickle cell anemia screening laws, it is well to identify their purpose. Persons afflicted with the disease are usually painfully aware of it from infancy. Individuals who are carriers of the sickle cell gene probably will not recognize their status unless they marry another carrier and produce an afflicted child or unless they are screened. Screening primarily discovers trait individuals. Trait is not a condition that requires medical care. Awareness of trait may be important in certain instances. For example, if a trait person is to undergo major surgery, the presence of the gene may influence the procedure of the anesthesiologist.[46] Nevertheless, the purpose of the sickle cell anemia screening laws can only be to warn a significant portion of black Americans that an unlucky mating choice offers a 25 per cent chance for a child with an incurable genetic disease.[47] The large number of premarital screening laws already written confirms this premise.

There is probably very little disagreement with a declaration that a program aimed at reducing the number of children born with an incurable genetic disease is valuable and welcome. It is the methodology of such a program that raises the difficult questions. A range of prophylactic alternatives are available to a technologically sophisticated and eugenically minded society. Compulsory amniocentesis coupled with selective abortion, sterilization, and mating prohibitions are options that are immediately apparent—and morally questionable.

Of course, a genetic screening program (even if compulsory) does no more than confront an individual with a biological fact. Yet, logically, a young person aware that he or she carries the sickling gene and educated about the implications for parenthood will be expected to be influenced in marital or procreative decisions. Thus, it is not inappropriate to characterize sickle cell anemia screening laws as eugenic legislation. A national web of such screening laws, coupled with a satisfactory educational program, could reasonably be expected to reduce the number of live births of children with sickle cell disease without invocation of more coercive measures.

The potential advent of large-scale genetic screening programs has recently generated interdisciplinary efforts to develop guidelines for their implementation. The focal concern has been the protection of the individual from the risk of misunderstanding and misuse of information derived from screening by the society at large.

A concomitant concern is that the individual not be intimidated by self-knowledge: "Several medical researchers have recently cautioned their colleagues of the potential for misinterpretation of the clinical meaning of sickle 'trait' and 'disease.' We are concerned about the dangers of societal misinterpretation of similar conditions and the possibility of widespread and undesirable labeling of individuals on a genetic basis. For instance, the lay public may incorrectly conclude that persons with sickle trait are seriously handicapped in their ability to function effectively in society. Moreover, protecting the confidentiality of test results will not shield all such subjects from a felt sense of stigmatization nor from personal anxieties stemming from their own misinterpretation of their carrier status."[48]

The latter of these concerns requires that any screening program include an extensive, sensitive plan for education and counseling of all subjects with particular attention to those with positive test results.

The former concern requires that a screening program maintain a posture of confidentiality to protect the privacy of those tested. The specter of social stigmatization argues against requiring the test of a specific group. Notably,

the literature thus far condemns compulsory genetic screening programs.

Of the 13 operational statutes, only that of Maryland expresses a clear concern for confidentiality. Only Georgia, Maryland, and Kentucky make provision for counseling persons screened. Only Maryland and Virginia provide for education of the public about sickle cell anemia. Only Arizona, Louisiana, and Maryland have clearly voluntary laws. An obvious, wide disparity exists between values proclaimed in the medical literature and the statutory language.

From the scientific perspective, the statutes are naive. Three states, Georgia, Louisiana, and Kentucky, provide for neonatal screening. Yet, during the first months of life a child with sickle cell disease (because of a high percentage of fetal hemoglobin still in the circulatory system) might not register a positive test result. Testing infants before they are six months of age is currently unwise.[49]

Further, the laws reflect a lack of understanding of the distribution of sickle cell gene. Kentucky and New York address their premarital screening laws to "Negroes"[50] and "persons not of the Caucasian, Indian, or Oriental races."[51] Yet, we have already seen that a significant number of persons of Middle Eastern and Mediterranean extraction will register the sickling gene.

Perhaps the most significant scientific error in the legislation is the failure to make the crucial distinction between sickle cell trait and sickle cell disease. Only Massachusetts, Maryland, and Virginia mention both conditions. Maryland alone troubles to define the words. An examination of the Arizona law, which has a typical "declaration of policy" section, illustrates the problem. That section reads: "It is the policy of this state to make every effort to detect, as early as possible, sickle cell anemia, a heritable disorder which leads to physical defects. The state department of health has the responsibility of designating tests and regulations to be used in executing this policy. Such tests shall be in accordance with accepted medical practice."[52]

In this provision, sickle cell anemia is understood to mean either the disease state or the sickling gene. Logically, it could not be the state's policy to detect the disease because it is usually readily manifest. Yet, trait does not lead to "physical defects." As written, the logical meaning of the Arizona law is that the state wishes to screen people for an affliction they already realize. The law is either the product of careless drafting or ignorance of biological facts pertaining to sickle cell anemia.

Unfortunately, most of the legislation could be similarly criticized. The federal law makes a similar error. "The Congress finds and declares . . . that sickle cell anemia is a debilitating, inheritable disease that afflicts approximately two million American citizens. . . ."[53] Two million persons may carry the trait; only about 50,000 suffer from the disease.

Sickle cell anemia legislation is also guilty of errors of omission. Not one law specifies the testing methods to be used in a screening program. It has already been noted that a number of such methods exist and that they are of varying efficiency. The state laws either completely fail to discuss testing or they defer to "accepted medical practices." A screening program that combined primary electrophoresis with secondary solubility tests of all abnormal hemoglobins would rarely yield a false test result.[54] The more rigorous electrophoretic method can be done at an acceptable cost.[55] Although no state has formally implemented an active screening program, private programs have utilized less efficient solubility testing.[56] It is incumbent upon any state considering screening legislation to insure accuracy in testing. This could be accomplished by requiring employment of the most accurate techniques available without regard to cost.

From the educational and counseling perspectives, the laws also are open to serious criticism. If the object of sickle cell screening is to forewarn carriers of potential danger to progeny, it is appropriate to screen and counsel at an age when such a message can be understood, perhaps early adolescence. Currently, many laws require the test for admission to public school. Clearly, a six-year-old cannot be taught the implications of his genetic makeup. Testimony at the several sickle cell anemia conferences illuminates the difficulties involved in teaching simple Mendelian laws to individuals. Counseling faces considerable anxiety in subjects. The most critical concern for the uninitiated

appears to be that the test results might injure otherwise normal sexual relationships and ultimately destroy a marriage.[57]

Perhaps the most egregious oversight of the sickle cell screening legislation is the paternity problem. A positive test result for trait immediately implies that one parent also has the trait. What happens when neither parent's test shows the sickling gene? The inference of maternal adultery is inescapable. One physician puts it bluntly: "This revelation can occur in, traumatize and even destroy otherwise stable families."[58] Another leading black physician categorically refuses to inform parents of test results when a paternity issue arises.[59]

A difficult question is posed: Should a physician screening pursuant to legislative mandate have the right of nondisclosure or false disclosure when he feels the test result will harm the patient?

Relevant case law deals with the duty of disclosure upon a physician seeking consent to treatment from his patient.[60] Nondisclosure is permitted if it is reasonable when compared to appropriate standards of practice.[61] Of course, such nondisclosure must be premised on harmful effects the information would have.[62]

The analogy to a physician seeking to treat a patient is limited. The screening program is not premised on treatment. It is questionable that a formal doctor-patient relationship exists in a mass screening situation.[63] It is probable that technicians and lay personnel will be screening in some situations.

The right of the screener to withhold test information (which might exacerbate an individual's suspicions) or to give false information (which could perhaps subject him to liability for fraud) has not yet been tested in court.

Two recent medical malpractice cases considered a similar problem. In *Gleitman v. Cosgove*[64] an action was brought against physicians for failure to explain the dangers of rubella for a first trimester fetus to a plaintiff who had been under their care during her pregnancy. The New Jersey Supreme Court affirmed the trial court's dismissal. It was held that there were no damages cognizable at law for the deformed child or the parents. Under tort law, damages are compensatory. Yet, the

defendants did not injure the fetus. The abortion law controversy current at decision appears to have clouded the issue of the validity of the plaintiff mother's cause of action. At least one justice found an actionable injury to the mother of the deformed child.[65] For two dissenting justices the question of the duty of disclosure upon the physicians was clear: "When Mrs. Gleitman told her obstetricians that she had German measles (rubella), they were placed under a clear duty to tell her of its high incidence of abnormal birth. That duty was not only a moral one but a legal one as well."[66]

Stewart v. Long Island College Hospital[67] arose out of a factual setting similar to the *Gleitman* case. The plaintiffs sued a hospital for failure to inform them that two out of four physicians reviewing the plaintiff mother's pregnancy recommended a therapeutic abortion because she had contracted rubella at a critical time. The court, following *Gleitman,* denied recovery to the infant plaintiff. But the jury awarded $10,000 to the mother because of the failure of the hospital physicians to indicate the disagreement among members of the abortion review committee. The damage award, a radical departure from the *Gleitman* decision a year earlier, was disallowed on appeal. The court was particularly concerned about the problem of damage measurement: "We note that it would be virtually impossible to evaluate as compensatory damages the anguish to the parents of rearing a malformed child as against the denial to them of the benefits of parenthood."[68]

The lower court in *Stewart* noted the existence of a line of cases holding that a "physician is under an obligation to disclose to his patient serious or statistically significant risks of the proposed treatment."[69]

Of course, there is a crucial distinction between a physician contemplating treatment and a screener performing a simple tissue test. Whether the latter situation requires a greater or lesser duty of truth telling remains an open question. Medical treatment may involve immediate physical risk. Concern for the patient's frame of mind may argue for nondisclosure.[70] No physical risk adheres to screening.

The compulsory sickle cell anemia legislation currently in force in nine states and the District of Columbia raises interesting questions for constitutional analysis. Is compulsory sickle cell anemia legislation a valid exercise of the police power? Demonstration of the invalidity of the legislative exercise is a burden upon the party attacking the statute.[71] A presumption of constitutionality favors the law.[72] Screening programs are not premised on availability of therapy. Sound reasoning, however, supports their passage. The acquisition of a solid body of statistical data on a genetic anomaly appears to be a reasonable justification for the public health measures. The possiblity that screening pursuant to legislation could reduce the number of persons born with sickle cell disease and thus lessen the medical case load offers further justification.

No Supreme Court decision offers an appropriate analogy for this argument. In *Jacobson v. Massachusetts*,[73] the high court did uphold a conviction of a man who refused compulsory smallpox vaccination even though he offered proof that, having suffered from the disease, he was immune to further attack. Two distinctions greatly dilute the importance of the decision. Smallpox is a highly contagious disease. Sickle cell anemia is communicated only by inheritance. An attempt to analogize the two forms of transmission must be rejected.[74] Epidemics of smallpox or venereal disease pose a much more immediate and larger threat to society than sickle cell anemia.

In *Zucht v. King*,[75] another assault was made on compulsory vaccination laws. Dismissing the case for want of a substantial federal question, the Supreme Court confirmed, *sub silentio*, its view of the broad health power of the state. Significantly, it agreed that the state could delegate authority to determine when health regulations should become operative. This implies that sections of sickle cell anemia laws that confer discretion on whom to test and what methodology to utilize are valid.[76]

Recently, the Supreme Court has commented on the propriety of employment criteria. In *Griggs v. Duke Power Company*,[77] the court addressed itself to the section of the Civil Rights Act that commands employment tests to be job related.[78] It found: "Congress has placed on the employer the burden

of showing that any given requirement must have a manifest relationship to the employment question."[79]

The same burden should be borne by employment physical testing. Thus, arguably, an employer who screens for sickle cell trait must prove, if he considers its presence cause for nonemployment, its relationship to incapacity to work. With the sole exception of aircraft pilots, there are insufficient data to exclude any persons from any job category. Supporting this contention is the recent finding that at least 39 players in the National Football League are trait carriers—without any apparent impediment to their athletic ability.

Discussion of compulsory eugenic legislation must note the case, *Buck v. Bell*,[80] which upheld a Virginia statute that provided for sterilization of institutionalized mental defectives. (A significant number of compulsory sterilization statutes are still to be found in the state codes.)[81] The *Buck* case was decided at the height of the American eugenics movement, and Justice Oliver Wendell Holmes, who wrote the opinion, was known to sympathize with principles of eugenics.[82] To the extent that *Buck* approves the proposition that the state can prohibit procreation where offspring would burden society, the decision arguably supports compulsory genetic screening. Indeed, proponents of screening legislation could argue that, in principle, *Buck* validates more serious intervention into personal freedoms than does testing.

Yet, the case is distinguishable in a number of important ways. Institutionalized mental defectives are a small, segregated group of individuals who put an obvious financial burden on the state. The progeny of such persons could never expect parental care. Persons with sickle cell trait lead normal lives. They are perfectly capable of parenthood. Indeed, their position is like that of numerous persons who carry autosomal recessive genes for other disorders and probably do not realize it.

Sickle cell anemia screening is performed on a significant segment of the population at large to uncover information about otherwise healthy persons

that will be of real importance in only about one in 100 marital decisions of black Americans. In itself a screening program offers no certainty of a reduction in trait matings or births of children with sickle cell disease, although such reduction would not be surprising.

Sickle cell anemia legislation raises a difficult equal protection issue. Classifications of persons cannot be expected to meet perfect definitions.[83] Certain classifications, including race, are suspect and will be carefully scrutinized by the courts.[84]

At least three state sickle cell anemia laws have made provision for screening a specific target subpopulation. A scrutiny of the relevant language uncovers serious constitutional defects. Virginia requires testing of inmates of state correctional institutions or mental hospitals at the discretion of the chief physician.[85] Awareness of trait is valuable to procreational decision making. Institutionalized persons are clearly not in a position to need such information. Further, the subpopulation of institutionalized persons probably is not large enough to be of significant statistical value for studies designed to increase knowledge of gene distribution. Thus, it seems that the Virginia statute mandating testing of incarcerated individuals fails to meet the requirement that the testing satisfy a rationally related state purpose.[86] Clearly, it could not pass muster under the more rigorous compelling state interest test if that were applied.

Current New York screening legislation, which can only be characterized as bizarre, poses the equal protection issue in a more insidious fashion. The law stipulates that urban public school children are required to test for sickle cell anemia. For children living in nonurban areas, testing is discretionary, and it is left to a physician to "determine whether a test for sickle cell anemia is necessary or desirable."[87]

Another section of the New York law states that the medical inspector who examines pupils who do not furnish public health certificates is now required to test for sickle cell anemia in children "between the ages of four and nine"[88] in a city school district. In nonurban areas, such a test is administered at the discretion of the physician.

Thus, in New York, locale has been made the determinative factor in sickle cell testing. Urban children must be tested; rural children may be tested. Residence would not seem to be an appropriate criterion. The urban/nonurban dichotomy is further weakened by the fact that the screening legislation does not apply to New York City, Buffalo, or Rochester.[89]

The classifications set up under New York law are confusing. It would seem that a law that required some, but not all, children to undergo a test prior to entry to public school, where that test was for a condition that each child faced at equal risk (that is, whites in cities with whites not in cities and blacks in cities with blacks not in cities), is irrational. The New York law may be an attempt to mask a racial classification. Black people predominantly live in cities.

Racial characterization also occurs in some premarital sickle cell screening laws. As noted previously, New York obliquely requires screening of those marriage license applicants not of the "Caucasian, Indian or Oriental" races. Kentucky bluntly requires screening of all "Negro" applicants. Given the scientifically documented prevalence of the sickling gene in non-Negro populations as well, and that failure to comply with the law precludes marriage in the state, an invidious discrimination is suggested.[90] Blacks cannot marry in the state if they are not tested. Whites who may have the gene need not be tested. New York does include a religious exemption in its premarital screening law. This, however, does not insulate the legislation from attack.[91] In an era of severe racial tensions, black marriage license applicants may refuse to undergo a test for sickle cell anemia on avowedly nonreligious grounds.

Most states require all marriage license applicants to undergo a blood test for venereal disease. (The power of the state to test for venereal disease is established.)[92] Blood drawn at that time can be used to test for sickle cell trait. It is important to understand that the objection to the genetic screening is not an objection to the taking of blood.

Indeed, for premarital screening, this is not the concern at all. The crucial issue is what effect knowledge of the trait condition will have on the individual. Some black persons see a new source for discrimination. This fear is exacerbated by knowledge that nonblack potential carriers need not be tested.

Arizona and California provide for testing for sickle cell anemia in any subgroup that is at unusual risk: "The state department of health may require that a test be given for sickle cell anemia to any identifiable segment of the population which the department determines is susceptible to sickle cell anemia at a disproportionately higher ratio than is the balance of the population."[93] This provision is cleverly drafted to avoid the immediate criticisms of the Kentucky law. It is reasonable on its face. Scrutiny of its application would be required before it could be attacked.

"The Constitution does not explicitly mention any right of privacy."[94] The roots of such a right have been found by the Supreme Court in the 1st,[95] 4th and 5th,[96] 9th,[97] and 14th[98] Amendments.

Compulsory sickle cell anemia legislation provokes a boundary analysis of the right to privacy. In *Griswold v. Connecticut*, the Supreme Court struck down a state statute prohibiting the use of contraceptive devices. The decision suggested that "specific guarantees in the Bill of Rights have penumbras, formed by emanations from these guarantees that help give them life and substance."[99] The right to marry, establish a home, and bring up children is within the protected area.[100] Procreation decisions pursuant to the right to marry are now, under *Griswold*, protected as private. The recent decisions on abortion laws confirm that procreative privacy is not peculiar to marriage.

"This right to privacy, whether it be founded in the Fourteenth Amendment's concept of personal liberty and restrictions upon state action, as we feel it is, or as the District Court determined, in the Ninth Amendment's reservation of rights to the people, is broad enough to encompass a woman's decision whether or not to terminate her pregnancy."[101]

Does the zone of privacy include the individual's genetic profile? Certain factors focus the question. Assuming that the state has a legitimate interest in preventing the birth of children afflicted with a fatal disease, the question remains whether that goal is properly pursued by compulsory legislation.

In principle, "a governmental purpose to control or prevent activities constitutionally subject to state regulation may not be achieved by means which sweep unnecessarily broadly and thereby invade the area of protected freedoms."[102] Balancing the governmental goal against the effect of the compulsory screening legislation, it appears the method is overly drastic. Voluntary screening legislation coupled with a sophisticated educational program is a more rational means to the same end.

The recent National Sickle Cell Anemia Control Act adheres to this view.[103] The law, which appropriates $85 million for screening programs and $30 million for diagnosis, research, and development of public education and counseling programs, is premised on voluntariness.[104] The promise of a chunk of federal money will probably stimulate amendment of compulsory legislation. With the exception of the inaccurate characterization of sickle cell anemia as an affliction burdening "two million American citizens," the federal legislation is laudable. It promises fund grants to screening programs that provide for strict confidentiality "and community representation."[105] It provides for counseling of persons who register positive test results.

The National Sickle Cell Anemia Control Act, premised as it is on voluntariness in screening programs, moots most of the problems posed by state compulsory screening legislation. States that wish to utilize federal money for screening will have to purge the compulsory element from their laws.

Yet, the development of amniocentesis and automated karyotype analysis as well as numerous genetic screening tests suggest that eugenic legislation will be considered again in the near future.[106] The advent of widespread routine selective therapeutic abortion to effect a reduction of deformed births is arguably imminent. Such a reduction is to be applauded. There is a lingering disaffection with the solution. Will therapeutic abortion deter research in the actual cure of genetic diseases?

The passage of ill-considered and poorly drafted sickle cell anemia laws should alert the legal and medical communities and the public at large that biomedical legislation must accurately incorporate scientific knowledge and reflect the ethical concerns of society. Future genetic screening legislation should not be specifically focused on a particular disease. Rather, the law should set up guidelines for testing in general that emphasize confidentiality, counseling, and test accuracy. Perhaps the crucial concern for such legislation should be to insure that public education includes a program to explain the mysteries of our genetic constitution.

Notes

1. Sickle cell anemia—improving the odds for your patient. *Patient Care* 6(3):104–129, 1972.

2. Nalbandian, R. M., Mass screening programs for sickle cell hemoglobin. *JAMA* 221:500, 1972.

3. Reference 1, at 105.

4. Green R. L., Huntsman, R. G., Serjeant, G. R., The sickle cell and altitude. *Br. Med. J.* 4:593, 1971.

5. Sickle cell trait has been associated with a sudden death syndrome. See Jones, S. R., Binder, R. A., Donowho, E. M., Jr.: Sudden death in sickle cell trait. *N. Engl. J. Med.* 282:323–324, 1970; see also The not so harmless sickle cell trait. *N. Engl. J. Med.* 286:377, 1972.

6. Weatherall, D. J., Clegg, J. B., *The Thalassaemia Syndromes*. London, Oxford Press (2d ed.), 1972, p. 48.

7. *Ibid.* at 49.

8. Reference 1.

9. Reference 6, at 53.

10. About one-half of the disease sufferers manifest the swelling of "hand and foot syndrome" in infancy. Nearly all have symptoms of chronic anemia. See reference 2.

11. Reference 6, at 55.

12. Binder, R. A., Jones, S. R., Prevalence and awareness of sickle cell hemoglobin in a military population. *JAMA* 214:909, 1970.

13. Livingstone, F. B., *Abnormal Hemoglobins in Human Populations; a Summary and Interpretation.* Chicago, Aldine Publishing Co., 1967.

14. Statement of Dr. Joseph Robinson, New York State Dept. of Health, Second Sickle Cell Anemia Conference, Harlem Hospital, New York City, Feb. 12, 1973.

15. A very small number of children with sickle cell disease could result from the mating of a person with the disease and a normal person.

16. The parents have only one chance in 121 of mating (1/11 × 1/11). The parents have one chance in four for a diseased child; thus, roughly ¼ × 1/121 = 1/484.

17. Bowman, J., "Sickle cell screening—medico-legal, ethical, psychological, and social problems: a sickle cell crisis" at 17. Paper presented at the National Conference on the Mental Health Aspects of Sickle Cell Anemia, Meharry Medical College, June 27, 1972. Dr. Bowman asserts that glucose phosphate dehydrogenase (G6PD) deficiency is the most common hereditary disorder among blacks.

18. King, J. W., Carson, G. ., Gardner, M., Sickling phenomenon as a basis for legal exclusion of paternity. *Cleve. Clin. Q.* 37:31, 1970.

19. Loh, W. P., A new solubility test for rapid detection of hemoglobin S. *J. Indiana State Med. Assoc.* 61:1651, 1968.

20. Kan, Y. W., Dozy, A. M., Alter, B. P., et al., Detecting the sickle cell gene in the human fetus, potential for intrauterine diagnosis of sickle cell anemia. *N. Engl. J. Med.* 287:1, 1972.

21. Reference 6, at Appendix A.

22. Nalbandian, R. M., Henry, R. L., Lusher, J. M., et al., Sickledex test for hemoglobin S . . . a critique. *JAMA* 218:1679, 1971.

23. [Bowman] J: Detecting sickle cell anemia. *Br. Med. J.* 3:644, 1972.

24. Nalbandian, R. M., An automated mass screening program for sickle cell disease. *JAMA* 281:1680, 1971.

25. *Ibid.* at 1681.

26. Mass. Ann. Laws, ch. 76, § 15A (1971).

27. Ariz. Public Health and Safety §§ 36–797, 41–42. Cal. Health and Safety Code art. 3.5, § 310–311 (West); note: another section of the same number was added by Stats. 1971, ch. 1029, p. 1028 (see art. 3.3). Ga. Laws 1972 No. 1258; Laws 1972 No. 1378. Ill. Public Act 77–1788, 77–1789 (1971). Ky. Reg. Sess. 1972 Bill No. 615. La. Rev. Stat. 40:1299.1. Md. art. 43, § 33A, art. 62, § 6A. Mass. Ann. Laws ch. 76, § 15A. Mississippi Bill No. 702. N.Y. Ed. Law §§ 903, 904 (McKinney Supp. 1972). N.Y. D. R. Law §§ 13aa (McKinney Supp. 1972). Va. Code Ann. §§ 32–112.10–19 (Additional Supp. 1972). District of Columbia City Council, Reg. No. 72–9, May 3, 1972.

28. New Jersey and Ohio have expressed legislative concern over sickle cell anemia. Because their laws are not specifically directed at screening, however, they will not be considered in the body of the paper.

New Jersey, in 1972, passed an act permitting county assistance for the care of children afflicted with sickle cell anemia (N.J. Ann. Stat. 9:14B–1). It permits an appropriation of "not more than $5,000 each year for the necessary expense incident to the diagnosis and treatment" of children with sickle cell anemia. Candidly, this must be regarded as a token gesture.

Ohio has mandated that the director of health "encourage and assist in the development of programs of education and research pertaining to the causes, detection, and treatment of sickle cell disease and provide for rehabilitation and counseling of persons possessing the trait of or afflicted with this disease" (Ohio Code Supp. 3701.131). Although trait screening programs could be carried on under this provision, they would seem to be incidental to a more comprehensive concern with the disease itself. The Ohio law represents a quick state response to funding provisions contained within the National Sickle Cell Anemia Control Act. Ohio authorizes the director of health to "accept and administer grants from the federal government" (Ohio Code Supp. 3701.131(c)).

29. See Swazey, Phenylketonuria: A Case Study in Biomedical Legislation, 48 *J. Urban L.* (1971).

30. 86 Stat. 136–139.

31. Ramsey, P., *Fabricated Man: The Ethics of Genetic Control.* New Haven, Yale University Press, 1970.

32. Powledge, T., Sickle cell anemia: The new ghetto hustle. *Sat. Rev. Sci.*, Feb. 1973, p. 38.

33. In conversation between the author and Sidney Von Luther, a black New York legislator who has proposed one version of a sickle cell screening law, this emerged as a factor.

34. *Newsweek*, Feb. 12, 1973, p. 63; also Kashif, D.C. fights sickle cell testing. *Muhammad Speaks*, Jan. 5, 1973.

35. Harlem Hospital's Comprehensive Sickle Cell Center hosted a conference on screening legislation, Jan. 12, 1973, and one on socioeconomic discrimination that results from being branded a sickle cell gene carrier, Feb. 23, 1973). On Feb. 24, 1973, a similar legislative conference was held at the United Hospitals Medical Center in Newark.

36. Dr. Joseph Robinson, at the second Harlem Hospital conference, named life insurance companies that charged higher premiums for trait individuals.

37. Rarely will a person with sickle cell disease reach employment age without being painfully aware of his affliction.

38. The recommendation to test for trait among all prospective black recruits was made recently by an ad hoc National Association of Scientists–National Research Council.

39. Statement at the second Harlem Hospital conference by Dr. Dorothy Holden, Downstate Medical Center, Brooklyn, N.Y.

40. A Pan American Airlines executive defended his company's screening policy at the second Harlem conference.

41. While it may be that a trait individual should not pilot an aircraft (although many probably have in the service), refusal of stewardess positions is difficult to justify.

42. J. Bowman at Harlem conference

43. Reference 32

44. Based on a Dept. of HEW survey, as of Feb. 26, 1973. The author is in some disagreement with the survey as to classification of legislation as mandatory.

45. Ky. Reg. Sess. 1972 House Bill No. 615, § 5. Indiana law on sickle cell anemia states that "any applicant for a license to marry . . . who shall knowingly and wilfully furnish any false information to the clerk . . . shall be guilty of a felony." Punishment includes a fine of $100 to $500 and up to five years in prison (Burn's Ind. Stat. 44–213 (e)).

46. Whitten, C. F., Sickle–cell programming—an imperiled promise. *N. Engl. J. Med.* 288:318–319, 1973. The author notes: "There is potential for intravascular sickling if hypoxia occurs under anesthesia. . . ."

47. Pearson, H. A., et al., Sickle cell testing programs. *J. Pediatr.* 81:1201, 1972.

48. Lappé, M., Gustafson, J. M., Roblin, R., et al., Ethical and social problems in screening for genetic disease. *N. Engl. J. Med.* 286:1132, 1972.

49. Agar gel electrophoresis will test neonatal subjects, but this procedure is much more expensive than solubility screening. See Pearson, reference 47.

50. Reference 45, at § 2.

51. N.Y. D. R. Law, § 13aa (McKinney Supp. 1972).

52. Ariz. Ann. Rev. Stat., § 36–797, 41–42.

53. 86 Stat. 137.

54. See reference 23.

55. Barnes, M. G., Komarmy, L., Novack, A. H., A comprehensive screening program for hemoglobinopathies. *JAMA* 219:701, 1972.

56. See reference 46.

57. Naomi Chamberlain, a consultant in community health care and preventive medicine in Washington, D.C., described practical problems a counselor faces in screening programs at the Harlem conference.

58. See reference 46.

59. See reference 17, at 19.

60. *Salgo v. Leland Stanford Univ.,* 154 Cal. App. 2d 560, 317 P.2d 170 (1957) is the leading case.

61. *Aiken v. Clary,* 396 S.W.2d 668 (Mo. 1965).

62. *Natanson v. Klein,* 186 Kan. 393, 350 P.2d 1093 (1960); *rehearing denied* 187 Kan. 186, 354 P.2d 670 (1960).

63. Sorenson, J. R., *Social Aspects of Applied Human Genetics,* New York, Russell Sage Foundation, 1971.

64. *Gleitman v. Cosgove,* 49 N.J. 22, 227 A.2d 689 (1967).

65. Weintraub, C. J., 49 N.J. 65.

66. 49 N.J. 49 (Jacobs, J. dissenting).

67. *Stewart v. Long Island College Hosp.,* 58 Misc. 2d 432, 296 N.Y.S.2d 41 (Sup. Ct. Nassau Co.), *rev'd* 35 A.D.2d 531, 313 N.Y.S.2d 502, *aff'd* 315 N.Y.S.2d 863 (1968).

68. 35 A.D.2d at 532.

69. 58 Misc. 2d at 438.

70. Cf. *Natanson v. Klein,* reference 62.

71. *United States v. Caroline Products Co.,* 304 U.S. 144 (1938).

72. 304 U.S. at 147.

73. 197 U.S. 12 (1905).

74. It is disturbing to note that the Washington, D.C., sickle cell screening regulation was passed pursuant to the power to "prevent and control the spread of communicable disease." 6–118 D.C. Code (1967 ed.) ch. 134, § 402.

75. 260 U.S. 174 (1922).

76. Cf. *Collins v. Texas,* 223 U.S. 288.

77. 401 U.S. 424 (1972).

78. 78 Stat. 255, § 703(h), title VII.

79. 401 U.S. 432.

80. 274 U.S. 200 (1927).

81. Fersterr, *Eliminating the Unfit—Is Sterilization the Answer?* 27 Ohio St. L. J. 591 (1966).

82. Haller, M. H., *Eugenics; Hereditarian Attitudes in American Thought.* New Brunswick, N.J., Rutgers University Press, 1963.

83. *Williamson v. Lee Optical of Oklahoma,* 348 U.S. 482 (1955).

84. *Loving v. Virginia,* 388 U.S. 1 (1967).

85. Va. Code, § 32–112.19 (Cum. Supp. 1972).

86. *Railway Express Agency v. New York,* 336 U.S. 106 (1949).

87. N.Y. Ed. Law § 903 (McKinney Supp. 1972).

88. N.Y. Ed. Law § 904 (McKinney Supp. 1972).

89. N.Y. Ed. Law § 901 (McKinney Supp. 1972).

90. *Ferguson v. Skrupa,* 372 U.S. 726 (1963).

91. Cf. *Dalli v. Board of Education,* Mass. Adv. Sh. 237, 242–3 (1971), 267 N.E.2d 919 (1917).

92. *Gould v. Gould,* 78 Conn. 242, 61 A.604 (1905); *cf.* 13 *St. John's L. Rev.* 199 (1938).

93. Ariz. Public Health and Safety, § 36–797.42; California has an identical section: Cal. Health and Safety Code, §§ 310, 311 (West 1972 Supp.).

94. *Roe v. Wade,* 41 L.W. 4213, 4225 (1973). [Reprinted as Chapter 68 of this volume.]

95. *Standley v. Georgia,* 394 U.S. 557, 564 (1969).

96. *Terry v. Ohio,* 392 U.S. 1, 8–9 (1968); *Katz v. United States,* 389 U.S. 347, 356 (1967).

97. *Griswold v. Connecticut,* 381 U.S. 479, 486 (Goldberg, J., concurring) (1965).

98. *Meyer v. Nebraska,* 262 U.S. 390, 392 (1923).

99. 381 U.S. 479, 481.

100. Reference 98, at 399.

101. Reference 94.

102. *N.A.A.C.P. v. Alabama,* 377 U.S. 288, 307.

103. 86 Stat. 136 et seq.

104. *Id.*

105. *Id.*

106. Milunsky, A., Littlefield, J. W., Kanfer, J. N., et al., Prenatal genetic diagnosis. *N. Engl. J. Med.* 283:1370, 1441, 1498, 1970.

30

John Stuart Mill
From *On Liberty*

Reprinted from John Stuart Mill, *On Liberty*, 2nd ed. (London: John W. Parker and Son, 1859), Chapter I, pp. 21–27; Chapter IV, pp. 134–148.

The object of this Essay is to assert one very simple principle, as entitled to govern absolutely the dealings of society with the individual in the way of compulsion and control, whether the means used by physical force in the form of legal penalties, or the moral coercion of public opinion. That principle is, that the sole end for which mankind are warranted, individually or collectively, in interfering with the liberty of action of any of their number, is self-protection. That the only purpose for which power can be rightfully exercised over any member of a civilized community, against his will, is to prevent harm to others. His own good, either physical or moral, is not a sufficient warrant. He cannot rightfully be compelled to do or forbear because it will be better for him to do so, because it will make him happier, because, in the opinions of others, to do so would be wise, or even right. These are good reasons for remonstrating with him, or reasoning with him, or persuading him, or entreating him, but not for compelling him, or visiting him with any evil in case he do otherwise. To justify that, the conduct from which it is desired to deter him, must be calculated to produce evil to some one else. The only part of the conduct of any one, for which he is amenable to society, is that which concerns others. In the part which merely concerns himself, his independence is, of right, absolute. Over himself, over his own body and mind, the individual is sovereign.

It is, perhaps, hardly necessary to say that this doctrine is meant to apply only to human beings in the maturity of their faculties. We are not speaking of children, or of young persons below the age which the law may fix as that of manhood or womanhood. Those who are still in a state to require being taken care of by others, must be protected against their own actions as well as against external injury. For the same reason, we may leave out of consideration those backward states of society in which the race itself may be considered as in its nonage. The early difficulties in the way of spontaneous progress are so great, that there is seldom any choice of means for overcoming them; and a ruler full of the spirit of improvement is warranted in the use of any expedients that will attain an end, perhaps otherwise unattainable. Despotism is a legitimate mode of government in dealing with barbarians, provided the end be their improvement, and the means justified by actually effecting that end. Liberty, as a principle, has no application to any state of things anterior to the time when mankind have become capable of being improved by free and equal discussion. Until then, there is nothing for them but implicit obedience to an Akbar or a Charlemagne, if they are so fortunate as to find one. But as soon as mankind have attained the capacity of being guided to their own improvement by conviction or persuasion (a period long since reached in all nations with whom we need here concern ourselves), compulsion, either in the direct form or in that of pains and penalties for non-compliance, is no longer admissible as a means to their own good, and justifiable only for the security of others.

It is proper to state that I forego any advantage which could be derived to my argument from the idea of abstract right, as a thing independent of utility. I regard utility as the ultimate appeal on all ethical questions; but it must be utility in the largest sense, grounded on the permanent interests of man as a progressive being. Those interests, I contend, authorize the subjection of individual spontaneity to external control, only in respect to those actions of each, which concern the interest of other people. If any one does an act hurtful to others, there is a *prima facie* case for punishing him, by law, or, where legal penalties are not safely applicable, by general disapprobation. There are also many positive acts for the benefit of others, which he may rightfully be compelled to perform; such as, to give evidence in a court of justice; to bear his fair share in the common defence, or in any other joint work necessary to the interest of the society of which he enjoys the protection; and to perform certain acts of individual beneficence, such as saving a fellow creature's life, or interposing to protect the defenceless against ill-usage, things which whenever it is obviously a man's duty to do, he may rightfully be made responsible to society for not doing. A person may cause evil to others not only by his actions but by his inaction, and in either case he is justly accountable to them for the injury. The latter case, it is true, requires a much more cautious exercise of compulsion than the former. To make anyone answerable for doing evil to others, is the rule; to make him answerable for not preventing evil, is, comparatively speaking, the exception. Yet there are many cases clear enough and grave enough to justify that exception. In all things which regard the external relations of the individual, he is *de jure* amenable to those whose interests are concerned, and if need be, to society as their protector. There are often good reasons for not holding him to the responsibility; but these reasons must arise from the special expediencies of the case: either because it is a kind of case in which he is on the whole likely to act better, when left to his own discretion, than when controlled in any way in which society have it in their power to control him; or because the attempt to exercise control would produce other evils, greater than those which it would prevent. When such reasons as these preclude the enforcement of responsibility, the conscience of the agent himself should step into the vacant judgment seat, and protect those interests of others which have no external protection; judging himself all the more rigidly, because the case does not admit of his being made accountable to the judgment of his fellow-creatures.

But there is a sphere of action in which society, as distinguished from the individual, has, if any, only an indirect interest; comprehending all that portion of a person's life and conduct which affects only himself, or if it also affects others, only with their free, voluntary, and undeceived consent and participation. When I say only himself, I mean directly, and in the first instance: for whatever affects himself, may affect others *through* himself; and the objection which may be grounded on this contingency, will receive consideration in the sequel. This, then, is the appropriate region of human liberty. It comprises, first, the inward domain of consciousness; demanding liberty of conscience, in the most comprehensive sense; liberty of thought and feeling; absolute freedom of opinion and sentiment on all subjects, practical or speculative, scientific, moral, or theological. The liberty of expressing

and publishing opinions may seem to fall under a different principle, since it belongs to that part of the conduct of an individual which concerns other people; but, being almost of as much importance as the liberty of thought itself, and resting in great part on the same reasons, is practically inseparable from it. Secondly, the principle requires liberty of tastes and pursuits; of framing the plan of our life to suit our own character; of doing as we like, subject to such consequences as may follow: without impediment from our fellow-creatures, so long as what we do does not harm them, even though they should think our conduct foolish, perverse, or wrong. Thirdly, from this liberty of each individual, follows the liberty, within the same limits, of combination among individuals; freedom to unite, for any purpose not involving harm to others: the persons combining being supposed to be of full age, and not forced or deceived.

No society in which these liberties are not, on the whole, respected, is free, whatever may be its form of government; and none is completely free in which they do not exist absolute and unqualified. The only freedom which deserves the name, is that of pursuing our own good in our own way, so long as we do not attempt to deprive others of theirs, or impede their efforts to obtain it. Each is the proper guardian of his own health, whether bodily, or mental and spiritual. Mankind are greater gainers by suffering each other to live as seems good to themselves, than by compelling each to live as seems good to the rest. . . .

Of the Limits to the Authority of Society over the Individual

What, then, is the rightful limit to the sovereignty of the individual over himself? Where does the authority of society begin? How much of human life should be assigned to individuality, and how much to society?

Each will receive its proper share, if each has that which more particularly concerns it. To individuality should belong the part of life in which it is chiefly the individual that is interested; to society, the part which chiefly interests society.

Though society is not founded on a contract, and though no good purpose

is answered by inventing a contract in order to deduce social obligations from it, everyone who receives the protection of society owes a return for the benefit, and the fact of living in society renders it indispensable that each should be bound to observe a certain line of conduct towards the rest. This conduct consists, first, in not injuring the interests of one another; or rather certain interests, which, either by express legal provision or by tacit understanding, ought to be considered as rights; and secondly, in each person's bearing his share (to be fixed on some equitable principle) of the labours and sacrifices incurred for defending the society or its members from injury and molestation. These conditions society is justified in enforcing, at all costs to those who endeavour to withhold fulfilment. Nor is this all that society may do. The acts of an individual may be hurtful to others, or wanting in due consideration for their welfare, without going the length of violating any of their constituted rights. The offender may then be justly punished by opinion, though not by law. As soon as any part of a person's conduct affects prejudicially the interests of others, society has jurisdiction over it, and the question whether the general welfare will or will not be promoted by interfering with it, becomes open to discussion. But there is no room for entertaining any such question when a person's conduct affects the interests of no persons besides himself, or needs not affect them unless they like (all the persons concerned being of full age, and the ordinary amount of understanding). In all such cases there should be perfect freedom, legal and social, to do the action and stand the consequences.

It would be a great misunderstanding of this doctrine, to suppose that it is one of selfish indifference, which pretends that human beings have no business with each other's conduct in life, and that they should not concern themselves about the well-doing or well-being of one another, unless their own interest is involved. Instead of any diminution, there is need of a great increase of disinterested exertion to promote the good of others. But disinterested benevolence can find other instruments to persuade people to their good, than whips and scourges, either of the literal or the metaphorical sort. I am the last person to undervalue the self-regarding virtues; they are only second in importance, if even second, to the social. It is equally the business of education to cultivate both. But even education works by conviction and persuasion as well as by compulsion, and it is by the former only that, when the period of education is past, the self-regarding virtues should be inculcated. Human beings owe to each other help to distinguish the better from the worse, and encouragement to choose the former and avoid the latter. They should be for ever stimulating each other to increased exercise of their higher faculties, and increased direction of their feelings and aims towards wise instead of foolish, elevating instead of degrading, objects and contemplations. But neither one person, nor any number of persons, is warranted in saying to another human creature of ripe years, that he shall not do with his life for his own benefit what he chooses to do with it. He is the person most interested in his own well-being: the interest which any other person, except in cases of strong personal attachment, can have in it, is trifling, compared with that which he himself has; the interest which society has in him individually (except as to his conduct to others) is fractional, and altogether indirect: while, with respect to his own feelings and circumstances, the most ordinary man or woman has means of knowledge immeasurably surpassing those that can be possessed by anyone else. The interference of society to overrule his judgment and purposes in what only regards himself, must be grounded on general presumptions; which may be altogether wrong, and even if right, are as likely as not to be misapplied to individual cases, by persons no better acquainted with the circumstances of such cases than those are who look at them merely from without. In this department, therefore, of human affairs, individuality has its proper field of action. In the conduct of human beings towards one another, it is necessary that general rules should for the most part be observed, in order that people may know what they have to expect; but in each person's own concerns, his individual spontaneity is entitled to free exercise. Considerations to aid his judgment, exhortations to strengthen his will, may be offered to

him, even obtruded on him, by others; but he himself is the final judge. All errors which he is likely to commit against advice and warning, are far outweighed by the evil of allowing others to constrain him to what they deem his good.

I do not mean that the feelings with which a person is regarded by others, ought not to be in any way affected by his self-regarding qualities or deficiencies. This is neither possible nor desirable. If he is eminent in any of the qualities which conduce to his own good, he is, so far, a proper object of admiration. He is so much the nearer to the ideal perfection of human nature. If he is grossly deficient in those qualities, a sentiment the opposite of admiration will follow. There is a degree of folly, and a degree of what may be called (though the phrase is not unobjectionable) lowness or depravation of taste, which, though it cannot justify doing harm to the person who manifests it, renders him necessarily and properly a subject of distaste, or, in extreme cases, even of contempt: a person could not have the opposite qualities in due strength without entertaining these feelings. Though doing no wrong to any one, a person may so act as to compel us to judge him, and feel to him, as a fool, or as a being of an inferior order: and since this judgment and feeling are a fact which he would prefer to avoid, it is doing him a service to warn him of it beforehand, as of any other disagreeable consequence to which he exposes himself. It would be well, indeed, if this good office were much more freely rendered than the common notions of politeness at present permit, and if one person could honestly point out to another that he thinks him in fault, without being considered unmannerly or presuming. We have a right, also, in various ways, to act upon our unfavourable opinion of any one, not to the oppression of his individuality, but in the exercise of ours. We are not bound, for example, to seek his society; we have a right to avoid it (though not to parade the avoidance), for we have a right to choose the society most acceptable to us. We have a right, and it may be our duty, to caution others against him, if we think his example or conversation likely to have a pernicious effect on

those with whom he associates. We may give others a preference over him in optional good offices, except those which tend to his improvement. In these various modes a person may suffer very severe penalties at the hands of others, for faults which directly concern only himself; but he suffers these penalties only insofar as they are the natural, and, as it were, the spontaneous consequences of the faults themselves, not because they are purposely inflicted on him for the sake of punishment. A person who shows rashness, obstinacy, self-conceit—who cannot live within moderate means—who cannot restrain himself from hurtful indulgences—who pursues animal pleasures at the expense of those of feeling and intellect—must expect to be lowered in the opinion of others, and to have a less share of their favourable sentiments; but of this he has no right to complain, unless he has merited their favour by special excellence in his social relations, and has thus established a title to their good offices, which is not affected by his demerits towards himself.

What I contend for is, that the inconveniences which are strictly inseparable from the unfavourable judgment of others, are the only ones to which a person should ever be subjected for that portion of his conduct and character which concerns his own good, but which does not affect the interests of others in their relations with him. Acts injurious to others require a totally different treatment. Encroachment on their rights; infliction on them of any loss or damage not justified by his own rights; falsehood or duplicity in dealing with them; unfair or ungenerous use of advantages over them; even selfish abstinence from defending them against injury—these are fit objects of moral reprobation, and, in grave cases, of moral retribution and punishment. And not only these acts, but the dispositions which lead to them, are properly immoral, and fit subjects of disapprobation which may rise to abhorrence. Cruelty of disposition; malice and ill-nature; that most antisocial and odious of all passions, envy; dissimulation and insincerity; irascibility on insufficient cause, and resentment disproportioned to the provocation; the love of domineering over others; the desire to engross more than one's share of advantages (the πλεον-εξία of the Greeks); the pride which derives gratification from the abasement of others; the egotism which thinks self and its concerns more important than everything else, and decides all doubtful questions in its own favour;—these are moral vices, and constitute a bad and odious moral character: unlike the self-regarding faults previously mentioned, which are not properly immoralities, and to whatever pitch they may be carried, do not constitute wickedness. They may be proofs of any amount of folly, or want of personal dignity and self-respect; but they are only a subject of moral reprobation when they involve a breach of duty to others, for whose sake the individual is bound to have care for himself. What are called duties to ourselves are not socially obligatory, unless circumstances render them at the same time duties to others. The term duty to oneself, when it means anything more than prudence, means self-respect or self-development; and for none of these is any one accountable to his fellow creatures, because for none of them is it for the good of mankind that he be held accountable to them.

The distinction between the loss of consideration which a person may rightly incur by defect of prudence or of personal dignity, and the reprobation which is due to him for an offence against the rights of others, is not a merely nominal distinction. It makes a vast difference both in our feelings and in our conduct towards him, whether he displeases us in things in which we think we have a right to control him, or in things in which we know that we have not. If he displeases us, we may express our distaste, and we may stand aloof from a person as well as from a thing that displeases us; but we shall not therefore feel called on to make his life uncomfortable. We shall reflect that he already bears, or will bear, the whole penalty of his error; if he spoils his life by mismanagement, we shall not, for that reason, desire to spoil it still further: instead of wishing to punish him, we shall rather endeavour to alleviate his punishment, by showing him how he may avoid or cure the evils his conduct tends to bring upon him. He may be to us an object of pity, perhaps of dislike, but not of anger or resentment; we shall not treat him like an enemy of society: the worst we

shall think ourselves justified in doing is leaving him to himself, if we do not interfere benevolently by showing interest or concern for him. It is far otherwise if he has infringed the rules necessary for the protection of his fellow-creatures, individually or collectively. The evil consequences of his acts do not then fall on himself, but on others; and society, as the protector of all its members, must retaliate on him; must inflict pain on him for the express purpose of punishment, and must take care that it be sufficiently severe. In the one case, he is an offender at our bar, and we are called on not only to sit in judgment on him, but, in one shape or another, to execute our own sentence: in the other case, it is not our part to inflict any suffering on him, except what may incidentally follow from our using the same liberty in the regulation of our own affairs, which we allow to him in his.

The distinction here pointed out between the part of a person's life which concerns only himself, and that which concerns others, many persons will refuse to admit. How (it may be asked) can any part of the conduct of a member of society be a matter of indifference to the other members? No person is an entirely isolated being; it is impossible for a person to do anything seriously or permanently hurtful to himself, without mischief reaching at least to his near connexions, and often far beyond them. If he injures his property, he does harm to those who directly or indirectly derived support from it, and usually diminishes, by a greater or less amount, the general resources of the community. If he deteriorates his bodily or mental faculties, he not only brings evil upon all who depended on him for any portion of their happiness, but disqualifies himself for rendering the services which he owes to his fellow creatures generally; perhaps becomes a burthen on their affection or benevolence; and if such conduct were very frequent, hardly any offence that is committed would detract more from the general sum of good. Finally, if by his vices or follies a person does no direct harm to others, he is nevertheless (it may be said) injurious by his example; and ought to be compelled to control himself, for

the sake of those whom the sight or knowledge of his conduct might corrupt or mislead.

And even (it will be added) if the consequences of misconduct could be confined to the vicious or thoughtless individual, ought society to abandon to their own guidance those who are manifestly unfit for it? If protection against themselves is confessedly due to children and persons under age, is not society equally bound to afford it to persons of mature years who are equally incapable of self-government? If gambling, or drunkenness, or incontinence, or idleness, or uncleanliness, are as injurious to happiness, and as great a hindrance to improvement, as many or most of the acts prohibited by law, why (it may be asked) should not law, so far as is consistent with practicability and social convenience, endeavour to repress these also? And as a supplement to the unavoidable imperfections of law, ought not opinion at least to organize a powerful police against these vices, and visit rigidly with social penalties those who are known to practise them? There is no question here (it may be said) about restricting individuality, or impeding the trial of new and original experiments in living. The only things it is sought to prevent are things which have been tried and condemned from the beginning of the world until now; things which experience has shown not to be useful or suitable to any person's individuality. There must be some length of time and amount of experience, after which a moral or prudential truth may be regarded as established: and it is merely desired to prevent generation after generation from falling over the same precipice which has been fatal to their predecessors.

I fully admit that the mischief which a person does to himself, may seriously affect, both through their sympathies and their interests, those nearly connected with him, and in a minor degree, society at large. When, by conduct of this sort, a person is led to violate a distinct and assignable obligation to any other person or persons, the case is taken out of the self-regarding class, and becomes amenable to moral disapprobation in the proper sense of the term. If, for example, a man, through intemperance or extravagance, becomes unable to pay his debts, or, having undertaken the moral responsibility of a family, becomes from the same cause incapable of supporting or educating them, he is deservedly reprobated, and might be justly punished; but it is for the breach of duty to his family or creditors, not for the extravagance. If the resources which ought to have been devoted to them, had been diverted from them for the most prudent investment, the moral culpability would have been the same. George Barnwell murdered his uncle to get money for his mistress, but if he had done it to set himself up in business, he would equally have been hanged. Again, in the frequent case of a man who causes grief to his family by addiction to bad habits, he deserves reproach for his unkindness or ingratitude; but so he may for cultivating habits not in themselves vicious, if they are painful to those with whom he passes his life, or who from personal ties are dependent on him for their comfort. Whoever fails in the consideration generally due to the interests and feelings of others, not being compelled by some more imperative duty, or justified by allowable self-preference, is a subject of moral disapprobation for that failure, but not for the cause of it, nor for the errors, merely personal to himself, which may have remotely led to it. In like manner, when a person disables himself, by conduct purely self-regarding, from the performance of some definite duty incumbent on him to the public, he is guilty of a social offence. No person ought to be punished simply for being drunk; but a soldier or a policeman should be punished for being drunk on duty. Whenever, in short, there is a definite damage, or a definite risk of damage, either to an individual or to the public, the case is taken out of the province of liberty, and placed in that of morality or law.

But with regard to the merely contingent, or, as it may be called, constructive injury which a person causes to society, by conduct which neither violates any specific duty to the public, nor occasions perceptible hurt to any assignable individual except himself; the inconvenience is one which society can afford to bear, for the sake of the greater good of human freedom. If grown persons are to be punished for not taking proper care of themselves, I would rather it were for their own sake, than under pretence of preventing them from impairing their capacity of rendering to society benefits which society does not pretend it has a right to exact. But I cannot consent to argue the point as if society had no means of bringing its weaker members up to its ordinary standard of rational conduct, except waiting till they do something irrational, and then punishing them, legally or morally, for it. Society has had absolute power over them during all the early portion of their existence: it has had the whole period of childhood and nonage in which to try whether it could make them capable of rational conduct in life. The existing generation is master both of the training and the entire circumstances of the generation to come; it cannot indeed make them perfectly wise and good, because it is itself so lamentably deficient in goodness and wisdom; and its best efforts are not always, in individual cases, its most successful ones; but it is perfectly well able to make the rising generation, as a whole, as good as, and a little better than, itself. If society lets any considerable number of its members grow up mere children, incapable of being acted on by rational consideration of distant motives, society has itself to blame for the consequences. Armed not only with all the powers of education, but with the ascendancy which the authority of a received opinion always exercises over the minds who are least fitted to judge for themselves; and aided by the *natural* penalties which cannot be prevented from falling on those who incur the distaste or the contempt of those who know them; let not society pretend that it needs, besides all this, the power to issue commands and enforce obedience in the personal concerns of individuals, in which, on all principles of justice and policy, the decision ought to rest with those who are to abide the consequences.

31

Gerald Dworkin
Paternalism

Reprinted with permission of the author and editors from *The Monist*, vol. 56, no. 1, January 1972, pp. 64–84.

Neither one person, nor any number of persons, is warranted in saying to another human creature of ripe years, that he shall not do with his life for his own benefit what he chooses to do with it.

Mill

I do not want to go along with a volunteer basis. I think a fellow should be compelled to become better and not let him use his discretion whether he wants to get smarter, more healthy or more honest.

General Hershey

I take as my starting point the "one very simple principle" proclaimed by Mill in *On Liberty* . . . "That principle is, that the sole end for which mankind are warranted, individually or collectively, in interfering with the liberty of action of any of their number, is self-protection. That the only purpose for which power can be rightfully exercised over any member of a civilized community, against his will, is to prevent harm to others. He cannot rightfully be compelled to do or forbear because it will be better for him to do so, because it will make him happier, because, in the opinion of others, to do so would be wise, or even right."[1]

This principle is neither "one" nor "very simple." It is at least two principles; one asserting that self-protection or the prevention of harm to others is sometimes a sufficient warrant and the other claiming that the individual's own good is *never* a sufficient warrant for the exercise of compulsion either by the society as a whole or by its individual members. I assume that no one with the possible exception of extreme pacifists or anarchists questions the correctness of the first half of the principle. This essay is an examination of the negative claim embodied in Mill's principle—the objection to paternalistic interferences with a man's liberty.

I

By paternalism I shall understand roughly the interference with a person's liberty of action justified by reasons referring exclusively to the welfare, good, happiness, needs, interests or values of the person being coerced. One is always well advised to illustrate one's definitions by examples but it is not easy to find "pure" examples of paternalistic interferences. For almost any piece of legislation is justified by several different kinds of reasons and even

if historically a piece of legislation can be shown to have been introduced for, purely paternalistic motives, it may be that advocates of the legislation with an anti-paternalistic outlook can find sufficient reasons justifying the legislation without appealing to the reasons which were originally adduced to support it. Thus, for example, it may be that the original legislation requiring motorcyclists to wear safety helmets was introduced for purely paternalistic reasons. But the Rhode Island Supreme Court recently upheld such legislation on the grounds that it was "not persuaded that the legislature is powerless to prohibit individuals from pursuing a course of conduct which could conceivably result in their becoming public charges," thus clearly introducing reasons of a quite different kind. Now I regard this decision as being based on reasoning of a very dubious nature but it illustrates the kind of problem one has in finding examples. The following is a list of the kinds of interferences I have in mind as being paternalistic.

II

1. Laws requiring motorcyclists to wear safety helmets when operating their machines.
2. Laws forbidding persons from swimming at a public beach when lifeguards are not on duty.
3. Laws making suicide a criminal offense.
4. Laws making it illegal for women and children to work at certain types of jobs.
5. Laws regulating certain kinds of sexual conduct, e.g. homosexuality among consenting adults in private.
6. Laws regulating the use of certain drugs which may have harmful consequences to the user but do not lead to anti-social conduct.
7. Laws requiring a license to engage in certain professions with those not receiving a license subject to fine or jail sentence if they do engage in the practice.
8. Laws compelling people to spend a specified fraction of their income on the purchase of retirement annuities. (Social Security)
9. Laws forbidding various forms of gambling (often justified on the grounds that the poor are more likely

to throw away their money on such activities than the rich who can afford to).
10. Laws regulating the maximum rates of interest for loans.
11. Laws against duelling.

In addition to laws which attach criminal or civil penalties to certain kinds of action there are laws, rules, regulations, decrees, which make it either difficult or impossible for people to carry out their plans and which are also justified on paternalistic grounds. Examples of this are:
1. Laws regulating the types of contracts which will be upheld as valid by the courts, e.g. (an example of Mill's to which I shall return) no man may make a valid contract for perpetual involuntary servitude.
2. Not allowing as a defense to a charge of murder or assault the consent of the victim.
3. Requiring members of certain religious sects to have compulsory blood transfusions. This is made possible by not allowing the patient to have recourse to civil suits for assault and battery and by means of injunctions.
4. Civil commitment procedures when these are specifically justified on the basis of preventing the person being committed from harming himself. (The D.C. Hospitalization of the Mentally Ill Act provides for involuntary hospitalization of a person who "is mentally ill, and because of that illness, is likely to injure *himself* or others if allowed to remain at liberty." The term injure in this context applies to unintentional as well as intentional injuries.)
5. Putting fluorides in the community water supply.

All of my examples are of existing restrictions on the liberty of individuals. Obviously one can think of interferences which have not yet been imposed. Thus one might ban the sale of cigarettes, or require that people wear safety belts in automobiles (as opposed to merely having them installed) enforcing this by not allowing motorists to sue for injuries even when caused by other drivers if the motorist was not wearing a seat belt at the time of the accident.

I shall not be concerned with activities which though defended on paternalistic grounds are not interferences with the liberty of persons, e.g. the giving of subsidies in kind rather than in cash on the grounds that the recipients would not spend the money on the goods which they really need, or not including a $1000 deductible provision in a basic protection automobile insurance plan on the ground that the people who would elect it could least afford it. Nor shall I be concerned with measures such as "truth-in-advertising" acts and the Pure Food and Drug legislation which are often attacked as paternalistic but which should not be considered so. In these cases all that is provided—it is true by the use of compulsion—is information which it is presumed that rational persons are interested in having in order to make wise decisions. There is no interference with the liberty of the consumer unless one wants to stretch a point beyond good sense and say that his liberty to apply for a loan without knowing the true rate of interest is diminished. It is true that sometimes there is sentiment for going further than providing information, for example when laws against usurious interest are passed preventing those who might wish to contract loans at high rates of interest from doing so, and these measures may correctly be considered paternalistic.

III

Bearing these examples in mind let me return to a characterization of paternalism. I said earlier that I meant by the term, roughly, interference with a person's liberty for his own good. But as some of the examples show the class of persons whose good is involved is not always identical with the class of person's whose freedom is restricted. Thus in the case of professional licensing it is the practitioner who is directly interfered with and it is the would-be patient whose interests are presumably being served. Not allowing the consent of the victim to be a defense to certain types of crime primarily affects the would-be aggressor but it is the interests of the willing victim that we are trying to protect. Sometimes a person may fall into both classes as would be the case if we banned the manufacture and sale of cigarettes and a given manufacturer happened to be a smoker as well.

Thus we may first divide paternalistic interferences into "pure" and "impure" cases. In "pure" paternalism the class of persons whose freedom is restricted is identical with the class of persons

whose benefit is intended to be promoted by such restrictions. Examples: the making of suicide a crime, requiring passengers in automobiles to wear seat belts, requiring a Christian Scientist to receive a blood transfusion. In the case of "impure" paternalism in trying to protect the welfare of a class of persons we find that the only way to do so will involve restricting the freedom of other persons besides those who are benefitted. Now it might be thought that there are no cases of "impure" paternalism since any such case could always be justified on non-paternalistic grounds, i.e. in terms of preventing harms to others. Thus we might ban cigarette manufacturers from continuing to manufacture their product on the grounds that we are preventing them from causing illness to others in the same way that we prevent other manufacturers from releasing pollutants into the atmosphere, thereby causing danger to the members of the community. The difference is, however, that in the former but not the latter case the harm is of such a nature that it could be avoided by those individuals affected if they so chose. The incurring of the harm requires, so to speak, the active co-operation of the victim. It would be mistaken theoretically and hypocritical in practice to assert that our interference in such cases is just like our interference in standard cases of protecting others from harm. At the very least someone interfered with in this way can reply that no one is complaining about his activities. It may be that impure paternalism requires arguments or reasons of a stronger kind in order to be justified since there are persons who are losing a portion of their liberty and they do not even have the solace of having it be done "in their own interest." Of course in some sense, if paternalistic justifications are ever correct then we are protecting others, we are preventing some from injuring others, but it is important to see the differences between this and the standard case.

Paternalism then will always involve limitations on the liberty of some individuals in their own interest but it may also extend to interferences with the liberty of parties whose interests are not in question.

IV

Finally, by way of some more preliminary analysis, I want to distinguish paternalistic interferences with liberty from a related type with which it is often confused. Consider, for example, legislation which forbids employees to work more than, say, 40 hours per week. It is sometimes argued that such legislation is paternalistic for if employees desired such a restriction on their hours of work they could agree among themselves to impose it voluntarily. But because they do not the society imposes its own conception of their best interests upon them by the use of coercion. Hence this is paternalism.

Now it may be that some legislation of this nature is, in fact, paternalistically motivated. I am not denying that. All I want to point out is that there is another possible way of justifying such measures which is not paternalistic in nature. It is not paternalistic because as Mill puts it in a similar context such measures are "required not to overrule the judgment of individuals respecting their own interest, but to give effect to that judgment: they being unable to give effect to it except by concert, which concert again cannot be effectual unless it receives validity and sanction from the law."[2]

The line of reasoning here is a familiar one first found in Hobbes and developed with great sophistication by contemporary economists in the last decade or so. There are restrictions which are in the interests of a class of persons taken collectively but are such that the immediate interest of each individual is furthered by his violating the rule when others adhere to it. In such cases the individuals involved may need the use of compulsion to give effect to their collective judgment of their own interest by guaranteeing each individual compliance by the others. In these cases compulsion is not used to achieve some benefit which is not recognized to be a benefit by those concerned, but rather because it is the only feasible means of achieving some benefit which *is* recognized as such by all concerned. This way of viewing matters provides us with another characterization of paternalism in general. Paternalism might be thought of as the use of coercion to achieve a good which is not recognized as such by those persons for whom the good is intended. Again while this formulation captures the heart of the matter—it is surely what Mill is objecting to in *On Liberty*—the matter is not always quite like that. For example when we force motorcyclists to wear helmets we are trying to promote a good—the protection of the person from injury—which is surely recognized by most of the individuals concerned. It is not that a cyclist doesn't value his bodily integrity; rather, as a supporter of such legislation would put it, he either places, perhaps irrationally, another value or good (freedom from wearing a helmet) above that of physical well-being or, perhaps, while recognizing the danger in the abstract, he either does not fully appreciate it or he underestimates the likelihood of its occurring. But now we are approaching the question of possible justifications of paternalistic measures and the rest of this essay will be devoted to that question.

V

I shall begin for dialectical purposes by discussing Mill's objections to paternalism and then go on to discuss more positive proposals.

An initial feature that strikes one is the absolute nature of Mill's prohibitions against paternalism. It is so unlike the carefully qualified admonitions of Mill and his fellow Utilitarians on other moral issues. He speaks of self-protection as the *sole* end warranting coercion, of the individuals own goals as *never* being a sufficient warrant. Contrast this with his discussion of the prohibition against lying in *Util*.

Yet that even this, rule, sacred as it is, admits of possible exception, is acknowledged by all moralists, the chief of which is where the with-holding of some fact . . . would save an individual . . . from great and unmerited evil.[3]

The same tentativeness is present when he deals with justice.

It is confessedly unjust to break faith with any one: to violate an engagement, either express or implied, or disappoint expectations raised by our own conduct, at least if we have raised these expectations knowingly and voluntarily. Like all the other obligations of justice already spoken of, this one is not regarded as absolute, but as capable of being overruled by a stronger obligation of justice on the other side.[4]

This anomaly calls for some explanation. The structure of Mill's argument is as follows:

1. Since restraint is an evil the burden of proof is on those who propose such restraint.
2. Since the conduct which is being considered is purely self-regarding, the normal appeal to the protection of the interests of others is not available.
3. Therefore we have to consider whether reasons involving reference to the individual's own good, happiness, welfare, or interests are sufficient to overcome the burden of justification.
4. We either cannot advance the interests of the individual by compulsion, or the attempt to do so involves evil which outweigh the good done.
5. Hence the promotion of the individual's own interests does not provide a sufficient warrant for the use of compulsion.

Clearly the operative premise here is (4) and it is bolstered by claims about the status of the individual as judge and appraiser of his welfare, interests, needs, etc.

With respect to his own feelings and circumstances, the most ordinary man or woman has means of knowledge immeasurably surpassing those that can be possessed by any one else.[5]

He is the man most interested in his own well-being: the interest which any other person, except in cases of strong personal attachment, can have in it, is trifling, compared to that which he himself has.[6]

These claims are used to support the following generalizations concerning the utility of compulsion for paternalistic purposes.

The interferences of society to overrule his judgment and purposes in what only regards himself must be grounded on general presumptions; which may be altogether wrong, and even if right, are as likely as not to be misapplied to individual cases.[7]

But the strongest of all the arguments against the interference of the public with purely personal conduct is that when it does interfere, the odds are that it interferes wrongly and in the wrong place.[8]

All errors which the individual is likely to commit against advice and warning are far outweighed by the evil of allowing others to constrain him to what they deem his good.[9]

Performing the utilitarian calculation by balancing the advantages and disadvantages we find that:

Mankind are greater gainers by suffering each other to live as seems good to themselves, than by compelling each other to live as seems good to the rest.[10]

From which follows the operative premise (4).

This classical case of a utilitarian argument with all the premises spelled out is not the only line of reasoning present in Mill's discussion. There are asides, and more than asides, which look quite different and I shall deal with them later. But this is clearly the main channel of Mill's thought and it is one which has been subjected to vigorous attack from the moment it appeared—most often by fellow Utilitarians. The link that they have usually seized on is, as Fitzjames Stephen put it, the absence of proof that the "mass of adults are so well acquainted with their own interests and so much disposed to pursue them that no compulsion or restraint put upon them by any others for the purpose of promoting their interest can really promote them."[11] Even so sympathetic a critic as Hart is forced to the conclusion that:

In Chapter 5 of his essay Mill carried his protests against paternalism to lengths that may now appear to us as fantastic. . . . No doubt if we no longer sympathise with this criticism this is due, in part, to a general decline in the belief that individuals know their own interest best.[12]

Mill endows the average individual with "too much of the psychology of a middle-aged man whose desires are relatively fixed, not liable to be artificially stimulated by external influences; who knows what he wants and what gives him satisfaction of happiness; and who pursues these things when he can."[13]

Now it is interesting to note that Mill himself was aware of some of the limitations on the doctrine that the individual is the best judge of his own interests. In his discussion of government intervention in general (even where the intervention does not interfere with liberty but provides alternative institutions to those of the market) after making claims which are parallel to those just discussed, e.g.

People understand their own business and their own interests better, and care for them more, than the government does, or can be expected to do.[14]

He goes on to an intelligent discussion of the "very large and conspicuous exceptions" to the maxim that:

Most persons take a juster and more intelligent view of their own interest, and of the means of promoting it than can either be prescribed to them by a general enactment of the legislature, or pointed out in the particular case by a public functionary.[15]

Thus there are things

of which the utility does not consist in ministering to inclinations, nor in serving the daily uses of life, and the want of which is least felt where the need is greatest. This is peculiarly true of those things which are chiefly useful as tending to raise the character of human beings. The uncultivated cannot be competent judges of cultivation. Those who most need to be made wiser and better, usually desire it least, and, if they desired it, would be incapable of finding the way to it by their own lights.

. . . A second exception to the doctrine that individuals are the best judges of their own interest, is when an individual attempts to decide irrevocably now what will be best for his interest at some future and distant time. The presumption in favor of individual judgment is only legitimate, where the judgment is grounded on actual, and especially on present, personal experience; not where it is formed antecedently to experience, and not suffered to be reversed even after experience has condemned it.[16]

The upshot of these exceptions is that Mill does not declare that there should never be government interference with the economy but rather that

. . . in every instance, the burden of making out a strong case should be thrown not on those who resist but on those who recommend government interference. Letting alone, in short, should be the general practice: every departure from it, unless required by some great good, is a certain evil.[17]

In short, we get a presumption, not an absolute prohibition. The question is why doesn't the argument against paternalism go the same way?

I suggest that the answer lies in seeing that in addition to a purely utilitarian argument Mill uses another as well. As a Utilitarian Mill has to show, in Fitzjames Stephen's words, that:

Self-protection apart, no good object can be attained by any compulsion which is not in itself a greater evil than the absence of the object which the compulsion obtains.[18]

To show this is impossible; one reason being that it isn't true. Preventing a man from selling himself into slavery (a

paternalistic measure which Mill himself accepts as legitimate), or from taking heroin, or from driving a car without wearing seat belts may constitute a lesser evil than allowing him to do any of these things. A consistent Utilitarian can only argue against paternalism on the grounds that it (as a matter of fact) does not maximize the good. It is always a contingent question that may be refuted by the evidence. But there is also a non-contingent argument which runs through *On Liberty*. When Mill states that "there is a part of the life of every person who has come to years of discretion, within which the individuality of that person ought to reign uncontrolled either by any other person or by the public collectively" he is saying something about what it means to be a person, an autonomous agent. It is because coercing a person for his own good denies this status as an independent entity that Mill objects to it so strongly and in such absolute terms. To be able to choose is a good that is independent of the wisdom of what is chosen. A man's "mode of laying out his existence is the best, not because it is the best in itself, but because it is his own mode."[19]

It is the privilege and proper condition of a human being, arrived at the maturity of his faculties, to use and interpret experience in his own way.[20]

As further evidence of this line of reasoning in Mill consider the one exception to his prohibition against paternalism.

In this and most civilised countries, for example, an engagement by which a person should sell himself, or allow himself to be sold, as a slave, would be null and void; neither enforced by law nor by opinion. The ground for thus limiting his power of voluntarily disposing of his own lot in life, is apparent, and is very clearly seen in this extreme case. The reason for not interfering, unless for the sake of others, with a person's voluntary acts, is consideration for his liberty. His voluntary choice is evidence that what he so chooses is desirable, or at least endurable, to him, and his good is on the whole best provided for by allowing him to take his own means of pursuing it. But by selling himself for a slave, he abdicates his liberty; he foregoes any future use of it beyond that single act.

He therefore defeats, in his own case, the very purpose which is the justification of allowing him to dispose of himself. He is no longer free; but is thenceforth in a position which has no longer

the presumption in its favour, that would be afforded by his voluntarily remaining in it. The principle of freedom cannot require that he should be free not to be free. It is not freedom to be allowed to alienate his freedom.[21]

Now leaving aside the fudging on the meaning of freedom in the last line it is clear that part of this argument is incorrect. While it is true that *future* choices of the slave are not reasons for thinking that what he chooses then is desirable for him, what is at issue is limiting his immediate choice; and since this choice is made freely, the individual may be correct in thinking that his interests are best provided for by entering such a contract. But the main consideration for not allowing such a contract is the need to preserve the liberty of the person to make future choices. This gives us a principle—a very narrow one—by which to justify some paternalistic interferences. Paternalism is justified only to preserve a wider range of freedom for the individual in question. How far this principle could be extended, whether it can justify all the cases in which we are inclined upon reflection to think paternalistic measures justified remains to be discussed. What I have tried to show so far is that there are two strains of argument in Mill—one a straight-forward Utilitarian mode of reasoning and one which relies not on the goods which free choice leads to but on the absolute value of the choice itself. The first cannot establish any absolute prohibition but at most a presumption and indeed a fairly weak one given some fairly plausible assumptions about human psychology; the second while a stronger line of argument seems to me to allow on its own grounds a wider range of paternalism than might be suspected. I turn now to a consideration of these matters.

VI

We might begin looking for principles governing the acceptable use of paternalistic power in cases where it is generally agreed that it is legitimate. Even Mill intends his principles to be applicable only to mature individuals, not those in what he calls "non-age." What is it that justifies us in interfering with children? The fact that they lack some of the emotional and cognitive capacities required in order to make fully rational decisions. It is an empirical question to just what extent children have an adequate conception of their own present and future interests but there is not much doubt that there are many deficiencies. For example it is very difficult for a child to defer gratification for any considerable period of time. Given these deficiencies and given the very real and permanent dangers that may befall the child it becomes not only permissible but even a duty of the parent to restrict the child's freedom in various ways. There is however an important moral limitation on the exercise of such parental power which is provided by the notion of the child eventually coming to see the correctness of his parent's interventions. Parental paternalism may be thought of as a wager by the parent on the child's subsequent recognition of the wisdom of the restrictions. There is an emphasis on what could be called future-oriented consent—on what the child will come to welcome, rather than on what he does welcome.

The essence of this idea has been incorporated by idealist philosophers into various types of "real-will" theory as applied to fully adult persons. Extensions of paternalism are argued for by claiming that in various respects, chronologically mature individuals share the same deficiencies in knowledge, capacity to think rationally, and the ability to carry out decisions that children possess. Hence in interfering with such people we are in effect doing what they would do if they were fully rational. Hence we are not really opposing their will, hence we are not really interfering with their freedom. The dangers of this move have been sufficiently exposed by Berlin in his *Two Concepts of Liberty.* I see no gain in theoretical clarity nor in practical advantage in trying to pass over the real nature of the interferences with liberty that we impose on others. Still the basic notion of consent is important and seems to me the only acceptable way of trying to delimit an area of justified paternalism.

Let me start by considering a case where the consent is not hypothetical in nature. Under certain conditions it is rational for an individual to agree that others should force him to act in ways in which, at the time of action, the individual may not see as desirable. If, for example, a man knows that he is

subject to breaking his resolves when temptation is present, he may ask a friend to refuse to entertain his requests at some later stage.

A classical example is given in the *Odyssey* when Odysseus commands his men to tie him to the mast and refuse all future orders to be set free, because he knows the power of the Sirens to enchant men with their songs. Here we are on relatively sound ground in later refusing Odysseus' request to be set free. He may even claim to have changed his mind but since it is just such changes that he wished to guard against we are entitled to ignore them.

A process analogous to this may take place on a social rather than individual basis. An electorate may mandate its representatives to pass legislation which when it comes time to "pay the price" may be unpalatable. I may believe that a tax increase is necessary to halt inflation though I may resent the lower pay check each month. However in both this case and that of Odysseus the measure to be enforced is specifically requested by the party involved and at some point in time there is genuine consent and agreement on the part of those persons whose liberty is infringed. Such is not the case for the paternalistic measures we have been speaking about. What must be involved here is not consent to specific measures but rather consent to a system of government, run by elected representatives, with an understanding that they may act to safeguard our interests in certain limited ways.

I suggest that since we are all aware of our irrational propensities, deficiencies in cognitive and emotional capacities and avoidable and unavoidable ignorance it is rational and prudent for us to in effect take out "social insurance policies." We may argue for and against proposed paternalistic measures in terms of what fully rational individuals would accept as forms of protection. Now, clearly since the initial agreement is not about specific measures we are dealing with a more-or-less blank check and therefore there have to be carefully defined limits. What I am looking for are certain kinds of conditions which make it plausible to suppose that rational men could reach agreement to limit their liberty

even when other men's interests are not affected.

Of course as in any kind of agreement schema there are great difficulties in deciding what rational individuals would or would not accept. Particularly in sensitive areas of personal liberty, there is always a danger of the dispute over agreement and rationality being a disguised version of evaluative and normative disagreement.

Let me suggest types of situations in which it seems plausible to suppose that fully rational individuals would agree to having paternalistic restrictions imposed upon them. It is reasonable to suppose that there are "goods" such as health which any person would want to have in order to pursue his own good—no matter how that good is conceived. This is an argument that is used in connection with compulsory education for children but it seems to me that it can be extended to other goods which have this character. Then one could agree that the attainment of such goods should be promoted even when not recognized to be such, at the moment, by the individuals concerned.

An immediate difficulty that arises stems from the fact that men are always faced with competing goods and that there may be reasons why even a value such as health—or indeed life—may be overridden by competing values. Thus the problem with the Christian Scientist and blood transfusions. It may be more important for him to reject "impure substances" than to go on living. The difficult problem that must be faced is whether one can give sense to the notion of a person irrationally attaching weights to competing values.

Consider a person who knows the statistical data on the probability of being injured when not wearing seat belts in an automobile and knows the types and gravity of the various injuries. He also insists that the inconvenience attached to fastening the belt every time he gets in and out of the car outweighs for him the possible risks to himself. I am inclined in this case to think that such a weighing is irrational. Given his life-plans which we are assuming are those of the average person, his interests and commitments already undertaken, I think it is safe to predict that we can find inconsistencies in his calculations at some point. I am assuming that this is not a man who for some conscious or unconscious reasons is trying to injure himself nor is he a man who just likes to "live dangerously." I am assuming that he is like us in all the relevant respects but just puts an enormously high negative value on inconvenience—one which does not seem comprehensible or reasonable.

It is always possible, of course to assimilate this person to creatures like myself. I, also, neglect to fasten my seat belt and I conceded such behavior is not rational but not because I weigh the inconvenience differently from those who fasten the belts. It is just that having made (roughly) the same calculation as everybody else I ignore it in my actions. (Note: a much better case of weakness of the will than those usually given in ethics texts.) A plausible explanation for this deplorable habit is that although I know in some intellectual sense what the probabilities and risks are I do not fully appreciate them in an emotionally genuine manner.

We have two distinct types of situation in which a man acts in a non-rational fashion. In one case he attaches incorrect weights to some of his values; in the other he neglects to act in accordance with his actual preferences and desires. Clearly there is a stronger and more persuasive argument for paternalism in the latter situation. Here we are really not—by assumption—imposing a good on another person. But why may we not extend our interference to what we might call evaluative delusions? After all in the case of cognitive delusions we are prepared, often, to act against the expressed will of the person involved. If a man believes that when he jumps out the window he will float upwards—Robert Nozick's example—would not we detain him, forcibly if necessary? The reply will be that this man doesn't wish to be injured and if we could convince him that he is mistaken as to the consequences of his action he would not wish to perform the action. But part of what is involved in claiming that a man who doesn't fasten his seat belts is attaching an irrational weight to the inconvenience of fastening them is that if he were to be involved in an accident and severely injured he would look back and admit that the inconvenience wasn't as bad as all that. So there is a sense in which if I could convince him

of the consequences of his action he also would not wish to continue his present course of action. Now the notion of consequences being used here is covering a lot of ground. In one case it's being used to indicate what will or can happen as a result of a course of action and in the other it's making a prediction about the future evaluation of the consequences—in the first sense—of a course of action. And whatever the difference between facts and values—whether it be hard and fast or soft and slow—we are genuinely more reluctant to consent to interferences where evaluative differences are the issue. Let me now consider another factor which comes into play in some of these situations which may make an important difference in our willingness to consent to paternalistic restrictions.

Some of the decisions we make are of such a character that they produce changes which are in one or another way irreversible. Situations are created in which it is difficult or impossible to return to anything like the initial stage at which the decision was made. In particular some of these changes will make it impossible to continue to make reasoned choices in the future. I am thinking specifically of decisions which involve taking drugs that are physically or psychologically addictive and those which are destructive of one's mental and physical capacities.

I suggest we think of the imposition of paternalistic interferences in situations of this kind as being a kind of insurance policy which we take out against making decisions which are far-reaching, potentially dangerous and irreversible. Each of these factors is important. Clearly there are many decisions we make that are relatively irreversible. In deciding to learn to play chess I could predict in view of my general interest in games that some portion of my free time was going to be pre-empted and that it would not be easy to give up the game once I acquired a certain competence. But my whole life-style was not going to be jeopardized in an extreme manner. Further it might be argued that even with addictive drugs such as heroin one's normal life-plans would not be seriously interfered with if an inexpensive and adequate supply were readily

available. So this type of argument might have a much narrower scope than appears to be the case at first.

A second class of cases concerns decisions which are made under extreme psychological and sociological pressures. I am not thinking here of the making of the decision as being something one is pressured into—e.g. a good reason for making duelling illegal is that unless this is done many people might have to manifest their courage and integrity in ways in which they would rather not do so—but rather of decisions such as that to commit suicide which are usually made at a point where the individual is not thinking clearly and calmly about the nature of his decision. In addition, of course, this comes under the previous heading of all-too-irrevocable decision. Now there are practical steps which a society could take if it wanted to decrease the possibility of suicide—for example not paying social security benefits to the survivors or as religious institutions do, not allowing such persons to be buried with the same status as natural deaths. I think we may count these as interferences with the liberty of persons to attempt suicide and the question is whether they are justifiable.

Using my argument schema the question is whether rational individuals would consent to such limitations. I see no reason for them to consent to an absolute prohibition but I do think it is reasonable for them to agree to some kind of enforced waiting period. Since we are all aware of the possibility of temporary states, such as great fear or depression, that are inimical to the making of well-informed and rational decisions, it would be prudent for all of us if there were some kind of institutional arrangement whereby we were restrained from making a decision which is (all too) irreversible. What this would be like in practice is difficult to envisage and it may be that if no practical arrangements were feasible then we would have to conclude that there should be no restriction at all on this kind of action. But we might have a "cooling off" period, in much the same way that we now require couples who file for divorce to go through a waiting period. Or, more far-fetched, we might imagine a Suicide Board composed of a psychologist and another member picked by the applicant. The Board would be required to meet and talk with the person proposing to take his life, though its approval would not be required.

A third class of decisions—these classes are not supposed to be disjoint—involves dangers which are either not sufficiently understood or appreciated correctly by the persons involved. Let me illustrate, using the example of cigarette smoking, a number of possible cases.

1. A man may not know the facts—e.g. smoking between 1 and 2 packs a day shortens life expectancy 6.2 years, the costs and pain of the illness caused by smoking, etc.

2. A man may know the facts, wish to stop smoking, but not have the requisite will power.

3. A man may know the facts but not have them play the correct role in his calculation because, say, he discounts the danger psychologically because it is remote in time and/or inflates the attractiveness of other consequences of his decision which he regards as beneficial.

In case 1 what is called for is education, the posting of warnings, etc. In case 2 there is no theoretical problem. We are not imposing a good on someone who rejects it. We are simply using coercion to enable people to carry out their own goals. (Note: There obviously is a difficulty in that only a subclass of the individuals affected wish to be prevented from doing what they are doing.) In case 3 there is a sense in which we are imposing a good on someone since given his current appraisal of the facts he doesn't wish to be restricted. But in another sense we are not imposing a good since what is being claimed—and what must be shown or at least argued for—is that an accurate accounting on his part would lead him to reject his current course of action. Now we all know that such cases exist, that we are prone to disregard dangers that are only possibilities, that immediate pleasures are often magnified and distorted.

If in addition the dangers are severe and far-reaching we could agree to allowing the state a certain degree of power to intervene in such situations. The difficulty is in specifying in advance, even vaguely, the class of cases in which intervention will be legitimate.

A related difficulty is that of drawing a line so that it is not the case that all ultra-hazardous activities are ruled out, e.g. mountain-climbing, bull-fighting, sports-car racing, etc. There are some risks—even very great ones—which a person is entitled to take with his life.

A good deal depends on the nature of the deprivation—e.g. does it prevent the person from engaging in the activity completely or merely limit his participation—and how important to the nature of the activity is the absence of restriction when this is weighed against the role that the activity plays in the life of the person. In the case of automobile seat belts, for example, the restriction is trivial in nature, interferes not at all with the use or enjoyment of the activity, and does, I am assuming, considerably reduce a high risk of serious injury. Whereas, for example, making mountain climbing illegal prevents completely a person engaging in an activity which may play an important role in his life and his conception of the person he is.

In general the easiest cases to handle are those which can be argued about in the terms which Mill thought to be so important—a concern not just for the happiness or welfare, in some broad sense, of the individual but rather a concern for the autonomy and freedom of the person. I suggest that we would be most likely to consent to paternalism in those instances in which it preserves and enhances for the individual his ability to rationally consider and carry out his own decisions.

I have suggested in this essay a number of types of situations in which it seems plausible that rational men would agree to granting the legislative powers of a society the right to impose restrictions on what Mill calls "self-regarding" conduct. However, rational men knowing something about the resources of ignorance, ill-will and stupidity available to the law-makers of a society—a good case in point is the history of drug legislation in the United States—will be concerned to limit such intervention to a minimum. I suggest in closing two principles designed to achieve this end.

In all cases of paternalistic legislation there must be a heavy and clear burden of proof placed on the authorities to demonstrate the exact nature of the harmful effects (or beneficial consequences) to be avoided (or achieved) and the probability of their occurrence. The burden of proof here is two-fold—what lawyers distinguish as the burden of going forward and the burden of persuasion. That the authorities have the burden of going forward means that it is up to them to raise the question and bring forward evidence of the evils to be avoided. Unlike the case of new drugs where the manufacturer must produce some evidence that the drug has been tested and found not harmful, no citizen has to show with respect to self-regarding conduct that it is not harmful or promotes his best interests. In addition the nature and cogency of the evidence for the harmfulness of the course of action must be set at a high level. To paraphrase a formulation of the burden of proof for criminal proceedings—better 10 men ruin themselves than one man be unjustly deprived of liberty.

Finally I suggest a principle of the least restrictive alternative. If there is an alternative way of accomplishing the desired end without restricting liberty then although it may involve great expense, inconvenience, etc. the society must adopt it.

Notes

1. J. S. Mill, *Utilitarianism* and *On Liberty* (Fontana Library Edition, ed. by Mary Warnock, London, 1962), p. 135. All further quotes from Mill are from this edition unless otherwise noted.

2. J. S. Mill, *Principles of Political Economy* (New York: P. F. Collier and Sons, 1900), p. 442.

3. Mill, *Utilitarianism* and *On Liberty*, p. 174.

4. *Ibid.*, p. 299.

5. *Ibid.*, p. 207.

6. *Ibid.*, p. 206.

7. *Ibid.*, p. 207.

8. *Ibid.*, p. 214.

9. *Ibid.*, p. 207.

10. *Ibid.*, p. 138.

11. J. F. Stephens, *Liberty, Equality, Fraternity* (New York: Henry Holt & Co., n.d.), p. 24.

12. H. L. A. Hart, *Law, Liberty and Morality* (Stanford: Stanford University Press, 1963), p. 32.

13. *Ibid.*, p. 33.

14. Mill, *Principles,* II, 448.

15. *Ibid.,* II, 458.

16. *Ibid.,* II, 459.

17. *Ibid.,* II, 451.

18. Stephen, p. 49.

19. Mill, *Utilitarianism* and *On Liberty,*
p. 197.

20. *Ibid.,* p. 186.

21. *Ibid.,* pp. 235–236.

Illustrative Cases

A 16-year-old girl, the child of retarded parents, is made a ward of the state when government authorities decide the parents cannot look after her adequately. Tests indicate that she is also retarded. Yet she has demonstrated a capacity for responsible behavior in her ability to help care for four younger siblings when the children lived with their parents. (The siblings are now also wards of the state.) She is very attractive and the authorities are concerned that she might become pregnant. Although she has no prior history of sexual contacts, the girl is forced by the authorities to have a small coil (IUD) implanted into the mouth of her uterus that would prevent conception. Insertion of the IUD in a woman who has never been pregnant is generally painful. Cramps and bleeding are common immediate side effects of insertion, but generally decrease over time. In about 2 to 20 percent of women, these symptoms require removal of the IUD. A more rare complication of wearing the IUD is severe pelvic infection, which in a few cases has resulted in death. Childbearing can be normally resumed when the coil is removed. However, in this case, the girl is greatly worried that this intervention will prevent her from ever having children. Moreover, other psychological harms that might befall her from being forced to wear the coil are unpredictable.

1. Was the action of the authorities warranted? Why?
2. Would your response be different if the girl had become pregnant while living with her family?

The following case is taken from a court decision:

. . . Mrs. Jones was brought to the hospital by her husband for emergency care, having lost two thirds of her body's blood supply from a ruptured ulcer. She had no personal physician, and relied solely on the hospital staff. She was a total hospital responsibility. It appeared that the patient, age 25, mother of a seven-month-old child, and her husband were both Jehovah's Witnesses, the teachings of which sect, according to their interpretation, prohibited the injection of blood into the body. When death without blood became imminent, the hospital sought the advice of counsel, who applied to the District Court in the name of the hospital for permission to administer blood. Judge Tamm of the District Court denied the application, and counsel immediately applied to me, as a member of the Court of Appeals, for an appropriate writ.

I called the hospital by telephone and spoke with Dr. Westura, Chief Medical Resident, who confirmed the representations made by counsel. I thereupon proceeded with counsel to the hospital, where I spoke to Mr. Jones, the husband of the patient. He advised me that, on religious grounds, he would not approve a blood transfusion for his wife. He said, however, that if the court ordered the transfusion, the responsibility was not his. I advised Mr. Jones to obtain counsel immediately. He thereupon went to the telephone and returned in 10 or 15 minutes to advise that he had taken the matter up with his church and that he had decided that he did not want counsel.

I asked permission of Mr. Jones to see his wife. This he readily granted. Prior to going into the patient's room, I again conferred with Dr. Westura and several other doctors assigned to the case. All confirmed that the patient would die without blood and that there was a better than 50 per cent chance of saving her life with it. Unanimously they strongly recommended it. I then went inside the patient's room. Her appearance confirmed the urgency which had been represented to me. I tried to communicate with her, advising her again as to what the doctors had said. The only audible reply I could hear was "Against my will." It was obvious that the woman was not in a mental condition to make a decision. I was reluctant to press her because of the seriousness of her condition and because I felt that to suggest repeatedly the imminence of death without blood might place a strain on her religious convictions. I asked her whether she would oppose the blood transfusion if the court allowed it. She indicated, as best I could make out, that it would not then be her responsibility . . . .

[I] signed the order allowing the hospital to administer such transfusions as the doctors should determine were necessary to save her life.

J. Skelly Wright, Circuit Judge

Application of President and Directors of Georgetown College
331 F.2d 1000 (D.C.Cir.).

1. As the physician to this patient, what are your obligations?
2. As physician, what would you do if you found your own ethical principles, or those of the medical profession, in conflict with the judge's ruling?

A physician is treating an adult patient for a respiratory disorder that causes the patient to cough and experience chest pain. The physician takes a history, examines the patient with his stethoscope, concludes he has a common viral disorder, and prescribes therapy. The patient is not satisfied with the examination and insists on a chest X ray. The physician asserts that his examination was adequate. He points out that cumulative X-ray exposures over long periods can be hazardous and that he believes unnecessary X rays are not warranted. The patient insists that it is his body, and that he will take the risk of an X ray at this time.

1. What considerations should the physician weigh in responding to the patient's request?

IV

Truth-Telling in the Physician-Patient Relationship

Introduction to Part IV

The medical relationship is based on an exchange of information that involves a double standard. The physician requires his patient to respond truthfully to questions; at the same time, the physician, in some instances, does not feel bound to respond completely truthfully to the patient's queries. This double standard is founded on a benevolent motive: truth is a good that may wound. This motive is discussed in some of the earliest medical documents. For example, in the selection "Decorum" from the *Hippocratic Corpus* (see Chapter 1 of this volume) the writer advises physicians of the dangers of telling patients about the nature of their illness, ". . . for many patients through this cause have taken a turn for the worse."

The essays in this section explore the problems physicians face in deciding what to reveal to patients about their illness. Thomas Percival, writing as the nineteenth century began, cites the opinions of several contemporaries on truth-telling before giving his own analysis, in which he asserts that the right of a patient to the truth in the medical relationship and the duty of the doctor to give it is suspended when the beneficial nature of truth might be reversed and become an agent of harm. Worthington Hooker, a half-century later, challenges Percival's stand. He is skeptical that truth is necessarily harmful to patients and argues that, though the physician may *withhold* truth for the sake of benefiting the patient, what the physician does say must be true.

Richard Cabot, a professor of medicine at the Harvard Medical School in the early twentieth century, who later also held a chair in social ethics at Harvard, writes of studies he conducted on the response of patients to truthful statements about their illness. He emphasizes the importance of method in truth-telling. The physician must explain the nuances of the clinical picture to a patient with care and consideration and not confront him with the blunt truth. This position is challenged by Joseph Collins, writing in *Harper's Magazine* in 1923. He insistently argues that patients usually do not want to know the truth about their serious illnesses: physicians should shield patients as long as possible from the despair such knowledge would bring through a therapeutic amalgam compounded of "falsehood and truth."

Collins' position appears to reflect the beliefs of many doctors. A study of the attitudes toward truth-telling of physicians treating cancer patients, conducted by the American psychiatrist Donald Oken in 1961, indicates physicians generally believe that patients with cancer do not want to be told the truth about their illness. Oken discusses the physician's clinical approach and attitudes toward concealing medical data and also analyzes surveys taken among cancer patients about their desire to know their diagnosis.

Our understanding of physicians' attitudes about information-sharing is also advanced by the study of Howard Waitzkin, a sociologist and physician, and John Stoeckle, a leader in the development of ambulatory care programs in the United States. They apply sociological analysis in examining the physician's need to preserve power in his relationship with patients as an important motive in withholding information from patients.

Lord Edmund-Davies, a judge, appraises the legal obligation of a physician to tell patients the truth. Cicely Saunders, director of the St. Christopher's Hospice in England, which is devoted to caring for incurable and dying patients, next explores the tribulations of patients who have gleaned the truth about their illness without being explicitly told, but who have nobody with whom to discuss their anxieties. She points out that a great deal of nonverbal communication passes between patient and doctor and suggests that the real question doctors face may well be, "What do you let your patients tell you?"

This section concludes with discussions by the physician Alan Leslie and the philosopher Sissela Bok about the ethics of giving patients placebos. The effects of these agents bear no intrinsic relation to their biological properties but stem from the patient's belief in their efficacy—a belief that is encouraged by the physician.

Communicating with patients is important in helping them cope with the anxiety and pain that accompany threats to health. Although how to reveal to patients the causes of their illness and the procedures being used to overcome it is fundamentally a matter of skillfully applying clinical technique, the question of what they should be told requires an understanding of ethics as well.

32

Thomas Percival

A Physician Should Be the Minister of Hope and Comfort to the Sick

Reprinted from Thomas Percival, *Medical Ethics*, 3rd ed. (Oxford: John Henry Parker, 1849), pp. 132–141.

Mr. Gisborne, in one of his interesting letters to me on the subject of Medical Ethics, suggests, that it would be advisable to add, *as far as truth and sincerity will admit.* "I know very well," says he," that the sentence, as it now stands, conveys to you, and was meant by you to convey to others, the same sentiment which it would express after the proposed addition. But, if I am not mistaken in my idea that there are few professional temptations to which Medical men are more liable (and frequently from the very best principles,) than that of unintentionally using language to the patient and his friends more encouraging than sincerity would vindicate on cool reflection, it may be right scrupulously to guard the avenues against such an error."

In the "Enquiry into the Duties of Men," the same excellent moralist thus delivers his sentiments more at large.[1] "A professional writer, speaking in a work already quoted respecting the performance of Surgical operations in hospitals, remarks, that it may be a salutary as well as an humane act in the attending Physician, occasionally to assure the patient that every thing goes on well, *if that declaration can be made with truth.* This restriction, so properly applied to the case in question, may with equal propriety be extended universally to the conduct of a Physician, when superintending operations performed, not by the hand of a Surgeon, but by Nature and Medicine. Humanity, we admit, and the welfare of the sick man, commonly require that his drooping spirits should be revived by every encouragement and hope which can honestly be suggested to him. But truth and conscience forbid the Physician to cheer him by giving promises, or raising expectations, which are known or intended to be delusive. The Physician may not be bound, unless expressly required, invariably to divulge at any specific time his opinion concerning the uncertainty or danger of the case; but he is invariably bound never to represent the uncertainty or danger as less than he actually believes it to be; and whenever he conveys, directly or indirectly, to the patient or to his family, any impression to that effect, though he may be misled by mistaken tenderness, he is guilty of positive falsehood. He is at liberty to say little; but let that little be true. St. Paul's direction, *not to do evil that good may come,* is clear, positive, and universal."[2]

Whether this subject be viewed as regarding general morality, or professional duty, it is of high importance; and we may justly presume that it involves considerable difficulty and intricacy, because opposite opinions have been advanced upon it by very distinguished writers. The ancients, though sublime in the abstract representations of virtue, are seldom precise and definite in the detail of rules for its observance. Yet in some instances they extend their precepts to particular cases; and Cicero, in the third book of his "Offices," expressly admits of limitations to the absolute and immutable obligation of fidelity and truth. (cc. 24, 25.)

The maxim of the poet, also, may be adduced as intended to be comprehensive of the moral laws, by which human conduct is to be governed:

Sunt certi denique fines,
Quos ultra citraque nequit consistere rectum.[3]

The early Fathers of the Christian Church, Origen, Clement, Tertullian, Lactantius, Chrysostom, and various others, till the period of St. Augustine, were latitudinarians on this point. But the holy father last mentioned, if I mistake not, in the warmth of his zeal, declared that he would not utter a lie, though he were assured of gaining Heaven by it.[4] In this declaration there is a fallacy, by which Augustine probably imposed upon himself: for a lie is always understood to consist in a *criminal* breach of truth, and therefore under no circumstances can be justified. It is alleged, however, that falsehood may lose the essence of lying, and become even praiseworthy, when the adherence to truth is incompatible with the practice of some other virtue of still higher obligation. This opinion almost the whole body of civilians adopt, with full confidence of its rectitude. The sentiments of Grotius may be seen at large in the satisfactory detail which he has given of the controversy relating to it.[5]

Puffendorff, who may be regarded as next to this great man in succession as well as authority, delivers the following observations in his "Law of Nature and Nations," which are pointedly applicable to the present subjects, yet carried assuredly to a very reprehensible extent: "Since those we talk to may often be in such circumstances, that, if we should tell them the downright truth of the matter, it would prejudice them, and would incapacitate us for procuring that lawful end we propose to ourselves for their good; we may in these cases use a fictitious or figurative way of speech, which shall not directly represent to our hearers our real thoughts and intentions: for, when a man is desirous, and it is his duty, to do a piece of service, he is not bound to take measures that will certainly render his attempts unsuccessful.[6]—"Those are by no means guilty of lying, who, for the better information of children, or other persons not capable of relishing the naked truth, entertain them with fictions and stories; nor those who invent something that is false, for the sake of a good end, which by the plain truth they could not have compassed; as, suppose, for protecting an innocent, for appeasing a man in his passion, for *comforting the afflicted*, for *animating the timorous*, for *persuading a nauseating patient to take his physic*, for overcoming an obstinate humour, for making an ill design miscarry."[7]

Several modern ethical writers of considerable celebrity have been no less explicit and indulgent on this question. Amongst these it may suffice to cite the testimony of the late Dr. Francis Hutcheson of Glasgow; of whom it is said by his excellent biographer, that "he abhorred the least appearance of deceit either in word or action."[8] "When in certain affairs," says he, "'tis known that men do not conceive it an injury to be deceived, there is no crime in false speech about such matters. . . . No man censures a Physician for deceiving a patient too much dejected, by expressing good hopes of him, or by denying that he gives him a proper medicine which he is foolishly prejudiced against: the patient afterwards will not reproach him for it. . . . Wise men allow this liberty to the Physician in whose skill and fidelity they trust: or if they do not, there may be a just plea from necessity."[9]—"These pleas of necessity some would exclude by a maxim of late received, *We must not do evil that good may come of it.* The author of this maxim is not well known. It seems, by a passage in St. Paul,[10] that Christians were reviled as

teaching, that, since the mercy and veracity of God were displayed by the obstinate wickedness of the Jews, they should continue in sin that this good might ensue from it. He rejects the imputation upon his doctrine; and hence some take up the contradictory proposition as a general maxim of great importance in morality. Perhaps it has been a maxim among St. Paul's enemies, since they upbraid him with counteracting it. Be the author who they please, the sentence is of no use in morals, as it is quite vague and undetermined. Must one do nothing for a good purpose, which would have been evil without this reference? 'Tis evil to hazard life without a view to some good; but, when 'tis necessary for a public interest, 'tis very lovely and honourable. 'Tis criminal to expose a good man to danger for nothing; but 'tis just even to force him into the greatest dangers for his country. 'Tis criminal to occasion any pains to innocent persons, without a view to some good; but for restoring of health we reward chirurgeons for scarifyings, burnings, and amputations. 'But,' say they, 'such actions, done for these ends, are not evil. The maxim only determines that we must not do, for a good end, such actions as are evil even when done for a good end.' But this proposition is identic and useless; for who will tell us next, what these actions, sometimes evil, are, which may be done for a good end? and what actions are so evil that they must not be done even for a good end? The maxim will not answer this question; and truly it amounts only to this trifle; *you ought not for any good end to do what is evil, or what you ought not to do, even for a good end.*"[11]

Dr. Johnson, who admits of some exception to the law of truth, strenuously denies the right of telling a lie to a sick man for fear of alarming him. "You have no business with consequences," says he; "you are to tell the truth. Besides, you are not sure what effect your telling him that he is in danger may have. It may bring his distemper to a crisis, and that may cure him. Of all lying I have the greatest abhorrence of this, because I believe it has been frequently practised on myself."[12]

If the Medical reader wishes to investigate this nice and important subject of casuistry, he may consult Grotius, *De Jure Belli ac Pacis*, Puffendorff, Grove's *Ethics*, Balguy's *Law of Truth*, Fénelon's *Telemachus*, Butler, Hutcheson, Paley, and Gisborne. Every practitioner must find himself occasionally in circumstances of very delicate embarrassment, with respect to the contending obligations of veracity and professional duty; and when such trials occur, it will behove him to act on fixed principles of rectitude, derived from previous information and serious reflection. Perhaps the following brief considerations, by which I have conscientiously endeavoured to govern my own conduct, may afford some aid to his decision.

Moral truth, in a professional view, has two references; one to the party to whom it is delivered, and another to the individual by whom it is uttered. In the first, it is a *relative* duty, constituting a branch of justice; and may be properly regulated by the Divine rule of equity prescribed by our Saviour, to do unto others, as we would (all circumstances duly weighed,) they should do unto us.[13] In the second, it is a *personal* duty, regarding solely the sincerity, the purity, and the probity of the Physician himself. To a patient, therefore, (perhaps the father of a numerous family, or one whose life is of the highest importance to the community,) who makes enquiries, which, if faithfully answered, might prove fatal to him, it would be a gross and unfeeling wrong to reveal the truth. His right to it is suspended, and even annihilated; because, its beneficial nature being reversed, it would be deeply injurious to himself, to his family, and to the public: and he has the strongest claim, from the trust reposed in his Physician, as well as from the common principles of humanity, to be guarded against whatever would be detrimental to him. In such a situation, therefore, the only point at issue is, whether the practitioner shall sacrifice that delicate sense of veracity, which is so ornamental to, and indeed forms a characteristic excellence of, the virtuous man, to this claim of Professional justice and social duty. Under such a painful conflict of obligations a wise and good man must be governed by those which are the most imperious; and will therefore generously relinquish every consideration referable only to himself. Let him be careful, however, not to do this, but in cases of real emergency, which happily seldom occur; and to guard his mind sedulously against the injury it may sustain by such violations of the native love of truth.

I shall conclude this long note with the two following very interesting biographical facts. The husband of the celebrated Arria, Caecina Paetus, was very dangerously ill. Her son was also sick at the same time, and died.[14] He was a youth of uncommon accomplishments, and fondly beloved by his parents. Arria prepared and conducted his funeral in such a manner, that her husband remained entirely ignorant of the mournful event which occasioned that solemnity. Paetus often enquired with anxiety about his son; to whom she cheerfully replied that he had slept well, and was better. But if her tears, too long restrained, were bursting forth, she instantly retired, to give vent to her grief; and when again composed, returned to Paetus with dry eyes and placid countenance, quitting, as it were, all the tender feelings of the mother at the threshold of her husband's chamber.

"Lady Russell's only son, Wriothesley, Duke of Bedford, died of the small-pox in May 1711, in the 31st year of his age.[15] . . . To this affliction succeeded, in Nov. 1711, the loss of her daughter, the Duchess of Rutland, who died in child-bed. Lady Russell, after seeing her in the coffin, went to her other daughter, married to the Duke of Devonshire, from whom it was necessary to conceal her grief, she being at that time in child-bed likewise; therefore she assumed a cheerful air, and with astonishing resolution, [verbally] agreeable to truth, answered her anxious daughter's enquiries with these words: 'I have seen your sister out of bed to-day.'"

Notes

1. Chap. 12. vol. ii. p. 159.

2. Rom. iii. 8.

3. Horace, *Sat.* i. 1. 106.

4. [Alluding perhaps to *De Mendac,* c. 21. § 42. tom. vi. p. 444. ed. Bened., or to *Cont. Mendac.* c. 20. § 40. tom. vi. p. 472; but if so, St. Augustine's meaning is not quite correctly given in the text.]

5. *De Jure Belli ac Pacis,* lib. iii. cap. 1. sect. 10 [9?] §§ 2–4. See also cap. 1. sect. 14–16.

6. Spavan's Puffendorff, vol. ii. chap. 1. p. 6.

7. *Ibid.* p. 9.

8. Leechman's biographical Preface to Hutcheson's *System of Moral Philosophy,* p. xxiv.

9. *System of Moral Philosophy,* bk. ii. ch. 10. § 4. vol. ii. p. 32.

10. Rom. iii. 8.

11. *System of Moral Philosophy,* bk. ii. ch. 17. § 7. vol. ii. p. 132.

12. See Boswell's *Life of Johnson,* June 13, 1784.

13. St. Matth. vii. 12.

14. Pliny, *Epist.* iii. 16.

15. Lady Rachel Russell's *Letters;* Note to Letter 149.

33

Worthington Hooker
Truth in Our Intercourse with the Sick

Reprinted from Worthington Hooker, *Physician and Patient* (New York: Baker and Scribner, 1849), pp. 357–382.

On the question, whether strict veracity should be adhered to, in every case and under all circumstances, in our intercourse with the sick, there is very great difference of opinion, as well among medical men, as in the community at large. Some are most scrupulosuly strict in their regard to truth; others, while they are generally so, make some few occasional exceptions in cases of great emergency and necessity; while others still (and I regret to say that they are very numerous) give themselves great latitude in their practice, if they do not in their avowed opinions.

In examining this subject, it is not so much my intention to discuss the abstract question, as to present the many practical considerations that present themselves, illustrating them, so far as is necessary, by facts and cases.

In order to introduce the subject, I will here quote a passage from Percival's *Medical Ethics,* which presents the views of those who are in favor of an occasional departure from truth, where the necessity of the case seems to demand it. [For material quoted, see p. 204, col. 3, "Every practitioner . . ." to end of selection.]

The falsehood in the two cases related by the author is of the most egregious character, and yet they are fair representations of that kind of deception which many feel authorized to use in the sick room. The equivocation which is practised, it is true, is not always as gross and as labored, but it is as real. And whatever be the degree or kind of deception, the same principles will apply to every case.

The question that presents itself is not, let it be understood, whether the truth shall in any case be *withheld,* but whether, in doing this, real falsehood is justifiable, in any form, whether direct or indirect, whether palpable or in the shape of equivocation.

And we may also remark, that the question is not, whether those who practice deception upon the sick are guilty of a criminal act. This depends altogether on the motive which prompts it, and it is certainly often done from the best and kindest motives. The question is stripped of all considerations of this nature, and comes before us as a simple practical question— whether there are any cases in which, for the sake of benefitting our fellow

men, perhaps even to the saving of life, it is proper to make an exception to the great general law of truth.

The considerations which will bring us to a clear and undoubted decision of this question, are not all to be drawn from the preciousness of the principle of truth, as an unbroken, invariable, and ever-present principle, the soul of all order, and confidence, and happiness, in the wide universe. But the principle of expediency also furnishes us with some considerations that are valuable in confirming our decision, if not in leading us to it. In truth, expediency and right always correspond, and would be seen to do so, if we could always see the end from the beginning.

I will remark upon each of the considerations as I present them.

First. It is erroneously assumed by those who advocate deception, that the knowledge to be concealed from the patient would, if communicated, be essentially injurious to him. Puffendorf remarks in relation to this point, that "when a man is desirous, and it is his duty, to do a piece of service, he is not bound to take measures that will *certainly* render his attempts unsuccessful." The certainty of the result, thus taken for granted, is far from being warranted by facts. Even in some cases where there was a strong probability (and this is all we can have in any case) that the effect would be hurtful, it has been found not to be so. I might here narrate some cases to prove the truth of this assertion, but it is not necessary. Suffice it to say, that it is confirmed by the experience of every physician who has pursued a frank and candid course in his intercourse with the sick.

Secondly. It is also erroneously assumed that concealment can always or generally be effectually carried out. There are so many ways by which the truth can be betrayed, even where concerted plans are laid, guarded at every point, that failure is much more common than success, so far as my observation has extended. Some unguarded expression or act, even on the part of those who are practising the concealment, or some information communicated by those who are not in the secret, perhaps by children, or some evidence casually seen, very often either reveals the truth, or awakens suspicion and prompts inquiry which the most skilful equivocation may not be able to elude. The very air that is assumed in carrying on the deception often defeats the object. In one instance where this was the case, the suspecting patient said very significantly, "How strangely you all seem—you act as if something dreadful had happened that you mean to keep from me." Even the little child often exhibits a most correct discrimination in detecting deception in the manner, the modes of expression, and even the very tone of the voice. And sometimes, nay very often, people so far undervalue the good sense and shrewdness of children, that their deception is even ridiculously bungling, and justly excites an honest indignation in the bosom of the deceived child.

I give the following scene as an illustration of the above remark.

"Come, take this," said a mother to her child, "it's something good."

The child was evidently a little suspicious that he was not dealt with candidly; but after a great many assurances from her on whom a child ought to be able to rely, if upon any body in the wide world, he was at length persuaded to take the spoon into his mouth. The medicine, which was really very bitter, was at once spit out, and the little fellow burst forth in reproaches upon his mother for telling him such a lie.

"No, my dear," said she, "I have told you no lie. The medicine *is* good—it is good to cure you. That is what I meant."

"Good to cure me!" cried he, with a look and an air of the most perfect contempt. "You cheated me. You *know* you did."

The contempt which this child manifested towards such barefaced equivocation was most justly merited, and yet this is a fair example of the deceptions which physicians are almost every day obliged to witness, and which, (may I not say?) some of them encourage both by precept and example.

Thirdly. If the deception be discovered or suspected, the effect upon the patient is much worse than a frank and full statement of the truth can produce. If disagreeable news, for example, be concealed from him, there is very great danger that it will in some way be revealed to him so abruptly and unexpectedly, as to give him a severe shock, which can for the most part be

avoided when the communication is made voluntarily. And then, too, the very fact that the truth has been withheld, increases, for obvious reasons, this shock. I will relate a case as an example. It occurred during the prevalence of an epidemic. A lady was taken sick and died. The fact of her death was studiously concealed from another lady of her acquaintance, who was liable to be attacked by the same disease. She was supposed by her to be doing well, until one day a child from a neighboring family accidentally alluded to the death of her friend in her presence. The shock which the sad news thus communicated produced upon her was almost overwhelming, and it was of course rendered more intense by the reflection, that her friends thought her to be exceedingly in danger of dying of the prevailing disease, and therefore had practised this concealment in order to quiet her apprehensions. She soon followed her friend, and it is not an improbable supposition, that the strong impression thus made upon her mind had some agency in causing her death.

In another case of a similar character, the first intimation which a lady had of the death of a friend was from seeing the husband of this friend pass in the street with a badge of mourning. She was immediately prostrated upon her bed, and was a long time in recovering from the shock.

In both of these cases the concealment of the truth was prompted by the best of motives—pure kindness; and yet nothing is more plain than that it was a *mistaken* kindness. Whatever may be true in other instances, the result showed this to be the fact in these two cases. And if it be true, as I think all experience will prove, that success, and not failure, in the attempt at concealment, is the exception to the general fact, it clearly follows that deception is impolitic as a measure of kindness, and therefore, aside from any other consideration, it should be wholly discarded in our intercourse with the sick.

I have a case in mind, which exhibits in contrast the influence of frankness and of deception.

A little girl, the daughter of a farmer, had her arm torn to pieces up to the

elbow in a threshing machine constructed very much like a picker. As her mother was confined to her bed with severe sickness, the child was carried into the house of a neighbor. When I arrived, I was told that her mother was in great distress, and fears were expressed that the accident would have a very bad influence upon her case. I asked if she knew what had happened. "No," said her husband, "not exactly. She found out by the children that Mary was hurt, and then sent for me, and asked me what was the matter. I told her at first that she had got her finger hurt. She said she knew that was not all, and I at length, after she had begged and begged me to tell all, told her that her hand was hurt badly. And now she is crying most piteously, and says that we are deceiving her, and that she knows that Mary is almost killed."

I immediately went in to see the mother, and found her indeed almost distracted with the great variety of dread visions that had suggested themselves to her fancy in regard to her darling child. As I entered the room she cried out, "Oh, she's dead, doctor, or dying—torn to pieces—in agony— Oh, isn't it so? tell me, tell me the truth!" "Be quiet," said I, "and I *will* tell you all the truth. I will not deceive you." I assured her that she need give herself no anxiety about the *life* of her child—that was safe. This announcement quieted her in a good measure, and I went on to tell her that the arm was badly torn, and that I must amputate it above the elbow. I told her that this would take but a minute or two, and then the child would be essentially well. It was necessary to go into these particulars in answer to her inquiries, (which were the more minute from the fact that she had been deceived,) or else I should forfeit her confidence, and thus commit the same error that had already been committed. She thanked me for being so frank with her, and said, that though it was hard to think of the operation, she could bear that, if the child's life was only spared. She grieved still, it is true; but there was none of that overwhelming distraction that results from vague apprehension.

Fourthly. The destruction of confidence, resulting from discovered deception, is productive of injurious consequences to the persons deceived. The moment that you are detected in deceiving the sick, you at once impair or even destroy their confidence in your veracity and frankness. Everything that you do afterward is suspected, and a full and unshrinking trust is not accorded to you even when you deserve it, though you may try to obtain it by the most positive and solemn assurances. If, for example, you wish to encourage a patient, and you tell him that though the bow of hope is dim to his eye, it is bright to your own: "Ah!" he will think, if he does not say, "how do I know but that it is as dim to him as it looks to me—he has deceived me once, and perhaps he does now."

Every physician has seen the injurious influence of deception upon children. Sometimes it is of a most disastrous character, and occasionally, I have not a doubt, it proves fatal. Deception is more frequently practiced upon children than upon adults, and many seem to think that they have not the same right to candor and honesty in our intercourse with them. But a child can appreciate fair and honest treatment as well as an adult can, and he has as good a right to receive it at our hands. He sometimes claims this right in terms, and by acts not to be mistaken. And when it is taken from him, he shows his sense of the wrong by remonstrances and retaliatory language, and by a system of rebellion to an authority which he despises, as well as fears, for its falsehood.

Suppose a mother succeeds in giving a dose of medicine by stratagem, the administration of every dose after it is accompanied with a fearful struggle. The strife which results from the spirit of resistance thus engendered, perhaps in the beginning of a long sickness, and which might in most cases have been avoided by frank and candid treatment, continues through the whole course of the disease to the last hour of life if the case prove fatal, the little creature feebly but obstinately resisting its mother, till the exhaustion of coming death puts an end to its struggles; and, though she plies every art that fondness can devise to win back the lost confidence of her darling child, it is all in vain.

If the reader have any adequate idea of the importance of quietness in the management of the sick, I need not spend time to prove, that this resistance of the sick child has an injurious effect upon the disease, and that in those cases where life has but a feeble trembling hold, where the silver cord is worn down almost to its last thread, such a struggle may break that thread by its violence. I have not a doubt that many a child has died under such circumstances, that might otherwise have recovered.

Let me not be understood to imply that the resistance made by children to the administration of medicine is invariably the result of deception practised upon them, though this is the cause undoubtedly in quite a large proportion of the cases, and those too of the worst and most unconquerable character. And it may be remarked, that in many cases this may be the cause of the difficulty where it is little suspected. For it is so common a habit to deceive children in this matter, that it is often done unconsciously. But though the parent may not remember it, the child does, and the cruel oppressive act (for so it may be properly called) locked up in the memory of the child, wakes up rebellion in his heart that is not easily quelled. Many a parent has thus in a moment, for the sake of a slight temporary advantage, sown the wind to reap the whirlwind.

Deception has very often been made use of in the management of the insane, though recently not to the same extent that it once was. The consideration which I have been illustrating and enforcing lies against the practice of it in our intercourse with this unfortunate class of patients, with the greater force, because in their case the mind is diseased, and any bad mental influence has therefore a worse effect than it would have upon a case of mere bodily disease. The reason is obvious—it acts directly upon the seat of the disease in the former case, but indirectly in the latter.

Besides, let the insane man once see that you have deceived him, and you lose the principal, perhaps we may say the only, moral means that you have for curing his malady. Confidence is essential to any good moral influence that you may exert upon him. I might cite many facts to prove this, but will advert to only one. The wife of an insane man was the only person among all his friends that had any control over him, and she could manage him with perfect ease. After his recovery she asked him the reason of this fact, and his reply was, "You was the only one that uniformly told me the truth."

The bad influence of deception upon the insane man is rendered the more certain and effectual from the fact that his insanity incapacitates him for appreciating the kind motives which may have prompted the deception. You cannot convince him as you can the sane sick man, that you have deceived him for his own good. His suspicious eye sees nothing but a sinister purpose in the cheat which you have practised upon him.

One of the most vivid recollections of my childhood is that of a scene which illustrates these remarks. A poor crazy man who wandered about the streets was thought to have become dangerous, and it was proposed to confine him in the common jail. A plan was laid to do it by stratagem. He fancied himself to own some large possessions, and talked much about going to Boston to see his friend the governor, and attend to his business there. A neighbor offered to go with him, and he accepted the offer. As they passed by the jail, his friend proposed to visit it. As they entered one of the cells he adroitly slipped out, and the door was closed upon the insane man. His dream of earthly happiness and wealth was in a moment at an end, and he beheld himself the victim of base treachery in the narrow cell of a prison. Never shall I forget how eloquently he pleaded for his release, how he asked what crime could be charged to his account, how he denounced those who had thus without cause shut him up like a felon, and especially with what sorrowful but burning indignation he spoke of the man, "who under the guise of friendship, had decoyed him into this snare of his enemies." Though a mere boy, I pitied him. I sympathised with him. I had known him only as a pleasant old man, who used to amuse us as we met him in the streets with stories of his immense wealth and of the splendid plans of building on which he loved to speculate. I felt that it was wrong to confine him among vile criminals, and wondered not that the keen sense of such injury prompted to the utterance of curses on those who inflicted it. But these natural feelings gave way in my bosom, as they did in older ones, to what was then supposed to be the necessity of the case—a necessity which, I rejoice to say, has since that been found not to exist in similar cases. A very great improvement has been effected in this as well as in other respects, in the management of the insane. Most of those whom it was once thought necessary to confine with bolts and bars, and perhaps chains, and upon whom deception was continually and systematically practised, thus adding poignancy to the pangs of the oppressed spirit, are now permitted to have so much liberty, that they are cheerful and happy, reposing entire confidence in their attendants, who are careful never to deceive them. And those whom it is thought necessary to confine, are not doomed to the cheerlessness and disgrace of the cell of the felon, but they are placed in as agreeable circumstances as is consistent with safety. And it has come to be an established rule with those who have the care of the insane, that force is always preferable to deception. But still, erroneous views are very prevalent in the community on this subject. It is common to this day, even among the excellent and well informed, to propose to send their insane friends to a Retreat by stratagem, and this has often been done even by the advice of physicians. So far as I recollect, in all the cases of insanity that have gone to Retreats from under my care, this mode of management has been spoken of by some, and generally by many, as the only proper mode. The public need to be instructed and reformed on this point.

It is a common observation that the insane are apt to look upon their best and most intimate friends as their enemies. Why is this? It is clear, that it is in part to be ascribed to the influence of deception, waking up, as might be expected, feelings of resentment and enmity in the bosom of the insane, which would not otherwise be there. . . .

The extent to which deception is practised upon the insane cannot be fully appreciated, except by those whose attention has been specially called to this subject. As I have already remarked in regard to children, so also it is with the insane—deception is so common, that people often make use

of it almost unconsciously. The whole course of management on the part of their friends, is often characterized throughout by an absence of candor and veracity.

The tendency of such a course is invariably to increase insanity, making it more intense and obstinate. And not only so, but it modifies to a greater or less degree its character. Deception prompts the insane man to exercise his ingenuity in forming plans to foil and circumvent his deceivers, whom he supposes very naturally to be his enemies. Of course, new feelings and thoughts are thus excited in his bosom, giving in some measure a new cast to his insanity.

I will here relate a case that illustrates these remarks.

The friends of an insane gentleman determined to send him to a Retreat by stratagem. For this purpose, he was induced by one of them to go a journey with him. On their way, his friend proposed to him to visit an Insane Retreat as a matter of curiosity. When they arrived there, he was given to understand that he was to remain as an inmate. Great was his rage at being so grossly deceived. After the first burst of indignation was passed, he saw that it was of no use to say anything or to make any resistance. He was a shrewd man, and therefore, as a matter of policy, he submitted with apparent cheerfulness to his new situation. He did not forget, as the insane sometimes fortunately do, the wrong which his friends had done him, and as he was decoyed there by stratagem, it is no wonder that he at length made his escape by stratagem also. He came out, as might have been expected, with his insanity more thoroughly fixed than it was when he went in, and he added to it a deep hatred of Retreats, and of course of the man who had betrayed him into one.

Another attempt was made to carry him to the same Retreat, which from mismanagement utterly failed. The insane man was victorious, and he felt himself to be so, over his friends, who he supposed were bent upon cheating and oppressing him. All this not only made him more crazy, but it gave a new shape to his insane ideas. In a conversation which I chanced to have with him, he said to me, "It is perfectly

evident, doctor, that these Insane Retreats are joint-stock institutions, and the stockholders are chiefly lawyers and doctors and ministers. And it's good stock too. Just see how much they charge for board—full double at least of the actual expenses. I need not tell you anything about it, however, for you own some of this stock, and you know how profitable it is to you."

"Oh no," said I, "this is all new to me." He looked at me as if he would look me through. He had been deceived so much, that he believed, he trusted no one. Although I gave him the most positive assurance that I owned no such stock, still, in spite of the confidence which he ordinarily reposed in me, he showed that he did after all suspect me on this point, so firmly was this notion about Retreats fastened in his mind. He went on to give his reasons for his opinion.

"I can look back," said he, "to my very childhood, and see that from that time to the present, there has been a series of efforts on the part of these stockholders to make me a crazy man; and they at length succeeded, and then contrived the mean plan of tricking me into one of their Retreats. The minister that I lived with when I was ten years old began this scheme, and all the ministers and lawyers and doctors, that I have had anything to do with since that time, have had a hand in it—have exerted their influence on me, all in relation to this one object. It's a regular money-making business. Of course the stockholders all want to see these Retreats well filled up. Just see how they have treated me lately. They have combined to cross my purposes, break up my plans, defeat my projects, ruin my business, and all this to irritate and disappoint me, and thus craze me. And then, to cap the whole, they lied to me and betrayed me into their prison to die a slow death, paying them all the time about twelve dollars a week. Good stock, doctor, but a cruel business," said he, with a most unearthly grin, and a shudder that shook his whole frame. "But thank heaven," cried he, "I've escaped their clutches. Though they have ruined me, they shall not have their twelve dollars a week out of me. No, I'll die first. Such systematic, cheating, lying oppression, I'll resist to the death."

It is evident that the treatment which this man received at the hands of his friends, tended to aggravate, instead of lessening his insanity. And I may remark, too, that the notion which he derived from this treatment, in relation to Retreats, false as it was, was founded on more plausible reasons as they were presented to his mind, than are some of the opinions that are adopted by some sane men in the community.

Fifthly. The *general* effect of deception, aside from the individual which it is supposed it will benefit, is injurious. The considerations on which I have already remarked, have had regard entirely to the person that is deceived, and I think that I have shown most clearly, that even taking this narrow view of the influence of deception, it is in almost all cases a bad influence: and therefore as we cannot tell in what cases this influence will be good, it is impolitic, and should be entirely discarded. Let us now go farther, and looking beyond the individuals who are the subjects of the deception, we shall see its influence extending all around from these individuals, as so many radiating points of influence, leavening the whole mass of society with a most poisonous leaven. It is not an influence that can be shut up in the case of any individual, in that one breast, or within that one chamber of sickness.

That confidence, which should always exist in the intercourse of the sick with their physicians and friends, and which may be made the channel of great and essential benefits to them, is materially impaired, often even destroyed by such deception. And this effect is unfortunately not confined to those who practice it, but the imputation rests upon others. The distrust thus produced often exerts a depressing influence in those cases, where the cordial influence of hope is most urgently needed, and where it can be administered in consonance with the most scrupulous veracity. It is well if, under such circumstances, the physician can appeal to the patient's own experience of his frankness in all his previous intercourse with him.

I call to mind an instance in which I was able to make this appeal with the most marked good effect. The patient was a lady who was in a great state of alarm in regard to the probable result of her sickness. She was indeed very sick, but there was good reason to hope that remedies would relieve her. At the same time I feared that the depressing effect of this state of alarm, if it should continue, would prove a serious obstacle to her recovery. But as I expressed to her the confident hope that she would get well, she said to me, "Physicians always talk in this way, and you do not really mean as you say. I shall die, I know that I shall die." I had been the physician of the family for many years, during which time they had gone through some trying scenes of sickness. Alluding to all this, I asked her if she could look back and call to mind a single instance in which I had not dealt candidly and frankly with her. She allowed that she could not. "Well," said I, "believe me *now*; I *am* in earnest; I do believe, and confidently, too, that you will recover." The tears were at once wiped away. Cheerfulness, the cheerfulness of hope, lighted up her countenance and the case went on to a speedy and full recovery.

Every day we see evidence of the fact that so large a proportion of the medical profession practice deception upon the sick, that the profession, as a whole, has to a greater or less degree the imputation fastened upon it. Indeed patients often, as a matter of course, make the distinction between the obligations to professional veracity, and those of the man, as a man, in his ordinary intercourse; and the physician, who has an established reputation for the strictest veracity everywhere else but in the sick chamber, has there the suspicion of deception put upon him; and it is supposed to be no imputation of which he should complain, because deception is allowed here almost by general permission. For this reason, whatever of frankness and honesty there may be in our intercourse with the sick, often fails to produce the effect intended, in part at least if not wholly. And this result follows just in proportion to the extent to which deception is made use of in the profession.

The indirect and collateral effects of deception are often manifest in a family of children. Its influence extends beyond the mind and character of the deceived child. If the other children witness the deception, what hinders them from believing that their parents can deceive them also whenever it suits their convenience? And if they do not witness it, the sick child will remember it when he recovers, and the rebellion which he has, in consequence, in his bosom towards an authority that rules by deceit, and is therefore deemed with good reason oppressive, is of course communicated to the other bosoms of the little flock. Many a parent, who supposed that he was doing nothing that would last beyond the present moment, has thus sown the seeds of rebellion among the little band of subjects, over whom God has placed him; and who can tell what the fruits will be, or to what extent or length of time they will grow!

I need barely say in concluding my remarks on this consideration, that the momentary good which occasionally results to *individual* cases from deception, is not to be put in comparison, for one moment, with the vast and permanent evils of a *general* character, that almost uniformly proceed from a breach of the great law of truth. And there is no warrant to be found for shutting our eyes to these general and remote results, in our earnestness to secure a particular and present good, however precious that good may be—a plain principle, and yet how often it is disregarded.

Sixthly. If it be adopted by the community as a common rule, that the truth may be sacrificed in urgent cases, the very object of the deception will be defeated. For why is it that deception succeeds in any case? It is because the patient supposes that all who have intercourse with him deal with him truthfully—that no such common rule has been adopted. There is even now, while the policy on this subject is unsettled and matter of dispute, enough distrust produced to occasion trouble. And if it should become a settled policy under an acknowledged common rule, the result would be *general* distrust, of course defeating deception at every point. And yet if it be proper to deceive, then most clearly is it proper to proclaim it as an adopted principle of action. Else we are driven to the absurd proposition, that while it is right to practice deception, it is wrong to say to the world that it is right.

It is in vain to say that the evil result which would attend this adoption of occasional deception, as the settled policy of the medical profession, would find a correction in the very terms of the rule which should be adopted, viz. that the case must be an urgent one to warrant deception, and there must be a fair prospect that it can be carried through without discovery. For every patient, that was aware of the adoption of such a rule, might and often probably would suspect that his own case is considered as coming within the terms of the rule.

Seventhly. Once open the door for deception, and you can prescribe for it no definite limits. Every one is to be left to judge for himself. And as present good is the object for which the truth is to be sacrified, the amount of good, for which it is proper to do it, can not be fixed upon with any exactness. Each one is left to make his own estimate, and the limit is in each one's private judgment, in each one's individual case as it arises. And the limit, which is at first perhaps quite narrow, is apt to grow wider, till the deception may get to be of the very worst and most injurious character. I will give a single illustration of this remark, which though not taken from the practice of medicine, is appropriate to my purpose. It has always been allowed in the laws of war, to deceive the enemy by stratagems, false lights, etc. At one time some English ships in two or three instances decoyed the enemy by counterfeiting signals of distress. The deception in this case is productive indirectly of the very worst consequences, for it manifestly tends to prevent relief from being afforded to those who are actually in a distressed condition. Our feelings of humanity instinctively condemn such a stratagem and yet it is only a mere extension of that deception, which has been by common consent allowed in war. It involves no different principles, and is only more objectionable, because it produces worse indirect results. It differs in degree only and not in kind.

So it is with deception always. Its indirect effects are always bad to some extent, and to what extent they will prove so we know not in each individual case. You can never know at the time how great is the sacrifice which you are making for a present good. While you may be thinking that you

are only sacrificing your own veracity, and that the influence of the act will not extend beyond the passing moment, you may be producing disastrous results upon the interests of others, and those results may be both lasting and accumulative. A man who was captured by some Indians, was asked by them if there were any white men in the neighborhood. He told them that there were, and directed them to a spot where he was very certain that there were none. They immediately started in pursuit, leaving him bound and in the charge of one of their number. When they were gone, he contrived to make his escape. Almost every one would say that this was a strong case, and that they could not blame him for telling a falsehood to Indians, in order to escape from their cruelty. Here was a great good to be obtained, the saving himself from torture, perhaps from death, and deceiving savages for such a purpose, it will be said, is not to be condemned. But mark the result of that deception. Five white men were found on the spot to which he directed them, and were captured.

In order to make out a justification of deception, on the ground of expediency in any case, all the possible results, direct and indirect, must be taken into the account. But this is impossible except to omniscience itself. Even in those cases which appear the most clear to us, there may be consequences of the most grave character utterly hidden from our view. In the instance just related, the captive was very certain, from some circumstances, that he directed his captors to a spot where there were no white men.

The uncertainty of our knowledge of the circumstances of each case prevents then our defining any limits, within which deception shall be bounded. We can make no accurate distinctions, which will enable us to say, that it can be beneficially employed in one case, while in another it will be inexpedient.

I have now finished the examination of the various considerations which have been suggested to my mind in relation to this subject. And I think that they settle the question as to the expediency of deception beyond all doubt. I think it perfectly evident, that the good,

which may be done by deception in a *few* cases, is almost as nothing, compared with the evil which it does in *many* cases, when the prospect of its doing good was just as promising as it was in those in which it succeeded. And when we add to this the evil which would result from a *general* adoption of a system of deception, the importance of a strict adherence to truth in our intercourse with the sick, even on the ground of expediency, becomes incalculably great.

In the passage, which I quoted in the beginning of this article from Percival's *Medical Ethics,* the writer makes, I conceive, a false issue on the question under consideration. He assumes that the injury, which results from a sacrifice of the truth for the good of the sick, comes upon him who practices the deception, and that in doing it, "he generously relinquishes every consideration referable only to himself." But the considerations that I have presented show, that the injury is very far from being thus confined. Often the very person intended to be benefited is injured, perhaps deeply, in some cases even fatally. And then the indirect effects can not be estimated.

There are many illustrations, used by those who advocate deception, which are plausible but fallacious. I will cite a single example. Dr. Hutcheson of Glasgow, as quoted by Dr. Percival, in remarking on the maxim, that we must not do evil that good may come, says, "Must one do nothing for a good purpose, which would have been evil without this reference? It is evil to hazard life without a view of some good; but when it is necessary for a public interest, it is very lovely and honorable. It is criminal to expose a good man to danger for nothing; but it is just even to force him into the greatest dangers for his country. It is criminal to occasion any pain to innocent persons, without a view to some good; but for restoring of health we reward chirurgeons for scarifyings, burnings, and amputations."

I would remark on this that the infliction of pain is not in itself a moral act, but the purpose for which it is done gives it all the moral character that it has. Aside from this, it affects no moral principle, as the infliction of an injury upon truth certainly does, independent of the object for which it is done. The infliction of pain then for a good purpose can not be said to be doing evil that good may come—it is doing good.

The sacrifice of life which the writer speaks of, is the sacrifice of a less good for a greater one simply, and not the sacrifice of any principle. But when the truth is sacrificed for what is deemed to be a greater good, it is in fact the sacrifice of a greater good, for not only a less, but an uncertain good—a sacrifice of the eternal principle, which binds together the moral universe in harmony, for a mere temporary good, which after all may prove to be a shadow instead of a reality.

I can not leave this subject without making some explanations of a few points, in order to guard against some erroneous inferences to which the sentiments that I have advanced might otherwise be liable.

I wish not to be understood as saying that we should never take pains to withhold knowledge from the sick, which we fear might be injurious to them. There are cases in which this should be done. All that I claim is this—that in withholding the truth no deception should be practised, and that if sacrifice of the truth be the necessary price for obtaining the object, no such sacrifice should be made. In the passage which I have quoted from Dr. Percival, he states a case in which he very properly says, that the patient's right to the truth is suspended; but I do not agree with him, that in withholding the truth we have the right to *put absolute falsehood in its place*.

It is always a question of expediency simply, whether the truth ought to be withheld. And it is a question that depends, for its proper decision, upon a variety of considerations in each individual case. It is very often decided injudiciously. There is generally too great a readiness to adopt an affirmative decision. It is too easily taken for granted, that the knowledge in question will do harm to the patient if it be communicated to him. The obvious rule on this subject is this—that the truth should not be withheld unless there be a reasonable prospect of effectually preventing a discovery of it, and that too by fair and honest means.

It has often been said that the physician has no right to excite too much hope in the mind of a patient by directing his attention, as is often done, to any favorable symptoms that may appear in his case. But I ask, how is it known that in the case in relation to which this remark is made, too much hope is excited? The physician is fallible, and is by no means answerable for putting just the right degree of hope into the patient's bosom. It is not to be expected of him that he shall always tell each patient just how his case stands. His own mind is often filled with conflicting hopes and fears, and he cannot decide clearly what the probabilities are in many cases. And if he thinks that he can do so, he may be very much mistaken. Estimates are often made most unwarrantably. An exactness is often aimed at which is impracticable. The patient in many cases has no right to such an estimate, for while it may be a mere guess, he may look upon it as a well-founded estimate, made upon a real knowledge of his case. He will therefore draw false inferences from it, and this the physician is bound to prevent, and in so doing he actually prevents deception.

The physician should always remember that though he may be aware himself of his liability to err in making any such estimate, the patient may have such confidence in his judgment, that he will consider the opinion which he may express to be of course a correct one—almost beyond the possibility of a mistake. So that however guarded he may be in expressing an unfavorable opinion of the probable issue of any case, that opinion may have too much weight in the patient's mind.

It is by no means true that all direct questions on the part of the sick must be directly and fully answered. For example, suppose the patient asks the physician, "Do you think on the whole that I shall recover"—a question that is sometimes asked under very embarrassing circumstances. If the physician thinks that he will probably not recover, he has no right to say to him that he will, for this would be falsehood. But he has a right, and it is his duty if he thinks it for the good of the patient, to withhold his opinion from him, if he can do it without falsehood or equivocation. He may say to him something like this: "It is difficult to decide that question. Perhaps it is not proper for me at this stage of your case to attempt to do it. You are very sick, and the issue of your sickness is known only to God. I hope that remedies will do so and so (pointing out somewhat the effects ordinarily to be expected) but I cannot tell." Something of this kind, varied according to the nature of each case, especially in the amount of hope communicated, it is perfectly consistent with truth and good faith to say; and very often when more is said, even in very dangerous cases, the physician goes beyond the limits which infinite wisdom has thought best to set to his knowledge. It is very common . . . for persons to recover, particularly in cases of acute disease, when the physician had supposed that they would die. This fact should make him somewhat cautious in giving definite opinions to the sick in relation to the probable final result of their sickness.

34

Richard C. Cabot

The Use of Truth and Falsehood in Medicine: An Experimental Study

Reprinted from *American Medicine*, vol. 5, 1903, pp. 344–349.

Two years ago, at the meeting of the Association of American Physicians at Washington, Dr. E. G. Janeway, then president of the association, chose for his presidential address the subject of "Truth in Medicine." Unfortunately, the address was never delivered, for President Janeway feeling keenly the responsibility of putting through the long schedule of papers assigned to the first morning session, omitted his own part of the program and contenting himself with a few introductory remarks started us at once on our morning's work. Only a hint of what he meant to say was vouchsafed to us. The subject, he said, "could have been handled under such heads as *truth in statistics; truth in diagnosis; truth in pathology; truth in therapeutics.*"

I have often regretted that Dr. Janeway's modesty and conscientiousness induced him to deprive us of this address. Still oftener I have speculated on what he would have said had the occasion seemed to him propitious. For the subject seems to me one that ought to be discussed by medical men. The results of experience should be compared according to the methods that have proved useful in the investigation of other topics. But as time has passed and Dr. Janeway has not returned to the topic, I have ventured to take up the hints and outlines which he furnished us and fill in, in my own fashion, the structure which I imagine he might have reared. Yet though he deserves credit for the plan of investigation which I have followed, it goes without saying that no one but myself is responsible for any opinion here expressed.

I approach the subject of truth in medicine, not from the point of view of scientific method, nor of metaphysic analysis, but of professional ethics. I do not ask "how can we find truth," nor "what is truth," but "how far should we speak the truth in dealing with our patients, our colleagues, or anyone else." "Are lies ever in place? If so, under what conditions?"

My method is experimental, the only one in which reasonable men place confidence, the only sound scientific method. I do not ask you to consider what, on general principles or according to authority or tradition, should be our course in this matter. As indicated in the title of my lecture I have made an experimental study of two different

hypotheses on the subject, submitting them to the test of experience, trying how they work, as any candid person must, if he wishes to make the fairest judgment in his power on any question. I have been working on this subject during a considerable part of the last eight years, and my conclusions, however faulty they may be, must be criticised like any other piece of scientific work only by those who have repeated the experiments on which they are based.

I began, as was natural, with the hypothesis on which I had been brought up. My medical training included some few lectures on medical ethics, but in matters of ethics, example far more than precept was the guide to the Harvard medical student of my day. Only once during my course was the rule for truth-speaking in medical matters directly stated.

"When you are thinking of telling a lie," said the teacher, "ask yourself whether it is simply and solely for the patient's benefit that you are going to tell it. If you are sure that you are acting for his good and not for your own profit, you can go ahead with a clear conscience."

The lies that the medical profession agree in condemning whenever the question arises are those told for personal and private gain. The magazine article representing work never performed and written solely for advertising purposes, is a lie that no one approves. The diagnosis of diphtheria when the physician knows the case is merely one of tonsillitis, is not justified by the increased fees which his frequent visits entail. There is no disagreement of opinion among physicians about such lies as these.

But the lies which are usually defended among physicians are of a different type and may be illustrated by the following quotations:

"The young physician in our day has some advantages in competition with older men. People sometimes consider a young man more up-to-date than his elders. Still there are some alleviations in growing old. When you don't know what's the matter with a patient you can enjoy the luxury of saying so. When you're young you have to know everything, for if you say you don't know, the patient is likely to chuck you out and send for some one else who does."

That *truth in diagnosis* is possible for the older physician, but not always for the younger, seems to be the moral of this quotation.

To speak the *truth in prognosis* is even harder. In the course of a lecture on the prognosis of heart disease, I once heard the following story:

A business man past middle life was found to be suffering from some form of heart disease. His wife inquired about the diagnosis and hearing it was heart disease she asked: "Isn't it true that he may drop dead suddenly?" The doctor had to confess that this was a possibility. "The consequence was," went on the story-teller, "that day after day she sat at her window about the time that her husband should be returning from business, watching to see whether he would come home on his feet or in an ambulance."

"Now," said the narrator, "when you get into practice, gentlemen, whatever you do, don't do that. Don't make a woman's life miserable because you can't keep a fact to yourself."

Surely it seems as if this is the place for a good straight lie. I thought so when I heard the story and made up my mind that whatever blunders I made in dealing with any patients I might have, this one I would avoid. But I found it more difficult than I had anticipated. It was not very many years before I saw in consultation a case the duplicate of that just described. Mr. B. had angina pectoris, aortic regurgitation, cardiac hypertrophy, in short, general arteriosclerosis affecting especially the heart and kidney. After I had talked over the case with the attending physician and was about to return and say a word to the family, my colleague said: "There's one thing I must warn you about. Mrs. B. is an excessively nervous, excitable woman, of no stamina at all. She gets hysterical on the slightest pretext, and when that happens she makes every one else in the house sick. If she heard what's the matter with her husband she'd go all to pieces. So you'll be very guarded in what you say, won't you?" To this I readily agreed. Remembering my lesson, and we went downstairs where Mrs. B. was waiting to hear the result

of our deliberations. She placed a chair for me and then planted herself in another, squarely facing me and very near. "Now, first of all," said she, "I want to know whether you are going to give me a straight and true answer to everything I ask you?" Having just promised the family physician that I would do nothing of the kind, I was so taken aback that I hesitated a moment. "That's enough," said Mrs. B., getting up. "I don't care to hear anything more."

I did not blame her. She had fairly caught us in our attempt to trick her. But the anecdote shows that the path of the medical man conscientiously trying to shield people from pain and trouble is sometimes a difficult and thorny one.

By means of these examples I hope I have succeeded in getting before you the problems that I wish to discuss.

I propose next to examine the matter more in detail, considering: (1) truth in diagnosis; (2) truth in prognosis; (3) truth in treatment.

By telling the truth I mean doing one's best to convey to another person the impression that one has about the matter in hand. One may do one's best and yet fail, but that is not lying. I once spent half an hour trying to convey to my parlor girl my impression about how to build a fire, but when she next tried to build one it appeared that the only idea she had received was that of packing kindling wood into the fireplace as tightly as she could and piling logs on top without a chink or cranny anywhere for a draught. Clearly I did not succeed in conveying my impression to her, yet I suppose no one would accuse me of lying to her. I had merited the cowboy's epitaph:

"He done his damndest; angels could do no more."

A *true impression*, not certain words literally true, is what we must try to convey. When a patient who has three fine rales at one apex and tubercle bacilli in his sputum asks, "Have I got tuberculosis?" it would be conveying a false impression to say "Yes, you have," and stop there. Ten to one his impression is that tuberculosis is a disease invariably and rapidly fatal. But that is not at all your impression of his case. To be true to that patient you must explain that what *he* means by

tuberculosis is the later stages of a neglected or unrecognized disease; that many people have as much trouble as he now has and get over it without finding it out; that with climatic and hygienic treatment he has a good chance of recovery, etc. To tell him simply that he has tuberculosis without adding any further explanation would convey an impression which in one sense is true, in the sense, namely, that to another physician it might sound approximately correct. What is sometimes called the simple truth, the "bald truth" or the "naked truth" is often practically false—as unrecognizable as Lear naked upon the moor. It needs to be explained, supplemented, modified.

Bearing in mind, then, that by truth speaking I mean the faithful attempt to convey a true impression, and by lying an *intentional deception,* however brought about, let us take up the question of

Truth and Falsehood in Diagnosis

The common conception of a doctor's duty in this matter, and one according to which I practised medicine for the first five or six years after graduation, is something as follows:

"Tell the truth so far as possible. But if you are young and not yet firmly established in practice it won't do to let the patient or his family know when you are in doubt about a diagnosis. If you do they will lose confidence in you and perhaps turn you out."

That is what is implied in the frank and refreshing confession of a middle aged and successful physician whose words I have already quoted: "The great advantage of getting old is that when you don't know, you can enjoy the luxury of saying so."

The first experience that made me doubt whether it was necessary for a young practitioner to pretend omniscience in order to retain his patients' confidence was the following: I had the opportunity of driving about a large town some 25 miles from Boston with a young physician only a year or two my senior. He took me on his regular rounds and we saw farmers and the grocer's wife, the hotel-keeper's daughter and the blacksmith's baby, as well as one or two well-to-do people. The great majority of the cases were in families of very limited education, the kind of folks that we think of as subsisting mostly on pies and patent medicine. But what made each case an eye-opener to me was the utter frankness of the doctor with the families. Diagnosis, prognosis, and treatment were given with an absence of subterfuge and of prevarication that astounded me, and what even more surprised me was to see the way the patients liked his frankness. I never have seen manifested more implicit confidence in a physician than during that drive. He never forced his doubts or his suspicions upon his patients, but when they asked a straight question they got a straight answer. A baby had a fever. "What's the baby got?" asked its mother. "Can't tell yet," said the doctor; "may be going to break out with something tomorrow or it may be all right in a day or two. We shall have to wait and see." There was no talk of "febricula" or "gastric fever." Not once did I hear him say that a patient was "threatened" with any disease. He knew that Nature makes no threats and that no honest doctor ever foists his ignorance upon "Nature" by charging her with making a "threat."

I asked him the obvious question: "How can you be so frank with your patients and yet keep their confidence?"

"Because they know," said he, "that whenever anything unusual comes up that I can't handle or that puzzles me I have a consultant. So when I say that I know, they believe me, and when I say I don't know and yet don't get in a consultant they understand that nothing of any seriousness is the matter, and that they don't need to worry. Lots of men are afraid to call a consultant because they're afraid the family will think the less of their ability. But it makes the family feel a great deal safer to know that I don't pretend to know everything and stand ready any moment to call in some one that knows more than I do. I've seen a man lose a family because he *didn't* have a consultant, but never because he did."

"Don't the families ever object to the expense of a consultant?" I asked. "No," said he, "it's perfectly easy to get good consultants at low prices if you explain the family's circumstances to them."

As a result of that conversation I began cautiously to try the experiment of telling the truth, whether I understood the case thoroughly or not. I never had reason to regret it, and I am every year more firmly convinced that the young doctor, even when practising chiefly among uneducated people, does not need to pretend omniscience merely because he is young and his patients ignorant. The truth works just as well for the pocket and a great deal better for the community and for our own self-respect.

"A certain profession of dogmatism," said Sir Frederick Treves in a recent address[1] to medical students, "is essential in the treatment of the sick. The sick man will allow of no hesitancy in the recognition of disease. He blindly demands that the appearance of knowledge shall be absolute, however shadowy and unsubstantial may be the basis of it."

This declaration has the great merit of frankness. But how would the doctor like to have his patients hear those words? How would he like to be caught by his patients in the act of passing on to medical students such little tricks of the trade as this? It is true that his address may never come to his patient's ears; he may never be found out. But is it good for us as professional men to have our reputations rest on the expectation of not being found out?

I doubt beside whether (as Dr. Gould[2] has pointed out in an admirable editorial) we "succeed in humbugging the patient's relations and friends by the devices which apparently suit the patient. Among intelligent laymen, far more frequently than is supposed, one finds that such sham certainty without the reality of knowledge and conviction is at once detected. Doctors make a great mistake when they think their deceits really deceive. Then there is the patient who recovers. When he is well the false diagnoses, the changes of dogmatic opinions, and of medicines, the blind alley of proved errors, these are thought over."

It is getting steadily harder to deceive the public. I recently heard a very prominent and representative citizen of Boston commenting upon the medical bulletins on President Roosevelt's leg. "Of course," he said, "no one ever believes these bulletins. The doctors give out only so much as they think fit, in order not to alarm the public unnecessarily. The result is that the public never believes the bulletins and is always more or less anxious."

Now, I do not believe that the truth was in any way tampered with in the bulletins either of President Roosevelt's or of President McKinley's illness. I believe these bulletins gave the strict and accurate truth. But I think it is generally admitted that such bulletins do not command the respect which they usually deserve. Business men and others to whom it may be of vital importance to get reliable information about the illness, are especially apt to "discount" the bulletins of the group of physicians in attendance on a man whose life is of great importance financially. We all remember how persistently the general public believed that King Edward's illness of last summer was due to malignant disease, and not to the "perityphlitis" mentioned in the bulletins. How can we blame the public for not believing the doctors in attendance on the King when one of them, Sir Frederick Treves, is willing publicly to advocate the systematic deception of patients? His words I have quoted. It is true that he does not advise deception under conditions like those of King Edward's illness, but how is the public to know just when and how far the doctor will think it best to deceive? Such discrimination is especially difficult in a country like England, where the public cannot help knowing that what is "given out" concerning foreign affairs, especially in matters of diplomacy and war, represents only so much of the truth as the officials think it best for the public to know.

I have been speaking of the disadvantages of trying to deceive a patient or those interested in him with regard to the diagnosis. I have argued so far that it is not necessary to assume absolute knowledge in order to impress the patient's mind and hold his confidence, and that owing to the increasing scepticism of the public, it is becoming more and more difficult to fool the patient at all.

Very few Americans like to lie. They would rather tell the truth if they could, but there are cases in which the voice of duty itself seems to tell us that we must lie. To prevent the breaking up of a family, to save a life, are we not to lie? A husband confesses to you the sin that has resulted in disease for him. The wife, suspecting something, catches you on your way out and asks you point blank what ails her husband. Can you tell her the truth? Well, suppose you tell her a good, round, well-constructed lie. What are the chances of her believing you? If she has got to the point of suspecting her husband, are her suspicions likely to be quieted permanently by your reassurances? Is there not a fair chance that she knows enough of the usual customs of physicians when placed in this position to discount what you say?

Then the truth in such matters very often comes to light sooner or later, and if it does, the wife is apt to let a number of persons know what kind of a trick you have played her. Of course; there are many such cases in which the truth never is found out, but I ask again, is it a good thing for us as professional men to be living in the hope of not being found out?

Truth and Falsehood in Prognosis

That it is a bad thing to lie about a prognosis we all admit, as a general rule, but there are cases when it is not easy to see what harm it does when the good that it does is very evident indeed.

A patient has gastric cancer. He is told that he has neuralgia of the stomach, and feels greatly relieved by the reassurance, for the effect of psychic influences is nowhere more striking than in gastric cancer (as the cases quoted in Osler's textbook show). Meantime the truth is told to the patient's wife, and she makes whatever preparations are necessary for the inevitable end. Now what harm can be done by such a lie as this? That sufferer is protected from those anticipations and forebodings which are often the worst portion of his misery, and yet his wife, knowing the truth and thoroughly approving of the deception, is able to see to it that her husband's financial affairs are straightened out and to prepare, as well as may be, for his death. Surely this seems a humane and sensible way to ease the patient's hard path, and who can be the worse off for it?

I answer, "Many may be worse off for it, and some must be." The patient himself is very possibly saved some suffering. But consider a minute. His wife

has now acquired, if she did not have it already, a knowledge of the circumstances under which doctors think it merciful and useful to lie. She will be sick herself some day, and when the doctors tell her that she is not seriously ill, is she likely to believe them?

I was talking not long ago on this subject with a girl of 22. "Oh, of course, I never believe what doctors say," was her comment, "for I've helped 'em lie too often and helped fix up the letters that were written so that no one should suspect the truth."

In other words, we have added to the lot of one person, the sufferings which we spare another. We rob Peter to pay Paul.

But it is not likely that the mischief will be so closely limited. There are almost always other members of the family who are let into the secret, and intimate friends, either before or after the patient's death, find out what is going on. Then there are nurses and servants from whom it is rarely wise or possible to keep hidden the actual state of affairs. All told, I doubt if there are less than a dozen souls on the average who are enlightened by such a case in regard to the standards of the physician in charge and so of the profession he represents. I have heard such things talked over among "the laity," and, as a rule, not one, but several cases are adduced to exemplify the prevailing customs of medical men in such circumstances.

We think we can isolate a lie as we do a case of smallpox, and let its effect die with the occasion that brought it about. But is it not common experience that such customs are infectious and spread far beyond our intention and beyond our control? They beget, as a rule, not any acute indignation among those who get wind of them (for "how," they say, "could the doctor do otherwise"), but rather a quiet, chronic incredulity which is stubborn, just in proportion as it is vitally important in a given case to get at the real truth, as in the case of King Edward before mentioned.

You will notice that I am not now arguing that a lie is, in itself and apart from its consequences, a bad thing. I am not saying that we ought to tell the truth in order to save our own souls or keep ourselves untainted. I am saying

that a lie saves present pain at the expense of greater future pain, and that if we saw as clearly the future harm as we see the present good, we could not help seeing that the balance is on the side of harm. It is intellectual short-sightedness.

I have told fully my share of lies, under the impression, shared I think, by many of the profession, that it is necessary in exceptional cases to do it for the good of the patient and his friends, but since I have been experimenting with the policy of telling the truth (at first cautiously, but lately with more confidence), I have become convinced that the necessity is a specious one, that the truth works better for all concerned, not only in the long run, but in relatively short spurts, and that its good results are not postponed to eternity, but are discernible within a short time.

In vindication of my belief let me tell you the sequel to one of the stories before related. You will recall that I prepared "to be very guarded in what I said" (as the technical phrase is) to a lady whose husband had angina. The attending physician, who had known the lady for years, and who represented entirely the views of her family, assured me that she was too delicate and too unstrung by neurasthenia to be capable of bearing the truth about her husband. If she knew that he might die suddenly and at any time, she would brood and fret over the knowledge until she became so querulous and unhinged that all the family, the sick husband included, would be made miserable. You remember how I made up my mind to conceal the truth from her if I could, and how she upset all my calculations by asking me suddenly whether or not I would tell her the whole truth so far as I knew it. Consider a moment the difficulties of that situation.

"Will you give me a true answer to every question I ask you?" I could scarcely be expected to pop out a prompt "yes" when I had just promised the family physician not to do anything of the sort. Of course I could not say "no," and if I hesitated an *instant*, I had betrayed my intention of deceiving her. What would you have done?

As a matter of fact I hesitated a bit, as I think anyone but a most practised liar or a hidebound truth-teller would have done. "That's enough," said she; "that's all I want to hear." But of course I couldn't leave it there, so I pulled myself together and made a clean breast of the whole thing. I told her just what I thought and what I expected, including all that I had promised the doctor not to tell. Now you will remember that the attending physician who had known her intimately for years had warned me that she could not bear this sort of news—that she would brood and worry over it, until she had made herself and everyone else in the house miserable. So when she cornered me and got the truth out of me, I made haste to get out of the house, and thanked my stars that I did not have to stay behind and pick up the pieces of the nervous wreck to which my plain, unvarnished tale must needs reduce the poor lady.

Several weeks after, I met the family physician and learned that for some mysterious reason the expected collapse on the part of the neurotic wife had never arrived. Everyone was still expecting her to go to pieces, but as yet she had got along about as usual. In point of fact she has never met their expectation. It is now nearly four years since the dreadful truth was told her and no breakdown has occurred.

After that most astonishing experience I began cautiously to tell the truth in similar cases, when intimate friends or relations of the patient declared that the truth could not be borne, and when I had no knowledge of the patient's character to set against that of his closest friends. It has been, on the whole, the most interesting and surprising experiment that I have ever tried. The astounding *innocuousness of the truth* when all reason and all experience would lead one to believe it must do harm, has surprised me even more than the remarkable tolerance of febrile patients for alcohol. It seems as if when the pinch comes and the individual has to face stern realities, some species of antitoxin is spontaneously and rapidly developed whereby the individual is rendered immune to the toxic and deleterious effects of the nervous shock!

Those of you who are familiar with Ehrlich's side-chain theory will remember that a group of cells, say those of the nervous system, acquires immunity against a given toxin, because the cells stimulated by the presence of the toxin, produce with great rapidity an *excess* of those very "receptors" or vulnerable points in virtue of which they are sensitive to toxic action. These new-fledged surplus "receptors" then break away from the parent cell, and swimming free in the blood-stream, meet the toxins, close with them before they reach the neural cells, save these precious cells from injury, and render the toxins harmless.

So may we not conceive that under the stimulus of the first sting and nettle of hard truth, the nervous system of the patient produces rapidly an overplus of free "receptors"—*rises to the emergency,* as we ordinarily say, and so is rendered immune against the otherwise depressing effects of full knowledge? Indeed, Ehrlich's theory might be described as an application to single groups of cells of that tendency to rise to an emergency, to fight when cornered, to supply an imperious demand, which we see often enough in men and in nations.

But whatever the theory, the fact has been brought home to me as it can only be brought home by actually trying the experiment; the fact, namely, that patients and patients' friends exhibit an astonishing power to stand the full truth, an amazing immunity against its depressing effects. No one ought to believe this who has not tried it, any more than you ought to believe what have said about the action of alcohol until you have repeated my experiments. All that my say-so ought to accomplish is to make someone ready to try the experiment; to take the risks which we must always face if we are to get ahead, and see whether he can verify my findings.

One precaution, however, must be borne in mind. Anyone who is familiar with experimental work knows that the difficulty of verifying another's experiment is often due to failure to repeat just that experiment and no other. A certain bloodstain is highly lauded. You try it and cannot get the results which its inventor claims for it. But very often you fail because you have not exactly followed the details of his technic.

So here, if you try to repeat my experiments I trust that you will notice just what it is that I recommended you to try. I am not recommending that we should explain to every mother in full detail the etiology, pathology, course, and prognosis of her baby's illness. I have never tried that experiment, and I should suppose it would be a very stupid, useless, and probably harmful thing to do. I do not believe in cramming information down peoples' throats or trying to tell them what they cannot understand properly, any more than I believe in button-holing every acquaintance in the street, and giving him a detailed account of what I consider his faults and failings.

But if my friend asks me for an opinion of his first literary productions, and if I think that they are dreadful rubbish, I do not consider it friendship to say pleasant things of his style and thereby encourage him to pursue literature as a calling. I do not give my opinion unless it is really asked for. But if it is, I do not believe in lying to save anyone's feelings. It does more harm in the end.

So in medicine, if a patient asks me a straight question I believe it works best to give him a straight answer, not a rough answer, but yet not a lie or a prevarication. I do not believe it pays to give an answer that would justify a patient in saying (in case he happened to find out the truth): "that doctor tried to trick me." I have heard a patient say that, apropos of a lie told by one of the most high-minded and honorable physicians I know, and I do not believe it advisable for any of us to expose ourselves to the chance of rousing that sort of indignation in a patient.

A straight answer to a straight question is what I am recommending, not an unasked presentation of the facts of the patient's case. He may not care to know those facts any more than I care to know the interesting details of dental pathology in which my dentist might wish to instruct me; I leave all that to him. Just so my patient may very properly prefer to be told nothing about his disease, trusting that I shall do my best and let him know when there is anything for him to do in the matter.

But a straight answer does not mean for me what is often called the "blunt truth," the "naked truth," the dry cold facts. The truth that I mean is a true *impression,* a fully drawn and properly shaded account such as is, as I well know, very difficult to give. I know one physician (and a splendid type of man he is, too), who, when he sees a case of rheumatic endocarditis, and is asked for a prognosis, is apt to say something like this: "Well, I'm mighty sorry for you, but your trouble is incurable. Your heart is damaged past repair and there is not much of anything to be done except to take salicylates during the acute attacks and hope that the process will become arrested spontaneously before long." "Is it likely to get worse?" asks the patient. "Yes, I'm afraid it is."

Now in one sense that is all true, but the impression that it will convey to the patient is not true, not at all what I mean by telling the truth. I would rather a physician would tell this sort of truncated, imperfect and very distressing truth, than give the patient a smooth and pleasant assurance that he can be cured and that all will go right provided he does so and so.

But better than either a misleading half truth or a pleasing lie, is an attempt so to answer the patient's question that he shall see not only what he can't do and can't hope for, but what he can do and what there is to *work* for hopefully. That his heart-valve is sclerosed and perhaps useless is true, and in that sense, to that extent, he is incurable; the sclerosed heart-valve is there once for all, and yet by accommodating himself to his diminished heart power, the patient can gradually educate to a considerable extent, both his heart and the rest of himself. His heart can be made to adjust itself to its maimed state and to put forth, in spite of it, a good deal more power than it would have done without the educational process; and the individual by learning to take the best advantage of all the power he has, can accomplish, not all that he *could* in health, yet perhaps as much as he actually *would* have done, allowing for the amount of wasted time and wasted opportunity that has often to be deducted from the effective power of a healthy man.

Because this kind of explanation is so difficult and takes so much time, we are apt to shirk it and give the patient either a rough half-truth or a smooth lie. In our free dispensaries one can witness any day a rich and varied assortment of these two methods of shirking a difficult and tedious explanation; the rough half-truth and the smooth lie

are dealt out by the shovelful and students watch and make their choice between these two pitiful makeshifts according to their temperaments, often in entire ignorance of any *tertium quid*. For it is particularly in dealing with uneducated people, such as frequent dispensaries, that we distrust the power of truth and the possibility of conveying it. In this field I have made many experiments both with lies and with the truth. I know very well that the truth is sometimes next to impossible to convey, owing to differences between the patient's vocabulary (or in habits of mind) and the physician's, but on the other hand the lie may do more harm, for there is more chance of its being implicitly believed.

To refuse to answer questions is now and then a necessity and need not involve any falsehood. For example, to baulk meddling inquiries by an outsider is often our business. Then there is the patient about to undergo an operation, who sometimes catechises us about the details of the operation and sometimes had better remain ignorant about it until after it is over. On the other hand, if the patient's mind is already occupying itself with a definite, but exaggerated picture of the horrors of the operation, a prosaic explanation of the real facts may act as a sedative.

Not infrequently we need to choose our time well, if a piece of painful truth has to be communicated and it may be necessary to avoid giving the patient a chance to cross-question us at a time when we consider him temporarily below par. I have heard a patient say: "The doctor didn't mean to let me get that out of him today," but without any bitterness or sense of being tricked by his physician, for the fact that the doctor avoided being questioned presaged that if cornered he would not tell a lie.

I have said that in my experience patients and their families often develop a most astonishing power to rise to the emergency and to bear the hard truth when it has to be told. But I cannot say that this is always so. There may be cases, I suppose there are such, when the patient does not react from the shock of a cruel truth, but is made worse by it. It is said that such a shock sometimes turns the scale and brings death.

Ought we to persist in telling the truth even when we believe it may kill

the patient? Could any effect produced by a lie be as bad as the loss of a human life?

Before answering this question directly, let me ask you to consider a somewhat fanciful hypothesis. Suppose it lay in our power to let loose into the atmosphere a poisonous gas which would vitiate the air of a whole town so that the whole community would gradually suffer in efficiency, in physical and moral fiber. Would it not be worth a human life to save a whole community from such a deterioration?

Now a lie seems to me to do something like that. By undermining the confidence of man in man it does its part in making not one but every human activity impossible. If we cannot trust one another, we cannot take a step in any direction. Business, social relations, science, everything worth doing depends on mutual confidence. It is the very air we breathe. To poison it is to do a far worse thing for society than could result from the loss of a single life. So that though I believe that it is extraordinarily rare to be able to save a life by a lie, it seems to me that the remedy, the lie, is worse than death.

Truth and Falsehood in Treatment

In discussing truth and falsehood in diagnosis and in prognosis I have dealt chiefly with spoken truth or spoken lies. In the domain of treatment the true or false impression is often conveyed without words.

I do not know who it was that defined a quack as "one who pretends to possess or to be able to use powers (either of diagnosis, prognosis or treatment) which in fact he *knows* he is without." If we think over the various forms of quacks familiar to us—Dr. Munyon, with all those specifics which he knows he does not possess; the cancer curers, those who advertise to cure "weak men," Francis Truth, who cheats his dupes with all-healing handkerchiefs sent through the mails at $5 apiece—we see that they all pretend to possess knowledge about valuable medicines or other remedies which they know they do not possess.

Now I was brought up, as I suppose every physician is, to use *placebos*, bread pills, water subcutaneously, and other devices for acting upon a patient's symptoms through his mind. How frequently such methods are used varies a great deal I suppose with individual practitioners, but I doubt if there is a physician in this room who has not used them and used them pretty often. It never occurred to me until I had given a great many placebos that if they are to be really effective they must deceive the patient. I had thought of them simply as a means of getting rid of a symptom and no more a lie than hypnotism or any other form of frankly mental therapeutics.

But one day a patient caught me in the attempt to put her to sleep by means of a subcutaneous injection of water. "I saw you get that ready," said she, "and there is no morphin in it; you were just trying to deceive me." I was fairly caught and there was no use trying to bluff it out, so I merely protested that my deception was well meant, that it profited me nothing, that it was simply intended to give her a night's rest without the depressing effects of morphia, etc.

"Of course I see that," she said, "but how am I to know in future what other tricks you will think it best to play me for my good? How am I to believe anything you say from now on?"

I did not know what answer to make at the time, and I have never been able to think of any since.

But water subcutaneously does not differ in principle from any other placebo. If the patient knows what you are up to when you give him a bread pill it will have no effect on him. If he is dyspeptic he must believe that you consider the medicine you give likely to act upon his stomach and *not merely upon his stomach through his mind*. Otherwise it will do him no good. Suppose you said to him: "I give you this pill for its mental effect. It has no action on the stomach," would he be likely to get benefit from it? In short, it is only when through the placebo one deceives the patient that any effect is produced. It is only when we act like quacks that our placebos work.

But what harm, you may ask, does a placebo do? Admitting that it is a form of deception and that if you are detected in it the patient and his friends are likely to lose confidence in you, what harm does it do so long as you are not found out?

Well, as previously said, I do not think it is a good thing for any man to succeed only so long as he is not found out, but there are other objections to the use of placebos which I will next try to explain.

The majority of placebos are given because we believe the patient will not be satisfied without them. He has learned to expect a medicine for every symptom, and without it he simply won't get well. True, but who taught him to expect a medicine for every symptom? He was not born with that expectation. He learned it from an ignorant doctor who really believed it, just as he learned that pimples are a disease of the blood, that shingles kills the patient whenever it extends clear round the body, and that in the spring the blood should be "purified" by this or that remedy. It is we physicians who are responsible for perpetuating false ideas about disease and its cure. The legends are handed along through nurses and fond mothers, but they originate with us, and with every placebo that we give we do our part in perpetuating error, and harmful error at that. If the patient did not expect a medicine for his attack (say of mumps) we should not give it, yet we do all we can to bolster up his expectation for another time, to deepen the error we deplore.

But here, as everywhere, experiment is the test. I have for the past few years been trying the experiment of explaining to the patient why he does not need a drug, when there is no drug known for his trouble. It takes a little more time at first, but one thorough explanation serves for many subsequent occasions. One has only to remind the patient of what we have gone over with him before. When the occasion for a drug really comes, the patient has far more confidence in its workings.

We feel these things acutely when a patient comes to us who has been previously under the care of another physician. How refreshing to hear the mother of a child sick with measles say, "Well, I don't suppose he needs any medicine, does he? The disease has to run its course, I suppose, and nursing is the main thing." That mother has been given the truth by her physician instead of placebos, and has become accustomed to realities as easily

as most people learn to believe outworn errors. On the other hand, we see now and then a patient into whose mind it has been carefully instilled by some physician that every draught of fresh air must be avoided like a plague, that every symptom needs a drug, and that a visit from the doctor every few days is a necessity to salvation.

But the habit of giving placebos has another evil result. It gives the patient indirectly a wrong idea, a harmful idea of the way disease is produced and avoided. If symptoms can be cured by drugs, it is impossible to bring to bear upon the patient the full force of that most fundamental principle of therapeutics: "to remove a symptom remove its cause." That a man can be made well "in spite of himself" as the patent-medicine advertisements say; that is, in spite of violating the laws of health, is a belief produced as one of the by-products of the way we hand out placebos, especially in our hospitals and dispensaries.

No patient whose language you can speak, whose mind you can approach needs a placebo. I give placebos now and then (I used to give them by the bushel) to Armenians and others with whom I cannot communicate, because to refuse to give them would then create more misunderstanding, a false impression, than to give them. The patient will think I am refusing to treat him at all; but if I can get hold of an interpreter and explain the matter, I tell him no lies in the shape of placebos.

Before I close this lecture I want to speak of one further point which my experiments with truth and falsehood have brought home to me. When I have plucked up courage and ventured to tell the truth in hard cases, I have been surprised again and again to find how the chances and accidents of nature have backed me up. Everything seems to conspire to help you out when you are trying to tell the truth, but when you are lying there are snares and pitfalls turning up everywhere and making your path a more and more difficult one.

I will sum up the results of my experiments with truth and falsehood, by saying that I have not yet found any case in which a lie does not do more harm than good, and by expressing my

belief that if anyone will carefully repeat the experiments he will reach
similar results. The technic of truth telling is sometimes difficult, perhaps
more difficult than the technic of lying,
but its results make it worth acquiring.

Notes

1. *British Medical Journal,* 1903.

2. *American Medicine,* November 1, 1902,
p. 681.

35

Joseph Collins
Should Doctors Tell the Truth?

Reprinted from the August 1927 issue
by special permission of *Harper's
Monthly Magazine,* vol. 155, 1927, pp.
320–326. Copyright © 1927 by
Harper's Magazine.

This is not a homily on lying. It is a
presentation of one of the most difficult
questions that confront the physician.
Should doctors tell patients the truth?
Were I on the witness stand and
obliged to answer the question with
"yes" or "no," I should answer in the
negative and appeal to the judge for
permission to qualify my answer. The
substance of this article is what that
qualification would be.

Though few are willing to make the
test, it is widely held that if the truth
were more generally told, it would
make for world-welfare and human
betterment. We shall probably never
know. To tell the whole truth is often
to perpetrate a cruelty of which many
are incapable. This is particularly true
of physicians. Those of them who are
not compassionate by nature are made
so by experience. They come to realize
that they owe their fellow-men justice,
and graciousness, and benignity, and it
becomes one of the real satisfactions of
life to discharge that obligation. To do
so successfully they must frequently
withhold the truth from their patients,
which is tantamount to telling them a
lie. Moreover, the physician soon
learns that the art of medicine consists
largely in skillfully mixing falsehood
and truth in order to provide the patient with an amalgam which will
make the metal of life wear and keep
men from being poor shrunken things,
full of melancholy and indisposition,
unpleasing to themselves and to those
who love them. I propose therefore to
deal with the question from a pragmatic, not a moral standpoint.

"Now you may tell me the truth," is
one of the things patients have frequently said to me. Four types of individuals have said it: those who honestly and courageously want to know
so that they may make as ready as possible to face the wages of sin while
there is still time; those who do not
want to know, and who if they were
told would be injured by it; those who
are wholly incapable of receiving the
truth. Finally, those whose health is
neither seriously disordered nor
threatened. It may seem an exaggeration to say that in forty years of contact
with the sick, the patients I have met
who are in the first category could be
counted on the fingers of one hand.
The vast majority who demand the
truth really belong in the fourth category, but there are sufficient in the

second—with whom my concern chiefly is—to justify considering their case.

One of the astonishing things about patients is that the more serious the disease, the more silent they are about its portents and manifestations. The man who is constantly seeking assurance that the vague abdominal pains indicative of hyperacidity are not symptoms of cancer often buries family and friends, some of whom have welcomed death as an escape from his burdensome iterations. On the other hand, there is the man whose first warning of serious disease is lumbago who cannot be persuaded to consult a physician until the disease, of which the lumbago is only a symptom, has so far progressed that it is beyond surgery. The seriousness of disease may be said to stand in direct relation to the reticence of its possessor. The more silent the patient, the more serious the disorder.

The patient with a note-book, or the one who is eager to tell his story in great detail, is rarely very ill. They are forever asking, "Am I going to get well?" and though they crave assistance they are often unable to accept it. On the other hand, patients with organic disease are very chary about asking point blank either the nature or the outcome of their ailment. They sense its gravity, and the last thing in the world they wish to know is the truth about it; and to learn it would be the worst thing that could happen to them.

This was borne in upon me early in my professional life. I was summoned one night to assuage the pain of a man who informed me that he had been for some time under treatment for rheumatism—that cloak for so many diagnostic errors. His "rheumatism" was due to a disease of the spinal cord called locomotor ataxia. When he was told that he should submit himself to treatment wholly different from that which he had been receiving, the import of which any intelligent layman would have divined, he asked neither the nature nor the probable outcome of the disease. He did as he was counselled. He is now approaching seventy and, though not active in business, it still engrosses him.

Had he been told that he had a disease which was then universally believed to be progressive, apprehension would have depressed him so heavily that he would not have been able to

offer the resistance to its encroachment which has stood him in such good stead. He was told the truth only in part. That is, he was told his "rheumatism" was "different"; that it was dependent upon an organism quite unlike the one that causes ordinary rheumatism; that we have preparations of mercury and arsenic which kill the parasite responsible for this disease, and that if he would submit himself to their use, his life would not be materially shortened, or his efficiency seriously impaired.

Many experiences show that patients do not want the truth about their maladies, and that it is prejudicial to their well-being to know it, but none that I know is more apposite than that of a lawyer, noted for his urbanity and resourcefulness in Court. When he entered my consulting room, he greeted me with a bonhomie that bespoke intimacy, but I had met him only twice—once on the golf links many years before, and once in Court where I was appearing as expert witness, prejudicial to his case.

He apologized for engaging my attention with such a triviality, but he had had pain in one shoulder and arm for the past few months, and though he was perfectly well—and had been assured of it by physicians in Paris, London, and Brooklyn—this pain was annoying and he had made up his mind to get rid of it. That I should not get a wrong slant on his condition, he submitted a number of laboratory reports furnished him by an osteopath to show that secretions and excretions susceptible of chemical examinations were quite normal. His determination seemed to be to prevent me from taking a view of his health which might lead me to counsel his retirement. He was quite sure that anything like a thorough examination was unnecessary but he submitted to it. It revealed intense and extensive disease of the kidneys. The pain in the network of nerves of the left upper-arm was a manifestation of the resulting autointoxication.

I felt it incumbent upon me to tell him that his condition was such that he should make a radical change in his mode of life. I told him if he would stop work, spend the winter in Honolulu, go on a diet suitable to a child

of three years, and give up exercise, he could look forward confidently to a recovery that would permit of a life of usefulness and activity in his profession. He assured me he could not believe that one who felt no worse than he did should have to make such a radical change in his mode of life. He impressed upon me that I should realize he was the kind of person who had to know the truth. His affairs were so diversified and his commitments so important that he *must* know. Completely taken in, I explained to him the relationship between the pain from which he sought relief and the disease, the degeneration that was going on in the excretory mechanisms of his body, how these were struggling to repair themselves, the procedure of recovery and how it could be facilitated. The light of life began to flicker from the fear that my words engendered, and within two months it sputtered and died out. He was the last person in the world to whom the truth should have been told. Had I lied to him, and then intrigued with his family and friends, he might be alive to-day.

The longer I practice medicine the more I am convinced that every physician should cultivate lying as a fine art. But there are many varieties of lying. Some are most prejudicial to the physician's usefulness. Such are: pretending to recognize the disease and understand its nature when one is really ignorant; asserting that one has effected the cure which nature has accomplished, or claiming that one can effect cure of a disease which is universally held to be beyond the power of nature or medical skill; pronouncing disease incurable which one cannot rightfully declare to be beyond cessation or relief.

There are other lies, however, which contribute enormously to the success of the physician's mission of mercy and salvation. There are a great number of instances in support of this but none more convincing than that of a man of fifty who, after twenty-five years of devotion to painting, decided that penury and old age were incompatible for him. Some of his friends had forsaken art for advertising. He followed their lead and in five years he was ready to gather the first ripe fruit of his labor. When he attempted to do so he was so immobilized by pain and rigidity that he had to forego work. One of those many persons who assume responsibility lightly assured him that if he would put himself in the hands of a certain osteopath he would soon be quite fit. The assurance was without foundation. He then consulted a physician who without examining him proceeded to treat him for what is considered a minor ailment.

Within two months his appearance gave such concern to his family that he was persuaded to go to a hospital, where the disease was quickly detected, and he was at once submitted to surgery. When he had recovered from the operation, learning that I was in the country of his adoption, he asked to see me. He had not been able, he said, to get satisfactory information from the surgeon or the physician; all that he could gather from them was that he would have to have supplementary X-ray or radium treatment. What he desired was to get back to his business which was on the verge of success, and he wanted assurance that he could soon do so.

He got it. And more than that, he got elaborate explanation of what surgical intervention had accomplished, but not a word of what it had failed to accomplish. A year of activity was vouchsafed him, and during that time he put his business in such shape that its eventual sale provided a modest competency for his family. It was not until the last few weeks that he knew the nature of his malady. Months of apprehension had been spared him by the deception, and he had been the better able to do his work, for he was buoyed by the hope that his health was not beyond recovery. Had he been told the truth, black despair would have been thrown over the world in which he moved, and he would have carried on with corresponding ineffectiveness.

The more extensive our field of observation and the more intimate our contact with human activity, the more we realize the finiteness of the human mind. Every follower of Hippocrates will agree that "judgment is difficult and experience fallacious." A disease may have only a fatal ending, but one does not know; one may know that certain diseases, such as general

paresis, invariably cause death, but one does not know that tomorrow it may no longer be true. The victim may be reprieved by accidental or studied discovery or by the intervention of something that still must be called divine grace.

A few years ago physicians were agreed that diabetes occurring in children was incurable; recently they held that the disease known as pernicious anemia always ended fatally; but now, armed with an extract from the pancreas and the liver, they go out to attack these diseases with the kind of confidence that David had when he saw the Philistine approach.

We have had enough experience to justify the hope that soon we shall be able to induce a little devil who is manageable to cast out a big devil who is wholly out of hand—to cure general paresis by inoculating the victim with malaria, and to shape the course of some varieties of sleeping sickness by the same means.

I am thankful for many valuable lessons learned from my early teachers. One of them was an ophthalmologist of great distinction. I worked for three years in his clinic. He was the most brutally frank doctor I have known. He could say to a woman, without the slightest show of emotion, that she was developing a cataract and would eventually be blind. I asked a colleague who was a co-worker in the clinic at that time and who has since become an eminent specialist, if all these patients developed complete opacity of the crystalline lens.

"Not one half of them," said he. "In many instances the process is so slow that the patient dies before the cataract arrives; in others it ceases to progress. It is time enough for the patient to know he has cataract when he knows for himself that he is going blind. Then I can always explain it to him in such a way that he does not have days of apprehension and nights of sleeplessness for months while awaiting operation. I have made it a practice not to tell a patient he has cataract."

"Yes, but what do you tell them when they say they have been to Doctor Smith who tells them they have cataract and they have come to you for denial or corroboration?"

"I say to them, 'You have a beginning cloudiness of the lens of one eye. I have seen many cases in which the

opacity progressed no farther than it has in your case; I have seen others which did not reach blindness in twenty years. I shall change your glasses, and I think you will find that your vision will be improved.'"

And then he added, "In my experience there are two things patients cannot stand being told: that they have cataract or cancer."

There is far less reason for telling them of the former than the latter. The hope for victims of the latter is bound up wholly in early detection and surgical interference. That is one of the most cogent reasons for bi-yearly thorough physical examination after the age of forty-five. Should we ever feel the need of a new law in this country, the one I suggest would exact such examination. The physician who detects malignant disease in its early stages is never justified in telling the patient the real nature of the disease. In fact, he does not know himself until he gets the pathologist's report. Should that indicate grave malignancy no possible good can flow from sharing that knowledge with the patient.

It is frequently to a patient's great advantage to know the truth in part, for it offers him the reason for making a radical change in his mode of life, sometimes a burdensome change. But not once in a hundred instances is a physician justified in telling a patient point blank that he has epilepsy, or the family that he has dementia præcox, until after he has been under observation a long time, unless these are so obvious that even a layman can make the diagnosis. We do not know the real significance of either disease, or from what they flow—we know that so many of them terminate in dementia that the outlook for all of them is bad. But we also know that many cases so diagnosticated end in complete recovery; and that knowledge justifies us in withholding from a patient the name and nature of his disorder until we are beyond all shadow of doubt.

Patients who are seriously ill are greedy for assurance even when it is offered half-heartedly. But those who have ailments which give the physician no real concern often cannot accept assurance. Not infrequently I have been unable to convince patients with nervous indigestion that their fears and concern were without foundation, and yet, years later when they developed organic disease, and I became really concerned about them, they assured me that I was taking their ailments too seriously.

There was a young professor whose acquaintance I made while at a German university. When he returned he took a position as professor in one of the well-known colleges for women. After several years he consulted me for the relief of symptoms which are oftentimes associated with gastric ulcer. It required no elaborate investigation to show that in this instance the symptoms were indicative of an imbalance of his nervous system. He refused to be assured and took umbrage that he was not given a more thorough examination each time that he visited me. Finally he told me that he would no longer attempt to conceal from me that he understood fully my reasons for making light of the matter. It was to throw him off the track, as it were. No good was to be accomplished from trying to deceive him; he realized the gravity of the situation and he was man enough to confront it. He would not show the white feather, and he was entitled to know the truth.

But the more it was proffered him, the greater was his resistance to it. He gave up his work and convinced his family and friends that he was seriously ill. They came to see me in relays; they also refused to accept the truth. They could understand why I told the patient the matter was not serious, but to them I could tell the facts. It was their right to know, and I could depend upon them to keep the knowledge from the patient and to work harmoniously with me.

My failure with my patient's friends was as great as with the patient himself. Fully convinced his back was to the wall, he refused to be looked upon as a lunatic or a hypochondriac and he decided to seek other counsel. He went from specialist to naturopath, from electrotherapist to Christian Scientist, from sanatorium to watering place and, had there been gland doctors and chiropractors in those days, he would have included them as well. Finally, he migrated to the mountains of Tennessee, and wooed nature. Soon I heard of him as the head of a school which was being run on novel pedagogic lines; character-building and health were the

chief aims for his pupils; scholastic education was incidental. He began writing and lecturing about his work and his accomplishments, and soon achieved considerable notoriety. I saw him occasionally when he came north and sometimes referred to his long siege of ill-health and how happily it had terminated. He always made light of it, and declared that in one way it had been a very good thing: had it not been for that illness he would never have found himself, never have initiated the work which was giving him repute, happiness, and competency.

One summer I asked him to join me for a canoe trip down the Allegash River. Some of the "carrys" in those days were rather stiff. After one of them I saw that my friend was semi-prostrated and flustered. On questioning him, I learned that he had several times before experienced disagreeable sensations in the chest and in the head after hard manual labor, such as chopping trees or prying out rocks. He protested against examination but finally yielded. I reminded myself how different it was fifteen years before when he clamored for examination and seemed to get both pleasure and satisfaction from it, particularly when it was elaborate and protracted. He had organic disease of the heart, both of the valve-mechanism and of the muscle. His tenure of life depended largely on the way he lived. To counsel him successfully it was necessary to tell him that his heart had become somewhat damaged. He would not have it. "When I was really ill you made light of it, and I could not get you interested. But now, when I am well, you want me to live the life of a dodo. I won't do it. My heart is quite all right, a little upset no doubt by the fare we have had for the past two weeks, but as soon as I get back to normal I shall be as fit as you are, perhaps more so."

We returned to New York and I persuaded him to see a specialist, who was no more successful in impressing him with the necessity of careful living than I was. In despair, I wrote to his wife. She who had been so solicitous, so apprehensive, and so deaf to assurance during the illness that was of no consequence wrote, "I am touched by your affectionate interest, but Jerome

seems so well that I have not the heart to begin nagging him again, and it fills me with terror lest he should once more become introspective and self-solicitous. I am afraid if I do what you say that it might start him off again on the old tack, and the memory of those two years frightens me still."

He died about four years later without the benefit of physician.

No one can stand the whole truth about himself; why should we think he can tolerate it about his health, and even though he could, who knows the truth? Physicians have opinions based upon their own and others' experience. They should be chary of expressing those opinions to sick persons until they have studied their psychology and are familiar with their personality. Even then it should always be an opinion, not a sentence. Doctors should be detectives and counsellors, not juries and judges.

Though often it seems a cruelty, the family of the patient to whom the truth is not and should not be told are entitled to the facts or what the physician believes to be the facts. At times, they must conspire with him to keep the truth from the patient, who will learn it too soon no matter what skill they display in deception. On the other hand, it is frequently to the patient's great advantage that the family should not know the depth of the physician's concern, lest their unconcealable apprehension be conveyed to the patient and then transformed into the medium in which disease waxes strong—fear. Now and then the good doctor keeps his own counsel. It does not profit the family of the man whose coronary arteries are under suspicion to be told that he has angina pectoris. If the patient can be induced to live decorously, the physician has discharged his obligation.

I recall so many instances when the truth served me badly that I find it difficult to select the best example. On reflection, I have decided to cite the case of a young man who consulted me shortly after his marriage.

He was sane in judgment, cheerful in disposition, full of the desire to attract those who attracted him. Anything touching on the morbid or "unnatural" was obviously repellent to him. His youth had been a pleasant one, surrounded by affection, culture, understanding, and wealth. When he graduated he had not made up his mind what he wanted to do in the world. After a year of loafing and traveling he decided to become an engineer. He matriculated at one of the technical schools, and his work there was satisfactory to himself and to his professors.

He astonished his intimates shortly after obtaining a promising post by marrying a woman a few years older than himself who was known to some of them as a devotee of bohemian life that did not tally with the position in society to which she was entitled by family and wealth. She had been a favorite with men but she had a reputation of not being the "marrying kind."

My friend fell violently in love with her, and her resistance went down before it. His former haunts knew him no more, and I did not see him for several months. Then, late one evening, he telephoned to say that it was of the greatest importance to him to consult me. He arrived in a state of repressed excitement. He wanted it distinctly understood that he came to me as a client, not as a friend. I knew, of course, that he had married. This, he confessed, had proved a complete failure, and now his wife had gone away and with another woman, one whom he had met constantly at her home during his brief and tempestuous courtship.

I attempted to explain to him that she had probably acted on impulse; that the squabbles of early matrimony which often appeared to be tragedies, were adjustable and, fortunately, nearly always adjusted.

"Yes," said he, "but you don't understand. There hasn't been any row. My wife told me shortly after marrying me that she had made a mistake, and she has told me so many times since. I thought at first it was caprice. Perhaps I should still have thought so were it not for this letter." He then handed me a letter. I did not have to read between the lines to get the full significance of its content. It set forth briefly, concretely, and explicitly her reasons for leaving. Life without her former friend was intolerable, and she did not propose to attempt it longer.

He knew there were such persons in the world, but what he wanted to know from me was, Could they not, if properly and prudently handled, be brought to feel and love like those the world calls normal? Was it not possible that her conduct and confession were the result of a temporary derangement and that indulgent handling of her would make her see things in the right light? She had not alienated his love even though she had forfeited his respect; and he did not attempt to conceal from me that if the tangle could not be straightened out he felt that his life had been a failure.

I told him the truth about this enigmatic gesture of nature, that the victims of this strange abnormality are often of great brilliancy and charm, and most companionable; that it is not a disease and, therefore, cannot be cured.

In this instance, basing my opinion upon what his wife had told him both in speech and in writing, I was bound to believe that she was one of the strange sisterhood, and that it was her birthright as well as her misfortune. Such being the case, I could only advise what I thought might be best for their mutual and individual happiness. I suggested that divorce offered the safest way out for both. He replied that he felt competent to decide that for himself; all that he sought from me was enlightenment about her unnatural infatuation. This I had only too frankly given him.

Two days later his body with a pistol wound in the right temple was found in a field above Weehawken.

That day I regretted that I had not lied to him. It is a day that has had frequent anniversaries.

36

Donald Oken

What to Tell Cancer Patients: A Study of Medical Attitudes

Reprinted with permission of author and editors from the *Journal of the American Medical Association*, vol. 175, 1961, pp. 1120–1128. Copyright © 1961, American Medical Association.

No problem is more vexing than the decision about what to tell the cancer patient. (Although the word cancer is neither a medical term nor a specific entity, common sense considerations provide a basis for use of this general term. As used in the present work, the term should be understood *to apply to all malignant neoplasms of characteristically grave prognosis.*) The situation is an ever recurring one and the questions involved are knotty. What should the patient be told? How and when should this be done? The manner in which such questions are handled is crucial for the patient and may determine his emotional status and capacity for function from that time on. It is easy enough to decide to follow a course which will "do least harm," but it is far from simple to determine just what course that is. The issues involved are complex factors which are difficult to assess, weigh, and place in proper perspective.

In his attempt to work out some solution, the doctor needs all the help he can get. The issues are a favorite and, often, heated topic of "corridor consultations." Often the opinion of a psychiatrist is sought: but psychiatric knowledge provides no clear and unequivocal answers. A considerable number of authors have attempted to provide assistance by describing their own views and approach. These writers, often wise and distinguished teachers drawing on long experience, offer solutions based on that experience. This too proves of insufficient help. Though many issues have become clarified, these experts differ widely about what to do. Opinions vary from one extreme to the other.[1-3] Careful review of this literature discloses a further lack: the almost complete absence of systematic research. There is a plethora of opinion but a minimum of dependable fact. This is a curious situation in an area of so great importance. The present paper represents an initial attempt to provide some research data which bear on this situation and on the general issue of "telling."

Earlier studies have utilized two approaches. One method involves questioning the public. Kelly and Friesen[4] queried 100 cancer patients and found 89 favored knowing their diagnosis. Interestingly, a somewhat smaller number (73) felt that others similarly afflicted

should be told. These authors also studied 100 clinic patients who were free of cancer, asking whether they would like to know if the examination revealed this disorder. Again, a large majority (82) said yes. Branch[5] questioned 105 patients, 51 of whom had cancer. Of the group which was cancer-free, 48 of 54 stated a preference for being told. Of the cancer patients, 39 knew the nature of their condition while 9 denied any illness whatsoever. Samp and Curreri[6] surveyed 560 cancer patients and their families, using a questionnaire covering attitudes about cancer and cancer education. Of their respondents, 87% felt that a patient should be told. Other responses indicated a favorable attitude about open dissemination of information and optimism about curability. There is a major drawback to a survey of cancer patients who have been told. Such patients cannot permit doubts about the wisdom of the policy of those whom they need to trust so desperately. Nor does one know what lurks unconsciously behind their overtly optimistic outlook. Similarly, one must be cautious about interpreting studies of persons who are cancer-free. They can "afford" to say they want to be told, since the question is only academic. Studies of patients with diagnosed but undisclosed malignancy would be of great interest.

A second approach is to see how large numbers of physicians cope with the problem. While such information *proves* nothing, it does furnish a wider frame of reference than individual opinion and provides a background of data on existing practice. Fitts and Ravdin[7] reported in 1953 on "What Philadelphia Physicians Tell Patients with Cancer," based on a mail survey of 442 physicians. Their questionnaire permitted 4 answers. Of the respondents, 3% said they "always tell," 28% "usually tell," 57% "usually do not tell," and 12% "never" do so. Thus, over two-thirds of the group infrequently or never disclosed the diagnosis. When the responses were broken down by specialty, dermatologists were at one end of the spectrum, 94% always or usually telling, and radiologists at the other, 12% doing so. Both, of course, see highly selected types of patients. Of the combined group of

specialists (surgeons, gynecologists, and internists) and general practitioners who care for the great bulk of cancer patients, only one quarter tended towards telling. The main reasons for telling, reported by those who usually did not, included refusal of necessary treatment and the need of patients to make plans. Those who tended to tell at times did not when requested not to by the family or if there was felt to be danger of an unfavorable reaction.

A nationwide mail survey of nearly 5,000 physicians was recently reported in a proprietary medical magazine.[8] The results indicated fewer physicians with a set policy. To a question about telling patients with an "established" diagnosis of "incurable cancer," 22% responded that they "never" told and 16% "always." The remainder indicated they "sometimes" told, giving as major determinants the stability of the patient, insistence by the patient or family, the necessity to put affairs in order, and the absence of anyone else who could be told. There was no indication about the proportion of this intermediate group who tended more towards telling or the reverse. General practitioners were less prone to tell than specialists, and physicians in large cities less likely to do so than their colleagues in smaller communities.

The Present Research

The research on which this report is based represents a further attempt to study physicians' approaches to the problem of what to tell cancer patients. The aim here has been not merely to learn what is done but, more importantly, to understand the attitudes which are underlying determinants of these strategies. Initially, a detailed questionnaire was sent to all of the 219 members of the staff of the departments of Internal Medicine, Obstetrics-Gynecology and Surgery (including Thoracic, Genito-Urinary and Neuro-Surgery, and Orthopedics) of the Michael Reese Hospital, a private non-profit teaching hospital in Chicago. This questionnaire included items concerned with (1) the policy with regard to "telling"; (2) factors involved in making a decision with an individual patient; (3) the sources from which the policy had been acquired; (4) the role of personal emotional factors; (5)

changes from a previous different policy and the possibility of future change; (6) attitudes about the research; and (7) personal choice, i.e., "if you were the patient, do you think you would want to be told?" A personal interview of 30 minutes' duration was held subsequently with 62 (30%) of the respondents, devoted to the intensive exploration of these and related areas and designed especially to elicit attitudes about cancer and its treatability. No attempt was made to probe for unconscious material. Interviews were unstructured and neutral in tone, but opposing arguments were raised to points of view expressed, in order to clarify the nature and intensity of determining attitudes. Interviewees were selected to represent a cross-section of each staff level within each specialty with regard to the policy about telling espoused on the questionnaire.

It is necessary to describe some of the characteristics of the group studied since these may bear on the findings. The great bulk of these physicians are in active private practice, in addition to taking a regular part in the teaching program. Most hold faculty positions at one or more medical schools. Though they are deeply involved in "academic medicine," for them the problem of dealing with the cancer patient is no academic matter; it is an everyday reality. Interest and cooperation was high, so that a 95% return of questionnaires was achieved, a level rarely attained. A group of general practitioners were included in the study, for a moderate number are members of the staff in the Department of Medicine, largely with "courtesy" (non-teaching) status. These, however, are probably the least representative group, for they are primarily older men. The remainder of the sample seems fairly typical of the larger specialty groups which are represented. The sample has, however, certain definite characteristics. The average age is 50. All practice in Chicago or surrounding suburban communities. Three-quarters received their medical education in Illinois. All but 6 are male. Almost all are Jewish; their private practices, correspondingly, include a predominance of middle-class Jewish patients. Balancing this is their wide experience, in this and other hospitals, working with ward service patients, the majority of whom are non-Jewish.

Questionnaire

The following questions apply to your policy about telling patients they have cancer. For the purpose of this questionnaire, assume that the diagnosis is certain and that though treatment may be possible the eventual prognosis is grave.

1. What is your usual policy about telling patients? (check one) A. Tell. Don't Tell.

2. How often do you make exceptions to your rule? (check one) A. Never. Very Rarely.

3. The following is a list of factors pertaining to the patient which may be relevant in your decision about telling a particular patient. Check *every* item which you would include in making your decision.
   a. Age
   b. Sex
   c. Religion
   d. Intelligence
   e. State of personal affairs
   f. Community standing
   g. Medical sophistication
   h. Patient a physician
   i. Length of expected survival
   j. Acceptance of recommended therapy
   k. Patient asking no questions
   l. Patient's expressed wish to be told
   m. Relatives wish (about telling patient)
   n. Emotional stability
   o. Other personality factors
   p. Other factors (specify)

4. Circle any item about which you feel is of *especial* importance.

5. For each item checked in 3, briefly explain how and in which direction it applies.

6. When you do not tell a patient, do you always tell a relative? (Yes or No).

7. How did you acquire your policy? (check *every* item which applies) A. Taught you in Med. School. B. Taught you during Clinical Training. C. Clinical experience. D. Non-professional experience with ill friends, family, etc. E. Other (specify).

8. Which of these was the single most important source?

9. Were you ever specifically taught some policy? (not necessarily your current one) (Yes or No)

10. A. Apart from your training, experience, etc., do you think that your *personal* attitudes about cancer, life illness, etc., are determinants of your policy? (Yes or No)*
    B. Do you think that such personal factors are more or less important than the others in determining your policy? (check one)

11. How likely do you think it is that your policy will change? (check one) A. No possibility. B. Very unlikely. C. Unlikely. D. Probably. E. Certainly.

12. A. Has your policy changed in the past? (Yes or No)
    B. If yes, how would you have previously answered Question 1? Question 2?

13. How do you think most surgeons would answer Question 1? Question 2?*

14. How do you think most psychiatrists would answer Question 1? Question 2?

15. Would your present policy be swayed by the results of research on this problem? (Yes or No)

16. Do you think research in this area should be done? (Yes or No)

17. Do you find it more difficult to tell a cancer patient than other patients who have another disease but the *same* prognosis? (Yes or No)*

18. If you were the patient, do you think you would want to be told? (Yes or No)*

Comments: (Any comments you can make on any question above, or related issues will be appreciated. If you can amplify or describe your personal policy or the reasons behind it this will be especially useful.)

Biographical Data: 1. Age. 2. Speciality or Sub-speciality. 3. Name of Medical School. 4. Year Graduated. 5. Board Certified (field(s) and year).

*This is the questionnaire submitted to Internists and Generalists. In the original version of the questionnaire submitted to surgeons, items 10, 17, and 18 were not included (these questions were asked, as worded, during interviews) and item 13 pertained to internists.

Table 36–1
Physicians' Policies About "Telling" Cancer Patients

Usual Policy	Exceptions Made	Internists		Surgeons[a]		Generalists		Total Group	
		No.	%	No.	%	No.	%	No.	%
Do not tell	Never	7	8	7	8	4	15	18	9
	Very rarely	36	43	44	53	10	37	90	47
	Occasionally	28	34	21	25	7	26	56	29
	Often	4	5	1	1	0	0	5	3
Subtotal		75	90	73	87	21	78	169	88
Tell	Often	3	4	4	5	1	4	8	4
	Occasionally	4	5	4	5	2	7	10	5
	Very rarely	1	1	2	2	3	11	6	3
	Never	0	0	0	0	0	0	0	0
Subtotal		8	10	10	12	7	22	24	12
Total		83	100	83	100[b]	27	100	193	100

[a]Includes gynecologists and thoracic, genito-urinary, orthopedic, and neurosurgeons as well as general surgeons.
[b]Sum appears to equal 99% because of rounding to nearest percentage.

A few comments regarding statistics are in order. All questionnaire results were subjected to analysis by standard procedures: chi square, analysis of variance, student's "t" test, and the sign test. For simplicity of presentation the details of each procedure and probability levels are not reported here. No finding reported fails to reach at least the generally accepted criterion ($p < .05$), unless specifically noted. Small discrepancies between the total figures reported for different items reflect variations in the numbers of subjects who failed to answer some questions.

"Telling"

The initial undertaking in this research was the determination of whether or not physicians tell their patients they have cancer. It is evident, as seen in Table 36–1, that there is a strong and general tendency to *withhold* this information. Almost 90% of the group is within this half of the scale. Indeed, a majority tell only very rarely, if ever. No one reported a policy of informing every patient. These findings are quite comparable to those of the Philadelphia study. No difference between specialities was uncovered; the small differences seen in Table 36–1, or involving the smaller groups of surgical subspecialties not detailed there, are far from significant statistically. (This lack of specialty differences was a consistent finding for all questionnaire items. Differences when present were small and off-set by wider divergencies within each specialty.) These findings

also cut across the hospital staff rank and age. Younger and less experienced men did not have any greater inclination to tell than their seniors.

Use of a questionnaire, of course, forces answers into an artificially rigid mold. But, information derived from the interviews strengthens the finding. Answers indicating that patients are told often turned out to mean telling the patient that he had a "tumor," with strict avoidance of the terms cancer, malignancy, and the like. These more specific words were almost never used unless the patient's explicit and insistent questioning pushed the doctor's back to the wall.

Euphemisms are the general rule. These may extend from the vaguest of words ("lesion," "mass"); to terms giving a general indication that the process is neoplastic ("growth," "tumor," "hyperplastic tissue")—often tempered by a false explicit statement that the process is benign; to somewhat more suggestive expression (a "suspicious" or "degenerated" tumor). Where major surgical or radiation therapy is involved, especially if the patient is hesitant about proceeding, recourse may be had to such terms as "precancerous," or a tumor "in the early curable stage." Some physicians avoid even the slightest suggestion of neoplasia and quite specifically substitute another diagnosis. Almost every one reported resorting such falsification on at least a few occasions, most notably

when the patient was in a far-advanced stage of illness at the time he was seen.

It is impossible to convey all the flavor of the diverse individual approaches. No two men use exactly the same technique. Each has his preferred plan, his select euphemisms, his favored tactics, and his own views about the optimal time for discussion and the degree of directness to be used. Some have a set pattern, while others vary their approach. But the general trend is consistent.

The modal policy is to tell as little as possible in the most general terms consistent with maintaining cooperation in treatment. Exceptions are made most commonly when the patient is in a position of financial responsibility which carries the necessity for planning. Questioning by the patient almost invariably is disregarded and considered a plea for reassurance unless persistent, and intuitively perceived as "a real wish to know." Even then it may be ignored. The vast majority of these doctors feel that almost all patients really do not want to know regardless of what people say. They approach the issue with the view that disclosure should be avoided unless there are positive indications, rather than the reverse. Intelligence and emotional stability are considered prerequisites for greater disclosure only if other "realistic" factors provide a basis for doing so. For the fewer physicians who tell with some frequency, these two factors assume more primary importance.

A few additional consistent themes emerge. Agreement was essentially unanimous that some family member must be informed if the patient is not made aware of the diagnosis. Legal and ethical considerations are by no means the only points of relevance here. Repeated instances were reported of patients who, dissatisfied with the progression of their disease in the face of treatment and desperate for help, were dissuaded from fruitless and unwise shifts to a new physician (or quack) only by the cooperation of an informed relative. Beyond this is the need to have someone to share the awful burden of knowledge. As one man put it, "I just can't carry the load alone." Few responsibilities are as heavy as knowing that someone is going to die; dividing it makes it easier to bear.

Variations in approach also converge to a single major goal: maintenance of hope. No inference was necessary to elicit this finding. Every single physician interviewed spontaneously emphasized this point and indicated his resolute and determined purpose is to sustain and bolster the patient's hope. Each in his own way communicates the possibility, even the likelihood, of recovery. Differences revolve about the range of belief about just how much information is compatible with the maintenance of hope. While some doctors believe "cancer means certain death and no normal person wants to die," others hold that "knowledge is power": power which can conquer fear. The crux of the divergence centers on two issues: whether cancer connotes certain death, and whether the expectation of death insurmountably deprives the patient of hope. The data indicate that an impressively large number of physicians would answer affirmatively to both.

Acquisition

The approach used by a physician may derive from many sources. Perhaps he acquired it as a result of teaching in medical school or while a house officer; maybe it grows out of his own clinical experience or is a result of personal experiences with afflicted friends and family; it may arise as a result of reading; or perhaps it is a personal conviction which stems from the deeper influences of his personality and individual philosophy. Information about this was specifically requested on the questionnaire. These results are available in Table 36–2.

Clinical experience would seem to be of overwhelming importance. Only 6% (12 of 203) failed to list this as a factor. Other sources are reported with far less frequency, and if reported at all, usually in addition to clinical experience, which is the factor accorded primary importance by more than three-quarters of the group. Medical school teaching apparently plays a minimal role. Internship and residency training is somewhat more often listed. Yet, only about one-third of the group did include this (and it was infrequently felt to be salient) when it might seem that the subject could not have failed to arise during training. The interviews confirmed this. Few people could remember hearing about the subject during their training. When someone did, usually there was no recall of anything specific said, other than the emphasis of the need of the physician to deal with the problem. This silence, like the lack of research, is striking. It is possible, of course, that what is reflected here is as much a failure of recall as the absence of teaching. Still, if this is true it requires explanation and points to some deficiency in the teaching process.

Personal factors are reported by only a moderate number of the group. The experience of seeing a close relative (most commonly a parent) die of cancer, was a decisive occurrence for some. This experience, however, did not lead to any difference in policy between these physicians and the group as a whole; they were neither more nor less likely to tell. Less concretely derived personal feelings were reported by a small group. These responses, comprising all but two of those listed as "other," were described in such terms as "my philosophy of life," "my personal conviction," or "projecting myself into the patient's situation." Interestingly, if such a feeling was reported at all, there was a strong likelihood that it was considered the determining factor.

Experience vs. Emotion

Results like these might seem to be anticipated. After all, why should we not expect clinical experience to provide the basis for action, and personal factors to play only a secondary role? Sound practice grows from experience. But is this actually the case here? Is this an area in which reason really prevails? There is much further data from the present research which suggests quite the opposite.

To begin with, experience can be acquired only over a span of time. A young group, whose graduation from medical school has taken place not many years earlier, might be expected to report that their policy stems largely from other sources. At least they should cite experience less often than their seniors. This is not the case. The group under 45 years of age, or those in the lower staff ranks, are just as likely to list experience as a factor as their older colleagues. Indeed, they are no less likely to cite it as the major determinant. The mean age and the staff level of those who reportedly based their policy on experience does not differ from those who do not. Nor do the policies of the two groups differ.

Experience, moreover, implies a state of knowledge based upon a range of earlier observation, with the opportunity to become familiar with the outcomes of various alternatives. Occasions for some such experience, of course, have been available to all these physicians. Yet only 27 (14%) have had the opportunity for first-hand knowledge based on their own trial of any policy different from their current one. More detailed exploration in the interviews cast a great deal of further doubt about the role of experience. It was the exception when a physician could report known examples of the unfavorable consequences of an approach which differed from his own. It was more common to get reports of instances in which different approaches had turned out satisfactorily. Most of the instances in which unhappy results were reported to follow a differing policy turned out to be vague accounts from which no reliable inference could be drawn.

Instead of logic and rational decision based on critical observation, what is found is opinion, belief, and conviction, heavily weighted with emotional justification. As one internist said: "I can't give a good reason except that I've always done it." Explanations are

Table 36–2
Sources from Which Policies Were Acquired

Source	Every Source		Major Source	
	No.	%	No.	%
Medical school teaching	11	7	0	0
Hospital training	72	35	10	5
Clinical experience	191	77	146	77
Illness in friends, family, etc.	61	30	15	8
Other	24	12	17	9
	362[a]	. . .	188	100[b]

[a]More than one answer can be given by a respondent.
[b]Sum appears to equal 99% because of rounding to nearest percentage.

begun characteristically with such phrases as "I feel . . ." or "It is my opinion. . . ." Personal convictions were stated flatly and dogmatically as if they were facts. Thus, "Most people do not want to know," "It is my firm belief that they always know anyway," or "No one can be told without giving up and losing all hope." Highly charged emotional terms and vivid expressions were the rule, indicating the intensity and nature of feelings present. Knowledge of cancer is "a death sentence," "a Buchenwald," and "torture." Telling is "the cruelest thing in the world," "awful," and "hitting the patient with a baseball bat." It is not necessary even to read the words on the questionnaires. Heavy underlinings and a peppering of exclamation points tell the story. These are hardly cool scientific judgments. It would appear that personal conviction is the decisive factor.

There is direct confirmation of this point. *Subsequent* to the general inquiry: "How did you acquire your policy?," it was specifically asked if personal issues were determinants. Nearly three-fourths (98 of 138) reported that personal elements were involved, in contrast to the much smaller number who listed this originally. These 98 were about equally divided as to whether these factors were the most important.

Inflexibility and Emotion

Attitudes to which much emotion is bound are characteristically modified only with great difficulty. Data has been presented indicating that little past change has occurred. What about the future? Here we can look at the question about the likelihood of policy change. Of 5 alternatives offered, "no

possibility" was indicated by a small group (6%). The response of these 11 is understandable since they are an older group (mean age 65.2). The remainder of the respondents showed a similar trend. The largest segment (78, 40%) felt that change was "very unlikely" and an additional third (70) "unlikely." Only a total of one-fifth felt that change was either "probable" (39) or "certain" (7). This group showed a significant tendency to be the same people who had reported earlier change. Apparently, there is a minority who tend to be generally flexible. Again, this was not a younger group.

Strong resistance to change is also evident in the responses to questions about research. Thirty of the group (16%) indicated that their policy would not be swayed by research. An additional 54 respondents (29%) felt sufficiently doubtful so that they were unable to answer yes or no, as requested (the only item in which this difficulty arose), and instead wrote in "perhaps" or "maybe." While this leaves a majority who answered yes, these negative answers are noteworthy. These are physicians who read assiduously and themselves conduct research. In what other area would they fail to be swayed by research? Many comments were made that "I wouldn't believe it" or "it couldn't be true," if research suggested a policy different from their own. Still more striking is the finding that 10% (19) of the group felt that research in this area should not be done at all! Small wonder so little has appeared.

Another relevant finding is the doctor's wish to be told if he were the patient. As expected, those who tend to

tell their patients wished to be told, themselves, more often than those who do not tell. But the total number of those who said they wished to be told (73 of 122) is far greater than those who tend to tell their patients. The explanation usually given was that, "I am one of those who can take it" or "I have responsibilities." That they did not feel this to be true for all physicians, however, is attested to by their treatment of other doctor-patients. Most of the group said they were neither more nor less likely to tell physicians than other patients. Of the group who did modify their policy, it was just as likely to find that they were *less* prone to tell doctors. It is impossible to draw any precise conclusion from this type of hypothetical question about one's self. But the inconsistency is characteristic of emotionally determined attitudes.

Depression and Suicide

The pros and cons of telling have been discussed so often that there is little point in doing so again. Whatever the reasons for telling, the argument against doing so centers on the anticipation of profoundly disturbing psychological effects. There is no doubt that this disclosure has a profound and potentially dangerous impact. Questions do arise about the capacity of human beings to make a satisfactory adaptation to the expectation of death. Can anyone successfully handle such news without paying a price which mitigates whatever value this knowledge brings? If so, how widespread is the ability to call forth the necessary psychological defenses? What about time: does this readjustment take place within some reasonable span? Can the emotional cost of such a shattering experience, or of the effort required for mastering it, be weighed and predicted? The truth is that we know very little about these matters.

It has been repeatedly asserted that disclosure is followed by fear and despondency which may progress into overt depressive illness or culminate in suicide. This was the opinion of the physicians in the present study. Quite representative was the surgeon who stated, "I would be afraid to tell and have the patient in a room with a window." When it comes to actually documenting the prevalence of such untoward reactions, it becomes difficult to find reliable evidence. Instances of depression and profound upsets came quickly to mind when the subject was raised, but no one could report more than a case or two, or a handful at most. This may merely follow from the rarity with which patients are told. Such an explanation must be reconciled with the fact that these same doctors could remember many instances in which the patient was told and seemed to do well. It may also reflect the selection of those told. Or perhaps the knowledge produces covert psychological changes which are no less malignant for their sublety. But actually, the incidence and severity of depression and other psychological reactions in cancer patients, and their relation to being told, is not known.

The same situation holds with regard to suicide. Only 6 doctors could report definite known cases of suicide (2 of these reported two cases and 1 "several"), although about one-third of the group had "heard of" suicides after being told. Further investigation indicated that at least 2 of these patients had never been told. (And it is not altogether inconceivable that they would have felt better, not worse, had this been done.) Actually, the circumstances surrounding all but one or two of these cases are quite vague; it is impossible to feel any certainty about what lay behind the suicide.

The Philadelphia study[7] failed also to uncover many instances of suicide. Only 3 cases were reported, two by one physician. Neither Finesinger and associates nor Calloway[9,10] could recall a suicide among their patients who had been told. Litin and Wilmer[11] reviewed all the records of suicide in one Minnesota county over 17 years. Only

one case was discovered which could be attributed to being informed of the diagnosis of cancer.

This by no means *proves* that telling is safe. The group who tell are equally vague in documenting that their patients do well. We simply do not have adequate data about the consequences of telling. As in any dreaded situation, emotion fills a vacuum with rumor, pseudofact, and projected fears. It is noteworthy that the question is posed: "can a patient stand not being told" is almost never heard, although it is equally valid from the scientific viewpoint.

A physician who tells some of his patients uses certain rules of thumb to guide his decisions. It is striking how inconsistently these guides vary from one physician to another. Thus, some are more likely to tell the very aged while others especially avoid telling this group. Some are inclined to tell patients with a better prognosis and others only when the prognosis is poor. The disagreement about doctor-patients has already been noted. Such discrepancies may portray quite accurately chance differences in experience. More intriguing is the possibility that they reflect the doctor's personality. In any event they are typical of a *priori* judgments unsubstantiated by facts.

Pessimism

Cancer has many unconscious meanings and fantasies associated with it. Whatever the unconscious feelings which it stirs, typically it is feared consciously as a process equated with suffering and certain death. There was good general agreement among the physicians interviewed that these are what patients primarily fear. Other connotations (for example, that cancer is dirty or shameful) were far less prevalent. Many patients mouth statements about curability, and "know" neither suffering nor death are inevitable. But the physicians here report that this knowledge is only skin deep. People continue to think of cancer as "the killer."

What is impressive is that the doctors themselves feel very much the same way. It was not patients who described the diagnosis as a "death warrant" or "a date of execution." The internist

who referred to cancer as an "incurable disease with an inevitable demise" expressed a view which was not atypical. The extent and intensity of this underlying pessimism stands out. The general feeling was that we can do very little to save lives and not a great deal to prevent suffering. Sighs and shrugging of the shoulders were the almost usual accompaniment of discussion in this area. Not that these men give up where the individual patient is concerned; on the contrary they fight ceaselessly and without compromise. But just below the surface is the feeling: "to me, it's like a stone wall—no prospects."

Early diagnosis is viewed with a not much more sanguine eye. Nearly all could remember a few cases, at least, where early diagnosis seemed of critical importance. (Breast and bowel lesions were singled out for special mention.) But a common feeling was that usually this makes no difference: "What's the use? You make an early diagnosis, the patient goes through a horrible operation and suffers, and two years later he's dead anyway." They are not convinced that it helps more than a handful.

"Death Shall Have No Dominion"[12]

Among the motivations for entering medicine, the wish to conquer suffering and death stands high on the list. Practicing physicians are not the kind of persons who can sit quietly by while nature pursues its course. One of the hardest things for a fledgling medical student to learn is watchful waiting. Few situations are as frustrating as sitting by impotently and "helplessly" in the face of illness. Fatal illness is felt as a major defeat. It is not uncommon to know at a glance that a colleague has recently lost a patient: it leaves its mark. Recently, Engel[13] has commented on the intensity of our feelings about death and our needs to deny its reality.

Perhaps herein lies some basis for the intense pessimism and despair and the emotional attitudes. Hollender[14] has also made this point. The many specific unconscious meanings of cancer converge on conscious ideas of pain, disintegration, dissolution, and death. If any group is constantly bombarded with the awful fact of death it is doctors—the same group which has such strong needs to conquer it. No wonder the feeling: "I'm upset emotionally by treating a (cancer) patient. I cry on the inside."

Situations of this kind, associated with intense charges of unpleasant emotions, call forth a variety of psychological defenses which reduce the intensity of feelings to manageable proportions. Among such defenses are those which involve the avoidance, negation, or denial of the existence of some unpleasant fact, and acting as if it were not real. These can be economical and effective mechanisms which find particular usefulness in dealing with situations in which no appropriate action is open. Unless they are given up at that point where something realistic and practical can be done, however, they become dangerous blocks to effective action.

Such mechanisms play a prominent role in the attitudes reported here. There is a strong tendency to avoid looking at the subject of cancer and the facts related to it. There is an avoidance of research and teaching, opposition to potential research, resistance to personal experimentation and change, and the projection of strongly held rationalizations into the vacuum of knowledge. To some extent, we do not *want* to know about what we are doing or why, because the subject is so upsetting. Unfortunately, in our denial we go beyond the limits of usefulness. By blocking off access to new knowledge, we cut ourselves off from the acquisition of facts which could be of real help.

The behavior of members of our own profession who develop cancer amply demonstrates the prevalence of these ostrich-like denial mechanisms. It is common to see colleagues with malignancies cling to an alternative diagnosis when their condition is obvious even to the untutored eye. (The tendency for physicians to ignore their illness of all types is also common knowledge.) Delay in the diagnosis of their own cancers by physicians is well documented.[15] Not only do physicians postpone seeking medical care, but their doctors delay further,[16] perhaps because the diagnostician must especially avoid recognition of cancer in a patient so like himself.

Withholding the diagnosis seems to represent a further manifestation of denial. This point has been made by

Finesinger et al.[9] and by Trawick.[17] If a physician wishes to avoid being confronted by his troubled feelings under ordinary circumstances, he will certainly not want to have these feelings stimulated when he is in the actual presence of a cancer patient. A fractured limb is kept splinted. Thus, the subject is not broached or is minimized and pushed aside from consideration. Failure of the patient to ask for his diagnosis under these circumstances is no corroboration that the doctor's avoidance is logically grounded. With his own tendencies to deny what he must greatly fear, the patient may take his cue from the doctor's silence as confirmation that the situation is hopeless and therefore better shunned. Tactful wishes to spare his distraught physician even may play a part.

Although avoidance of telling reflects the psychological problems of the doctor, this by no means implies that such a policy is therapeutically incorrect. It would be entirely erroneous if this study were interpreted to mean that patients should be told. This must be emphasized. Telling the patient may have no less emotional basis as a "counterphobic" denial that cancer is a terribly serious disease. The data indicate that equally irrational and affect-laden attitudes lie behind *both* tendencies.

Intuitive understanding of what the patient experiences is a time proven and essential guide for the physician. Our own dread and concern about cancer mirrors what patients feel. Anxiety about death is ubiquitous. (Beigler[18] has pointed out how its development may actually herald a fatal outcome.) To ignore wisdom based on insight into ourselves and to go about blithely telling patients they have cancer, obviously would be senseless. Intuitively derived insights are important and legitimate scientific data about psychological processes. Instinctive judgments, however, can be terribly misleading. In matters of life and death, personal intuition is far too likely to be subject to personal unconscious distortions and thus prove a false guide which clouds experience and hides truth.

Delay in Diagnosis

Cancer authorities have been greatly concerned with the problem of delay in diagnosis and treatment. Much of

the delay is due to patients themselves, but many studies have revealed a significant proportion which is ascribable to physicians. A recently published critical survey of this literature documents the importance of attitudinal factors such as pessimism and insensitivity (low index of suspicion).

The American Cancer Society has devoted vast effort and sums of money to public information campaigns. Publicity about the "danger signals" of cancer has led to howls of protest by some physicians who feel that such campaigns stimulate cancerophobia. Leaving aside any possible correctness of such contentions, why has the issue been so heated? Perhaps, we have here another manifestation of the wish to keep cancer out of sight and mind. For the most part, officials of the Society have responded to such complaints with defensive statements that the majority of the medical profession agrees that their approach has merit which exceeds the harm. The interviews here tend to support this view, although agreement was usually lukewarm. Reservations centered less on the problem of cancerophobia than on the positive value of public education. Part of this reflects the pessimism already described, but more is involved. The view expressed was that patients who respond to publicity are usually complaint (and cancer) free, while those with symptoms requiring attention are dominated by their irrational fears and are unaffected. The general conclusion was that education utilizing only a rational appeal is insufficient. New techniques must be developed which will modify emotional attitudes.

The same conclusion can be drawn about the education programs directed towards physicians. Cancer authorities cannot be lulled into complacency by the overt agreement of the profession with their goals or by their successes in providing technical information. Much more ingenuity and effort will be required to alter and surmount the formidable psychological barriers of physicians' covert attitudes. The medical profession plays a pivotal role in cancer control far beyond its direct functions in diagnosis and treatment. When doctors lose hope their patients know it. If doctors communicate the feeling that cancer is dreadful and irremediable, how can patients fail to despair? And frightened and despairing, how can they deal with the possibility that they have cancer? Their only recourse is to keep the possibility hidden—from themselves as well as their doctors. Thus, they court the very fate which they most fear. No physician, no matter how skillful, can treat the patient who stays away. Unwittingly, our own feelings reinforce the anxieties which keep them away, the very opposite of our intent. Perhaps the doctor, more than the patient, should be a target for emotional reeducation.

Summary and Conclusions

Medicine is a difficult and exacting profession making heavy psychological as well as physical demands. Our personalities, feelings, and attitudes play a major role in determining the manner in which we communicate with and treat patients. They can constitute a tool of incalculable value: the art of medicine. But they can also interfere. No area in which we work makes heavier claims than the treatment of cancer patients, with the suffering, pain, and death which are its frequent attendants. Pressed by these demands, we turn away in order to blunt their awful impact. In doing so, we sap the strength of our most potent asset, the ability to concentrate the full force of our reason. We fail to apply our scientific skills or do adequate research. Thus we block our own efforts. Only by conquering our irrational attitudes, proceeding to acquire knowledge, and acting on the basis of reason can we advance. Awareness of these attitudes is the first step. Knowing of our deep pessimism about cancer and of our avoidance of research and teaching regarding communications with the cancer patient, we can advance to develop new knowledge of more sensitive and skilled approaches. We will know then how to be *truly* kind to our patients.

References

1. Cabot, R., *Meaning of Right and Wrong,* New York: The Macmillan Company, 1933.

2. Seelig, M. C., Should Cancer Patients Be Told Truth? *Missouri Med.* 40:33–35 (Feb.) 1943.

3. Wangensteen, O., Should Patients Be Told They Have Cancer, *Surgery* 27:944–947 (June) 1950.

4. Kelly, W. D., and Friesen, S. R., Do Cancer Patients Want to Be Told? *Surgery* 27:822–826 (June) 1950.

5. Branch, C. H. H., Psychiatric Aspects of Malignant Disease, *CA, Bull. Can. Prog.* 6:102–104 (May) 1956.

6. Samp, R. J., and Curreri, A. R., Questionnaire Survey on Public Cancer Education Obtained from Cancer Patients and Their Families, *Cancer* 10:382–384 (March–April) 1957.

7. Fitts, W. T. Jr., and Ravdin, I. S., What Philadelphia Physicians Tell Patients with Cancer, *JAMA* 153:901–904 (Nov. 7) 1953.

8. Rennick, D., editor, What Should Physician Tell Cancer Patient?, *New Medical Materia* 2:51–53 (March) 1960.

9. Finesinger, J. E., Shands, H. C., and Abrams, R. P., Managing Emotional Problems of Cancer Patient, *CA, Bull. Can. Prog.* 3:19–31 (Jan.) 1953.

10. Calloway, E., Psychological Care of Cancer Patient, *J. Med. Ass. Georgia* 41:503–504 (Nov.) 1952.

11. Litin, E. M., and Wilmer, H. D., unpublished data (personal communication from Litin, E. M.).

12. Thomas, D., And Death Shall Have No Dominion, in *Collected Poems of Dylan Thomas,* New York: New Directions, 1957.

13. Engel, G. L., Is Grief Disease? Challenge for Medical Research, *Psychosom. Med.* 23:18 (Jan.–Feb.) 1961.

14. Hollender, M. H., Psychology of Medical Practice, Chap. 4 in: *Patient With Carcinoma,* Philadelphia: W. B. Saunders and Company, 1958.

15. Alvarez, W. C., How Early Do Physicians Diagnose Cancer of Stomach in Themselves? *JAMA* 97:77–83 (July 11) 1931.

16. Robbins, G. F., MacDonald, J. D., and Pack, G. T., Delay in Diagnosis and Treatment of Physicians with Cancer, *Cancer* 6:624–626 (May) 1953.

17. Trawick, J. D.: Psychiatrist and Cancer Patient, *Dis. Nerv. Syst.* 11:278–280 (Sept.) 1950.

18. Beigler, J. C., Anxiety as Aid to Prognostication of Impending Death, *Arch. Neurol. Psychiat.* 77:171–177 (Feb.) 1957.

37

Howard Waitzkin and John D. Stoeckle

From "The Communication of Information about Illness"

Reprinted by permission of the editors from *Advances in Psychosomatic Medicine,* vol. 8, 1972, pp. 185–189.

The Problem of Uncertainty and the Problem of Power

Several sociologists have discussed the uncertainty inherent in medical practice. In his theoretical exposition of the doctor-patient relationship, Parsons points out that uncertainty regarding the outcome of illness increases physicians' frustration.[1] Fox documents the uncertainty experienced by medical students in their education and by both physicians and patients involved in medical research. In addition, she analyzes the frequently nonrational and quasi-magical mechanisms which patients and doctors use to come to terms with uncertainty in the medical sphere.[2] Although both physician and patient experience uncertainty, there remains a "competence gap" between them which derives from a discrepancy in technical knowledge. The competence gap means that uncertainty generally is greater for the patient than for the physician.

From a slightly different perspective, several economists have pointed out that uncertainty is one characteristic which distinguishes the medical sector from other sectors of the economy.[3,4] Fuchs states, for example, that "very few industries could be named where the consumer is so dependent upon the producer for information concerning the quality of the product." According to Fuchs, consumer ignorance in the health field derives from three causes. First, there is an inherent uncertainty regarding the effect of service on any individual. The lay person cannot know the value of a particular procedure or treatment, especially in cases when the medical profession is far from agreed within itself. Secondly, since medical services are infrequently purchased, consumers tend not to develop expertise about treatment or where to go for it. Thirdly, the medical profession does little to inform consumers. In fact, through restrictions on advertising and price competition, the profession appears to take positive action to keep consumers uninformed.[5]

The competence gap between producers and consumers of health care leads to unique problems of social control. Because of ignorance, the consumer can exert little control over the quality of services he purchases from his physician. Under conditions of consumer ignorance and uncertainty, Par-

sons believes, professional groups must be self-regulating, taking responsibility (through regulatory mechanisms such as examinations and licensure) for the technical standards of its members. Moreover, from the patient's point of view, the competence gap "must be bridged by something like what we call trust."[6] Because of his own uncertainty, the patient tends to relinquish control over his physician's actions and assumes that control will emerge from more generalized regulatory mechanisms within the medical profession.

Yet even when doctors are certain about the course of disease or the outcome of therapy, they tend to prolong patients' uncertainty. Davis has found, for example, that physicians delay the communication of prognosis to the families of children with poliomyelitis, long after the physicians have a clear understanding of the children's residual deficits.[7,8] Similarly, as Roth has demonstrated, physicians treating patients with tuberculosis refrain from divulging the expected date of discharge from the hospital.[9,10] Numerous studies of dying patients have shown that although the vast majority desire to know the facts concerning their condition, most of their physicians (69–90%, depending on the study) favor the withholding of information from them.[11,12]

How can one explain the observed tendency of physicians to maintain patients' uncertainty, even when patients prefer to be informed and when the physicians' own uncertainty is reduced? The most obvious answer is based on individual psychology: relating bad news can be an emotionally upsetting experience. Recent experimental evidence suggests that, as a general phenomenon, individuals hesitate to communicate bad news as opposed to good news.[13] Physicians may refrain from such communication more than other groups because of a greater fear of death: several studies have reported a higher fear of death among physicians and medical students than among members of other professions.[14] Such psychological reasons might explain the withholding of information from dying patients or the parents of children with polio, but they do not seem to apply to situations in which information is withheld from patients

who are improving over the course of therapy.[15-22]

To explain physicians' inclination to maintain uncertainty in their patients, we offer a theoretical proposition concerning the source of a physician's power: *a physician's ability to preserve his own power over the patient in the doctor-patient relationship depends largely on his ability to control the patient's uncertainty.* The physician enhances his power to the extent that he can maintain the patient's uncertainty about the course of illness, efficacy of therapy, or specific future actions of the physician himself.

In proposing this theoretical statement, we are extending a theory applied in general sociology to the study of bureaucracy. Crozier's comparative studies of bureaucracy have led to the following formulation concerning the relationship between power and uncertainty:

In such a context, the power of A over B depends on A's ability to predict B's behavior and on the uncertainty of B about A's behavior. As long as the requirements of action create situations of uncertainty, the individuals who have to face them have power over those who are affected by the results of their choice.[23]

Using data from observations of supervisor-subordinate relationships, Crozier supports his theoretical proposition that supervisory personnel enhance their own power by maximizing their subordinates' uncertainty regarding the future actions of the supervisors. It should be noted that Crozier employs Dahl's definition of power: "The power of a person A over a person B is the ability of A to obtain that B do something he would not have done otherwise."[24] However, Crozier's formulation seems equally consistent with Parsons' definition of power as a generalized medium of exchange, which he has used to describe power relationships in several social institutions:

Hence the power of A over B is, in its legitimized form, the "right" of A, as a decision making unit involved in collective process, to make decisions which take precedence over those of B, in the interest of the effectiveness of the collective operation as a whole.[25]

Incorporating Parsons' definition into Crozier's formulation, one would expect that A's ability to make decisions taking precedence over B depends on A's ability to maintain B's uncertainty regarding A's behavior.

These considerations are readily applicable to the doctor-patient relationship. Just as the bureaucratic supervisor enhances his own power by maximizing his subordinate's uncertainty, the physician increases his power by maintaining the patient's uncertainty about illness and treatment. This theoretical statement does not imply that the maintenance of uncertainty is intrinsically dysfunctional. As Parsons points out, the physician and patient can be conceptualized as a collectivity, working toward the common goal of therapy.[26] From this viewpoint, the physician's ability to make necessary therapeutic decisions may depend on his power position vis-à-vis that of the patient. The less uncertain the patient becomes about the nature of his illness and the effects of treatment, the less willing he may be to relinquish decision-making power to the physician. At other times, however, the physician's maintenance of uncertainty may serve no concrete collective function and may merely satisfy the physician's psychological need for power. Since physicians probably vary in their need for power, one would expect that this variation among physicians would reflect itself in different tendencies to maintain uncertainty in patients. That is, a physician's need for power, apart from the specific characteristics of a particular patient, may affect the way he communicates information regarding illness and therapy.

Others also have commented on the relationship between power and the manipulation of information. In a discussion of the social functions of ignorance, Moore and Tumin point out that ignorance on the part of the consumer of specialized services helps to preserve the privileged position of the dispenser of the services. The implication here is that ". . . the specialist's position may be endangered by 'the patient's becoming his own physician.' "[27] In a report of participant observation in tuberculosis hospitals, Roth states that the more closely a patient's experience and knowledge approach that of a physician, the greater becomes the patient's resistance to giving up control of the service to the physician.[28] In this way, reduced uncertainty of tuberculosis patients concerning the course of their illness appears to diminish the power of physicians within the doctor-patient relationship.

The postulated association between uncertainty and power may help explain physicians' reluctance to reveal information to dying patients. A physician's disclosure of fatal illness is equivalent to a declaration of his own powerlessness. What need has a dying patient for a physician? Perhaps the patient may rely on a physician for palliative therapy or for supportive concern. But the physician's technical ability to cure has vanished, and admission of this fact implies loss of power. Glaser and Strauss describe a unique situation in cancer wards of a Veterans Administration hospital, where patients are poor and possess no alternative to the free care they receive at the hospital. In contrast to the usual reluctance of physicians to inform cancer patients about their illness,[29] physicians on these particular wards do not hesitate to disclose terminality to patients directly. Glaser and Strauss comment, "Since the captive lower class patients cannot effectively threaten the hospital or the doctors, the rule at this hospital is to disclose terminality regardless of the patient's expected reaction."[30] Thus, when physicians' power is assured because of patients' low socioeconomic status, the control of uncertainty becomes less crucial.

Finally, information itself yields power. In the quite different contexts of both psychological and information theory, Maslow and Cherry point out that information allows the recipient to select his own future action from a wider range of possible alternatives. Maslow puts the matter succinctly, "What you *don't* know has power over you; knowing it brings it under your control, and makes it subject to your choice. Ignorance makes real choice impossible."[31,32]

To summarize our argument to this point: Uncertainty, though an inherent feature of medical practice, is experienced to a greater extent by patients than by physicians. Information transmitted from physician to patient, by reducing the patient's uncertainty, also reduces the physician's power within the doctor-patient relationship.

Notes

1. Parsons, T., *The Social System* (New York: Free Press, 1951).

2. Fox, R. C., Training for uncertainty, in Merton, Reader, and Kendall, eds.. *The Student Physician* (Cambridge: Harvard University Press, 1957); Fox, R.C. "A sociological perspective on organ transplantation and dialysis. *Ann. N.Y. Acad. Sci.* 169:406–428 (1970).

3. Arrow, K. J., Uncertainty and the welfare economics of medical care. *Amer. Econ. Rev.* 53:941–973.

4. Fuchs, V. R., The contribution of health services to the American economy. *Milbank Mem. Fund Quart.* 44:65–101 (1966).

5. Ibid.

6. Parsons, T., Research with human subjects and the professional complex. *Daedalus* 8:325–360 (1969).

7. Davis, F., Uncertainty in medical prognosis: Clinical and functional. *Amer. J. Sociol.* 66:41–48 (1960).

8. Davis, F., *Passage through Crisis* (Indianapolis: Bobbs-Merrill, 1963).

9. Roth, J. A., Information and the control of treatment in tuberculosis hospitals; in Friedson, *The Hospital in Modern Society* (Glencoe: Free Press, 1963).

10. Roth, J. A., *Timetables* (Indianapolis: Bobbs-Merrill, 1963).

11. Feifel, H., Death, in Farberow, *Taboo Topics* (New York: Atherton, 1966).

12. Oken, D., What to tell cancer patients: A study of medical attitudes. *J. Amer. Med. Assn.* 175:1120–1128 (1961). [Reprinted as Chapter 36 of this volume.]

13. Rosen, S., and Tesser, A., On reluctance to communicate undesirable information: The MUM effect. *Sociometry* 33:253–263 (1970).

14. White, L. P. the self-image of the physician and the care of dying patients. *Ann. N.Y. Acad. Sci.* 164:822–831 (1969).

15. Cartwright, A., *Human Relations and Hospital Care* (London: Routledge & Kegan Paul, 1964).

16. McGhee, A., *The Patient's Attitude to Nursing Care* (Edinburgh: Livingstone, 1961).

17. Duff, R. S., and Hollingshead, A. B., *Sickness and Society* (New York: Harper & Row, 1968).

18. Skipper, J. K., and Leonard, R. C. (eds.), Social interaction and patient care (Philadelphia: Lippincott, 1965).

19. Titmuss, R. M., Essays on *"The Welfare State"* (London: Unwin, 1963).

20. Frank, D. A., Hospitals and me don't take. A participant observation study of physically ill adolescents. (Thesis, Cambridge, Mass., 1970.)

21. Roth, Information and control.

22. Roth, *Timetables*.

23. Crozier, M. *The Bureaucratic Phenomenon* (Chicago: University of Chicago Press, 1964).

24. Dahl, R., The concept of power. *Behav. Sci.* 2:201–215 (1957).

25. Parsons, T., On the concept of political power; in Bendix and Lipset, *Class, Status and Power* (New York: Free Press, 1966).

26. Davis, *Passage through Crisis.*

27. Roth, Information and control.

28. See Oken, note 12, and Rosen and Tesser, note 13.

29. Moore, W. E., and Tumin, M. M., Some social functions of ignorance. *Amer. Sociol. Rev.* 14:787–795 (1949).

30. Glaser, B., and Strauss, A., *Awareness of Dying* (Chicago: Aldine, 1965).

31. Maslow, A., The need to know and the fear of knowing. *J. Gen. Psychol.* 68:111–125 (1963).

32. Cherry, C., *On Human Communication* (Cambridge: MIT Press, 1966).

38

Lord Edmund-Davies
The Patient's Right to Know the Truth

Reprinted with permission of the author and editors from *Proceedings of the Royal Society of Medicine*, vol. 66, June 1973, pp. 533–536.

We are bidden to discuss the patient's "right." We therefore begin with a word of common currency in the law. But the only rights known to the lawyer are those which the law recognizes by condemning the wrongdoer and compensating the party wronged. There exists no legal right without its corresponding legal duty, for when a man claims something as his right, he claims it as something due to him.

I therefore propose to consider whether a doctor is under any legal duty to tell his patients the truth about their condition. Putting the matter in that broad way, with one solitary exception to be mentioned later, I know of no judicial authority for the general proposition that he is. And I have heard of no case in which a doctor has [been] sued or could have been sued for failing to tell a patient the truth about himself. Equally, I have never heard of the converse case of a doctor being sued because he did tell his patient the truth.

The reason for this dearth of authority is not far to seek. A doctor may be sued by his patient either for breach of contract or for negligence or for both; but he will not be the loser unless the patient proves that he suffered damage as a result of the doctor's breach. This necessity can create difficulties even in straightforward medicolegal cases based on negligent treatment. But to establish that a patient has been injured in person or pocket simply by the withholding of the truth is indeed a daunting task.

Let us, however, assume that the patient can somehow prove that damage flowed from his medical adviser's failure to tell him the truth. He still has to establish that by his omission the doctor failed in his legal duty. Does the duty exist? For the sake of prudence, I hasten to stress that of course, I now speak extrajudicially and, were I hereafter called upon to consider the problem in judicial proceedings, I should regard myself as wholly unfettered by anything I say tonight. Having provided myself with that escape clause, I answer the question by saying: "In general, no such legal duty exists."

Particular circumstances may, however, create a duty. For example, I may make clear to my doctor that I am consulting him about my condition because I contemplate making certain property dispositions, or giving directions to my lawyer dependent on his diagnosis. In this way I may confront my doctor with a cruel dilemma. But, having made my position clear to him, it is up to him to decide whether or not to act as my adviser. If he does, he is legally obliged to tell me the whole truth and nothing but the truth. Accordingly, if he says that in his opinion I am good for quite a few years when he knows in fact that I am in a very bad way, and if, relying on his diagnosis, I take steps which I would not otherwise have taken, he is liable to compensate me or my estate for any consequential damage. And in those special circumstances it would afford him no defence to say that he was doing what he thought was best for me.

Again, if a patient contemplates bringing legal proceedings for personal injuries, the decision whether to sue at all, or, having started the action, whether to pursue it to finality or to settle it, may well turn upon the plaintiff's present condition, as compared with his condition before his accident. His lawyer is there to advise him, but nevertheless the ultimate decision is that of the injured party himself. He therefore has a legal right to be told by his doctor what the true position is, so that he can view the problem in an informed manner. If the doctor conceals the truth from him he breaches his legal duty and would be liable if, as a result, the plaintiff fared worse in his litigation than he would had the truth been told.

There are cases, too, where the doctor or surgeon acts unlawfully unless he does so with the patient's consent. Since there can be no true consent without knowledge, there must in those cases be no withholding the truth, whether the patient has specifically asked for it or not. We must consider that aspect of our topic a little later.

But, apart from such special circumstances, I do not think that the law recognizes any obligation in the doctor to tell the truth. Indeed, it has been known to withhold condemnation even when the doctor told his patient a lie. In a case tried in 1954 (*Hatchard* v. *Black*; see *British Medical Journal* 1954) a doctor diagnosed a toxic goitre; he discussed with the patient the alternative treatments of an operation or a course of drugs. He pointed out that drugs would take a long time.

The patient then chose the operation. As a result, her left recurrent laryngeal nerve was injured and her left vocal cord paralysed. The patient sued both doctor and surgeon. She alleged that the doctor had advised her that the operation involved no risk to her voice and that the surgeon had operated negligently. The doctor denied having told the patient that no risk was involved, but the surgeon admitted that he had told her just that. The case was tried with a jury and this is what Denning, L. J., said to them when he summed up:

What should a doctor tell a patient? (The surgeon) has admitted that on the evening before the operation he told (the plaintiff) that there was no risk to her voice when he knew that there was some slight risk; but that he did it for her own good because it was of vital importance that she not worry. . . . He told a lie, but he did it because in the circumstances it was justifiable. . . . The law does not condemn the doctor when he only does what a wise doctor so placed would do. And none of the doctors called as witnesses have suggested that (the surgeon) was wrong. All agreed that it was a matter for his own judgment. If they do not condemn him, why should you? It is for you to say whether you think that (the doctor) told her that there was no risk whatever, or he may have prevaricated to put her off, as many a good doctor would, rather than worry her. But even if you think he did tell her, is that a cause for censure?

And, having heard that, the jury returned verdicts in favour of both defendants.

I wonder whether your stillness while I quoted those words was due to your respect for a great Judge and Christian gentleman, or whether you have simply been reduced to stunned silence. At least some of you, I feel sure, will take the opposite view. I recall that in a lecture to surgeons Mr. Rodney Smith (1969) said that they must *never* lie, adding:

Although we may edit the truth in the sense that favourable aspects are discussed at more length than the unfavourable, we should answer a patient's questions with the truth and never with a lie. The fact that his surgeon has lied almost invariably at some stage becomes clear to the patient and from then onwards the chances of helping him have gone.

But Lord Denning was dealing with the law, and what the law requires is

no more (and no less) than reasonable care and skill in the treatment of each particular patient. Beyond that, it refuses to generalize, and this for what we regard as good reasons. For just as the medicine a doctor prescribes and the surgeon advises will vary with each patient, so will the extent to which the doctor lifts the veil. At the threshold there arises the question: What patient and what truth? To tell the truth to some may be brutal, despite their entreaties; to withhold it from others may be a massive mistake. In deciding what is the proper course in the particular case lies the art of medicine. And what was a right decision six months ago may be wrong today, for the fearful patient of earlier days may have acquired an inner tranquillity enabling him to bear with fortitude what would formerly have left him terror-stricken.

The position is, of course, particularly difficult if the patient is dying. Whether or not there is any legal duty to warn the patient of this fact, Professor John Hinton is surely right in saying that:

Most doctors will bear in mind how far a person needs to set his affairs in order, when considering what they should tell a dying patient. Imparting advice to a man that it might be a wise precaution to tidy up business arrangements serves more than that single function. Conveyed with tact, it is a hint that an ill man can discuss further with his doctor, if he is of a mind to know more, or it is advice he can just accept at its face value (Hinton 1967).

But *one* legal right in relation to truth the patient most assuredly possesses. It is that his medical adviser will take all proper steps to learn for himself what the truth is about his patient. This, at least, he must do, whether or not he then proceeds to impart it; and if he fails to do it he is both morally wrong and legally liable for any harm which befalls the patient as a result.

Let me now say a few words about the one case I know of where in this country a doctor was held legally liable for failing to tell his patient the truth (*Gerber* v. *Pines*, 1935, 79 Sol. J. 13). In the course of a hypodermic injection for rheumatism the needle broke and part remained in the patient's body. The doctor was unable to get it out and it remained there until removed by operation five days later. In an action brought by the patient, Mr. Justice du

Parcq held that no lack of skill had been established, but he said that the other question to be decided was whether the doctor should have told the patient at once what had happened. The Judge said that, though there were exceptions, as a general rule a patient in whose body a doctor knew he had left some foreign substance was entitled to be told at once. In the particular case he held that there was a breach of duty amounting to negligence in not at once informing the plaintiff or her husband on the day of the accident what had happened. But the Judge considered that in the circumstances the damages must be very small and he awarded the plaintiff five guineas.

That decision is, as I have said, a lone ranger in our law. And in Ireland they declined to follow it in another broken needle case (*Daniels* v. *Heskin*, 1953, Ir.L.T.189). Mr. Justice Kingsmill-Moore there said:

I cannot admit any abstract duty to tell patients what is the matter with them or, to particularize, to say that a needle has been left in their tissue. All depends on the circumstances, the character of the patient, her health . . . the nature of the tissue in which the needle is embedded, the possibility of subsequent infection or other danger, the arrangements which are being made for future observation and care, and innumerable other considerations.

There remain to be dealt with those cases where the lawyer joins with the priest in holding that truth must out, although according to Holy Writ, "He that hath knowledge spareth his words" (Proverbs xvii.27). These cases have a common link. They are cases in which the plaintiff's consent is necessary before a proposed course of medical or surgical treatment is embarked upon. In such circumstances he must be adequately informed of what is involved, for if the truth is withheld the layman is in no proper position to give his consent. What the doctor must tell him will vary with the circumstances, but a distinguished Australian doctor put the matter with helpful clarity. He said:

When the patient's condition is diagnosed, he needs to be told three things, in words that he can understand. He needs to be told what is wrong with him, what it may possibly mean in the future, and what medical science has

to offer him. If these three things are advanced carefully, the patient can make some reasonable arrangements and may also bring his usual defences to the situation at whatever level he finds necessary (Elland 1968).

A surgical operation is lawful only with the consent of the person operated upon, otherwise the surgeon risks being sued for assault. Indeed, one legal writer expresses the view that he might open himself to a *criminal* charge of assault occasioning actual bodily harm (Clerk & Lindsell on Torts, 12th edn, para. 88), but I must not be taken necessarily to accept the correctness of that alarming statement. Even if the patient consents to an exploratory operation, the surgeon has no defence if he performs a major one, except in an unforeseeable emergency requiring an immediate decision in order to save life or prevent grave injury to health. And the necessity for consent is not in principle confined to surgical operations. It extends to every other form of medical treatment, for it is technically an assault even to administer a drug secretly and against the patient's wishes.[1] But there are few reported cases in this country, owing to the wise practice of surgeons here to demand of their patients written authorization of any necessary treatment.

In transplant cases the donor is to be regarded as one of the two patients involved—though never, one hopes, of the same surgeon. However eager the donor is to play out his self-sacrificial role, the surgeon is under a legal duty to make clear to him the risks involved, both in the operation itself and in the resultant impairment of his corpus. He may not want the truth, but in this case the truth must be forced upon him. A man may declare himself ready to die for another, but the surgeon must never take him at his word. For in general, as Lord Devlin (1962) has said, "The Good Samaritan is a character unesteemed in English law." And the patient must be capable of comprehending the truth when it is told him. If mentally debilitated, his consent is worthless. And a risk is also involved if the would-be donor is a minor.

Then what of patients who are in no fit condition to comprehend the truth even were it told them, and who are therefore incapable of giving or withholding their consent? What, for example, is to be done in a dire emergency

such as calls for an organ transplant to the badly injured? I know of no reported decision in this country, but I think I do know what would happen if a surgeon operated with proper skill upon such a patient who later sued him for assault simply because he had not consented to become a transplant donee. I predict that the patient would lose, though I decline to prophesy tonight what the precise *ratio decidendi* would be. For the present I am content to adopt the words of the Canadian Chief Justice who said:

I think it is better . . . to put consent altogether out of the case where a great emergency which could not be anticipated arises, and to rule that it is the surgeon's duty to act in order to save the life or preserve the health of the patient; and that in the honest execution of that duty he should not be exposed to legal liability (Chisholm, C. J., in *Marshall* v. *Curry*, 1933, 3 D.L.R. 260).

And there I must stop. But not in the arid terms of a lawyer. Let me instead leave you with the memorable words of an American physician (Henderson 1935). Writing on the issue of truth, he said:

Far older than the precept, "the truth, the whole truth, and nothing but the truth," is another that originates within our profession, that has always been the guide of the best physicians, and, if I may venture a prophecy, will always remain so. So far as possible, "do no harm." You can do harm by the process that is quaintly called telling the truth. You can do harm by lying. . . . It will arise also from what you say and what you fail to say. But try to do as little harm as possible, not only in treatment with drugs, or with the knife, but also in treatment with words, with the expression of your sentiments and emotions. Try at all times to act upon the patient so as to modify his sentiments to his own advantage, and remember that, to this end, nothing is more effective than arousing in him the belief that you are concerned wholeheartedly and exclusively for *his* welfare.

If a doctor fits his actions to these words, his patient can have no cause for complaint and the doctor need fear neither the law nor his own conscience, whatever be the truth told or withheld.

Note

1. *See* a case reported in the *British Medical Journal* (1949). But contrast the Canadian decision in *Male* v. *Hopmans* (1967) 64 D.L.R. (2d) 105, where a patient with an

injured knee gave his consent to general treatment for it. The doctor, fearing infection or even fatal results, decided without first obtaining the patient's specific consent to use a drug with known possible side-effects. He failed to carry out the recommended tests to discover whether such side-effects were happening, and the patient in fact suffered immediately from them. It was held that, having obtained incipient consent to general treatment, the doctor had used his discretion properly in deciding to use the drug without first obtaining the patient's specific consent, but was negligent in omitting the recommended known tests.

References

British Medical Journal (1949)i, 1100.

British Medical Journal (1954)ii, 106.

Devlin, Lord, *Samples of Lawmaking* (Oxford, 1962), p. 90.

Elland, J. *Medical Journal of Australia* (1968)i, 979.

Henderson, L. J. *New England Journal of Medicine* #112 (1935), 819.

Hinton, J. *Dying* (Penguin Books, Harmonsworth, 1967), p. 127.

Smith, R. *Journal of the Royal College of Surgeons of Edinburgh* #15 (1969), 63.

39

Cicely M. S. Saunders
Telling Patients

Reprinted with permission of the editor from *District Nursing* (now *Queens Nursing Journal*), September 1965, pp. 149–150, 154.

Every patient needs an explanation of his illness that will be understandable and convincing to him if he is to co-operate in his treatment or be relieved of the burden of unknown fears. This is true whether it is a question of giving a diagnosis in a hopeful situation or of confirming a poor prognosis.

The fact that a patient does not ask does not mean that he has no questions. One visit or one talk is rarely enough. It is only by waiting and listening that we can gain an idea of what we should be saying. Silences and gaps are often more revealing than words as we try to learn what a patient is facing as he travels along the constantly changing journey of his illness and his thoughts about it. The help he needs at each stage may be quite different. The real question is perhaps best expressed simply as "What do you let your patients tell you?"

The alternatives are not merely silence, bland denial, or stark fatal truth. There are many different truths just as there are many ways of imparting them. We have to try and learn to give the one the individual needs at that moment in the simplest and kindest way we can offer it, leaving him the choice to take it or leave it as he wishes. One patient may be anxiously preventing us from assaulting him with information that he is not able or willing to handle; while another has already come to terms with a hopeless prognosis but needs reassurance to dispel inaccurate and often horrible apprehensions. So much of the communication will be without words or given indirectly. This is true of all real meeting with people but especially true with those who are facing, knowingly or not, difficult or threatening situations. It is also particularly true of the very ill.

The main argument against a policy of deliberate, invariable denial of unpleasant facts is that it makes such communication extremely difficult, if not impossible. Once the possibility of talking frankly with a patient has been admitted it does not mean that this will always take place but the whole atmosphere is changed. We are then free to wait quietly for clues from each patient, seeing them as individuals from whom we can expect intelligence, courage and individual decisions. They will feel secure enough to give us these clues when they wish. Such a process is described in the story that follows.

Mrs. D. was forty-two when she was admitted with terminal ovarian cancer. This had been diagnosed first as laparotomy six months previously when it was already widespread. She had an exceedingly devoted husband and two children, twelve and nine years old. She had not been told either her diagnosis or prognosis and her husband said that he did not know how much she really knew.

She was a friendly person and was quickly on easy terms with everyone in the ward but she had a courteous reserve which made it impossible to be certain what she was thinking about herself or her illness. She kept her own counsel and although I noted ten days after her admission "She is realising a little, I think," this was from her attitude rather than from any words. She needed frequent examinations and discussions to enable us to maintain control over increased pain and vomiting, so we knew each other quite well and, like all the ward staff, I enjoyed spending time with her.

Even so it was nearly two months before she suddenly said to me in a new tone of voice which made me pull the curtain round to ensure privacy,

"Doctor, where did all this begin?"

"It began in an ovary."

"That's bad, isn't it?"

"Sometimes it is."

She waited in silence for a moment and then said, "It's my mother I'm sorry for, my sister died of the same thing two years ago."

After another pause she went on, "What I really wanted to ask you, doctor . . . is it wrong for me to let my children go on visiting me now that I am getting so thin?"

"While you are smiling and talking I am sure that is what your children will see and when you don't feel like it . . . then I don't think your husband will bring them."

She accepted this and then went on talking, obviously ready to do so at last. Gradually it came out that she had heard some doctors talking at the end of her bed after her operation and had known her diagnosis and prognosis from then on. She went on "I haven't been able to discuss it with my husband and I'm so afraid that it will be very hard for him when he realises that

I have been carrying this alone all this time."

"Love doesn't need words. I think you will find that you have really been sharing it together and you will just find yourselves talking about it one day." Next day this happened and when Mr. D. came out afterwards to Sister he wept but was deeply relieved that they had shared in words at last.

Mrs. D. lived another nine days after this. She told me that during the past months it had somehow come to be "all right" and that as she had asked God for help each day it had always been possible to get through just that one day. Gradually the parting from her family, that she had thought she could not face, had somehow become possible and even quiet. Her simply expressed faith meant a great deal to her but here too she seemed best able to find what she needed within herself and she did not wish to see her Presbyterian minister again at this stage. She kept her usual outward calm which expressed an inner serenity of unusual depth and reality.

I have a photograph taken a week before her death which shows this and also shows that she was able to read a book with concentrated attention in spite of the fairly large doses of diamorphine and promazine she needed to control physical distress. This was taken with her ready permission to use it for lectures and to tell her story to anyone who might be helped by it. She died very peacefully in an atmosphere of readiness and fulfilment. I think that each of us grieved for her in a personal way but I know that our main feeling was one of great admiration. She had done all she could to help her family to accept her death with as much hope and peace as she had found herself and I believe that her manner through her whole illness and the sharing with her husband at the end must still be a strength to them.

She Overheard

Mrs. D. came to know her diagnosis by overhearing a discussion. If we consider that no patient can bear such knowledge, how do we feel about those who discover it in such ways, unable because officially they do not "know" to hear of good hopes of cure

or palliation, of the unlikelihood of distress for them or of possibilities of help should it occur? No wonder that many retreat into open denial or hidden despair or both. The patient quoted at the head of this article is not unique in her knowledge and in the way she gained it. Silence can tell as much or more than words. The isolation in which she faced it is also all too common.

A very ill patient can feel desperately lonely in a ward, but loneliness may be just as acute for the patient at home. The family, having rushed round at the first news, now seems to avoid him and to be unable to talk of anything but superficialities or obviously empty reassurances. At times they may make his increasing weakness, of which he is all too conscious, even more of a burden by their well-meant encouragement. Their anxiety can make a real vacuum round him.

Geoffrey Gorer[1] noted that nineteen patients in his survey who had died of cancer had without exception been kept in ignorance. He found much regret and bitterness about this among the bereaved and thought that good marriages had been reduced to "unkindness and falsity" by this deception. On the other side, Hinton[2] found that the great majority of 102 dying patients in a general ward knew that death was more than likely although they had not been "told." These two facts look very disturbing when put together, for the truth from which the patient is being "protected" is the truth with which he is being forced to live in isolation.

I am not suggesting that there should be any universal policy, certainly not one of routine "telling" but only that there seems to be some need for rethinking. Nurses may sometimes be able to give information about a patient's attitude to his doctor, who may well not know him as well as they do. Both families and nurses can also go a long way in relieving this loneliness without using direct words at all.

Listen

Most patients are far more eager that we should know what they think than that we should tell them what we think. They often need little encouragement to help them unburden themselves and there is always something to be done to express our interest and concern. To persevere with the practical is both a way to relieve an intolerable grief and to communicate awareness of it. Talk of symptoms can indeed be a way to avoid more difficult questions but can also be carried on in such a way as to bring reassurance on deeper levels. By such means a patient can be helped into that feeling of security that will enable him to face the future, whatever it may hold.

Two months of concentrating on the prevention of all the physical distress of Mrs. D's illness had produced an atmosphere in which she first handled her own thoughts and then voiced the question to which she needed an answer. Concern for a person and his symptoms, not obvious pity or indulgence (attitudes very enfeebling to both parties), can give him the feeling of warm acceptance we all need if we are to feel secure.

In such a setting people come to the place where they know they are free to talk as and when they are ready. When they are, they may seem to hold two quite incompatible views of their illness or to change from day to day. Often they will wait until long after the processes of illness themselves have revealed to them what is happening (and so often it is the loss of weight that seems to bring this home to them). They may only talk when they have some specific question such as Mrs. D's about her family. Other questions are the following, "Will it be very long? Will I get pain? Will it be in my sleep? What will it be like at the end?" Fear may be drained out of these questions even as they are voiced but we can also be reassuring about each one of them or answer them indirectly even before they are asked. If we are not there to listen how much anguish may go unrelieved?

We learn to come to terms with the fact of death ourselves from such people as Mrs. D. If we fail to do so we will not be able to hand on that essential feeling of security to our patients and to their families, often the more frightened of the two. They have most likely never thought of the achievements that can make this part of a life of such memorable importance, they do not know that the final coming of death to a patient with terminal cancer can and should be immensely quiet and peaceful even when the illness has been very different. They do not know the calmness with which the approach of death is often watched by the very ill or the very old. We can lift much of their apprehension by our own confidence about these things. We learn such confidence and an assurance that "all manner of things shall be well" from our patients themselves.

A patient needs the chance to handle his experiences in a way that will make them significant or at least bearable to him and it is he who should decide how he will do this. We cannot impose our own beliefs upon him but if we believe that there is a meaning, our silent steadiness will help him find his own way through. This is not a situation for dogmatic statements or general rules. Trust and faith in life and death are not two different attitudes but different aspects of the same attitude and he who appears to have little conscious knowledge of death's imminence may be well prepared. The body has a wisdom of its own and will help the strong instinct to fight for life to change into an active kind of acceptance that may never be expressed in words. In this, and in many other things, we cannot hurry the dying but we must let them teach us.

Notes

1. Hinton, J. M. (1963), The Physical and Mental Distress of the Dying. *Quart. J. Med.*, 32, 1.

2. Gorer, Geoffrey (1965), *Death, Grief and Mourning in Contemporary Britain*. Cresset Press, London.

40

Alan Leslie
Ethics and Practice of Placebo Therapy

Reprinted with permission of author and publisher from the *American Journal of Medicine*, vol. 16, 1954, pp. 854–862.

Medicine, often called the healing art, has in the course of events and especially during recent years made striking scientific advances. The art of medicine, in contrast to the science of medicine, was highly developed long ago and consequently has had less room for advancement. The early maturity of this important facet of the practice of medicine was natural enough since prior to the advent of scientific medicine the doctor had a small specific armamentarium and, consciously or not, depended on art for many of his cures. Fortunately for him, patients usually recovered despite such medicaments as the flesh of vipers, the spermatic fluid of frogs, horns of deer, animal excretions, holy oil and many other colorful and often disgusting substances of mystical attributes. These substances could have mitigated suffering only by virtue of their placebo effects.

The placebo is as potent today as it was during medical antiquity. Witness the success of witch doctors and other present day practitioners of bizarre forms of healing art who add little more than suggestion to Nature's potent healing processes. Since these "doctors" are usually unaware that their devices are essentially without intrinsic therapeutic value, they have faith in their methods, which results in a reinforcing of the suggestion with which they treat their followers.

Because medicine has been so concerned with its scientific growth too little attention has been paid to advancing the art of medicine, to which therapy with placebos belongs, and consequently knowledge of the use of placebos has not progressed significantly. Nevertheless, placebos are employed by most physicians who treat patients. The paucity of medical writing on the subject, noted by Pepper[1] in 1945, constitutes a conspicuous absence particularly if, as concluded by Findley,[2] the placebo is the most important therapeutic weapon in the hands of even the modern physician. This anomalous state of affairs is at last being corrected. An excellent Cornell Conference on Therapy[3] in which placebos were discussed was published in transcription form in 1947 and significant scientific studies of placebos have been reported by Wolf and his associates.[4-6]

It is surprising that in the light of their importance and everyday use placebos have until so recently been all but neglected in medical curricula and writings. The reasons for this seemingly protracted indifference to so fascinating a topic as the placebo can only be conjectural. If we assume that early healers knew naught of placebos as such (a possibly unjustified assumption), and by consequence did not write about them, why then do we have such a paucity of writings on the subject from latter day medical authors who should be fully aware of the nature of placebos? There is an ethical consideration, current even today, with sharp divergence of opinion concerning the use of the placebo. This in itself should have led to a plethora of spirited writing pro and con but surprisingly has not. Weiss and English[7] wrote, "The physician who prescribes placebos, in whatever form, is not consciously dishonest." The implication that the physician is in any wise dishonest is a serious one but probably not the authors' intent. They also noted, "The most frequent method of psychotherapy is the giving of placebos," combined with assurance. As noted by Hyman,[8] in view of the possible failure of psychotherapy the addition of suggestion to placebo medication is not without danger. It is difficult to see how placebos, because of their very nature, can act independently of suggestion. Perhaps it is merely a matter of degree. Hyman's approach to the ethics of the question appears rational in his observation that, although such methods have been attacked by dwellers in ivory towers, they serve a beneficial role in the hands of the modern physician but should be no more than a temporary expedient. I, with many others, believe that the prime roles of the placebo are in the adjuvant therapy of those cases of constitutional disease in which psychic factors play an important contributory part and in research.

Pepper[1] concerned himself at some length with the etymology and definition of the word, "placebo." He called it a "humble humbug" and stated that it must be a "medicine without any pharmacologic action whatever." It is perhaps a humble humbug which, however, requires consummate skill in its administration. But can an effective placebo be without measurable effect?

Wolf[4] and Wolf and Wolff[5] demonstrated measurable changes at end-organs after the administration of placebo drugs. What sets off the neurohumoral mechanism presumably responsible for these changes? It would seem that suggestion is the *sine qua non* of placebo therapy, the effectiveness of the placebo being directly proportional to the degree of associated suggestion and receptivity of the patient. Conversely, as also shown by Wolf and Wolff,[5] the suggestible patient under-reacts to large doses of a potent drug when under the impression that he is receiving a "placebo." Even noxious effects have been observed after placebo administration.[6] Wolf's subjects reported drowsiness, anorexia, nausea, palpitation, weakness and epigastric pain. Toxic manifestations, including a skin rash, diarrhea, urticaria and angioneurotic edema were objective phenomena illustrating how extremely potent the factor of suggestion can be.

The American Illustrated Medical Dictionary[9] defines placebo as "an inactive substance or preparation, formerly given to please or gratify a patient, now also used in controlled studies to determine the efficacy of medicinal substances." Webster[10] says that it is a "medicine or preparation, esp. an inactive one, given merely to satisfy a patient." These definitions are still less than satisfactory but both include the important limitation to administered, apparently medicinal substances, and exclude psychotherapeutic physical procedures. In other words, although all placebos are psychotherapy, the converse is manifestly not so. The former definition includes one important use of placebos but is still too limited. In the light of the more modern concept of placebos our definition must be extended, and might be stated somewhat as follows: A placebo is a medicine or preparation which has no inherent pertinent pharmacologic activity but which is effective only by virtue of the factor of suggestion attendant upon its administration. The substance may be ingested, injected, inserted, inhaled or applied.

Why do the dwellers in ivory towers decry the use of placebos, if indeed they do? Their opposition appears to stem from a personal philosophy rather than from any objective consideration of carefully documented scientific data. If this is so the controversy cannot be regarded as one of different interpretations placed on freely available scientific evidence but rather as one of differing subjective moralities. This is an unacceptable state of affairs. We admit freely that the caliber of medical practice is not standardized but is variable and ever changing in the direction of improvement. On the other hand, there has long been a high standard of morality among physicians. The Hippocratic Oath embodies it. In the Book of Ecclesiasticus the reader is told to "Honour a physician . . . for of the most high cometh healing."

Physicians of high principles may have misgivings over giving placebos because their use entails the practice of deception on a patient. Although several physicians with whom I have discussed this point honestly believe that the use of placebos is not deception but merely one form of psychotherapy, I am convinced that this opinion could not have been attained without rationalization. My thesis acknowledges that placebo therapy entails deception, since the patient is led to believe that he has been given a substance of inherent therapeutic value. The abiding question is whether or not such a practice of deception is justifiable on ethical grounds. There is a fine line of distinction between the words, deception and deceit. They are not entirely synonymous since deceit implies blameworthiness whereas deception does not necessarily do so. For example, a sleight-of-hand entertainer practices deception on his audience but only for their amusement, certainly a laudable activity. Can an outright lie be justified by circumstance? As members of society we have been taught that to lie is wrong, but this teaching is not necessarily absolute. For example, if a dangerous paranoiac carrying a gun asks the whereabouts of his fancied persecutor, it is propitious and right to misdirect him.

The most pointed occasion when the physician must decide whether or not to lie is in the case of the patient with incurable cancer. As individuals, physicians are reluctant to lie but as physicians we must maintain an elasticity of attitude. Plato,[11] who dwelt at some length on the deportment of

physicians, wrote, "A lie is useful only as a medicine to men. The use of such medicines should be confined to physicians." Parkinson[12] embodied a strong defense of the physician's integrity in his succinct observation, "The facts are that in clinical science there is devotion to truth and conformity to scientific standards as scrupulous as anywhere, but in practising the art truth has often to be softened." Incidentally, as Henderson[13] suggested, what the doctor believes to be true sometimes isn't; the patient may thereby be misinformed, albeit unwittingly on the part of the doctor. Also according to Henderson, what the doctor actually says is not in itself important, but rather what the patient comprehends and what it does to him. A physician can usually evade a possibly harmful truth and still satisfy his patient. Such an evasion is on practical grounds preferable to an unequivocal lie, because a lie can be uncovered, and if this should happen the physician will lose the patient's confidence and respect. If the patient is insistent, there is of course no alternative to the truth. Hippocrates, whose precepts[14] are widely considered to be as good today as they were nearly 2,500 years ago, wrote as follows: "Naught should be betrayed to the patient of what may happen or of what may eventually threaten him, because many patients have been driven in this way to extreme measures." In general, honesty is the best policy, subject to modification according to circumstances. This question in the case of incurable cancer is still moot, and being tangential to the present discussion will not be considered further.

Returning to the consideration of deception as applied in medical practice, I will state that I believe deception is completely moral when it is used for the welfare of the patient. If this is admitted, who then is to decide what constitutes the patient's welfare? Omniscience would be an attribute desirable in any individual responsible for the welfare of another. Being human, however, the physician lacks this quality, but, by the very nature of his position, is the best arbiter of this question when it concerns a patient. Therefore, when the patient's welfare dictates the use of a placebo there can be no detrimental reflection on the physician

who prescribes it. In fact, the physician who in an appropriate situation refuses to order a placebo, implying in effect that, "I can't help you because there is no medicine for your disease," is cruel and is surely not to be praised for his morality. If, in order to avoid giving a placebo, he is so misguided as to prescribe a potent medicament which is not specifically indicated, his position is completely without justification. Neither is it necessary in such a case for the physician to prescribe an "impure" placebo, which in contradistinction to a "pure" placebo contains a substance of some inherent pharmacologic activity not relevant to the immediate problem in order to relieve a tacit feeling of guilt at resorting to placebo therapy. Whether the placebo is pure or impure is of no consequence. What is important is the humane and understanding use of the placebo itself.

It is poor practice for the physician to prescribe an impure placebo by virtue of the loose reasoning that the preparation can do no harm and may do some good. Vitamin therapy without specific indication, for example, may actually be good placebo therapy because of the conditioning of the general public to the thought that vitamins have superlative esoteric medicinal properties. Unfortunately, but not uncommonly, the physician himself becomes deluded. After prescribing substances as placebos and observing dramatic (but none the less psychotherapeutic) improvement, he may after repeated successes begin to think, "Maybe we have something here, after all." Here lies danger, for although by his belief in the potency of his one-time placebo the physician unconsciously reinforces its psychotherapeutic value, the way may be cleared for such impotent therapy to be prescribed in situations calling for specific and potent medicine.

Physicians are also subject to a form of mass delusion, which is rarely more than transitory. Our credulity is importuned and exploited by manufacturers of drugs and therapeutic products who enthusiastically bombard us with glowing reports on new remedies. The number of substances which have gone from popularity to oblivion attests to their placebo nature and illustrates the need for the critical evaluation of new agents.

Before proceeding to delineate situations in which deception in the form of placebo therapy is indicated, it can be stated almost categorically that it is impossible to divorce the component of suggestion, in either favorable or unfavorable direction, from the final therapeutic effect even when avowedly potent substances are administered. The final therapeutic effect is the resultant of the inherent effect of the drug and the effect of suggestion attendant on its administration. By the same token, the regularly observed variation in the effect of any given drug in any individual may depend on the effectiveness of the factor of associated suggestion, conditioned by such variables as the immediate receptivity of the patient, the technic of administration and the environment.

Indications

There are circumstances in which placebos constitute the therapy of choice. In the management of some patients who need support for strong dependency feelings, medication, which is ever the symbol of the doctor, may well have its purpose served by a placebo if no more specific effect is desired. In other circumstances placebos can be important adjuvants to more specific therapy and in fact placebo effects are often gratuitous attributes of specific therapy.

Clearly, the placebo is a research tool of prime importance. There is no substitute for the placebo in the "double-blind" evaluation of new drugs. The investigator in such an experiment is naturally aware that a calculated deception is being practiced upon his subject. The subject also may be aware of the game being played; at the discretion of the investigator, however, such information may be withheld. Of real importance in insuring the objectivity of the study is keeping both subject and investigator "blind" so that neither knows whether at any given moment the drug under study or the placebo control is being given. This will minimize the factor of suggestion, either subjective on the part of the patient or unconsciously interjected by the investigator.

Another clear indication for placebo therapy occurs in patients who have

received sedatives or narcotics in whom the indication for these drugs no longer exists. Following surgery most people require narcotics for variable durations for the control of pain. During periods of stress many people require sedation to relieve anxiety by day and to induce sleep at night. It is quite easy for patients to become dependent on, if not addicted to, these agents. They continue to call for them, perhaps as a mild withdrawal manifestation. At this stage the substitution of a placebo for a short time is usually all that is necessary for the transition to no medicine.

In incurable neoplastic disease there can be no objection to the administration of sufficient sedative and narcotic medication to control all pain and apprehension. There is, nevertheless, the drawback of undesirable associated pharmacologic effects such as constipation and respiratory depression. Since it is possible to raise the pain threshold of most individuals by the use of placebos, it would seem likely that the judicious interpolation of placebos would decrease the narcotic-sedative requirements. The over-all comfort of the patient would thereby be enhanced.

Occasionally when a doctor sees a patient for the first time he finds that the patient has been taking a conglomerate assortment of drugs which have confused the picture by cumulative or additive effects. The dependency of such a patient on his medicines can be transferred to a placebo, so that these confusing, cumulative or additive effects may be dissipated. It thus becomes possible to make a more rational evaluation of the problem which can then be treated directly and more specifically. Oberndorf[15] reported a typical case in point. An asthmatic woman who was nearly moribund when first seen had, as is so frequent in individuals with asthma, received a superabundance of medication. Placebos were substituted for epinephrine and sedatives, with salutary effects on the course of the illness.

Some people are temperamentally impatient and demand results before they normally would be forthcoming. Occasionally, during a period of diagnostic observation or testing, a placebo will provide a gentle sop to their impatience and keep them under control while the important business is being

conducted. The office administration of a placebo injection can serve as the reason to bring a patient for regular, more specific psychotherapy.

Now let us examine some situations in which the indications for the use of placebos are perhaps less clear. The management of chronic disease taxes the imagination of the most experienced clinician. Patients with crippling arthritis, paraplegia, hemiplegia, chronic cardiac or pulmonary dyspnea all require prolonged medical attendance. Occasionally, in addition to specific medication an analgesic or sedative drug may be required. Such a drug should not be administered for indefinite periods without interruption because there is a remarkably quick conditioning of patients to the sedative or analgesic effect, the associated psychic effect, or a combination of the two. Unless these drugs are given for strictly limited periods, such chronically ill individuals, like the postoperative patient, may become dependent on them. This should not be permitted because of the tolerance developed with consequently increased requirements, as well as undesirable associated pharmacologic effects. Placebos may be helpful in the transition to the acceptable discontinuation of the drug. But we must beware of another real pitfall, which is the development, by conditioning, of dependency on the placebo itself. Whether or not this is undesirable may be argued but in general it is preferable that the patient be well enough adjusted to his disease so he need not depend even on a placebo. From another but practical point of view, in our understaffed institutions for the care of the chronically ill the time needed for the administration of placebos might interfere with more urgent nursing activities. Special situations require special consideration. I am thinking of a sixty year old man with a cardiac aneurysm which developed following a coronary occlusion. After some years of auricular fibrillation and bare maintenance of compensation at absolute rest this man had an aortic saddle embolization which led to gangrene and required amputation of first one then the other leg. During active treatment he received narcotics for which placebo injections were later substituted. Severe unremitting phantom limb pain was unrelieved by local measures and the neurosurgeon could offer only radical neurosurgery, which the patient declined. This man continued to take two daily injections of sterile saline solution, which satisfied him. He had become so dependent on them that he experienced great pain when they were omitted. Because of this man's underlying chronic disability it was decided to continue the placebos until such time as he might voluntarily relinquish them.

There is no unanimity of opinion among psychiatrists about the use of placebos in psychiatry. Some reject them altogether while others believe that they are invaluable in certain instances. In the section on the psychoneuroses in a standard textbook of medicine Rennie[16] states that, "Even the placebo, which has no place in psychiatry, can work miracles." In reference to the psychoses, Whitehorn[17] states that, "Placebo medication has a legitimate diagnostic purpose, but the use of placebos as a regular therapy is of dubious propriety and is unjustified when good psychotherapy is available." Alvarez[18] advises taking away a diagnostic placebo before commencing psychotherapy. Weiss and English[7] stated that the answer to the problem of psychogenic illness is correct diagnosis and expressive psychotherapy rather than suppressive psychotherapy, as exemplified by the use of placebos. This might be interpreted as a disavowal of the use of placebos in psychogenic disease, in agreement with one group of psychiatrists. No one will question the importance of correct diagnosis and it is true that the use of placebos is not ideal in many instances of psychogenic disease. It must be remembered, however, that even with a correct diagnosis to to work from, it is for manifold reasons frequently impossible to offer a patient the ideal of expressive psychotherapy. If suppressive psychotherapy offers relief but no cure to some of these patients, should it be denied them? If circumstance precludes cure a compromise is obligatory, if without it the idealist turns his back on the reality of a patient seeking relief. I hesitate to enter this controversy and prefer to take a sideline position, hoping meanwhile that our psychiatrist colleagues will debate the technical aspects of the

issue. Nevertheless, there is a place for an expression of opinion by the general physician, and as Shaw[19] cautioned in 1936, we must avoid overemphasis of either empiricism or rationalism in medicine. Both can contribute to the balanced judgment which will accrue to the patient's benefit. This principle should apply equally well in psychiatry as it does in medicine, if indeed the two fields can be separated.

Whether or not placebos have a role in the therapy of psychotic patients when the psychosis is active, I will also leave for the psychiatrists to decide but I suspect that placebos will be ineffectual and harmless. In the psychoneuroses and occasionally in psychoses in remission, placebos may be of value. Watts and Wilbur[20] in discussing the treatment of functional disorders notice that the psychotherapeutic effect of drugs or placebos may be great. If we agree, as I believe we should, that much good can be accomplished and little harm result from properly administered placebo therapy, we will be acting for the welfare of the patient which, after all, is our primary objective. Naturally, there must be a good diagnostic evaluation before placebo therapy is selected.

The prolonged use of the placebo merely to pacify a patient whose problem is not thoroughly understood cannot be condemned too harshly. Diagnosis often requires observation and repeated examination. The physician who relaxes his diagnostic efforts because the patient appears to respond to a placebo may miss the opportunity to treat a remediable condition. Properly used, the placebo, by allaying fear and providing hope, may help a patient adjust to a conflict situation that cannot be resolved. Since placebos may lose their potency unless periodic reinforcing psychotherapy is forthcoming, the physician must be prepared to provide skillful, long-range care.

The symptoms associated with relatively acute organic disease are frequently modified by a greater or lesser degree of psychogenic overlay. This ordinarily does not call for separate handling, since the inseparable beneficial psychic effects of potent medication would also be operative. On occasion, however, it may be desirable to

employ some psychotherapeutic potentiation by the use of an appropriate placebo. With a self-limited indication this may be worthwhile adjuvant therapy. For instance, the use of a "tonic," such as the elixir of iron, quinine and strychnine, may strengthen a patient convalescing from a febrile or wasting illness if, presumably through a placebo effect, it convinces him that he is hungry and leads to a desirably high calorie intake. Intermittent use of this sort of placebo has a place in the care of the chronically ill person if the patient is not allowed to become dependent and then later disillusioned.

The use of the placebo as a diagnostic tool has been a subject of considerable debate. There is no question about the diagnostic value of specific therapeutic tests but in light of Wolf and Wolff's observations of measurable physiologic effects of placebos, opinions concerning the diagnostic value of therapeutic testing with placebos must be modified. Unless responses to placebos used diagnostically are carefully evaluated, serious errors will be made. The absence of response to a placebo favors an organic basis for complaints but positive responses may well be devoid of diagnostic significance and not indicative of psychogenic disease.

In principle, therefore, it would appear that placebos properly used have a limited role in diagnosis and an important one in the management of somatic disease and the psychoneuroses at any time that the affective state of the patient may be beneficially conditioned by this form of suggestion.

No doubt there are indications for placebo therapy which have not been specifically considered herein. If so, I implore the indulgence of the critical reader. One repeated word of caution: Placebo therapy should not be ordered unless the physician has examined the indications even more carefully than if he were about to order specific therapy.

Technic

In our approach to technics of administration we will assume that we have demonstrated that placebo therapy is justified and has fairly specific indications. The discussion will be simpler if we limit ourselves to our conception of placebo, which predicates that placebos may be ingested, inserted, injected, inhaled or applied. Here there is a wide latitude for individuality of methods so I will not attempt to do more than offer a few illustrative examples, as well as some general "do's and don'ts."

Ingested medicines are in the form of liquids, tablets, capsules, pills or powders. Except for gastric antacids, and to a certain extent even here, powders are almost obsolete. Since pills offer no particular advantage over tablets and capsules, which are both easier to swallow and to manufacture, these, too, are being used infrequently. This leaves tablets, capsules and liquids as the oral medications in everyday use. It is only fitting that oral placebos should also be in these forms.

People tend to be skeptical of medications which do not look, taste or smell like "medicine." We have come to associate the warm red-yellow-brown colors with liquids for oral use and the colors blue and green with poisonous or external-use-only liquids. This, of course, is not absolute but, other things being equal, our liquid placebo should be red, yellow or brown rather than blue or green.

The addition of red coloring agents to many liquid medicines is a long-standing, widespread, innocent practice which, incidentally, is officially sanctioned by the U.S.P. and the N.F. in such commonly prescribed preparations as the elixir of phenobarbital which contains 1 per cent of amaranth solution, a red dye, and the alkaline aromatic solution which contains the same dye in 1.4 per cent concentration. Similarly, a liquid placebo can be given an appropriate taste. Most people over the age of thirty remember how bad tasting medicine used to be. Cod liver oil and the expectorants containing ammonium chloride are two which come quickly to mind. The tinctures of valerian and asafetida were bitter, and in fact were standard placebo medications. Bitterness, rather than ordinary nastiness, carries a strong placebo effect. Modern pharmacies may not stock the old stand-bys but will be pleased to prepare 0.1 per cent solutions of sodium dehydrocholate which, because of its current use in the determination of circulation time, is available everywhere. This may be colored red, if desired, with something like

amaranth solution or tincture of cudbear.

When we decide to prescribe a placebo capsule we need not be concerned over the taste, since gelatin capsules are considered to be tasteless. Color, however, is important. A capsule colored red, blue or yellow suggests specific attributes which a transparent, colorless capsule containing a white powder might seem to lack. Furthermore, when it is a question of weaning a patient from barbiturate medication it is relatively simple to substitute a starch or lactose capsule for a barbiturate capsule of identical appearance.

Size of medication should be a consideration. Tiny or oversize tablets and capsules may be more impressive than average sized ones, the tiny one suggesting great strength, the jumbo one impressing by its heroic size. Aspirin, although a valuable drug, by being available without prescription has come to be regarded by the public as only a mild remedy. A tablet which resembles aspirin, even if quite potent, will therefore appear undistinguished and consequently lose much of its psychotherapeutic punch.

The cutaneous application of placebo substances is an everyday practice. Whereas patients may be reluctant to apply a cold water wet dressing to an inflamed area, they will be perfectly agreeable to applying one containing a dissolved substance. When Epsom salts are added to water, the patient will be properly impressed by the healing virtues of the solution. Although magnesium sulfate is not significantly absorbed through intact skin and does not exert any specific cutaneous effect, cooling evaporation from a dressing open to the air or the moist heat of a hot soak, whichever effect is desired by the physician, still occurs when there is magnesium sulfate in the water. A sore muscle group will more readily be kept at a desired rest if methyl salicylate has been applied to the overlying skin and the region wrapped in flannel, preferably red. If salicylate absorption is desired, aspirin by mouth would be preferable, for there is no evidence that methyl salicylate applied to the skin is concentrated in the underlying muscle. But the

sensation of cutaneous warmth which is due to the irritative erythema, plus the definitive odor, are impressive to all but the most skeptical. I do not mean to belittle all liniments: they provide lubrication helpful in massage and may just as well smell of wintergreen. Similarly, while a plain hot water mouth wash or gargle would not be respected, a colored one containing a few drops of aromatic oil would be accepted without question. The odor of tincture of benzoin will make the inhalation of steam comprehensible to the average patient. People have by association come to expect this odor and without it they will be reluctant to inhale the steam which alone has the therapeutic value. So we see that the "humble humbug" of Pepper is valuable to induce the patient to take beneficial treatment which otherwise might be neglected.

All dermatologists have seen young patients with warts which respond well to the application of almost any substance. This is presumably a placebo effect, since other forms of psychotherapy are equally effective. The spunk water of Huckleberry Finn and Tom Sawyer was undoubtedly as potent as any authoritative prescription preparation.

The use of suppositories as placebos should ordinarily be avoided for the same reasons that potent medication given for systemic effect is also better administered by other routes. Conceivably, however, a cocoa butter suppository might be temporarily substituted for one containing aminophyllin if indications for the latter cease to exist and the patient has become dependent.

Of these four avenues of drug administration certainly the oral route is for many reasons the simplest and the best for the placebo. But for universal patient acceptance nothing can approach the psychotherapeutic impressiveness of puncture of the integument by a hollow needle. The placebo substance introduced via the needle is usually second in importance to the needle stick. Sherlock Holmes called for the needle. Addicts take narcotics by the needle. Pre- and postoperative sedatives and narcotics are injected. Blood is transfused and various solutions are infused through needles. Little wonder that there is an association of the injection with powerful medication. The injection requires little or no reinforcing psychotherapy, even with relatively prolonged use. I recall the case of the addict with severe rheumatoid arthritis who "required" 30 mg. of morphine every two hours. After a program of narcotic reduction the patient continued to present himself every two hours for 0.5 cc. of sterile water, saying, "I know you're not giving me much, Doc, but I'll take what I can get."

The injected placebo may by pharmacologic action impart subjective sensations to the recipient, without any specific therapeutic action. Irritating substances may cause local pain, aside from the trauma of the injection. Even if we grant that there is no danger of tissue necrosis the practice of injecting materials for the specific production of pain as part of the act is to be condemned. We should not allow therapy to be confused with punishment, nor should we appeal to any masochistic individual tendencies. The practice of injecting irritating concentrated solutions of vitamins, in the absence of clear-cut signs of vitamin deficiency, is widespread but usually ill advised. But occasionally the indication is specific for just this placebo and when the patient tastes it shortly after the painful injection, he feels doubly benefited. A placebo may carry with it the production of other subjective sensations which may potentiate the placebo effect. For example, one action of nicotine acid is the production of a flush and sensation of heat, desirable therapeutic effects under certain circumstances, undesirable "side" effects under others, but psychotherapeutic when used for that purpose. The intravenous administration of placebo substances is to be criticized since untoward effects sometimes are observed.

The type of placebo chosen by the physician depends not only on the situation presented by the patient but on the physician himself and the inescapable patient-doctor relationship or temperamental rapport. As noted by Houston,[21] the doctor himself is an important therapeutic agent. It is hard for a doctor to avoid being part actor no matter how he may try. In times past

doctors grew beards and wrote prescriptions in Latin, using the apothecary system. This awed a credulous populace and covered some of the gaps in medical knowledge. As we progress it becomes less necessary to resort to this sort of thing. But without carrying it to the point of charlatanism the doctor is more or less effective by his demeanor, whether this is called personality, bedside manner or anything else, and by the way he does and should modify this for each and every patient in order to establish rapport. Whereas the quiet executive is impressed by quiet efficiency, the folksy farmer's wife might respond only to a warmer, more personal touch. Essentially, there should be provided an atmosphere in which the patient will be receptive to therapy so that the psychotherapeutic aspect of specific medication is not lost and the psychotherapeutic effect of placebo medication is enhanced.

Substances which may be harmful or toxic should never be used as placebos. Because of the wide choice of harmless placebos it is unnecessary to court danger. Inorganic arsenical compounds such as Fowler's solution by mouth or cacodylates by needle have dwindling indications, if indeed indications still remain at all. Physicians formerly believed firmly in their inherent therapeutic value but with more accurate knowledge of pharmacology this belief has been shaken. There is certainly no specific benefit to be anticipated from the administration of inorganic arsenical preparations. They are described as "alteratives" in our older books of materia medica. This is defined as an "obsolete term originally used for drugs said to reestablish healthy functions of the system." Some dermatologists continue to use Fowler's solution in the treatment of recalcitrant dermatoses, claiming occasionally dramatic improvement, without knowing the modus operandi. But we should no longer use these potentially toxic compounds in a confused way as a sort of impure placebo.

It is desirable in patients who respond well to placebo therapy to prevent their becoming dependent on placebos. These individuals, considered as a group, are more dependent than most people. The use of placebos supplies a socially acceptable substitute dependency when more profound

psychotherapy is not available. Consequently these patients are frequently content to take placebos almost indefinitely. If placebo administration is prolonged, dependency becomes physiologic, as well as psychologic, as illustrated by characteristic withdrawal phenomena when a placebo narcotic-substitute is discontinued. Since, as already noted, dependency on placebos is undoubtedly less undesirable than addiction to narcotics, there is justification for their prolonged administration in some cases. But in addition to the question of the propriety of allowing a patient to become dependent on the placebo there is always the question of the feasibility of maintaining him satisfactorily on a placebo regimen. This must be resolved on an individual basis and requires careful evaluation and perhaps a period of trial.

When the decision has been reached to discontinue placebo medication, the procedure to be employed depends on the relationship of doctor and patient. The patient's dependency is divided between the doctor and the placebo doctor-symbol. If the former predominates, the problem is relatively simple; if the latter predominates, the difficulty may be very great. The technic employed must be adapted to the specific situation. One warning is in order. The doctor who gives a placebo should never allow himself to appear hostile to a patient at the proposed time of discontinuing it by triumphantly telling him that he wasn't getting anything but water, lactose or whatever the substance might have been. The man who has used a wheelchair and is being encouraged to walk would fall flat if not given crutches or a cane for support. Similarly, the patient who has leaned on a placebo must not have this support rudely knocked out from under him without some transitional device. Some individuals may be told, if circumstances warrant their being given this information, that they had received placebos to help them away from narcotics or sedatives. Others should never be told that their precious medicine was a hoax. No rule of preselection of patients can be laid down; each doctor treats each patient in his own most effective way.

Concluding Remarks

In our discussion we have attempted first to establish that the use of the placebo entails the use of deception, then that this deception is permissible since it is for the benefit of the patient. We have defined placebo as "a medicine or preparation which has no inherent pertinent pharmacologic activity but which is effective only by virtue of the factor of suggestion attendant upon its administration." Placebos are useful in diagnosis, therapy and research.

When a placebo is indicated as principal or associated psychotherapy it should not be withheld, but the physician must be alert to the limitations of this form of therapy. The specific technic is largely a matter of personal choice, depending on the physician's rapport with the patient. The physician should be sensitive to changes in his patient which would point to a change in or discontinuation of such therapy.

The principles set forth are not intended as inviolate rules but only as guides to be modified according to the needs of the individual patient as appraised by the individual physician. The proper use of the placebo requires, in addition to broad medical knowledge, a depth of human understanding not requisite to the purely materialistic approach to medicine.

References

1. Pepper, O. H. P., A note on the placebo. *Tr. & Stud., Coll. Physicians, Philadelphia,* 13: 81, 1945.

2. Findley, T., The placebo and the physician. *M. Clin. North America,* 37: 1821, 1953.

3. Cornell Conferences on Therapy. The use of placebos in therapy. 2: 1, 1947.

4. Wolf, S., Effects of suggestion and conditioning on the action of chemical agents in human subjects—the pharmacology of placebos. *J. Clin. Investigation,* 29: 100, 1950.

5. Wolf, S. and Wolff, H. G., *Human Gastric Function,* 2nd ed., p. 170. New York and London, 1947. Oxford.

6. Wolf, S., Toxic effect of placebo administration *Clin. Research Proc.,* 1: 117, 1953.

7. Weiss, E., and English, O. S., *Psychosomatic Medicine.* Philadelphia, 1947. W. B. Saunders & Co.

8. Hyman, H. T., *An Integrated Practice of Medicine.* Philadelphia, 1947. W. B. Saunders & Co.

9. Dorland, W. A. N., *The American Illustrated Medical Dictionary,* 22nd ed. Philadelphia, 1951. W. B. Saunders & Co.

10. *Webster's New International Dictionary of the English Language,* 2nd ed. Springfield, Mass., 1947. G. C. Merriam Co.

11. Plato, *The Republic.*

12. Parkinson, J., The patient and the physician. *Ann. Int. Med.,* 35: 307, 1951.

13. Henderson, L. J., Quoted by Means, J. H., Evolution of the doctor-patient relationship. *Bull. New York Acad. Med.,* 29: 725, 1953.

14. Hippocrates. Quoted by Castiglioni, A., *A History of Medicine,* 2nd ed. New York, 1947. Alfred A. Knopf.

15. Oberndorf, C. P. Psychogenic factors in asthma. *New York State J. Med.,* 35: 41, 1935.

16. Rennie, T. A. C., in *A Textbook of Medicine,* 8th ed. (Cecil, R. A., and Loeb, R. F.) Philadelphia, 1951. W. B. Saunders & Co.

17. Whitehorn, J. C., in *A Textbook of Medicine,* 8th ed. (Cecil, R. A., and Loeb, R. F.). Philadelphia, 1951. W. B. Saunders & Co.

18. Alvarez, W. C., *The Neuroses.* Philadelphia, 1951. W. B. Saunders & Co.

19. Shaw, M. E. Medical facts and fallacies. *Brit. M. J.,* 1: 515, 1936.

20. Watts, M. S. M., and Wilbur, D. L., Treatment of functional disorders. *J.A.M.A.,* 152: 1192, 1953.

21. Houston, W. R., The doctor himself as a therapeutic agent. *Ann. Int. Med.,* 11: 1416, 1938.

41

Sissela Bok
The Ethics of Giving Placebos

In 1971 a number of Mexican-American women applied to a family-planning clinic for contraceptives. Some of them were given oral contraceptives and others were given placebos, or dummy pills that looked like the real thing. Without knowing it the women were involved in an investigation of the side effects of various contraceptive pills. Those who were given placebos suffered from a predictable side effect: 10 of them became pregnant. Needless to say, the physician in charge did not assume financial responsibility for the babies. Nor did he indicate any concern about having bypassed the "informed consent" that is required in ethical experiments with human beings. He contented himself with the observation that if only the law had permitted it, he could have aborted the pregnant women!

The physician was not unusually thoughtless or hardhearted. The fact is that placebos are so widely prescribed for therapeutic reasons or administered to control groups in experiments, and are considered so harmless, that the fundamental issues they raise are seldom confronted. It appears to me, however, that physicians prescribing placebos cannot consider only the presumed benefit to an individual patient or to an experiment at a particular time. They must also take into account the potential risks, both to the patient or the experimental subject and to the medical profession. And the ethical dilemmas that are inherent in the various uses of placebos are central to such an estimate of possible benefits and risks.

The derivation of "placebo," from the Latin for "I shall please," gives the word a benevolent ring, somehow placing placebos beyond moral criticism and conjuring up images of hypochondriacs whose vague ailments are dispelled through adroit prescriptions of beneficent sugar pills. Physicians often give a humorous tinge to instructions for prescribing these substances, which helps to remove them from serious ethical concern. One authority wrote in a pharmacological journal that the placebo should be given a name previously unknown to the patient and preferably Latin and polysyllabic, and "it is wise if it be prescribed with some assurance and emphasis for psychotherapeutic effect. The older physicians each had his favorite placebic prescriptions—one

chose tincture of Condurango, another the Fluid-extract of *Cimicifuga nigra*." After all, are not placebos far less dangerous than some genuine drugs? As another physician asked in a letter to *The Lancet:* "Whenever pain can be relieved with two milliliters of saline, why should we inject an opiate? Do anxieties or discomforts that are allayed with starch capsules require administration of a barbiturate, diazepam or propoxyphene?"

Before the 1960's placebos were commonly defined as just such pharmacologically inactive medications as salt water or starch, given primarily to satisfy patients that something is being done for them. It has only gradually become clear that any medical procedure has an implicit placebo effect and, whether it is active or inactive, can serve as a placebo whenever it has no specific effect on the condition for which it is prescribed. Nowadays fewer sugar pills are prescribed, but X rays, vitamin preparations, antibiotics and even surgery can function as placebos. Arthur K. Shapiro defines a placebo as "any therapy (or component of therapy) that is deliberately or knowingly used for its nonspecific, psychologic or psycho-physiologic effect, or that . . . , unknown to the patient or therapist, is without specific activity for the condition being treated."

Clearly the prescription of placebos is intentionally deceptive only when the physician himself knows they are without specific effect but keeps the patient in the dark. In considering the ethical issues attending deception with placebos I shall exclude the many procedures in which physicians have had—or still have—misplaced faith; that includes most of the treatments prescribed until this century and a great many still in use but of unproved or even disproved value.

Considering that in the past most therapies had little or no specific effect (yet sometimes succeeded thanks to faith on the part of healers and sufferers) and that we now have more effective remedies, it might be thought that the need to resort to placebos would have decreased. Improved treatment and diagnosis, however, have raised the expectations of patients and health professionals alike and consequently the incidence of reliance on placebos has risen. This is true of placebos given both in experiments and for therapeutic effect.

Modern techniques of experimentation with humans have vastly expanded the role of placebos as controls. New drugs, for example, are compared with placebos in order to distinguish the effects of the drug from chance events or effects associated with the mere administration of the drug. They can be tested in "blind" studies, in which the subjects do not know whether they are receiving the experimental drug or the placebo, and in "double-blind" studies, in which neither the subjects nor the investigators know.

Experiments involving humans are now subjected to increasingly careful safeguards for the people at risk, but it will be a long time before the practice of deceiving experimental subjects with respect to placebos is eradicated. In all the studies of the placebo effect that I surveyed in a study initiated as a fellow of the Interfaculty Program in Medical Ethics at Harvard University, only one indicated that those subjected to the experiment were informed that they would receive placebos; indeed, there was frequent mention of intentional deception. For example, a study titled "An Analysis of the Placebo Effect in Hospitalized Hypertensive Patients" reports that "six patients . . . were asked to accept hospitalization for approximately six weeks . . . to have their hypertension evaluated and to undertake a treatment with a new blood pressure drug. . . . No medication was given for the first five to seven days in the hospital. Placebo was then started."

As for therapeutic administration, there is no doubt that studies conducted in recent decades show placebos can be effective. Henry K. Beecher studied the effects of placebos on patients suffering from conditions including postoperative pain, angina pectoris and the common cold. He estimated that placebos achieved satisfactory relief for about 35 percent of the patients surveyed. Alan Leslie points out, moreover, that "some people are temperamentally impatient and demand results before they normally would be forthcoming. Occasionally, during a period of diagnostic observation or testing, a placebo will provide a

gentle sop to their impatience and keep them under control while the important business is being conducted."

A number of other reasons are advanced to explain the continued practice of prescribing placebos. Physicians are acutely aware of the uncertainties of their profession and of how hard it is to give meaningful and correct answers to patients. They also know that disclosing uncertainty or a pessimistic prognosis can diminish benefits that depend on faith and the placebo effect. They dislike being the bearers of uncertain or bad news as much as anyone else. Sitting down to discuss an illness with a patient truthfully and sensitively may take much-needed time away from other patients. Finally, the patient who demands unneeded medication or operations may threaten to go to a more cooperative doctor or to resort to self-medication; such patient pressure is one of the most potent forces perpetuating and increasing the resort to placebos.

There are no conclusive figures for the extent to which placebos are prescribed, but clearly their use is widespread. Thorough studies have estimated that as many as 35 to 45 percent of all prescriptions are for substances that are incapable of having an effect on the condition for which they are prescribed. Kenneth L. Melmon and Howard F. Morrelli, in their textbook *Clinical Pharmacology*, cite a study of treatment for the common cold as indicating that 31 percent of the patients received a prescription for a broad-spectrum or medium-spectrum antibiotic, 22 percent received penicillin and 6 percent received sulfonamides— "none of which could possibly have any beneficial specific pharmacological effect on the viral infection per se." They point out further that thousands of doses of vitamin B-12 are administered every year "at considerable expense to patients without pernicious anemia," the only condition for which the vitamin is specifically indicated.

In view of all of this it is remarkable that medical textbooks provide little analysis of placebo treatment. In a sample of 19 popular recent textbooks in medicine, pediatrics, surgery, anesthesia, obstetrics and gynecology only three even mention placebos, and none of them deal with either the medical or the ethical dilemmas placebos present.

Four out of six textbooks on pharmacology consider placebos, but with the exception of the book by Melmon and Morrelli they mention only the experimental role of placebos and are completely silent on ethical issues. Finally, four out of eight standard texts on psychiatry refer to placebos, again without ever mentioning ethical issues.

Yet little thought is required to see the dilemma placebos should pose for physicians. A placebo can provide a potent, although unreliable, weapon against suffering, but the very manner in which it can relieve suffering seems to depend on keeping the patient in the dark. The dilemma is an ethical one, reflecting contrary views about how human beings ought to deal with each other, an apparent conflict between helping patients and informing them about their condition.

This dilemma is pointed up by the concept of informed consent: the idea that the individual has the right to give prior consent to, and even to refuse, what is proposed to him in the way of medical care. The doctrine is recognized in proliferating "bills of rights" for patients. The one recommended by the American Hospital Association states, for example, that the patient has the right to complete, understandable information on his diagnosis, treatment and prognosis; the right to whatever information is needed so that he can give informed consent to any treatment; the right to refuse treatment to the extent permitted by law.

Few physicians appear to consider the implications of informed consent when they prescribe placebos, however. One reason is surely that the usefulness of a placebo may be destroyed if informed consent is sought, since its success is assumed to depend specifically on the patient's ignorance and suggestibility. Then too the substances employed as placebos have been considered so harmless, and at the same time so potentially beneficial, that it is easy to assume that the lack of consent cannot possibly matter. In any case health professionals in general have not considered the possibility that the prescription of a placebo is so intrinsically misleading as to make informed consent impossible.

Some authorities have argued that there need not be any deception at all.

Placebos can be described in such a way that no outright verbal lie is required. For example: "I believe these pills may help you." Lawrence J. Henderson went so far as to maintain that "it is meaningless to speak of telling the truth, the whole truth and nothing but the truth to a patient . . . because it is . . . a sheer impossibility. . . . Since telling the truth is impossible, there can be no sharp distinction between what is false and what is true."

Can one really think of prescribing placebos as not being deceptive at all as long as the words are sufficiently vague? In order to answer this question it is necessary to consider the nature of deception. When someone intentionally deceives another person, he causes that person to believe what is false. Such deception may be verbal, in which case it is a lie, or it may be nonverbal, conveyed by gestures, false visual cues or the myriad other means human beings have devised for misleading one another. What is common to all intentional deception is the intent to deceive and the providing of misleading information, whether that information is verbal or nonverbal.

The statement that a placebo may help a patient is not a lie or even, in itself, deceitful. Yet the circumstances in which a placebo is prescribed introduce an element of deception. The setting in a doctor's office or hospital room, the impressive terminology, the mystique of the all-powerful physician prescribing a cure—all of these tend to give the patient faith in the remedy; they convey the impression that the treatment prescribed will have the ingredients necessary to improve the patient's condition. The actions of the physician are therefore deceptive even if the words are so general as not to be lies. Verbal deception may be more direct, but all kinds of deception can be equally misleading.

The view that merely withholding information is not deceptive is particularly inappropriate in the case of placebo prescriptions because information that is material and important is withheld. The crucial fact that the physician may not know what the patient's problems are is not communicated. Information concerning the prognosis is vague and information about the specific way in which the treatment may affect the condition is not provided. Henderson's view fails to

make the distinction between such relevant information, which it is usually feasible to provide, and infinite details of decreasing importance, which to be sure can never be provided with any completeness. It also fails to distinguish between two ways in which the information reaching the patient may be altered: it may be withheld or it may be distorted. Often the two are mingled. Consider the intertwining of distortion, mystification and failure to inform in the following statement, made to unsuspecting recipients of placebos in an experiment performed in a psychiatric outpatient clinic: "You are to receive a test that all patients receive as part of their evaluation. The test medication is a nonspecific autonomous nervous system stimulant."

Even those who recognize that placebos are deceptive often dispel any misgivings with the thought that they involve no serious deception. Placebos are regarded as being analogous to the innocent white lies of everyday life, so trivial as to be quite outside the realm of ethical evalution. Such liberties with language as telling someone that his necktie is beautiful or that a visit has been a pleasure, when neither statement reflects the speaker's honest opinion, are commonly accepted as being so trivial that to evaluate them morally would seem unduly fastidious and, from a utilitarian point of view, unjustified. Placebos are not trivial, however. Spending for them runs into millions of dollars. Patients incur greater risks of discomfort and harm than is commonly understood. Finally, any placebo uses that are in fact trivial and harmless in themselves may combine to form nontrivial practices, so that repeated reliance on placebos can do serious harm in the long run to the medical profession and the general public.

Consider first the cost to patients. A number of the procedures undertaken for their placebo effect are extremely costly in terms of available resources and of expense, discomfort and risk of harm to patients. Many temporarily successful new surgical procedures owe their success to the placebo effect alone. In such cases there is no intention to deceive the patient; physician and patient alike are deceived. On occasion, however, surgery is deliberately

performed as a placebo measure. Children may undergo appendectomies or tonsillectomies that are known to be unnecessary simply to give the impression that powerful measures are being taken or because parents press for the operation. Hysterectomies and other operations may be performed on adults for analogous reasons. A great many diagnostic procedures that are known to be unnecessary are undertaken to give patients a sense that efforts are being made on their behalf. Some of these carry risks; many involve discomfort and the expenditure of time and money. The potential for damage by an active drug given as a placebo is similarly clear-cut. Calvin M. Kunin, T. Tupasi and W. Craig have described the ill effects—including death— suffered by hospital patients as a result of excessive prescription of antibiotics, more than half of which they found had been unneeded, inappropriately selected or given in incorrect dosages.

Even inactive placebos can have toxic effects in a substantial proportion of cases; nausea, dermatitis, hearing loss, headache, diarrhea and other symptoms have been cited. Stewart Wolf reported on a double-blind experiment to test the effects of the drug mephenesin and a placebo on disorders associated with anxiety and tension. Depending on the symptom studied, roughly 20 to 30 percent of the patients were better while taking the pills and 50 to 70 percent were unchanged, but 10 to 20 percent were worse—"whether the patient was taking mephenesin or placebo." A particularly serious possible side effect of even a harmless substance is dependency. In one case a psychotic patient was given placebo pills and told they were a "new major tranquilizer without any side effects." After four years she was taking 12 tablets a day and complaining of insomnia and anxiety. After the self-medication reached 25 pills a day and a crisis had occurred, the physician intervened, talked over the addictive problem (but not the deception) with the patient and succeeded in reducing the dose to two a day, a level that was still being maintained a year later. Other cases have been reported of patients' becoming addicted or habituated to these substances to the point of not being able to function without them, at times even requiring that they be stepped up to very high dosages.

Most obvious, of course, is the damage done when placebos are given in place of a well-established therapy that is clearly indicated for the patient's condition. The Mexican-American women I mentioned at the outset, for example, were actually harmed by being given placebo pills in the guise of contraceptive pills. In 1966 Beecher, in an article on the ethics of experiments with human subjects, documented a case in which 109 servicemen with streptococcal respiratory infections were given injections of a placebo instead of injections of penicillin, which was already known to prevent the development of rheumatic fever in such patients and which was being given to a larger group of patients. Two of the placebo subjects developed rheumatic fever and one developed an acute kidney infection, whereas such complications did not occur in the penicillin-treated group.

There have been a number of other experiments in which patients suffering from illnesses with known cures have been given placebos in order to study the course of the illness when it is untreated or to determine the precise effectiveness of the known therapy in another group of patients. Because of the very nature of their aims the investigators have failed to ask subjects for their informed consent. The subjects have tended to be those least able to object or defend themselves: members of minority groups, the poor, the institutionalized and the very young.

A final type of harm to patients given placebos stems not so much from the placebo itself as from the manipulation and deception that accompany its prescription. Inevitably some patients find out that they have been duped. They may then lose confidence in physicians and in bona fide medication, which they may need in the future. They may even resort on their own to more harmful drugs or other supposed cures. That is a danger associated with all deception: its discovery leads to a failure of trust when trust may be most needed. Alternatively, some people who do not discover the deception and are left believing that a placebic remedy works may continue to rely on it under the

wrong circumstances. This is particularly true with respect to drugs, such as antibiotics, that are used sometimes for their specific action and sometimes as placebos. Many parents, for example, come to believe they must ask for the prescription of antibiotics every time their child has a fever.

The major costs associated with placebos may not be the costs to patients themselves that I have discussed up to this point. Rather they may be costs to new categories of patients in the future, to physicians who do not abuse placebo treatment and to society in general.

Deceptive practices, by their very nature, tend to escape the normal restraints of accountability and so can spread more easily. There are many instances in which an innocuous-seeming practice has grown to become a large-scale and more dangerous one; warnings against "the entering wedge" are often rhetorical devices but may sometimes be justified when there are great pressures to move along the undesirable path and when the safeguards against undesirable developments are insufficient. In this perspective there is reason for concern about placebos. The safeguards are few or nonexistent against a practice that is secretive by its very nature. And there are ever stronger pressures—from drug companies, patients eager for cures and busy physicians—for more medication, whether it is needed or not. Given such pressures the use of placebos can spread along a number of dimensions.

The clearest danger lies in the gradual shift from pharmacologically inert placebos to more active ones. It is not always easy to distinguish completely inert substances from somewhat active ones and these in turn from more active ones. It may be hard to distinguish between a quantity of an active substance so low that it has little or no effect and quantities that have some effect. It is not always clear to physicians whether patients require an inert placebo or possibly a more active one, and there can be the temptation to resort to an active one just in case it might also have a specific effect. It is also much easier to deceive a patient with a medication that is known to be "real" and to have power. One recent textbook in medicine goes so far as to advocate the use of small doses of effective compounds as placebos rather

than inert substances—because it is important for both the doctor and the patient to believe in the treatment! The fact that the dangers and side effects of active agents are not always known or considered important by the physician is yet another factor contributing to the shift from innocuous placebos to active ones.

Meanwhile the number of patients receiving placebos increases as more and more people seek and receive medical care and as their desire for instant, push-button alleviation of symptoms is stimulated by drug advertising and by rising expectations of what "science" can do. Reliance on placebic therapy in turn strengthens the belief that there really is a pill or some other kind of remedy for every ailment. As long ago as 1909 Richard C. Cabot wrote, in a perceptive paper on the subject of truth and deception in medicine: "The majority of placebos are given because we believe the patient . . . has learned to expect medicine for every symptom, and without it he simply won't get well. True, but who taught him to expect a medicine for every symptom? He was not born with that expectation. . . . It is we physicians who are responsible for perpetuating false ideas about disease and its cure. . . . With every placebo that we give we do our part in perpetuating error, and harmful error at that."

A particularly troubling aspect of the spread of placebos is that it now affects so many children. Parents increasingly demand pills, such as powerful stimulants, to modify their children's behavior with a minimum of effort on their part; there are some children who may need such medication but many receive it without proper diagnosis. As I have mentioned, parents demand antibiotics even when told they are unnecessary, and physicians may give in to the demands. In these cases the very meaning of "placebo" has shifted subtly from "I shall please the patient" to "I shall please the patient's parents."

Deception by placebo can also spread from therapy and diagnosis to experimental applications. Although placebos can be given nondeceptively in experimentation, someone who is accustomed to prescribing placebos therapeutically without consent may not take the precaution of obtaining such consent when he undertakes an experiment on human subjects. Yet therapeutic deception is at least thought to be for the patient's own good, whereas experimental deception may not benefit the subject and may actually harm him; even the paternalistic excuse that the investigator is deceiving the patient for his own good then becomes inapplicable.

Finally, acceptance of placebos can encourage other kinds of deception in medicine such as failure to reveal to a patient the risks connected with an operation, or lying to terminally ill patients. Medicine lends itself with particular ease to deception for benevolent reasons because physicians are so clearly more knowledgeable than their patients and the patients are so often in a weakened or even irrational state. As Melvin Levine has put it, "the medical profession has practiced as if the truth is, in fact, a kind of therapeutic instrument [that] . . . can be altered or given in small doses . . . [or] not used at all when deemed detrimental to the patients. . . . Many physicians have utilized truth distortion as a kind of anesthetic to promote comfort and ease treatment." Such practices are presumably for the good of patients. No matter how cogent and benevolent the reasons for resorting to deception may seem, when those reasons are considered in secret, without the consent of the doctored, they tend to be reinforced by less benevolent pressures, self-deception begins to blur nice distinctions and occasions for giving misleading information multiply.

Because of all these ways in which placebo usage can spread it is impossible to look at each incident of manipulation in isolation. There are no watertight compartments in medicine. When the costs and benefits of any therapeutic, diagnostic or experimental procedure are weighed, not only the individual consequences but also the cumulative ones must be taken into account. Reports of deceptive practices inevitably filter out, and the resulting suspicion is heightened by the anxiety that threats to health always create. And so even the health professionals who do not mislead their patients are injured by those who do and the entire institution of medicine is threatened by practices lacking in candor, however

harmless the results may appear to be in some individual cases.

What should be the profession's attitude with regard to placebos? In the case of most experimental applications there are ways of avoiding deception without abandoning placebo controls. Subjects can be informed of the nature of the experiment and of the fact that placebos will be administered; if they then consent to the experiment, the use of placebos cannot be considered surreptitious. Although the subjects in a blind or double-blind experiment will not know exactly when they are receiving placebos or even whether they are receiving them, the initial consent to the experimental design, including placebos, removes the ethical problems having to do with deception. If, on the other hand, there are experiments of such a nature that asking subjects for their informed consent to the use of placebos would invalidate the results or cause too many subjects to decline, then the experiment ought not to be performed and the desired knowledge should be sought by means of a different research design.

As for the diagnostic and therapeutic use of placebos, we must start with the presumption that it is undesirable. By and large, given the principle of informed consent as well as concern for human integrity, no measures that affect someone's health should be undertaken without explanation and permission. Placebos are not so trivial as to be unworthy of ethical evaluation; they carry a definite possibility of harm and discomfort to patients as well as high collective costs; as a result placebo prescriptions present a more serious inroad on patient decision making than has been appreciated up to now. Surreptitious diagnostic and therapeutic administration of placebos should therefore be ruled out whenever possible.

The prohibition should not be absolute, however. In some cases the balance of benefit over cost is so overwhelming that reasonable people would choose to be deceived. There is no clear formula that will quickly reveal in each case whether the benefits will greatly outweigh the possible harm. Much of the problem can be avoided if care is taken to avoid placebos if possible and to observe the following principles in the remaining cases: (1) Placebos should be used

only after a careful diagnosis; (2) no active placebos should be employed, merely inert ones; (3) no outright lie should be told and questions should be answered honestly; (4) placebos should never be given to patients who have asked not to receive them; (5) placebos should never be used when other treatment is clearly called for or all possible alternatives have not been weighed.

If placebo medicine is to be thus limited, the information provided to both medical personnel and patients will have to change radically. Placebos, so often resorted to and yet so rarely mentioned, will have to be discussed from scientific as well as ethical points of view during medical training. Textbooks will have to confront the medical and ethical dilemmas analytically and exhaustively. Similarly, much education must be provided for the public. There must be greater stress on the autonomy of the patient and on his right to consent to treatment or to refuse treatment after being informed of its nature. Understanding of the normal courses of illnesses should be stressed, including the fact that most minor conditions clear up by themselves rather quickly. The great pressure patients exert for more medication must be countered by limitations on drug advertising and by information concerning the side effects and dangers of drugs.

I have tried to show that the benevolent deception exemplified by placebos is widespread, that it carries risks not usually taken into account, that it represents an inroad on informed consent, that it damages the institution of medicine and contributes to the erosion of confidence in medical personnel.

Honesty may not be the highest social value; at exceptional times, when survival is at stake, it may have to be set aside. To permit a widespread practice of deception, however, is to set the stage for abuses and growing mistrust. Augustine, considering the possibility of giving official sanction to white lies, pointed out that "little by little and bit by bit this will grow and by gradual accessions will slowly increase until it becomes such a mass of wicked lies that it will be utterly impossible to find any means of resisting such a plague grown to huge proportions through small additions."

Illustrative Cases

A physician is treating a 19-year-old woman afflicted with serious kidney disease. She first came to see the physician about six weeks earlier because of the onset of severe headaches. Tests revealed that her kidneys were seriously damaged. She was placed on a kidney dialysis machine, which cleansed the substances from her blood that her failing kidneys could no longer remove.

Before her condition declined further, and while she was relatively strong, the physician suggested that a kidney be transplanted to replace one of her damaged kidneys. Because organ transplants have proved most successful when the donor is closely related to the recipient, tests for tissue compatibility were run on the patient's immediate family—her mother, father, and 16-year-old brother. Only the brother showed a degree of compatibility high enough to consider a transplant.

The physician met alone with the brother to tell him that he was the only candidate immediately available to donate a kidney. He outlined the risks of the operation that the brother would have to undergo to remove his kidney, and the risks that he faced in the future living with one kidney. He also explained the benefits that his sister could expect from the transplant. The physician urged the brother to agree to the operation because of the serious nature of his sister's illness. But he said that if the brother declined the procedure, he would tell the family that none of their kidneys were biologically suited for a transplant in this case.

The brother decided not to offer his kidney to his sister: the procedure appeared to carry too many risks for him. Moreover, he revealed to the physician that he never really felt close to his sister. The physician met with all members of the family, told them their tissues were biologically incompatible with that of the patient's, and that none of them were possible donors.

1. From an ethical viewpoint, should the physician have chosen this course?
2. Why?

An accountant, age 47, with a wife and three children develops mild respiratory complaints and periods of unusual fatigue. He consults the physician, whom he has been seeing for twenty years. Unable to explain the symptoms, the doctor hospitalizes the person. A series of tests definitely establishes the existence of a fatal illness whose symptoms would continue relatively mild probably for two to three years, then become severe, with death likely to occur in five years.

1. Should the patient be told the facts?
2. If not, should anyone?
3. Should the patient's emotional state influence the doctor's decision?

A physician performing a routine check-up on a 2-year-old child gives her a vaccine to protect her against mumps. Before the child leaves the doctor's office with her mother, the doctor discovers in his record that he had given a mumps immunization to the child last year. He realizes that this second immunization against mumps was unnecessary but will have no adverse medical consequences.

1. Should he tell the child's mother about his error and risk undermining the confidence the family has in him?

V

Medical Experimentation on Human Subjects

Introduction to Part V

The search for knowledge and for improved methods of diagnosis and treatment have been a part of the professional and scientific concerns of medicine at least since the time of Hippocrates. In earlier centuries little distinction was made between medical treatment and clinical investigation. In the writings of Claude Bernard and particularly in his 1865 work, *An Introduction to the Study of Experimental Medicine* we find some of the beginnings of modern clinical investigation. Bernard was a scientific pioneer, a worldly philosopher of medical experimentation as a distinct endeavor in medicine. He saw the effort as an ethical demand on the professional physician and surgeon.

The material in this section that follows Bernard is arranged chronologically. It displays the sophistication of the medical writing of the late nineteenth and early twentieth centuries that dealt with issues now considered quite new—such as protecting the welfare of subjects, distinguishing experimental techniques from proved or accepted therapy, and weighing risks and benefits of each particular investigation.

With the writings of Andrew Ivy, R. A. McCance, Austin Bradford Hill, and Henry Beecher, we reach the modern era of both professional and public concern for the dangers of uncontrolled medical experimentation. Dr. Ivy was a key consultant during the preparation of the so-called Nuremberg Code of Ethics in Medical Research developed by the Allies after World War II and applied at the War Crimes Trials in Germany. R. A. McCance draws a careful picture of what is involved in the practice of experimental medicine, and Austin Bradford Hill explores the methodology and ethical problems of the clinical trial. These essays, and the statement on human experimentation made by the Medical Research Council of Great Britain, demonstrate a growing concern in the post–World War II era with the ethical problems generated by

the rapid expansion of biomedical research.

Yet Henry Beecher's writings must be recognized as the most significant contemporary effort to alert the medical profession and the public to the errors of judgment and the overstepping of ethical boundaries in otherwise important and commendable medical research in the United States. His article, which is included in this chapter, struck the medical research community in the United States like an exploding fragmentation bomb. All manner of investigators and research projects, from the military and government laboratories to the university centers, were hard hit by his very specific and well-documented illustrations. The reprinted letters to the editor of the *New England Journal of Medicine* indicate the scope of the reaction to it.

The remaining selections in this section are a part of the still-continuing aftermath of Beecher's writings and of a few highly publicized specific instances in which research subjects were exposed to dangers without their knowledge or informed consent, such as occurred in the Tuskegee Syphilis Study.

As a result of these disclosures, the federal government of the United States has moved broadly into a regulatory program designed to ensure protection of the welfare of research subjects in medical and behavioral scientific investigation. In very recent years, state governments as well have begun to enact laws controlling and sometimes prohibiting different types of medical and behavioral research or curtailing the utilization of certain types of research subjects such as prisoners and mental patients.

This section is the most dramatic example in our collection of the results of increased public attention to issues of medical ethics. From the idea of an ethical call to do clinical research, we have moved in less than two decades to medical research viewed in the public eye as a suspect activity that should require the prior approval of a governmentally constituted authority for each project. Furthermore, it has become an activity that, if not conducted in accordance with specific control laws for each type of research, can result in criminal imprisonment of the investigator even when no harm has come to his research subjects.

At this point in our history, the movement for legal controls and prohibition in areas of medical research has not yet reached its apex. We cannot yet measure the public gains and losses that may be produced from these programs of legal control. Our overall concern must be for achieving a proper balance between effective and equitable safeguards of the welfare of research subjects and the continued encouragement and support of meritorious scientific inquiry in the interest of the improved health of all the peoples of the world.

42

Claude Bernard
Vivisection

We have succeeded in discovering the laws of inorganic matter only by penetrating into inanimate bodies and machines; similarly we shall succeed in learning the laws and properties of living matter only by displacing living organs in order to get into their inner environment. After dissecting cadavers, then, we must necessarily dissect living beings, to uncover the inner or hidden parts of the organisms and see them work; to this sort of operation we give the name of vivisection, and without this mode of investigation, neither physiology nor scientific medicine is possible; to learn how man and animals live, we cannot avoid seeing great numbers of them die, because the mechanisms of life can be unveiled and proved only by knowledge of the mechanisms of death.

Men have felt this truth in all ages; and in medicine, from the earliest times, men have performed not only therapeutic experiments but even vivisection. We are told that the kings of Persia delivered men condemned to death to their physicians, so that they might perform on them vivisections useful to science. According to Galen, Attalus III (Philometor), who reigned at Pergamum, one hundred thirty-seven years before Jesus Christ, experimented with poisons and antidotes on criminals condemned to death.[1] Celsus recalls and approves the vivisection which Herophilus and Erasistratus performed on criminals with the Ptolemies' consent. It is not cruel, he says, to inflict on a few criminals, sufferings which may benefit multitudes of innocent people throughout all centuries.[2] The Grand Duke of Tuscany had a criminal given over to the professor of anatomy, Fallopius, at Pisa, with permission to kill or dissect him at pleasure. As the criminal had a quartan fever, Fallopius wished to investigate the effects of opium on the paroxysms. He administered two drams of opium during an intermission; death occurred after the second experiment.[3] Similar instances have occasionally recurred, and the story is well known of the archer of Meudon[4] who was pardoned because a nephrotomy was successfully performed on him. Vivisection of animals also goes very far back. Galen may be considered its founder. He performed his experiments especially on monkeys and on young pigs and described the instruments and methods used in experimenting. Galen performed almost no other kind of experiment than that which we call disturbing experiments, which consist in wounding, destroying or removing a part, so as to judge its function by the disturbance caused by its removal. He summarized earlier experiments and studied for himself the effects of destroying the spinal cord at different heights, of perforating the chest on one side or both sides at once; the effects of section of the nerves leading to the intercostal muscles and of section of the recurrent nerve. He tied arteries and performed experiments on the mechanism of deglutition.[5] Since Galen, at long intervals in the midst of medical systems, eminent vivisectors have always appeared. As such, the names of Graaf, Harvey, Aselli, Pecquet, Haller, etc., have been handed down to us. In our time, and especially under the influence of Magendie, vivisection has entered physiology and medicine once for all, as an habitual or indispensable method of study.

The prejudices clinging to respect for corpses long halted the progress of anatomy. In the same way, vivisection in all ages has met with prejudices and detractors. We cannot aspire to destroy all the prejudice in the world; neither shall we allow ourselves here to answer the arguments of detractors of vivisection; since they thereby deny experimental medicine, i.e., scientific medicine. However, we shall consider a few general questions, and then we shall set up the scientific goal which vivisection has in view.

First, have we a right to perform experiments and vivisections on man? Physicians make therapeutic experiments daily on their patients, and surgeons perform vivisections daily on their subjects. Experiments, then, may be performed on man, but within what limits? It is our duty and our right to perform an experiment on man whenever it can save his life, cure him or gain him some personal benefit. The principle of medical and surgical morality, therefore, consists in never performing on man an experiment which might be harmful to him to any extent, even though the result might be highly advantageous to science, i.e., to the health of others. But performing experiments and operations exclusively from the point of view of the patient's own advantage does not prevent their turning out profitably to science. It cannot indeed be otherwise; an old physician who has often administered drugs and treated many patients is more experienced, that is, he will experiment better on new patients, because he has learned from experiments made on others. A surgeon who has performed operations on different kinds of patients learns and perfects himself experimentally. Instruction comes only through experience; and that fits perfectly into the definitions given at the beginning of this introduction.

May we make experiments on men condemned to death or vivisect them? Instances have been cited, analogous to the one recalled above, in which men have permitted themselves to perform dangerous operations on condemned criminals, granting them pardon in exchange. Modern ideas of morals condemn such actions; I completely agree with these ideas; I consider it wholly permissible, however, and useful to science, to make investigations on the properties of tissues immediately after the decapitations of criminals. A helminthologist had a condemned woman without her knowledge swallow larvæ of intestinal worms, so as to see whether the worms developed in the intestines[6] after her death. Others have made analogous experiments on patients with phthisis doomed to an early death; some men have made experiments on themselves. As experiments of this kind are of great interest to science and can be conclusive only on man, they seem to be wholly permissible when they involve no suffering or harm to the subject of the experiment. For we must not deceive ourselves, morals do not forbid making experiments on one's neighbor or on one's self; in everyday life men do nothing but experiment on one another. Christian morals forbid only one thing, doing ill to one's neighbor. So, among the experiments that may be tried on man, those that can only harm are forbidden, those that are innocent are permissible, and those that may do good are obligatory.

Another question presents itself. Have we the right to make experiments on animals and vivisect them? As for me, I think we have this right, wholly and absolutely. It would be strange indeed if we recognized man's right to make use of animals in every walk of life, for domestic service, for food, and then forbade him to make use of them for his own instruction in one of the sciences most useful to humanity. No hesitation is possible; the science of life can be established only through experiment, and we can save living beings from death only after sacrificing others. Experiments must be made either on man or on animals. Now I think that physicians already make too many dangerous experiments on man, before carefully studying them on animals. I do not admit that it is moral to try more or less dangerous or active remedies on patients in hospitals, without first experimenting with them on dogs; for I shall prove, further on, that results obtained on animals may all be conclusive for man when we know how to experiment properly. If it is immoral, then, to make an experiment on man when it is dangerous to him, even though the result may be useful to others, it is essentially moral to make experiments on an animal, even though painful and dangerous to him, if they may be useful to man.

After all this, should we let ourselves be moved by the sensitive cries of people of fashion or by the objections of men unfamiliar with scientific ideas? All feelings deserve respect, and I shall be very careful never to offend anyone's. I easily explain them to myself, and that is why they cannot stop me. I understand perfectly how physicians under the influence of false ideas, and lacking the scientific sense, fail to appreciate the necessity of experiment and vivisection in establishing biological science. I also understand perfectly how people of fashion, moved by ideas wholly different from those that animate physiologists, judge vivisection quite differently. It cannot be otherwise. Somewhere in this introduction we said that, in science, ideas are what give facts their value and meaning. It is the same in morals, it is everywhere the same. Facts materially alike may have opposite scientific meanings, according to the ideas with which they are connected. A cowardly assassin, a hero and a warrior each plunges a dagger into the breast of his fellow. What differentiates them, unless it be

the ideas which guide their hands? A surgeon, a physiologist and Nero give themselves up alike to mutilation of living beings. What differentiates them also, if not ideas? I therefore shall not follow the example of LeGallois,[7] in trying to justify physiologists in the eyes of strangers to science who reproach them with cruelty; the difference in ideas explains everything. A physiologist is not a man of fashion, he is a man of science, absorbed by the scientific idea which he pursues: he no longer hears the cry of animals, he no longer sees the blood that flows, he sees only his idea and perceives only organisms concealing problems which he intends to solve. Similarly, no surgeon is stopped by the most moving cries and sobs, because he sees only his idea and the purpose of his operation. Similarly again, no anatomist feels himself in a horrible slaughter house; under the influence of a scientific idea, he delightedly follows a nervous filament through stinking livid flesh, which to any other man would be an object of disgust and horror. After what has gone before we shall deem all discussion of vivisection futile or absurd. It is impossible for men, judging facts by such different ideas, ever to agree; and as it is impossible to satisfy everybody, a man of science should attend only to the opinion of men of science who understand him, and should derive rules of conduct only from his own conscience.

The scientific principle of vivisection is easy, moreover, to grasp. It is always a question of separating or altering certain parts of the living machine, so as to study them and thus to decide how they function and for what. Vivisection, considered as an analytic method of investigation of the living, includes many successive steps, for we may need to act either on organic apparatus, or on organs, or on tissue, or on the histological units themselves. In extemporized and other vivisections, we produce mutilations whose results we study by preserving the animals. At other times, vivisection is only an autopsy on the living, or a study of properties of tissues immediately after death. The various processes of analytic study of the mechanisms of life in living animals are indispensable, as we shall see, to physiology, to pathology and to therapeutics. However, it would not do to believe that vivisection in itself can constitute the whole experimental method as applied to the study of vital phenomena. Vivisection is only anatomical dissection of the living; it is necessarily combined with all the other physico-chemical means of investigation which must be carried into the organism. Reduced to itself, vivisection would have only a limited range and in certain cases must even mislead us as to the actual rôle of organs. By these reservations I do not deny the usefulness or even the necessity of vivisection in the study of vital phenomena. I merely declare it insufficient. Our instruments for vivisection are indeed so coarse and our senses so imperfect that we can reach only the coarse and complex parts of an organism. Vivisection under the microscope would make much finer analysis possible, but it presents much greater difficulties and is applicable only to very small animals.

But when we reach the limits of vivisection we have other means of going deeper and dealing with the elementary parts of organisms where the elementary properties of vital phenomena have their seat. We may introduce poisons into the circulation, which carry their specific action to one or another histological unit. Localized poisonings, as Fontana and J. Müller have already used them, are valuable means of physiological analysis. Poisons are veritable reagents of life, extremely delicate instruments which dissect vital units. I believe myself the first to consider the study of poisons from this point of view, for I am of the opinion that studious attention to agents which alter histological units should form the common foundation of general physiology, pathology and therapeutics. We must always, indeed, go back to the organs to find the simplest explanations of life.

To sum up, dissection is a displacing of a living organism by means of instruments and methods capable of isolating its different parts. It is easy to understand that such dissection of the living presupposes dissection of the dead.

Notes

1. Daniel Leclerc. *Histoire de la médecine*, p. 338.

2. Celsus, *De Medicina*.

3. Astruc, *De Morbis Venereis*. Vol. II, pp. 748 and 749.

4. Rayer, *Traité des maladies des reins*. Vol. III, p. 213. Paris, 1841.

5. Dezeimeris, *Dictionnaire historique*, Vol. II, p. 444. Daremberg. *Exposition des connaissances de Galien sur l'anatomie pathologique et la pathologie du système nerveux*. Thesis, 1841, pp. 13 and 80.

6. Davaine, *Traité des entozoaires*. Paris, 1860. Synopsis, xxvii.

7. LeGallois, *Œuvres*. Paris, 1824. Preface, p. xxx.

43

Charles Francis Withington

The Possible Conflict between the Interests of Medical Science and Those of the Individual Patient, and the Latter's Indefeasible Rights

Reprinted from Charles Francis Withington, *The Relation of Hospitals to Medical Education* (Boston: Cupples, Uphman and Company, 1886), pp. 14–17.

While it is true . . . that in many respects there is an identity of interest between practitioner and patient in the advancement of medical science, and while any gains so made are for the benefit of the whole race, it may nevertheless be admitted that these advantages are not equally distributed among all persons, and that it is occasionally at the expense of the individual that truths of the greatest general utility have been learned. A surgeon's first operation of ovariotomy, for instance, is not so skilfully performed as his one hundredth, yet through the former he gains a facility in the operation which enhances his subsequent capacity to save life. Yet somebody must be his first patient. So in the development and establishment of any new method of surgical procedure; the later subjects profit from experiences obtained at the expense of the earlier subjects. If it be an injustice that the individual should sometimes suffer for the welfare of the race, it is one that is not confined to the development of medical science, but exists throughout the constitution of things. Everywhere it is true of Nature, in the words of Tennyson,

So careful of the type she seems
So careless of the single life.

In the matter under consideration it is the clear duty of those who are charged with the administration of charitable trusts to adjudicate between what are at times the conflicting claims of medical science and of individual welfare so that neither interest may receive more than the least possible detriment. In the older countries of Europe especially, where the life and happiness of the so-called lower classes are perhaps held more cheaply than with us, enthusiastic devotees of science are very apt to encroach upon the rights of the individual patient in a manner which cannot be justified. In this country we are less likely to fall into this error than those living under monarchical institutions, but even with us it may be well to draw up, as it were, a Bill of Rights which shall secure patients against any injustice from the votaries of science. The occupants of hospital wards are something more than merely so much clinical material during their lives and so much pathological material after their death.

Subjection To Experiments

The first matter to be referred to, namely the extent to which a patient may rightfully be made the subject of experimentation, is one in which it is impossible to draw a definite line. On the one hand, every practitioner must admit that the treatment which he adopts in every case that comes under his charge is to a certain extent experimental. That is to say, the result of the treatment is a matter of greater or less probability, but never of certainty. Whatever course is decided upon, an alternative has usually presented itself, and in the event, whether favorable or otherwise, the question usually suggests itself, "what would have happened if I had followed the alternative course?" Again, a physician reads a plausible account of a new method of treatment for some disease in which his own previous experience has been unfavorable. He decides that the next case that presents itself shall be treated in accordance with the new method. This is purely an experiment, yet it may be perfectly legitimate, and is equally so whether the patient comes to him in private or in hospital practice. To go a step further: it may devolve upon the physician to test for himself and for the good of science some new and hitherto untried remedy in a certain disease. There is here the puzzling ethical fact that he would be unwilling, were the patient one of his own family, to subject him to the risk of the proposed novelty. Yet if what is known of the physiological action of the drug makes its employment reasonable, it may be proper for him in the interests of medical science to establish its usefulness or the reverse. This can only be done by making trial of it in appropriate cases. The individuals upon whom that trial chances to fall are then exactly in the position of those alluded to a moment ago, whose lot was cast in the early days of ovariotomy. Like the men who have lived in times of political crisis and turmoil, their environment was their misfortune. Responsibilities were devolved upon them whose discharge was of greater profit to their posterity than to themselves. Hospital patients, then, cannot complain if they have to bear a part in the solution of the medical problems of the day, in so far, at least, as a similar obligation rests upon the sick who are outside of such institutions.

They have, however, a right to immunity from experiments merely *as such,* and outside of therapeutic application. This right is one that is especially liable to violation by enthusiastic investigators. Its violation may, on the one hand, involve no pain, discomfort or other harm, as when anthropometrical observations are sought, a collection of sphygmographic tracings is desired, or the facts regarding the normal condition of the reflexes are wished for. If the investigator were to ask these things as a favor, few, if any, of the patients would refuse him; and if as a matter of convenience he takes them as a right, no harm is done. On the other hand, however, there are experiments, pure and simple, which do involve harm and pain to their subjects. Within a year or two, two prominent English therapeutists who were studying the action of nitrite of sodium, administered the drug to a large number of hospital patients in doses designed to show its physiological action. The vaso-motor symptoms produced were uncomfortable and in some cases, to the subjects at least, alarming. To perfect the demonstration the administrations were repeated again and again in the same and in new subjects. The whole affair was an egregious usurpation. There was no pretense that the drug was given for any therapeutic purpose. If the experimenters wished to investigate the physiological action of the drug they should have called for volunteers; they had no right to make any man the unwilling victim of such an experiment.

A temptation kindred to the above is the recommendation of hopeless surgical operations. When the patient demands such an operation the surgeon should set the chances fairly before him and if it is still insisted upon, he is then justified in undertaking an operation which gives but small chances of success. But he has no right to take advantage of the patient's extremity to *recommend* a procedure which can have no other advantage than to enhance the operator's reputation for boldness.

44

Patrick Manson
Experimental Proof of the Mosquito-Malaria Theory

Reprinted with deletion of pictures and graphs from *British Medical Journal,* vol. 2, 1900, pp. 949–951.

Although the theory that the malaria parasite is transmitted from man to man by particular species of mosquito is now accepted by all biologists and medical men who have given adequate attention to the subject, it cannot be said that the general public (including those Europeans who in malarious countries might benefit by the practical application of the theory) unreservedly believe in, much less practically apply it. Endless objections, the outcome of an imperfect acquaintance with the subject and, perhaps, of a disinclination to admit that a pathological puzzle of so many centuries standing could receive so simple an explanation, have been raised by the amateur biologist and sanitarian, so much so that it seemed not improbable that a great principle, pregnant with important issues, might remain barren and unutilised.

Impressed with this fear, and being anxious to see some fruit from a theory which I knew to be true and for which I was in a measure responsible, I cast about for means by which the conversion and co-operation of the public might be secured. I felt that unless the public believed in the efficiency of the sanitary measures so definitely indicated by the mosquito-malaria theory, and, understood the principles on which these measures should be founded, they would not adopt them nor, what is so necessary to the success of all such measures, co-operate heartily in carrying them out. As the histological, biological, and experimental evidence which had satisfied men of science was not understood by the public, it seemed to me that some simple demonstration, such as would be unanswerable and at the same time readily comprehended by laymen, was required.

Grassi in conjunction with Bignami had succeeded in conveying malaria by mosquito bite. Although these experimenters took every care to exclude fallacy, the fact that the experiments were made in Rome, itself of fever repute and in the middle of a highly-malarial district, had an undoubted influence in preventing due appreciation by the public of the conclusive nature of their work. Furthermore, things occurring at a distance and in a strange land do not appeal so strongly as do things happening in our midst. It occurred to me, therefore, that if I repeated Grassi and Bignami's experiments in a more dramatic and crucial manner, that if I fed laboratory-reared mosquitos on a malarial patient in a distant country and subsequently carried the mosquitos to the centre of London, and there set them to bite some healthy individual free from any suspicion of being malarial, and if this individual within a short period of being bitten developed malarial fever and showed in his blood the characteristic parasite, the conclusion that malaria is conveyed by the mosquito would be evident to every understanding, and could not possibly be evaded.

It also occurred to me that if a certain number of Europeans who had never suffered from malaria kept in good health and free from malaria during an entire malarial season in an intensely malarial locality, where all inhabitants and visitors suffered from malaria, and if they kept well without the use of quinine or other medicinal prophylactic, simply by avoiding mosquito bite, the above conclusion would be accounted; and, also, that if this immunity were attained by inexpensive means—means which did not interfere seriously with comfort, pleasure, or business—the mosquito-malaria theory would not only be proved to the satisfaction of the public, but the public would be willing to accept the sanitary measures which the theory and experiments indicated.

After having obtained promises of support from the Colonial Office and from the London School of Tropical Medicine, and having secured volunteers for the experiments, still further to accentuate my object and to arrest the attention of those principally interested, I publicly announced in a popular lecture at the Colonial Institute that the above experiments were about to be undertaken, and with the same object in view I ventured to forecast their issue.

Experiment I—London

Drs. Bignami and Bastianelli very kindly undertook to send me relays of infected mosquitos from Rome. I have to thank these gentlemen for the great care exercised in this somewhat responsible matter. Every case of malaria coming to a general hospital is not suitable for experiment. To have sent mosquitos infected with malignant tertian parasites might have endangered the life of the subject of the experiment; and quartan-infected insects might have conferred a type of disease which, though not endangering life, is extremely difficult to eradicate. The cases, therefore, on which the experimental insects were fed, had to be examples of pure benign tertian—a type of case not readily met with in Rome during the height of the malarial season; the absolute purity of the infection could be ascertained only by repeated and careful microscopic examination of the blood of the patient.

When the insects had fed, Dr. L. Sambon, who had gone to Rome on Experiment No. 2, placed them in small cylindrical cages made of mosquito netting stretched on a wire frame. Four such cylinders were packed in a well ventilated box and forwarded to the London School of Tropical Medicine through the British Embassy in Rome. The box was 9 inches in depth and 8½ inches on the sides. The wire openings were 3 inches square on each side. The cages were each 8 inches in length and 3½ inches in diameter. By the courtesy of the Postmaster-General they came forward by the Indian mail so that they arrived in London some 48 hours after leaving Rome. A good many of the mosquitos died on the journey or soon after arrival; a fair proportion survived and appeared to be healthy and vigorous. We are indebted to Dr. Sambon for the method employed of caging mosquitos. Future experimenters will find it very useful. To infect the insect, or to become infected by them, the experimenter has merely to place his hand in the cage after carefully untying the netting at one end or, better, by laying the closed cage on his damped hand.

Notes of Experiment

I am 23 years of age, was born in China, but have lived in this country since I was 3; have never been abroad since, nor in any district in this country reputed to be malarial. I am healthy.

The first consignment of mosquitos arrived at the London School of Tropical Medicine on July 5th. Only some half-dozen had survived the journey. They were in a languid condition, and would not feed satisfactorily. One may have bitten me. By July 7th they were all dead. The second consignment arrived on August 29th. They had been infected in Rome on August 17th, 20th, and 23rd, by being fed upon a patient with a double benign tertian infection. The patient was reported to have had numerous parasites, including many gametes, in his blood. On arrival twelve insects were lively and healthy-looking. I fed five of them on August 29th, three on August 31st, one on September 2nd, and one on September 4th. They bit my fingers and hands readily. The bites were followed by a considerable amount of irritation, which persisted for two days.

The third consignment arrived on September 10th. They had been fed in Rome on September 6th and 7th on a patient suffering from a simple tertian infection, but with very few parasites in his blood. There were some 50 to 60 mosquitos in good condition. Twenty-five bit me on September 10th, and 10 on September 12th.

Up till September 13th I had been perfectly well. On the morning of the 13th I rose feeling languid and out of sorts with a temperature of 99°F. By midday I was feeling chilly and inclined to yawn. At 4.30 P.M. I went to bed with severe headache, sensation of chilliness, lassitude, pains in the back and bones, and a temperature of 101.4°. Repeated examinations failed to discover any malarial parasites in my blood.

September 14th.—I slept fairly well but woke at 3 A.M. with slight sweating and a temperature of 101°. During the day my temperature ranged between 101° and 102°. The symptoms of September 13th were exaggerated and anorexia was complete. Several examinations of the blood were made again with negative result. To relieve headache 10 grs. of phenacetin were given at 6 P.M.; I perspired profusely but slept indifferently.

September 15th.—Woke at 7 A.M. feeling distinctly better, with a temperature of 100.4°. No malaria parasites were discovered on repeated examinations of my blood by my father. About 2 P.M. I commenced to feel slightly chilly; this soon wore off, and I became hot and restless. By 4.30 P.M. temperature was 103.6°. It remained about 103° till 9 P.M., when profuse sweating set in. I am told there was some delirium.

September 16th.—I woke at 8 A.M. feeling quite well; temperature 98.4°. I made several blood examinations and found one doubtful half-grown tertian parasite. In the afternoon and evening there was a recurrence of fever (temperature 102.8°), relieved by sweating.

September 17th.—Again felt quite well on waking after a good night's sleep; temperature 99°. At 10 A.M. several half-grown parasites, a gamete, and two pigmented leucocytes were discovered in the first blood film examined. During the day many tertian parasites were found. Their presence was verified by my father, Dr. Frederick Taylor, Lieutenant-Colonel Oswald Baker, I.M.S., Dr. Galloway, Mr. Watson Cheyne, F.R.S., and Mr. James Cantlie, some of whom saw the films prepared.

About 2 P.M. the sensation of chilliness returned. Temperature 101.8°. By 5 P.M. temperature had reached 103°. There was then copious sweating. The edge of the spleen could be felt on deep inspiration, and there was a slight feeling of discomfort in the region of that organ. Dr. Frederick Taylor and Mr. Watson Cheyne confirmed the presence of splenic enlargement. By 9 P.M. the temperature had fallen to 99.2°, and I was feeling better. Quinine (10 grs.) was given.

September 18th.—Woke after a good night feeling perfectly well (temperature 97°). Ten grains of quinine were taken, and subsequently five grains every eight hours. I continued perfectly well all day. A few three-quarter grown tertian parasites and some gametes were found during the forenoon and afternoon; they were seen by Dr. Oswald Browne, my father, and myself. At 10 P.M. the parasites had disappeared, the last being found at 5 P.M.

September 19th.—No parasites discovered. Temperature normal. Feeling quite well. There is no splenic enlargement, and no tenderness. Appetite returned.

September 25th.—In good health. No recurrence of malarial symptoms.

Experiment II—The Roman Campagna

A wooden hut, constructed in England, was shipped to Italy and erected in the Roman Campagna at a spot ascertained by Dr. L. Sambon, after careful inquiry, to be intensely malarial, where the permanent inhabitants all suffer from malarial cachexia, and where the field labourers who come from healthy parts of Italy to reap the harvest after a short time all contract fever. This fever-haunted spot is in the King of Italy's hunting ground near Ostia, at the mouth of the Tiber. It is waterlogged and jungly, and teems with insect life.

The only protection against mosquito bite and fever employed by the experimenters who occupied this hut was mosquito netting, wire screens in doors and windows, and, by way of extra precaution, mosquito nets around their beds. Not a grain of quinine was taken. Drs. Sambon and Low, Signor Terzi, and their two Italian servants, entered on residence in the hut early in July. They go about the country quite freely—always, of course, with an eye on *Anopheles*—during the day, but are careful to be indoors from sunset to sunrise. Up to September 21st, the date of Dr. Sambon's last letter to me, the experimenters and their servants had enjoyed perfect health, in marked contrast to their neighbors, who were all of them either ill with fever or had suffered malarial attacks.

For the present I content myself with announcing this result. Complete details of their experiences will doubtless be made public by Drs. Sambon and Low at the termination of the malarial season, and of their experiment, at the end of October. Suffice it to say that these gentlemen express themselves as satisfied that protection from mosquito bite protects from malaria, and that protection from mosquito bite is perfectly compatible with active outdoor occupation during the day.

Application of the Experiments

It remains for the public to apply the lesson taught by these experiments. Will this be done? Already I have heard objections and difficulties mooted. I saw it advanced recently that it is impossible to avoid mosquito bite in the tropics, and that it was useless trying to do so. One has sometimes to go out in the evening; a doctor, for example, must visit his patient at any hour. This is quite true; but surely because we cannot escape a risk altogether this is no reason why we should not try to minimise it. Dr. Daniels, who has recently returned from British Central Africa, tells me that not one mosquito in a thousand in that country carries malarial zygotes, that is to say, is infective. If a man exposes himself therefore in British Central Africa to mosquito bite habitually, so that he gets bitten say ten times every night, the chances are that he is effectually inoculated with malaria some four times a year; but if the same man systematically protected himself from mosquito bite, and, in consequence of his care reduced the chances of being bitten to once a month, he might be a hundred years in British Central Africa before he became infected. This minimising of risk is certainly worth striving for.

The question of expense cannot for a moment be entertained in discussing the means for protection. One life saved, one invaliding obviated, would, even in a pecuniary sense, pay for all the wire gauze and mosquito netting requisite to protect every European house in West Africa.

These experiments, together with the work of Ross, Grassi, Celli, Bignami, Bastianelli, and other Italians, the recent observations on native malaria by Koch, and the representatives of the Malaria Commission of the Royal Society and Colonial Office, plainly indicate that the practical solution of the malaria problem lies in:

1. Avoiding the neighbourhood of native houses—the perennial source of malaria parasites.

2. The destruction, so far as practicable, of *Anopheles'* breeding pools.

3. And principally: Protection from mosquito bite.

45

Alphonse M. Schwitalla

The Real Meaning of Research and Why It Should Be Encouraged

Research is a bugbear to some people; a shibboleth to others. Some have found it an incubus; others have found it the guiding torch of truth. Some regard it as a gift of the gods; others find it the millstone on the neck of progress. Misunderstandings on this score have been beyond number.

And yet the fact is definite and clear, simple and unmistakable, that research among all human agencies has been the outstanding factor in the material development of our civilization. Research is after all nothing but the quest for truth. Without that quest we cannot uncover the mysteries of nature; we cannot delve into the meaning of life; we cannot envisage the hopes of the future, and we cannot draft programs for the betterment of mankind. Misunderstandings have arisen, it is true, regarding the types of research. In the minds of many, research evokes a vision of complicated machinery, elaborate equipment, huge laboratories, large personnel, extravagant budgets. Yet none of these things is essential to the concept of research or to its success. A photographic plate and a piece of tungsten were the equipment from which radiography was developed and from this the whole theory of radiant energy was contributed to theoretical and practical physics. A test tube in the hands of one may be a more powerful instrument than the most complicated set-up in the hands of another.

When we come to speak of research in the hospital, we carry into the hospital world the prejudices, predilections, the bigotry and the allegiance of the people at large. For after all superintendents of hospitals, members of boards, members of the lay and professional staffs and nurses are human beings and they share the ideas as well as the psychoses of the popular mind. They may under favorable circumstances have lifted themselves above the general convictions, the general fears and hopes, but we must not expect from them, taken as a large group, the highest manifestations of scientific idealism.

And so while it seems a truism to say that the hospital must encourage research, there still remains the large task of making the implications of that statement clear to the individual hospital administrator, to the board member, to the staff member, to the nurse. Research is a process but it is also an atmosphere. Let me speak of it first of all as the latter, an atmosphere that pervades an institution, that fills with a lifegiving influence the hospital activities, that stimulates thought and actuates policies.

The hospital is a depository of human problems. Each patient that passes the admission desk comes into the hospital as a living question mark, which theoretically at least is to be erased before the dismissal blank has been filled out. In regard to each patient, the complex mechanism of the hospital is set in motion in the quest for the truth behind the question mark and when that truth is discovered, a contribution is made to the sum total of human knowledge.

The research atmosphere is unescapable in an institution seeking to view its problem in such a light. The problem may be an oft repeated one, a million-times-told tale, yet with our modern concept of individualization and disease, it becomes progressively clear that each patient is a law to himself, presenting phases of a disease, complications, indications and contraindications without number. A fundamental principal of the law of variation as interpreted by science statistics is that the uniformities in a varied assembly of things can be discovered adequately only when the individual cases have reached a sufficiently large number. In this sense every hospital, be it large or small, can make its contribution to the sum total of human knowledge by developing in the members of its staff, medical as well as nursing and administrative, the feeling of responsibility, first, for discovering the meaning of a particular disease and second for making this accumulated knowledge accessible to the professions at large through reports and publications.

Saving Many Lives

In a hospital in which this quest for truth is active, its effect is noticeable in the general tone of the administrative and professional personnel. In fact if there is one feature that differentiates a lethargic from an enthusiastic institution, a hospital that does its duty as contrasted with a hospital that enjoys its duty, it is the fact that the latter type of institution considers its patients as human problems to be solved by the full expenditure of energy and resources. A human life saved is more than one human life saved, it may mean the lives of countless others saved through the accumulated and integrated experience gained through that process of saving. Surely, then, a hospital must encourage research.

Must a hospital also encourage research as a process—formal research? In answering this question we may again subdivide our problem into two, for statistical research differs from experimental research. I might grant for the sake of argument that all hospitals, especially those that are limited in resources, may not be able to undertake some of the larger programs of experimental research, but I cannot grant that even the smallest and the poorest hospital can be excused from accepting the privilege of making at least a minimum contribution to the sum total of knowledge concerning the human organism through the statistical research it is able to carry on.

What we ordinarily understand by clinical research often takes the form of a report of so many cases of a particular class of disease. Has this value? Surely, speaking generally, we shall all agree that it has. Therapeutics, again speaking generally, can be evaluated only when we know whether the success of a certain procedure exceeds the average of success in the control of cases of that particular kind. One physician or one group of physicians cannot supply such data. The statistics must be gathered from every known quarter and the more agencies that contribute to the accumulation, the safer becomes the application of a method or a process to the treatment of human beings. This kind of research even the smallest hospital can conduct.

There is, however, another form of clinical research regarding which question might arise. The twilight zone of human knowledge becomes progressively illuminated through the shafts of light that are pushed into the darkness. A new discovery, a new application of an old discovery, a modification of an old method, these and many similar processes may hold untold possibilities for saving the lives and preserving the health of human beings. Surely the

hospital may encourage this sort of research and should encourage it if the hospital is to make available to its patients the benefits of scientific discovery. Perhaps the term research is stretched too far in its meaning as applied to such a state and condition but an example will illustrate my meaning. Suppose that after the first announcements concerning the efficacy of insulin the hospitals the country over had waited until insulin treatment had been tried under the rigid condition that obtained in the larger hospitals and in some university hospitals, surely many a diabetic would have lost his chance to regain health. Instead, medical men in every quarter of our land undertook the application of the new discovery to all available cases of diabetes. It is true mistakes might have been made and perhaps the history of failures in this field might form an illuminating chapter, but without doubt alleviation of suffering was brought to many.

Taking Advantage of Scientific Discoveries

And what is true of insulin is just as true of countless less sensational procedures of which our research journals and our medical publications bring almost monthly record. I am not making a plea here for rashness or for misguided scientific zeal or for precipitancy, but every hospital administrator can enumerate cases that would undoubtedly have profited by the application of new procedures and perhaps might have been completely cured if the staff of the hospital had been quick to avail themselves of the latest contributions to science. While this may not be creative research, it is applied research, research into the limits of applicability of a given procedure to individual variations of a given type of disease.

There is another form of research to which I wish to call especial attention. Our hospitals have ceased to be merely institutions for the restoration of health and for the preservation of health; they have become schools, of a specialized kind to be sure, but still schools— schools for patients, schools for interns, schools for nurses, postgraduate schools for practitioners. Some hospitals by their public pronouncements have manifested their consciousness of

these educational responsibilities and all modern hospitals, even the smallest, are alive to them.

In this sense the hospital affords an experimental population in which to solve countless problems in adult and child health education, in methods of teaching theoretical and practical medicine and nursing, hospital administration, hospital interrelationships, public health, community, civic, state and national health responsibility. Practically every hospital, whether it be situated at the crossroads or in the midst of the bustle of the city, can make a contribution towards one phase or another of the numerous ramifications of hospital influence. None of these problems will find a final solution, it is true, because changing circumstances and changing times will continue to modify many seemingly final conclusions, but out of the welter of opinion and partial experience, there may develop a general psychological attitude and some principle may be adopted that will mark a turning point in hospital history.

Man Is Not a Laboratory Animal

Now let us consider the highest type of research possible in a hospital—formal, experimental, creative research. This, I am willing to concede, is not possible in all types of hospitals. There may be restrictions of budget and of personnel that will prevent the pushing onward of scientific thought through such types of research as are ordinarily performed in research laboratories. Even in this field, however, those hospitals that can afford the facilities, must and should be encouraged to enter upon a project proportionate to their means. The sick human being, it is true, is not a laboratory animal but neither is he so isolated in his human glory that he must be regarded as completely outside the possibilities of sane, carefully controlled, watchfully supervised experimentation, which may bring health to himself and health to countless other beings. I am aware that this question must be approached with the utmost delicacy, but I can well imagine circumstances arising in which, given the knowledge and skill of the physician and adequate facilities, a reasonable experimentation might well be regarded by the patient himself as a privilege that he would not, were the matter carefully explained, care to forego.

There is another form of research that cannot be too strongly insisted upon. Every autopsy is a solution of a research problem. The unknown factors in a disease are often uncovered by a carefully conducted postmortem examination. If the contributions made to the knowledge of medicine through autopsies could be heaped together, surely they would prove to be greater than those that came through many of the other forms of medical research. The responsibilities of hospitals in this field have been extensively stressed in the last few years and they will receive an added emphasis through the recent demands of the American Medical Association. But autopsies will be useful only insofar as they are conducted by men adequately trained and are reported by men equally well versed in the various medical sciences upon the knowledge of which an autopsy may draw. We may insist upon autopsies but that insistence alone will not advance medicine. We must stress the responsibilities for making the knowledge gained through autopsies accessible to ever widening circles of students.

Upon whom do the responsibilities for research in the hospital finally rest? The answer to this question, it seems to me, must be unequivocally given—it rests squarely upon the chief of staff, and in hospitals in which there is departmental organization, upon the directors of departments. In my opinion this is not a matter in which the superintendent of the hospital can play a leading rôle. It is well enough to talk about research in the hospital, but research cannot be conducted by inadequately trained men who cannot see a problem or who having seen the problem are blind to its implications or to the avenues by which it may be approached.

When Tact Is Essential

I know that this matter is beset with difficulties. Departmental directors are frequently men of an older school, men who held sacred the healing functions of medicine and men to whom the teaching function of the practitioner was a self-gratifying luxury. Such a man may have under him a subordinate who comes from a modern medical school, himself vibrant with the verve of discovery, himself perhaps an author of no small achievement. Even in this case, I believe organization demands the mutual subordination of viewpoints, psychological and social adjustments, without stifling the ambition of the subordinate. The medical man who has graduated within the last fifteen years has been trained, at least in a rudimentary way, in the intricacies of research. Given the chance and the environment, he will allow his investigative powers their legitimate exercises and I would bespeak for the ardent tyro, the paternal guidance and helpful encouragement of an enlightened director. Lucky the hospital in which the entire staff is imbued with the enthusiasm for contributing to our knowledge of human disease.

And what is the role of the superintendent and of the board of directors in this undertaking? They should, first of all, become keenly alive to the hospital's responsibility for making contributions to knowledge. These contributions may have merely local significance, they may afford stimulation for the local medical society and its members or for the local population. But they have greater value if in addition they extend the influence of their hospital to ever widening circles. Secondly, I would say that it is the function of the superintendent and of the board of directors to see to it that the staff includes as many men imbued with the spirit of research as the geographical location of the hospital, the available finances and the facilities allow.

Hospitals Can Learn from Schools

Thirdly, the superintendent and the board of directors should try to create better and better facilities for the prosecution of research and should seek to rise from one level to a still higher level of scientific achievement. Fourthly, the superintendent and the board of directors should make it their business to point out problems from time to time as they are suggested by the conditions in the institution. Schools, colleges and universities have learned the importance of self-surveys, exhaustive or partial, periodically conducted. It is amazing how much such self-surveys have contributed to pedagogical theory and to school science. Hospitals, if they wish to meet their responsibilities should adopt similar methods.

Fifthly, the superintendent and the board of trustees should give the opportunity for research, and without invading the field of professional medicine, should wisely and cautiously direct the minds of the members of the staff to a deeper and fuller appreciation of the research attitude. They should put at the disposal of their staff members, libraries and laboratories, books, instruments, personnel, which will, by their very availability, galvanize scientific indolence into industrious activity.

Will the patient be lost sight of in all of this? Emphatically, no. The patient must ever remain the center of the hospital. It is, after all, for his sake that scientific achievement must be pushed to the ultimate limits of professional knowledge. The patient's life, his health, his safety are foremost, but none of these can be secured unless someone, somewhere, sometime is engaged in the type of activity I am here advocating.

46

Andrew C. Ivy
Nazi War Crimes of a Medical Nature

Reprinted with permission of the editors from *Federation Bulletin,* vol. 33, 1947, pp. 133–146. Copyright 1947, Federation of State Medical Boards of the United States, Inc.

In my capacity as consultant of the Bureau of Medicine and Surgery of the Navy, I first came into contact with the nazi war crimes of a medical nature. As our troops advanced into Germany, a number of trained scientists accompanied the advanced patrols to obtain information that might be of assistance in completing the war against Japan. The experimental data of Dr. Rascher had been obtained and required evaluation. Dr. Rascher had cooled human subjects to a temperature of 75 and 80 F. to ascertain the best way to resuscitate them. Some of the data in Rascher's reports were obviously good and conformed with evidence obtained in animals. Other data were obviously unreliable and labeled Dr. Rascher not only as an unethical and atrocious person but also as a pseudo-scientist and seeker of political preferment.

In August 1946 I went to Germany at the request of the Secretary of War to visit the various sections of the War Crimes Branch of the Adjutant General's Office. I reviewed and analyzed the documents they had collected, and discussed the ethical principles under which experiments on human subjects are justified. The attorneys had a number of questions in mind, such as: Were the experiments necessary? Were they properly designed? Were the results of any value? Is it legal or ethical to experiment on human subjects? Since some of the victims were condemned prisoners was it not proper to use such prisoners in experiments? Some of the attorneys knew we had performed a great number of experiments on ourselves, and volunteer human subjects during the war. Some had heard about the experiments of Walter Reed, Goldberger, and others. The attorneys appeared somewhat confused regarding the ethical and legal aspects as well as the scientific aspects of the question. These questions had to be answered in order to determine whom to indict and the degree of guilt.

In January 1947 I returned to review about 2,000 pages of transcript of the prosecution and about 250 documents that had been introduced by the prosecution.

In other words, I have served in the same capacity that a physician and scientist serves in this country in a trial which has medical and scientific aspects.

In dealing with these crimes of a medical nature, it is first necessary to separate those which are experimental in nature, or those which were done with the idea of answering a scientific question from those in which no scientific question was involved. This is necessary in order to clarify our thinking and to prevent emotions from swaying judgment.

The nonexperimental crimes were different in nature. I shall cite a few of these. First, the mass killings started out with so-called euthanasia or mercy killings or the extermination of the useless life. This was first practiced on the insane by a secret edict of Hitler published in 1939. It is interesting, in this connection, that in the Haddemar trials which occurred late last Spring, the German defense attorneys did not even know of this secret edict of Hitler. Our investigators had uncovered it. It is also interesting that there was so much talk against euthanasia in certain areas of Germany, particularly in the region of Wiesbaden, that Hitler in 1943 asked Himmler to stop it. But, it had gained so much impetus by 1943 and was such an easy way in crowded concentration camps to get rid of undesirables and make room for newcomers, that it could not be stopped. The wind had become a whirlwind.

A second type of mass killing consisted in the extermination of poor workers. This consisted of placing poor producing persons on a low caloric or "hunger diet." It was easy to sell the idea that since food was scarce, those that did the most work should have the most calories. Hence a lot of people were placed on diets containing first a thousand and then 800 and then finally when they had contracted some disease or became so weak that they could no longer stand, they were considered to be living a useless life, and were according to their terminology "mercifully killed."

A third type of mass killing was obviously genocidal (race killing) in nature. This pertained to gypsies, Jews, Poles, and Russians in the order given. That is, these individuals were frequently referred to in the nazi documents as belonging to the subhuman species and were considered to be primates somewhere between the range of the human being or the Herrenvolk and a chimpanzee. There was one instance where 120 murders were committed to provide skeletons of Russian Jews for an anthropological museum at the University of Strasbourg. Professor Hirt, the director of a museum, wrote a letter to Himmler in which he used the sales talk pertaining to race, nazi racial theory. He said that he had representative skeletons of various races and species in his museum but he did not have any specimens of the "subhuman species" represented by the Jewish Russian Commissar, and he wanted specimens of that sort. The bodies were supplied by the Institute for the Study of Races but when the Allies landed in Normandy, Professor Hirt became skittish and manifested his criminal culpability by writing to Mr. Sievers, one of the men who worked under Himmler, and inquiring what he should do with the unused specimens. He said that he could say they were bodies the French had left behind in 1940. He was told that he had better wait a while, since the material was quite valuable. However, by the time our troops reached Metz, a letter was written to the effect that all of the material had been destroyed.

Another type of nonexperimental crime was committed in operations performed on prisoners without apparently any purpose except practice, and which represented the crime of mutilation. In several places, definite evidence has been obtained showing that the prisoners were used for experimental surgical material to train senior students and recent graduates in surgical technic in the same way that dogs are used in this country. For example, one morning on one patient a surgical team would perform a subtotal gastrectomy, a cholecystectomy and a choledochoenterostomy. Sometimes six to ten prisoners would be scheduled for the students to practice on.

The experimental crimes were crimes; first, they were crimes because they were performed on prisoners without their consent and in complete disregard for their human rights. They were not conducted so as to avoid unnecessary pain and suffering, death being the premeditated outcome in a number of these experiments. Second, they were crimes because they were

contrary to the Hague Conventions and the Rules of Land Warfare. In some of the experiments, the data were obviously faked and unreliable. Fortunately, for the sake of respect to our own profession, only about seventy of the nazi physicians were concerned in this work, only a few of them were well known and none were outstanding physicians and scientists.

One of the experiments they performed, which was particularly atrocious, was the typhus experiment. I copied from one of the notebooks a protocol of one of these typhus experiments. These experiments were performed under the supervision of Dr. Mrugowski, Director of the Hygienic Institute of the Waffen SS, which was not a part of the Robert Koch Institute for the Study of Contagious Diseases. This is the protocol.

"Typhus fever vaccine experiments series 7, May 28, 1943, dates of vaccination: Group 1, 20 persons; vaccine—acid; Group 2, 20 persons; vaccine—acid absorbate; Group 3, 20 persons; vaccine Weigl."

"August 27, 1943: Group 1, 20 persons; Group 2, 20 persons; Group 3, 20 persons; Group 4, 10 persons as a control. Each was injected intravenously with one quarter of a c.c. of whole blood from a typhus fever patient."

"September 7, charts and histories completed. The experimental series were concluded. Total, fifty-three deaths, eighteen in Group 1 with vaccine acid; eighteen in Group 2 with vaccine acid absorbate; nine in Group 3 with Weigl vaccine; eight with control." Eight of the ten controlled subjects died.

"September 9, 1943, charts and case histories delivered to Berlin." This is a protocol of one of the series of experiments conducted at Buchenwald Concentration Camp between January 1942 to January 1943. During this period at least 729 persons were subjected to such experimentation and 154 died. This does not include the so-called "passage group." In order to keep the typhus virus alive and virulent, they would take two prisoners and inject the virus. At the height of the disease they would take another prisoner and inject the blood from the acutely ill typhus fever patient. Thus they kept the virus alive and handy. In other words, these

prisoners were used just as rats, guinea pigs and rabbits are used in the laboratory and sometimes without showing them as much consideration as we show our animals in the laboratory.

I desire to show you what frequently resulted when persons having the nazi-SS type of training were placed in charge of experimental work under conditions where the aim was to seek political preferment or to follow orders, rather than to seek the scientific truth.

The following statement refers to Dr. Ding who was the physician actually in charge of doing the typhus experiments at Buchenwald and who later committed suicide. "Dr. Ding, being placed under pressure by the Hygienic Institute in Berlin, demanded that we produce large quantities of typhus vaccine for the fighting troops. From that moment, we produced systematically two types of vaccine. One type was perfectly harmless but had no value. This was produced in large quantities and sent to the front. A second type was produced in small quantities by the American method and was highly effective. It—the American vaccine—was used only for special cases and we too who worked in Block 50 were repeatedly vaccinated with the potent vaccine."

This is just one of several examples present in the documents showing what the nazi-SS training and political pressure caused these people to do. At least ten other experiments just as atrocious could be cited and established as having occurred.

I should like to cite an experiment with an objective which had no bearing on the welfare of the German Army, Navy, or Air Force. The Nazi party, in order to promote the master race by genocide, desired to find a secret or quiet way of sterilizing large populations. To this end they had three experiments in progress when the war closed. One experiment consisted of putting the dried juice of a plant in the flour fed the population. The dried juice was supposed to sterilize both males and females, particularly the female. A second experiment . . . consisted in having them stand at a counter and fill out the forms while being exposed without their knowledge to a castration dose of X ray. A third experiment consisted in calling the women of a population in for a routine physical examination. While being examined, an intra-uterine injection was made. As well as could be determined, a silver nitrate solution was used.

After Himmler and his cohorts had sterilized the undesirable population he planned to repopulate the territory with the master race. But he was not satisfied to do this at the normal average rate of one birth every fifteen months, so he had some scientists work on multiple ovulation. An endocrinologist from Denmark was sent to Ravensbruk. There he injected into women an extract of the anterior lobe of the pituitary gland to produce multiple ovulation so as to obtain multiple pregnancies.

This should give one some idea of the extent to which the ideology of the Herrenvolk, Lebensraum, and genocide was being developed.

Political prisoners, the citizens of Germany or other countries, were used for any sort of experiments. For example, it was reported, according to the documents, that the Russians had used a poison bullet. This report was not authenticated. The nazis wondered what the poison might be and they calculated it might be aconite. So they put aconite in some bullets and shot some prisoners in various places with the poison bullets. They then described the symptomatology of aconite poisoning and gave the length of life after the shooting of the individual depending on where the wound had been produced. There were two subjects in the experiment in whom the bullet had pierced the leg completely and these prisoners survived the experiment.

The sea water experiments teach a very interesting lesson and bring up some familiar names. In 1943 at the Naval Medical Research Institute there was developed an effective and efficient method for desalting sea water. By June of that year this and other apparatus for prolonging life on a raft at sea was tested in the field. Then the information was released to the newspapers and magazines. Life Magazine published a picture of a sailor in a rubber raft drinking this desalted sea water. The picture was turned over to Himmler early in 1944 who sent it to his technical bureau

with the statement: Why haven't you done something like this? The technical bureau replied: "The technical bureau, the RLM reports to the Fuehrer that two processes are available to render sea water potable, one the I.G. method using mainly silver nitrate which gets rid of the chloride from the salt in the sea water and requires the resulting water to be sucked through a filter which requires bulky equipment and silver which is scarce. The second is the Berka method which involves only the addition of (fruit acid) citric acid to sea water." Reading further, "German technical science has actually succeeded in rendering sea water potable for people in distress at sea but naturally the office is very much interested in ascertaining how, above all, the United States have solved this problem and it is requested that this information be sought."

It was argued by Berka that citric acid made a combination of salt which was not metabolized. A physiologist was called in and told that the Berka method was of no value. The physiologist of course was right because citric acid only counteracts a salty taste. Because the physiologist did not have an inside political track in the hierarchy his statement was discounted. Dr. Eppinger and Dr. Heubner were called in. It was agreed that some experiments should be made and Dr. Bligelboeck was asked to perform the experiments and was told that they were to be performed on gypsies and a few other persons at Dachau. I saw his data books during my last trip to Germany, and I interrogated him. You could easily observe from the data that the prisoner-subjects had stolen water and were otherwise very uncooperative.

I asked him what sort of assistants he had helping to determine blood potassium, sodium, specific gravity, and so forth. I found they were all well-trained chemists. Then I said, "Do you believe that the data which you have here are worthy of publication in a medical journal?" He said immediately, "No, by no means." I said, "You had well trained assistants." He replied, "Yes, sir." I said, "Well, why didn't you choose reliable subjects to work on?" He said, "Well, I wrote to Professor

Eppinger to the effect that these experiments should be performed only on myself and my corpsmen, or on convalescent soldiers about to be returned to the front; but I received a reply that these experiments were to be done at Dachau on the prisoners. I had to go there and perform them."

In other words, we have here a well-trained scientific physician who knew what constituted a scientific experiment. The design of his experiment was excellent, very much like the experiments we performed in Bethesda in 1942 and 1943. He knew that the data that he was collecting were valueless from a scientific standpoint. This is to be kept in mind because it emphasizes one of the ethical points pertaining to human experimentation. That is, in studies on human subjects the cooperation of the subjects is practically always essential.

The tragedy of all of these experiments of this blotch on the history of medicine is that nothing of significance was added to medical knowledge.

These were crimes against German laws and international law. As late as 1945, a review of German criminal law stated that euthanasia of any degree was criminal. It was stated that the law must take care not to shatter the confidence of the sick in the medical profession. The extermination of a worthless life, for instance killing of incurable idiots, could be made unpunishable solely by change of legislation. That was the status of German law. A German criminal court recently executed four doctors who took part in euthanasia experiments. These experiments were crimes in relation to international law for the following reason: I quote from the Hague Conventions and the Rules of Land Warfare which were signed by Germany and were known to German military officers. "The inhabitants and belligerents remain under the protection and the rule of the principles of the law of nations as they result from the usages established among civilized peoples and from the laws of humanity. Family honor and rights, the lives of persons and private property, as well as religious convictions, and practice must be respected." These experiments were all performed contrary to the ethics under which legitimate human experimentation is performed and has been performed throughout the world even in Germany before and during the war.

On my last trip to Germany I took affidavits and legal documents showing the conditions under which human beings were used as experimental subjects in the U.S.A. during the war. These are the conditions: (1) Consent of the subject must be obtained. All subjects have been volunteers in the absence of coercion in any form. Before volunteering, the subjects have been informed of the hazards, if any. (2) The experiment to be performed must be so designed and based on the results of animal experimentation and the knowledge of the natural history of the disease under study that the anticipated results will justify the performance of the experiment. That is, the experiment must be such as to yield results for the good of society unprocurable by other methods of study and must not be random and unnecessary in nature. (3) The experiment must be conducted only by scientifically qualified persons to avoid all unnecessary physical and mental suffering and injury so that on the basis of the results of previous animal experimentation there is no a *priori* reason to believe that death or disabling injury will occur except in such experiments as those of Walter Reed on yellow fever where the experimenters served as subjects along with the nonscientific personnel. In other words, whenever there has been danger attached to any experiment, any a *priori* hazard, it has been honorable medically for the experimenters also to serve as subjects. Such rules are required to insure the human rights of the individual, to avoid the debasement of a method for doing good, and the loss of the faith of the public in the profession.

Here are some of the arguments that the nazis used to condone experiments on human subjects without their consent. They have been offered during interrogation of medical prisoners. The first argument is superior orders. They say, "We had a gun at our head." That is true in many instances. They had a gun at their head, but from the standpoint of law if someone has a gun at my head, puts a gun in my hand and tells me they will shoot me unless I shoot a certain individual, if I shoot the individual I am a murderer under mitigation. I have no right to murder under

the law even though I might be killed if I did not commit the murder. A second argument is that the experiments were performed only on prisoners who were condemned to die by the nazi-SS leaders. That is wrong. Some of these prisoners had and others had not been condemned to die. It was also argued that since they would die in the concentration camp sooner or later one might as well obtain some good for humanity out of them. This particular argument has been advanced many times for doing experiments on prisoners condemned to die; and, on the surface, it appears to be justified. Its error will be indicated later.

The third argument was presented by those nazi scientists who were not pseudo-scientists. They argued that since the experiments were to be done anyway under orders of the nazi-SS, they should be done by qualified and trained scientists so the data would be reliable.

The fourth argument was based on the argument of euthanasia. If it is right to take the life of useless and incurable persons, which as they point out has been suggested in England and the United States, then it is right to take the lives of persons who are destined to die for political reasons. Good, they say, is accomplished in both instances.

To analyze these arguments logically one must review the principles of ethics. There are three views regarding the source of power of ethical and moral principles. One of these is called the intuitive view, according to which the power is derived from a divine person or is revealed to holy men. The second source of power of ethical principles is referred to as the traditional view, according to which the power is derived from custom, social or political usage or the law. The third is referred to as the scientific view, according to which the power of ethical rules is derived from the happiness and social welfare or ultimate good which follows their obedience.

On the basis of these views, human experimentation can be justified by the results, provided (1) the experimenters make certain the reason for performing the experiment is adequate; (2) provided unnecessary pain and distress is avoided; (3) provided human rights of the subject are not transgressed, and (4)

provided the indirect effects on the public and experimenters are not such as to promote a spirit of inhumanity or cruelty. Those provisions are very important because otherwise one argues, like the nazis, that the end justifies the means. They are provisions which prevent the debasement of a method for doing good.

Let us refer to the Oath of Hippocrates which has served as the ethical guide for our profession for twenty-two centuries. This oath pledges us to teach our science and art; to manifest good conduct; to honor the physician-patient relationship, and to demonstrate a reverence for life. In the interpretation of biology, there is one important thread that runs throughout and that is, as Schopenhauer pointed out, "the will-to-live." If we apply the golden rule to the will-to-live, we derive therefrom a reverence for life. The Oath of Hippocrates is the golden rule of the physician.

Except for such rules enforced by the profession itself, how can the public have confidence in the individual physician and the profession? The attitude of the physician towards the patient must conform to the golden rule and the public must realize that this rule of conduct is guarded and enforced by the profession. Enforcement by law is not enough.

When the nazi-SS administrators and physicians were asked if they would want their children, wives and themselves experimented on without their consent in the way these prisoners were used, they all said no.

The crux of the ethical question pertaining to the Nürnberg trials from the medical viewpoint is whether condemned prisoners should be experimented on without their consent if such were allowed by law. My answer to that question is no. I should refuse to experiment on any prisoner condemned to die or group of prisoners condemned to die without their consent. This conviction is based on the following very pragmatic reasons: (1) It has not been shown to be necessary to use human beings without their consent. Prisoners in our own country and elsewhere have volunteered when told of the good that the results of the experiment might produce. (2) In most experiments the interest and cooperation of the subject is necessary. In the presence of coercion, the reliability of the results may be questioned. That is exactly what occurred in at least three of the nazis' experiments as documented by unchallengeable evidence. (3) The performance of experiments on human subjects without their consent though they were condemned to die would undermine the faith ordinary patients have in the profession. It would make hangmen in my opinion out of physicians. (4) The weakening of one moral principle favors the weakening of another until the individual or a profession becomes immoral or amoral.

I tried in my reading of documents and discussion with the prisoners and physicians in Germany to ascertain the background of these atrocities. Some of these individuals were pseudo-scientists who were trying to gain political preferment in the Nazi party. This was an important factor. However, there were other factors. One was a debased regard of the duty of a physician toward poor and underprivileged patients. That was the start. I have talked to doctors who have received some postgraduate education in Vienna and Germany, and who said they could not condone the way the poor and underprivileged patients were treated in the clinics. A second factor was the practice of euthanasia for the extermination of useless persons by secret edict and subterfuge. This led to the development of ways and means for killing large groups of people. These breaches of ethics nurtured by a third factor of the ideology of the Herrenvolk and the means of killing en masse facilitated the practice of genocide and the killing of anyone who was undesirable to an official. A fourth factor played an important role in many minds. Namely, the welfare of the armed forces is the supreme good. Some believe solely in the last explanation: that is, to most nazis and most of the German people the welfare of the armed forces was the supreme good and anything that helped the armed forces was right.

It is important to know and to realize that there was a small group of physicians in Germany who knew that these things were going on and protested. I saw a letter which Himmler wrote to Rascher. It stated, "Please provide me with a list of those individuals with Christian medical ideas who believe

that these experiments we are performing on the human beings are wrong." He said, "They are traitors." In other words, he wanted the list so as to bring the critics to justice.

I agree with the statement which was made by Dr. Enloe of New York in the Journal of the American Medical Association in December to the effect that many German physicians did not know what was going on in these camps and that if those who knew had protested, they would have been placed in a concentration camp themselves. Nevertheless, Professor Rose in one of the meetings where the results of the typhus experiments were first reported is said to have criticized the experiments by saying that they were superfluous, that everything determined by them could have been found out on animals, and that in his opinion murder was being committed. He was soon silenced apparently because he did not speak up again. Also, there were two physiologists who were asked to take part in the freezing experiments who refused and were able to get away with it.

I have said in a previous discussion that there is a very serious aspect to the fact that the German medical profession and German medical science permitted these things to happen. I should like to emphasize this statement, though it is subject to a double interpretation. On the one hand, it is subject to the interpretation that I would seriously criticize and condemn the whole German profession for not protesting, for not fighting the nazis, and for permitting these things to occur. It was too late, of course, for physical comfort to protest during the war when these crimes happened. In fact, by that time the Nazi party had destroyed medical organizations and had converted what was left into political gangs. On the contrary, when I made that statement I made it with the idea in mind that it showed how a political gang, how an ideology such as that of totalitarianism, can insidiously take over a profession which has high ideals and finally subvert that profession or at least some members of it into performing atrocities, and place that profession in such a position where it is unable to protest effectively.

Before the war occurred, the German medical profession had been placed by

Hitler and Himmler under nazi political control under Dr. Conti. He was the leader and iron-handed ruler of the German medical profession. This is what he taught: The German physician should not consider only the sick individual but he should always see beyond the sick individual the heredity stream of the German people flowing according to eternal laws. It will be the business of the German physician not only to aid the German individual physically but to guide him psychologically according to the credo of the national socialist ideology, and so forth. In order to enter medical school the student had to be trained in the nazi ideology. It was necessary to pass examinations in nazi racial theory. The medical curriculum was broken with party drills, rallies and raids on anti-nazis.

Today in the American-occupied zone there are five medical schools in operation. They have a total enrollment of 8,154. About 20 per cent of them are females. The curriculum is much like that in the United States. The faculties have been denazified. They consist of teachers who, as I came into contact with them at the University of Erlanger, are competent, but who are very short of materials, supplies, textbooks and literature.

In this connection I should like to read a statement: "There is a large medical proletariat ready to swing into any ideological camp that is ready to offer them some measure of security and social recognition; by assuming an altruistic attitude toward these people, helping them out with some teaching materials, by letting them know of American technics and achievements, it may be possible to make these men susceptible to our ideas rather than to those of other political and national groups whose views we would prefer not to see spread further." I should like to support that statement. I found on discussing the status of medical science in Germany the extent to which recent medical information has permeated medical circles in Germany, that it would be very worthwhile for us to get our medical journals and periodicals into the hands of these teachers.

These considerations teach me that it is dangerous to stray from the ethical code of Hippocrates. It is dangerous to interfere with or to jeopardize the doctor-patient relationship. We must oppose any political theory which would regiment the profession under a totalitarian authority or insidiously strangle its independence. The profession must have foresight and courage to fight those proposals which would destroy or place in jeopardy the ethics of the profession. The doctor-patient relationship and the ultimate health and welfare of the society must be kept foremost. Medicine as first recognized by Hippocrates has a moral and social philosophy as well as a scientific and technical philosophy to maintain.

47

The Nuremberg Code

Reprinted from *Trials of War Criminals before the Nuernberg Military Tribunals under Control Council Law No. 10,* vol. 2 (Washington, D.C.: U.S. Government Printing Office, 1949), pp. 181–182.

The Proof as to War Crimes and Crimes against Humanity

Judged by any standard of proof the record clearly shows the commission of war crimes and crimes against humanity substantially as alleged in counts two and three of the indictment. Beginning with the outbreak of World War II criminal medical experiments on non-German nationals, both prisoners of war and civilians, including Jews and "asocial" persons, were carried out on a large scale in Germany and the occupied countries. These experiments were not the isolated and casual acts of individual doctors and scientists working solely on their own responsibility, but were the product of coordinated policy-making and planning at high governmental, military, and Nazi Party levels, conducted as an integral part of the total war effort. They were ordered, sanctioned, permitted, or approved by persons in positions of authority who under all principles of law were under the duty to know about these things and to take steps to terminate or prevent them.

Permissible Medical Experiments

The great weight of evidence before us is to the effect that certain types of medical experiments on human beings, when kept within reasonably well-defined bounds, conform to the ethics of the medical profession generally. The protagonists of the practice of human experimentation justify their views on the basis that such experiments yield results for the good of society that are unprocurable by other methods or means of study. All agree, however, that certain basic principles must be observed in order to satisfy moral, ethical and legal concepts:

1. The voluntary consent of the human subject is absolutely essential.

This means that the person involved should have legal capacity to give consent; should be so situated as to be able to exercise free power of choice, without the intervention of any element of force, fraud, deceit, duress, over-reaching, or other ulterior form of constraint or coercion; and should have sufficient knowledge and comprehension of the elements of the subject matter involved as to enable him to make an understanding and enlightened decision. This latter element requires that before the acceptance of an affirmative decision by the experimental subject there should be made known to him the nature, duration, and purpose of the experiment; the method and means by which it is to be conducted; all inconveniences and hazards reasonably to be expected; and the effects upon his health or person which may possibly come from his participation in the experiment.

The duty and responsibility for ascertaining the quality of the consent rests upon each individual who initiates, directs or engages in the experiment. It is a personal duty and responsibility which may not be delegated to another with impunity.

2. The experiment should be such as to yield fruitful results for the good of society, unprocurable by other methods or means of study, and not random and unnecessary in nature.

3. The experiment should be so designed and based on the results of animal experimentation and a knowledge of the natural history of the disease or other problem under study that the anticipated results will justify the performance of the experiment.

4. The experiment should be so conducted as to avoid all unnecessary physical and mental suffering and injury.

5. No experiment should be conducted where there is an a *priori* reason to believe that death or disabling injury will occur; except, perhaps, in those experiments where the experimental physicians also serve as subjects.

6. The degree of risk to be taken should never exceed that determined by the humanitarian importance of the problem to be solved by the experiment.

7. Proper preparations should be made and adequate facilities provided to protect the experimental subject against even remote possibilities of injury, disability, or death.

8. The experiment should be conducted only by scientifically qualified persons. The highest degree of skill and care should be required through all stages of the experiment of those who conduct or engage in the experiment.

9. During the course of the experiment the human subject should be at liberty to bring the experiment to an end if he has reached the physical or mental state where continuation of the experiment seems to him to be impossible.

10. During the course of the experiment the scientist in charge must be prepared to terminate the experiment at any stage, if he has probable cause to believe, in the exercise of the good faith, superior skill and careful judgment required of him that a continuation of the experiment is likely to result in injury, disability, or death to the experimental subject.

48

R. A. McCance
The Practice of Experimental Medicine

Reprinted with permission of author and editors from *Proceedings of the Royal Society of Medicine,* vol. 44, 1951, pp. 189–194.

We have most of us a picture in our minds of what we mean by medical practice, both in its broader aspects, and in its narrower fields of general practice, consulting practice and so on. Each of these phrases conjures up something very real. To most of us the doctor comes to heal and we can picture his work: we appreciate the disciplines, responsibilities and the ethical background of the life of anyone who dedicates himself to such a service. Few people have such a clear picture of what the practice of experimental medicine involves; yet broadly speaking, those who set out to advance our knowledge of disease and treatment must sooner or later have recourse to experiment, for in the biological sciences experiment is the only sure way by which any advance can be established.

Claude Bernard's writings entitle him to be regarded as the father of experimental medicine but Harvey, Jenner and John Hunter were brilliant exponents of its possibilities long before his time, and the practice was already well established by the middle of the last century. Many of Claude Bernard's writings on the subject of experimental medicine do not require to be brought up to date. They are ageless. Changing customs and the passage of time, however, have created new situations and fresh problems and it is with these that I propose to deal.

Let us start with the word experiment, which most biologists use very loosely to cover any investigation, however trifling, made to advance knowledge. The term generally implies some deliberate change of conditions without foreknowledge of the results but with subsequent observation of them. It may be used, however, even when the conditions are not being deliberately changed, when the term observation would be more correct. Many doctors would not regard the attempt to cure an individual patient as an experiment, yet it undoubtedly may be, if the results are observed and followed up, for the essence of treatment is to do something positive to a patient, i.e. alter his conditions, in the hope that the effect will be of benefit to him.

People who are sick are often apprehensive. They long for reassurance which they do not find in the word "experiment." Worse still, the word may conjure up alarming possibilities in their minds. This is partly due to the activities of the antivivisection societies, partly to the casual use of terms such as "human guinea-pigs," partly to the atrocities which were perpetrated in concentration camps, and partly to the investigators themselves. The only comment made by a member of the governing body of the hospital when our department was being formed was that the name [Department of Experimental Medicine] was an unfortunate one. I hope it was not, for I think it was the correct name, and we shall certainly do our best to prove it.

There is one fundamental difference between the investigator and the physician. A good investigator may be as full of bedside charm and therapeutic ability as a good physician, but he must primarily be interested in his problem. The physician is interested first, last and all the time in his patients, and he has little sympathy with the attitude of the man who appears from time to time in the wards with a request to be allowed to disturb in some way one of his patients who may just be turning the corner after a critical illness. It goes against the grain to allow his patients to be used for a controlled therapeutic experiment if it means deliberately withholding from half of them the treatment which he believes, albeit unjustifiably, will do them good. He forgets, indeed he may not even know, that what he would have regarded as an "unjustifiable experiment" five years ago may have become one of his standard diagnostic or therapeutic procedures. The investigator finds it equally difficult to see eye to eye with a colleague who can alter a patient's treatment in the middle of one of his experiments without even letting him know, so nullifying two or three weeks of his work. Tact and a spirit of mutual co-operation and understanding are the only solutions. Taking a little trouble to develop new micro-methods often gives the entrée to a children's department, and placing a few beds at the disposal of an investigator often allows him to organize and complete good work to everyone's satisfaction and benefit.

Patients provide the problems, and disease may produce conditions which could never have been achieved experimentally and which demand detailed investigation, but if the illness is acute and treatable it is usually unjustifiable to withhold the remedy for long enough to make all the observations desirable in a satisfactory experiment. Chronic disease offers greater opportunity, but the basis of all successful experimentation is control of the conditions, and in the wards this may be very difficult. It is often much more satisfactory to work on normal men and women. Normal men and women are ideal for all physiological experiments when the "stress" originates in the environment, and some of the metabolic disease states can be reproduced in normal people. I have never had much difficulty in obtaining the co-operation of normal subjects. It is always a great help to have made the same experiment on oneself first and to be prepared if necessary to do so again. This is certainly true of metabolism experiments. Students make good subjects for some tests and they have frequently been employed, but in my experience they are not the best subjects for most experimental work. They can seldom give the necessary time for metabolism experiments, and they are often so overcome by the sight of blood that the complication of a faint is introduced into any test involving its removal. An experienced laboratory worker, male or female, is infinitely preferable. Subjects can, I believe, be hired for experimental work in some countries, and this may be a satisfactory arrangement, but I should be sorry to see this kind of service placed upon a commercial basis in this country. In the United States the patient is expected to contribute materially towards the expenses of his stay in hospital and he is generally anxious, therefore, to make this as short as possible. The hospital, in fact, may have to be reimbursed if a patient's discharge is delayed for experimental work, or if a special admission is made for such purposes. Valuable work was done by groups of conscientious objectors during and just after the war, and this is a form of national service which might very well be encouraged if the volunteers have the necessary mental and physical balance. Service personnel are now being employed for some experimental work on the physiological effects of heat and cold, high and low atmospheric and other gas pressures, and the stresses and strains of warfare.

These men volunteer for the work and for some purposes they may be excellent.

Those who practise experimental medicine are naturally most interested in human disease and physiology and, as Claude Bernard put it: "Il est bien certain que pour les questions d'application immédiate à la pratique médicale, les expériences faites sur l'homme sont toujours les plus concluantes." Nevertheless, the advantages of turning to animals are numerous, and the greater part of the work of a department of experimental medicine is often carried out on them. They can be obtained as and when required; their size is often convenient; they can be killed if necessary. Greater numbers of small animals than of human beings can be used and a better statistical result obtained. Their rapid rate of reproduction and short life span are invaluable for work on nutrition, genetics and carcinogenesis. In fact, once the investigator has posed his problem to himself he generally looks around for the most suitable animal on which to study it, and his choice often makes for success or failure. "Le choix intelligent d'un animal présentant une disposition anatomique heureuse est souvent la condition essentielle du succès d'une expérience et de la solution d'un problème physiologique très important." Claude Bernard was right but it is not always possible to reproduce in animals the set of conditions which have been under observation in man, and many since his time have forgotten that what has been proved for one species may not hold for another, and one of the attributes that makes for success in experimental medicine is the instinct which tells a man when to check his results on a second species, and above all when to turn from animals to man, or *vice versa*.

There is no difficulty about working with animals in this country, provided suitable accommodation can be found for them. One must comply with the Law relating to experiments on animals, but few people would wish to do otherwise. A licence is obtainable for any justifiable work on living animals. The investigator then has to make an annual return of his experiments and his animals are periodically inspected, but he benefits in that he is protected

from unauthorized interference. The Authorities at the Home Office have always been most helpful to me. A licence is not required to kill animals, so that any of their tissues may be obtained immediately after death for chemical, metabolic or pathological work without let or hindrance.

There is no difficulty about making some kinds of experiments on one's fellow creatures, and they are the only mammals for which a vivisection licence is not required in this country, but the use of man as one's experimental material raises all kinds of issues, moral, ethical and legal which have never really been faced and which, in my opinion, should be faced. A hundred years ago the issue was clear. "On a le devoir et par conséquent le droit de pratiquer sur l'homme une expérience toutes les fois qu'elle peut lui sauver la vie, le guérir ou lui procurer un avantage personnel. La principe de moralité médicale . . . consiste donc à ne jamais pratiquer sur un homme une expérience qui ne pourrait que lui être nuisible à un degré quelconque, bien que le résultat pût intéresser beaucoup la science, c'est-à-dire la santé des autres."

We should, I think, for present purposes, regard anything done to a patient, which is not generally accepted as being for his direct therapeutic benefit or as contributing to the diagnosis of his disease, as constituting an experiment, and falling, therefore, within the scope of the term experimental medicine. The definition, however, should not include all those unplanned experiments which are inseparable from the admission of any child or adult to a hospital, and which are often attended with considerable physical and psychological dangers, nor should it include the administration of established prophylactic remedies, even though some of them, particularly the attenuated viruses, may involve risk. The experiment visualized may be one of omission and consist of withholding treatment from a "control," or it may be one of commission and consist of making some test on a patient for which there is no obvious and immediate need. Whatever the problem interesting the investigator, however, it is, of course, true to say that the results of such tests must always help to characterize the diseased state and when known may sometimes be of benefit to the patient on whom the tests have been made. There is a case to be made out for regarding all these tests as being "investigations" conducted in the sufferer's best interests and therefore not constituting an experiment made solely for the advancement of knowledge. Wassermann reactions are carried out on every patient admitted to some hospitals and every patient entering the Mayo Clinic is, I believe, subjected to an elaborate series of investigations. The real distinction is a subtle one and may depend upon the mental approach of the man who makes the tests. Nevertheless, I regard collecting an extra specimen of urine or taking an extra 5 c.c. of blood from a vein puncture, made purely for established diagnostic or therapeutic purposes, as falling within the range of the term "experiment." I would certainly regard weighing a baby "unnecessarily" as an experiment. Some people may think I am taking up a ridiculous attitude over this, but if an experiment is not defined in this way, where is the line to be drawn?

All experiments involve some risk. It may be an infinitesimally small one, but it is always there—you, or the nurse, may drop the baby for instance. If the experiment involves special vein punctures, or perhaps infusions, the risk is considerably enhanced, but it still remains immeasurably small in the hands of an experienced operator. Nevertheless, I have myself seen and experienced the most alarming effects from pyrogens and I think it is quite likely that the virus which gave me a mild attack of jaundice in 1939 reached me through a syringe. In assessing the risks involved in any experiment and therefore the justification for doing it, there are many factors which require consideration. The skill and experience of the investigator are important ones, but so is the place where the experiment is to be performed. A procedure which would be perfectly safe in a well-equipped and well-staffed establishment might be quite unjustifiable somewhere else. A well-trained person is much less likely to make a mistake over a drug or its dosage than an untrained technician in a badly staffed hospital. I have recently given this question a good deal of thought in connexion with our work in Germany and other "field" work.

The mention of assistants brings me to another point. Many experimental workers are not qualified in medicine, and yet they take part in hospital work and experiments on normal people. Could they conceivably be regarded as "unqualified assistants," and what would be the position if an accident were found to be due to one of them? If a foreign medical man has come to this country to work in a department of experimental medicine it has, since 1947, been possible for him under the Medical Practitioners and Pharmacists Act to have his name placed temporarily on the Medical Register. This legalizes his position and if he can then join one of the Medical Defence Unions he and the department should be fully covered.

If an experiment is the first of a series it involves much more risk than one which has been made many times before by the same people out of the same bottles. I never worry at all, however, about trying out an unknown substance on man, for with a little patience one can work up the dose on oneself or other normal people so gradually that the risk can be reduced to vanishing point, but I do not think I would ever have had the temerity to carry out the first hepatic biopsy or cardiac catheterization. Our pioneer studies of renal function in newborn infants were made on babies which had been born with inoperable meningomyeloceles. Hundreds of these experiments have now been made on normal newborn and on premature infants in other countries—yet I am still hesitating about doing so.

The risk involved in any experiment depends very much on whether the investigator knows that he will always retain control of the situation. An experiment on salt deficiency or dehydration can be pushed till the subject is showing severe effects, because the remedy is available all the time. To inoculate someone with icterogenic serum is a risk that I personally would never take, nor would I ever have cared to take it even before the risks were so well known, for once the inoculation had been made, I would have lost control. Everyone working experimentally with normal human subjects or with patients must remember not only his responsibility to the subject or patient but also

his responsibility to the discipline of experimental medicine. One irresponsible experimenter can do great harm to medical science.

No experiments can be carried out on a healthy colleague without his co-operation and consent and any elaborate experiment should be preceded by a medical examination; the same thing applies to a healthy child. It would also, I believe, be regarded as an offence under common law to make any investigation upon a child which involved the removal of hair, skin or blood without its parents' consent. In consequence of this, school children are so well protected by their teachers and other officials that it is often a very elaborate affair arranging for an experiment on a group of them. When a person comes into hospital, however, many investigations are made, and necessarily made, for direct diagnostic or therapeutic purposes, and patients expect a certain number of "tests." These are part of the hospital routine, and although patients have the right to refuse, it is extremely rare in this country for anyone to do so, and, as a matter of fact, many appreciate the attention. Hence, many experiments, even quite elaborate ones, can be made on patients, within the therapeutic routine of the hospital so to speak, without anyone thinking anything of it. Many experiments are made on this basis, and all help to define the effects of disease on function but the results seldom get recorded on the patients' notes. If the experiment is more elaborate and demands considerable co-operation, the investigator may feel it desirable to ask the patient for his "permission." It is often difficult for an investigator to explain the nature and object of his work to a non-scientific colleague and generally quite impossible to a patient. The investigator can only tell the patient in very general terms what his experiment will involve, explain the nature of the risks and ask for his co-operation. Experiments on children and infants are carried out on exactly the same basis except that parents have to be approached for permission, and the whole procedure becomes much more formal and tricky, for it is generally possible to size up a prospective subject before asking him for his co-operation, whereas it is a very different matter to go up to an unknown parent on visiting day and make your request.

It is still more difficult to approach a newly delivered mother about an experiment on her baby, even if this only involves a study of how it breathes, and the inclination to make the experiment without doing so is very great. Patients and parents, however, rarely refuse, and in my experience opposition to experimental work in hospital generally comes from colleagues under whom the patients have been admitted, and from the nursing staff who are, in general, antagonistic to research, especially on children, unless maybe it is being carried out by their own particular "chief." An experimental study always involves them in extra work the reason for which they do not fully understand and which often appears to them to run counter to their ideas about the comfort and care of the patient. They are on the whole satisfied with the knowledge of to-day. They forget that nothing in this world is static and that knowledge can be lost as well as gained. Research has made our knowledge great and can make it greater, but without research knowledge would fall away as it did in the Middle Ages. All our triumphs of to-day would be forgotten—they may be anyway—but without continuous research there would be nothing to take their place. Those who educate medical students and nurses should therefore emphasize to them the value of the experimental approach, and encourage them at some point in their careers to do something for the medical science of to-day and to-morrow by taking an active interest in experimental work.

No doubt the practice differs from one hospital to another, but the principles just outlined about "permission" seem to hold generally throughout this country. In some continental countries the position is rather different and the co-operation of the patient or parent is seldom sought and in some places it is generally assumed that it would be refused. This is an unfortunate state of affairs. A little thought shows that the whole position in this country depends upon trust. The patient trusts the staff of the hospital, and the investigator, knowing this, usually dispenses with the formality of asking for "permission," when his experiments simply involve procedures which are the commonplaces of clinical practice but he

generally prefers to take the patient or parent into his confidence over anything more elaborate, and this is where his conscience and judgment become so important.

This seems a happy arrangement and one which we are fortunate to have evolved. Some other nations have not been so successful. The whole atmosphere of trust would be destroyed if patients had to be asked to fill in a printed form of consent for experiment as they are as a rule for an operation. I would feel happier, however, for the future, if patients could be made more aware that at some hospitals—the best hospitals—experimental work is carried out not only for the benefit of the immediate sufferers, but also for the benefit of mankind, and that they themselves owe incalculable advantages to work of this kind which has already been done on others; furthermore, that if they or their children are privileged to be admitted to these hospitals, they may be expected to co-operate. In the form given to patients on admission to one hospital I know, there is a small paragraph and the addition of a few words to it illustrates the sort of thing I have in mind. The additions proposed are in italics. "The hospital staff seeks your assistance in carrying out the hospital's duty to the community in the *investigation of disease and in the* training of doctors and nurses: if a member of the staff wishes to *make a special study of your condition or to* explain it to a medical student, doctor or nurse, it is hoped that we may have your co-operation."

Although it is legal to kill an animal without any vivisection licence and tissues can be taken immediately after death without any formalities whatever, it is extremely difficult to obtain fresh human tissues for experimental work unless they have been removed by a biopsy, for once a person has died a post-mortem examination may only be made with the permission of the next of kin or the person in lawful possession of the body (unless of course the coroner or the official referee under the Cremation Acts orders a post-mortem to be carried out to ascertain the cause of death). These manoeuvres all take time during which the chemistry of the cells becomes completely disorganized,

but, the law being as it is, it would, I feel sure, be unlawful to remove any part of the body for purposes of research immediately after the death of the patient without the previous consent of the nearest relative. This makes it very difficult to carry out many desirable investigations, and even the gross composition of the human body is still only known to us in very vague terms because of the legal obstacles which prevent a *bona fide* investigator from obtaining the complete body of a human being for analysis. With the co-operation of an anatomy school it can be done, and we have ourselves done it, but the removal for examination must not take place until forty-eight hours after death, and it is necessary to comply with other legal formalities. There is much more work to be carried out on the metabolism of fresh human tissues and on the chemical composition of the organs of whole bodies by people with the necessary interests and opportunities.

A great deal more might be said about the practice of experimental medicine, and its place in medical practice as a whole. Almost every statement I have made could have been greatly enlarged but it would be better for others to do this in the light of their own experiences. As I see it, however, the medical profession has a responsibility not only for the cure of the sick and for the prevention of disease but for the advancement of knowledge upon which both depend. This third responsibility can only be met by investigation and experiment, and from the nature of things it is always likely to remain the task of a few men and women specially gifted and/or trained for the purpose. Some of these people have in the past sacrificed considerable wealth for the mental satisfaction of their work. This may not have to be so in the future but all such practitioners have a right to expect the fullest co-operation from their medical colleagues, from nurses and other assistants, from hospital managements, from patients and relatives and from the community at large.

49

Austin Bradford Hill
Medical Ethics and Controlled Trials

Reprinted with permission of the editor from *British Medical Journal,* vol. 1, 1963, pp. 1043–1049.

In commemorating the work and character of Marc Daniels it is only natural that this yearly lecture should almost invariably be related to some aspect of the epidemiology, prevention, or treatment of tuberculosis. For herein lay his most memorable contributions to medicine, and herein he displayed at their best his talent and his personality. However—and I think very fortunately—the conditions of the lecture do not limit the speaker to the field of tuberculosis. They permit him to explore any subject in public health, epidemiology, or therapeutics that can be regarded as apposite to Dr. Daniels's own research interests. I need therefore make no apology for departing so far from custom and for devoting myself to a quite general problem in clinical medicine—the trial of a new (or old) treatment.

More important perhaps than terms and conditions, I know well that I am embarking upon a theme which in the early trials of the new drugs in tuberculosis was often in Marc Daniels's thoughts. Not only had he an urge for perfection and accuracy, not only had he a patience and capacity for hard work that enabled him to seek that perfection in every detail—characteristics which are so necessary for the success of an organized controlled trial—but (as I wrote almost 10 years ago) he had an outlook upon the ethical problem which made him pause and reflect at every step. With all his eagerness for the experimental approach no one could have been more humane, more careful of the patient's well-being. These characteristics were fortunately linked with an unusual organizing ability and an unusual share of that statistical common sense that is anything but common.

In a review (*British Medical Journal,* 1948) of the Medical Research Council's first controlled trial of streptomycin in the treatment of pulmonary tuberculosis it was suggested that the trial might well become a model in this field. The prediction was right. Many therapeutic trials in many branches of medicine have been founded upon this early essay. And it is in this development that lies the true memorial to Marc Daniels.

Treatment of Pulmonary Tuberculosis with Streptomycin

When, in 1946, the Medical Research Council's Streptomycin in Tuberculosis Trials Committee set out to investigate the effect of that drug in pulmonary tuberculosis it was faced with no serious ethical problem. The antibiotic had been discovered two years previously, its striking powers *in vitro* and in experimental tuberculous infection in guinea-pigs had been reported; the published clinical results were distinctly encouraging though not conclusive. Yet overriding all this evidence in favour of the drug was the fact that at that time exceedingly little of it was available in Great Britain, nor were dollars available for any wide-scale purchase of it from the U.S.A. Except for that situation it would certainly on ethical grounds have been impossible to withhold the drug from desperately ill patients. *With* that situation, however, it would, the Committee believed, have been unethical *not* to have seized the opportunity to design a strictly controlled trial which could speedily and effectively reveal the value of the treatment. There was no dearth of patients with the type of disease defined (acute progressive bilateral pulmonary tuberculosis of presumably recent origin, bacteriologically proved, unsuitable for collapse therapy, age-group 15–30). There was no possibility of obtaining sufficient streptomycin for them all. There was no other suitable form of treatment for them but bed rest.

Thus, knowing that all the streptomycin available in this country was being effectively used—much of it for two rapidly fatal forms of the disease, the miliary and meningeal—the Committee (1948) could proceed not only without qualms of conscience but with a sense of duty to do so.

It is perhaps not often that such a situation exists—though it recurred in this country a few years later with the introduction of the inactivated vaccine against poliomyelitis—but whenever a newly introduced drug or vaccine is scarce in its early days, then there presents an opportunity of which immediate advantage should, if possible, be taken. With a serious disease in which the old offers very little hope of benefit the new cannot be withheld. The chance of adequately and quickly assessing the value of the latter, if any, may never again occur.

In spite of circumstances so favourable to the therapeutic experiment the Tuberculosis Trials Committee had nevertheless two ethical problems to resolve. About the first—the doctor's responsibility to the patient in his care—there was, of course, no real difficulty. In this trial, as *in all controlled trials,* it was implicit that the doctor must do for his patient whatever he really believes to be essential for that patient to restore him to health. If he believes that it is essential for the patient's well-being that he remove him from a comparative group on an orthodox treatment to a group on a new and unproved treatment (or vice versa), then surely it is his basic duty so to remove him. While such removals may seriously weaken, or even destroy, the value of a trial there can be no other means of meeting the ethical situation. For example, in the specific trial to which I refer, the cases accepted were by definition unsuitable for collapse therapy. Yet it was axiomatic that the clinicians were free to adopt collapse therapy if the course of the disease so changed that they believed such a measure was indispensable and urgent (and it was, indeed, adopted in 11 of the 52 cases).

The second ethical problem was this. All the patients on streptomycin were given four injections of the drug daily for (mainly) four months. What should be the parallel treatment of the control group? The Committee again had no difficulty. It immediately rejected any idea of corresponding injections of saline, so frequently and for so long a time, and relied upon a clear answer emerging in so serious a situation from two groups, both on bed-rest, but one injected and one not. It could not for ethical reasons insist upon an exact equality between the groups, the full double-blind procedure. Nor in this instance do I myself believe that procedure to have been required when the success or failure of the treatment rested upon life or death, or in the assessment of X-ray changes by persons kept unaware of the treatment given to the patient.

In a controlled trial, as in all experimental work, there is no need in the search for precision to throw common sense out of the window.

The Experimental Approach

In the assessment of a treatment medicine always has proceeded, and always must proceed, by way of experiment. The experiment may merely consist in giving the treatment to a particular patient or series of patients, and of observing and recording what follows—with all the difficulty of interpretation, of distinguishing the *propter hoc* from the *post hoc.* Nevertheless, even in these circumstances and in face of the unknown a question has been asked of Nature, and it has been asked by means of trial in the human being. There can be no possible escape from that. This is *human* experimentation—of one kind at least. *Somebody* must be the first to exhibit a new treatment in man. *Some patient,* whether for good or ill, must be the first to be exposed to it.

What, therefore, is new in the development of the last 20 years is, I would suggest, the most careful *planning* of the experiment in advance, and an experiment that usually, though not invariably, makes the following demands: (a) the construction of two (or more) closely similar *groups* of patients observed at the same time and differing in their treatment; (b) the construction of these groups by some process of *random* allocation; and (c) the *withholding* of a form of treatment from one or other of these groups.

In other words, we have the familiar controlled trial of to-day in which group A is given the new drug or other treatment under test and group B is not given that treatment, and the progress of their illness is then assessed and compared. As an additional, and occasional, feature we may (d) use a placebo as the treatment of the control group.

It is by means of such *comparisons* that we hope to avoid the dangers of deduction described so well by a writer in the *Boston Medical and Surgical Journal* a trifle over 100 years ago (Cheever, 1861). "Effects are ascribed to drugs which really flow from natural causes, and are but the usual succession of the morbid phenomena; sequences are taken for consequences, and all just conclusions confused. From the want of this knowledge [of the natural history of the disease]; from defective observation, rash generalizations, and hasty conclusions a *priori,*

have arisen the thousand conflicting theories which have degraded Medicine from its true position as a science, and interfered with its advancement as a practical art."

To be fair to Dr. Cheever I should add that he thought the experimental approach to be of "doubtful application in the therapeutical art" and had this to say of statisticians in 1861: "All the theorists say to the practitioner at the bedside, 'Do not try, but think; reason, argue, deduce!' Empirical Hunter said, 'Do not think, but try!' So the modern disciples of the numerical method would say to us, 'Neither think, nor try; but calculate!' Meanwhile the patient dies."

However that may be (and Dr. Cheever offers no alternative), the object of the present-day numerical method is to ensure that the patient will die rather less often. Let me return to the planned experiment designed to this very end.

The Controlled Trial

Customarily the situation is this, that from pharmacological and other tests there is reason to believe that a new drug is safe and likely to be beneficial. Neither belief, however, is established and neither can be established without some form of trial in man. Yet a very little experience of medicine shows that very often the beliefs are accepted without adequate trial and that very often they are wrong.

To take, almost at random, a quite simple and recent example from the literature. Thulbourne and Young (1962) point out that "in surgical wards antibiotics are commonly administered prophylactically to patients known to have chronic chest disease, and to those who for some other reason are thought to run a special risk of post-operative chest infection." Critical of this routine, they conducted a clinical trial with 65 patients given a course of penicillin before and after operation and 70 not so treated. It appears that the drug neither reduced the incidence of post-operative chest infections nor lessened their severity. Was it, one may ask in passing, more ethical to continue to use unquestioningly a powerful antibiotic, day in, day out, with no measure of its benefit than deliberately to withhold it from a specific group of patients in an attempt to find out?

A similar question may be posed of the trial by Fraser, Hatch, and Hughes (1962) of aspirin and antibiotics in the treatment of minor respiratory infections. The three randomly constructed groups treated with (1) potassium phenoxymethyl penicillin, (2) oxytetracycline, and (3) calcium aspirin, show no appreciable differences in the number of patients who developed complications, nor in the duration of their illness, fever, and headache. In short, there is no evidence that the antibiotics influenced either the course of the disease or the number or quality of the complications; and the authors are led to conclude that the indiscriminate exhibition of antibiotics has no advantage over aspirin in treating these uncomplicated minor illnesses in young adults.

A more difficult and complex situation was revealed in a trial of long-term anticoagulant therapy in cerebrovascular disease (Hill, Marshall, and Shaw, 1960, 1962). In previous uncontrolled studies there was a distinct if inconclusive suggestion in favour of their use, and sufficient, indeed, to make a trial difficult. Yet when put to the test of a controlled trial with the comparison of a fully treated group and a group given a dose insufficient to interfere with the clotting mechanism, it not only appeared that no protection was afforded against the recurrence of cerebrovascular accident, but there was a small but definite risk of cerebral haemorrhage in the fully treated cases.

Here we have an instance—and by no means unique—of the wheel turning full circle. At the start of the trial was it ethical to withhold the treatment? At its end was it ethical to give it? It is very easy to be wise (and critical) *after* the event; the problem is to be wise (and ethical) *before* the event.

In all walks of life, I fancy, we are not always wise in our reluctance to depart from the *status quo,* our established and yet unproved beliefs. In medicine, to give an example, Sir George Pickering (1949) described how he was taught that iron and arsenic each had a specific effect on blood formation in man. "As a student and house-physician I saw nearly all patients with anaemia treated with a mixture containing 5 grains of iron and

ammonium citrate, 2 minims of liquor arsenicalis, and other ingredients to supply taste and colour, which were given long Latin names. This was a time-honoured treatment used in my hospital and generally in this country for many years. I never saw any improvement of anaemia result from this treatment, though the patients were no doubt pleased to be seen from time to time by a considerate doctor. We now know as a result of applying the experimental method that the dose of iron used was quite inadequate, that there is a very common form of anaemia which responds readily to adequate dosage of iron, and which is in fact due to iron deficiency. As a result of applying the experimental method, we are not only now able to help patients that we could not help before, but by having learned the specific nature of the malady we are now able to prevent it in people who would probably have developed it but for our intervention. As far as I know arsenic has never been shown to benefit any form of anaemia."

Sometimes, of course, the difficulties of experiment are very much graver than in that example. When the benefits of streptomycin had been clearly established in young adult phthisis it was not at all easy to devise trials which would measure the relative value of *para*-aminosalicylic acid and isoniazid. Yet whether the experiment was well- or ill-designed it had *somehow* to be made. In looking back, and forward, it is proper to remember McCance's (1951) comment that the physician "forgets, indeed he may not even know, that what he would have regarded as an 'unjustifiable experiment' five years ago may have become one of his standard diagnostic or therapeutic procedures." To take a gloomier view, some of his standard diagnostic and therapeutic procedures of to-day may in five years' time be entirely obsolete.

In short, medical literature abounds with examples to show that the belief that an unproved treatment (new or old) *must* for ethical reasons be exhibited is unwarranted. Some treatments are valueless, some are hazardous. The whole question is how best can we discover those facts. If the clinical trial is the method of choice then

the question becomes in what circumstances can the doctor withhold (or give) a treatment while preserving the high ethical standards demanded of his profession?

There is no easy answer. In my own experience of collaboration with doctors the problem calls for close and careful consideration in the *specific circumstances of each proposed trial.* No doubt, of course, one can enunciate some very broad principles of ethical behaviour, principles which are an intrinsic part of the doctor's training. But I do not myself believe that it is possible to go very much beyond that, that one can reduce the broad principles to precise rules of action that are applicable in all circumstances.

A Draft Code of Ethics

This, however, is not the view of such an authoritative body as the Ethical Committee of the World Medical Association (1962). The results of their deliberations have been set out in a preliminary draft code of ethics on human experimentation which should serve as a guide to doctors.

In criticizing this code and in setting out subsequently my own views on medical ethics in controlled trials I am deeply conscious of the fact that I am a layman. My excuse is that I have participated and studied in some branch of medicine throughout my working life, and in clinical trials for nearly the last 20 years. In the planning and conduct of these trials I have had the good fortune to be associated with a very large number of medically qualified men and women, including many of the leaders of the profession. I have endeavoured to absorb their ways of thinking as well as their knowledge. I have spent many hours reflecting on these critical problems of ethics, and it is my hope that this account of those reflections may be of value. I would beg the reader to keep that in mind when I invade what may appear to be the very special province of the profession itself.

The code of the Ethical Committee of the World Medical Association starts with a precise definition of an experiment on a human being: "an act whereby the investigator deliberately changes the internal or external environment in order to observe the effects of such a change." Such change in the environment, it continues, should be made only if certain conditions are observed, and one of these conditions is that the experiment should be conducted "under the supervision of a qualified medical man." Even as a layman invited to this *sanctum sanctorum* of British Medicine I cannot let that pass. In an exceedingly rash experiment that I have so far very carefully avoided I decide to measure the effects of my methods of teaching. I divide the class into two and I instruct these halves in quite different ways. I assess the effects of such a change in the *external* environment. An even rasher experiment—on randomly determined nights I persuade my wife to drink a cup of hot milk before going to bed; I record her subsequent complaints of insomnia—that is, the effects of a change in the *internal* environment. Am I to be supervised in either of these pursuits of knowledge by a medically qualified man? Without being facetious (and basically neither of my experiments is facetious) there are scores of experiments—for example, in industrial psychology—which are not the prerogative, or even within the special competence, of the medically qualified.

It may be retorted that such researches are not intended here. Maybe not, but it is what the words say. And if the code is to be helpful to your profession, surely it must be clear as to what it does mean? Surely it must not be open to argument as to *intention* regarding who, what, when, or where? If it is thus open to argument and individual interpretation what is its value?

Another of the general principles that the code sets out in relation to the change in the environment is this: "That the nature, the reason, and the risks of the experiment are fully explained to the subject of it, who should have complete freedom to decide whether or not to take part in the experiment." It is quite clear that this provision applies to my present subject-matter, since under the heading "experiments for the benefit of the patient" it is said that "controlled trials in therapeutic and preventive medicine should be conducted according to the general and special ethical rules concerning experiments on the individual."

Personally, and speaking as a patient, I have no doubt whatever that there are circumstances in which the patient's consent to taking part in a controlled trial should be sought. I have equally no doubt that there are circumstances in which it need not—and even should not—be sought. My quarrel is again with a code that takes no heed—and in dealing with generalities can take no heed—of the enormously varying circumstances of clinical medicine. Surely it is often quite impossible to tell ill-educated and sick persons the pros and cons of a new and unknown treatment versus the orthodox and known? And, in fact, of course one does not know the pros and cons. The situation implicit in the controlled trial is that one has two (or more) possible treatments and that one is wholly, or to a very large extent, ignorant of their relative values (and dangers). Can you describe that situation to a patient so that he does not lose confidence in you—the essence of the doctor/patient relationship—and in such a way that he fully understands and can therefore give an *understanding* consent to his inclusion in a trial? In my opinion nothing less is of value. Just to ask the patient does he mind if you try some new tablets on him does nothing, I suggest, to meet the problem. That is merely paying lip-service to it. If the patient cannot really grasp the whole situation, or without upsetting his faith in your judgment cannot be made to grasp it, then in my opinion the ethical decision still lies with the doctor, whether or no it is proper to exhibit, or withhold, a treatment. He cannot divest himself of it simply by means of an illusory or uncomprehending consent.

Another general principle of this code lays down firmly "that children in institutions and not under the care of relatives should not be the subject of human experiments." Does pasteurized milk contribute less than raw milk to the promotion of health and growth? Does sugar in the diet influence the incidence of caries? Is gammaglobulin more, or less, effective than convalescent serum in the prevention of measles? Was it unethical to find out in the very circumstances in which it was possible (as well as important for the subjects) to do so? The guide says Yes.

It also asserts that "persons retained in mental hospitals or hospitals for

mental defectives should not be used for human experiment," and this would seem to me automatically to condemn as unethical clinical trials in psychiatry. Again, that may not be the intention; but it certainly has that result.

These are just a handful of examples of the proposed "should and should not" that come from high authority. It is said that they are only a "guide to doctors in different parts of the world," but once so formulated and promulgated it would, I suggest, be difficult, if not even sometimes legally hazardous, for a doctor to act counter to them. It is my belief that they may hamper, if not prevent, much research through clinical trials that not only is entirely ethical but can, indeed, be more ethical than the unthinking use—that is, *experiment*—of unproved treatments.

It is, however, easy to be destructive. Let me attempt to be constructive.

The Specific Approach

With every proposed clinical trial there is, in my experience, a whole series of ethical problems that have to be closely considered and solved before the trial is set in train and *within the particular circumstances of that trial*. In other words, my philosophy embodies *general* questions answered in a *specific* setting. Included in these questions will be the following.

Is the Proposed Treatment Safe or, in Other Words, Is It Unlikely to Do Harm to the Patient?

There can be no categorical answer Yes or No. No one of the enormously beneficial treatments that have revolutionized therapeutics over the last 20 years is free of undesired side-effects or without any hazard to the patient. None could have been introduced if complete safety had been demanded. Similarly, no operative procedure is without its mortality, however small.

With a known hazard of a proved effective treatment the decision to take that risk would obviously be influenced by the risk of *not* giving the treatment; for example, the doctor might well decide to [prescribe] chloramphenicol in typhoid fever and be reluctant to do so in uncomplicated whooping-cough. The same reasoning will be needed in facing the unknown. With no knowledge of a danger it would be proper to explore the potentialities of a new treatment in a disease of some severity, but not with a mild self-limiting condition.

Similarly, the possible nature and degree of the hazard itself calls for reflection. Taking again the known case, the physician might legitimately accept the transient nausea of P.A.S., but, in given circumstances, reject the irreversible vestibular damage that may follow certain treatments with streptomycin. With the unknown, using as guide all the available pharmacological information, he will need, I suggest to think of similar lines.

In all clinical trials worthy of the name careful and precise observations are a *sine qua non*. Where any risk from a treatment may be anticipated one will need to think whether any special observations can be made to bring it to light—and possibly more rapidly than by means of haphazard uses of the treatment. Here indeed, I would argue, is one of the advantages—practical and ethical—of the controlled trial, that by its exact comparisons it may more rapidly pinpoint the unsuspected undesirable side-effects of a treatment. I would add, however, that no trial is likely to reveal the rare and disastrous effect that occurs only once in many hundreds of cases.

Can a New Treatment Ethically Be Withheld from Any Patients in the Doctor's Care?

The basis of the controlled trial of a new treatment compared with the old is, of course, that we are entirely ignorant of the relative values of these treatments. Presumably, however, we shall know something of the absolute value of the older treatment, and the question, therefore, may well be *not* can the doctor withhold the new, but can he withhold the established in favour of what is then quite unproved?

Let us again consider some possible circumstances. At one extreme we may have an orthodox treatment that offers nothing in a disease that is lethal—for example, cancer. It would seem to me that the doctor cannot withhold any new treatment that appears to offer a hope of success. At the other end of the scale we have an orthodox treatment that offers nothing in a mild self-limiting disease—for example, the common cold. Can we not, at the very

least in young adults who are unlikely to suffer complications or to die from a running nose, withhold the latest wonder drug from one group to measure adequately its alleged effects?

In between these extremes there will be an enormous diversity of circumstances—a diversity both in diseases and their severity and in established treatments and their values, proved or accepted. Surely the question can be answered *only* in terms of those circumstances?

What Patients May Be Brought into a Controlled Trial and Allocated Randomly to Different Treatments?

The essential feature of a controlled trial that determines an answer to this question is that it must be possible ethically to give *every* patient admitted to a trial any of the treatments involved. The doctor accepts, in other words, that he really has no knowledge at all that one treatment will be better or worse, safer or more dangerous, than another. I have already briefly illustrated above how often that is true. If the doctor does not believe that, if he thinks even in the absence of any evidence that for the patient's benefit he ought to give one treatment rather than another, then that patient should not be admitted to the trial. Only if, in his state of ignorance, he believes the treatment given to be a matter of indifference can he accept a random distribution of the patients to the different groups.

In that situation I would, as a statistician, point out that there is nothing unethical in the use of random sampling numbers, though to the uninitiated they may appear a trifle inhuman. If the treatment is a matter of indifference, then how we distribute the patients to each treatment is equally a matter of indifference. It happens that the use of random sampling numbers is usually a better method than the more traditional alternate patient technique.

I would argue, too, that ethically the doctor is in very much the same situation if, more traditionally, he measures the relative effects of treatments by ''ringing the changes'' *within* patients rather than *between* patients. It was, wrote Lord MacMillan (1937), a wise statesman who said of the law that

''where it is not necessary to change it is necessary not to change.'' The same dictum will apply to controlled trials within the patient, and so, *mutatis mutandis,* we will have to answer just the same questions as I am posing here in relation to trials between patients.

Returning to my question what patients may be brought into a trial, we shall need to think whether certain types should be omitted even though there may be no evidence whatever that one treatment rather than another will be to their benefit—for example, pregnant women with whom in the light of recent knowledge we should obviously deal with ultracaution, patients with complicating conditions and diseases, the very old and frail or the very young to whom any specially required observations and measurements (of, say, the blood) will be unduly vexatious, etc.

All this must be thought upon. By certain omissions from a trial we may limit the generality of the answer given by it, but on ethical grounds that, in my experience, must be accepted. While on this question of omissions I would repeat, and with the utmost emphasis, what I pointed out in reference to the first trial of streptomycin in pulmonary tuberculosis—namely, that it is implicit in all the trials with which I have been concerned that omissions must take place *after* the admission of the patients if the doctor in charge of a patient believes it to be necessary for that patient. This indeed may make extremely difficult the effective trial of treatments in chronic diseases. If the patient does not recover at the exhibition of one treatment, the doctor may feel it necessary to exhibit the other and thus nullify the required strictly controlled comparison. But that, of course, has been accepted at the outset in every controlled trial—that the ethical obligation always and entirely outweighs the experimental. The doctor in practice testing—that is, experimenting with—a new treatment can always change back to the old and orthodox if he thinks fit. Controlled trials should be equally fluid—though they may rightly demand very much more careful observation and reflection before the change back is made.

It is pertinent, too, to point out that the controlled trial almost invariably demands the follow-up and study of *every* patient admitted to it whether on the allocated treatment or not. Once again, therefore, it may be, to my mind, more ethical in its concepts and execution than the uncontrolled haphazard observations of patients, many of whom are quite unconcernedly lost to sight.

Is It Necessary to Obtain the Patient's Consent to His Inclusion in a Controlled Trial?

I have already made clear that in my opinion this question should really be worded, *When* is it necessary to ask the patient's consent to his inclusion in a controlled trial? At one extreme is the situation in which the patient will be subjected to discomfort or pain on one or more occasions—for example, by an inoculation, or a series of inoculations, with normal saline to measure the value of inoculation with a believed efficacious agent. Here, in face of pain and discomfort which is not an inevitable concomitant of the patient's disease or of its treatment, I would myself wish to have a full and understanding consent.

Going further, I would in particular wish to seek it in the trial of a prophylactic inoculation in which the doctor is not concerned merely to do his best for the patients already in his care, but in which he is *inviting* well persons voluntarily to enter an experiment. In making the invitation it would be proper, as well as prudent, to explain the circumstances to those you endeavour to attract. It is, however, clear that the results of such experiments (for example, the use of an influenza vaccine in patients with chronic bronchitis) may not only contribute to knowledge but be of considerable benefit subsequently to the participants themselves. Trials are frequently made with both motives, and should be thought upon in both respects.

Returning to the problem of the treatment of patients in the doctor's care, the customary situation of the controlled trial is, as I have already described, an ignorance of the relative merits of two (or more) treatments. To dispel that ignorance you decide to give one treatment to one of your patients and the other treatment to

another of your patients—for example, corticosteroids and aspirin in some form of rheumatoid arthritis. Having made up your mind that you are not in any way subjecting either patient to a recognized and unjustifiable danger, pain, or discomfort, can anything be gained ethically by endeavouring to explain to them your own state of ignorance and to describe the attempts you are making to remove it? And what is true of two patients is equally true of 20 or 200. Once you have decided that either treatment *for all you know* may be equally well exhibited to the patient's benefit, and without detriment, is there any real basis for seeking consent or refusal?

Does the doctor invariably seek the patient's consent before using a new drug alleged to be efficacious and safe? If the answer is No, then what process, one may ask, makes it needful for him to do so if he chooses to test the drug in such a way that he can compare its effects with those of the previous orthodox treatment?

Is it Ethical to Use a Placebo, or Dummy Treatment?

The answer to this question will depend, I suggest, upon whether there is already available an orthodox treatment of proved or accepted value. If there is such an orthodox treatment the question hardly arises, for the doctor will wish to know whether a new treatment is more, or less, effective than the old, not that it is more effective than nothing. For instance, the U.K./U.S. international trial of corticosteroids in the treatment of rheumatic fever in children contrasted their effects with those following the administration of aspirin, the accepted treatment of the day. Those in charge of the trial believed that it would have been unethical to withhold aspirin, however tenuous its claims may have been. On the other hand, if there is no orthodox treatment, then surely in certain circumstances one may ethically invent one?

In the treatment of the common cold in young adults the trial was designed to contrast the antihistamine compound with an inert substance. Since the measure of the effects of the drug would inevitably lie in the subjective impressions of the patients, this form of control was essential and no trial could have been usefully instituted without it.

Having made it clear to the patients that they would not all get the drug our own consciences were clear.

Indeed, in this connexion I believe a useful question to ask oneself is to what extent is an exact control essential? The answer certainly is not that one of the group must *always* be a mirror-image of the other. The ethical problem may sometimes, I believe, be met in realizing that and in not making the best the enemy of the good. As I described earlier, the M.R.C. Committee did not regard it as at all needful to mimic the injections of streptomycin in its early trial in pulmonary tuberculosis. Many such occasions will arise in this field of controlled trials.

In this setting the doctor will also wish to consider the doctor/patient relationship. Harm may be done if the public comes to believe that doctors are constantly using them as guineapigs. In exhibiting new treatments they are, it is my belief, doing that willynilly, but the public does not realize it. But they need not go out of their way to make it obvious by an *unnecessary* use of dummy pills. On the other hand, I do not myself believe the argument that it is never ethical knowingly to use a placebo in a controlled trial. Though they may not always be doing so knowingly, doctors are surely using placebos every day in exhibiting drugs of which they do not know the value, and many of which will disappear in the course of time.

Is It Proper for the Doctor Not to Know the Treatment Being Administered to His Patient?

The so-called "double-blind" procedure in a controlled trial requires that neither patient nor doctor should know the nature of the treatment being given in the individual case. By such means it is hoped that unbiased subjective impressions and judgments of the course of the illness can be obtained. Sometimes one can escape the issue merely by taking a little thought and trouble. There can be no ethical objection to one doctor treating the patient and another, without knowledge of the treatment, making the assessments.

Thus in many trials of drugs in the treatment of pulmonary tuberculosis the X-ray evidence has been assessed by independent experts who had nothing to do with the treatment of the patients and were never in the individual case informed of its nature. Similarly, in a trial of an alleged active agent in rheumatoid arthritis one doctor injected the concoction (or its control) into the patient and knew the nature of the injection. Another doctor assessed the relief of pain, stiffness, etc., and did not know the nature of the injection. However, there are occasions when it is difficult to use such methods and when, therefore, it is needful to consider whether the doctor in charge of the patient can himself be kept in ignorance of the treatment.

If a trial of this nature is set up, it is axiomatic, of course, that the code can be broken at any moment if the doctor thinks necessary. The question, therefore, is rather whether it is proper for the doctor ever to start that way and to endeavour to maintain his ignorance. The issue, I suggest, turns as usual upon what may conceivably happen to the detriment of the patient if the doctor does not know the treatment. That is what calls for reflection in the special circumstances of each trial.

The answer may be that *nothing whatever* is likely to happen to the detriment of the patient—and this, I believe, was the case in our trial of a short course of an antihistamine for the common cold. On the other hand, it may be that some harm could occur, particularly in a trial of long duration, through, for example, the doctor failing to adjust the dose of a drug finely enough to meet the individual patient's needs. In such a situation it would seem that the double-blind procedure could not be used at all.

It is, however, in terms such as these applicable to the specific disease and its treatment that the answer to the question must be sought.

Conclusion

It is my experience that these six questions will cover the main ethical problems of a controlled clinical trial, and it is to them that the answers in every variety of circumstances must be pursued. One thing, however, I would in conclusion make very clear. In this lecture I have been concerned *entirely* with controlled trials, and the philosophy and arguments that I have put forward apply only to such trials. I have

not concerned myself with a quite different problem, what one may perhaps term exploratory observations—for example, cardiac catheterization, liver biopsy, and the like. Such observations, I would believe, may call for a different approach, and, indeed, one of the problems that the profession will have to face in the proposals of the World Medical Association is the inclusion within one and the same code of such diverse pursuits as controlled trials and exploratory observations.

I admit, as I said earlier, that it may appear impertinent for an unqualified camp follower to air such views, and particularly in this environment. There are just two things I would add in extenuation, and I hope that they may prove to be the only really categorical assertions of which I have been guilty in this lecture. The first is that from my associations with doctors in controlled trials I have learned that the better the statistician understands the doctor/patient relationship and the doctor's very real and unique ethical problem the better can he help to devise a trial that may be less than ideal experimentally but yet likely to be of some, and perhaps considerable, value to medicine.

Secondly, and still more important, I have learned that though the statistician may himself never see a patient—though indeed like Tristram Shandy's Uncle Toby he may live his life in doubt which is the right and which the wrong end of a woman—nevertheless, he cannot sit in an armchair, remote and Olympian, comfortably divesting himself of all ethical responsibility. As a partner in a combined endeavour a full share of that responsibility will always lie with him. He must endeavour to acquire the ethical perception and code of honour that is second nature of those qualified in medicine. And above all he must learn to blend the objectivity and humanity that this lecture commemorates.

References

Brit. Med. J., 1948, 2, 791.

Cheever, D. W. (1861). *Boston Med. Surg. J.,* 63, 449.

Fraser, P. K., Hatch, L. A., and Hughes, K. E. A. (1962). *Lancet,* 1, 614.

Hill, A. Bradford, Marshall, J., and Shaw, D. A. (1960). *Quart. J. Med.,* 29, 597.

———. *Brit. Med. J.,* 2, 1003.

McCance, R. A. (1951). *Proc. Roy. Soc. Med.,* 44, 189. [Reprinted as Chapter 48 of this volume.]

MacMillan, Lord (1937). *Law and Other Things.* Cambridge Univ. Press.

Medical Research Council Streptomycin in Tuberculosis Trials Committee (1948). *Brit. Med. J.,* 2, 769.

Pickering, G. W. (1949). *Proc. Roy. Soc. Med.,* 42, 229.

Thulbourne, T., and Young, M. H. (1962). *Lancet,* 2, 907.

World Medical Association (1962). *Brit. Med. J.,* 2, 1119.

50

Responsibility in Investigations on Human Subjects: Statement by the Medical Research Council [of Great Britain]

Reprinted by permission of the Medical Research Council and publisher from the *British Medical Journal,* vol. 2, 1964, pp. 178–180.

During the last 50 years medical knowledge has advanced more rapidly than at any other period in its history. New understandings, new treatments, new diagnostic procedures, and new methods of prevention have been, and are being, introduced at an ever-increasing rate; and if the benefits that are now becoming possible are to be gained these developments must continue.

Undoubtedly the new era in medicine upon which we have now entered is largely due to the marriage of the methods of science with the traditional methods of medicine. Until the turn of the century the advancement of clinical knowledge was in general confined to that which could be gained by observation, and means for the analysis in depth of the phenomena of health and disease were seldom available. Now, however, procedures that can safely, and conscientiously, be applied to both sick and healthy human beings are being devised in profusion, with the result that certainty and understanding in medicine are increasing apace.

Yet these innovations have brought their own problems to the clinical investigator. In the past, the introduction of new treatments or investigations was infrequent, and only rarely did they go beyond a marginal variation on established practice. To-day far-ranging new procedures are commonplace, and such are their potentialities that their employment is no negligible consideration. As a result, investigators are frequently faced with ethical and sometimes even legal problems of great difficulty. It is in the hope of giving some guidance in this difficult matter that the Medical Research Council issue this statement.

A distinction may legitimately be drawn between procedures undertaken as part of patient-care which are intended to contribute to the benefit of the individual patient, by treatment, prevention, or assessment, and those procedures which are undertaken either on patients or on healthy subjects solely for the purpose of contributing to medical knowledge and are not themselves designed to benefit the particular individual on whom they are performed. The former fall within the ambit of patient-care and are governed by the ordinary rules of professional conduct in medicine; the latter fall within the ambit of investigations on volunteers.

Important considerations flow from this distinction.

Procedures Contributing to the Benefit of the Individual

In the case of procedures directly connected with the management of the condition in the particular individual, the relationship is essentially that between doctor and patient. Implicit in this relationship is the willingness on the part of the subject to be guided by the judgment of his medical attendant. Provided, therefore, that the medical attendant is satisfied that there are reasonable grounds for believing that a particular new procedure will contribute to the benefit of that particular patient, either by treatment, prevention, or increased understanding of his case, he may assume the patient's consent to the same extent as he would were the procedure entirely established practice. It is axiomatic that no two patients are alike and that the medical attendant must be at liberty to vary his procedures according to his judgment of what is in his patients' best interests. The question of novelty is only relevant to the extent that in reaching a decision to use a novel procedure the doctor, being unable to fortify his judgment by previous experience, must exercise special care. That it is both considerate and prudent to obtain the patient's agreement before using a novel procedure is no more than a requirement of good medical practice.

The second important consideration that follows from the distinction is that it is clearly within the competence of a parent or guardian of a child to give permission for procedures intended to benefit that child when he is not old or intelligent enough to be able himself to give a valid consent.

A category of investigation that has occasionally raised questions in the minds of investigators is that in which a new preventive, such as a vaccine, is tried. Necessarily, preventives are given to people who are not, at the moment, suffering from the relevant illness. But the ethical and legal considerations are the same as those that govern the introduction of a new treatment. The intention is to benefit an individual by protecting him against a future hazard; and it is a matter of professional judgment whether the procedure in question offers a better chance of doing so than previously existing measures.

In general, therefore, the propriety of procedures intended to benefit the individual—whether these are directed to treatment, to prevention, or to assessment—are determined by the same considerations as govern the care of patients. At the frontiers of knowledge, however, where not only are many procedures novel but their value in the particular instance may be debatable, it is wise, if any doubt exists, to obtain the opinion of experienced colleagues on the desirability of the projected procedure.

Control Subjects in Investigations of Treatment or Prevention

Over recent years the development of treatment and prevention has been greatly advanced by the method of the controlled clinical trial. Instead of waiting, as in the past, on the slow accumulation of general experience to determine the relative advantages and disadvantages of any particular measure, it is now often possible to put the question to the test under conditions which will not only yield a speedy and more precise answer but also limit the risk of untoward effects remaining undetected. Such trials, are, however, only feasible when it is possible to compare suitable groups of patients and only permissible when there is a genuine doubt within the profession as to which of the two treatments of preventive regimes is the better. In these circumstances it is justifiable to give to a proportion of the patients the novel procedure on the understanding that the remainder receive the procedure previously accepted as the best. In the case when no effective treatment has previously been devised then the situation should be fully explained to the participants and their true consent obtained.

Such controlled trials may raise ethical points which may be of some difficulty. In general, the patients participating in them should be told frankly that two different procedures are being assessed and their co-operation invited. Occasionally, however, to do so is contraindicated. For example, to awaken patients with a

possibly fatal illness to the existence of such doubts about effective treatment may not always be in their best interest; or suspicion may have arisen as to whether a particular treatment has any effect apart from suggestion, and it may be necessary to introduce a placebo into part of the trial to determine this. Because of these and similar difficulties it is the firm opinion of the Council that controlled clinical trials should always be planned and supervised by a group of investigators and never by an individual alone. It goes without question that any doctor taking part in such a collective controlled trial is under an obligation to withdraw a patient from the trial, and to institute any treatment he considers necessary, should this, in his personal opinion, be in the better interests of his patient.

Procedures Not of Direct Benefit to the Individual

The preceding considerations cover the majority of clinical investigations. There remains, however, a large and important field of investigations on human subjects which aim to provide normal values and their variation so that abnormal values can be recognized. This involves both ill persons and "healthy" persons, whether the latter are entirely healthy or patients suffering from a condition that has no relevance to the investigation. In regard to persons with a particular illness, such as metabolic defect, it may be necessary to know the range of abnormality compatible with the activities of normal life or the reaction of such persons to some change in circumstances, such as an alteration in diet. Similarly it may be necessary to have a clear understanding of the range of a normal function and its reaction to change in circumstances in entirely healthy persons. The common feature of this type of investigation is that it is of no direct benefit to the particular individual and that, in consequence, if he is to submit to it he must volunteer in the full sense of the word.

It should be clearly understood that the possibility or probability that a particular investigation will be of benefit to humanity or to posterity would afford no defence in the event of legal

proceedings. The individual has rights that the law protects and nobody can infringe those rights for the public good. In investigations of this type it is therefore always necessary to ensure that the true consent of the subject is explicitly obtained.

By true consent is meant consent freely given with proper understanding of the nature and consequences of what is proposed. Assumed consent or consent obtained by undue influence is valueless, and, in this latter respect, particular care is necessary when the volunteer stands in special relationship to the investigator, as in the case of a patient to his doctor, or a student to his teacher.

The need for obtaining evidence of consent in this type of investigation has been generally recognized, but there are some misunderstandings as to what constitutes such evidence. In general, the investigator should obtain the consent himself in the presence of another person. Written consent unaccompanied by other evidence that an explanation has been given, understood, and accepted, is of little value.

The situation in respect of minors and mentally subnormal or mentally disordered persons is of particular difficulty. In the strict view of the law parents and guardians of minors cannot give consent on their behalf to any procedures which are of no particular benefit to them and which may carry some risk of harm. Whilst English law does not fix any arbitrary age in this context, it may safely be assumed that the Courts will not regard a child of 12 years or under (of 14 years or under for boys in Scotland) as having the capacity to consent to any procedure which may involve him in an injury. Above this age the reality of any purported consent which may have been obtained is a question of fact, and as with an adult the evidence would, if necessary, have to show that irrespective of age the person concerned fully understood the implications to himself of the procedures to which he was consenting.

In the case of those who are mentally subnormal or mentally disordered the reality of the consent given will fall to be judged by similar criteria to those which apply to the making of a will, contracting a marriage, or otherwise taking decisions which have legal force as well as moral and social implications. When true consent in this sense cannot be obtained, procedures which are of no direct benefit and which might carry a risk of harm to the subject should not be undertaken.

Even when true consent has been given by a minor or a mentally subnormal or mentally disordered person, considerations of ethics and prudence still require that, if possible, the assent of parents or guardians or relatives, as the case may be, should be obtained.

Investigations that are of no direct benefit to the individual require, therefore, that his true consent to them shall be explicitly obtained. After adequate explanation, the consent of an adult of sound mind and understanding can be relied upon to be true consent. In the case of children and young persons the question whether purported consent was true consent would in each case depend upon facts such as the age, intelligence, situation, and character of the subject, and the nature of the investigation. When the subject is below the age of 12 years, information requiring the performance of any procedure involving his body would need to be obtained incidentally to and without altering the nature of a procedure intended for his individual benefit.

Professional Discipline

All who have been concerned with medical research are aware of the impossibility of formulating any detailed code of rules which will ensure that irreproachability of practice which alone will suffice where investigations on human beings are concerned. The law lays down a minimum code in matters of professional negligence and the doctrine of assault. But this is not enough. Owing to the special relationship of trust that exists between a patient and his doctor, most patients will consent to any proposal that is made. Further, the considerations involved in a novel procedure are nearly always so technical as to prevent their being adequately understood by one who is not himself an expert. It must therefore be frankly recognized that, for practical purposes, an inescapable moral responsibility rests with the doctor concerned for determining what investigations are, or

are not, proposed to a particular patient or volunteer. Nevertheless, moral codes are formulated by man, and if, in ever-changing circumstances of medical advance, their relevance is to be maintained, it is to the profession itself that we must look, and in particular to the heads of departments, the specialized Societies, and the editors of medical and scientific journals.

In the opinion of the Council, the head of a department where investigations on human subjects take place has an inescapable responsibility for ensuring that practice by those under his direction is irreproachable.

In the same way the Council feel that, as a matter of policy, bodies like themselves that support medical research should do everything in their power to ensure that the practice of all workers whom they support shall be unexceptionable and known to be so.

So specialized has medical knowledge now become that the profession in general can rarely deal adequately with individual problems. In regard to any particular type of investigation, only a small group of experienced men who have specialized in this branch of knowledge are likely to be competent to pass an opinion on the justification for undertaking any particular procedure. But in every branch of medicine specialized scientific societies exist. It is upon these that the profession in general must mainly rely for the creation and maintenance of that body of precedents which shall guide individual investigators in case of doubt, and for the critical discussion of the communications presented to them on which the formation of the necessary climate of opinion depends.

Finally, it is the Council's opinion that any account of investigations on human subjects should make clear that the appropriate requirements have been fulfilled, and, further, that no paper should be accepted for publication if there are any doubts that such is the case.

The progress of medical knowledge has depended, and will continue to depend, in no small measure upon the confidence which the public has in those who carry out investigations on human subjects, be these healthy or sick. Only in so far as it is known that such investigations are submitted to

the highest ethical scrutiny and self-discipline will this confidence be maintained. Mistaken, or misunderstood, investigations could do incalculable harm to medical progress. It is our collective duty as a profession to see that this does not happen and so to continue to deserve the confidence that we now enjoy.

51

Henry K. Beecher
Ethics and Clinical Research

Reprinted with permission of the publisher from the *New England Journal of Medicine*, vol. 274, 1966, pp. 1354–1360.

Human experimentation since World War II has created some difficult problems with the increasing employment of patients as experimental subjects when it must be apparent that they would not have been available if they had been truly aware of the uses that would be made of them. Evidence is at hand that many of the patients in the examples to follow never had the risk satisfactorily explained to them, and it seems obvious that further hundreds have not known that they were the subjects of an experiment although grave consequences have been suffered as a direct result of experiments described here. There is a belief prevalent in some sophisticated circles that attention to these matters would "block progress." But, according to Pope Pius XII,[1] "... science is not the highest value to which all other orders of values ... should be subordinated."

I am aware that these are troubling charges. They have grown out of troubling practices. They can be documented, as I propose to do, by examples from leading medical schools, university hospitals, private hospitals, governmental military departments (the Army, the Navy and the Air Force), governmental institutes (the National Institutes of Health), Veterans Administration hospitals and industry. The basis for the charges is broad.[2]

I should like to affirm that American medicine is sound, and most progress in it soundly attained. There is, however, a reason for concern in certain areas, and I believe the type of activities to be mentioned will do great harm to medicine unless soon corrected. It will certainly be charged that any mention of these matters does a disservice to medicine, but not one so great, I believe, as a continuation of the practices to be cited.

Experimentation in man takes place in several areas: in self-experimentation; in patient volunteers and normal subjects; in therapy; and in the different areas of *experimentation on a patient not for his benefit but for that, at least in theory, of patients in general.* The present study is limited to this last category.

Table 51–1
Money Available for Research Each Year

	Massachusetts General Hospital	National Institutes of Health[a]
1945	$ 500,000[b]	$ 701,800
1955	2,222,816	36,063,200
1965	8,384,342	436,600,000

[a]National Institutes of Health figures based upon decade averages, excluding funds for construction, kindly supplied by Dr. John Sherman, of National Institutes of Health.
[b]Approximation, supplied by Mr. David C. Crockett, of Massachusetts General Hospital.

Reasons for Urgency of Study

Ethical errors are increasing not only in numbers but in variety—for example, in the recently added problems arising in transplantation of organs.

There are a number of reasons why serious attention to the general problem is urgent.

Of transcendent importance is the enormous and continuing increase in available funds, as shown in Table 51–1.

Since World War II the annual expenditure for research (in large part in man) in the Massachusetts General Hospital has increased a remarkable 17-fold. At the National Institutes of Health, the increase has been a gigantic 624-fold. This "national" rate of increase is over 36 times that of the Massachusetts General Hospital. These data, rough as they are, illustrate vast opportunities and concomitantly expanded responsibilities.

Taking into account the sound and increasing emphasis of recent years that experimentation in man must precede general application of new procedures in therapy, plus the great sums of money available, there is reason to fear that these requirements and these resources may be greater than the supply of responsible investigators. All this heightens the problems under discussion.

Medical schools and university hospitals are increasingly dominated by investigators. Every young man knows that he will never be promoted to a tenure post, to a professorship in a major medical school, unless he has proved himself as an investigator. If the ready availability of money for conducting research is added to this fact, one can see how great the pressures are on ambitious young physicians.

Implementation of the recommendations of the President's Commission on Heart Disease, Cancer and Stroke means that further astronomical sums of money will become available for research in man.

In addition to the foregoing three practical points there are others that Sir Robert Platt[3] has pointed out: a general awakening of social conscience; greater power for good or harm in new remedies, new operations and new investigative procedures than was formerly the case; new methods of preventive treatment with their advantages and dangers that are now applied to communities as a whole as well as to individuals, with multiplication of the possibilities for injury; medical science has shown how valuable human experimentation can be in solving problems of disease and its treatment; one can therefore anticipate an increase in experimentation; and the newly developed concept of clinical research as a profession (for example, clinical pharmacology)—and this, of course, can lead to unfortunate separation between the interests of science and the interests of the patient.

Frequency of Unethical or Questionably Ethical Procedures

Nearly everyone agrees that ethical violations do occur. The practical question is, how often? A preliminary examination of the matter was based on 17 examples, which were easily increased to 50. These 50 studies contained references to 186 further likely examples, on the average 3.7 leads per study; they at times overlapped from paper to paper, but this figure indicates how conveniently one can proceed in a search for such material. The data are suggestive of widespread problems, but there is need for another kind of information, which was obtained by examination of 100 consecutive human studies published in 1964, in an excellent journal; 12 of these seemed to be unethical. If only one quarter of them is truly unethical, this still indicates the existence of a serious situation.

Pappworth,[4] in England, has collected, he says, more than 500 papers based upon unethical experimentation. It is evident from such observations that unethical or questionably ethical procedures are not uncommon.

The Problem of Consent

All so-called codes are based on the bland assumption that meaningful or informed consent is readily available for the asking. As pointed out elsewhere,[5] this is very often not the case. Consent in any fully informed sense may not be obtainable. Nevertheless, except, possibly, in the most trivial situations, it remains a goal toward which one must strive for sociologic, ethical and clear-cut legal reasons. There is no choice in the matter.

If suitably approached, patients will accede, on the basis of trust, to about any request their physician may make. At the same time, every experienced clinician investigator knows that patients will often submit to inconvenience and some discomfort, if they do not last very long, but the usual patient will never agree to jeopardize seriously his health or his life for the sake of "science."

In only 2 of the 50[6] examples originally compiled for this study was consent mentioned. Actually, it should be emphasized in all cases for obvious moral and legal reasons, but it would be unrealistic to place much dependence on it. In any precise sense statements regarding consent are meaningless unless one knows how fully the patient was informed of all risks, and if these are not known, that fact should also be made clear. A far more dependable safeguard than consent is the presence of a truly *responsible* investigator.

Examples of Unethical or Questionably Ethical Studies

These examples are not cited for the condemnation of individuals; they are recorded to call attention to a variety of ethical problems found in experimental medicine, for it is hoped that calling attention to them will help to correct abuses present. During ten years of study of these matters it has become apparent that thoughtlessness and carelessness, not a willful disregard of the patient's rights, account for most of the cases encountered. Nonetheless,

it is evident that in many of the examples presented, the investigators have risked the health or the life of their subjects. No attempt has been made to present the "worst" possible examples; rather, the aim has been to show the variety of problems encountered.

References to the examples presented are not given, for there is no intention of pointing to individuals, but rather, a wish to call attention to widespread practices. All, however, are documented to the satisfaction of the editors of the *Journal*.

Known Effective Treatment Withheld
Example 1. It is known that rheumatic fever can usually be prevented by adequate treatment of streptococcal respiratory infections by the parenteral administration of penicillin. Nevertheless, definitive treatment was withheld, and placebos were given to a group of 109 men in service, while benzathine penicillin G was given to others.

The therapy that each patient received was determined automatically by his military serial number arranged so that more men received penicillin than received placebo. In the small group of patients studied 2 cases of acute rheumatic fever and 1 of acute nephritis developed in the control patients, whereas these complications did not occur among those who received the benzathine penicillin G.

Example 2. The sulfonamides were for many years the only antibacterial drugs effective in shortening the duration of acute streptococcal pharyngitis and in reducing its suppurative complications. The investigators in this study undertook to determine if the occurrence of the serious nonsuppurative complications, rheumatic fever and acute glomerulonephritis, would be reduced by this treatment. This study was made despite the general experience that certain antibiotics, including penicillin, will prevent the development of rheumatic fever.

The subjects were a large group of hospital patients; a control group of approximately the same size, also with exudative Group A streptococcus, was included. The latter group received only nonspecific therapy (no sulfadiazine). The total group denied the effective penicillin comprised over 500 men.

Rheumatic fever was diagnosed in 5.4 per cent of those treated with sulfadiazine. In the control group rheumatic fever developed in 4.2 per cent.

In reference to this study a medical officer stated in writing that the subjects were not informed, did not consent and were not aware that they had been involved in an experiment, and yet admittedly 25 acquired rheumatic fever. According to this same medical officer *more than 70* who had had known definitive treatment withheld were on the wards with rheumatic fever when he was there.

Example 3. This involved a study of the relapse rate in typhoid fever treated in two ways. In an earlier study by the present investigators chloramphenicol had been recognized as an effective treatment for typhoid fever, being attended by half the mortality that was experienced when this agent was not used. Others had made the same observations, indicating that to withhold this effective remedy can be a life-or-death decision. The present study was carried out to determine the relapse rate under the two methods of treatment; of 408 charity patients 251 were treated with chloramphenicol, of whom 20, or 7.97 per cent, died. Symptomatic treatment was given, but chloramphenicol was withheld in 157, of whom 36, or 22.9 per cent, died. According to the data presented, 23 patients died in the course of this study who would not have been expected to succumb if they had received specific therapy.

Study of Therapy
Example 4. TriA (triacetyloleandomycin) was originally introduced for the treatment of infection with gram-positive organisms. Spotty evidence of hepatic dysfunction emerged, especially in children, and so the present study was undertaken on 50 patients, including mental defectives or juvenile delinquents who were inmates of a children's center. No disease other than acne was present; the drug was given for treatment of this. The ages of the subjects ranged from thirteen to thirty-nine years. "By the time half the patients had received the drug for four weeks, the high incidence of significant hepatic dysfunction . . . led to the discontinuation of administration to the remainder of the group at three weeks." (However, only two weeks

after the start of the administration of the drug, 54 per cent of the patients showed abnormal excretion of bromsulfalein.) Eight patients with marked hepatic dysfunction were transferred to the hospital "for more intensive study." Liver biopsy was carried out in these 8 patients and repeated in 4 of them. Liver damage was evident. Four of these hospitalized patients, after their liver-function tests returned to normal limits, received a "challenge" dose of the drug. Within two days hepatic dysfunction was evident in 3 of the 4 patients. In 1 patient a second challenge dose was given after the first challenge and again led to evidence of abnormal liver function. Flocculation tests remained abnormal in some patients as long as five weeks after discontinuance of the drug.

Physiologic Studies
Example 5. In this controlled, double-blind study of the hematologic toxicity of chloramphenicol, it was recognized that chloramphenicol is "well known as a cause of aplastic anemia" and that there is a "prolonged morbidity and high mortality of aplastic anemia" and that ". . . chloramphenicol-induced aplastic anemia can be related to dose. . . ." The aim of the study was "further definition of the toxicology of the drug. . . ."

Forty-one randomly chosen patients were given either 2 or 6 gm. of chloramphenicol per day; 12 control patients were used. "Toxic bone-marrow depression, predominantly affecting erythropoiesis, developed in 2 of 20 patients given 2.0 gm. and in 18 of 21 given 6 gm. of chloramphenicol daily." The smaller dose is recommended for routine use.

Example 6. In a study of the effect of thymectomy on the survival of skin homografts 18 children, three and a half months to eighteen years of age, about to undergo surgery for congenital heart disease, were selected. Eleven were to have total thymectomy as part of the operation, and 7 were to serve as controls. As part of the experiment, full-thickness skin homografts from an unrelated adult donor were sutured to the chest wall in each case. (Total thymectomy is occasionally, although not usually part of the primary cardiovascular surgery involved, and

whereas it may not greatly add to the hazards of the necessary operation, its eventual effects in children are not known.) This work was proposed as part of a long-range study of "the growth and development of these children over the years." No difference in the survival of the skin homograft was observed in the 2 groups.

Example 7. This study of cyclopropane anesthesia and cardiac arrhythmias consisted of 31 patients. The average duration of the study was three hours, ranging from two to four and a half hours. "Minor surgical procedures" were carried out in all but 1 subject. Moderate to deep anesthesia, with endotracheal intubation and controlled respiration, was used. Carbon dioxide was injected into the closed respiratory system until cardiac arrhythmias appeared. Toxic levels of carbon dioxide were achieved and maintained for considerable periods. During the cyclopropane anesthesia a variety of pathologic cardiac arrhythmias occurred. When the carbon dioxide tension was elevated above normal, ventricular extrasystoles were more numerous then when the carbon dioxide tension was normal, ventricular arrhythmias being continuous in 1 subject for ninety minutes. (This can lead to fatal fibrillation.)

Example 8. Since the minimum blood-flow requirements of the cerebral circulation are not accurately known, this study was carried out to determine "cerebral hemodynamic and metabolic changes . . . before and during acute reductions in arterial pressure induced by drug administration and/or postural adjustments." Forty-four patients whose ages varied from the second to the tenth decade were involved. They included normotensive subjects, those with essential hypertension and finally a group with malignant hypertension. Fifteen had abnormal electrocardiograms. Few details about the reasons for hospitalization are given.

Signs of cerebral circulatory insufficiency, which were easily recognized, included confusion and in some cases a nonresponsive state. By alteration in the tilt of the patient "the clinical state of the subject could be changed in a matter of seconds from one of alertness to confusion, and for the remainder of the flow, the subject was maintained in the latter state." The femoral arteries were cannulated in all subjects, and the internal jugular veins in 14.

The mean arterial pressure fell in 37 subjects from 109 to 48 mm. of mercury, with signs of cerebral ischemia. "With the onset of collapse, cardiac output and right ventricular pressures decreased sharply."

Since signs of cerebral insufficiency developed without evidence of coronary insufficiency the authors concluded that "the brain may be more sensitive to acute hypotension than is the heart."

Example 9. This is a study of the adverse circulatory responses elicited by intra-abdominal maneuvers:

When the peritoneal cavity was entered, a deliberate series of maneuvers was carried out [in 68 patients] to ascertain the effective stimuli and the areas responsible for development of the expected circulatory changes. Accordingly, the surgeon rubbed localized areas of the parietal and visceral peritoneum with a small ball sponge as discretely as possible. Traction on the mesenteries, pressure in the area of the celiac plexus, traction on the gallbladder and stomach, and occlusion of the portal and caval veins were the other stimuli applied.

Thirty-four of the patients were sixty years of age or older; 11 were seventy or older. In 44 patients the hypotension produced by the deliberate stimulation was "moderate to marked." The maximum fall produced by manipulation was from 200 systolic, 105 diastolic, to 42 systolic, 20 diastolic; the average fall in mean pressure in 26 patients was 53 mm. of mercury.

Of the 50 patients studied, 17 showed either atrioventricular dissociation with nodal rhythm or nodal rhythm alone. A decrease in the amplitude of the T wave and elevation or depression of the ST segment were noted in 25 cases in association with manipulation and hypotension or, at other times, in the course of anesthesia and operation. In only 1 case was the change pronounced enough to suggest myocardial ischemia. No case of myocardial infarction was noted in the group studied although routine electrocardiograms were not taken after operation to detect silent infarcts. Two cases in which electrocardiograms were taken after operation showed T-wave and ST-segment changes that had not been present before.

These authors refer to a similar study in which more alarming electrocardiographic changes were observed. Four patients in the series sustained silent myocardial infarctions; most of their patients were undergoing gallbladder surgery because of associated heart disease. It can be added further that in the 34 patients referred to above as being sixty years of age or older, some doubtless had heart disease that could have made risky the maneuvers carried out. In any event, this possibility might have been a deterrent.

Example 10. Starling's law—"that the heart output per beat is directly proportional to the diastolic filling"—was studied in 30 adult patients with atrial fibrillation and mitral stenosis sufficiently severe to require valvulotomy. "Continuous alterations of the length of a segment of left ventricular muscle were recorded simultaneously in 13 of these patients by means of a mercury-filled resistance gauge sutured to the surface of the left ventricle." Pressures in the left ventricle were determined by direct puncture simultaneously with the segment length in 13 patients and without the segment length in an additional 13 patients. Four similar unanesthetized patients were studied through catheterization of the left side of the heart transeptally. In all 30 patients arterial pressure was measured through the catheterized brachial artery.

Example 11. To study the sequence of ventricular contraction in human bundle-branch block, simultaneous catheterization of both ventricles was performed in 22 subjects; catheterization of the right side of the heart was carried out in the usual manner; the left side was catheterized transbronchially. Extrasystoles were produced by tapping on the epicardium in subjects with normal myocardium while they were undergoing thoracotomy. Simultaneous pressures were measured in both ventricles through needle puncture in this group.

The purpose of this study was to gain increased insight into the physiology involved.

Example 12. This investigation was carried out to examine the possible effect of vagal stimulation on cardiac arrest. The authors had in recent years transected the homolateral vagus nerve immediately below the origin of the recurrent laryngeal nerve as palliation

against cough and pain in bronchogenic carcinoma. Having been impressed with the number of reports of cardiac arrest that seemed to follow vagal stimulation, they tested the effects of intrathoracic vagal stimulation during 30 of their surgical procedures, concluding, from these observations in patients under satisfactory anesthesia, that cardiac irregularities and cardiac arrest due to vagovagal reflex were less common than had previously been supposed.

Example 13. This study presented a technic for determining portal circulation time and hepatic blood flow. It involved the transcutaneous injection of the spleen and catheterization of the hepatic vein. This was carried out in 43 subjects, of whom 14 were normal; 16 had cirrhosis (varying degrees), 9 acute hepatitis, and 4 hemolytic anemia.

No mention is made of what information was divulged to the subjects, some of whom were seriously ill. This study consisted in the development of a technic, not of therapy, in the 14 normal subjects.

Studies to Improve the Understanding of Disease

Example 14. In this study of the syndrome of impending hepatic coma in patients with cirrhosis of the liver certain nitrogenous substances were administered to 9 patients with chronic alcoholism and advanced cirrhosis: ammonium chloride, di-ammonium citrate, urea or dietary protein. In all patients a reaction that included mental disturbance, a "flapping tremor" and electroencephalographic changes developed. Similar signs had occurred in only 1 of the patients before these substances were administered:

The first sign noted was usually clouding of the consciousness. Three patients had a second or a third course of administration of a nitrogenous substance with the same results. It was concluded that marked resemblance between this reaction and impending hepatic coma, implied that the administration of these [nitrogenous] substances to patients with cirrhosis may be hazardous.

Example 15. The relation of the effects of ingested ammonia to liver disease was investigated in 11 normal subjects, 6 with acute virus hepatitis,

26 with cirrhosis, and 8 miscellaneous patients. Ten of these patients had neurologic changes associated with either hepatitis or cirrhosis.

The hepatic and renal veins were cannulated. Ammonium chloride was administered by mouth. After this, a tremor that lasted for three days developed in 1 patient. When ammonium chloride was ingested by 4 cirrhotic patients with tremor and mental confusion the symptoms were exaggerated during the test. The same thing was true of a fifth patient in another group.

Example 16. This study was directed toward determining the period of infectivity of infectious hepatitis. Artificial induction of hepatitis was carried out in an institution for mentally defective children in which a mild form of hepatitis was endemic. The parents gave consent for the intramuscular injection or oral administration of the virus, but nothing is said regarding what was told them concerning the appreciable hazards involved.

A resolution adopted by the World Medical Association states explicitly: "Under no circumstances is a doctor permitted to do anything which would weaken the physical or mental resistance of a human being except from strictly therapeutic or prophylactic indications imposed in the interest of the patient." There is no right to risk an injury to 1 person for the benefit of others.

Example 17. Live cancer cells were injected into 22 human subjects as part of a study of immunity to cancer. According to a recent review, the subjects (hospitalized patients) were "merely told they would be receiving 'some cells'"—". . . the word cancer was entirely omitted. . . ."

Example 18. Melanoma was transplanted from a daughter to her volunteering and informed mother, "in the hope of gaining a little better understanding of cancer immunity and in the hope that the production of tumor antibodies might be helpful in the treatment of the cancer patient." Since the daughter died on the day after the transplantation of the tumor into her mother, the hope expressed seems to have been more theoretical than practical, and the daughter's condition was described as "terminal" at the time the mother volunteered to be a recipient. The primary implant was widely excised on the twenty-fourth day after it

had been placed in the mother. She died from metastatic melanoma on the four hundred and fifty-first day after transplantation. The evidence that this patient died of diffuse melanoma that metastasized from a small piece of transplanted tumor was considered conclusive.

Technical Study of Disease
Example 19. During bronchoscopy a special needle was inserted through a bronchus into the left atrium of the heart. This was done in an unspecified number of subjects, both with cardiac disease and with normal hearts.

The technic was a new approach whose hazards were at the beginning quite unknown. The subjects with normal hearts were used, not for their possible benefit but for that of patients in general.

Example 20. The percutaneous method of catheterization of the left side of the heart has, it is reported, led to 8 deaths (1.09 per cent death rate) and other serious accidents in 732 cases. There was, therefore, need for another method, the transbronchial approach, which was carried out in the present study in more than 500 cases, with no deaths.

Granted that a delicate problem arises regarding how much should be discussed with the patients involved in the use of a new method, nevertheless where the method is employed in a given patient for *his* benefit, the ethical problems are far less than when this potentially extremely dangerous method is used "in 15 patients with normal hearts, undergoing bronchoscopy for other reasons." Nothing was said about what was told any of the subjects, and nothing was said about the granting of permission, which was certainly indicated in the 15 normal subjects used.

Example 21. This was a study of the effect of exercise on cardiac output and pulmonary-artery pressure in 8 "normal" persons (that is, patients whose diseases were not related to the cardiovascular system), in 8 with congestive heart failure severe enough to have recently required complete bed rest, in 6 with hypertension, in 2 with aortic insufficiency, in 7 with mitral stenosis and in 5 with pulmonary emphysema.

Intracardiac catheterization was carried out, and the catheter then inserted into the right or left main branch of the pulmonary artery. The brachial artery was usually catheterized; sometimes, the radial or femoral arteries were catheterized. The subjects exercised in a supine position by pushing their feet against weighted pedals. "The ability of these patients to carry on sustained work was severely limited by weakness and dyspnea." Several were in severe failure. This was not a therapeutic attempt but rather a physiologic study.

Bizarre Study
Example 22. There is a question whether ureteral reflux can occur in the normal bladder. With this in mind, vesicourethrography was carried out on 26 normal babies less than forty-eight hours old. The infants were exposed to X rays while the bladder was filling and during voiding. Multiple spot films were made to record the presence or absence of ureteral reflux. None was found in this group, and fortunately no infection followed the catheterization. What the results of the extensive X-ray exposure may be, no one can yet say.

Comment on Death Rates

In the foregoing examples a number of procedures, some with their own demonstrated death rates, were carried out. The following data were provided by 3 distinguished investigators in the field and represent widely held views.

Cardiac catheterization: right side of the heart, about 1 death per 1000 cases; left side, 5 deaths per 1000 cases. "Probably considerably higher in some places, depending on the portal of entry." One investigator had 15 deaths in his first 150 cases. It is possible that catheterization of a hepatic vein or the renal vein would have a lower death rate than that of catheterization of the right side of the heart, for if it is properly carried out, only the atrium is entered en route to the liver or the kidney, not the right ventricle, which can lead to serious cardiac irregularities. There is always the possibility, however, that the ventricle will be entered inadvertently. This occurs in at least half the cases, according to 1 expert— "but if properly done is too transient to be of importance."

Liver biopsy: the death rate here is estimated at 2 to 3 per 1000, depending in considerable part on the condition of the subject.

Anesthesia: the anesthesia death rate can be placed in general at about 1 death per 2000 cases. The hazard is doubtless higher when certain practices such as deliberate evocation of ventricular extrasystoles under cyclopropane are involved.

Publication

In the view of the British Medical Research Council[7] it is not enough to ensure that all investigation is carried out in an ethical manner: it must be made unmistakably clear in the publications that the proprieties have been observed. This implies editorial responsibility in addition to the investigator's. The question rises, then, about valuable data that have been improperly obtained.[8] It is my view that such material should not be published.[9] There is a practical aspect to the matter: failure to obtain publication would discourage unethical experimentation. How many would carry out such experimentation if they *knew* its results would never be published? Even though suppression of such data (by not publishing it) would constitute a loss to medicine, in a specific localized sense, this loss, it seems, would be less important than the far reaching moral loss to medicine if the data thus obtained were to be published. Admittedly, there is room for debate. Others believe that such data, because of their intrinsic value, obtained at a cost of great risk or damage to the subjects, should not be wasted but should be published with stern editorial comment. This would have to be done with exceptional skill, to avoid an odor of hypocrisy.

Summary and Conclusions

The ethical approach to experimentation in man has several components; two are more important than the others, the first being informed consent. The difficulty of obtaining this is discussed in detail. But it is absolutely essential to *strive* for it for moral, sociologic and legal reasons. The statement that consent has been obtained has little meaning unless the subject or his guardian is capable of understanding what is to be undertaken and unless all hazards are made clear. If these are not known this, too, should be stated. In such a situation the subject at least knows that he is to be a participant in an experiment. Secondly, there is the more reliable safeguard provided by the presence of an intelligent, informed, conscientious, compassionate, responsible investigator.

Ordinary patients will not knowingly risk their health or their life for the sake of "science." Every experienced clinician investigator knows this. When such risks are taken and a considerable number of patients are involved, it may be assumed that informed consent has not been obtained in all cases.

The gain anticipated from an experiment must be commensurate with the risk involved.

An experiment is ethical or not at its inception; it does not become ethical *post hoc*—ends do not justify means. There is no ethical distinction between ends and means.

In the publication of experimental results it must be made unmistakably clear that the proprieties have been observed. It is debatable whether data obtained unethically should be published even with stern editorial comment.

Notes

1. Pope Pius XII. Address. Presented at First International Congress on Histopathology of Nervous System, Rome, Italy, September 14, 1952.

2. At the Brook Lodge Conference on "Problems and Complexities of Clinical Research" I commented that "what seem to be breaches of ethical conduct in experimentation are by no means rare, but are almost, one fears, universal." I thought it was obvious that I was by "universal" referring to the fact that examples could easily be found in *all* categories where research in man takes place to any significant extent. Judging by press comments, that was not obvious; hence, this note.

3. Platt (Sir Robert), 1st bart. *Doctor and Patient: Ethics, morals, government.* 87 pp. London: Nuffield provincial hospitals trust, 1963. Pp. 62 and 63.

4. Pappworth, M. H. Personal communication.

5. Beecher, H. K. Consent in clinical experimentation: Myth and reality. J.A.M.A. 195:34, 1966.

6. Reduced here to 22 for reasons of space.

7. Great Britain, Medical Research Council, *Memorandum*, 1953.

8. As far as principle goes, a parallel can be seen in the recent Mapp decision by the United States Supreme Court. It was stated there that evidence unconstitutionally obtained cannot be used in any judicial decision, no matter how important the evidence is to the ends of justice.

9. Great Britain, Medical Research Council, *Memorandum*, 1953.

52

Letters to the Editor in Response to Beecher's Essay

Reprinted with permission of the publisher from the *New England Journal of Medicine,* vol. 275, October 1966, pp. 790–791.

Human Experimentation

To the Editor: Using arbitrary judgments, Beecher, in the issue of June 16, has made an attempt to estimate the frequency of sins of commission in human experimentation. But how does this compare with the number of sins of omission? I suggest that the evils of *failure* to conduct human investigation predominate, and, not recorded in medical journals, they are hidden from view like the submerged mass of an iceberg.

It is interesting that the question of ethical propriety seems to arise in connection with planned studies in man, and not in relation to informal observations during the everyday practice of the modern equivalents of cupping, bleeding and purging. Green noted,[1] "... when the value of a treatment, new or old, is doubtful, there may be a higher moral obligation to test it critically than to continue to prescribe it year-in, year-out with the support merely of custom or of wishful thinking." Beecher cites a study in which a known effective remedy for typhoid fever, chloramphenicol, was withheld from 157 and administered to 251 patients. The group receiving symptomatic treatment alone had a higher mortality, and he pronounced the study questionable. We might speculate that if such a study had been conducted in prematurely born infants, the group receiving chloramphenicol might have suffered a higher mortality because of an unsuspected hazard in newborn patients unable to dispose of this drug efficiently. The phrase "known effective treatment" sounds formidable and concrete; we must remember that many of our treatments rest on rather shaky foundations of evidence, and the act of withholding such mixed blessings is not always unethical.

I also fear that some may interpret Beecher's article as a blanket condemnation of nontherapeutic human studies because his examples of unethical or questionably ethical studies are placed under such headings as "Physiologic Studies" and "Studies to Improve the Understanding of Disease." Beecher once quoted[2] McCance's advice: "... The medical profession has a responsibility not only for the cure of the sick and for the prevention of disease but for the advancement of knowledge upon which both depend. This ... re-sponsibility can only be met by investigation and experiment. ..." It will be particularly unfortunate for patients if physicians are not encouraged to improve their understanding of disease by properly safeguarded human studies. What is needed is not less human experimentation but more good investigation in man. Emphasis should be placed on the word "good," in both the ethical and the scientific connotations of this word.

William A. Silverman, M.D.
New York City

References

1. Green, F. H. K. Quoted by Jackson, D. Mac G. Moral responsibility in clinical research. *Lancet* 1:902, 1958.

2. Beecher, H. K. *Experimentation in Man.* Springfield, Ill.: Thomas, 1958.

To the Editor: In appreciation of Dr. Beecher's courageous paper on "Ethics and Clinical Research," I should like to contribute two comments to the discourse so forthrightly reopened by him. The first is that it would be unfortunate if data "improperly obtained" were not published. Such an editorial policy would maintain the low visibility of "unethical experimentation" and preclude not only review but also careful and constant appraisal of the conflicting values inherent in experimentation. Indeed, to make these problems even more visible and subject to our collective scrutiny, all clinical research papers submitted for publication should include in the section on *methods* a clear statement of how consent was obtained. Secondly, the implementation of Dr. Beecher's second safeguard,— "the presence of an intelligent, informed, conscientious, compassionate, responsible investigator,"—a difficult challenge at best, might be facilitated by establishing in medical schools intensive seminars on the ethical problems in clinical investigations. Here, I have not in mind occasional lectures but searching and extended discussions of such questions as when, how and to what extent there is a duty and obligation to obtain consent, under what conditions and to what extent members of which group (such as normal volunteers, prisoners, dying patients, children and incompetent patients) should be asked and allowed to participate in experimentation, by what means if any (for example, codes, medical review boards, federal agencies, legislatures or courts) what kinds of medical experimentation should be supervised and controlled. Our medical education in the past has not prepared us for coping with questions that depart from our traditional concerns with the physician-patient relation and extend to broader scientific and societal issues. Dr. Beecher's article highlights the need for such inquiries.

Jay Katz, M.D.
Associate Professor of Law
Associate Clinical Professor of Psychiatry
Yale Law School
New Haven, Connecticut

To the Editor: Henry K. Beecher's article, "Ethics and Clinical Research," focuses attention on a crucial issue confronting every physician who assumes professional responsibility for the care of a *fellow human being*.

A patient in pain or discomfort, worried about his health, comes to a physician with the implicit faith that the doctor will make use of all available scientific knowledge and skill to diagnose and cure, if possible, and, above all, will offer comfort. The suffering human being believes this to be the case; otherwise, he cannot accept the discomfort of laboratory procedures and surgical treatment.

For a physician, or a group of physicians in a medical center, to act otherwise without full discussion with the patient, his family and referring doctor betrays the inherent moral responsibility assumed by any doctor who participates in the care of a patient.

The private practitioner who refers his patient to a medical center for expert diagnosis and therapy, needs to be constantly aware of the studies and treatment involved in the care of his patient. He must interpret to the patient and his family what is taking place. He must also be ready, at times, to exert strong pressure to limit the extent of experimental procedures that may be life threatening without sufficient beneficial value to justify the risk.

The *Journal* and Dr. Beecher offer a great service by calling this issue to the attention of readers.

Morris A. Wessel, M.D.
New Haven, Connecticut

To the Editor: In the June 16 issue of the *Journal* Dr. Beecher quotes out of context, oversimplifies and otherwise distorts the purpose and findings of our investigation of the hematologic toxicity of chloramphenicol, reported in the *New England Journal of Medicine* (272:1137, 1965). In our opinion these practices, particularly when unaccompanied by bibliographic reference to the work cited, are inappropriate in a scientific journal. Our investigation was carried out in 1961 and 1962 as part of a larger study of the therapy of infections due to relatively resistant organisms. The maximum dose of chloramphenicol used in our study approximates that recommended then and now in the drug-package insert for infections due to less susceptible organisms. Before its initiation the research proposal was approved by a local committee composed of University and Veterans Administration investigators and administrators, fulfilling a requirement of the National Institutes of Health not instituted until 1966. We believe that our conduct of the investigation also complies with the *Code of Ethics of the World Medical Association* set forth in the Declaration of Helsinki in 1964 (*Brit. M. J.* 2:177, 1964). The interested reader is asked to review these publications and form an independent judgment.

James L. Scott, M.D.
Gerald A. Belkin, M.D.
Sydney M. Finegold, M.D.
John S. Lawrence, M.D.
Los Angeles, California

To the Editor: In the considerable correspondence evoked by the paper, "Ethics and Clinical Research," two or three misunderstandings have emerged: a few writers have construed the paper as a sweeping indictment of all human experimentation. It is impossible for me to understand how they could have arrived at this view. Certainly, any such conclusion is utterly foreign to my belief as well as to statements made in the paper ("... American medicine is sound and most progress in it soundly attained"), and also not in keeping with my entire career in the field of

human experimentation, stretching back as it does thirty-six years and recorded in several books and 200 articles involving human studies made on myself as well as on others.

Another puzzling misunderstanding is the fairly frequent failure to grasp the distinction between experimentation carried out for the direct benefit of the subject (nearly all therapy involves some experimentation, as I mentioned) and experimentation not for the specific benefit of the subject involved but for science in general. The study was explicitly limited to the latter area.

Several critics have thought that references to the case material should have been given. Fortunately, the editor agreed wholeheartedly that these should not be published. All references were, of course, deposited in his office and checked for accuracy of statement by the editor and 2 of his associates. I had no wish to point to individuals but rather to what I believed to be widespread practices. And, secondly, I was assured by a distinguished lawyer that a number of the investigators involved could be held on criminal charges if discovered by their subjects. I wanted no part in such an action.

I appreciate Professor Katz's letter and respect his opinion concerning the publication of unethically obtained data, although my views differ as I mentioned in the article. It *is* debatable whether such publication should or should not be carried out. I at least have the support of the parallel case of the United States Supreme Court in which the Mapp Decision held that evidence unconstitutionally obtained shall not be used in any judicial decision, however important it may be to the ends of justice.

I agree with Dr. Silverman's desire to know the frequency of "failure to conduct human investigation," to know the "price of omission." He will have to tell me how to get at the problem; I do not know how to do it. Most of what he had to say concerns therapy, specifically not the subject of my inquiry (as indicated above). I agree with his comments on the need for constant re-examination of old remedies and examination of new. I have striven to do this for thirty-six years.

Dr. Wessel's thoughtful comments are to the point and appreciated.

Drs. Scott et al. charge distortion of their study of the hematologic toxicity of chloramphenicol. I do not believe this is so, and obviously neither did the 3 editors who checked my cases, and themselves inserted into my manuscript the statement: "All," they said, "are documented to the satisfaction of the editor of the *Journal*."

Henry K. Beecher, M.D.

Boston

53

William J. Curran

Current Legal Issues in Clinical Investigation with Particular Attention to the Balance between the Rights of the Individual and the Needs of Society

Reprinted from *Psychopharmacology: A Review of Progress 1957–1967* (Washington: U.S. Public Health Service Publication No. 1836, 1968), pp. 337–343.

As the only lawyer and, in fact, the only discipline other than medicine speaking on this program, I have a special responsibility. By also being last on the program, the opportunity has been afforded me to hear all of the other papers and to listen to the many fine and penetrating comments on these papers during this morning's program.

What I have heard has been disturbing. The general tone of the papers and comments has been one of severe uneasiness and frustration with the current trend of governmental and legal controls on experimental medicine and psychology. There have been some vigorous attacks on both the statutes and the regulations of the Federal Food and Drug Administration. There has been confusion and uncertainty expressed about the meaning of the new laws and their eventual effect upon the research community and the drug industry.

It seems to me that this program has spotlighted a lack of understanding in the clinical research community of these changes in law and changes in attitude on the part of the regulatory agencies. It would seem to the researcher that for what was a feeling of mutual cooperation there has been substituted a series of publicly imposed and publicly policed *obstacles* to research. And at the center of all this seem to be the lawyers, watching and waiting for every misstep and for every chance to promulgate a new law or regulation in a scientific field they don't understand and upon a research community whose values they don't appreciate.

This may be a true assessment. But true or not, it is here and it is upon us. As a lawyer, it is my job to live with the law as you who are researchers live with science and nature. I "make" very little of the law I practice. Few lawyers do. We represent not only the government but researchers, drug companies, and research organizations. One thing we learn very quickly: there is little sense in merely fighting against change in the law. If we are to represent our clients properly we must understand the law and why it has been enacted. We must be able to predict the attitude, the direction, the trend in the law in our fields of specialization.[1] Only in this way will we be able to advise our clients properly.

The clinical research community itself needs to understand the public attitudes, the social trends, that are shaping the law today. Otherwise you are fighting blindly against a force you cannot see. Your frustration will echo Matthew Arnold's armies clashing by night:

"Swept with confused alarms of struggle and flight."

Purpose of This Paper

It is my objective in this paper to examine some of the social and legal mechanisms which are at work currently in developing the law concerning clinical investigation, particularly that involving the use of experimental drugs. In drawing this picture, I by no means intend to convey the impression that I necessarily favor these developments in the law or the social movements which I see as forming them. I am merely trying to put them before you in the perspective of another professional, a lawyer, who wants very much to help to accommodate the demands of our American legal system to the healthy progress of scientific research in this country.

The Setting: The Balancing of Interests

Modern legal systems are devoted in large measure to seeking a peaceful balance in a given society between competing social interests. In so doing, the law, and particularly the courts, weigh these interests one against another, giving values to each, quantifying them on a crude scale of civic worth. We know that this is not a scientifically valid enterprise, we are constantly counting apples and oranges, but we must do it if we are to keep the settlement of differences from being fought out in the streets.

In the area of clinical research, it seems to me we must examine three major social interests or values. The first is the protection of the individual, here the research subject or patient. The second is the need of society for the fruits of the research, which might also be said to be the justification for conducting the research. The third and last interest to be considered is the need to foster, promote, and encourage research. This requires an examination of the needs of the researcher.

This kind of balancing of interests in the law courts has been called by Roscoe Pound "social engineering." It is at the heart of Pound's theory of Sociological Jurisprudence developed in his years as Dean of the Harvard Law School. (Pound was a philosopher of the law. To show how we accommodate to the changes in legal demands, our Dean of the past twenty years at Harvard was an income-tax law authority.) With this method, our courts developed the law of property in the early years of this country, protecting industrial growth and the spread of the railroads through the west. In later years, the courts had to accommodate older values to the rise of the labor unions and the rights of labor to unite against property interests. In most recent years, the courts have been most concerned with the clash, not of people against property, but people against people in the civil rights cases of the 1950's and 1960's.

It will not be unusual, therefore, for the courts to weigh the interests we have described in clinical investigation. I would like to consider each of these interests separately in the next pages.

Protection of the Individual

Up to the 1960's we had no "law" in the United States which specifically concerned protecting the rights of the subject of medical research. Nearly all of the activity in this field was international,[2] with the Nuremberg Code in 1947 and the United Nations Covenant on Civil and Political Rights in 1958. (Codification efforts continued on the international scene during the 1960's, of course, with the Declaration of Helsinki by the World Medical Association in 1964.)

In the United States, those of us who were interested in this subject during the 1950's—and there were very few of us then—expected the law to grow as most American law in fields such as this develops, i.e., through cases in the courts involving the rights of research subjects or patients. It would be a Common-Law development, or the studied laying down of principles over a period of time, the best method of balancing the interests discussed earlier. We expected that the model for construction of standards in the field

would be that of the medical-practice field, drawn mainly from medical malpractice cases. The standard of care in this field is the accepted practice of qualified practitioners in the "community" under study.[3] In other words, medicine has been allowed, within margins not here relevant, to set its own standards of quality of medical care. Those of us interested in developing legal standards for medical research attempted during the 1950s to encourage the best research groups and organizations all over the country to establish and to articulate "good practices" in the use of human subjects which could be used as a basis for determining some commonly accepted principles in the research community. One of the first interdisciplinary legal studies undertaken at the Law-Medicine Institute at Boston University when I was director was a project to explore and to develop such practices.[4] We had only very limited success in this ambitious undertaking. We were working at a time somewhat before the researchers were ready to believe such action was necessary. Our *Final Report* predicted much of what was to come in the way of government regulation, however, and many of our recommendations are still worth examining.[5]

The Doctrine of Informed Consent

There was a jarring note which we should acknowledge in the malpractice litigation of the 1950's. This was the growth of the concept of "informed consent."[6] It arose out of cases where plaintiffs' attorneys, having difficulty proving negligence by the community standard, alleged that their clients had not been fully informed of the forseeable risks which normally accompany the kind of treatment or procedure that they had undergone. The plaintiff-patient, in these cases, was the unfortunate victim of this statistically predictable bad result. The legal claim was based in battery, not in negligence, for, the court said, the patient would not have consented had he known of the risk. The doctor therefore had no effective consent and had treated or operated upon the plaintiff in an unlawful manner. Plaintiffs' lawyers seized upon this theory because of the difficulty of obtaining doctors to act as witnesses against other doctors in negligence-based malpractice cases. In the "informed consent cases," lawyers thought that the suit could be won without the testimony of another physician to support the claim. There was much discussion about this doctrine of informed consent in the medical literature, particularly in the popular medical press. Most American doctors came to know and fear the term.

But the courts were still making adjustment, as they always do, in the Common-Law doctrine. The courts determined that this requirement of informed consent was also to be measured by the community standard of medical practitioners. The doctor need only tell the patient of the risks inherent in the treatment or procedure to the extent that other qualified physicians would have done in a similar case in his, the defendant doctor's, own medical community.[7]

I take some time to outline the basic law in this area because the concept of informed consent was adopted in part in both Federal regulatory systems imposed on the research community in the middle 1960's.

Federal Action on Clinical Investigation Standards

The slow development of legal standards for protecting research subjects and patients in clinical research in the United States just did not happen. We had no cases, no suits against researchers, or drug companies, or research organizations during these years upon which such principles could be built. Regulation did come, however, and it arose in the two fields of Federal activity related to clinical investigation, i.e., the regulation of new drugs by the FDA and the financial support of research projects by the NIH.

The Different Approaches

These two Federal agencies have taken entirely different approaches to exercising their responsibilities of surveillance over research practices. The FDA is engaged in direct regulation of the field, setting its own standards by rule-making from Washington. The NIH, on the other hand, has embarked upon a program to stimulate and to encourage self-regulation by the research community based upon "peer review" of actual practices.

FDA Regulation

Federal activity began with the 1962 amendments to the Federal Food, Drug, and Cosmetic Act. During debate, the U.S. Senate added to the legislation a requirement that the investigator obtain the consent of the subject to receive an experimental drug. A great furor was created when this was done and researchers succeeded in getting the Senate to modify the requirement and to dispense with it under certain conditions. As the legislation was enacted it requires consent "except where they [the investigators] deem it not feasible or, in their professional judgment, contrary to the best interests of such human beings."[8]

There is no doubt but that this addition to the legislation was a by-product of the general thrust of the civil rights movement on the national level. Constitutional protections are being added to every major piece of legislation in Washington. The requirement of consent is a part of this bundle of personal rights which the courts and the Congress are so sensitive about in these days. This requirement in the 1962 Amendments was not a part of the original bill. It was not advocated by the industry or by expert witnesses coming before the hearings. It was the brainchild of civil rights-conscious, law-trained senators led particularly by Senator Jacob Javits of New York.

After the legislation was passed, it was the responsibility of the FDA to promulgate administrative rules to spell out the meaning in detail of the new law, including this added requirement of patient consent. This latter would be no easy job for the agency. They did not have a "legislative history" on the requirement to guide them. That is, there was no discussion and testimony at the hearings, no detailed debate,[9] no industrial practices, upon which they could base their interpretive rulings. Perhaps understandably, the FDA of that period took no action to interpret further this requirement. They adopted regulations which merely repeated the language of the statute. It took a new regime under Dr. James Goddard to move the FDA on this requirement. In August, 1966, the FDA adopted regulations in this area. The regulations

could be described as follows:
1. They do purport to define the terms of the 1962 law.
2. They use the *Helsinki Declaration* and the *Nuremberg Code* as guidelines for the definitions adopted.
3. The requirements distinguish between therapeutic and non-therapeutic investigations. They allow no exceptions from the consent requirement in non-therapeutic studies.
4. They use a combination of *Helsinki* and *Nuremberg* to form the definition of the term, "consent."
5. They allow the use of controls and double blind studies as long as the subject is told he "may" receive a placebo or otherwise be used as a control.
6. They define the key "loophole" phrases, "not feasible" and "contrary to the best interests of such human beings."

The above list is my own. Others, including the FDA and Dr. Goddard, might describe the regulations differently and feature other aspects of the agency action. However, I believe this list highlights the basic intentions behind the regulations.

On the whole, from a strictly legal standpoint, the regulations are a good professional piece of work. By using the *Helsinki Declaration* in particular, the agency adopted guidelines already sanctioned by the medical community on a world-wide basis. In making a distinction between therapeutic and non-therapeutic studies (and not using for this distinction the poorer phrases "direct" and "indirect" benefit) the agency achieved a flexibility and sophistication which should prove helpful in later regulations.

If I were to criticize the regulations, it would be in regard to the interpretations given to the "loophole phases." Here the agency had no international or national guidelines to follow. Neither of these phrases appear in any of the codifications or legal commentaries. The definitions adopted are quite narrow and allow very little deviation from the general requirement of informed consent of the research subject. Very important from the researcher's viewpoint is the fact that "not feasible" is *not* interpreted to allow deviation based upon non-feasibility within the research design or the convenience of the research team. Deviation is allowed only on grounds directly related to the subject himself in individual cases, the wording being that consent is "not feasible" where it cannot be obtained "because of inability to communicate with the patient or his representative; for example, where the patient is in a coma or is otherwise incapable of giving informed consent, his representative cannot be reached, and it is imperative to administer the drug without delay."

Certainly this is a narrow exception. It indicates clearly the agency's determination to allow deviation from the consent requirement only in the most extraordinary of circumstances. However, this definition, by its very strictness, seems to sanction experimentation on the seriously ill and even on unconscious people, a questionable ethical position at best.

The other "loophole" definition gets the FDA into another ethical weakness. The term "contrary to the best interests of such human beings" is interpreted as applying when "the communication of information to obtain consent would seriously affect the patient's disease status and the physician has exercised a professional judgment that under the particular circumstances of this patient's case the patient's best interests would suffer if consent were sought." This definition seems to sanction experimentation on patients who are either unaware of the nature of their illness (e.g., cancer) or are unaware or are misled about its seriousness. It is difficult to give the phrase any other application to a clinical situation. Consent is dispensed with because getting his *informed* consent would require telling the patient some *truth* which had been kept from him up to that point. The physician (note the use of the role-identification here of therapist, not "investigator") is allowed to exercise his "professional judgment" concerning the particular circumstances of "this patient's case." The circumstances must concern the patient's illness and the physician's handling of that illness in that person. He is exercising a therapeutic judgment, not an experimental or investigative judgment. He is assumed to be wearing two hats, one as attending physician to his patient and the other as investigator to his subject. Here he is allowed to base his judgment to eliminate a research requirement upon his *therapy* role, not his investigator's role. I would say that

the FDA has made another questionable ethical assumption here. It has assumed that such a patient can be used *at all* in an experimental situation. The question first to be answered is whether such a patient who does not know these facts about his illness should be used in an experiment. Secondly, this regulation allows the investigator to wear both hats, which has many ethical implications, and allows him to make judgments about the research requirements while wearing the therapist's hat.

It should be said, however, that the FDA, in making these interpretations, was following the tenor of Congressional debate on these terms. As noted earlier, however, this debate was conducted very late in the legislative process of this legislation and without the benefit of earlier testimony or findings at the hearing on the bill.

Again, however, on the whole these regulations are, in my opinion, a step forward in defining the responsibility of the FDA under the law imposed by the United States Congress. Before determining to act, the FDA found that, in at least 25% of the New Drug Applications it was receiving, there had been no patient-subject consents sought or obtained. The FDA was determined to reduce this percentage or it could expect Congress to tighten the statutory requirements even further.

Controls by the National Institutes of Health

At the National Institutes of Health, which are themselves in the research business, the reluctance to attempt regulation of the research community regarding patient rights and safety was even greater than at FDA. It was professional concern which moved the officials at NIH to take some action. On December 3, 1965, the National Advisory Council to NIH announced that guidelines would be prepared to require "prior review" of the judgment of principal investigators concerning the welfare of human beings used in clinical and behavioral studies. In short order, these requirements were set down by memorandum from the Surgeon General in February, 1966, and revised in July and December 1966.

In general, these requirements could be described as follows:
1. They set up a system primarily of self-regulation in the research organizations funded by PHS. Of course, this does not mean any abdication of responsibility for these areas on the part of NIH, its staff, or advisory groups.
2. They provide broad guidelines for action rather than detailed controls.
3. The guidelines are three in number:
a. protection of the rights and welfare of the subject,
b. obtaining "informed consent," and
c. assessment of the risks and potential medical benefits of the investigation.
4. The actual surveillance of these guidelines for the protection of subjects is vested in a review panel of peers of the investigator within his own university or research organization.
5. The review is of the "judgment" of the principal investigator, not an independent judgment of the peer review panel.
6. By the revision of July, 1966, the NIH moved the requirement of compliance with the guidelines from an individual requirement on each research-grant application to a general institutional assurance for all projects funded by NIH in that institution.

All of these principles, which are again my own list and not that of NIH, are consistent with the NIH philosophy of decentralization of decision-making to the research community in matters of technical and creative significance.

I am sure that all of us hope that this NIH method of control can be made to work. It is much closer to what those of us who were interested in this field prior to the 1960's had hoped would be developed than any strict regulatory or codification scheme could achieve. As of July, 1967, the NIH was operating this method through over 1,000 institutional assurances filed in Bethesda and Washington covering over 25,000 investigators.

The Needs of Society
The second interest to be weighed in these scales of social values is a much more broadly identified concern, the needs of the society in general for the benefits to be derived from research. This could also be said, as noted earlier, to be the justification for engaging in the research on human beings in the

first place. The types of issues to be considered would be as follows:

1. This would require arriving at a quantification of the social worth of the particular field of research as compared to other enterprises and other areas of research.

2. This weighing of social worth would be used to justify the allocation of scarce resources (of professional manpower and medical facilities, for example) to research enterprises.

3. And lastly, this weighing of social worth in the research would justify (or not justify) a particular degree of risk or inconvenience for the selected research subjects or patients. This latter weighing of research worth directly against subject risk is specifically sanctioned in the *Nuremberg Code* and in the NIH guidelines.

Consideration of the needs of society for the fruits of research and its weighing against the rights of the individual is consistent with Roscoe Pound's Sociological Jurisprudence mentioned earlier in this paper. It *also* corresponds to Marxist and ancient Chinese social philosophies in its conscious willingness to subjugate the rights and welfare of the individual man to the demands of society. In quite up-to-date manner it also fits smoothly into the cost-benefit analysis techniques of modern American management specialists. However, it is *not* consistent with the current mood of this country to protect civil rights and the individual in all possible circumstances and the current trend of the U.S. Supreme Court to give predominence to civil rights under a Natural Law philosophy, which emphasizes human values, rather than under more pragmatic philosophies such as that of Pound.

The Promotion of Research

The last of the three interests to be weighed in the scale of social values is the promotion and encouragement of clinical research. This might be said to be a part of the second value discussed above in that the social worth of medical research would have to be determined in positive terms in order to justify the promotion and encouragement of such research. I list it as a separate value, however, in order to stress the

different factors which would be considered in order to achieve it. Also, it is quite legitimate as a separate value in the courts or in the legislature where promotion of an enterprise or an industry as such is a quite common motivation for action or decision. The courts in particular are in the habit of weighing the legitimate interest of industry (such as the railroads in the west or the mills in New England) to operate and to prosper in the general interests of the community.

This interest could also be described as a consideration of the needs of the researcher or research enterprise as contrasted to the needs of society or the needs of the individual subject or patient. These needs should not be thought of as necessarily in conflict. In most situations they will be mutually supportive. A "weighing" operation may often take place only outside the field with priorities of societal need or desirability come into play, as in determining a Federal or State budget allocation.

The particular issues to be considered in the social setting (as a court or legislature) when this third value is examined would be:

1. The need to establish an environment which will encourage creativity in the research enterprise or in the individual investigator.

2. The allocation of resources to enable the research to prosper. (Similar to the determination of priorities for the allocation of resources examined under the second value.)

3. The need to recruit and to retain investigators and other personnel in the research field.

In examining this interest, we find that a typically American approach to it is to allocate money to the existing researchers and to expect all of the other needs to fall into line behind it. Many people, even in the highest places, seem to think that as long as the money keeps coming, our society can:

1. Regulate, regulate, regulate the very devil out of the researcher,

2. Subject him to public scrutiny in all of his activities,

3. Chastize him for not getting "results" quickly and efficiently in every project which "our money" supports, and

4. Attempt to "coordinate" his research in order to eliminate "unnecessary duplication."

From a legal viewpoint, we must consider what the impact of laws and regulations in favor of protecting the individual may be upon the researcher and the research enterprise. We must realize that strict regulations may stifle initiative and discourage researchers from entering the field or staying in it. We must realize that scientists and research clinicians cannot be treated in the same manner as entrepreneurs in industries such as the railroads or manufacturing. What would not deter the entrepreneur may well demoralize the clinical investigator. Also from a legal standpoint, controls on the use of human subjects may in practice eliminate some sources of research subjects entirely, not a desirable result if the law wishes to encourage research enterprise. Lastly, the threat, as well as the actuality, of law suits against researchers can act as a significant inhibiting factor in regard to initiative and boldness in research. We cannot deny that the rate of medical malpractice cases is increasing, though suits against researchers are rare, if not non-existent at present.

The law certainly can protect physicians and scientists in favored activities. In recent years the law has granted immunities from suits against physicians and others in areas such as rendering emergency medical aid (the so-called "good Samaritan Laws"), child-abuse reporting, mental hospital commitment certifications, Medicare hospital-utilization committee decisions, and the taking of blood samples from automobile drivers suspected of drunken driving. The law has barred suits against physicians in these situations because, had it not done so, there was a fear that the physicians would not continue to perform these essential professional services. Perhaps there will be situations in clinical research where such legal protection of investigators will be desirable.

Conclusion: The Trends in American Law

In the above paper I have attempted to examine the social forces and legal philosophy behind the recent quite revolutionary intrusions of law and governmental regulation into the field of clinical research, especially research involving the use of new drugs. It has been pointed out that the legal system is engaged in the weighing and balancing of societal interests which may be in conflict. In this situation, the interests being weighed would seem to be three in number: (1) the protection of the individual research subject; (2) the needs of society for the fruits of clinical research; and (3) the promotion and encouragement of medical research enterprise. Each of these three interests has been examined in some detail.

There can be no doubt but that the first of these interests, protection of the individual research subject, is receiving the greatest legal attention at present. This is a part of the current trend in American law-making in the courts and in the legislatures. This is the mood of the country. You who are in clinical research must realize this. If there is any clash of interests in the courts, it is individual rights, civil rights, consumer protection which is carrying the day. The Supreme Court of the United States is directing massive changes in our fundamental law. The changes are not only in criminal-law procedures, but in many other life situations demanding "due process of law." And it is not only the highest Federal court which is taking such action, but the Supreme Courts of the various states. For example, in a recent case, the New York State Court of Appeals ordered the application of due process of law to the punishing of a high-school pupil accused of cheating, with a lawyer representing the pupil's interest. President James A. Perkins of Cornell University made a speech just last weekend to an educational group warning them of what he described as a dangerous trend in America to take educational issues into court instead of allowing educators to decide them. What Perkins, who is not an alarmist or an ultraconservative educator, was seeing is what you researchers, mental hospital administrators, and drug company investigators and medical directors have been experiencing in your fields.[10]

You are not alone. The legal revolution is going on all around you. I implore you not to ignore it, but to study it and to try to understand it. There are many of us in the legal profession who are willing and eager to help you to communicate effectively in this new environment of Law, Medicine, and Science in the latter third of the Twentieth Century.

Notes

1. "The prophecies of what the court will do in fact, and nothing more pretentious, are what I mean by the law." Oliver Wendell Holmes, *The Path of the Law* (1897).

2. See my paper reviewing the international codes: Curran, Legal Codes in Scientific Research Involving Human Subjects, *Lex et Scientia*, vol. 2, p. 341 (1966).

3. Curran, Problems of Establishing a Standard of Care, *Medical Malpractice* (University of Michigan, 2d edition, 1966).

4. "Administrative Practices in Clinical Research," NIH Research Grant No. 7039, January 1, 1960–March 31, 1963. The original principal investigator was Irving Ladimer, S.J.D. The final report was prepared with Donald A. Kennedy, Ph.D., as principal investigator.

5. See particularly Chapter X, Findings and Recommendations, in the *Final Report*.

6. Plant, Informed Consent—A New Area of Malpractice Liability, *Medical Malpractice*, supra, note 3.

7. The most significant recent case in this field is *Wilson v. Scott,* 412 S.W. 2d 299 (Texas, 1967), a case where the doctor defendant admitted that he did not tell his patient about the 1% chance of loss of hearing in a delicate ear operation. He admitted further, surprisingly, that it was the practice of other physicians in his area to tell their patients of such risks. Understandably, the doctor was held liable in damages when his patient suffered the hearing loss.

8. FFDCA, Section 505 (i).

9. Except on the "loophole phrases," as noted later.

10. As anyone could judge from his recent book, Perkins, *The University in Transition*, (1966).

54

Walsh McDermott

Opening Comments: A Colloquium on Ethical Dilemmas from Medical Advances

Reprinted with permission of author and publisher from the *Annals of Internal Medicine,* vol. 67, September 1967, pp. 39–42.

When the needs of society come in head-on conflict with the rights of an individual, someone has to play God. We can avoid this responsibility so long as the power to decide the particular case-in-point is clearly vested in someone else, for example, a duly elected government official. But in clinical investigation, the power to determine this issue of "the individual versus society" is clearly vested in the physician. Both the power itself and, above all, *our awareness that we are wielding it* are increasing every day and can be expected to increase much further. It is this inescapable *awareness* that we are wielding power that has us so deeply troubled, for we are a generation nurtured on the slogan "the end does not justify the means" in matters concerning the individual and his society. Yet as a society we enforce the social good over the individual good across a whole spectrum of nonmedical activities every day, and many of these activities ultimately affect the health or the life of an individual.

Traditionally in our Judeo-Christian culture we have handled this issue by one of two mechanisms. When, as in our racial problem, for example, the conflict contains no built-in contradiction, we publicly and officially subscribe to a set of ideals. We can work privately and publicly toward the attainment of these ideals, and with their attainment would come the solution of the problem. This mechanism works when the forces in conflict are intrinsically reconcilable even though the reconciliation might take many decades or a century. But we use another mechanism when the conflict is head on, when the group interest and the individual interest are basically irreconcilable.

In circumstances like these, such as the decision to impose capital punishment or the selection of only a minority of our young men to become soldiers, the issue is decided by a judgment that is arbitrary as it affects the individual. In short, we play God. When we take away an individual's life or liberty by one of these arbitrary judgments we try to depersonalize the process by spreading responsibility for the decision throughout a framework of legal institutions. Thus, it is usually a jury, not a judge, that determines the death penalty; a local draft board, not a bureaucrat, that decides who goes to

Vietnam. This second type of mechanism works only because there is widespread public acceptance that society has rights too and that it is preferable that the power to enforce these rights over the rights of the individual be institutionalized.

I submit that the core of this ethical issue as it arises in clinical investigation lies in this second category—the one wherein, to ensure the rights of society, an arbitrary judgment must be made against an individual.

This is not to say that all ethical problems in clinical investigation fall into the irreconcilable category. On the contrary, in numerical terms most of them probably do not.

Without question, a considerable portion of the lapses in fully protecting individual rights in clinical investigation can be avoided by more careful and open attention to the subject and by our ingenuity in developing new practices to attain some of the same old ends. This will prove quite costly in financial terms, but what is being accomplished in this way is very much to the good and is to be strongly encouraged. But there remains that hard core of the problem: the kind of situation in which it clearly seems to be in the best interests of society that the information be obtained. It can be obtained only from studies on certain already unlucky individuals, and no convincing case can be made that they can expect much in the way of benefits except those accruing to them as members of society.

Clearly there are three questions here: (1) From where does society get its rights or interest that makes it imperative to perform biomedical studies on an individual?; (2) how is the individual subject selected?; and (3) how are the social priorities decided?

The social priorities are easy; any small group of certified medical statesmen can settle them in an afternoon. As we all know, however, it is the other two questions that are so thorny.

Without too deep reflection it seems to me that society's actually having a right here is a relatively new phenomenon that is chiefly derived from the demonstration that knowledge gained by studies in a few humans can show us how to operate programs of great practical benefit to the group. Until the late nineteenth century, as I understand it, most human experimentation expanded knowledge but did not increase the power to control disease. The physicians of that day thus had no problem in maintaining the double ethical charge still preserved in the Helsinki Declaration: to "safeguard the health of the people," on the one hand, and to make the health of "my patient" the first consideration, on the other hand. But starting, I suppose, with the yellow fever studies in Havana, we have seen large social payoffs from certain experiments in humans, and there is no reason to doubt that the process could continue. It is by this demonstration, analogous to the great "invention of invention" of Newton's era, that medicine has given to society the case for its rights in the continuation of clinical investigation. Once this demonstration was made, we could no longer maintain, in strict honesty, that in the study of disease the interests of the individual are invariably paramount.

Yet we are temperamentally incapable of leaving it at that. Our reflex action here is to try to imitate what we do when the same conflict arises in irreconcilable form elsewhere in our society. That is to say, we are willing to concede that some judgments must be arbitrary, but we attempt to clothe them with institutional forms so that at least the judgments are not made solely by one person. We will play God, but we would like to do it by group effort.

I am deeply convinced that such efforts provide no real solution because our culture has not yet faced up to the irreconcilable nature of the conflict at the heart of this particular issue. And until it does so, there exists no recognized consensus or article in the "social contract," if you will, to provide that base on which any law or regulation must rest if it is to be viable.

Conventional juridical procedures including the traditional jury system are too slow to fit the urgent nature of many clinical decisions. Any peer group committee we might set up, let us say from law, theology, and medicine, would have credentials that are obviously suspect. It has been chosen neither by the society nor by the individual whose conflicting rights are to be arbitrated; more importantly, it lacks

that widespread social consensus that supports trial by jury or your local draft board. Therefore, such a peer committee cannot, in fact, dilute and hence dissipate the ethical responsibility of the clinical investigator although it may give the superficial image of doing so. Thus, by the terms of our culture, as may be seen in the Declaration of Helsinki, no matter who the investigator takes into partnership when he acts, he acts alone.

What can we do to solve this agonizing dilemma? Obviously we cannot convene a constitutional convention of the Judeo-Christian culture and add a few amendments to it. Yet, in a figurative sense, until we can do something very much like that, I believe deeply that the problem, at its roots, is unsolvable and that we must continue to live with it.

To be sure, by careful attention we can cut down the number of instances in which the problem presents itself to us in its starkest form. But there is no escape from the fact that, if the future good of society is to be served, there will be times when the clinical investigator must make an arbitrary judgment with respect to an individual. The necessity for such arbitrary judgments has had *tacit* social recognition and approval for some time. Because the approval *was* tacit, however, there was an imbalance of actions and words, in effect, a hypocrisy, that marvelous human invention by which we are enabled to adapt to problems judged to be not yet ripe for solution. By this hypocrisy society had its future medical interests fully protected. At the same time the attitude could be maintained that in medical matters, *as contrasted with those in many other walks of life,* the sole public interest was in the inviolability of the individual.

Now, most unfortunately, these essentially harmless hypocrisies of our culture have been codified. For both the Helsinki Declaration and the new Food and Drug Administration regulations handed down this week are honest reflections of our culture complete with all its hypocrisies. As such, if they were followed to the letter, they would produce the curious situation in which the only stated public interest is that of the individual. The future interest of society and its sometime conflict

with the interest of the individual, in effect, are ignored. I believe it has been most unwise to try to extend the principle of "a government of laws and not men" into areas of such great ethical subtlety as clinical investigation.

When in our cultural evolution it has not yet been possible to develop an institutional framework for a particular kind of arbitrary decision that may affect an individual, there is only one basis on which to proceed, and that is on the basis of trust. My position may sound paternalistic, as indeed it is. Making arbitrary decisions concerning an individual in conflicts as yet unsolved by our society is one of the major responsibilities of a parent.

Society may not have given us a clear blueprint for clinical investigation, but it has long given us immense trust to handle moral dilemmas of other sorts, including many in which, in effect, we have to play God. Thus, the moral dilemma of clinical investigation is not something new; what is new about the problem is its rapid increase in size. This rapid increase in size is no help to us now, but it may hasten the day, still far off, when in medical investigations we can institutionalize this making of arbitrary decisions between an individual and his society.

In the meantime we can do no more than carry on under the mantle of the trust we now possess. To continue to receive that trust we must be ever conscious that the issue of the individual vis-à-vis society is always *there,* and we can try our best to create an environment of awareness of it on our clinical services. For once a moral dilemma has become clearly recognized; whenever each person *acts* within that dilemma, his act can be seen for what it is, and the extent to which he has seemed to act with acceptable propriety can be judged.

But the hard core of our moral dilemma will not yield to the approaches of "Declarations" or "Regulations"; for as things stand today such statements must completely ignore the fact that society, too, has rights in human experimentation. Somehow, somewhere, in this question of human experimentation, as in so many other aspects of our society, we will have to learn how to institutionalize "playing God" while still maintaining the key elements of a free society.

55

Hans Jonas
Philosophical Reflections on Experimenting with Human Subjects

In Paul A. Freund, ed., *Experimentation with Human Subjects* (New York: George Braziller, 1969), pp. 1–31. Reprinted by permission of the American Academy of Arts and Sciences.

Experimenting with human subjects is going on in many fields of scientific and technological progress. It is designed to replace the over-all instruction by natural, occasional experience with the selective information from artificial, systematic experiment which physical science has found so effective in dealing with inanimate nature. Of the new experimentation with man, medical is surely the most legitimate; psychological, the most dubious; biological (still to come), the most dangerous. I have chosen here to deal with the first only, where the case *for* it is strongest and the task of adjudicating conflicting claims hardest. When I was first asked[1] to comment "philosophically" on it, I had all the hesitation natural to a layman in the face of matters on which experts of the highest competence have had their say and still carry on their dialogue. As I familiarized myself with the material,[2] any initial feeling of moral rectitude that might have facilitated my task quickly dissipated before the awesome complexity of the problem, and a state of great humility took its place. The awareness of the problem in all its shadings and ramifications speaks out with such authority, perception, and sophistication in the published discussions of the researchers themselves that it would be foolish of me to hope that I, an onlooker on the sidelines, could tell those battling in the arena anything they have not pondered themselves. Still, since the matter is obscure by its nature and involves very fundamental, transtechnical issues, anyone's attempt at clarification can be of use, even without novelty. And even if the philosophical reflection should in the end achieve no more than the realization that in the dialectics of this area we must sin and fall into guilt, this insight may not be without its own gains.

The Peculiarity of Human Experimentation

Experimentation was originally sanctioned by natural science. There it is performed on inanimate objects, and this raises no moral problems. But as soon as animate, feeling beings become the subjects of experiment, as they do in the life sciences and especially in medical research, this innocence of the search for knowledge is lost and questions of conscience arise.

The depth to which moral and religious sensibilities can become aroused over these questions is shown by the vivisection issue. Human experimentation must sharpen the issue as it involves ultimate questions of personal dignity and sacrosanctity. One profound difference between the human experiment and the physical (beside that between animate and inanimate, feeling and unfeeling nature) is this: The physical experiment employs small-scale, artificially devised substitutes for that about which knowledge is to be obtained, and the experimenter extrapolates from these models and simulated conditions to nature at large. Something deputizes for the "real thing"—balls rolling down an inclined plane for sun and planets, electric discharges from a condenser for real lightning, and so on. For the most part, no such substitution is possible in the biological sphere. We must operate on the original itself, the real thing in the fullest sense, and perhaps affect it irreversibly. No simulacrum can take its place. Especially in the human sphere, experimentation loses entirely the advantage of the clear division between vicarious model and true object. Up to a point, animals may fulfill the proxy role of the classical physical experiment. But in the end man himself must furnish knowledge about himself, and the comfortable separation of noncommittal experiment and definitive action vanishes. An experiment in education affects the lives of its subjects, perhaps a whole generation of schoolchildren. Human experimentation for whatever purpose is always *also* a responsible, nonexperimental, definitive dealing with the subject himself. And not even the noblest purpose abrogates the obligations this involves.

This is the root of the problem with which we are faced: Can both that purpose and this obligation be satisfied? If not, what would be a just compromise? Which side should give way to the other? The question is inherently philosophical as it concerns not merely pragmatic difficulties and their arbitration, but a genuine conflict of values involving principles of a high order. May I put the conflict in these terms. On principle, it is felt, human beings *ought not* to be dealt with in that way (the "guinea pig" protest); on the other hand, such dealings are increasingly urged on us by considerations, in turn appealing to principle, that claim to override those objections. Such a claim must be carefully assessed, especially when it is swept along by a mighty tide. Putting the matter thus, we have already made one important assumption rooted in our "Western" cultural tradition: The prohibitive rule is, to that way of thinking, the primary and axiomatic one; the permissive counter-rule, as qualifying the first, is secondary and stands in need of justification. We must justify the infringement of a primary inviolability, which needs no justification itself; and the justification of its infringement must be by values and needs of a dignity commensurate with those to be sacrificed.

Before going any further, we should give some more articulate voice to the resistance we feel against a merely utilitarian view of the matter. It has to do with a peculiarity of human experimentation quite independent of the question of possible injury to the subject. What is wrong with making a person an experimental subject is not so much that we make him thereby a means (which happens in social contexts of all kinds), as that we make him a thing—a passive thing merely to be acted on, and passive not even for real action, but for token action whose token object he is. His being is reduced to that of a mere token or "sample." This is different from even the most exploitative situations of social life: there the business is real, not fictitious. The subject, however much abused, remains an agent and thus a "subject" in the other sense of the word. The soldier's case is instructive: Subject to most unilateral discipline, forced to risk mutilation and death, conscripted without, perhaps against, his will—he is still conscripted with his capacities to act, to hold his own or fail in situations, to meet real challenges for real stakes. Though a mere "number" to the High Command, he is not a token and not a thing. (Imagine what he would say if it turned out that the war was a game staged to sample observations on his endurance, courage, or cowardice.)

These compensations of personhood are denied to the subject of experimentation, who is acted upon for an extraneous end without being engaged in a real relation where he would be the counterpoint to the other or to circumstance. Mere "consent" (mostly amounting to no more than permission) does not right this reification. Only genuine authenticity of volunteering can possibly redeem the condition of "thinghood" to which the subject submits. Of this we shall speak later. Let us now look at the nature of the conflict, and especially at the nature of the claims countering in this matter those on behalf of personal sacrosanctity.

"Individual Versus Society" as the Conceptual Framework

The setting for the conflict most consistently invoked in the literature is the polarity of individual versus society—the possible tension between the individual good and the common good, between private and public welfare. Thus, W. Wolfensberger speaks of "the tension between the long-range interests of society, science, and progress, on one hand, and the rights of the individual on the other."[3] Walsh McDermott says: "In essence, this is a problem of the rights of the individual versus the rights of society."[4] Somewhere I found the "social contract" invoked in support of claims that science may make on individuals in the matter of experimentation. I have grave doubts about the adequacy of this frame of reference, but I will go along with it part of the way. It does apply to some extent, and it has the advantage of being familiar. We concede, as a matter of course, to the common good some pragmatically determined measure of precedence over the individual good. In terms of rights, we let some of the basic rights of the individual be overruled by the acknowledged rights of society—as a matter of right and moral justness and not of mere force or dire necessity (much as such necessity may be adduced in defense of that right). But in making that concession, we require a careful clarification of what the needs, interests, and rights of society are, for society—as distinct from any plurality of individuals—is an abstract and, as such, is subject to our definition, while the individual is the

primary concrete, prior to all definition, and his basic good is more or less known. Thus the unknown in our problem is the so-called common or public good and its potentially superior claims, to which the individual good must or might sometimes be sacrificed, in circumstances that in turn must also be counted among the unknowns of our question. Note that in putting the matter in this way—that is, in asking about the right of society to individual sacrifice—the consent of the sacrificial subject is no necessary part of the *basic* question.

"Consent," however, is the other most consistently emphasized and examined concept in discussions of this issue. This attention betrays a feeling that the "social" angle is not fully satisfactory. If society has a right, its exercise is not contingent on volunteering. On the other hand, if volunteering is fully genuine, no public right to the volunteered act need be construed. There is a difference between the moral or emotional appeal of a cause that elicits volunteering and a right that demands compliance—for example, with particular reference to the social sphere, between the *moral claim* of a common good and society's *right* to that good and to the means of its realization. A moral claim cannot be met without consent; a right can do without it. Where consent is present anyway, the distinction may become immaterial. But the awareness of the many ambiguities besetting the "consent" actually available and used in medical research[5] prompts recourse to the idea of a public right conceived independently of (and valid prior to) consent; and, vice versa, the awareness of the problematic nature of such a right makes even its advocates still insist on the idea of consent with all its ambiguities: an uneasy situation either way.

Nor does it help much to replace the language of "rights" by that of "interests" and then argue the sheer cumulative weight of the interest of the many over against those of the few or the single individual. "Interests" range all the way from the most marginal and optional to the most vital and imperative, and only those sanctioned by particular importance and merit will be admitted to count in such a calculus—which simply brings us back to the question of right or moral claim.

Moreover, the appeal to numbers is dangerous. Is the number of those afflicted with a particular disease great enough to warrant violating the interest of the nonafflicted? Since the number of the latter is usually so much greater, the argument can actually turn around to the contention that the cumulative weight of interest is on *their* side. Finally, it may well be the case that the individual's interest in his own inviolability is itself a public interest, such that its publicly condoned violation, irrespective of numbers, violates the interest of all. In that case, its protection in *each* instance would be a paramount interest, and the comparison of numbers will not avail.

These are some of the difficulties hidden in the conceptual framework indicated by the terms "society-individual," "interest," and "rights." But we also spoke of a moral call, and this points to another dimension—not indeed divorced from the social sphere, but transcending it. And there is something even beyond that: true sacrifice from highest devotion, for which there are no laws or rules except that it must be absolutely free. "No one has the right to choose martyrs for science" was a statement repeatedly quoted in the November, 1967, *Dædalus* conference. But no scientist can be prevented from making himself a martyr for his science. At all times, dedicated explorers, thinkers, and artists have immolated themselves on the altar of their vocation, and creative genius most often pays the price of happiness, health, and life for its own consummation. But no one, not even society, has the shred of a right to expect and ask these things in the normal course of events. They come to the rest of us as a *gratia gratis data*.

The Sacrificial Theme

Yet we must face the somber truth that the *ultima ratio* of communal life is and has always been the compulsory, vicarious sacrifice of individual lives. The primordial sacrificial situation is that of outright human sacrifices in early communities. These were not acts of blood-lust or gleeful savagery; they were the solemn execution of a supreme, sacral necessity. One of the fellowship of men had to die so that all could live, the earth be fertile, the cycle of nature renewed. The victim

often was not a captured enemy, but a select member of the group: "The king must die." If there was cruelty here, it was not that of men, but that of the gods, or rather of the stern order of things, which was believed to exact that price for the bounty of life. To assure it for the community, and to assure it ever again, the awesome *quid pro quo* had to be paid over again.

Far should it be from us to belittle, from the height of our enlightened knowledge, the majesty of the underlying conception. The particular *causal* views that prompted our ancestors have long since been relegated to the realm of superstition. But in moments of national danger we still send the flower of our young manhood to offer their lives for the continued life of the community, and if it is a just war, we see them go forth as consecrated and strangely ennobled by a sacrificial role. Nor do we make their going forth depend on their own will and consent, much as we may desire and foster these. We conscript them according to law. We conscript the best and feel morally disturbed if the draft, either by design or in effect, works so that mainly the disadvantaged, socially less useful, more expendable, make up those whose lives are to buy ours. No rational persuasion of the pragmatic necessity here at work can do away with the feeling, a mixture of gratitude and guilt, that the sphere of the sacred is touched with the vicarious offering of life for life. Quite apart from these dramatic occasions, there is, it appears, a persistent and constitutive aspect of human immolation to the very being and prospering of human society—an immolation in terms of life and happiness, imposed or voluntary, of few for many. What Goethe has said of the rise of Christianity may well apply to the nature of civilization in general: *"Opfer fallen hier, / Weder Lamm Noch Stier, / Aber Menschenopfer uner-hoert."* [6] We can never rest comfortably in the belief that the soil from which our satisfactions sprout is not watered with the blood of martyrs. But a troubled conscience compels us, the undeserving beneficiaries, to ask: Who is to be martyred? in the service of what cause and by whose choice?

Not for a moment do I wish to suggest that medical experimentation

on human subjects, sick or healthy, is to be likened to primeval human sacrifices. Yet something sacrificial is involved in the selective abrogation of personal inviolability and the ritualized exposure to gratuitous risk of health and life, justified by a presumed greater, social good. My examples from the sphere of stark sacrifice were intended to sharpen the issues implied in that context and to set them off clearly from the kinds of obligations and constraints imposed on the citizen in the normal course of things or generally demanded of the individual in exchange for the advantages of civil society.

The "Social Contract" Theme

The first thing to say in such a setting-off is that the sacrificial area is not covered by what is called the "social contract." This fiction of political theory, premised on the primacy of the individual, was designed to supply a rationale for the *limitation* of individual freedom and power required for the existence of the body politic, whose existence in turn is for the benefit of the individuals. The principle of these limitations is that their *general* observance profits all, and that therefore the individual observer, assuring this general observance for his part, profits by it himself. I observe property rights because their general observance assures my own; I observe traffic rules because their general observance assures my own safety; and so on. The obligations here are mutual and general; no one is singled out for special sacrifice. Moreover, for the most part, *qua* limitations of my liberty, the laws thus deducible from the hypothetical "social contract" enjoin me from certain actions of my liberty, the laws thus detive actions (as did the laws of feudal society). Even where the latter is the case, as in the duty to pay taxes, the rationale is that I am myself a beneficiary of the services financed through these payments. Even the contributions levied by the welfare state, though not originally contemplated in the liberal version of the social contract theory, can be interpreted as a personal insurance policy of one sort or another—be it against the contingency of my own indigence, be it against the dangers of disaffection from the laws in consequence of widespread unrelieved destitution, be it even against the disadvantages of a diminished consumer market. Thus, by some stretch, such contributions can still be subsumed under the principle of enlightened self-interest. But no complete abrogation of self-interest at any time is in the terms of the social contract, and so pure sacrifice falls outside it. Under the putative terms of the contract alone, I cannot be required to die for the public good. (Thomas Hobbes made this forcibly clear.) Even short of this extreme, we like to think that nobody is entirely and one-sidedly the victim in any of the renunciations exacted under normal circumstances by society "in the general interest"—that is, for the benefit of others. "Under normal circumstances," as we shall see, is a necessary qualification. Moreover, the "contract" can legitimitize claims only on our overt, public actions and not on our invisible private being. Our powers, not our persons, are beholden to the common weal. In one important respect, it is true, public interest and control do extend to the private sphere by general consent: in the compulsory education of our children. Even there, the assumption is that the learning and what is learned, apart from all future social usefulness, are also for the benefit of the individual in his own being. We would not tolerate education to degenerate into the conditioning of useful robots for the social machine.

Both restrictions of public claim in behalf of the "common good"—that concerning one-sided sacrifice and that concerning the private sphere—are valid only, let us remember, on the premise of the primacy of the individual, upon which the whole idea of the "social contract" rests. This primacy is itself a metaphysical axiom or option peculiar to our Western tradition, and the whittling away of its force would threaten the tradition's whole foundation. In passing, I may remark that systems adopting the alternative primacy of the community as their axiom are naturally less bound by the restrictions we postulate. Whereas we reject the idea of "expendables" and regard those not useful or even recalcitrant to the social purpose as a burden that society must carry (since their individual claim to existence is as absolute as that of the most useful), a

truly totalitarian regime, Communist or other, may deem it right for the collective to rid itself of such encumbrances or to make them forcibly serve some social end by conscripting their persons (and there are effective combinations of both). We do not normally—that is, in nonemergency conditions—give the state the right to conscript labor, while we do give it the right to "conscript" money, for money is detachable from the person as labor is not. Even less than forced labor do we countenance forced risk, injury, and indignity.

But in time of war our society itself supersedes the nice balance of the social contract with an almost absolute precedence of public necessities over individual rights. In this and similar emergencies, the sacrosanctity of the individual is abrogated, and what for all practical purposes amounts to a near-totalitarian, quasi-communist state of affairs is *temporarily* permitted to prevail. In such situations, the community is conceded the right to make calls on its members, or certain of its members, entirely different in magnitude and kind from the calls normally allowed. It is deemed right that a part of the population bears a disproportionate burden of risk of a disproportionate gravity; and it is deemed right that the rest of the community accepts this sacrifice, whether voluntary or enforced, and reaps its benefits—difficult as we find it to justify this acceptance and this benefit by any normal ethical categories. We justify it transethically, as it were, by the supreme collective emergency, formalized, for example, by the declaration of a state of war.

Medical experimentation on human subjects falls somewhere between this overpowering case and the normal transactions of the social contract. On the one hand, no comparable extreme issue of social survival is (by and large) at stake. And no comparable extreme sacrifice or foreseeable risk is (by and large) asked. On the other hand, what is asked goes decidedly beyond, even runs counter to, what it is otherwise deemed fair to let the individual sign over of his person to the benefit of the "common good." Indeed, our sensitivity to the kind of intrusion and use involved is such that only an end of transcendent value or overriding urgency can make it arguable and possibly acceptable in our eyes.

Health as a Public Good

The cause invoked is health and, in its more critical aspect, life itself—clearly superlative goods that the physician serves directly by curing and the researcher indirectly by the knowledge gained through his experiments. There is no question about the good served nor about the evil fought—disease and premature death. But a good to whom and an evil to whom? Here the issue tends to become somewhat clouded. In the attempt to give experimentation the proper dignity (on the problematic view that a value becomes greater by being "social" instead of merely individual), the health in question or the disease in question is somehow predicated on the social whole, as if it were society that, in the persons of its members, enjoyed the one and suffered the other. For the purposes of our problem, public interest can then be pitted against private interest, the common good against the individual good. Indeed, I have found health called a national resource, which of course it is, but surely not in the first place.

In trying to resolve some of the complexities and ambiguities lurking in these conceptualizations, I have pondered a particular statement, made in the form of a question, which I found in the *Proceedings* of the earlier *Dædalus* conference: "Can society afford to discard the tissues and organs of the hopelessly unconscious patient when they could be used to restore the otherwise hopelessly ill, but still salvageable individual?" And somewhat later: "A strong case can be made that society can ill afford to discard the tissues and organs of the hopelessly unconscious patient; they are greatly needed for study and experimental trial to help those who can be salvaged."[7] I hasten to add that any suspicion of callousness that the "commodity" language of these statements may suggest is immediately dispelled by the name of the speaker, Dr. Henry K. Beecher, for whose humanity and moral sensibility there can be nothing but admiration. But the use, in all innocence, of this language gives food for thought. Let me, for a moment, take the question literally. "Discarding" implies proprietary rights—nobody can discard what does not belong to him in the first place. Does society then own my body? "Salvaging" implies the same and, moreover, a use-value to the owner. Is the life-extension of certain individuals then a public interest? "Affording" implies a critically vital level of such an interest—that is, of the loss or gain involved. And "society" itself—what is it? When does a need, an aim, an obligation become social? Let us reflect on some of these terms.

What Society Can Afford

"Can Society afford . . . ?" Afford what? To let people die intact, thereby withholding something from other people who desperately need it, who in consequence will have to die too? These other, unfortunate people indeed cannot afford not to have a kidney, heart, or other organ of the dying patient, on which they depend for an extension of their lease on life; but does that give them a right to it? And does it oblige society to procure it for them? What is it that *society* can or cannot afford—leaving aside for the moment the question of what it has a *right* to? It surely can afford to lose members through death; more than that, it is built on the balance of death and birth decreed by the order of life. This is too general, of course, for our question, but perhaps it is well to remember. The specific question seems to be whether society can afford to let some people die whose death might be deferred by particular means if these were authorized by society. Again, if it is merely a question of what society can or cannot afford, rather than of what it ought or ought not to do, the answer must be: Of course, it can. If cancer, heart disease, and other organic, non-contagious ills, especially those tending to strike the old more than the young, continue to exact their toll at the normal rate of incidence (including the toll of private anguish and misery), society can go on flourishing in every way.

Here, by contrast, are some examples of what, in sober truth, society cannot afford. It cannot afford to let an epidemic rage unchecked; a persistent excess of deaths over births, but neither—we must add—too great an excess of births over deaths; too low

an average life expectancy even if demographically balanced by fertility, but neither too great a longevity with the necessitated correlative dearth of youth in the social body; a debilitating state of general health; and things of this kind. These are plain cases where the whole condition of society is critically affected, and the public interest can make its imperative claims. The Black Death of the Middle Ages was a *public* calamity of the acute kind; the life-sapping ravages of endemic malaria or sleeping sickness in certain areas are a public calamity of the chronic kind. Such situations a society as a whole can truly not "afford," and they may call for extraordinary remedies, including, perhaps, the invasion of private sacrosanctities.

This is not entirely a matter of numbers and numerical ratios. Society, in a subtler sense, cannot "afford" a single miscarriage of justice, a single inequity in the dispensation of its laws, the violation of the rights of even the tiniest minority, because these undermine the moral basis on which society's existence rests. Nor can it, for a similar reason, afford the absence or atrophy in its midst of compassion and of the effort to alleviate suffering—be it widespread or rare—one form of which is the effort to conquer disease of any kind, whether "socially" significant (by reason of number) or not. And in short, society cannot afford the absence among its members of *virtue* with its readiness for sacrifice beyond defined duty. Since its presence—that is to say, that of personal idealism—is a matter of grace and not of decree, we have the paradox that society depends for its existence on intangibles of nothing less than a religious order, for which it can hope, but which it cannot enforce. All the more must it protect this most precious capital from abuse.

For what objectives connected with the medico-biological sphere should this reserve be drawn upon—for example, in the form of accepting, soliciting, perhaps even imposing the submission of human subjects to experimentation? We postulate that this must be not just a worthy cause, as any promotion of the health of anybody doubtlessly is, but a cause qualifying for transcendent social sanction. Here one thinks first of those cases critically affecting the whole condition, present and future, of the community we have illustrated.

Something equivalent to what in the political sphere is called "clear and present danger" may be invoked and a state of emergency proclaimed, thereby suspending certain otherwise inviolable prohibitions and taboos. We may observe that averting a disaster always carries greater weight than promoting a good. Extraordinary danger excuses extraordinary means. This covers human experimentation, which we would like to count, as far as possible, among the extraordinary rather than the ordinary means of serving the common good under public auspices. Naturally, since foresight and responsibility for the future are of the essence of institutional society, averting disaster extends into long-term prevention, although the lesser urgency will warrant less sweeping licenses.

Society and the Cause of Progress

Much weaker is the case where it is a matter not of saving but of improving society. Much of medical research falls into this category. As stated before, a permanent death rate from heart failure or cancer does not threaten society. So long as certain statistical ratios are maintained, the incidence of disease and of disease-induced mortality is not (in the strict sense) a "social" misfortune. I hasten to add that it is not therefore less of a human misfortune, and the call for relief issuing with silent eloquence from each victim and all potential victims is of no lesser dignity. But it is misleading to equate the fundamentally human response to it with what is owed to society: it is owed by man to man—and it is thereby owed by society to the individuals as soon as the adequate ministering to these concerns outgrows (as it progressively does) the scope of private spontaneity and is made a public mandate. It is thus that society assumes responsibility for medical care, research, old age, and innumerable other things not originally of the public realm (in the original "social contract"), and they become duties toward "society" (rather than directly toward one's fellow man) by the fact that they are socially operated.

Indeed, we expect from organized society no longer mere protection against harm and the securing of the conditions of our preservation, but active and constant improvement in all the domains of life: the waging of the battle against nature, the enhancement of the human estate—in short, the promotion of progress. This is an expansive goal, one far surpassing the disaster norm of our previous reflections. It lacks the urgency of the latter, but has the nobility of the free, forward thrust. It surely is worth sacrifices. It is not at all a question of what society can afford, but of what it is committed to, beyond all necessity, by our mandate. Its trusteeship has become an established, ongoing, institutionalized business of the body politic. As eager beneficiaries of its gains, we now owe to "society," as its chief agent, our individual contributions toward its *continued pursuit*. I emphasize "continued pursuit." Maintaining the existing level requires no more than the orthodox means of taxation and enforcement of professional standards that raise no problems. The more optional goal of pushing forward is also more exacting. We have this syndrome: Progress is by our choosing an acknowledged interest of society, in which we have a stake in various degrees; science is a necessary instrument of progress; research is a necessary instrument of science; and in medical science experimentation on human subjects is a necessary instrument of research. Therefore, human experimentation has come to be a societal interest.

The destination of research is essentially melioristic. It does not serve the preservation of the existing good from which I profit myself and to which I am obligated. Unless the present state is intolerable, the melioristic goal is in a sense gratuitous, and this not only from the vantage point of the present. Our descendants have a right to be left an unplundered planet; they do not have a right to new miracle cures. We have sinned against them, if by our doing we have destroyed their inheritance—which we are doing at full blast; we have not sinned against them, if by the time they come around arthritis has not yet been conquered (unless by sheer neglect). And generally, in the matter of progress, as humanity had no claim on a Newton, a Michelangelo, or a St. Francis to appear, and no right to the blessings of their unscheduled deeds, so progress,

with all our methodical labor for it, cannot be budgeted in advance and its fruits received as a due. Its coming-about at all and its turning out for good (of which we can never be sure) must rather be regarded as something akin to grace.

The Melioristic Goal, Medical Research, and Individual Duty

Nowhere is the melioristic goal more inherent than in medicine. To the physician, it is not gratuitous. He is committed to curing and thus to improving the power to cure. Gratuitous we called it (outside disaster conditions) as a *social* goal, but noble at the same time. Both the nobility and the gratuitousness must influence the manner in which self-sacrifice for it is elicited, and even its free offer accepted. Freedom is certainly the first condition to be observed here. The surrender of one's body to medical experimentation is entirely outside the enforceable "social contract."

Or can it be construed to fall within its terms—namely, as repayment for benefits from past experimentation that I have enjoyed myself? But I am indebted for these benefits not to society, but to the past "martyrs," to whom society is indebted itself, and society has no right to call in my personal debt by way of adding new to its own. Moreover, gratitude is not an enforceable social obligation; it anyway does not mean that I must emulate the deed. Most of all, if it was wrong to exact such sacrifice in the first place, it does not become right to exact it again with the plea of the profit it has brought me. If, however, it was not exacted, but entirely free, as it ought to have been, then it should remain so, and its precedence must not be used as a social pressure on others for doing the same under the sign of duty.

Indeed, we must look outside the sphere of the social contract, outside the whole realm of public rights and duties, for the motivations and norms by which we can expect ever again the upwelling of a will to give what nobody—neither society, nor fellow man, nor posterity—is entitled to. There are such dimensions in man with trans-social wellsprings of conduct, and I have already pointed to the paradox,

or mystery, that society cannot prosper without them, that it must draw on them, but cannot command them.

What about the moral law as such a transcendent motivation of conduct? It goes considerably beyond the public law of the social contract. The latter, we saw, is founded on the rule of enlightened self-interest: *Do ut des*—I give so that I be given to. The law of individual conscience asks more. Under the Golden Rule, for example, I am required to give as I wish to be given to under like circumstances, but not in order that I be given to and not in expectation of return. Reciprocity, essential to the social law, is not a condition of the moral law. One subtle "expectation" and "self-interest," but of the moral order itself, may even then be in my mind: I prefer the environment of a moral society and can expect to contribute to the general morality by my own example. But even if I should always be the dupe, the Golden Rule holds. (If the social law breaks faith with me, I am released from its claim.)

Moral Law and Transmoral Dedication

Can I, then, be called upon to offer myself for medical experimentation in the name of the moral law? *Prima facie*, the Golden Rule seems to apply. I should wish, were I dying of a disease, that enough volunteers in the past had provided enough knowledge through the gift of their bodies that I could now be saved. I should wish, were I desperately in need of a transplant, that the dying patient next door had agreed to a definition of death by which his organs would become available to me in the freshest possible condition. I surely should also wish, were I drowning, that somebody would risk his life, even sacrifice his life, for mine.

But the last example reminds us that only the negative form of the Golden Rule ("Do not do unto others what you do not want done unto yourself") is fully prescriptive. The positive form (Do unto others as you would wish them to do unto you"), in whose compass our issue falls, points into an infinite, open horizon where prescriptive force soon ceases. We may well say of somebody that he ought to have come to the succor of B, to have shared with him in his need, and the like. But we may not say that he ought to have given his life for him. To have done so would be praiseworthy; not to have done so is not blameworthy. It cannot be asked of him; if he fails to do so, he reneges on no duty. But *he* may say of himself, and only he, that he ought to have given his life. *This* "ought" is strictly between him and himself, or between him and God; no outside party—fellow man or society—can appropriate its voice. It can humbly receive the supererogatory gifts from the free enactment of it.

We must, in other words, distinguish between moral obligation and the much larger sphere of moral value. (This, incidentally, shows up the error in the widely held view of value theory that the higher a value, the stronger its claim and the greater the duty to realize it. The highest are in a region beyond duty and claim.) The ethical dimension far exceeds that of the moral law and reaches into the sublime solitude of dedication and ultimate commitment, away from all reckoning and rule—in short, into the sphere of the *holy*. From there alone can the offer of self-sacrifice genuinely spring, and this—its source—must be honored religiously. How? The first duty here falling on the research community, when it enlists and uses this source, is the safeguarding of true authenticity and spontaneity.

The "Conscription" of Consent

But here we must realize that the mere issuing of the appeal, the calling for volunteers, with the moral and social pressures it inevitably generates, amounts even under the most meticulous rules of consent to a sort of *conscripting*. And some soliciting is necessarily involved. This was in part meant by the earlier remark that in this area sin and guilt can perhaps not be wholly avoided. And this is why "consent," surely a non-negotiable minimum requirement, is not the full answer to the problem. Granting then that soliciting and therefore some degree of conscripting are part of the situation, who may conscript and who may be conscripted? Or less harshly expressed: Who should issue appeals and to whom?

The naturally qualified issuer of the appeal is the research scientist himself, collectively the main carrier of the impulse and the only one with the technical competence to judge. But his being very much an interested party (with vested interests, indeed, not purely in the public good, but in the scientific enterprise as such, in "his" project, and even in his career) makes him also suspect. The ineradicable dialectic of this situation—a delicate incompatibility problem—calls for particular controls by the research community and by public authority that we need not discuss. They can mitigate, but not eliminate the problem. We have to live with the ambiguity, the treacherous impurity of everything human.

Self-Recruitment of the Community

To whom should the appeal be addressed? The natural issuer of the call is also the first natural addressee: the physician-researcher himself and the scientific confraternity at large. With such a coincidence—indeed, the noble tradition with which the whole business of human experimentation started—almost all of the associated legal, ethical, and metaphysical problems vanish. If it is full, autonomous identification of the subject with the purpose that is required for the dignifying of his serving as a subject—here it is; if strongest motivation—here it is; if fullest understanding—here it is; if freest decision—here it is; if greatest integration with the person's total, chosen pursuit—here it is. With the fact of self-solicitation the issue of consent in all its insoluble equivocality is bypassed *per se*. Not even the condition that the particular purpose be truly important and the project reasonably promising, which must hold in any solicitation of others, need be satisfied here. By himself, the scientist is free to obey his obsession, to play his hunch, to wager on chance, to follow the lure of ambition. It is all part of the "divine madness" that somehow animates the ceaseless pressing against frontiers. For the rest of society, which has a deep-seated disposition to look with reverence and awe upon the guardians of the mysteries of life, the profession assumes with this proof of its devotion the role of a self-chosen, consecrated

fraternity, not unlike the monastic orders of the past, and this would come nearest to the actual, religious origins of the art of healing.

It would be the ideal, but is not a real solution, to keep the issue of human experimentation within the research community itself. Neither in numbers nor in variety of material would its potential suffice for the many-pronged, systematic, continual attack on disease into which the lonely exploits of the early investigators have grown. Statistical requirements alone make their voracious demands; and were it not for what I have called the essentially "gratuitous" nature of the whole enterprise of progress, as against the mandatory respect for invasion-proof selfhood, the simplest answer would be to keep the whole population enrolled, and let the lot, or an equivalent of draft boards, decide which of each category will at any one time be called up for "service." It is not difficult to picture societies with whose philosophy this would be consonant. We are agreed that ours is not one such and should not become one. The specter of it is indeed among the threatening utopias on our own horizon from which we should recoil, and of whose advent by imperceptible steps we must beware. How then can our mandatory faith be honored when the recruitment for experimentation goes outside the scientific community, as it must in honoring another commitment of no mean dignity? We simply repeat the former question: To whom should the call be addressed?

"Identification" as the Principle of Recruitment in General

If the properties we adduced as the particular qualifications of the members of the scientific fraternity itself are taken as general criteria of selection, then one should look for additional subjects where a maximum of identification, understanding, and spontaneity can be expected—that is, among the most highly motivated, the most highly educated, and the least "captive" members of the community. From this naturally scarce resource, a descending order of permissibility leads to greater abundance and ease of supply, whose use should become proportionately more hesitant as the exculpating criteria are relaxed. An inversion of normal "market" behavior is demanded here—namely, to accept the lowest quotation last (and excused only by the greatest pressure of need); to pay the highest price first.

The ruling principle in our considerations is that the "wrong" of reification can only be made "right" by such authentic identification with the cause that it is the subject's as well as the researcher's cause—whereby his role in its service is not just permitted by him, but *willed*. That sovereign will of his which embraces the end as his own restores his personhood to the otherwise depersonalizing context. To be valid it must be autonomous and informed. The latter condition can, outside the research community, only be fulfilled by degrees; but the higher the degree of the understanding regarding the purpose and the technique, the more valid becomes the endorsement of the will. A margin of mere trust inevitably remains. Ultimately, the appeal for volunteers should seek this free and generous endorsement, the appropriation of the research purpose into the person's own scheme of ends. Thus, the appeal is in truth addressed to the one, mysterious, and sacred source of any such generosity of the will—"devotion," whose forms and objects of commitment are various and may invest different motivations in different individuals. The following, for instance, may be responsive to the "call" we are discussing: compassion with human suffering, zeal for humanity, reverence for the Golden Rule, enthusiasm for progress, homage to the cause of knowledge, even longing for sacrificial justification (do not call that "masochism," please). On all these, I say, it is defensible and right to draw when the research objective is worthy enough; and it is a prime duty of the research community (especially in view of what we called the "margin of trust") to see that this sacred source is never abused for frivolous ends. For a less than adequate cause, not even the freest, unsolicited offer should be accepted.

The Rule of the "Descending Order" and Its Counter-Utility Sense

We have laid down what must seem to be a forbidding rule to the number-hungry research industry. Having faith

in the transcendent potential of man, I do not fear that the "source" will ever fail a society that does not destroy it—and only such a one is worthy of the blessings of progress. But "elitistic" the rule is (as is the enterprise of progress itself), and elites are by nature small. The combined attribute of motivation and information, plus the absence of external pressures, tends to be socially so circumscribed that strict adherence to the rule might numerically starve the research process. This is why I spoke of a descending order of permissibility, which is itself permissive, but where the realization that it is a *descending* order is not without pragmatic import. Departing from the august norm, the appeal must needs shift from idealism to docility, from high-mindedness to compliance, from judgment to trust. Consent spreads over the whole spectrum. I will not go into the casuistics of this penumbral area. I merely indicate the principle of the order of preference: The poorer in knowledge, motivation, and freedom of decision (and that, alas, means the more readily available in terms of numbers and possible manipulation), the more sparingly and indeed reluctantly should the reservoir be used, and the more compelling must therefore become the countervailing justification.

Let us note that this is the opposite of a social utility standard, the reverse of the order by "availability and expendability": The most valuable and scarcest, the least expendable elements of the social organism, are to be the first candidates for risk and sacrifice. It is the standard of *noblesse oblige*; and with all its counterutility and seeming "wastefulness," we feel a rightness about it and perhaps even a higher "utility," for the soul of the community lives by this spirit.[8] It is also the opposite of what the day-to-day interests of research clamor for, and for the scientific community to honor it will mean that it will have to fight a strong temptation to go by routine to the readiest sources of supply—the suggestible, the ignorant, the dependent, the "captive" in various senses.[9] I do not believe that heightened resistance here must cripple research, which cannot be permitted; but it may indeed slow it down by the smaller numbers fed into experimentation in consequence. This price—a possibly slower rate of progress—may

have to be paid for the preservation of the most precious capital of higher communal life.

Experimentation on Patients

So far we have been speaking on the tacit assumption that the subjects of experimentation are recruited from among the healthy. To the question "Who is conscriptable?" the spontaneous answer is: Least and last of all the sick—the most available of all as they are under treatment and observation anyway. That the afflicted should not be called upon to bear additional burden and risk, that they are society's special trust and the physician's trust in particular—these are elementary responses of our moral sense. Yet the very destination of medical research, the conquest of disease, requires at the crucial stage trial and verification on precisely the sufferers from the disease, and their total exemption would defeat the purpose itself. In acknowledging this inescapable necessity, we enter the most sensitive area of the whole complex, the one most keenly felt and most searchingly discussed by the practitioners themselves. No wonder, it touches the heart of the doctor-patient relation, putting its most solemn obligations to the test. There is nothing new in what I have to say about the ethics of the doctor-patient relation, but for the purpose of confronting it with the issue of experimentation some of the oldest verities must be recalled.

The Fundamental Privilege of the Sick

In the course of treatment, the physician is obligated to the patient and to no one else. He is not the agent of society, nor of the interests of medical science, nor of the patient's family, nor of his co-sufferers, or future sufferers from the same disease. The patient alone counts when he is under the physician's care. By the simple law of bilateral contract (analogous, for example, to the relation of lawyer to client and its "conflict of interest" rule), the physician is bound not to let any other interest interfere with that of the patient in being cured. But manifestly more sublime norms than contractual ones are involved. We may speak of a sacred trust; strictly by its terms, the doctor is, as it were, alone with his patient and God.

There is one normal exception to this—that is, to the doctor's not being the agent of society vis-à-vis the patient, but the trustee of his interests alone: the quarantining of the contagious sick. This is plainly not for the patient's interest, but for that of others threatened by him. (In vaccination, we have a combination of both: protection of the individual and others.) But preventing the patient from causing harm to others is not the same as exploiting him for the advantage of others. And there is, of course, the abnormal exception of collective catastrophe, the analogue to a state of war. The physician who desperately battles a raging epidemic is under a unique dispensation that suspends in a nonspecifiable way some of the strictures of normal practice, including possibly those against experimental liberties with his patients. No rules can be devised for the waiving of rules in extremities. And as with the famous shipwreck examples of ethical theory, the less said about it the better. But what is allowable there and may later be passed over in forgiving silence cannot serve as a precedent. We are concerned with non-extreme, non-emergency conditions where the voice of principle can be heard and claims can be adjudicated free from duress. We have conceded that there are such claims, and that if there is to be medical advance at all, not even the superlative privilege of the suffering and the sick can be kept wholly intact from the intrusion of its needs. About this least palatable, most disquieting part of our subject, I have to offer only groping, inconclusive remarks.

The Principle of "Identification" Applied to Patients

On the whole, the same principles would seem to hold here as are found to hold with "normal subjects": motivation, identification, understanding on the part of the subject. But it is clear that these conditions are peculiarly difficult to satisfy with regard to a patient. His physical state, psychic preoccupation, dependent relation to the doctor, the submissive attitude induced by treatment—everything connected with his condition and situation makes the sick person inherently less of a sovereign person than the healthy

one. Spontaneity of self-offering has almost to be ruled out; consent is marred by lower resistance or captive circumstance, and so on. In fact, all the factors that make the patient, as a category, particularly accessible and welcome for experimentation at the same time compromise the quality of the responding affirmation that must morally redeem the making use of them. This, in addition to the primacy of the physician's duty, puts a heightened onus on the physician-researcher to limit his undue power to the most important and defensible research objectives and, of course, to keep persuasion at a minimum.

Still, with all the disabilities noted, there is scope among patients for observing the rule of the "descending order of permissibility" that we have laid down for normal subjects, in vexing inversion of the utility order of quantitative abundance and qualitative "expendability." By the principle of this order, those patients who most identify with and are cognizant of the cause of research—members of the medical profession (who after all are sometimes patients themselves)—come first; the highly motivated and educated, also least dependent, among the lay patients come next; and so on down the line. An added consideration here is seriousness of condition, which again operates in inverse proportion. Here the profession must fight the tempting sophistry that the hopeless case is expendable (because in prospect already expended) and therefore especially usable; and generally the attitude that the poorer the chances of the patient the more justifiable his recruitment for experimentation (other than for his own benefit). The opposite is true.

Nondisclosure as a Borderline Case

Then there is the case where ignorance of the subject, sometimes even of the experimenter, is of the essence of the experiment (the "double blind"-control group-placebo syndrome). It is said to be a necessary element of the scientific process. Whatever may be said about its ethics in regard to normal subjects, especially volunteers, it is an outright betrayal of trust in regard to the patient who believes that he is receiving treatment. Only supreme importance of the objective can exonerate it, without making it less of a transgression. The

patient is definitely wronged even when not harmed. And ethics apart, the practice of such deception holds the danger of undermining the faith in the *bona fides* of treatment, the beneficial intent of the physician—the very basis of the doctor-patient relationship. In every respect, it follows that concealed experiment on patients—that is, experiment under the guise of treatment—should be the rarest exception, at best, if it cannot be wholly avoided.

This has still the merit of a borderline problem. The same is not true of the other case of necessary ignorance of the subject—that of the unconscious patient. Drafting him for nontherapeutic experiments is simply and unqualifiedly impermissible; progress or not, he must never be used, on the inflexible principle that utter helplessness demands utter protection.

When preparing this paper, I filled pages with a casuistics of this harrowing field, but then scrapped most of it, realizing my dilettante status. The shadings are endless, and only the physician-researcher can discern them properly as the cases arise. Into his lap the decision is thrown. The philosophical rule, once it has admitted into itself the idea of a sliding scale, cannot really specify its own application. It can only impress on the practitioner a general maxim or attitude for the exercise of his judgment and conscience in the concrete occasions of his work. In our case, I am afraid, it means making life more difficult for him.

It will also be noted that, somewhat at variance with the emphasis in the literature, I have not dwelt on the element of "risk" and very little on that of "consent." Discussion of the first is beyond the layman's competence; the emphasis on the second has been lessened because of its equivocal character. It is a truism to say that one should strive to minimize the risk and to maximize the consent. The more demanding concept of "identification," which I have used, includes "consent" in its maximal or authentic form, and the assumption of risk is its privilege.

No Experiments on Patients Unrelated to Their Own Disease

Although my ponderings have, on the whole, yielded points of view rather than definite prescriptions, premises rather than conclusions, they have led me to a few unequivocal yeses and noes. The first is the emphatic rule that patients should be experimented upon, if at all, *only* with reference to *their disease.* Never should there be added to the gratuitousness of the experiment as such the gratuitousness of service to an unrelated cause. This follows simply from what we have found to be the *only* excuse for infracting the special exemption of the sick at all—namely, that the scientific war on disease cannot accomplish its goal without drawing the sufferers from disease into the investigative process. If under this excuse they become subjects of experiment, they do so *because,* and only because, of *their* disease.

This is the fundamental and self-sufficient consideration. That the patient cannot possibly benefit from the unrelated experiment therapeutically, while he might from experiment related to his condition, is also true, but lies beyond the problem area of pure experiment. I am in any case discussing nontherapeutic experimentation only, where *ex hypothesi* the patient does not benefit. Experiment as part of therapy—that is, directed toward helping the subject himself—is a different matter altogether and raises its own problems, but hardly philosophical ones. As long as a doctor can say, even if only in his own thought: "There is no known cure for your condition (or: You have responded to none); but there is promise in a new treatment still under investigation, not quite tested yet as to effectiveness and safety; you will be taking a chance, but all things considered, I judge it in your best interest to let me try it on you"—as long as he can speak thus, he speaks as the patient's physician and may err, but does not transform the patient into a subject of experimentation. Introduction of an untried therapy into the treatment where the tried ones have failed is not "experimentation on the patient."

Generally, and almost needless to say, with all the rules of the book, there is something "experimental" (because tentative) about every individual treatment, beginning with the diagnosis itself; and he would be a poor doctor who would not learn from every case for the benefit of future cases, and a poor member of the profession who would not make any new insights gained from his treatments available to the profession at large. Thus, knowledge may be advanced in the treatment of any patient, and the interest of the medical art and all sufferers from the same affliction as well as the patient himself may be served if something happens to be learned from his case. But this gain to knowledge and future therapy is incidental to the *bona fide* service to the present patient. He has the right to expect that the doctor does nothing to him just in order to learn.

In that case, the doctor's imaginary speech would run, for instance, like this: "There is nothing more I can do for you. But you can do something for me. Speaking no longer as your physician but on behalf of medical science, we could learn a great deal about future cases of this kind if you would permit me to perform certain experiments on you. It is understood that you yourself would not benefit from any knowledge we might gain; but future patients would." This statement would express the purely experimental situation, assumedly here with the subject's concurrence and with all cards on the table. In Alexander Bickel's words: "It is a different situation when the doctor is no longer trying to make [the patient] well, but is trying to find out how to make others well in the future."[10]

But even in the second case, that of the nontherapeutic experiment where the patient does not benefit, at least the patient's own disease is enlisted in the cause of fighting that disease, even if only in others. It is yet another thing to say or think: "Since you are here—in the hospital with its facilities—anyway, under our care and observation anyway, away from your job (or, perhaps, doomed) anyway, we wish to profit from your being available for some other research of great interest we are presently engaged in." From the standpoint of merely medical ethics, which has only to consider risk, consent, and the worth of the objective, there may be no cardinal difference between this case and the last one. I hope that the medical reader will not think I am making too fine a point when I say that from the standpoint of the subject and his dignity there is a cardinal difference that crosses the line between the permissible and the impermissible, and this by the same principle of "identification" I have been invoking all along. Whatever the rights and wrongs of any experimentation on any patient—in the one case, at least that residue of identification is left him that it is his own affliction by which he can contribute to the conquest of that affliction, his own kind of suffering which he helps to alleviate in others; and so in a sense it is his own cause. It is totally indefensible to rob the unfortunate of this intimacy with the purpose and make his misfortune a convenience for the furtherance of alien concerns. The observance of this rule is essential, I think, to at least attenuate the wrong that nontherapeutic experimenting on patients commits in any case.

On the Redefinition of Death

My other emphatic verdict concerns the question of the redefinition of death—that is, acknowledging "irreversible coma as a new definition for death,"[11] I wish not to be misunderstood. As long as it is merely a question of when it is permitted to cease the artificial prolongation of certain functions (like heartbeat) traditionally regarded as signs of life, I do not see anything ominous in the notion of "brain death." Indeed, a new definition of death is not even necessary to legitimize the same result if one adopts the position of the Roman Catholic Church, which here at least is eminently reasonable—namely that "when deep unconsciousness is judged to be permanent, extraordinary means to maintain life are not obligatory. They can be terminated and the patient allowed to die."[12] Given a clearly defined negative condition of the brain, the physician is allowed to allow the patient to die his own death by *any* definition, which of itself will lead through the gamut of all possible definitions. But a disquietingly contradictory purpose is combined with this purpose in the quest for a new definition of death—that is, in the will to *advance* the moment of declaring him dead: Permission not to turn off the respirator, but, on the contrary, to keep it on and thereby maintain the body in a state of what would have been "life" by the older definition (but is only a "simulacrum" of life by the new)—so as to get at his organs and tissues under the ideal conditions of what would previously have been "vivisection."[13]

Now this, whether done for research or transplant purposes, seems to me to overstep what the definition can warrant. Surely it is one thing when to cease delaying death, another when to start doing violence to the body; one thing when to desist from protracting the process of dying, another when to regard that process as complete and thereby the body as a cadaver free for inflicting on it what would be torture and death to any living body. For the first purpose, we need not know the exact borderline between life and death—we leave it to nature to cross it wherever it is, or to traverse the whole spectrum if there is not just one line. All we need to know is that coma is irreversible. For the second purpose we must know the borderline with absolute certainty; and to use any definition short of the maximal for perpetrating on a *possibly* penultimate state what only the ultimate state can permit is to arrogate a knowledge which, I think, we cannot possibly have. *Since we do not know the exact borderline between life and death,* nothing less than the maximum definition of death will do—brain death plus heart death plus any other indication that may be pertinent—before final violence is allowed to be done.

It would follow then, for this layman at least, that the use of the definition should itself be defined, and this in a restrictive sense. When only permanent coma can be gained with the artificial sustaining of functions, by all means turn off the respirator, the stimulator, any sustaining artifice, and let the patient die; but let him die all the way. Do not, instead, arrest the process and start using him as a mine while, with your own help and cunning, he is still kept this side of what may in truth be the final line. Who is to say that a shock, a final trauma, is not administered to a sensitivity diffusely situated elsewhere than in the brain and still vulnerable to suffering a sensitivity that we ourselves have been keeping alive. No fiat of definition can settle this question.[14] But I wish to emphasize that the question of possible suffering (easily brushed aside by a sufficient

show of reassuring expert consensus) is merely a subsidiary and not the real point of my argument; this, to reiterate, turns on the indeterminacy of the boundaries between *life and death,* not between sensitivity and insensitivity, and bids us to lean toward a maximal rather than a minimal determination of death in an area of basic uncertainty.

There is also this to consider: The patient must be absolutely sure that his doctor does not become his executioner, and that no definition authorizes him ever to become one. His right to this certainty is absolute, and so is his right to his own body with all its organs. Absolute respect for these rights violates no one else's rights, for no one has a right to another's body. Speaking in still another, religious vein: The expiring moments should be watched over with piety and be safe from exploitation.

I strongly feel, therefore, that it should be made quite clear that the proposed new definition of death is to authorize *only* the one and *not* the other of the two opposing things: only to break off a sustaining intervention and let things take their course, not to keep up the sustaining intervention for a final intervention of the most destructive kind.

Conclusion

There would now have to be said something about nonmedical experiments on human subjects, notably psychological and genetic, of which I have not lost sight. But I must leave this for another occasion. I wish only to say in conclusion that if some of the practical implications of my reasonings are felt to work out toward a slower rate of progress, this should not cause too great dismay. Let us not forget that progress is an optional goal, not an unconditional commitment, and that its tempo in particular, compulsive as it may become, has nothing sacred about it. Let us also remember that a slower progress in the conquest of disease would not threaten society, grievous as it is to those who have to deplore that their particular disease be not yet conquered, but that society would indeed be threatened by the erosion of those moral values whose loss, possibly

caused by too ruthless a pursuit of scientific progress, would make its most dazzling triumphs not worth having. Let us finally remember that it cannot be the aim of progress to abolish the lot of mortality. Of some ill or other, each of us will die. Our mortal condition is upon us with its harshness but also its wisdom—because without it there would not be the eternally renewed promise of the freshness, immediacy, and eagerness of youth; nor would there be for any of us the incentive to number our days and make them count. With all our striving to wrest from our mortality what we can, we should bear its burden with patience and dignity.

Notes

1. In preparation for the Conference from which this volume originated.

2. G. E. W. Wolstenholme and Maeve O'Connor (editors), *CIBA Foundation Symposium, Ethics in Medical Progress: With Special Reference to Transplantation* (Boston, 1966); "The Changing Mores of Biomedical Research," *Annals of Internal Medicine* (Supplement 7), Vol. 67, No. 3 (Philadelphia, September, 1967); *Proceedings of the Conference on the Ethical Aspects of Experimentation on Human Subjects,* November 3–4, 1967 (Boston, Massachusetts; hereafter called *Proceedings*); H. K. Beecher, "Some Guiding Principles for Clinical Investigation," *Journal of the American Medical Association,* Vol. 195 (March 28, 1966), pp. 1135–36; H. K. Beecher, "Consent in Clinical Experimentation: Myth and Reality," *Journal of the American Medical Association,* Vol. 195 (January 3, 1966), pp. 34–35; P. A. Freund, "Ethical Problems in Human Experimentation," *New England Journal of Medicine,* Vol. 273 (September 23, 1965), pp. 687–92; P. A. Freund, "Is the Law Ready for Human Experimentation?," *American Psychologist,* Vol. 22 (1967), pp. 394–99; W. Wolfensberger, "Ethical Issues in Research with Human Subjects," *World Science,* Vol. 155 (January 6, 1967), pp. 47–51; See also a series of five articles by Drs. Schoen, McGrath, and Kennedy, "Principles of Medical Ethics," which appeared from August to December in Volume 23 of *Arizona Medicine.* The most recent entry in the growing literature is E. Fuller Torrey (editor), *Ethical Issues in Medicine* (New York, 1968), in which the chapter "Ethical Problems in Human Experimentation" by Otto E. Guttentag should be especially noted.

3. Wolfensberger, "Ethical Issues in Research with Human Subjects," p. 48.

4. *Proceedings,* p. 29.

5. Cf. M. H. Pappworth, "Ethical Issues in Experimental Medicine" in D. R. Cutler (editor), *Updating Life and Death* (Boston, 1969), pp. 64–69.

6. *Die Braut von Korinth:* "Victims do fall here, / Neither lamb nor steer, Nay, but human offerings untold."

7. *Proceedings,* pp. 50–51.

8. Socially, everyone is expendable relatively—that is, in different degrees; religiously, no one is expendable absolutely: The "image of God" is in all. If it can be enhanced, then not by anyone being expended, but by someone expending himself.

9. This refers to captives of circumstance, not of justice. Prison inmates are, with respect to our problem, in a special class. If we hold to some idea of guilt, and to the supposition that our judicial system is not entirely at fault, they may be held to stand in a special debt to society, and their offer to serve—from whatever motive—may be accepted with a minimum of qualms as a means of reparation.

10. *Proceedings,* p. 33. To spell out the difference between the two cases: In the first case, the patient himself is meant to be the beneficiary of the experiment, and directly so; the "subject" of the experiment is at the same time its object, its end. It is performed not for gaining knowledge, but for helping him—and helping him in the *act* of performing it, even if by its results it also contributes to a broader testing process currently under way. It is in fact part of the treatment itself and an "experiment" only in the loose sense of being untried and highly tentative. But whatever the degree of uncertainty, the motivating anticipation (the wager, if you like) is for success, and success here means the subject's own good. To a pure experiment, by contrast, undertaken to gain knowledge, the difference of success and failure is not germane, only that of conclusiveness and inconclusiveness. The "negative" result has as much to teach as the "positive." Also, the true experiment is an act distinct from the uses later made of the findings. And, most important, the subject experimented on is distinct from the eventual beneficiaries of those findings: He lets himself be used as a means toward an end external to himself (even if he should at some later time happen to be among the beneficiaries himself). With respect to his own present needs and his own good, the act is gratuitous.

11. "A Definition of Irreversible Coma," Report of the *Ad Hoc* Committee of Harvard Medical School to Examine the Definition of Brain Death, *Journal of the American Medical Association,* Vol. 205, No. 6 (August 5, 1968), pp. 337–40. [Reprinted as Chapter 79 of this volume.]

12. As rendered by Dr. Beecher in *Proceedings,* p. 50.

13. The Report of the *Ad Hoc* Committee no more than indicates this possibility with the second of the "two reasons why there is need for a definition": "(2) Obsolete criteria for the definition of death can lead to controversy in obtaining organs for transplantation." The first reason is relief from the burden of indefinitely drawn out coma. The report wisely confines its recommendations on application to what falls under this first reason—namely, turning off the respirator—and remains silent on the possible use of the definition under the second reason. But when "the patient is declared dead on the basis of these criteria," the road to the other use has theoretically been opened and will be taken (if I remember rightly, it has even been taken once, in a much debated case in England), unless it is blocked by a special barrier in good time. The above is my feeble attempt to help doing so.

14. Only a Cartesian view of the "animal machine," which I somehow see lingering here, could set the mind at rest, as in historical fact it did at its time in the matter of vivisection: But its truth is surely not established by definition.

56

From *Final Report of the Tuskegee Syphilis Study Ad Hoc Advisory Panel*

Reprinted from the Report (Washington, D.C.: U.S. Public Health Service, 1973), pp. 5–15.

Report on Charge I-A—Determine Whether the Study Was Justified in 1932

Background Data

The Tuskegee Study was one of several investigations that were taking place in the 1930's with the ultimate objective of venereal disease control in the United States. Beginning in 1926, the United States Public Health Service, with the cooperation of other organizations, actively engaged in venereal disease control work.[1] In 1929, the United States Public Health Service entered into a cooperative demonstration study with the Julius Rosenwald Fund and state and local departments of health in the control of venereal disease in six southern states[2]: Mississippi (Bolivar County); Tennessee (Tipton County); Georgia (Glynn County); Alabama (Macon County); North Carolina (Pitt County); Virginia (Albermarle County). These syphilis control demonstrations took place from 1930–1932 and disclosed a high prevalence of syphilis (35%) in the Macon County survey. Macon County was 82.4% Negro. The cultural status of this Negro population was low and the illiteracy rate was high.

During the years 1928–1942 the Cooperative Clinical Studies in the Treatment of Syphilis[3] were taking place in the syphilis clinics of Western Reserve University, Johns Hopkins University, Mayo Clinic, University of Pennsylvania, and the University of Michigan. The Division of Venereal Disease, USPHS provided statistical support, and financial support was provided by the USPHS and a grant from the Milbank Memorial Fund. These studies included a focus on effects of treatment in latent syphilis which had not been clinically documented before 1932. A report issued in 1932 indicated a satisfactory clinical outcome in 35% of untreated latent syphilitics.

The findings of Bruusgaard of Oslo on the results of untreated syphilis became available in 1929.[4] The Oslo study was a classic retrospective study involving the analysis of 473 patients at three to forty years after infection. For the first time, as a result of the Oslo study, clinical data were available to suggest the probability of spontaneous cure, continued latency, or serious or fatal outcome. Of the 473 patients included in the Oslo study, 309 were living and examined and 164 were deceased. Among the 473 patients, 27.7 percent were clinically free from symptoms and Wassermann negative; 14.8 percent had no clinical symptoms with Wassermann positive; 14.1 percent had heart and vessel disease; 2.76 percent had general paresis and 1.27 percent had tabes dorsalis. Thus in 1932, as the Public Health Service put forth a major effort toward control and treatment, much was still unknown regarding the latent stages of the disease especially pertaining to its natural course and the epidemiology of late and latent syphilis.

Facts and Documentation Pertaining to Charge I-A

1. There is no protocol which documents the original intent of the study. None of the literature searches or interviews with participants in the study gave any evidence that a written protocol ever existed for this study. The theories postulated from time to time include the following purposes either by direct statement or implication.[5-7]

a. Study of the natural history of the disease.

b. Study of the course of treated and untreated syphilis (Annual Report of the Surgeon General of the Public Health Service of the United States 1935–36).

c. Study of the differences in histological and clinical course of the disease in black versus white subjects.

d. Study with an "acceptance" of the postulate that there was a benign course of the disease in later stages vis-a-vis the dangers of available therapy.

e. Short term study (6 months or longer) of the incidence and clinical course of late latent syphilis in the Negro male (From letter of correspondence from T. Clark, Assistant Surgeon General, to M. M. Davis of the Rosenwald Fund, October 29, 1932)—Original plan of procedure is stated herein.

f. A study which would provide valuable data for a syphilis control program for a rural impoverished community.

In the absence of an original protocol, it can only be assumed that between 1932 and 1936 (when the first report[5] of the study was made) the decision was made to continue the study as a long-term study. The Annual Report of the Surgeon General for 1935–36 included the statement: "Plans for the continuation of this study are underway. During the last 12 months, success has been obtained in gaining permission for the performance of autopsies on 11/15 individuals who died."

2. There is no evidence that informed consent was gained from the human participants in this study. Such consent would and should have included knowledge of the risk of human life for the involved parties and information re possible infections of innocent, nonparticipating parties such as friends and relatives. Reports such as "Only individuals giving a history of infection who submitted voluntarily to examination were included in the 399 cases" are the only ones that are documentable.[5] Submitting voluntarily is not informed consent.

3. In 1932, there was a known risk to human life and transmission of the disease in latent and late syphilis[26] was believed to be possible. Moore[3] 1932 reported satisfactory clinical outcome in 85% of patients with latent syphilis that were treated in contrast to 35% if no treatment is given.

4. The study as announced and continually described as involving "untreated" male Negro subjects was not a study of "untreated" subjects. Caldwell[8] in 1971 reported that: All but one of the originally untreated syphilitics seen in 1968–1970 have received therapy, although heavy metals and/or antibiotics were given for a variety of reasons by many non-study physicians and not necessarily in doses considered curative for syphilis. Heller[6] in 1946 reported "about one-fourth of the syphilitic individuals received treatment for their infection. Most of these, however, received no more than 1 or 2 arsenical injections; only 12 received as many as 10." The "untreated" group in this study is therefore a group of treated and untreated male subjects.

5. There is evidence that control subjects who became syphilitic were transferred to the "untreated" group. This data is present in the patient files at the Center for Disease Control in Atlanta. Caldwell[8] reports 12 original controls either acquired syphilis or were found

to have reactive treponemal tests (unavailable prior to 1953). Heller,[6] also, reported that "It is known that some of the control group have acquired syphilis although the exact number cannot be accurately determined at present." Since this transfer of patients from the control group to the syphilitic group did occur, the study is not one of late latent syphilis. Also, it is not certain that this group of patients did in fact receive adequate therapy.

6. In the absence of a definitive protocol, there is no evidence or assurance that standardization of evaluative procedures, which are essential to the validity and reliability of a scientific study, existed at any time. This fact leaves open to question the true scientific merits of a longitudinal study of this nature. Standardization of evaluative procedures and clinical judgment of the investigators are considered essential to the valid interpretation of clinical data.[9] It should be noted that, in 1932, orderly and well planned research related to latent syphilis was justifiable since (a) Morbidity and mortality had not been documented for this population and the significance of the survey procedure had just been reported in findings of the prevalence studies for 6 southern counties;[1] (b) Epidemiologic knowledge of syphilis at the time had not produced facts so that it could be scientifically documented "just how and at what stage the disease is spread."[27] (c) There was a paucity of knowledge re clinical aspects and spontaneous cure in latent syphilis[3] and the Oslo study[4] had just reported spontaneous remission of the disease in 27.7% of the patients studied. If perhaps a higher "cure" rate could have been documented for the latent syphilitics, then the treatment priorities and recommendations may have been altered for this community where funds and medical services were already inadequate.

The retrospective summary of the "Scientific Contributions of the Tuskegee Study" from the Chief, Venereal Disease Branch, USPHS (dated November 21, 1972) includes the following merits of the study:

Knowledge already gained or potentially able to be gained from this study may be categorized as contributing to

improvements in the following areas:
1. Care of the surviving participants,
2. Care of all persons with latent syphilis,
3. The operation of a national syphilis control program,
4. Understanding of the disease of syphilis,
5. Understanding of basic disease producing mechanisms.

Panel Judgments on Charge 1-A
1. In retrospect, the Public Health Service Study of Untreated Syphilis in the Male Negro in Macon County, Alabama, was ethically unjustified in 1932. This judgment made in 1973 about the conduct of the study in 1932 is made with the advantage of hindsight acutely sharpened over some forty years, concerning an activity in a different age with different social standards. Nevertheless one fundamental ethical rule is that a person should not be subjected to avoidable risk of death or physical harm unless he freely and intelligently consents. There is no evidence that such consent was obtained from the participants in this study.

2. Because of the paucity of information available today on the manner in which the study was conceived, designed and sustained, a scientific justification for a short term demonstration study cannot be ruled out. However, the conduct of the longitudinal study as initially reported in 1936 and through the years is judged to be scientifically unsound and its results are disproportionately meager compared with known risks to human subjects involved. Outstanding weaknesses of this study, supported by the lack of written protocol, include lack of validity and reliability assurances; lack of calibration of investigator responses; uncertain quality of clinical judgments between various investigators; questionable data base validity and questionable value of the experimental design for a long term study of this nature.

The position of the Panel must not be construed to be a general repudiation of scientific research with human subjects. It is possible that a scientific study in 1932 of untreated syphilis, properly conceived with a clear protocol and conducted with suitable subjects who fully understood the implications of their involvement, might have been justified in the pre-penicillin era.

This is especially true when one considers the uncertain nature of the results of treatment of late latent syphilis and the highly toxic nature of therapeutic agents then available.

Report on Charge I-B—Determine Whether the Study Should Have Been Continued when Penicillin Became Generally Available

Background Data

In 1932, treatment of syphilis in all stages was being provided through the use of a variety of chemotherapeutic agents including mercury, bismuth, arsphenamine, neoarsphenamine, iodides and various combinations thereof. Treatment procedures being used in the early 1930's extended over long periods of time (up to two years) and were not without hazard to the patient.[10] As of 1932, also, treatment was widely recommended and treatment schedules specifically for late latent syphilis were published and in use.[3, 10] The rationale for treatment at that time was based on the clinical judgment "that the latent syphilitic patient must be regarded as a potential carrier of the disease and should be treated for the sake of the Community's health."[3] The aims of treatment in the treatment of latent syphilis were stated to be: (1) to increase the probability of "cure" or arrest, (2) to decrease the probability of progression or relapse over the probable result if no treatment were given and (3) the control of potential infectiousness from contact of the patient with adults of either sex, or in the case of women with latent syphilis, for unborn children.

According to Pfeiffer (1935),[11] treatment of late syphilis is quite individualistic and requires the physician's best judgment based upon sound fundamental knowledge of internal medicine and experience, and should not be undertaken as a routine procedure. Thus, treatment was being recommended in the United States for all stages of syphilis as of 1932 despite the "spontaneous" cure concept that was being justified by interpretations of the Oslo study, the potential hazards of treatment due to drug toxicity and to possible Jarisch-Herxheimer reactions in acute late syphilis.[12]

Documented reports of the effects of penicillin in the 1940's and early 1950's vary from outright support and endorsement of the use of penicillin in late and latent syphilis,[13-15] to statements of possible little or no value,[16-17] to expressions of doubts and uncertainty[18-19] related to its value, the potency of penicillin, absence of control of the rate of absorption, and potential hazard related to severe Herxheimer effects.

Although the mechanism of action of penicillin is not clear from available scientific reports of late latent syphilis, the therapeutic benefits were clinically documented by the early 1950's and have been widely reported from the mid 1950's to the present. In fact, the Center for Disease Control of the USPHS has reported treatment of syphilitic mothers in all stages of infection with penicillin as of 1953[20] and has demonstrated that penicillin is the most effective treatment yet known for neurosyphilis (1960).[21]

Facts and Documentation re Charge I-B

1. Treatment schedules recommending the use of arsenicals and bismuth in the treatment of late latent syphilis were available in 1932.[3] Penicillin therapy was recommended for treatment of late latent syphilis in the late 1940's[14-15] which was *before* it became readily available for public use (estimated to have been 1952–53).

2. It was "known as early as 1932 that 85% of patients treated in late latent syphilis would enjoy prolonged maintenance of good health and freedom from disease as opposed to 35 percent if left untreated."[3] Scientists in this study,[5] reported in 1936, that morbidity in male Negroes with untreated syphilis far exceeds that in a comparable nonsyphilitic group and that cardiovascular and central nervous system involvements were two to three times as common. Moreover, Wenger,[22] in 1950, reported: "We know now, where we could only surmise before, that we have contributed to their ailments and shortened their lives. I think the least we can say is that we have a high moral obligation to those that have died to make this the best study possible." The effect of syphilis in shortening life was published from observations made by Usilton et al. in 1937.[23] The study by Rosahn[24] at Yale in 1947

reported strong clinical evidence that syphilis ran a more fatal course in Negroes than in Caucasians.

3. Reports regarding the withholding of treatment from patients in this study are varied and are still subject to controversy. Statements received from personal interviews conducted by Panel members with participants in this study cannot be considered as conclusive since there are varied opinions concerning what actually happened. In written letters and in open interviews, the panel received reports that treatment was deliberately withheld on the one hand and on the other, we were told that individuals seeking treatment were not denied treatment (in transcript and correspondence documents).

What is clearly documentable (in a series of letters between Vonderlehr and Health officials in Tuskegee taking place between February 1941 and August 1942) is that known seropositive, untreated males under 45 years of age from the Tuskegee Study had been called for army duty and rejected on account of a positive blood. The local board was furnished with a list of 256 names of men under 45 years of age and asked that these men be excluded from the list of draftees needing treatment! According to the letters, the board agreed with this arrangement in order to make it possible to continue this study on an effective basis. It should be noted that some of these patients had already received notices from the Local Selective Service Board "to begin their antisyphilitic treatment immediately."

According to Wenger,[22] the patients in the study "received no treatment on our recommendation." At the present time, we know that most of the participants in this study received some form of treatment with heavy metals and/or antibiotics.[8] Although the adequacy of treatment received is not known, it is clear that the treatment received was provided by physicians who were not a part of the study and who were individually sought by the individual patients related to their own medical symptoms and pursuit of treatment.

4. The five survey periods in this study occurred in 1932, 1938–39, 1948, 1952–53 and 1968–70.[8-25] This study lacks continuity except through the public health nurse and at these isolated survey periods. In 1969 an Ad Hoc Committee reviewed the Tuskegee

Study with the purpose: to examine data from the Tuskegee Study and offer advice on continuance of this study. . . . A summary report of the meeting includes the following:

The purpose of the meeting was to determine if the Tuskegee Study should be terminated or continued. Considerations were:
1. How the study was set up in 1932
2. Are the participants all available
3. How are the survivors faring

At the time of this study there were only seven patients whose primary cause of death was ascribed to syphilis.

It was determined that benefits to be achieved from the study at this time were:
1. Relationship of serology to morbidity from syphilis
2. Relationship of known pathology to syphilis
3. Various epidemiological considerations.

Full treatment of the survivors was also considered and the following liabilities listed.

Danger of late Herxheimer's reaction which would worsen or possibly kill those syphilitic patients suffering from cardiovascular or neurological conditions.

At this time it was mentioned that both Macon County Health Department and Tuskegee Institute were cognizant of the study.

The meeting was terminated with several salient points.
1. This type of study would never be repeated.
2. There were certain medical facts to be learned by continuing the present study.
3. Treatment for these patients was not indicated unless they had signs of active syphilitic disease.
4. More contact should be established between PHS and Macon County Health Department and Medical Society so they would cooperate in the continuance of the study.

It should be noted that the Committee was eminently represented from the medical community. However, legal representatives and others from the non-medical community of scholars were not adequately represented for so sensitive a study. This is especially true since the Tuskegee Study was being continued at a time when Department of Health, Education, and Welfare guidelines for the Protection of Human Subjects were being widely disseminated for compliance by all institutions receiving grant support. The three hours and ten minutes were not adequate for in-depth study of the broad issues, implications and ramifications of this study.

In 1970, Drs. Anne Yobs and Arnold L. Schroeter in separate memoranda (to the Director, Center for Disease Control and to the Chief, Venereal Disease Branch) recommended procedures for orderly termination of this study. Dr. James Lucas, Assistant Chief of the Venereal Disease Branch, in a memorandum to the Chief of the Venereal Disease Branch dated September 10, 1970 states: It must be fully realized that the remaining contribution from this study will be largely of *historical* interest. Nothing learned will prevent, find, or cure a single case of infectious syphilis or bring us closer to our basic mission of controlling venereal disease in the United States.

5. There is a crucial absence of evidence that patients were given a ''choice'' of continuing in the study once penicillin became readily available. This fact serves to amplify the magnitude of encroachment on the human lives and well-being of the participants in this study. This is especially significant when there is uncertainty as to the whole issue of ''consent'' of the participants.

Panel Judgments on Charge I-B

The ethical, legal and scientific implications which are evoked from the facts presented in the previous section led the Panel to the following judgment:

That penicillin therapy should have been made available to the participants in this study especially as of 1953 when penicillin became generally available.

Withholding of penicillin, after it became generally available, amplified the injustice to which this group of human beings had already been subjected. The scientific merits of the Tuskegee Study are vastly overshadowed by the violation of basic ethical principles pertaining to human dignity and human life imposed on the experiment subjects.

Report on Charge I—Summary

This section of the Advisory Panel's report deals specifically with Charge Codes I-A and I-B.

Statement of Charge Codes

Charge I-A.
Determine whether the study was justified in 1932, and
Charge I-B.

Determine whether it should have been continued when penicillin became generally available.

Introduction

The Background Paper on the Tuskegee Study, prepared by the Venereal Disease Branch of the Center for Disease Control, July 27, 1972, included the following statements:

Because of the lack of knowledge of the pathogenesis of syphilis, a long-term study of untreated syphilis was considered desirable in establishing a more knowledgeable syphilis control program.

A prospective study was begun late in 1932 in Macon County, Alabama, a rural area with a static population and a high rate of untreated syphilis. An untreated population such as this offered an unusual opportunity to follow and study the disease over a long period of time. In 1932, a total of 26 percent of the male population tested, who were 25 years of age or older, were serologically reactive for syphilis by at least two tests, usually on two occasions. The original study group was composed of 399 of these men who had received no therapy and who gave historical and laboratory evidence of syphilis which had progressed beyond the infectious stages. A total of 201 men comparable in age and environment and judged by serology, history, and physical examination to be free of syphilis were selected to be the control group.

Panel Conclusions re Charge I-A and I-B of the Tuskegee Study

After extensive review of the available documents, interviews with associated parties and pursuit of various other avenues of documentation, the Panel concludes that:

1. In retrospect, the Public Health Service Study of Untreated Syphilis in the Male Negro in Macon County, Alabama was ethically unjustified in 1932.

2. Because of the paucity of information available today on the manner in which the study was conceived, designed and sustained, scientific justification for a short-term demonstration study in 1932 cannot be ruled out. However, the conduct of the longitudinal study as initially reported in 1936 and through the years is judged to be scientifically unsound and its results are disproportionately meager compared with known risks to the human subjects involved.

3. Penicillin therapy should have been made available to the participants in this study not later than 1953.

The Panel qualifies its conclusions with several position statements summarized as follows [see also "Panel Judgments," pp. 317–318]:

History has shown that certain people under psychological, social or economic duress are particularly acquiescent. These are the young, the mentally impaired, the institutionalized, the poor and persons of racial minority and other disadvantaged groups. These are the people who may be selected for human experimentation and who, because of their station in life, may not have an equal chance to withhold consent.

The Tuskegee Syphilis Study, placed in the perspective of its early years, is not an isolated event in terms of the generally accepted conditions and practices that prevailed in the 1930's.

To: The Assistant Secretary for Health and Scientific Affairs

From: Jay Katz, M.D.
Yale Law School
New Haven, Connecticut

Topic: Reservations about the Panel Report on Charge I

I should like to add the following findings and observations to the majority opinion:

1. There is ample evidence in the records available to us that the consent to participation was not obtained from the Tuskegee Syphilis Study subjects, but that instead they were exploited, manipulated, and deceived. They were treated not as human subjects but as objects of research. The most fundamental reason for condemning the Tuskegee Study at its inception and throughout its continuation is not that all the subjects should have been treated, for some might not have wished to be treated, but rather that they were never fairly consulted about the research project, its consequences for them, and the alternatives available to them. Those who for reasons of intellectual incapacity could not have been so consulted should not have been invited to participate in the study in the first place.

2. It was already known before the Tuskegee Syphilis Study was begun, and reconfirmed by the study itself, that persons with untreated syphilis have a higher death rate than those who have been treated. The life expectancy of at least forty subjects in the study was markedly decreased for lack of treatment.

3. In addition, the untreated and the "inadvertently" (using the word frequently employed by the investigators) but inadequately treated subjects suffered many complications which could have been ameliorated with treatment. This fact was noted on occasion in the published reports of the Tuskegee Syphilis Study and as late as 1971. However the subjects were not apprised of this possibility.

4. One of the senior investigators wrote in 1936 that since "a considerable portion of the infected Negro population remained untreated during the entire course of syphilis . . . an unusual opportunity (arose) to study the untreated syphilitic patient from the beginning of the disease to the death of the infected person." Throughout, the investigators seem to have confused the study with an "experiment in nature." But syphilis was not a condition for which no beneficial treatment was available, calling for experimentation to learn more about the condition in the hope of finding a remedy. The persistence of the syphilitic disease from which the victims of the Tuskegee Study suffered resulted from the unwillingness or incapacity of society to mobilize the necessary resources for treatment. The investigators, the USPHS, and the private foundations who gave support to this study should not have exploited this situation in the fashion they did. Unless they could have guaranteed knowledgeable participation by the subjects, they all should have disappeared from the research scene or else utilized their limited research resources for therapeutic ends. Instead, the investigators believed that the persons involved in the Tuskegee Study would *never* seek out treatment; a completely unwarranted assumption which ultimately led the investigators deliberately to obstruct the opportunity for treatment of a number of the participants.

5. In theory if not in practice, it has long been "a principle of medical and surgical mortality (never to perform) on man an experiment which might be harmful to him to any extent, even though the result might be highly advantageous to science" (Claude Bernard 1865), at least without the knowledgeable consent of the subject. This was one basis on which the German physicians who had conducted medical experiments in concentration camps were tried by the Nuremberg Military Tribunal for crimes against humanity. Testimony at their trial by official representatives of the American Medical Association clearly suggested that research like the Tuskegee Syphilis Study would have been intolerable in this country or anywhere in the civilized world. Yet the Tuskegee study was continued after the Nuremberg findings and the Nuremberg Code had been widely disseminated to the medical community. Moreover, the study was not reviewed in 1966 after the Surgeon General of the USPHS promulgated his guidelines for the ethical conduct of research, even though this study was carried on within the purview of his department.

6. The Tuskegee Syphilis Study finally was reviewed in 1969. A lengthier transcript of the proceedings, not quoted by the majority, reveals that one of the five members of the reviewing committee repeatedly emphasized that a moral obligation existed to provide treatment for the "patients." His plea remained unheeded. Instead the Committee, which was in part concerned with the possibility of adverse criticism, seemed to be reassured by the observation that "if we established good liaison with the local medical society, there would be no need to answer criticism."

7. The controversy over the effectiveness and the dangers of arsenic and heavy metal treatment in 1932 and of penicillin treatment when it was introduced as a method of therapy is beside the point. For the real issue is that the participants in this study were never informed of the availability of treatment because the investigators were never in favor of such treatment. Throughout the study the responsibility rested heavily on the shoulders of the investigators to make every effort to apprise the subjects of what could be done for them if

they so wished. In 1937 the then Surgeon General of the USPHS wrote: "(f)or late syphilis no blanket prescription can be written. Each patient is a law unto himself. For every syphilis patient, late and early, a careful physical examination is necessary before starting treatment and should be repeated frequently during its course." Even prior to that, in 1932, ranking USPHS physicians stated in a series of articles that adequate treatment "will afford a practical, if not complete guaranty of freedom from the development of any late lesions. . . ."

In conclusion, I note sadly that the medical profession, through its national association, its many individual societies, and its journals, has on the whole not reacted to this study except by ignoring it. One lengthy editorial appeared in the October 1972 issue of the *Southern Medical Journal* which exonerated the study and chastised the "irresponsible press" for bringing it to public attention. When will we take seriously our responsibilities, particularly to the disadvantaged in our midst who so consistently throughout history have been the first to be selected for human research?

References

1. Clark, T., *The Control of Syphilis in Southern Rural Areas*. Julius Rosenwald Fund, Chicago, 1932, p. 27.

2. Ibid. pp. 6–36.

3. Moore, Joseph Earle. Latent Syphilis Cooperative Clinical Studies in the Treatment of Syphilis. Reprint No. 45 from *Venereal Disease Information*, Vol. XIII, Nos. 8–12, 1932 and Vol. XIV, No. 1, 1933, pp. 1–56.

4. Bruusgaard, E., The Fate of Syphilitics Who Are Not Given Specific Treatment. *Archiv tur Dermatologie und Syphilis* 1929, 157, p. 309.

5. Vonderlehr, R. A., et al., Untreated Syphilis in the Male Negro. *Venereal Disease Information* 17:260–265, 1936.

6. Heller, J. R. and Bruyere, P. T., Untreated Syphilis in Male Negro: II. Mortality During 12 Years of Observation. *Venereal Disease Information* 27:34–38, 1946.

7. Shafer, J. K., Usilton, L. J., and Gleason, G. A., Untreated Syphilis in Male Negro: Prospective Study of Effect on Life Expectancy. *Public Health Reports* 69:684–690, 1954; *Milbank Memorial Fund Quarterly*. 32:262–274, July 1954.

8. Caldwell, J. G., Price, E. V., Schroeter, A. L., and Fletcher, G. F., Aortic Regurgitation in a Study of Aged Males with Previous Syphilis. Presented in part at American Venereal Disease Association Annual Meeting, 22 June 1971.

9. Feinstein, A. R., *Clinical Judgment*. Baltimore, William and Wilkins Co., 1967, pp. 45–48.

10. Gaupin, C. E., The Treatment of Latent Syphilis. *Kentucky Medical Journal* 30: 74–77, February 1932.

11. Pfeiffer, A., Medical Aspects in the Prevention and Managment of Late and Latent Syphilis. *Psychiatric Quarterly* 9: 185–193, April 1935.

12. Greenbaum, S. C., The "Bismuth Approach" in the Treatment of Acute (Late) Syphilis. *Journal of Chemotherapy* 13: 5–8, April 1936.

13. Stokes, J. H., et al., The Action of Penicillin in Late Syphilis. *J.A.M.A.* 126: 73–79, September 1944.

14. Dexter, D. C., and Tucker, H. A., Penicillin Treatment of Benign Late Gummatous Syphilis, Report of Twenty-one Cases. *American Journal of Syphilis, Gonorrhea, and Venereal Disease* 30: 211–226, May 1946.

15. Committee on Medical Research, The Changing Character of Commercial Penicillin with Suggestions as to the Use of Penicillin in Syphilis. U.S. Health Service and Food and Drug Administration. *J.A.M.A.* 131: 271–275, May 1946.

16. Barnett, C. W., The Public Health Aspects of Late Latent Syphilis. *Stanford Medical Bulletin* 10: 152–156, August 1952.

17. Reynolds, F. W., Treatment Failures Following the Use of Penicillin in Late Syphilis. *American Journal of Syphilis, Gonorrhea, and Veneral Disease* 32: 233–242, May 1948.

18. McElligott, G. L. M., The Management of Late and Latent Syphilis. *British Medical Journal* 1:829–830, April 1953.

19. Barnett, C. W., Epstein, N. J., Brewer, A. F., et al., Effect of Treatment in Late Latent Syphilis. *Arch Dermat Syph* 69: 91–99, January 1954.

20. *VD Fact Sheet*. No. 10. U.S. Public Health Service Publication, December 1953, p. 20.

21. *VD Fact Sheet*. No. 17. U.S. Public Health Service Publication, December 1960, p. 19.

22. Wenger, O. C., Untreated Syphilis in Negro Male. Hot Springs Seminar, 9-18-50 (From CDC Files).

23. Usilton, L., et al., A Tentative Death Curve for Acquired Syphilis in White and Colored Males in the United States, *Venereal Disease Information* 18: pp. 231–234, 1937.

24. Rosahn, P. D., Autopsy Studies in Syphilis. *Journal of Venereal Disease Information* 28: Supplement No. 21, pp. 32–39, 1949.

25. Rivers, E., Schuman, S., Simpson, L., and Olansky, S., Twenty Years of Follow-up Experience in a Long-Range Medical Study. *Public Health Reports* 68: (4), 391–395, April 1953.

26. Vonderlehr to T. Clark—Memorandum—June 10, 1932.

27. Letter from L. Usilton, VD Program 1930–32 and memorandum from Vonderlehr to T. Clark (Assistant Surgeon General) June 10, 1932.

57

Bernard Barber

The Ethics of Experimentation with Human Subjects

Reprinted with deletion of charts by permission of author and publisher from *Scientific American*, vol. 234, no. 2, February 1976, pp. 25–31.

The power, scope and funding of biomedical research have expanded enormously in the past 40 years. So also, inevitably, has clinical research with human subjects. That expansion has led in the past decade to widespread reflection on what is increasingly perceived as a new social problem: the abuse of human subjects of medical experimentation. In particular it is alleged that human subjects are not always protected from undue risk and do not always have the opportunity to voluntarily give their adequately informed consent to participation in experiments.

A social problem is defined in part by the concern it arouses, and this one has clearly aroused concern. Members of the medical profession itself led the way, with increasing numbers of journal articles, books and seminars on the issues. The public has become aroused, largely through popular accounts of dramatic incidents—genuine scandals in certain cases—involving the violation of the dignity and rights of patients. And the Federal Government has moved to protect human subjects, potential or actual. Beginning in 1966 the National Institutes of Health, the Food and Drug Administration and the Department of Health, Education, and Welfare have issued increasingly detailed regulations governing experimentation with human subjects in projects they support, which means in most of the biomedical research done in the country. In 1974 a National Commission for the Protection of Human Subjects of Biomedical and Behavioral Research was established to advise the Department of Health, Education, and Welfare, and it is to be replaced by a long-term National Advisory Council that is to deal with the same issues.

The regulations, commissions and councils and the very fact of interference in medical activities by outsiders are viewed by many investigators as being onerous and even dangerous. On the other hand, many outsiders believe far more social control is required. The debate on the issue has been conducted without much reference to objective evidence. In 1970 our Research Group on Human Experimentation undertook two studies of investigators' attitudes and practices. On the basis of our results I would argue that there is indeed inadequate ethical concern among biomedical investigators, that it

is reflected in excessively risky procedures and that better internal and external controls are essential.

There are two major reasons for the general recognition that experimentation with humans is a subject for concern, one of which I alluded to at the outset: the increased power, scope and funding of biomedical research. The other reason is a change in values: increased emphasis on equality, participation and the challenging of arbitrary authority.

It is easy to forget how new scientific medicine is. The revolutionary advances based on knowledge of physiology and biochemistry have come in the past 40 years, and they came from research. The basic work could be done with test-tube preparations and laboratory animals, but eventually human subjects had to be involved. Man is "the final test site," as Henry K. Beecher, a pioneer among physicians concerned about the ethics of research, once put it. Unfortunately there are no statistics on the number of people who are subjects in medical experiments or even on how many projects involve human subjects; the National Institutes of Health keeps records according to area of research (a disease or a physiological process, for example) rather than according to species of experimental subject; the NIH can say only that recently about a third of the projects it approves involve human subjects. It is clear, however, that the number of human subjects is larger than it used to be and that some small but significant minority of those subjects are involved in risky experiments. If more people have been put at more risk, then there is a rational basis for concern about the satisfactory balancing of risks and benefits, about adequate protection from unnecessary risk and about some groups being put at more risk than other groups.

Over and beyond this utilitarian basis for the new social concern with medical experimentation is the value factor, which arises from recent social changes. All over the world individuals have been demanding more equality of treatment and the right to be informed about and to participate in decisions affecting them and have been challenging the right of experts to make those decisions unilaterally. People who define themselves as being unequal, underprivileged or exploited are demanding better treatment and better protection, whether it is underdeveloped countries as against developed ones, blacks as against whites, women as against men, young as against old, patients as against doctors—or subjects as against investigators. This moral revolution of rising value-expectations has combined with the revolution in medicine to focus attention on the ethics of experimentation with human subjects.

Public awareness of the problem is too much the result of headlined scandals, but the scandals do illustrate some of the possible abuses. In the 1960's two respected cancer investigators who were studying the immune response to malignancies injected live cancer cells into a number of geriatric patients at the Jewish Hospital and Medical Center of Brooklyn without first obtaining the patients' informed consent. A few years later a leading virologist conducted an experiment at Willowbrook, a New York State institution for the severely retarded. Reasoning that a serious liver infection, hepatitis, was in effect endemic in the hospital anyway, he deliberately exposed some children to hepatitis virus in an attempt to achieve controlled conditions for testing a vaccine. The accusation was that the children's parents were not given enough information on which to base informed consent, and that in some cases consent was given perfunctorily by administrators of the institution.

More recently there was the exposure by the press of the ongoing syphilis experiment in Tuskegee, Ala. Since the 1930's a group of black subjects with syphilis had been kept under observation in an effort to study the course of the disease. That was not considered wrong in the 1930's, when the known treatments for the disease were only marginally effective, but by 1945 penicillin had become available as a safe and extremely effective cure for syphilis. Yet somehow the experiment was continued, and presumably some men died of the disease who could have been cured.

How significant are such scandals? We do not know, because no one has been doing the kind of social bookkeeping about numbers of subjects, degree of risk, adequacy of consent and efficacy of protective mechanisms that would yield an overall view of experimentation with human beings and that might contradict the more extreme allegations of abuse elicited by the publicized scandals. In the absence of such intensive record keeping it remains for social research to fill the gap by sampling the total range of experimentation with human subjects. To that end our group conducted first a national mail survey of nearly 300 biomedical research institutions and then an intensive interview study of 350 individual investigators at two institutions.

Our national survey questionnaire was answered by 293 teaching and nonteaching hospitals and other research institutions that, our analysis showed, constituted a national representative sample of all such institutions. Those who filled out the questionnaire were generally themselves active researchers and members of their institution's review committee, set up to pass on research proposals. We asked the investigators to give us their response to six simulated proposals such as those that might come before a review committee. The proposals were detailed research protocols designed to measure the degree of the investigators' concern about informed consent and their willingness to approve of studies involving various levels of risk. We could be confident that the protocols were "hypothetical-actual" rather than "hypothetical-fantastic" because we constructed them with careful attention to the research literature, checked them with specialists and pretested them with a dozen chiefs of research at medical centers, who found them to be convincingly real.

One protocol described a study of chromosome breakage in users of hallucinogenic drugs; blood samples (for chromosomes) and urine samples (for evidence of drug use) were to be taken, at no risk but also without notification of the experimental purpose, from students routinely visiting the university health center. Another protocol proposed that the thymus gland, which is a component of the immune system, be removed unnecessarily from a random sample of children undergoing heart surgery; the objective was to learn the effect of the thymectomy on the survival of an experimental skin graft made at the same time. The other protocols dealt with a random test of alternative treatments for a congenital heart defect in children; with an evaluation of the efficacy of a new drug for severe depression (placebos were given to some patients); with a study of lung function in patients kept under unnecessarily prolonged anesthesia after undergoing a routine hernia repair, and with an investigation of the effect of radioactive calcium on bone metabolism in children.

The answers to the thymectomy, anesthesia and radioactive-calcium protocols in particular gave us measures of the respondents' attitudes toward the balancing of risks and benefits. A clear pattern emerged. In the case of the high-risk thymectomy, for example, 72 percent of the respondents said the project should not be approved no matter how high the probability was that it would establish the efficacy of thymectomy in promoting transplant survival. On the other hand, 28 percent of the respondents said they would approve the experiment; 6 percent said they would approve it even if the chance of significant results was no better than one in 10. Similarly, 54 percent were against doing the calcium study at all—but 14 percent said they would approve it even if the odds were only one in 10 that it would lead to an important medical discovery. Our basic finding was that whereas the majority of the investigators were what we called "strict" with regard to balancing risks against benefits, a significant minority were "permissive," that is, they were much more willing to accept an unsatisfactory risk-benefit ratio.

The same general pattern of a strict majority and a permissive minority emerged from our second study, in which we interviewed 350 investigators actively engaged in research with human subjects. The investigators were at institutions to which we gave the synthetic names University Hospital and Research Center and Community and Teaching Hospital. The institutions were picked (by a technique known as cluster analysis) as being representative of two kinds of medical center that do considerable amounts of research. The interviewees told us about 424 different studies involving human subjects, and

44.   It has been shown that the thymus has an important bearing on the development and maintenance of immunity. For this reason the researcher proposes an investigation to determine the effect of thymus removal on the survival of tissue transplants, a very timely and important problem. In a sample of children and adolescents admitted for surgery to correct congenital heart lesions, he would randomly select an experimental group for thymectomy. Though the thymectomy will prolong the heart surgery by a few minutes, there is otherwise extremely little additional surgical risk from this procedure. At the conclusion of each heart operation, a full-thickness skin graft, approximately one cm. in diameter and obtained from an unrelated adult donor, would be sutured in place on the chest wall of both the experimental and control groups. He would then compare the survival of the skin grafts in each of the groups. It has been shown in a number of investigations of neonatal rats and other animals that those whose thymus had been removed were much less likely to reject skin grafts. The possible long-term immunological problems that might result are as yet not completely known, but a number of studies in animals indicate significant immunological deficiencies after thymectomy. Studies done in humans with myasthenia gravis, some of whom had undergone thymectomy, have not definitively demonstrated that the immunological abnormalities discovered in these patients were the result of thymectomies. To quote one authority: "There were no immunologic abnormalities that could be attributed to the effect of thymectomy per se."

The research will result in no therapeutic benefits for the patients involved. The researcher plans to obtain the consent of his potential patient-volunteers and/or their parents after explaining the procedures involved in the investigation as well as the possible short-term surgical and long-term immunological hazards for the subjects.

for each study they estimated the risk for subjects, the potential benefit for subjects, the potential benefit for future patients and the potential scientific importance of the study. It was reassuring to find that the investigators considered that only 56 percent of the clinical investigations graded for risk and benefits involved any risk for the subjects. We went on, however, to cross-tabulate the estimated risks and benefits, and we concluded that in 18 percent of the studies the risk was not adequately counterbalanced by the benefits. We called those studies the "less favorable" ones, and we proceeded to classify them further according to their potential benefits for other patients or for medical science. Even when these compensating justifications were taken into account, tabulation revealed a "least favorable" category of studies in which the poor immediate risk-benefit ratio was not compensated for by possible future benefits. These "least favorable" investigations constituted 8 percent of the investigations in our analysis.

The concept of informed consent is a troublesome one. The investigator wants to have enough subjects and is afraid of scaring them off. Patients are likely to be concerned about their own condition, may feel powerless with respect to the physician or hospital and often have difficulty understanding medical language or concepts. Even established medical procedures can have somewhat unpredictable consequences, so that physicians feel there is a limit to how completely "informed" a patient can be. The fact remains that regulations of Government funding agencies and most institutions now require that the human subject of an experiment (or his guardian, in the case of small children and mentally incompetent patients) understand that something is being done (or some treatment is being withheld) for reasons other than immediate therapeutic ones; the subject or guardian must be informed of any risks and must give consent voluntarily.

With regard to informed consent, our questionnaires and interviews again revealed a minority with "permissive" views and practices, although that minority was smaller than it was for unfavorable risk-benefit ratios. For example, 23 percent of the questionnaire respondents said they would approve the chromosome-break proposal, which presented the informed-consent issue clearly and in effect by itself. The situation was more complex in the heart-defect protocol. Here other dubious elements competed with the fact that the investigator would not inform the parents that his decision whether or not to operate would be a random one, not based on therapeutic considerations. Only 12 percent of our respondents said they would approve of the study without requiring any revisions, but only 65 percent specifically mentioned the lack of informed consent as a problem.

The best available research evidence on informed consent comes from a study conducted by Bradford H. Gray, who was then a graduate student at Yale University, at a distinguished university hospital and research center (not the one in our interview study). With the consent of the responsible investigator, Gray interviewed 51 women who were the subjects in a study of the effects of a new labor-inducing drug. Although the women had signed a consent form, often in the hectic course of the admitting procedure or in the labor room itself, 20 of them (39 percent) learned only from Gray's interview, which was held after the drug infusion had been started or even after the delivery, that they were the subjects of research. Among those who did know, most of them did not understand at least one aspect of the study: that there might be hazards, that it was a double-blind experiment, that they would be subjected to special monitoring and test procedures or that they were not required to participate; four of the women said they would have refused to participate if they had known there was any choice. Many of the women had been referred for the study by their private physician, but instead of being informed that an experimental drug was to be administered they were told that it would be a "new" drug; they trusted their doctor and assumed that "new" meant "better."

How does it happen that the treatment of human subjects is sometimes less than ethical, even in some of the most respected university-hospital centers? We think the abuses can be traced to defects in the training of

45. A researcher plans to study bone metabolism in children suffering from a serious bone disease. He intends to determine the degree of appropriation of calcium into the bone by using radioactive calcium. In order to make an adequate comparison, he intends to use some healthy children as controls, and he plans to obtain the consent of the parents of both groups of children after explaining to them the nature and purposes of the investigation and the short and long-term risks to their children. Evidence from animals and earlier studies in humans indicates that the size of the radioactive dose to be administered here would only very slightly (say, by 5-10 chances in a million) increase the probability of the subjects involved contracting leukemia or experiencing other problems in the long run. While there are no definitive data as yet on the incidence of leukemia in children, a number of doctors and statistical sources indicate that the rate is about 250/million in persons under 18 years of age. Assume for the purpose of this question that the incidence of the bone disease being discussed is about the same as that for leukemia in children under 18 years of age. The investigation, if successful, would add greatly to medical knowledge regarding this particular bone disease, but the administration of the radioactive calcium would not be of immediate therapeutic benefit for either group of children. The results of the investigation may, however, eventually benefit the group of children suffering from the bone disease. Please assume for the purposes of this question that there is no other method that would produce the data the researcher desires. The researcher is known to be highly competent in this area.

45A. Hypothetically assuming that you constitute an institutional review "committee of one," and that the proposed investigation has never been done before, please check the lowest probability that you would consider acceptable for your approval of the proposed investigation. (Check only one)

( ) 1. If the chances are 1 in 10 that the investigation will lead to an important medical discovery.

( ) 2. If the chances are 3 in 10 that the investigation will lead to an important medical discovery.

( ) 3. If the chances are 5 in 10 that the investigation will lead to an important medical discovery.

( ) 4. If the chances are 7 in 10 that the investigation will lead to an important medical discovery.

( ) 5. If the chances are 9 in 10 that the investigation will lead to an important medical discovery.

( ) 6. Place a check here if you feel that, as the proposal stands, the researcher should not attempt the investigation, no matter what the probability that an important medical discovery will result. (IF YOU CHECKED HERE, please explain): _____

45B. Which of the above responses comes closest to what you feel the existing institutional review committee in your institution would make? _____ (Please write in the number of the response.)

45C. Which of the above responses comes closest to what you feel the majority of the researchers in your institution would make, acting in their role as researcher rather than as a "committee of one"? _____ (Please write in the number of the response.)

physicians and in the screening and monitoring of research by review committees, and also to a fundamental tension between investigation and therapy. We have data bearing on each of these causative factors.

It is in medical school that the profession's central and most serious concerns are presumably given time and place and that its basic knowledge and values are instilled. Yet the evidence from our interviews shows that there is not much training in research ethics in medical school. Of the more than 300 investigators who responded to questions in this area, only 13 percent reported they had been exposed in medical school to part of a course, a seminar or even a single lecture devoted to the ethical issues involved in experimentation with human subjects; only one respondent said he had taken an entire course dealing with the issues. Another 13 percent reported that the subject had come to their attention when, as students, they did practice procedures on one another; for 24 percent it was in the course of experiments with animals; 34 percent remembered discussion of ethical issues in specific research projects. One or more of these learning experiences were reported by 43 percent of the respondents—but the remaining 57 percent reported not a single such experience. The figures were about the same whether the investigators were graduates of elite U.S. medical schools, other U.S. schools or foreign schools. The figures were a little better, however, for those who had graduated since 1950 than for older investigators.

What little ethics training there is is apparently not very effective: the investigators who reported having learned something about research ethics were only slightly less permissive in response to protocols presenting the risk-benefit issue than those who reported no such experiences. It would appear that both the amount and the quality of medical-school training in the ethics of research could be improved. In this connection it is worth remembering that the many physicians who are not engaged in investigation at all also need some background in experimentation ethics, if only so they can evaluate requests that they direct their patients toward a colleague's research project.

Scientific "peer review" is a keystone of scientific inquiry, operating implicitly in many ways and explicitly in the case of professional journals, grant-awarding committees and many institutional reviewing boards such as the "tissue committees" that assess the results of surgery in hospitals. Ethical peer review of experimentation with human beings should be the counterpart of scientific peer review, but until the mid-1960's such activity received limited support among biomedical researchers. Even after 1966, when the NIH mandated ethical peer review for all its grantees, effective review did not become universal. Our questionnaire went to hospitals and other research centers that had filed with the NIH formal assurances that the required institutional review committee had been established, but 10 percent of the respondents said their institution's committee reviewed only proposals for outside funds and 5 percent reported that only formal proposals to the NIH were reviewed. The two institutions in our interview study were among the 85 percent that stated they were reviewing all research proposals, and yet 8 percent of our interviewees volunteered the information that at least one of their own investigations with human subjects had not been reviewed.

How effective are the review committees in handling the protocols that do come before them? Our questionnaire respondents told us that in 34 percent of the institutions the committees had never required any revisions, rejected any proposals or had any proposals withdrawn in anticipation of rejection for ethical reasons; 31 percent reported revisions, 32 percent outright rejections and 19 percent withdrawals. Either some of these committees have very few ethical problems coming before them or they are ineffective. Gray's study in an institution with an active and strong committee suggests that they are ineffective rather than underworked. The committee whose performance he examined found relatively few proposals that did not need some kind of modification, and he thinks "a record of few actions by committees is an indication that their members are indifferent or that their standards are loose."

The peer-review groups seemed weak in other ways. In some institutions there was no face-to-face discussion among the reviewers. Only 22 percent of the committees had members from outside the institution, something that was then recommended and has since been mandated by the Department of Health, Education, and Welfare. In practically none of the institutions was there continuous monitoring of studies that were approved, although this was even then required by Government regulations. In general ethical peer review is hampered by the fact that each committee operates in isolation and must consider every new issue on its own and without benefit of precedent. A case-reporting system, such as operates in the law, would make that unnecessary and would promote both equity among institutions and high standards. The major weakness in the system is the lack of keen interest in and support of the review committees on the part of most working biomedical investigators. Research is their business; research is their mission and predominant interest, not applied ethics or active advocacy of patients' rights.

Most biomedical investigators are, however, interested in taking care of patients and making them well. As a result medical institutions and individual investigators operate today with two powerful sets of values and goals. On the one hand there is the pursuit and advancement of scientific knowledge. On the other there is the provision of humane and effective therapy for patients. Through a broad range of complex interactions these two sets of values and goals are harmonious, even complementary and mutually reinforcing. Occasionally, however, scientific research and humane therapy can be in conflict. When that happens, there is sometimes a tendency to choose the pursuit of knowledge at the expense of the ethical treatment of patients. An irreducible minimum of conflict may be inevitable. The ethical task now is to come as close as possible to that minimum—and to resolve unavoidable conflict in favor of humane therapy.

There is evidence that the enhanced excitement attending scientific achievement and the rewards bestowed on it in recent decades have skewed the decision-making process in many cases of conflict. As our data show, the medical schools have been largely indifferent to training their students in the ethics of research. Moreover, their record in peer review has been inferior to that of other institutions. Answers to our questionnaire showed they were less likely than other research centers to have set up a review committee before the NIH required one, less likely to have one that met the first NIH guidelines in 1966, less likely to have a committee that reviews all clinical research and less likely to include on their committee medical or nonmedical members from outside the institution. Medical schools, the Association of American Medical Colleges and professional associations of clinical investigators have been much quicker to seek research funds or to protest funding cuts than to organize seriously for the purpose of studying the ethics of research and making policy in that area.

The same emphasis on the pursuit of knowledge rather than on ethics is apparent among individual biomedical investigators. Ethical concern for the subjects of their research is not a major factor when they select their collaborators; at least it is not often mentioned as a characteristic they look for in collaborators. Scientific ability is a major concern. When we asked our 350 interview subjects, "What three characteristics do you most want to know about another researcher before entering into a collaborative relationship with him?" 86 percent of the respondents mentioned scientific ability, 45 percent mentioned motivation to work hard and 43 percent mentioned personality. Only 6 percent of them listed anything we could classify as "ethical concern for research subjects."

The tension between investigation and ethical concern is perhaps best illustrated by indications that the struggle for scientific priority and recognition exerts pressure on ethical considerations. Our data show that the social structure of competition and reward is one of the sources of permissive behavior in experimentation with human subjects; the relatively unsuccessful scientist, striving for recognition, was most likely to be permissive both in his approval of hypothetical protocols and in his own investigative work. We divided our respondents into four

categories based on the number of papers they had published and the number of times their work had been cited by other workers; the frequency of citation has been shown to be a good measure of scientific excellence. We called the most-cited investigators the "high quality" scientists and those who had published a great deal but were never cited the "extreme mass-producer" scientists. It was the extreme mass-producers who were most often engaged in investigations with less favorable risk-benefit ratios, who approved of the protocols with poorer risk-benefit ratios and who least often expressed awareness of the importance of consent. Caught up in the socially structured competitive system of science, unsuccessful in it but still pursuing the prize of peer recognition, they appear to be more likely to overvalue scientific work as against humane therapy.

It is not only the mass-producers, contending for recognition among peers in their discipline, who are apt to be more permissive. We also weighed the rank achieved by each worker within his own institution against various measures of his effectiveness compared with that of his colleagues. We found that the "underrewarded" investigators tended to be the more permissive. There is also a quite different kind of medical investigator who we think is likely to be pushed toward permissive practices by scientific competition: some of the professionally esteemed, highly successful medical scientists who are engaged in intense competition for priority and recognition in well-publicized areas of research. There are not many of those people, and they did not emerge in our sample, although some workers who refused to be interviewed may belong in that category. In the absence of real data we can only point to such evidence as published discussions concerning the worldwide heart-transplant competition of a few years ago, which raised questions about the premature exposure of human subjects to what were then still experimental procedures.

Given the fact that there are ethical defects in current medical-research standards and practices, do the resulting abuses strike particularly, as is

often alleged, at certain social groups: at the poor, at children and at institutionalized patients (prisoners in particular)?

The evidence from our interviews with 350 investigators indicates that the poorer patients in hospitals are indeed at a disadvantage as subjects of research. For each of the 424 studies our respondents reported, they told us whether fewer than 50 percent, between 50 and 75 percent or more than 75 percent of the subjects were ward or clinic patients (as opposed to patients in private or semiprivate rooms and under the care of their own physician). We found first of all that ward and clinic patients were more likely to be subjects of experiments. Moreover, when we examined the cases we had previously identified as having "less favorable" and "least favorable" risk-benefit ratios, we found that both categories were almost twice as likely to involve subjects more than three-quarters of whom were ward and clinic patients as the studies with the more favorable ratios were.

The ward and clinic patients are, of course, vulnerable to that kind of discrimination. They can most readily be channeled into an experimental group by admitting physicians and clerks without interference from a personal physician. They tend to be less knowledgeable about hospitals, more readily intimidated and less likely to understand what they are told about an experimental project, and therefore less likely to be able to withhold their consent or to give genuinely informed consent. In sum, they are the least likely to be able to protect themselves.

Many institutionalized patients are poor and perhaps incompetent, and they may feel completely dependent on the institution's administrators and physicians. Prisoners are a special case: they are institutionalized in an implicitly coercive situation, so that genuinely informed consent may be a logical impossibility. On the other hand, a prison population is by definition a good source of experimental and control subjects living under controllable conditions, and there have been instances where prison studies have been conducted humanely, with good scientific results and apparently with good effect on the prisoners' morale. Experimentation with prisoners is nevertheless subject to grave abuses. Last summer the head of the Food and Drug Administration told a Senate committee that a review of experimentation in 19 prisons revealed abuses ranging from unprofessional supervision of drug tests to inadequate medical care and follow-up treatment.

Children constitute still another special group. Small children cannot give consent for their own participation in experiments; older children, who could, are often not asked. As the Willowbrook incident demonstrated, parents are not always adequately protective of their children's interests. In the case of institutionalized patients, prisoners and children, new regulations of the Department of Health, Education, and Welfare call for special protective committees and procedures. These will only be effective, however, in a context of better ethical training for investigators and more effective peer review.

The ethical problems that attend medical research with human subjects are representative of an entire class of problems created by the impact of professionals and professional power on the general public and on public policy. In the area of research with human subjects the medical investigators are not alone; there is a tendency in other fields too for humane concerns to be left at the laboratory door. Psychologists and sociologists have often been accused of circumventing the requirement for consent and of applying unethical manipulative techniques in their investigations of human behavior, and neither profession has welcomed scrutiny from outsiders or restrictive regulation. The issue goes beyond research ethics, however. Many professions now command knowledge that has great potential usefulness for human welfare but bestows power that can be abused. Because professional power is largely based on knowledge that has not yet diffused to the general public it must to a considerable degree be self-regulated, but because professional power is of such major public consequence it must also be subject to significant public control. The medical-research profession does not have a proud record of self-regulation or acceptance of public controls.

58

World Medical Association

Declaration of Helsinki: Recommendations Guiding Medical Doctors in Biomedical Research Involving Human Subjects

Reprinted with permission of the World Medical Association.

Adopted by the 18th World Medical Assembly, Helsinki, Finland, 1964 and as revised by the 29th World Medical Assembly, Tokyo, Japan, 1975.

Introduction

It is the mission of the medical doctor to safeguard the health of the people. His or her knowledge and conscience are dedicated to the fulfillment of this mission.

The Declaration of Geneva of the World Medical Association binds the doctor with the world, "The health of my patient will be my first consideration," and the International Code of Medical Ethics declares that, "Any act or advice which could weaken physical or mental resistance of a human being may be used only in his interest."

The purpose of biomedical research involving human subjects must be to improve diagnostic, therapeutic and prophylactic procedures and the understanding of the aetiology and pathogenesis of disease.

In current medical practice most diagnostic, therapeutic or prophylactic procedures involve hazards. This applies a fortiori to biomedical research.

Medical progress is based on research which ultimately must rest in part on experimentation involving human subjects.

In the field of biomedical research a fundamental distinction must be recognized between medical research in which the aim is essentially diagnostic or therapeutic for a patient, and medical research, the essential object of which is purely scientific and without direct diagnostic or therapeutic value to the person subjected to the research.

Special caution must be exercised in the conduct of research which may affect the environment, and the welfare of animals used for research must be respected.

Because it is essential that the results of laboratory experiments be applied to human beings to further scientific knowledge and to help suffering humanity, the World Medical Association has prepared the following recommendations as a guide to every doctor in biomedical research involving human subjects. They should be kept under review in the future. It must be stressed that the standards as drafted are only a guide to physicians all over the world. Doctors are not relieved from criminal, civil and ethical responsibilities under the laws of their own countries.

I. Basic Principles

1. Biomedical research involving human subjects must conform to generally accepted scientific principles and should be based on adequately performed laboratory and animal experimentation and on a thorough knowledge of the scientific literature.

2. The design and performance of each experimental procedure involving human subjects should be clearly formulated in an experimental protocol which should be transmitted to a specially appointed independent committee for consideration, comment and guidance.

3. Biomedical research involving human subjects should be conducted only by scientifically qualified persons and under the supervision of a clinically competent medical person. The responsibility for the human subject must always rest with a medically qualified person and never rest on the subject of the research, even though the subject has given his or her consent.

4. Biomedical research involving human subjects cannot legitimately be carried out unless the importance of the objective is in proportion to the inherent risk to the subject.

5. Every biomedical research project involving human subjects should be preceded by careful assessment of predictable risks in comparison with foreseeable benefits to the subject or to others. Concern for the interests of the subject must always prevail over the interest of science and society.

6. The right of the research subject to safeguard his or her integrity must always be respected. Every precaution should be taken to respect the privacy of the subject and to minimize the impact of the study on the subject's physical and mental integrity and on the personality of the subject.

7. Doctors should abstain from engaging in research projects involving human subjects unless they are satisfied that the hazards involved are believed to be predictable. Doctors should cease any investigation if the hazards are found to outweigh the potential benefits.

8. In publication of the results of his or her research, the doctor is obliged to preserve the accuracy of the results. Reports of experimentation not in accordance with the principles laid down in this Declaration should not be accepted for publication.

9. In any research on human beings, each potential subject must be adequately informed of the aims, methods, anticipated benefits and potential hazards of the study and the discomfort it may entail. He or she should be informed that he or she is at liberty to abstain from participation in the study and that he or she is free to withdraw his or her consent to participation at any time. The doctor should then obtain the subject's freely given informed consent, preferably in writing.

10. When obtaining informed consent for the research project the doctor should be particularly cautious if the subject is in a dependent relationship to him or her or may consent under duress. In that case the informed consent should be obtained by a doctor who is not engaged in the investigation and who is completely independent of this official relationship.

11. In case of legal incompetence, informed consent should be obtained from the legal guardian in accordance with national legislation. Where physical or mental incapacity makes it impossible to obtain informed consent, or when the subject is a minor, permission from the responsible relative replaces that of the subject in accordance with national legislation.

12. The research protocol should always contain a statement of the ethical considerations involved and should indicate that the principles enunciated in the present Declaration are complied with.

II. Medical Research Combined with Professional Care (Clinical Research)

1. In the treatment of the sick person, the doctor must be free to use a new diagnostic and therapeutic measure, if in his or her judgment it offers hope of saving life, reestablishing health or alleviating suffering.

2. The potential benefits, hazards and discomfort of a new method should be weighed against the advantages of the best current diagnostic and therapeutic methods.

3. In any medical study, every patient—including those of a control group, if any—should be assured of the best proven diagnostic and therapeutic method.

4. The refusal of the patient to participate in a study must never interfere with the doctor-patient relationship.

5. If the doctor considers it essential not to obtain informed consent, the specific reasons for this proposal should be stated in the experimental protocol for transmission to the independent committee (I, 2).

6. The doctor can combine medical research with professional care, the objective being the acquisition of new medical knowledge, only to the extent that medical research is justified by its potential diagnostic or therapeutic value for the patient.

III. Nontherapeutic Biomedical Research Involving Human Subjects (Nonclinical Biomedical Research)

1. In the purely scientific application of medical research carried out on a human being, it is the duty of the doctor to remain the protector of the life and health of that person on whom biomedical research is being carried out.

2. The subjects should be volunteers—either healthy persons or patients for whom the experimental design is not related to the patient's illness.

3. The investigator or the investigating team should discontinue the research if in his/her or their judgment it may, if continued, be harmful to the individual.

4. In research on man, the interest of science and society should never take precedence over considerations related to the well-being of the subject.

Illustrative Cases

You are a physician in a government hospital. Your patient, a veteran, has an incurable disease of a rare nature, always fatal within a year after onset. Another physician, who is studying the disease in the same hospital, has gone as far as he can with laboratory experiments and requests the use of your patient to complete what he believes to be the final tests of his theory about the cause, not cure, of the patient's ailment. Because his disease is rare, the chance of getting another patient so well located to help in the experiment is slim. When approached, the patient is reluctant to consent to participating unless you can convince him of the justifications for his cooperation.

1. What might the justifications be?
2. If he still refuses, should he be coerced, subtly or actively, to participate?
3. Should small actions of a research nature that could be helpful to the experiment, and not harmful to him, be taken (for example, collecting extra blood or urine specimens) without telling him?
4. Would it make a difference if this fatal disease were common and its potential cure rested on this patient's consent to participate in the experiment?

Medical authorities at an institution for the retarded, housing 1,000 children aged 5 to 15, have had to contend with periodic outbreaks of infectious hepatitis, a viral disorder that strikes the liver and causes the child afflicted with it to be ill for several weeks with such symptoms as fever, nausea, jaundice, abdominal pain, and general malaise. For several months after the acute symptoms disappear, the child may still complain of fatigue. In a very small number of cases, acute massive necrosis of the liver may occur, which can result in death. Infectious hepatitis has its highest incidence among young people, particularly those living together at close quarters such as in institutions. Between 50,000 to 70,000 cases are reported each year in the United States, which one pediatric textbook estimates represent no more than 10 percent of the cases that actually occur. The medical authorities in this institution decide to conduct experiments that involve giving the disease

to groups of newly admitted children and carefully observing them. Only children whose parents or guardian had given consent are used. The knowledge that the physicians hope to acquire from these experiments might someday prevent outbreaks of this disorder.

1. What moral considerations would you introduce in deciding for or against the conduct of this experiment?

VI

Procreative Decisions

Introduction to Part VI

A number of topics that are often treated separately and pursued in their own right are combined in this section. All these somewhat different topics are at least in part interrelated in a significant way. For several reasons, including increased awareness of rapid human population growth, advanced knowledge in genetics, increased concern about the quality of our individual and collective lives, and a move toward equal rights and autonomy for women, a whole range of decisions are being asked of us as individuals and collectivities, decisions about whether or when or why to conceive children, and when or whether or why to carry a developing human conceptus or fetus to term and bring it into the world.

Concerns about the quality of the lives of those who are to be born and the quality of the environment into which they are born has surely been one side of this increasing preoccupation with the reasonableness and the nature of our procreative decisions. Concerns about our freedom as to when, how, and why to make these decisions, particularly the freedom of women, has been another major source of heightening the self-consciousness with which we approach procreative decisions and their impact. All these themes pervade the literature on policies in population, genetics, abortion, and fetal experimentation.

Population Policy

Population growth is widely discussed in the media, the schools, and in daily conversation. Environmental degradation, starvation, poverty, crowding, and unplanned pregnancies are among the serious problems that have been associated with population growth. These problems affect not only the decisions of policy makers and a variety of professionals, but those of individuals and couples as well. For example, some couples say they do not plan to have any children because there are enough children in the world already. Regardless of whether their worry about population growth in

the world is the primary or sole reason such couples may have for deciding not to have children, and regardless of whether their decision is based on careful analysis, individuals or couples who seriously accept such a rationale for their decisions are assuming or acting exactly as if they have sufficient expertise in population matters as well as in ethics to feel that they know what is right or wrong. No one should be greatly surprised, then, to find that medical professionals as well as their patients are making procreative decisions based on such moral judgments but often without considering existing analyses of the nature and seriousness of population-related problems and policies.

At least three of the major policy positions in the population field are represented in the selections in this anthology, knowledge of which is useful both for those who provide medical advice and for those who seek it. In this section, Garrett Hardin presents a crisis orientation that views the growth of population as an imminently disastrous phenomenon of our modern era. According to Hardin, the problems generated by population growth are so serious and the desire for more children than our world can hold is so strong certain forms of societal coerciveness will be needed to curb population growth.

Michael S. Teitelbaum writes in the spirit and tradition of those who have favored voluntary family-planning programs as a way to bring births into equilibrium with deaths and to achieve zero population growth. Influenced by the first world meeting of governments held at Bucharest in 1974 for planning population policy, Teitelbaum emphasizes socioeconomic development, an element of population policy for which family planners have often argued. Teitelbaum seeks to bring together those who see only socioeconomic development as population policies and those who see only family-planning programs as population policies.

In his analysis of population policy alternatives, Arthur J. Dyck not only identifies and analyzes the crisis-oriented and family-planning program positions, but also examines and offers some support for the argument that socioeconomic development emphasizing benefits for the poorest members of any given society is the most important kind of population policy.

Genetic Dimensions

Procreative decisions, influenced by advanced knowledge and techniques of human genetics, are also being made with some anxiety as to how we can maintain and advance the quality of life for individuals and communities. As a scientist, Marc Lappé critically examines some of the scientific and moral assumptions in literature advocating various forms of genetic control. John Fletcher's essay is a study of how parents and children are affected by decisions to abort fetuses diagnosed as genetically deviant.

Using the methods and concepts of ethics, Karen Lebacqz analyzes the factual and moral thinking that goes into the justification of making prenatal diagnoses of genetic abnormalities and what it means from a moral perspective to justify decisions to abort fetuses on the basis of speculation about their future happiness and well-being as developing human beings. Joseph Fletcher is an ethicist who gives strong support to making highly selective judgments about who should and who should not be born, depending on the genetic potential for a certain quality of life.

Abortion

Whatever else it may be, the decision to interrupt a pregnancy by removing the fetus from the womb is a medical intervention. It is important, therefore, to include at the very outset, as in the first two articles in this section, some indication of the thinking and practices of the medical profession itself. No discussion of abortion would be complete without providing the two quite divergent landmark decisions on abortion of the U.S. Supreme Court and the Federal Constitutional Court of the Federal Republic of Germany. In both of these decisions, the extent

to which procreative decisions, particularly by women, should be private and unregulated by the state was carefully weighed in the context of the state's interest and obligations in developing human life. But whereas the U.S. Supreme Court concluded that decisions to abort in the first three months of pregnancy are to be considered private and beyond state regulation, the West German court did not, and specified the circumstances under which the law could permit abortions.

With these medical and legal discussions as background, the section on abortion now turns to a consideration of the very complex and vexing philosophical and religious issues that are raised in arguing for and against abortion under a variety of circumstances. The philosopher Judith Jarvis Thomson defends the autonomy of decisions regarding abortion as a form of justifiable killing. Sissela Bok develops her arguments for abortions under a certain range of circumstances by providing reasons why individuals and societies will not undermine the value they place on human life provided that they are clear as to when, to what degree, and under what circumstances human life in its various stages of development is to be valued. The essay by John Badertscher, although it is an excellent portrayal of the subtle way in which religion enters debates about abortion, is also a very sensitive analysis of major differing viewpoints on abortion, one that leads Badertscher to argue for certain policies for regulating abortion decisions.

Fetal Experimentation

Although the Supreme Court decision (*Roe* v. *Wade*) had a great deal to say about the freedom of decisions to abort fetuses, it left doubtful and uncertain what freedom there was to make use of living fetuses whose destiny is abortion and dead fetuses who are aborted, whether spontaneously or purposely. And although the fetus can be argued to be dependent on the woman in whose womb it exists, in the context of making decisions about abortion, the fetus takes on a

certain independent status in arguments for making it the subject of biological or medical experimentation. In any event, questions have been asked about the relation between procreative decisions and decisions regarding fetuses that have no further future. These questions and their moral implications are well illustrated in the documents provided in this subsection as well as the other arguments regarding the moral bases of procreative decisions in Part VI.

Population Policy

59

Garrett Hardin

The Tragedy of the Commons

Reprinted with permission of author and publisher from *Science*, vol. 162, December 1968, pp. 1243–1248. Copyright © 1968 by the American Association for the Advancement of Science.

At the end of a thoughtful article on the future of nuclear war, Wiesner and York[1] concluded that: "Both sides in the arms race are . . . confronted by the dilemma of steadily increasing military power and steadily decreasing national security. *It is our considered professional judgment that this dilemma has no technical solution.* If the great powers continue to look for solutions in the area of science and technology only, the result will be to worsen the situation."

I would like to focus your attention not on the subject of the article (national security in a nuclear world) but on the kind of conclusion they reached, namely that there is no technical solution to the problem. An implicit and almost universal assumption of discussions published in professional and semipopular scientific journals is that the problem under discussion has a technical solution. A technical solution may be defined as one that requires a change only in the techniques of the natural sciences, demanding little or nothing in the way of change in human values or ideas of morality.

In our day (though not in earlier times) technical solutions are always welcome. Because of previous failures in prophecy, it takes courage to assert that a desired technical solution is not possible. Wiesner and York exhibited this courage; publishing in a science journal, they insisted that the solution to the problem was not to be found in the natural sciences. They cautiously qualified their statement with the phrase, "It is our considered professional judgment. . . ." Whether they were right or not is not the concern of the present article. Rather, the concern here is with the important concept of a class of human problems which can be called "no technical solution problems," and, more specifically, with the identification and discussion of one of these.

It is easy to show that the class is not a null class. Recall the game of tick-tack-toe. Consider the problem, "How can I win the game of tick-tack-toe?" It is well known that I cannot, if I assume (in keeping with the conventions of game theory) that my opponent understands the game perfectly. Put another way, there is no "technical solution" to the problem. I can win only by giving a radical meaning to the word "win." I can hit my opponent over the head; or

I can drug him; or I can falsify the records. Every way in which I "win" involves, in some sense, an abandonment of the game, as we intuitively understand it. (I can also, of course, openly abandon the game—refuse to play it. This is what most adults do.)

The class of "No technical solution problems" has members. My thesis is that the "population problem," as conventionally conceived, is a member of this class. How it is conventionally conceived needs some comment. It is fair to say that most people who anguish over the population problem are trying to find a way to avoid the evils of overpopulation without relinquishing any of the privileges they now enjoy. They think that farming the seas or developing new strains of wheat will solve the problem—technologically. I try to show here that the solution they seek cannot be found. The population problem cannot be solved in a technical way, any more than can the problem of winning the game of tick-tack-toe.

What Shall We Maximize?

Population, as Malthus said, naturally tends to grow "geometrically," or, as we would now say, exponentially. In a finite world this means that the per capita share of the world's goods must steadily decrease. Is ours a finite world?

A fair defense can be put forward for the view that the world is infinite; or that we do not know that it is not. But, in terms of the practical problems that we must face in the next few generations with the foreseeable technology, it is clear that we will greatly increase human misery if we do not, during the immediate future, assume that the world available to the terrestrial human population is finite. "Space" is no escape.[2]

A finite world can support only a finite population; therefore, population growth must eventually equal zero. (The case of perpetual wide fluctuations above and below zero is a trivial variant that need not be discussed.) When this condition is met, what will be the situation of mankind? Specifically, can Bentham's goal of "the greatest good for the greatest number" be realized?

No—for two reasons, each sufficient by itself. The first is a theoretical one. It is not mathematically possible to maximize for two (or more) variables at the same time. This was clearly stated by von Neumann and Morgenstern[3], but the principle is implicit in the theory of partial differential equations, dating back at least to D'Alembert (1717–1783).

The second reason springs directly from biological facts. To live, any organism must have a source of energy (for example, food). This energy is utilized for two purposes: mere maintenance of life requires about 1600 kilocalories a day ("maintenance calories"). Anything that he does over and above merely staying alive will be defined as work, and is supported by "work calories" which he takes in. Work calories are used not only for what we call work in common speech; they are also required for all forms of enjoyment, from swimming and automobile racing to playing music and writing poetry. If our goal is to maximize population it is obvious what we must do: We must make the work calories per person approach as close to zero as possible. No gourmet meals, no vacations, no sports, no music, no literature, no art. . . . I think that everyone will grant, without argument or proof, that maximizing population does not maximize goods. Bentham's goal is impossible.

In reaching this conclusion I have made the usual assumption that it is the acquisition of energy that is the problem. The appearance of atomic energy has led some to question this assumption. However, given an infinite source of energy, population growth still produces an inescapable problem. The problem of the acquisition of energy is replaced by the problem of its dissipation, as J. H. Fremlin has so wittily shown.[4] The arithmetic signs in the analysis are, as it were, reversed; but Bentham's goal is still unobtainable.

The optimum population is, then, less than the maximum. The difficulty of defining the optimum is enormous; so far as I know, no one has seriously tackled this problem. Reaching an acceptable and stable solution will surely require more than one generation of hard analytical work—and much persuasion.

We want the maximum good per person; but what is good? To one person it is wilderness, to another it is ski lodges for thousands. To one it is estuaries to nourish ducks for hunters to shoot; to another it is factory land. Comparing one good with another is, we usually say, impossible because goods are incommensurable. Incommensurables cannot be compared.

Theoretically this may be true; but in real life incommensurables *are* commensurable. Only a criterion of judgment and a system of weighting are needed. In nature the criterion is survival. Is it better for a species to be small and hideable, or large and powerful? Natural selection commensurates the incommensurables. The compromise achieved depends on a natural weighting of the values of the variables.

Man must imitate this process. There is no doubt that in fact he already does, but unconsciously. It is when the hidden decisions are made explicit that the arguments begin. The problem for the years ahead is to work out an acceptable theory of weighting. Synergistic effects, nonlinear variation, and difficulties in discounting the future make the intellectual problem difficult, but not (in principle) insoluble.

Has any cultural group solved this practical problem at the present time, even on an intuitive level? One simple fact proves that none has: there is no prosperous population in the world today that has, and has had for some time, a growth rate of zero. Any people that has intuitively identified its optimum point will soon reach it, after which its growth rate becomes and remains zero.

Of course, a positive growth rate might be taken as evidence that a population is below its optimum. However, by any reasonable standards, the most rapidly growing populations on earth today are (in general) the most miserable. This association (which need not be invariable) casts doubt on the optimistic assumption that the positive growth rate of a population is evidence that it has yet to reach its optimum.

We can make little progress in working toward optimum population size until we explicitly exorcize the spirit of Adam Smith in the field of practical demography. In economic affairs, *The Wealth of Nations* (1776) popularized the "invisible hand," the idea that an individual who "intends only his own gain," is, as it were, "led by an invisible hand to promote . . . the public interest."[5] Adam Smith did not assert that this was invariably true, and perhaps neither did any of his followers. But he contributed to a dominant tendency of thought that has ever since interfered with positive action based on rational analysis, namely, the tendency to assume that decisions reached individually will, in fact, be the best decisions for an entire society. If this assumption is correct it justifies the continuance of our present policy of laissez-faire in reproduction. If it is correct we can assume that men will control their individual fecundity so as to produce the optimum population. If the assumption is not correct, we need to reexamine our individual freedoms to see which ones are defensible.

Tragedy of Freedom in a Commons

The rebuttal to the invisible hand in population control is to be found in a scenario first sketched in a little-known pamphlet in 1833 by a mathematical amateur named William Forster Lloyd (1794–1852).[6] We may well call it "the tragedy of the commons," using the word "tragedy" as the philosopher Whitehead used it: "The essence of dramatic tragedy is not unhappiness. It resides in the solemnity of the remorseless working of things."[7] He then goes on to say, "This inevitableness of destiny can only be illustrated in terms of human life by incidents which in fact involve unhappiness. For it is only by them that the futility of escape can be made evident in the drama."

The tragedy of the commons develops in this way. Picture a pasture open to all. It is to be expected that each herdsman will try to keep as many cattle as possible on the commons. Such an arrangement may work reasonably satisfactorily for centuries because tribal wars, poaching, and disease keep the numbers of both man and beast well below the carrying capacity of the land. Finally, however, comes the day of reckoning, that is, the day when the long-desired goal of social stability becomes a reality. At this point, the inherent logic of the commons remorselessly generates tragedy.

As a rational being, each herdsman seeks to maximize his gain. Explicitly or implicitly, more or less consciously, he asks, "What is the utility to me of adding one more animal to my herd?" This utility has one negative and one positive component.

1. The positive component is a function of the increment of one animal. Since the herdsman receives all the proceeds from the sale of the additional animal, the positive utility is nearly +1.

2. The negative component is a function of the additional overgrazing created by one more animal. Since, however, the effects of overgrazing are shared by all the herdsmen, the negative utility for any particular decision-making herdsman is only a fraction of −1.

Adding together the component partial utilities, the rational herdsman concludes that the only sensible course for him to pursue is to add another animal to his herd. And another; and another. . . . But this is the conclusion reached by each and every rational herdsman sharing a commons. Therein is the tragedy. Each man is locked into a system that compels him to increase his herd without limit—in a world that is limited. Ruin is the destination toward which all men rush, each pursuing his own best interest in a society that believes in the freedom of the commons. Freedom in a commons brings ruin to all.

Some would say that this is a platitude. Would that it were! In a sense, it was learned thousands of years ago, but natural selection favors the forces of psychological denial.[8] The individual benefits as an individual from his ability to deny the truth even though society as a whole, of which he is a part, suffers. Education can counteract the natural tendency to do the wrong thing, but the inexorable succession of generations requires that the basis for this knowledge be constantly refreshed.

A simple incident that occurred a few years ago in Leominster, Massachusetts, shows how perishable the knowledge is. During the Christmas shopping season the parking meters downtown were covered with plastic bags that bore tags reading: "Do not open until after Christmas. Free parking courtesy of the mayor and city council." In other words, facing the prospect of an increased demand for already scarce space, the city fathers reinstituted the system of the commons. (Cynically, we suspect that they gained more votes than they lost by this retrogressive act.)

In an approximate way, the logic of the commons has been understood for a long time, perhaps since the discovery of agriculture or the invention of private property in real estate. But it is understood mostly only in special cases which are not sufficiently generalized. Even at this late date, cattlemen leasing national land on the western ranges demonstrate no more than an ambivalent understanding, in constantly pressuring federal authorities to increase the head count to the point where overgrazing produces erosion and weed-dominance. Likewise, the oceans of the world continue to suffer from the survival of the philosophy of the commons. Maritime nations still respond automatically to the shibboleth of the "freedom of the seas." Professing to believe in the "inexhaustible resources of the oceans," they bring species after species of fish and whales closer to extinction.[9]

The National Parks present another instance of the working out of the tragedy of the commons. At present, they are open to all, without limit. The parks themselves are limited in extent—there is only one Yosemite Valley—whereas population seems to grow without limit. The values that visitors seek in the parks are steadily eroded. Plainly, we must soon cease to treat the parks as commons or they will be of no value to anyone.

What shall we do? We have several options. We might sell them off as private property. We might keep them as public property, but allocate the right to enter them. The allocation might be on the basis of wealth, by the use of an auction system. It might be on the basis of merit; as defined by some agreed-upon standards. It might be by lottery. Or it might be on a first-come, first-served basis, administered to long queues. These, I think, are all the reasonable possibilities. They are all objectionable. But we must choose—or acquiesce in the destruction of the commons that we call our National Parks.

Pollution

In a reverse way, the tragedy of the commons reappears in problems of pollution. Here it is not a question of taking something out of the commons, but of putting something in—sewage, or chemical, radioactive, and heat wastes into water; noxious and dangerous fumes into the air; and distracting and unpleasant advertising signs into the line of sight. The calculations of utility are much the same as before. The rational man finds that his share of the cost of the wastes he discharges into the commons is less than the cost of purifying his wastes before releasing them. Since this is true for everyone, we are locked into a system of "fouling our own nest," so long as we behave only as independent, rational, free-enterprisers.

The tragedy of the commons as a food basket is averted by private property, or something formally like it. But the air and waters surrounding us cannot readily be fenced, and so the tragedy of the commons as a cesspool must be prevented by different means, by coercive laws or taxing devices that make it cheaper for the polluter to treat his pollutants than to discharge them untreated. We have not progressed as far with the solution of this problem as we have with the first. Indeed, our particular concept of private property, which deters us from exhausting the positive resources of the earth, favors pollution. The owner of a factory on the bank of a stream—whose property extends to the middle of the stream—often has difficulty seeing why it is not his natural right to muddy the waters flowing past his door. The law, always behind the times, requires elaborate stitching and fitting to adapt it to this newly perceived aspect of the commons.

The pollution problem is a consequence of population. It did not much matter how a lonely American frontiersman disposed of his waste. "Flowing water purifies itself every 10 miles," my grandfather used to say, and the myth was near enough to the truth when he was a boy, for there were not too many people. But as population became denser, the natural chemical and biological recycling processes became overloaded, calling for a redefinition of property rights.

How To Legislate Temperance?

Analysis of the pollution problem as a function of population density uncovers a not generally recognized principle of morality, namely: *the morality of an act is a function of the state of the system at the time it is performed.*[10] Using the commons as a cesspool does not harm the general public under frontier conditions, because there is no public; the same behavior in a metropolis is unbearable. A hundred and fifty years ago a plainsman could kill an American bison, cut out only the tongue for his dinner, and discard the rest of the animal. He was not in any important sense being wasteful. Today, with only a few thousand bison left, we would be appalled at such behavior.

In passing, it is worth noting that the morality of an act cannot be determined from a photograph. One does not know whether a man killing an elephant or setting fire to the grassland is harming others until one knows the total system in which his act appears. "One picture is worth a thousand words," said an ancient Chinese; but it may take 10,000 words to validate it. It is as tempting to ecologists as it is to reformers in general to try to persuade others by way of the photographic shortcut. But the essense of an argument cannot be photographed: it must be presented rationally—in words.

That morality is system-sensitive escaped the attention of most codifiers of ethics in the past. "Thou shalt not . . ." is the form of traditional ethical directives which make no allowance for particular circumstances. The laws of our society follow the pattern of ancient ethics, and therefore are poorly suited to governing a complex, crowded, changeable world. Our epicyclic solution is to augment statutory law with administrative law. Since it is practically impossible to spell out all the conditions under which it is safe to burn trash in the back yard or to run an automobile without smog-control, by law we delegate the details to bureaus. The result is administrative law, which is rightly feared for an ancient reason—*Quis custodiet ipsos custodes?*—"Who shall watch the watchers themselves?" John Adams said that we must have "a government of laws and not men." Bureau administrators, trying to evaluate the morality of acts in the total system, are singularly liable to corruption, producing a government by men, not laws.

Prohibition is easy to legislate (though not necessarily to enforce); but how do we legislate temperance? Experience indicates that it can be accomplished best through the mediation of administrative law. We limit possibilities unnecessarily if we suppose that the sentiment of *Quis custodiet* denies us the use of administrative law. We should rather retain the phrase as a perpetual reminder of fearful dangers we cannot avoid. The great challenge facing us now is to invent the corrective feedbacks that are needed to keep custodians honest. We must find ways to legitimate the needed authority of both the custodians and the corrective feedbacks.

Freedom To Breed Is Intolerable

The tragedy of the commons is involved in population problems in another way. In a world governed solely by the principle of "dog eat dog"—if indeed there ever was such a world—how many children a family had would not be a matter of public concern. Parents who bred too exuberantly would leave fewer descendants, not more, because they would be unable to care adequately for their children. David Lack and others have found that such a negative feedback demonstrably controls the fecundity of birds.[11] But men are not birds, and have not acted like them for millenniums, at least.

If each human family were dependent only on its own resources; *if* the children of improvident parents starved to death; *if*, thus, overbreeding brought its own "punishment" to the germ line—*then* there would be no public interest in controlling the breeding of families. But our society is deeply committed to the welfare state,[12] and hence is confronted with another aspect of the tragedy of the commons.

In a welfare state, how shall we deal with the family, the religion, the race, or the class (or indeed any distinguishable and cohesive group) that adopts overbreeding as a policy to secure its own aggrandizement?[13] To couple the concept of freedom to breed with the belief that everyone born has an equal right to the commons is to lock the world into a tragic course of action.

Unfortunately this is just the course of action that is being pursued by the United Nations. In late 1967, some 30 nations agreed to the following:

The Universal Declaration of Human Rights describes the family as the natural and fundamental unit of society. It follows that any choice and decision with regard to the size of the family must irrevocably rest with the family itself, and cannot be made by anyone else.[14]

It is painful to have to deny categorically the validity of this right; denying it, one feels as uncomfortable as a resident of Salem, Massachusetts, who denied the reality of witches in the 17th century. At the present time, in liberal quarters, something like a taboo acts to inhibit criticism of the United Nations. There is a feeling that the United Nations is "our last and best hope," that we shouldn't find fault with it; we shouldn't play into the hands of the archconservatives. However, let us not forget what Robert Louis Stevenson said: "The truth that is suppressed by friends is the readiest weapon of the enemy." If we love the truth we must openly deny the validity of the Universal Declaration of Human Rights, even though it is promoted by the United Nations. We should also join with Kingsley Davis[15] in attempting to get Planned Parenthood-World Population to see the error of its ways in embracing the same tragic ideal.

Conscience Is Self-Eliminating

It is a mistake to think that we can control the breeding of mankind in the long run by an appeal to conscience. Charles Galton Darwin made this point when he spoke on the centennial of the publication of his grandfather's great book. The argument is straightforward and Darwinian.

People vary. Confronted with appeals to limit breeding, some people will undoubtedly respond to the plea more than others. Those who have more children will produce a larger fraction of the next generation than those with more susceptible consciences. The difference will be accentuated, generation by generation.

In C. G. Darwin's words: "It may well be that it would take hundreds of generations for the progenitive instinct to develop in this way, but if it should

do so, nature would have taken her revenge, and the variety *Homo contracipiens* would become extinct and would be replaced by the variety *Homo progenitivus*."[16]

The argument assumes that conscience or the desire for children (no matter which) is hereditary—but hereditary only in the most general formal sense. The result will be the same whether the attitude is transmitted through germ cells, or exosomatically, to use A. J. Lotka's term. (If one denies the latter possibility as well as the former, then what's the point of education?) The argument has here been stated in the context of the population problem, but it applies equally well to any instance in which society appeals to an individual exploiting a commons to restrain himself for the general good—by means of his conscience. To make such an appeal is to set up a selective system that works toward the elimination of conscience from the race.

Pathogenic Effects of Conscience

The long-term disadvantage of an appeal to conscience should be enough to condemn it; but has serious short-term disadvantages as well. If we ask a man who is exploiting a commons to desist "in the name of conscience," what are we saying to him? What does he hear?—not only at the moment but also in the wee small hours of the night when, half asleep, he remembers not merely the words we used but also the nonverbal communication cues we gave him unawares? Sooner or later, consciously or subconsciously, he senses that he has received two communications, and that they are contradictory: (i) (intended communcation) "If you don't do as we ask, we will openly condemn you for not acting like a responsible citizen"; (ii) (the unintended communication) "If you *do* behave as we ask, we will secretly condemn you for a simpleton who can be shamed into standing aside while the rest of us exploit the commons."

Everyman then is caught in what Bateson has called a "double bind." Bateson and his co-workers have made a plausible case for viewing the double bind as an important causative factor in the genesis of schizophrenia.[17] The double bind may not always be so damaging, but it always endangers the

mental health of anyone to whom it is applied. "A bad conscience," said Nietzsche, "is a kind of illness."

To conjure up a conscience in others is tempting to anyone who wishes to extend his control beyond the legal limits. Leaders at the highest level succumb to this temptation. Has any President during the past generation failed to call on labor unions to moderate voluntarily their demands for higher wages, or to steel companies to honor voluntary guidelines on prices? I can recall none. The rhetoric used on such occasions is designed to produce feelings of guilt in noncooperators.

For centuries it was assumed without proof that guilt was a valuable, perhaps even an indispensable, ingredient of the civilized life. Now, in this post-Freudian world, we doubt it.

Paul Goodman speaks from the modern point of view when he says: "No good has ever come from feeling guilty, neither intelligence, policy, nor compassion. The guilty do not pay attention to the object but only to themselves, and not even to their own interests, which might make sense, but to their anxieties."[18]

One does not have to be a professional psychiatrist to see the consequences of anxiety. We in the Western world are just emerging from a dreadful two-centuries-long Dark Ages of Eros that was sustained partly by prohibition laws, but perhaps more effectively by the anxiety-generating mechanisms of education. Alex Comfort has told the story well in *The Anxiety Makers*;[19] it is not a pretty one.

Since proof is difficult, we may even concede that the results of anxiety may sometimes, from certain points of view, be desirable. The larger question we should ask is whether, as a matter of policy, we should ever encourage the use of a technique the tendency (if not the intention) of which is psychologically pathogenic. We hear much talk these days of responsible parenthood; the coupled words are incorporated into the titles of some organizations devoted to birth control. Some people have proposed massive propaganda campaigns to instill responsibility into the nation's (or the world's) breeders. But what is the meaning of the word responsibility in this context? Is it not merely a synonym for the word conscience? When we use the word responsibility in the absence of substantial sanctions are we not trying to browbeat a free man in a commons into acting against his own interest? Responsibility is a verbal counterfeit for a substantial *quid pro quo*. It is an attempt to get something for nothing.

If the word responsibility is to be used at all, I suggest that it be in the sense Charles Frankel uses it.[20] "Responsibility," says this philosopher, "is the product of definite social arrangements." Notice that Frankel calls for social arrangements—not propaganda.

Mutual Coercion Mutually Agreed upon

The social arrangements that produce responsibility are arrangements that create coercion, of some sort. Consider bank-robbing. The man who takes money from a bank acts as if the bank were a commons. How do we prevent such action? Certainly not by trying to control his behavior solely by a verbal appeal to his sense of responsibility. Rather than rely on propaganda we follow Frankel's lead and insist that a bank is not a commons; we seek the definite social arrangements that will keep it from becoming a commons. That we thereby infringe on the freedom of would-be robbers we neither deny nor regret.

The morality of bank-robbing is particularly easy to understand because we accept complete prohibition of this activity. We are willing to say "Thou shalt not rob banks," without providing for exceptions. But temperance also can be created by coercion. Taxing is a good coercive device. To keep downtown shoppers temperate in their use of parking space we introduce parking meters for short periods, and traffic fines for longer ones. We need not actually forbid a citizen to park as long as he wants to; we need merely make it increasingly expensive for him to do so. Not prohibition, but carefully biased options are what we offer him. A Madison Avenue man might call this persuasion; I prefer the greater candor of the word coercion.

Coercion is a dirty word to most liberals now, but it need not forever be so. As with the four-letter words, its dirtiness can be cleansed away by exposure to the light, by saying it over and over without apology or embarrassment. To many, the word coercion implies arbitrary decisions of distant and irresponsible bureaucrats; but this is not a necessary part of its meaning. The only kind of coercion I recommend is mutual coercion, mutually agreed upon by the majority of the people affected.

To say that we mutually agree to coercion is not to say that we are required to enjoy it, or even to pretend we enjoy it. Who enjoys taxes? We all grumble about them. But we accept compulsory taxes because we recognize that voluntary taxes would favor the conscienceless. We institute and (grumblingly) support taxes and other coercive devices to escape the horror of the commons.

An alternative to the commons need not be perfectly just to be preferable. With real estate and other material goods, the alternative we have chosen is the institution of private property coupled with legal inheritance. Is this system perfectly just? As a genetically trained biologist I deny that it is. It seems to me that, if there are to be differences in individual inheritance, legal possession should be perfectly correlated with biological inheritance—that those who are biologically more fit to be the custodians of property and power should legally inherit more. But genetic recombination continually makes a mockery of the doctrine of "like father, like son" implicit in our laws of legal inheritance. An idiot can inherit millions, and a trust fund can keep his estate intact. We must admit that our legal system of private property plus inheritance is unjust—but we put up with it because we are not convinced, at the moment, that anyone has invented a better system. The alternative of the commons is too horrifying to contemplate. Injustice is preferable to total ruin.

It is one of the peculiarities of the warfare between reform and the status quo that it is thoughtlessly governed by a double standard. Whenever a reform measure is proposed it is often defeated when its opponents triumphantly discover a flaw in it. As Kingsley Davis has pointed out,[21] worshippers of the status quo sometimes imply that no reform is possible without unanimous agreement, an implication contrary to historical fact. As nearly as I can make out, automatic rejection of proposed reforms is based on one of two unconscious assumptions: (i) that the status quo is perfect; or (ii) that the choice we face is between reform and no action; if the proposed reform is imperfect, we presumably should take no action at all, while we wait for a perfect proposal.

But we can never do nothing. That which we have done for thousands of years is also action. It also produces evils. Once we are aware that the status quo is action, we can then compare its discoverable advantages and disadvantages with the predicted advantages and disadvantages of the proposed reform, discounting as best we can for our lack of experience. On the basis of such a comparison, we can make a rational decision which will not involve the unworkable assumption that only perfect systems are tolerable.

Recognition of Necessity

Perhaps the simplest summary of this analysis of man's population problems is this: the commons, if justifiable at all, is justifiable only under conditions of low-population density. As the human population has increased, the commons has had to be abandoned in one aspect after another.

First we abandoned the commons in food gathering, enclosing farm land and restricting pastures and hunting and fishing areas. These restrictions are still not complete throughout the world.

Somewhat later we saw that the commons as a place for waste disposal would also have to be abandoned. Restrictions on the disposal of domestic sewage are widely accepted in the Western world; we are still struggling to close the commons to pollution by automobiles, factories, insecticide sprayers, fertilizing operations, and atomic energy installations.

In a still more embryonic state is our recognition of the evils of the commons in matters of pleasure. There is almost no restriction on the propagation of sound waves in the public medium. The shopping public is assaulted with mindless music, without its consent. Our government is paying out billions of dollars to create supersonic transport which will disturb 50,000 people for every one person who is whisked from coast to coast 3 hours faster. Advertisers muddy the airwaves of radio and television and pollute the view of travelers. We are a long way from outlawing the commons in matters of pleasure. Is this because our Puritan inheritance makes us view pleasure as something of a sin, and pain (that is, the pollution of advertising) as the sign of virtue?

Every new enclosure of the commons involves the infringement of somebody's personal liberty. Infringements made in the distant past are accepted because no contemporary complains of a loss. It is the newly proposed infringements that we vigorously oppose; cries of "rights" and "freedom" fill the air. But what does "freedom" mean? When men mutually agreed to pass laws against robbing, mankind became more free, not less so. Individuals locked into the logic of the commons are free only to bring on universal ruin; once they see the necessity of mutual coercion, they become free to pursue other goals. I believe it was Hegel who said, "Freedom is the recognition of necessity."

The most important aspect of necessity that we must now recognize, is the necessity of abandoning the commons in breeding. No technical solution can rescue us from the misery of overpopulation. Freedom to breed will bring ruin to all. At the moment, to avoid hard decisions many of us are tempted to propagandize for conscience and responsible parenthood. The temptation must be resisted, because an appeal to independently acting consciences selects for the disappearance of all conscience in the long run, and an increase in anxiety in the short.

The only way we can preserve and nurture other and more precious freedoms is by relinquishing the freedom to breed, and that very soon. "Freedom is the recognition of necessity"—and it is the role of education to reveal to all the necessity of abandoning the freedom to breed. Only so, can we put an end to this aspect of the tragedy of the commons.

References

1. J. B. Wiesner and H. F. York, *Sci. Amer.* 211 (No. 4), 27 (1964).

2. G. Hardin, *J. Hered.* 50, 68 (1959); S. von Hoernor, *Science* 137, 18 (1962).

3. J. von Neumann and O. Morgenstern, *Theory of Games and Economic Behavior* (Princeton Univ. Press, Princeton, N.J., 1947), p. 11.

4. J. H. Fremlin, *New Sci.*, No. 415 (1964), p. 283.

5. A. Smith, *The Wealth of Nations* (Modern Library, New York, 1937), p. 423.

6. W. F. Lloyd, *Two Lectures on the Checks to Population* (Oxford Univ. Press, Oxford, England, 1833), reprinted (in part) in *Population, Evolution, and Birth Control*, G. Hardin, Ed. (Freeman, San Francisco, 1964), p. 37.

7. A. N. Whitehead, *Science and the Modern World* (Mentor, New York, 1948), p. 17.

8. G. Hardin, Ed. *Population, Evolution, and Birth Control* (Freeman, San Francisco, 1964), p. 56.

9. S. McVay, *Sci. Amer.* 216 (No. 8), 13 (1966).

10. J. Fletcher, *Situation Ethics* (Westminster, Philadelphia, 1966).

11. D. Lack, *The Natural Regulation of Animal Numbers* (Clarendon Press, Oxford, 1954).

12. H. Girvetz, *From Wealth to Welfare* (Stanford Univ. Press, Stanford, Calif. 1950).

13. G. Hardin, *Perspec. Biol. Med.* 6, 366 (1963).

14. U. Thant, *Int. Planned Parenthood News*, No. 168 (February 1968), p. 3.

15. K. Davis, *Science* 158, 730 (1967).

16. S. Tax, Ed., *Evolution after Darwin* (Univ. of Chicago Press, Chicago, 1960), vol. 2, p. 469.

17. G. Bateson, D. D. Jackson, J. Haley, J. Weakland, *Behav. Sci.* 1, 251 (1956).

18. P. Goodman, *New York Rev. Books* 10(8), 22 (23 May 1968).

19. A. Comfort, *The Anxiety Makers* (Nelson, London, 1967).

20. C. Frankel, *The Case for Modern Man* (Harper, New York, 1955), p. 203.

21. J. D. Roslansky, *Genetics and the Future of Man* (Appleton-Century-Crofts, New York, 1966), p. 177.

60

Michael S. Teitelbaum

Population and
Development:
Is a Consensus
Possible?

Reprinted by permission from *Foreign Affairs*, July 1974. Copyright © 1974 by Council on Foreign Relations, Inc.

Concern about population growth is only one of many issues on the world's agenda, and it is fair to say that as compared with immediate problems such as energy, food supplies and monetary reform it ranks low among priorities of statesmen. However, as Canute learned in his confrontation with the tide, some processes have an inexorable force and will neither disappear on their own nor cease on request. Population growth is one such process. Over the past few years discussion of what actions are appropriate to confront the flow of human reproduction has entered the arena of international affairs, and 1974 will mark the first worldwide intergovernmental conference on the subject, to be held in Bucharest in August.

While in the past there has been extensive debate concerning the virtues and disadvantages of population growth, there is today hardly any responsible spokesman who would argue that it can logically continue forever. All agree that in the long term the necessity for "zero population growth" will be seen as a truism rather than a slogan, for the alternative of unending population growth in a finite world is patently absurd.

There are ramifying debates, however, as to (1) the process by which such growth will decline and eventually cease, (2) the time perspective which is appropriate for this to take place, and (3) the need for efforts directed specifically toward reducing population growth as contrasted with general economic and social development. Advocates of exaggerated positions have joined the fray with gusto and have often taken center-stage, leading to a political and ideological polarization of major proportion. On the one hand, the so-called "population bomb" is blamed for most of the ills of the world, including hunger, poverty, pollution, crime, and even mental illness. From this perspective such problems could be resolved via voluntary or coercive population programs if only the political will and financial resources were available. On the other hand, advocates of the contrary polar view repeatedly rise to deny the salience of current population growth as a problem, and to decry what they view as its increasing overemphasis among the purveyors of development assistance.

Even within the ranks of those most concerned over world population growth, there is a growing current of doubt about the effectiveness of deliberate governmental population policies. By "population policies" here we mean only those deliberate governmental actions intended to affect fertility behavior (though policies affecting mortality and migration may also properly be considered population policies). Such population policies include programs and laws affecting information and education, family planning services, and incentives directed toward fertility behavior, as well as efforts to alter the frequency and age of marital unions. Many commentators are now vigorously proclaiming the ineffectiveness of such special policies, asserting that only through improvements in health, nutrition, income, social justice, status of women, or other such general factors will the issue of population growth ever be resolved.

The debate is increasingly one of international politics, crosscut by the currents of academic theories, ethical principles, and religious and ideological doctrines. Mere data cannot be expected to resolve such debates, which derive more from perception than from fact. But if the debate *were* a rational one, what *could* the data tell us? To what extent can the strongly held positions on "the population problem" be supported by fact, and to what extent is agnosticism in the absence of factual data an appropriate posture?

II

There can be no doubt as to the factually extraordinary nature of the current population situation of the world. From the appearance of mankind to early modern times the human population grew at a rate averaging very close to zero. For short periods local populations might have grown relatively rapidly, but then disease or famine would set in and the population would stop growing or would decline. The overall human growth rate cannot have averaged more than two-thousandths of a percent (0.002 percent or 20 per million) annually up to early modern times. The average birthrate was high but so was the death rate, and the result was near-equilibrium. Merely to survive as a species, humankind had to maximize its reproductivity to compensate for its devastating mortality, and strongly pro-natalist social institutions were therefore by definition characteristic of all human societies which survived through this epoch into the modern world.

With the appearance of scientific, political, social and economic institutions capable of reducing human mortality, mankind's equilibrium began to change, first gradually and then dramatically. As the then-developing countries of eighteenth- and nineteenth-century Europe pursued their processes of modernization, industrialization, and urbanization, their death rates began to decline, while birthrates remained at the high levels supported by millennia-old social practices favoring high fertility. The result was a major acceleration in population growth, with sustained growth rates many hundreds of times greater than previously. Annual population growth rates of 0.5 to 1.5 percent (5,000 to 15,000 per million) became common, and sustained growth rates for Europe as a whole averaged about 0.7 percent. While such figures may not sound high when compared to current rates of economic growth and inflation, they resulted in a doubling of the European population during the nineteenth century. In the context of these increases and of the periodic economic and agricultural setbacks of nineteenth-century Europe, waves of European migrants flowed to colonies on other continents. Only after many decades did these rates of population growth begin to moderate, not through a return to previous high mortality rates, but through a decline in fertility.

This process of change from high-mortality/high-fertility to low-mortality/high-fertility, and finally to low-mortality/low-fertility came to be called the Demographic Transition. It was an historical process easier to describe than to explain. The causes of the mortality decline are variously held to reside in improved sanitation and health measures, in new and more productive agricultural crops (such as the potato) introduced into Europe from the New World, in improved communication and transport of foodstuffs to reduce localized famine, and in an

inexplicable decline in the virulence of epidemic diseases such as bubonic plague and smallpox. The causes of the fertility decline are even more in dispute. Concepts such as urbanization, industrialization, modernization, compulsory education, recognition of the decline in infant mortality rates, and even a growth in "rationality" and "hope" are variously employed to explain the course of fertility decline. Yet as one examines all available data a satisfying explanation becomes more and more evanescent. For example, England, the pioneer of the Industrial Revolution, with her rapid urbanization and modernization, did not experience a decline in fertility until the late 1800s, while France, with her tepid pace of development, her Catholicism, and her large peasant population, was the pioneer of the fertility decline.

If one cannot be confident as to the causes of fertility decline, there can be no doubt as to its reality and persistence. The long-term trend of fertility in developed countries has been downward throughout the twentieth century, with the post-World War II "baby boom" (which in fact characterized only a few developed countries) representing merely a temporary aberration from this trend. By the 1970s fertility rates in nearly all developed countries had dropped to levels very close to "replacement" (that number of children required simply to replace the present population of reproductive age), and the prospect arose of a new equilibrium being established.

The population history of the developing countries of the twentieth century is markedly different. The decline in mortality began only four or five decades ago and has been far more precipitous than the earlier decline in Europe. In large part these later declines have been unrelated to economic development—due instead to the importation and rapid implementation of modern and relatively inexpensive public health measures and medical technologies which had been developed only gradually during the nineteenth and early twentieth centuries. At the same time birthrates in the developing countries at the onset of the mortality decline were substantially higher than those of pre-industrial Europe, due primarily to the prevalence of earlier and more nearly universal marriage in the developing countries.[1]

While birthrates have subsequently declined in some developing countries, typically they have remained higher than those of pre-industrial Europe, while mortality declines have been dramatic. The result has been population growth rates in the developing countries which dwarf the previously unprecedented rates of nineteenth-century Europe. Some developing countries are currently experiencing growth rates approaching 3.5 percent (35,000 per million), fully twice as great as the highest experienced during Europe's most rapid growth. The average of all developing countries, including those which have experienced unmistakable fertility declines, is still about 2.5 percent. A difference of such magnitude has enormous implications when one is dealing with population processes. The disequilibrium of birthrates and death rates in the developing countries over the past four decades has been literally extraordinary—quite unprecedented in the history of the human species, including that of nineteenth-century Europe.

If the pace of both mortality decline and population growth has quickened among the twentieth-century developing countries as compared with those of the previous centuries, so there are modest signs of a quickened pace of fertility decline. In the case of England, for example, fertility did not show an unambiguous decline until fully 100 years after mortality began to fall. In contrast, as we see in Table 60–1 below, at least a dozen developing countries of small to moderate size can unambiguously document a substantial decline in birthrates only a few decades after the onset of substantial declines in mortality.

In addition, as the table indicates, another group of countries may have experienced such declines, but limitations of available data preclude any firm conclusions. In some cases changes in age structure and marital patterns were important factors in declining birthrates, but in many there is unmistakable evidence that fertility within marriage is undergoing downward revision.[2]

As in the case of the European Demographic Transition, an explanation of the above declines in birthrates in developing countries is a matter of almost continuous academic disputation.

Table 60-1
Declines in Crude Birthrate (Live Births per 1,000 Population) in 1960s

Area	Certain decline	Possible decline
Asia	Hong Kong (15 or more) Singapore (15 or more) Taiwan (10–14) South Korea (10–14) Sri Lanka (5–9) W. Malaysia (5–9)	China (5–9) Turkey (5–9)
Latin America	Barbados (10–14) Chile (10–14) Costa Rica (10–14) Trinidad & Tobago (10–14) Jamaica (5–9) Puerto Rico (5–9)	Brazil (5–9) Colombia (5–9) Cuba (5–9) El Salvador (5–9) Guatemala (5–9) Venezuela (5–9)
Africa	Mauritius (10–14) Egypt (5–9) Tunisia (5–9)	

( ) = approximate number of points decline.
Source: Berelson, *World Population: Status Report 1974*.

Some argue that most of the countries with clear declines in fertility have experienced rapid economic development, industrialization, and urbanization, and it is the impact of these socioeconomic forces which explains the declining birthrates. Others point to the intensive population and family planning programs in most of these countries and argue that declining birthrates may be explained at least partially in terms of the high effectiveness and acceptability of these programs.

Whatever the truth of various explanatory positions, the present world distribution of birthrates is so closely related to development status that the birthrate itself can be used as an efficient way of distinguishing developing from developed countries. There are few exceptions to the rule of thumb that developing countries have birthrates above 30 per thousand while developed countries have birthrates well below 30 per thousand. Indeed the few notable exceptions to this rule are themselves instructive, for they are developing countries, such as South Korea and Taiwan, which are well along the roads of both development and their own demographic transitions.

III

Perhaps the least widely understood aspect of population growth is its tendency to continue even after fertility has declined. Rapid population growth can be said to have the property of

momentum, much like the tendency of a fast-moving vehicle to continue its motion long after its brakes are applied. There are two components of this population momentum, one obvious and the other more subtle. The obvious factor is that the social and economic forces encouraging high fertility have been established over the millennia of mankind's existence on earth, and simply cannot be eliminated overnight. We know from the European experience that such changes can take many decades, and even if the process is greatly accelerated in today's developing countries it can still take many years. The more subtle basis for the momentum of population growth resides in the age structure of a rapidly growing population. Such a population is distinguishable from a slow-growing population by the former's very "young" age structure, i.e., by its large proportion of children and adolescents. In such a country there are many more young people than adults, and as the young enter the reproductive ages there inevitably will be more potential parents. The implications for future growth of this population momentum are often overlooked. Government officials, even some well versed in economics, often view population growth rates as amenable to the same type of short-term manipulation as other societal rates such as investment rates, interest rates,

and unemployment rates. Such perceptions are factually incorrect; the momentum of population growth is determined not by government policies but by the inexorable logic of mathematics.

Let us assume, for example, that development and population efforts will be exceedingly successful over the next decade, and that by the period 1980–85 fertility in developing countries will decline to the "replacement" level now characteristic of developed countries. Under such an exceptionally optimistic assumption the population of the developing world would nonetheless continue to grow for many decades, and would eventually reach a size fully 88 percent greater than its 1970 level. All large developing countries would experience very substantial population increases due to their built-in momentum for further growth, although there would be differences in the magnitude of these increases.

If we now relax our extreme assumption of a fertility decline to "replacement" level by 1980–85 and assume that this level will be reached 20 years later in 2000–2005 (which would still represent a rapid fertility decline when compared to the experience of Europe), another set of figures emerges. The difference in eventual growth indicated by the two sets of figures illustrates how important to eventual population size is the date by which fertility declines to low levels. In the present example a difference of "only" 20

Table 60-2

Country	Population circa 1970 (in millions)	Eventual population size (in millions)		Percent increase from 1970 level	
		Replacement by 1980–85	Replacement by 2000–05	Replacement by 1980–85	Replacement by 2000–05
China	734	1,270	1,622	+ 73%	+121%
India	534	1,002	1,366	+ 88	+156
Brazil	94	192	266	+104	+183
Bangladesh	69	155	240	+125	+248
Nigeria	65	135	198	+108	+205
Pakistan	57	112	160	+ 96	+181
Mexico	51	111	168	+118	+229
Philippines	38	79	119	+108	+213
Egypt	34	64	92	+ 88	+171
Developing World	2,530	4,763	6,525	+ 88	+158
World	3,652	6,245	8,135	+ 71	+123

Source: Tomas Frejka, *Reference Tables to "The Future of Population Growth,"* New York: The Population Council, 1973.

years implies an eventual population increase in developing countries of nearly four billion instead of the 2.2 billion resulting from the early fertility reduction. The point is shown dramatically in Table 60-2.

These illustrations demonstrate not only the power of population momentum but also the degree to which most developing countries are already virtually assured of major population increases, whatever happens to fertility levels. In most cases the focus of present policy decisions directed toward fertility behavior need not be on the next 75 to 125 percent increase; such growth is coming, welcome or not. The issue at hand is the desirability of subsequent increases of even greater magnitude. The momentum of population growth thus requires that policy-makers think beyond the next development decade, beyond the next election, and even beyond the next 50 years—into the next century. In an age when officials must necessarily concentrate upon the coming harvest or the rates of price increases of raw or manufactured goods, such a perspective requires statesmanship of an impressive dimension.

IV

Faced with such a problem and imbued with farsightedness and vision, what should a policy-maker actually do? If it is true that our understanding of fertility decline in both nineteenth-century Europe and twentieth-century developing countries is at best merely tentative and at worst almost nil, one

may well ask how anyone could be justified in asserting that any particular policy is *the* "correct" one. Unfortunately, such scientific ambiguities have not been reflected in humility on the part of discussants of these issues. A policy-maker seeking to find a sensible way to deal with population issues will find himself assaulted on all sides by strongly held and aggressively asserted positions as to why he ought (or ought not) adopt specific policy approaches. As the issue of population has become more and more one of policy rather than science, political considerations have naturally become more determinant in the elaboration of these positions. Furthermore, the near identity between high fertility and low development status (for which there may be causal connections in both directions) has meant that international discussions of population have increasingly taken on the flavor of a debate between the developing and developed worlds, in the same category as such debates regarding raw materials, colonialism, and the terms of international trade.

The result of all this can only be confusion, particularly on the part of the intelligent and concerned policy-maker who is seeking the best possible advice on what if anything should be his government's policy regarding population growth. In the interest of clarification it is possible to dissect analytically the various positions one from another, but with two important

caveats. First, limitation of space makes it inevitable that descriptions of these positions will be oversimplified distillations of what are often subtle and eloquent arguments. Second, it must be noted that these positions are distinct from one another only in analytical terms; in the real world a person or country will usually adopt several of the positions which are mutually supportive of a particular perspective on population issues. A list of extant analytical positions ought to include at least the following:

Positions against the Need for Special Population Programs and Policies

1. The Pro-natalist position
Rapid population growth in a particular country or region is a positive force on grounds of (a) economic development, in that a larger population provides necessary economies of scale and a sufficient labor supply; (b) protection of currently underpopulated areas from covetous neighbors; (c) differentials in fertility among ethnic, racial, religious, or political population segments; (d) military and political power and the vitality of a younger age structure.
2. The Revolutionist position
Population programs are mere palliatives to fundamental social and political contradictions which will inevitably lead to a just revolution, and may therefore be viewed as inherently counterrevolutionary.
3. The Anti-colonial and Genocide positions

The motives of rich countries which are pushing poor developing countries to adopt aggressive population programs are open to suspicion. These rich countries went through a period of rapid population growth as a component of their own development processes, and their current efforts to restrain population growth in the developing countries are an attempt to maintain the status quo by retarding the development of these countries. One can also see the undue emphasis on population as an attempt on the part of the rich developed countries to "buy development cheaply."

Finally, a person who is very suspicious of the motives of the developed countries could see in their population efforts an attempt to limit or reduce the relative or absolute size of poor and largely nonwhite populations. Such a practice could be seen as a subtle form of genocide deriving from racist or colonialist motives.

4. The Over-consumption position
So-called "population problems" are actually problems of resource scarcity and environmental deterioration which derive primarily from activities of the rich developed countries, and not from high fertility in the developing countries.

Even if fertility is too high in the developing countries, this is a consequence of their poverty, which in turn results from over-consumption of the world's scarce resources by rich countries.

5. The Accommodationist position
As in the past, growing numbers can be readily accommodated by improvements in agricultural and industrial technologies.

The world has already shown that Malthus' predictions were incorrect; the same is true of the neo-Malthusian predictions and solutions.

That which is termed "overpopulation" in a given situation is really a matter of underemployment. A humane and properly structured economy can provide employment and the means of subsistence for all people, no matter what the size of the population.

6. The Problem-is-Population-Distribution position
It is not numbers per se which are causing population problems, but their distribution in space. Many areas of the world (or country) are underpopulated; others have too many people in too small an area.

Instead of efforts to moderate the rate of numbers growth, governments should undertake efforts to reduce rural-urban flows and bring about a more even distribution of population on the available land.

7. The Mortality and Social Security position
High fertility is a response to high mortality and morbidity; bring these levels down and fertility will decline naturally.

Living children are the primary means by which poor people can achieve security in old age. Hence a reduction in infant and child mortality levels or provision of alternative forms of social security would lead to a reduction in fertility.

8. The Status and Roles of Women position
High fertility levels are perpetuated by norms and practices which define women primarily as procreative agents. As long as women's economic and social status depend largely or solely upon the number of children they bear, there is little possibility that societal fertility will decline substantially.

9. The Religious Doctrinal position
In one form this position holds that population is not a serious problem. Be fruitful and multiply, God will provide. In another form this position holds that while current rates of population growth are a serious problem, the primary instruments to deal with them are morally unacceptable, e.g., modern contraception and surgical sterilization are "unnatural," abortion is "murder."

10. The Medical Risk position
The goal of fertility reduction is not worth the medical risks of the primary instruments of population programs. Oral contraceptives and intrauterine devices have measurable, if small, short-term risks, and some people fear their long-term effects. Sterilization and abortion are operative procedures, all of which have an element of risk, particularly when performed outside the hospital.

11. The Holistic Development position
Fertility decline is a natural concomitant of social and economic development, as proven by the European Demographic Transition.

Most of the fertility decline in developing countries with family planning programs therefore derives from the impact of social and economic development rather than from the programs themselves.

International assistance for development is too heavily concentrated upon population programs, and is short-changing general development programs.

12. The Social Justice position.
Neither population programs nor economic development as presently pursued will bring about necessary fertility declines.

Fertility will not decline until the basic causes of high fertility—poverty, ignorance, fatalism, etc.—are eliminated through social policies which result in a redistribution of power and wealth among the rich and poor, both within and among nations.

Positions Supporting the Need for Special Population Programs and Policies

1. The Population Hawk position
Unrestrained population growth is the principal cause of poverty, malnutrition, environmental disruption, and other social problems. Indeed we are faced with impending catastrophe on food and environmental fronts.

Such a desperate situation necessitates draconian action to restrain population growth, even if coercion is required. "Mutual coercion, mutually agreed upon."

Population programs are fine as far as they go, but they are wholly insufficient in scope and strength to meet the desperate situation.

2. The Provision of Services position
Surveys and common sense show that there is a great unmet demand for fertility control in all countries; hence the main problem is to provide modern fertility control to already motivated people.

Some proponents also hold that the failure of some service programs is due to inadequate fertility control technologies, and that the need for technological improvements is urgent.

3. The Human Rights position
As recognized in the U.N. Tehran Convention (1968), it is a fundamental human right for each person to be able to determine the size of his or her own family.

Furthermore, some argue that each woman has the fundamental right to the control of her own bodily processes. (This position usually leads to support for abortion as well as contraception.)

Health is also a basic human right, which population programs help to achieve through a variety of direct and indirect pathways, including the direct medical benefits of increased child spacing on maternal and child health, and the indirect effects of reducing the incidence of dangerous illegal abortions.

4. The Population-Programs-Plus-Development position

Social and economic development are necessary but not sufficient to bring about a new equilibrium of population at low mortality and fertility levels. Special population programs are also required.

Too rapid population growth is a serious intensifier of other social and economic problems, and is one, though only one, of a number of factors behind lagging social and economic progress in many countries.

Some countries might benefit from larger populations, but would be better served by moderate rates of growth over a longer period than by very rapid rates of growth over a shorter period. An effective population program therefore is an essential component of any sensible development program.

As has been noted, these analytically separable positions are by no means mutually exclusive in the real world. Typically a given proponent will adopt an array of these positions which are found to be mutually reinforcing of the conclusion being put forward. For example, a common argument heard from representatives of Third World countries might include elements of the Pro-natalist, the Anti-colonial and Genocide, the Over-consumption, the Accommodationist, the Medical Risk, and the Holistic Development positions. Two countries might agree in their overall posture toward population programs, but might at the same time disagree strongly on the specific positions supporting the common posture. It is little wonder that international debates on population programs often fail even to define the issues, much less resolve disagreements. Such difficulties

are compounded by the incendiary nature of some of the rhetorical positions; terms such as "counterrevolutionary," "genocide," "population bomb," and "population crisis" are hardly conducive to sober reflection on empirical realities.

V

Despite such centrifugal tendencies, which often seem to send international meetings careening off onto tangential paths, it is encouraging that one can now perceive a fragile but growing consensus coalescing about a small number of arguments which are firmly rooted in the best available evidence. The central core of this consensus is the Population-Programs-Plus-Development position described earlier, but amended importantly by incorporation of major elements of disparate other positions. Partial elements of this view may be discerned in the writings and speeches of a number of statesmen, economists, demographers, educators, and family planners.

The consensus position begins with a frank recognition that population growth is not the only, or even the primary, source of the poverty, disease, illiteracy, and gross inequality which now characterize the world. The ultimate solution to such problems depends on the true social and economic development of the poor countries and regions of the world. Such development cannot be "bought cheaply" through concentration on population as the major problem. Second, the consensus position recognizes that whatever the population problem may be it is not uniform throughout the world, nor can a single characterization be correctly applied to all countries or even to all developing countries. In some areas it is evident that the population is already too large for indigenous resources, while in others resources are available in abundance, and development might be served by substantial increases in population size. Third, it is recognized that many of the problems arising from population concentrations derive from patterns of distribution and rural-urban migration as well as from overall rates of population increase. Fourth, the consensus position explicitly recognizes that, barring catastrophe, the population of the world and particularly of the developing countries will increase dramatically

no matter what population policies are adopted; hence the world's technological and economic resources must be mobilized to assure that these sharply increased numbers can be accommodated and provided with opportunities for lives of dignity. Fifth, the consensus notes the happy convergence of most voluntary population programs with the goal of maximizing the basic human right of each individual to determine his or her own fertility.

The advocates of the consensus then go on to recognize the reflexive importance of rapid population growth upon the prospects for true social and economic development. While reductions in population growth rates are by no means sufficient to bring about such development, the very rapid growth rates of some countries stand as serious impediments to such progress. This is true both in areas in which population size is already taxing available resources and in those which could benefit by very substantial population increases. In the first case both the absolute size of the population and its rate of increase are important, while in the latter case attention is drawn to the benefits of moderate as opposed to rapid rates of increase. Hence population programs are seen as necessary but not sufficient components of all development programs. In no case is the goal in the short term a cessation of population growth, for the momentum of growing populations for further growth is well recognized in the consensus position. Indeed it is the force and duration of this momentum which provides a powerful argument for early attention to population policy, even in those fortunate countries for which substantial further growth may be a positive development.

The mechanism by which fertility is to be moderated combines strenuous efforts at accelerating social and economic development with vigorous programs directed specifically to population concerns. The consensus position recognizes that the overall level of social and economic development has effects on fertility levels which are largely independent of and distinct from the effects of population programs. But the converse proposition is also recognized as true: that population programs providing modern methods of fertility control have effects upon fertility levels which are independent and distinct from the effects of the overall level of economic and social development.

After more than a decade of experience with population programs in a variety of developmental settings, we now have convincing empirical evidence of the validity of both of these propositions. If all countries for which data are available are categorized simultaneously in terms both of the strength of their family planning programs and of their relative levels of social and economic development, the data show that *both* factors are important in explaining declines in birthrates and differences in contraceptive use. In a study done at the Population Council,[3] 26 developing countries were categorized simultaneously in terms of their development status[4] and the strength of their family planning programs.[5] Each country was then characterized by two indicators of fertility control: the proportion of married women of reproductive age who are family planning users, and the change in the crude birthrate over the decade of the 1960s. The study documents the importance of both development status and program strength. For example, in countries with high development status, those with strong programs (such as South Korea, Taiwan, Singapore and Hong Kong) show much higher contraceptive use and much sharper birthrate declines than do those with moderate and weak programs (such as Chile, Jamaica and the Philippines). By the same token, of those countries with moderate program strength, those with high development status (such as Chile and Jamaica) show much higher contraceptive use and much sharper birthrate declines than do those with middle and low development status (such as Colombia, Pakistan and India). Hence more than a decade of experience is available to document the proposition that programs directed to economic development and to population growth *are* mutually supportive; there is no empirical warrant for the "either/or" type of argument.

In view of such considerations, the consensus holds that policies and programs are required *both* for general development *and* for specific population

concerns, and that these complementary efforts ought to be components of all international development assistance. Thus population programs are seen to justify the investment of a proportion of the resources available for development, though their requirements tend to be small relative to other development needs. While some critics argue that population programs today are claiming a disproportionate share of such resources, the available data indicate otherwise. Of the $6.15 billion available for official development assistance from 12 developed countries in 1971, only two percent was expended on population activities. Similarly, the 1972–1976 plan of the World Bank calls for about one percent of its available funds to be expended on population programs. Hence the present allocation of development funds to population activities is very small indeed, and even a substantial increase in such allocations would not alter the status of population activities as minor claimants upon international development resources.

VI

The consensus opinion outlined here represents an unlikely amalgam of major elements of at least the following analytically separable positions: Population-Programs-Plus-Development; Accommodationist; Pro-natalist; Holistic Development; Social Justice; Provision of Services; and Human Rights.

It is particularly notable that the consensus position explicitly accepts many of the major propositions of those who argue strongly against separate population programs, but concludes on the basis of the best available evidence that vigorous population programs are nonetheless a necessary component of enlightened development efforts. Thus the consensus seeks to integrate the critical evaluations of current population programs with the principal arguments favoring population programs as part of development efforts. If the consensus position thereby advances the discussion about population issues in both scientific and political terms, it may represent a happy example of a true Hegelian synthesis.

The consensus position asserts that there is no one population policy appropriate for all countries or even for

all developing countries. In such a setting it is of central importance that each government examine its own country's situation in an objective manner and adopt population policies which are consistent with that analysis. This is equally true for developed countries as for developing countries. In this regard it is notable that in recent years explicit policies on population have been most common in the developing countries. Most of the large developing countries have adopted official policies to reduce population growth rates, though the degree of commitment and implementation of these policies varies from high to nil. In developed countries population policies have been less explicitly demographic and are seen as part of general social policy. While concern has been expressed in some developed countries about excessive population growth (particularly in the United States, Great Britain, and the Netherlands), the generally very low fertility levels of developed countries has sometimes led to concern about too little population growth. Some have adopted policies intended to encourage fertility, though none of these policies has been notably successful in the long term. (Ironically the one possible exception is that of the pro-natalist policies of Romania, the site of the World Population Conference.) Most developed countries still are characterized by limitations on the availability of some effective means of fertility control, both pre-conception and post-conception. Such facts make awkward the posture of developed countries urging fertility reduction upon developing countries. Nonetheless, it remains true that fertility in developed countries is everywhere low and generally declining, and the issue of population has been taken seriously enough in 14 developed countries to bring about the establishment of official commissions to study and advise on population policies.[6]

Hence it may be seen that consideration of population policies is increasingly the province of governments, both in developing and developed countries. In all such deliberations, the emphasis must be on the objective and informed nature of the discussion.

Crisis-mongering and doom-saying have no place in such a process; but neither do apathy, self-deception, or suspicion. While there may be no universally applicable population policies, a summary of the several points raised in this paper suggests that there are a number of universal propositions which are appropriate in the development of population policies tailored to each specific situation:

Current population growth as such is not necessarily a problem. It becomes a problem to the extent that it is in conflict with human values. Such conflicts arise if population growth is too rapid to be effectively provided for, or to the extent that growth in a particular situation represents additional population for which resources for a decent and productive life are not available. In some countries it is evident that additional population will be very difficult to accommodate (though such increases are inevitable due to the momentum of population growth). In other countries resources are adequate to provide for substantial further growth, but very rapid growth rates pose serious problems of short- and medium-term accommodation. Such countries would be better served by more moderate growth rates over a longer period.

Great caution must be exercised in accepting (explicitly or implicitly) the European experience as a model for policies on either economic development or fertility reduction in developing countries. Both economic growth and population growth have been far more rapid in the developing countries than in Europe. In the case of economic development there is increasing concern that the capital-intensive European model may be inappropriate for population-rich but capital-poor countries. Similarly, the long lags between economic development and fertility reduction which characterized much of the European experience may be unacceptably long for currently developing countries, especially given their much higher rates of population increase. This is particularly true in view of the sharply reduced opportunities for international migration as a "release valve" for excessive population growth. Hence total reliance upon so-called "natural"

fertility declines following economic and social development may be as unwise for developing countries as would be a total reliance upon "laissez-faire" economic growth patterns. In both areas there is a central role for governments in guiding the process toward ends they view as desirable.

The effects of population policies are characterized by exceptionally long lag-times. This is particularly true in the case of the momentum for further growth of countries which have experienced very rapid growth in recent years. No matter what happens to fertility trends in such countries, all will grow very substantially over the coming decades. The momentum for a population increase on the order of 75 to 125 percent from 1970 levels is already built into the age structure of most developing countries. Even if fertility in these countries were to decline in a few years to the "replacement" levels of the rich countries (obviously a near impossibility), growth of such magnitudes would still occur before equilibrium was reestablished. This means that whatever population policy or program is adopted, all developing countries must plan to accommodate very substantial population increases with adequate food, employment, education, and housing. It also indicates that what may appear to be short-term delays in the onset of fertility decline today will have important multiplier effects in the decades ahead. Finally it demonstrates that, barring catastrophe, countries which could benefit from substantial further growth are virtually assured of it, even if they begin strenuous population programs at once.

Population programs are a necessary but not sufficient component of an enlightened strategy for economic and social development. The accumulated evidence of over two decades of such programs clearly demonstrates that they can have significant effects on fertility if they are effectively implemented. In the first place it is self-evident that no fertility declines can take place in the absence of the means of fertility control; the provision of the most effective fertility control methods through a population program should result in greater realization of motivations to reduce fertility which arise from sources outside the program itself. In addition,

the presence of an effective and visible program can itself serve to increase the motivation to reduce fertility. This is not to say that fertility will not decline in the absence of an effective program. Folk methods of contraception which have moderate effectiveness (such as withdrawal) and illegal abortion are available to highly motivated people of all strata, and modern methods are available through private sources to most of the elite. Nonetheless, it is abundantly clear that enlightened population programs can serve both to encourage such motivations and to maximize their realization, while being fully consistent with basic human rights recognized by all international bodies.

A phenomenon such as continuing rapid population growth, with its long-term momentum and widespread ramifications, requires farsighted statesmanship of uncommon proportion. The need to reject the simplistic "either/or" in favor of vigorous efforts on both the development and population fronts is strongly supported by the best available evidence. Policy-makers may ignore such empirical realities only at their nations' peril.

Notes

1. The pattern of late marriage and non-marriage which characterized industrializing Western Europe is so unusual that it is known as "the European marriage pattern." See John Hajnal, "European marriage patterns in perspective," in *Population in History,* edited by David V. Glass and D. E. C. Eversley, Chicago: Aldine, 1965.

2. John A. Ross, et al., "Findings from family planning research," *Reports on Population/Family Planning,* 12, October 1972, Table 2; Robert J. Lapham and W. Parker Mauldin, "National family planning programs: review and evaluation," *Studies in Family Planning,* 3 (3), March 1972.

3. Bernard Berelson, "An evaluation of the effects of population control programs," in H. B. Parry (ed.), *Population and Its Problems,* Oxford: Oxford University Press, 1974 and *Studies in Family Planning,* 5 (1), January 1974.

4. Development status is classified as high, middle, or low on the basis of three major socioeconomic indicators which are generally considered to be related to motivation for a small family: per capita gross domestic product as an indicator of general standard of living; infant mortality as an indicator of health and general mortality conditions; and female enrollment in formal schooling as an indicator of the level of both popular education and the status of women.

5. Family planning programs are classified as strong, moderate, or weak based upon their coverage of the country's population, the continuity and duration of effort, the vigor with which the program is actually pursued, etc.

6. These are, in alphabetical order: Argentina, Australia, Bulgaria, Canada, Czechoslovakia, France, Greece, Great Britain, Hungary, Israel, Japan, Netherlands, Romania, and the United States.

61

Arthur J. Dyck
Assessing the Population Debate

Reprinted by permission of the publisher from *The Monist,* January, 1977.

Debates over the nature of population problems and the kinds of population policies that are needed to respond to these problems generate a great deal of heat. Deep differences of opinion are not in themselves surprising or disturbing when complex social problems and policies designed to alleviate them are under discussion. However, there is an especially urgent need to analyze population policy debates because of the serious nature of the disagreements that exist and the serious consequences either of choosing the wrong policies or of choosing none.

In this essay, we will seek to describe as clearly as possible significant sources of agreement and disagreement about population policy. This will involve a description of three major groups whose population policy recommendations vie for acceptance: (1) crisis environmentalists, (2) family planners, and (3) developmental distributivists. These three groups represent distinct policy orientations and priorities. The recommendations that are associated with these orientations are not mutually exclusive. For example, family planners may also favor policies being recommended by developmental distributivists. At the same time, there are family planners who are sympathetic to some of the analyses of crisis environmentalists. We are not concerned here with these overlapping allegiances, but rather with how these three distinct orientations within debates concerning population policy shape our understanding of population problems and of what responses to them are morally appropriate. After analyzing these views, we will briefly assess what appear to be the most cogent moral priorities for guiding population policy.

When we speak here of "policy recommendations," we are referring to recommendations that specify a responsible agency, a goal, and appropriate means for its realization.[1] In the population field, one can distinguish between population-influencing policies and population-responsive policies. Population-responsive policies are those that seek to ameliorate problems that arise as a consequence of population growth, population loss, or problems associated with migration. Population-influencing policies are those that seek directly to influence populations to increase or decrease in number and/or to induce changes in location. In this essay our focus is on three different orientations toward what are considered to be population-influencing policies.

No attempt will be made to specify in advance what makes a policy a population policy nor what makes a problem a population problem. Delineations of population policy and population problems are at the very heart of the debates about population policy. As we shall see, each of these major groups under consideration defines population problems and population policies quite differently.

Crisis Environmentalists

There is a group of thinkers who take the view that rapid population growth has already produced a serious crisis for the human species and the planet earth. Sometimes, as in Paul Ehrlich, the emphasis is on resource depletion, pollution, and environmental degradation.[2] Others, like William and Paul Paddock, concentrate more specifically on depletion of food resources and, in 1967, predicted widespread famine in 1975.[3] Garrett Hardin has stressed all of these themes as consequences of rapid population growth.[4] These four thinkers and those who share their viewpoint assume that population growth is likely to continue and even escalate in the absence of explicit governmental constraint or mutually agreed-upon coercion. There is complete agreement that resources needed for the survival of the human species are finite and will be depleted unless population is held at a level that establishes a favorable balance between numbers of people and available resources.

The key empirical assumption that characterizes crisis environmentalists is that as population increases, pollution, resource depletion, and environmental damage increase. Indeed, this group is virtually convinced that the number of people on the earth already exceeds the optimal level. The environmental threats to human survival are exacerbated, therefore, by every increase in the number of people, and the problems associated with these increases may, at any time, become irreversibly lethal because of the finite nature of the earth. Ehrlich expresses this in a

very simple and clear formula: the environment is sick, the disease is overpopulation, the remedy is population control, using coercion as necessary.[5]

It is not immediately evident that population density is the only or the most important factor in bringing about environmental degradation. Why then, the reader may ask, do crisis environmentalists focus on overpopulation as the critical factor in environmental problems, and why also does coercion of a societal or governmental variety appear to be necessary? In Ehrlich's writings, it is assumed that economic interests and pollution on the part of large corporations are more difficult to change or control than individual fertility behavior. Even so, the interest that people take in having children is strong and may require governmental sanctions if birth rates are to be reduced. Kingsley Davis[6] and Garrett Hardin[7] have contended that there is no logical reason to expect individual couples to decide on an average family size that will be congruent with societal expectations or needs. Davis bases his argument largely on the discrepancy between family size desired and achieved on the one hand, and the family size norm necessary for approaching and achieving zero population growth. However, there is an assumption, explicitly articulated by Hardin, that the kind of self-interest that individuals invest in their children is such that the interest of the larger society in children is not and cannot be congruent with those of individuals. Hardin's argument bears scrutiny.

According to Hardin, childbearing can be compared with sheep raising. In his imaginative essay, he has us visualize a small group of sheep herders who share a common plot of ground for grazing. Each sheep herder desires to raise and nurture, for economic reasons, as many sheep as possible. Left to their own choices, individual sheep herders will increase their flocks to the point where the grazing land available will no longer sustain its ever increasing use. To avoid this inevitable outcome, mutually agreed-upon coercion is required. According to Hardin, the desire for children is comparable enough to the desire for more sheep to warrant the claim that

as in the case of the sheep herders, individual couples will only be constrained at the level that societal survival demands by mutually agreed-upon coercion. In a modern state, that means governmental intervention.

As Hardin's argument indicates, crisis environmentalists make the definite anthropological or even quasi-theological assumption that individual interests and societal interests are in a number of critical ways, and certainly in matters of procreation, in conflict with one another. Hence the need for coercion. Furthermore, the appeal to the finitude of the earth and its resources makes it seem self-evident that the moral argument for coercive population policies is justified because the very survival of the human species is at stake. This appeal to an ultimate threat to human life makes it understandable why there is very little discussion of questions of justice and liberty in the literature of crisis environmentalists, and that when there is mention of these moral values, they are easily swallowed up by appeals to the urgent necessity to avert ultimate disaster. The appeal to survival, therefore, is at the heart of the moral justifications that crisis environmentalists offer for coercive population policies. Some of the policies mentioned in this literature include economic incentives,[8] both positive and negative, compulsory abortion in certain cases,[9] triage in matters of food policy,[10] and antifertility chemicals in water supplies.[11]

If one asks what loyalties are shared by crisis environmentalists, deep commitments to the continuation of all animal species and of the ecological systems that support life on this planet are very much in evidence. It is also true that many crisis environmentalists are biologists. (By no means are biologists as such necessarily crisis environmentalists: some are definitely not.) Among other things, there is, therefore, an understandable conception of what kinds of things count as resources to be held precious and irreplaceable. Wilderness and other animal species are often singled out as such. Given these priorities, space becomes virtually as important a problem as environmental degradation by reason of industrial pollutants and the like. Even if consumption and pollution were greatly limited and altered in ways that would conserve resources, the sheer density of population would remain an issue with regard to how much wilderness and plant and animals species are to be preserved.[12] For this reason alone, crisis environmentalists would continue to speak of overpopulation as an immediate threat to the quality of life, if not to the survival of the human species, in spite of progress that does and may occur in pollution abatement and food production.

Family Planners

Although crisis environmentalists have received considerable publicity, certainly in this country, it is family planners who have had the ear of governments in the United States and in numerous countries throughout the world.[13] The family planning movement in the United States has a history that can be traced to the work of Margaret Sanger and others who are founders of the family planning movement in this country, a movement that has been exported all over the world by various planned parenthood organizations.[14] The thinking of family planners is well represented within the Report of the U.S. Commission on Population Growth and the American Future and within the official global policies of the Population Division of the U.S. Agency for International Development.[15] What, then, are the major tenets of family planners and what are their specific objections to the views of crisis environmentalists?

Family planners, like crisis environmentalists, sometimes speak of overpopulation, but more often focus upon unwanted fertility or rapid population growth. They have gathered data in many regions of the world which, on the face of it, lend support for the view that in every country and in most families, parents have children that they do not want; these data also allegedly indicate favorable attitudes toward the use of birth control methods.[16] Family planners have concluded that if governments make birth control methods and the knowledge of their use readily and freely available to everyone, people would have less children.[17]

Sometimes family planners, particularly within the context of the Population Commission Report and the publications of USAID, amass arguments which are specifically designed to persuade people to have small families and to consider them ideal. Hence, such literature discusses the undesirability of large families: the larger the family, the more difficult it is to deal with poverty, to provide education for one's children, to accumulate savings for investments, and to maintain the health of mothers and of the children who might be born. All of these empirical claims argue that it is in the interest of each family to practice family planning and to stay small.

The Population Commission Report and USAID documents also stress the societal interest in curbing rapid population growth and in keeping average family size small. In the words of the Population Commission Report,

There is hardly any social problem confronting this nation whose solution would be easier if our population were larger. . . . After two years of concentrated effort, we have concluded that no substantial benefits would result from continued growth of the nation's population.

The "population problem" is long run and requires long-run responses. It is not a simple problem. . . .

It is a problem which can be interpreted in many ways. It is the pressure of population reaching out to occupy open spaces and bringing with it a deterioration of the environment. It can be viewed as the effect on natural resources of increased numbers of people in search of a higher standard of living. It is the impact of population fluctuations in both growth and distribution upon the orderly provision of public services. It can be seen as the concentration of people in metropolitan areas and depopulation elsewhere, with all that implies for the quality of life in both places. It is the instability over time of proportions of the young, the elderly, and the productive. For the family and the individual, it is the control over one's life with respect to the reproduction of new life—the formal and informal pronatalist pressures of an outmoded tradition, and the disadvantages of and to the children involved.[18]

The Population Commission set zero population growth as a desirable goal for the United States. Despite the alleged seriousness of population-related problems and a goal of zero population growth, however, family planners, unlike crisis environmentalists, do not recommend coercive government policies. On the contrary, they favor complete voluntarism in the form of government investment in free-standing birth control clinics to offer all the available methods of birth control to those who would not otherwise be able to afford them. The Population Commission proposed an expenditure of $1,800,000,000 for the fiscal years 1974–1978 inclusive for that purpose, more than ten times as much as the $150,000,000 it recommended for continuing the governmental provision of maternal and child health clinics.[19] In the light of their research on unwanted fertility, family planners expect individuals to use these governmental services for reducing family size and, hence, population growth in the United States and throughout the world.

There are two additional, significant reasons why family planners do not advocate coercion and why they trust that governmental provision of birth control services will be efficacious to approach zero population growth. The first is that family planners assume that there is no serious conflict between individuals and society, in that couples are expected to have fewer children and so to move in the direction of zero population growth. This strongly held assumption is partially supported by the data collected on unwanted fertility and on favorable attitudes toward the use of birth control methods. The belief that individual interests and societal interests will ultimately harmonize is completely at odds with the assumption of crisis environmentalists that such interests ultimately conflict. This difference provides one important rationale for the tendency of family planners to reject a crisis orientation.

The second reason that family planners disavow coercion is that they put a strong value on freedom. Freedom for family planners largely means absence of governmental constraints. The Population Commission Report, in the chapter on resources and the environment, observes that,

Population growth forces upon us slow but irreversible changes in life style. Imbedded in our traditions as to what constitutes the American way of life is freedom from public regulation —virtually free use of water; access to uncongested; unregulated roadways; freedom to do as we please with what we own; freedom from permits, licenses, fees, red tape, and bureaucrats; and freedom to fish, swim, and camp where and when we will.[20]

In keeping with this view of freedom from regulation, the Population Commission and family planners generally advocate the removal of any existing impediments, including monetary costs, which would hinder anyone from access to abortion, sterilization, and contraceptive services.[21]

Family planners, as their name implies, began historically with a distinct loyalty to families. But increasingly, the family planning movement is focussing on the individual. In the Population Commission Report, it is definitely the individual and not the family whose welfare is of primary concern. The recommendations of the Population Commission to increase government expenditures for making birth control knowledge and methods freely available include specific recommendations to remove all barriers, legal or customary, that would prevent unmarried individuals and minors from receiving these same services. No individual is to be excluded from government subsidized birth control services, including sterilization and abortion, on the basis of age, marital status, or lack of consent from parents or other parties. Whereas, then, family planners used to focus on the welfare of families and the nation states in which they were found, now the focus is on individuals and their nation states. Global concern is present but not emphasized as it is in the crisis environmentalists.

Developmental Distributivists

This group is characterized by its belief that certain kinds of improvements in socioeconomic conditions lead to lower birth rates as observed in the "demographic transition" experienced in Western countries. Although developmental distributivists include individuals and groups with a wide variety of religious and political affiliations, such as Roman Catholicism and Marxism, they are united in their opposition to the way in which crisis environmentalists and family planners depict the relationship between population growth and serious societal problems. The World Plan of Action forged at the Population Conference held at Bucharest in August 1974 largely reflects the thinking and policies of developmental distributivists.[22]

To begin with, developmental distributivists have analyzed the complexity of the relationships between population variables and environmental problems. As Roger Revelle has noted,

More than half of the environmental deterioration in the United States since 1940 . . . has resulted from our growing affluence and changes in consumption patterns—from our increasingly filthy habits. For example, one of the major sources of pollution is the growth of electric power generation from the burning of sulfur-containing coal and oil, which rose about fivefold between 1940 and 1965, while the population was growing by 47 percent. With the per capita power consumption of 1970, . . . our population would have to be reduced to 20 million souls to arrive at the same total power consumption as in 1940.[23]

The point of this analysis is that pollution and affluence grow much faster than the population, and that pollution grows as affluence grows. If, as many population experts assert, decreasing population growth will increase affluence, then decreasing population growth will increase environmental deterioration unless, of course, our present modes of production, consumption, and waste disposal are changed. Developmental distributivists and others have argued, therefore, that our current habits and not population growth by itself are at the heart of those environmental problems that can be considered serious.

How do developmental distributivists view the availability of food and the problem of famine? One of the favorite examples of overpopulation according to crisis environmentalists is the country of India. There is, however, scholarly research on famines in India claiming that in the nineteenth century famines were due to genuine food shortages, but that in the twentieth century, famines are due to distribution problems and to the tendency for the price of food to rise sharply in periods of relative scarcity.[24] In India, as in many economically developing countries, food production is increasing at a greater rate than population.[25] But poor people starve or are malnourished in India, as in other countries, because they do not always have the money or the knowledge to feed themselves properly. For example, a widely practiced feeding habit, withholding solid foods from infants in their first two years of life, is a major cause of infant

mortality.[26] No reduction in population size and no reduction in family size will by itself affect these causes of malnutrition.

Revelle has calculated that it is technically possible to feed up to 38 to 48 billion people in this world, ten to thirteen times the present population.[27] He has also argued that the world has never had so much food and so small a proportion of starving people.[28] This is not to say that he or any other developmental distributivist is contending for a world of 30 to 40 billion people. The point is rather that people starve because of the policies their governments pursue, their poverty, and their lack of knowledge rather than because of a general lack of food or the lack of potential for producing it.

Whereas crisis environmentalists and family planners particularly stress the unfavorable socioeconomic consequences of large families and rapid population growth, developmental distributivists have seen unfavorable socioeconomic conditions as major factors in bringing about large families and rapid population growth. Developmental distributivists take the view that illiteracy, especially of women, high infant mortality rates, extremely unjust distributions of income, lack of governmental social security systems, and underemployment and poor production in agriculture are among some of the most important socioeconomic conditions that contribute to high fertility rates and rapid population growth. These are precisely the causal links stressed in the World Plan of Action adopted at Bucharest.[29]

Developmental distributivists are not arguing that general improvements in socioeconomic conditions as measured by levels of per capita income or per capita GNP will by themselves bring about lower fertility rates. The key to lowering fertility lies in the extensiveness of the distribution of income and of social services. After analyzing considerable data, William Rich concluded that,

Development policies that focus on participation and increased access to benefits for the population as a whole do seem to produce a major impact on family size. In countries which have a relatively equitable distribution of health and education services, and which provide land, credit, and other income opportunities, the cumulative effect of such policies seems to be that the poorest half of the population is vastly better off than it is in countries with equal or higher levels of per capita GNP but poor distribution patterns. The combined effect of such policies has made it possible for some countries to reduce birth rates despite their relatively low levels of national production.[30]

Demographers have long theorized that the change to low birth rates in Western countries (the demographic transition) was associated with low infant mortality rates, high literacy rates, and processes of modernization that included such developments as higher income and better income distribution, improved agriculture, and the provision of social security. Furthermore, there is evidence that the demographic transition that occurred in the more affluent countries of the West will also occur as a result of socioeconomic development in currently less affluent nations. Dudley Kirk's analysis concludes that a growing number of countries are entering a demographic transition at a somewhat faster rate than was true of Western countries.[31] Family planners have cited a number of countries that are experiencing significant declines in birth rates. They attribute these declines to the introduction of family planning programs.[32] Developmental distributivists, however, examining the same data, point out that every one of these countries is experiencing important gains in distributing socioeconomic benefits and that it is precisely under these conditions that people use family planning programs for the purpose of reducing birth rates.

Recently, Michael Teitelbaum has spoken of a new consensus that population policies should combine family planning programs and socioeconomic development.[33] It should be recognized, however, that from the point of view of developmental distributivists, it is not just any kind of socioeconomic development, whether or not it is combined with family planning programs, which will yield lower birth rates. Countries like Brazil and Mexico with much higher per capita income continue to have high birth and growth rates, whereas countries like Sri Lanka and Taiwan have had falling birth and growth rates with considerably lower levels of per capita income.[34] The difference lies in the type of socioeconomic development. Sri Lanka

and Taiwan have raised the employment and income of the very poorest sectors of their societies, and have greatly increased the distribution of income and social services as well. It should be noted also that where we do have controlled studies, family planning programs by themselves have not proved efficacious for lowering birth rates. John Wyon, in a carefully controlled field study conducted in the Punjab area of India from 1953–60, found that although a high proportion of couples could be induced to accept birth control methods, no appreciable change in birth rates resulted.[35] Johns Hopkins University did a similar study in Pakistan for five years with identical results.[36] In the late 1960s, Wyon returned to the same villages in the Punjab which he had studied earlier. Now he found that birth rates were lower. Why? The most visible reason seemed to be that with the coming of the Green Revolution to that area, people there were experiencing higher income, more education, especially for girls, and fewer infant deaths.[37]

Developmental distributivists do agree with the family planners that in procreative matters it is reasonable to expect that the interests of individuals and couples will more or less correspond with the interests of their societies. However, unlike the family planners, developmental distributivists do not expect this to happen by itself or through policies that make all existing birth control methods and birth control information freely available to everyone. From the standpoint of developmental distributivists, the interests of individuals and of their societies can only be expected to harmonize when some reasonable degree of social justice has been realized. Developmental distributivists do not accept a notion of freedom that focusses exclusively on absence of constraint. If people are to be free, they must also have the ability and the means to make choices and to participate in the opportunities available within a given society. Having a small family, for example, makes sense if one can be relatively certain that one's children will have opportunities for health care, education, and future employment.

Social justice as a requisite of population policy is the moral outlook

characteristic of developmental distributivists. Marx, Engels, and subsequent Marxists rejected Malthus and subsequent Malthusians precisely in the name of social justice.[38] At Bucharest, Marxists, Roman Catholics, and the great majority of representatives from various countries found themselves allied against the family planning ideology reflected in the views of the United States and its supporters.[39] What united these groups was the view that social justice in the form of better health care, better income distribution, better status for women, provision for the aged, and the like constitute population policies. What is more, policies that strive to realize justice in these forms are not to be construed simply as responses to problems caused by population growth but are to be seen as policies that help to lower birth rates. It was not surprising, therefore, that crisis environmentalists did not even get a hearing at Bucharest.

Developmental distributivists represent a wide range of loyalties. Roman Catholics and others have a central focus on strengthening familial life. Marxists, of course, have a special interest in the working class. However diverse their other loyalties may be, developmental distributivists have a strong concern for human welfare on a global scale. Nothing less than regard for the fate of the whole human race unites them. All of these loyalties, however, are very much conditioned and shaped by strong national loyalties and interests.

Conclusions: The Vital Role of Moral Values

What do we learn from the analysis of differing views of population problems and policy responses to them? There is no space here to do more than make some brief suggestions as to the direction in which I think the debate over population policy ought to go.

It should be evident that there is no clear agreement as to what are to be considered population-related problems, nor as to how serious these are. There is considerable consensus that environmental degradation is a serious matter, but the solutions to this problem require considerably more than changes in the numbers and concentrations of people. It is not difficult to make the point that the earth cannot sustain an indefinite number of people and that, therefore, there is a hypothetical condition that could be identified as "overpopulation." But there is not agreement as to how societies achieve and maintain zero population growth where this seems to be a reasonable goal for a given society.

To answer this kind of question, it is necessary to initiate and study population-influencing policies designed to solve some problem considered to be population-related. One of the frustrations of the current analyses of family planning programs is that these programs do not, by and large, include sufficient data collection and the use of controls that would assist us in the debates over the successes and failures of these programs. Nor do we have any evidence, even if there were a consensus that serious social ills are population-related, that the kinds of incentive programs and various forms of compulsion being suggested by some crisis environmentalists would actually work if they were adopted. No programs of this sort were recommended or even mentioned in the World Plan of Action forged at Bucharest.

A simple call for more research is not enough in this circumstance. The research most needed, namely controlled studies of population-influencing policies, are precisely under debate, and the evidence as to which of these is most efficacious and most feasible would only be known once a number of them were tried. How, then, does one choose the social experiments that will deal with some of the serious problems that are thought to be population-related? It seems to me that the decision should rest on strictly moral grounds.

At this very point, crisis environmentalists would tend to object. What is characteristic of crisis environmentalists is the view that population-related problems have put us into an immediate crisis and threaten what is surely the most basic moral value on which all of us would agree, namely the value of life itself and the survival of the whole human species. Now I agree that the value of life is fundamental and will assume that readers and the other population orientations share the desire to secure as far as is

humanly possible the survival of the human species. But is it population growth as such that poses an immediate threat to human survival?

Although there is considerable debate about the imminence of serious, even irreversible threats to the ecosphere, it is clear that constraints on our wastefulness and pollution will need to become part of modern industrial life. Scientists contribute to human welfare and survival by documenting these necessities and constraints. However, crisis environmentalists have done us a disservice by giving us simplified, even factually false accounts of the way in which population and environmental variables interact. Indeed, some scientists, like Ehrlich and Ehrlich, have made astounding factual errors in their calculations of strains on our environment.[40] A number of these have been documented by Revelle, such as miscalculations of how long it will take for silt to fill Lake Nasser, misstatements of the need for water in the United States, errors in estimating annual fish production, large overstatements of the existence of DDT in the environment, etc.[41] If biologists and other scientists of the environment are to have credibility with the public, with their peers, and with political decision-makers, they will have to maintain the high standards of science in what is admittedly an area in which values other than truth-telling and precision are creeping to the fore. J. Bronowski states "the scientist's moral" as one which brooks "no distinction between ends and means."[42] He clearly sees this as the practice of scientists and cites with approval this description of scientific practice and morality:

In like manner, if I let myself believe anything on insufficient evidence, there may be no great harm done by the mere belief; it may be true after all, or I may never have occasion to exhibit it in outward acts. But I cannot help doing this great wrong towards Man, that I make myself credulous. The danger to society is not merely that it should believe wrong things, though that is great enough; but that it should become credulous.[43]

Garrett Hardin[44] is another crisis environmentalist who has strained the usual limits of credibility. There is no need in the present essay to repeat and elaborate the very cogent arguments by

Murdoch and Oaten directed against the use by Hardin of the lifeboat metaphor.[45] The crux of the matter is that we are hardly in a lifeboat situation with respect to population-related problems. As Murdoch and Oaten point out, taking a lifeboat stance at this present time for the U.S. would not only be politically detrimental, it would also worsen the current situation of some nations and would actually, so far as our best evidence indicates, contribute to maintaining high birth rates through exacerbating conditions of poverty. It should be noted also that environmental scientists are going to have to become much clearer about whether they really mean to argue as though environmental resources are finite and nonrenewable. Limiting population growth in any given generation is not nearly so important an issue if the basic necessities of human existence are finite and nonrenewable. If we do have enough renewable resources to keep the human species viable for a great number of subsequent generations, then it is of course important to consider our responsibilities over many generations. Furthermore, the exhaustion of certain finite and nonrenewable resources becomes a matter of the loss of a particular pattern of consumption or life-style, and not a matter of life or death for the species where the basic necessities of life are seen as renewable.

Family planners have stressed the value of freedom in the form of absence of constraint. They have collected data that lend credence to the possibility of maintaining voluntarism in population policy. I have no quarrel with this aim and the value that propels it. However, family planning programs and the moral basis on which they are predicated are inadequate.

Consider certain insufficiencies in the moral basis of current family planning policies of the United States. On the face of it, these policies would seem to be beneficial and to some degree, where they meet definite needs, they are. But family planners have not given ample attention to the special conditions associated with poverty which make the free availability of birth control methods something less than a clear benefit. As developmental distributivists have indicated, there are many circumstances under which the poor need children for labor and for security in old age. Also, it is the poor who will lose some of their children through disease and malnutrition. These conditions of poverty are not eliminated by having small families. As one poverty-stricken black mother has eloquently put it:

Even without children my life would still be bad—they're not going to give us what *they* have, the birth control people. They just want us to be a poor version of them only without our children and our faith in God and our tasty fried food, or anything.[46]

It can be argued, therefore, that the provision of birth control techniques and knowledge for the poor without changing their circumstances in any other respect may fail to improve, or may even worsen their situation. Is such a policy, then, a violation of justice?

From a certain utilitarian perspective, one could argue that justice will have been obtained if family planning policies serve to bring about the greatest good for the greatest number, even though some of those who are least well off in the society may not directly benefit. But even if family planning policies were efficacious in lowering birth rates, the fact that for some these policies were disadvantageous could be construed as a violation of the basic principles of justice. As the philosopher John Rawls has argued, the fairness of a policy depends on whether at least in part the implementation of that policy is advantageous to everyone, not simply the greatest number of persons affected by the policy.[47]

Applying Rawls's theory of justice, a policy that seeks to be advantageous for society as a whole through reducing its population growth will only be a just policy to the extent that it is advantageous to every member of that society and not simply advantageous for the greatest number or for the society as a whole. Even if, therefore, the government provision of free-standing birth control clinics to serve the poor, who could not otherwise afford them, were to achieve some social benefit for the majority of a society, it would on this principle be unjust because it is not clearly advantageous to the poor unless something else is done to assure a better life for poor people who reduce their family size. Among the unemployed, where their unemployment is

not eliminated or adequately compensated and there is aid to dependent children, there is no predictable advantage to childlessness. This is exactly one reason why blacks in the United States have seen genocidal overtones in government sponsorship of clinics almost exclusively devoted to birth control. And as we have indicated before, in a number of circumstances, as in subsistence agriculture, children are clearly economic assets, not liabilities, even on economic grounds.

This is not to argue against the provision of family planning services. Maternal and child health clinics in the United States have provided such services and the poor have in this context requested such services. When contraceptive services are accompanied by maternal and child health services, they begin to create the conditions under which the poor see some hope that their children will live and that the government is concerned with their present and future welfare. Contraceptive services without facilities for reducing infant and maternal deaths provide little basis for such a hope, certainly not from the perspective of the poor.

From the standpoint of justice, and also from the standpoint of what appear to be population-related variables, the following types of policies suggested at Bucharest deserve a chance in countries that are concerned about population growth, as well as in countries where these policies have not as yet been implemented to any significant degree:
1. Good health services available to all, including contraceptive services in the context of providing care for the whole family.
2. Literacy and nutritional education, especially for women, where there are inequalities in this respect. (This policy along with the policy above would have the effect of reducing infant and maternal mortality.)
3. Labor-intensive development, particularly in the agricultural sphere.
4. Equality for women.
5. Social security systems that provide for the aged in ways that do not make them dependent upon the survival and prosperity of their children.
6. Improvements in the distribution of income and income earning opportunities.
Each one of these policies is in itself

advantageous to those who are now disadvantaged. Each one of them is also potentially a population-influencing policy in the direction of lowering birth rates. Each and every one of these has its own moral justification, although the specific form this would take is subject to debate and would need to be elaborated. The extent to which any or all of these can be implemented will, of course, depend upon the resources available to any government that seeks to do so.

What I have tried to argue in only a preliminary and suggestive way is that these policies have relevance to what are considered to be population-related issues, and at the same time are ingredients in the realization of social justice by providing advantages to the relatively disadvantaged. There is no decisive evidence that they will or will not work as population policies. There is evidence, however, that the notion of justice implicit in them is one which the large bulk of the world's population clearly understands and endorses.

Notes

1. Ralph B. Potter, *War and Moral Discourse* (John Knox Press, 1969), p. 23. Throughout this essay I am making use of certain descriptive categories developed by Potter and delineated in his book. Each major school of thought, therefore, is examined as to its *empirical* assumptions, *quasi-theological* assumptions, modes of *moral reasoning,* and *loyalties.*

2. Paul Ehrlich, *The Population Bomb* (New York: Ballantine Books, 1968). See also Paul Ehrlich and Anne Ehrlich, *Population, Resources, and Environment: Issues in Human Ecology* (San Francisco: W. H. Freeman, 1970).

3. W. Paddock and P. Paddock, *Famine 1975* (Boston: Little, Brown, 1967).

4. Garrett Hardin, "The Tragedy of the Commons," *Science* 162 (1969), pp. 1243–1248. [Reprinted as Chapter 59 of this volume.]

5. Ehrlich, *The Population Bomb.*

6. Kingsley Davis, "Population Policy: Will Current Programs Succeed?" *Science* 158 (1969), pp. 730–739.

7. Hardin, "The Tragedy of the Commons."

8. Edward Pohlman, "Incentives: Not Ideal, But Necessary," in J. Philip Wogaman (ed.), *The Population Crisis and Moral Responsibility* (Washington, D.C.: Public Affairs Press, 1973), pp. 225–232. For a noncrisis-oriented, careful sorting out of ethical issues raised by incentive policies, see Robert M. Veatch, "Governmental Incentives: Ethical Issues at Stake," pp. 207–224, in the same book.

9. Davis, "Population Policy: Will Current Programs Succeed?," and Ehrlich and Ehrlich, *Population, Resources, and Environment: Issues in Human Ecology.*

10. Paddock and Paddock, *Famine 1975.* See also Wade Greene, "Triage: Who Shall Be Fed? Who Shall Starve?" *New York Times Magazine,* January 9, 1975. This essay cites the Paddocks, Hardin, and Ehrlich, among others.

11. Melvin M. Ketchel, "Fertility Control Agents as a Possible Solution to the World Population Problem," *Perspect. Biol. Med.* 11 (1968), pp. 687–703.

12. See Ralph B. Potter, *The Simple Structure of the Population Debate: The Logic of the Ecology Movement* (Hastings-on-Hudson, New York: Institute of Society, Ethics and the Life Sciences, August, 1971) for a fuller discussion of these issues.

13. Phyllis Tilson Piotrow, *World Population Crisis: The United States Response* (New York: Praeger, 1973). Annually since 1969, the Population Council has published reviews of family planning activities in governments around the world. See, for example, Dorothy Nortman and Ellen Hofstatter, "Population and Family Planning Programs: A Factbook," *Reports on Population/Family Planning,* December 1974.

14. Piotrow, *World Population Crisis: The United States Response.*

15. *Population and the American Future: The Report of the Commission on Population Growth and the American Future* (New York: Signet Books, New American Library, 1972); Philander P. Claxton, Jr., and Marjorie A. Costa, *Statement by the Delegation of the United States of America,* Second Asian Population Conference, Tokyo, November 1–13, 1972; *U.S. Aid to Population/Family Planning in Asia,* Report of a Staff Survey Team to the Committee on Foreign Affairs, U.S. House of Representatives, 93rd Congress, 1st Session, February 25, 1973 (Washington, D.C.: U.S. Government Printing Office, 1973); *United States of America Country Statement,* in response to the United Nations Second Inquiry Among Governments on Population Growth and Development (submitted by the Department of State, June 1973); "United Nations World Population Year and Conference, 1974," draft of pamphlet prepared by U.S. State Department, 1973.

16. There are numerous articles in the various publications of the Population Council, particularly discussions of KAP (Knowledge, Attitudes and Practices) studies that seek to document these contentions. See also *Population and the American Future.*

17. This is what KAP studies purport to show. For a criticism of these studies and the conclusions drawn from them, see Anthony Marino, "K.A.P. Surveys and the Politics of Family Planning," *Concerned Demography* 3(1) (Fall 1971), pp. 36–75.

18. *Population and the American Future,* pp. 1–2.

19. *Population and the American Future,* p. 188.

20. *Population and the American Future,* pp. 72–73.

21. *Population and the American Future,* Chapter 11.

22. The Bucharest World Plan of Action has been reprinted in an appendix to "A Report on Bucharest," *Studies in Family Planning* 5 (12), December 1974 (New York: The Population Council).

23. Roger Revelle, "Paul Ehrlich: New High Priest of Ecocatastrophe," *Family Planning Perspectives* 3 (2), April 1971, p. 68. Revelle has calculated how many people would have been needed in the United States in 1965 to keep pollution levels precisely where they were in 1940:
Other things being equal, the number of automobiles and the amount of gasoline and paper consumed would have remained about constant over the quarter century if our population had declined from 133 million people in 1940 to 67 million in 1965. To maintain a constant flow of sulphur dioxide in the air from electric power plants, the population would have had to decrease to only 40 million people. Presumably the amount of nitrogen fertilizers would not have increased, if all but 17 million Americans had reemigrated to the homes of their ancestors. Only 17 million people in the country would use the same amount of nitrogen in 1965 as we used in 1940. The national parks would have remained as uncrowded in 1965 as they were in 1940 if our population during the interval had gone down from 130 million people in 1940 to 30 million people in 1965, instead of going up to 195 million as, of course, it actually did.
Roger Revelle, (Testimony), *Effects of Population Growth on Natural Resources and the Environment,* Hearings before the Reuss Subcommittee on Conservation and Natural Resources (Washington, D.C.: U.S. Government Printing Office, 1969).

24. B. M. Bhatia, *Famines in India: 1860–1965* (New York: Asia Publishing House, 1967).

25. James Gavan and John Dixon, "The Food Situation in India: A Perspective" (unpublished Essay, Harvard Center for Population Studies, October 1974); see also Roger Revelle, "Food and Population," in *Scientific American,* 231 (3), September 1974.

26. J. B. Wyon and J. E. Gordon, *The Khanna Study* (Cambridge: Harvard University Press, 1971).

27. Roger Revelle, "Food and Population."

28. Roger Revelle, "Paul Ehrlich: New High Priest of Ecocatastrophe."

29. Appendix to "A Report on Bucharest," *Studies in Family Planning.*

30. William Rich, *Smaller Families Through Social and Economic Progress,* Monograph No. 7 of the Overseas Development Council, Washington, D.C., January 1973, p. 37. See also James Kocher, *Rural Development, Income Distribution and Fertility Decline,* an occasional paper of the Population Council (Bridgeport, Conn.: Key Book Service, 1973).

31. Dudley Kirk, "A New Demographic Transition?," in *Rapid Population Growth: Consequences and Policy Implications* (Baltimore: Johns Hopkins Press, 1971), pp. 123–147.

32. Population Council literature contains many such articles. See also R. T. Ravenholt, James W. Brackett, and John Chao, "Family Planning Programs and Fertility Patterns," *Family Planning Programs,* Population Report, Series J, No. 1, August 1973 (Department of Medical and Public Affairs, The George Washington University Medical Center).

33. Michael S. Teitelbaum "Population and Development: Is a Consensus Possible?," *Foreign Affairs,* July 1974, pp. 742–760. [Reprinted as Chapter 60 of this volume.]

34. Rich, *Smaller Families Through Social and Economic Progress;* Kocher, *Rural Development, Income Distribution and Fertility Decline;* William W. Murdoch and Allen Oaten, "Population and Food: Metaphors and the Reality," *BioScience* 25 (1975), pp. 561–567.

35. Wyon and Gordon, *The Khanna Study.*

36. John C. Cobb, Harry M. Roulet, and Paul Harper, "An I.U.D. Field Trial in Lulliani, West Pakistan" (paper presented at the American Public Health Association), October 21, 1965.

37. Wyon and Gordon, *The Khanna Study.* See also Robert Repetto, "The Interaction of Fertility and the Size Distribution of Income" (Research Paper No. 8, Harvard Center for Population Studies, October 1974), and William Rich, *Smaller Families Through Social and Economic Progress.*

38. See, e.g., the discussion of Marx and Marxism in Warren S. Thompson and David T. Lewis, *Population Problems* (New York: McGraw-Hill, 1965), pp. 48–51.

39. Official Roman Catholic affinity for stressing the centrality of social justice as a population policy can best be gleaned from Pope Paul VI's Encyclical, *Populorum Progressio* (Boston: Daughters of St. Paul, 1967).

40. Ehrlich and Ehrlich, *Population, Resources, and Environment: Issues in Human Ecology.*

41. Revelle, "Paul Ehrlich: New High Priest of Ecocatastrophe."

42. J. Bronowski, *Science and Human Values* (New York: Harper & Row, Revised Edition, 1965), p. 65.

43. Bronowski, *Science and Human Values,* p. 66.

44. Garrett Hardin, "The Tragedy of the Commons"; see also "Living on a Lifeboat," *BioScience* 24, 1974, pp. 561–568.

45. Murdoch and Oaten, "Population and Food: Metaphors and the Reality."

46. Robert Coles, *Children of Crisis* (Boston: Atlantic–Little, Brown, 1964), pp. 368–369.

47. John Rawls, *A Theory of Justice* (Cambridge: Harvard University Press, 1971), p. 60.

Genetic Dimensions

62

Marc Lappé

Moral Obligations and the Fallacies of "Genetic Control"

Reprinted with permission of the editor from *Theological Studies,* vol. 33, 1972, pp. 411–427.

Chance Events and the Myth of Genetic Certainty

The sciences of molecular biology and human genetics emerged within my own lifetime. Partly as a consequence of the development of these two sciences, my generation was the first to become swept up in what we now recognize as "The Biological Revolution." What made genetics "revolutionary" is that it was transformed from a science whose content was discernible only by inference, to one which seemingly could be known with certainty: the discovery which made the unknown knowable was made the year I was born.

In 1943, Oswald Avery wrote his brother Roy to describe his findings about a physiological principle which appeared to be able to confer the properties of virulence to a bacterium. The excited tone of his letter reflected the utter incredulity that Avery must have felt upon learning the outcome of his experiments: a *chemical* had made it possible to induce predictable and hereditable changes in living cells. Genes were molecules! As such they were subject to human control and manipulation. Avery wrote: "This is something which has long been the dream of geneticists. . . . [Up until now] the mutations they induced . . . are always unpredictable and random and chance changes."[1]

Although Avery was mistaken in his assumption that this knowledge would allow us generally to control where and when mutations occur, he was correct in concluding that his discovery revolutionized our ability potentially to control what specific genetic information a cell contained or expressed. Thus, when he discovered the molecular basis for a "transforming principle," he simultaneously acquired the ability to effect genetic transformations. The phenomenon by which the acquisition of knowledge per se changes that which has become known (or affords the potential for such change) represents a subtle mechanism by which genetic information (as well as much other knowledge in science) escapes the moral scrutiny of its possessors. Hans Jonas perceptively observed:

Effecting changes in nature as a means and as a result of knowing it are inextricably interlocked, and once this combination is at work it no longer matters whether the pragmatic destination of theory is expressly accepted . . . or not. The very process of attaining knowledge leads through manipulation of the things to be known, and this origin fits of itself the theoretical results of an application whose possibility is irresistible . . . whether or not it was contemplated in the first place.[2]

In Avery's case, he might well have foreseen that transformation could be used to confer virulence to normally nonpathogenic bacteria, but he certainly could not have anticipated that his principle, in conjunction with the later to be discovered "R" factors, would be used to make potent, antibiotic resistant biological warfare agents![3] But the prospect of nefarious application is *not* what makes genetic knowledge unique. Rather, its uniqueness lies in the manner in which "knowing" the genetics of something changes it.

For example, the simple act of acquiring prenatal genetic information about a fetus—whether or not he is carrying a particular gene, or if he will develop a genetically determined disease later in his life—automatically sets into motion a train of events which themselves change that individual's future. At the very moment you acquire a "bit" of genetic information about a fetus (or any person, for that matter), you have begun to define him in entirely novel terms. You tell him (and sometimes others) something about where he came from and who is responsible for what he is now. You project who he may or may not become in the future. You set certain limits on his potential. You say something about what his children will be like, and whether or not he will be encouraged or discouraged to think of himself as a parent. In this way the information you obtain changes both the individual who possesses it, and in turn the future of that information itself.

In addition to the potential for individual stigmatization, there is also sufficient ambiguity in genetic "facts" themselves to seriously question the judiciousness of massive operations designed to ascertain the genetic composition of whole populations. In contrast to the simplistic views of genetics in Avery's time, we now know that genetic information, by its very nature, tends to confound rational analysis. It is *redundant,* such that a flaw in replication or a mutational event need not

irrevocably distort or destroy (as had previously been assumed) the information contained in the genetic material. It is *self-correcting,* containing enzymes whose sole function is to recognize damaged segments of DNA molecules, excise them, and faithfully reconstruct the whole (thereby compelling reconsideration of estimations of mutation rates and their causes). It is *heterogeneous,* with most seemingly "single" genes being in fact clusters of genes with related functions ("pleiotrophy") or products ("alleles," or "pseudalleles"), each gene having the potential property of producing different effects in different organs at different times in development (frustrating any simplistic analysis of whether or not a single gene or many is responsible for a given complex constellation of developmental defects).

These observations begin to explain why at the human level, for example, medical researchers have been at a loss to explain why some individuals who by all measurements have the defective genes for phenylketonuria[4] do *not* in fact show the physical stigmata of the condition. If, as appears likely, this genetic "defect" (and perhaps the one responsible for the related condition galactosemia) is not an "all or none" phenomenon, but can actually be compensated for by the operation of other genes, all of our assumptions about the nature of such genes, *and* our moral decisions of what should be done in the event that an individual is discovered with them, have to be seriously reassessed. The fact that this reassessment is *not* currently going on reflects, I believe, an underlying cultural bias that affects our analyses of genetic problems. It is not just that we want simple answers to complex questions; it is that we would like to be able to *control* a material whose nature eludes our dominion.

Intolerance for Uncertainty and the Quest for Genetic Control

If genetic systems are so inherently difficult to understand, why do we feel impelled to seek to control them? The problem appears to be rooted in our Western psyche and philosophical assumptions about the use of knowledge. Avery's letter gives us a sense of the

deep-seated aversion most Western scientists (and philosophers) feel towards the chance events that appear to govern genetic systems. (Recall Avery's mistaken assumption that he had discovered the means to *control* the class of events we call "random mutations," when in fact he had merely discovered an analogue for one specific mutational event.)

Joseph Fletcher, an ethicist, echoes this profound disquiet towards uncertainty in genetic systems when he states: "We cannot accept the 'invisible hand' of blind chance or random nature in genetics."[5] An implicit assumption in Fletcher's remarks is that the reduction of uncertainty is equivalent to progress, a view widely held in the West.[6] In genetic systems, the paradox is that progress (in this sense evolutionary progress) is accomplished *because of* genetic instability and susceptibility to chance events, not in spite of it.

James Crow, a renowned population geneticist, has described the operation of chance in sexual reproduction by pointing out that "In a sexual population, genotypes are formed and broken up by recombination every generation, and a particular genotype is therefore evanescent: what is transmitted to the next generation is a sample of genes, not a [whole] genotype."[7] It is difficult to reconcile evolutionary progress with this image alone, since Crow omits (by intention, I am sure) discussion of the mechanisms by which variation is introduced into sexual populations. Faced with the reality of incessant fluctuation and change of genetic systems, the Nobel laureate geneticist Joshua Lederberg asked at one point: "If a superior individual . . . is identified, why not copy it directly, rather than suffer all the risks of recombinational disruption, including those of sex? . . . Leave sexual reproduction for experimental purposes; when a suitable type is ascertained, take care to maintain it by clonal propagation."[8]

If from Avery's day scientists believed they had discovered the means to control the transmission of hereditary information, why does Joshua Lederberg believe that the only real means of control for man would be to clone him? The answer in part is that the kinds of control which were possible in bacteria thirty years ago remain an illusive quest for human organisms today. Not only is cloning a distant and limited prospect for man, but so is the much-vaunted genetic engineering which would precede it. Mammalian cells, unlike bacterial ones, appear to be extraordinarily resistant to the introduction of most forms of genetic information. Although reports have appeared indicating that bacterial viral genes will function after being introduced into human cells in tissue culture[9] (a feat proving difficult to replicate), enormous difficulties remain in attempting to use the same techniques actually to treat individuals with the genetic defect that the virus appears to correct. Another technique for correcting "defective genes" also appears to pose currently insuperable problems for human application. It entails fusing or "hybridizing" a cell lacking a particular gene with one containing the active equivalent.[10] This technique may prove to be limited to tissue-culture studies, since the number of cells needed to correct the same defect in a person would be astronomically large and the problem of immunologic acceptance of the cells a thorny one.

While tantalizing in the control that such techniques appear to promise for the future, there is a danger in their seductiveness in the present. In the first place, they obfuscate the need for solving current problems which do not need novel technical solutions, such as general health care. Secondly, they pose the threat of dehumanization that Jacques Ellul identifies with technique per se. Ellul observes that "When technique enters into every area of life, including the human, it ceases to be external to man and becomes his very substance. It is no longer face to face with man but is integrated with him, and it progressively absorbs him."[11] In the context of the above examples, Ellul would envision man's existence becoming dependent upon and inevitably indistinguishable from the vast array of artificially engineered genes and tissue-culture support systems needed to sustain him. More importantly, such techniques do not offer permanent solutions to human problems but merely transiently replace one technique (e.g., insulin for treating diabetes) with another (genetic engineering of Islets of Langerhans cells in the pancreas) for coping with man's medicogenetic dilemmas. Since none

of these projected genetic techniques offer the prospect of the permanent change that can only be accomplished by changing the germ plasm itself, they offer only the illusion of changing man.

The "New" Eugenics and the "Old"

In presenting a scenario of genetically "engineering" man,[12] Lederberg and Fletcher believe that current knowledge of genetics mandates a new eugenics to meet pressing human needs. There are two points to be made about any such proposal: (1) Concern about effecting widespread genetic changes in a population is unwarranted, given existing demographic trends; but (2) the general *motivation* for proposing cloning or other engineering of man must be taken seriously, because it reveals a tacit approval by some of the best minds of the country for both the legitimacy and the need for introducing genetic controls.

To some geneticists, the recrudescence of a social concern for applied human genetics is mandated by an assumed or projected deterioration of the genetic quality of the species. They frankly admit that this concern must be properly construed as a "eugenic" one, but insist that it is based on hard facts. They maintain that their concern is not tainted with the racial connotation that irrational eugenicists had applied in the past. Nevertheless, both the basis for this concern—a progressive "genetic deterioration" of man—and the proposed remedy—a humane form of "genetic counseling" or at an extreme "negative eugenics"—actually are synonymous with the analyses of a hundred years ago.

While Galton is the name usually associated with the "eugenics" movement of the late 1800's, it is actually Darwin whose ideas have endured. Galton described the aim of eugenics[13] (a word he coined) in blatantly racist, class-society terms. Its purpose was "to give the more suitable races or strains of blood a better chance of prevailing speedily over the less suitable [races] than they otherwise would have had."[14] Darwin, not Galton, represented the more representative and "morally enlightened" tone of the eugenics movement:

With savages, the weak in body or mind are soon eliminated; and those that survive commonly exhibit a vigorous state of health. We civilized men, on the other hand, do our utmost to check the process of elimination; we build asylums for the imbecile, the maimed, and the sick; we institute poor-laws; and our medical men exert their utmost skill to save the life of everyone to the last moment. There is reason to believe that vaccination has preserved thousands, who from a weak constitution would formerly have succumbed to small pox. Thus the weak members of civilized society propagate their kind. No one who has attended to the breeding of domestic animals will doubt that this must be highly injurious to the race of man. It is surprising how soon want of care, or care wrongly directed leads to the degeneration of a domesticated race; but excepting in the case of man himself, hardly anyone is so ignorant as to allow his worst animals to breed. . . .

The aid which we feel impelled to give to the helpless is mainly an incidental result of the instinct of sympathy, which was originally acquired as part of the social instincts, but subsequently rendered, in the manner previously indicated, more tender and more widely diffused. Nor could we check our sympathy, even at the urging of hard reason, without deterioration in the noblest part of our nature . . . if we were to neglect the weak and helpless, it could only be for a contingent benefit, with an overwhelming present evil. *We must therefore bear the undoubtedly bad effects of the weak surviving and propagating their kind; but there appears to be at least one check in steady action, namely that the weaker and inferior members of society do not marry so freely as the sound; and this check might be indefinitely increased by the weak in body or mind refraining from marriage, though this is more to be hoped for than expected.*[15]

"Expecting" the weak to refrain from marriage may strike us as a quaint nineteenth-century idea; but it faithfully echoes some contemporary statements of the value of "quasi-coercive" genetic counseling. These are some today who no longer "hope" but "expect" the weak in body and mind to refrain from marriage or its genetic equivalent childbearing. A growing number of people use moral arguments to urge those who are genetically "handicapped" (and this may only mean individuals who *carry* but do not express aberrant genes) to fulfil their social responsibility by refraining from procreation.[16] This moral suasion is mistakenly based on the assumption that genetic deterioration of the species will be the inevitable consequence of the "unbridled" procreation of the unfit.

Moral Obligations in the Face of Genetic Realities

Darwin's focus on the moral dilemmas facing those who think they recognize a genetic basis for human suffering and feel impelled to act on this assumption has a contemporary ring. Theodosius Dobzhansky assessed the eugenic situation in 1961 in this Darwinian tradition: "We are then faced with a dilemma—if we enable the weak and the deformed to live and to propagate their kind, we face the prospect of a genetic twilight; but if we let them die or suffer when we can save them, we face the certainty of a moral twilight. How to escape this dilemma?"[17] Thus ten years ago, the moral problems were not posed in terms of the need for genetic improvement, but rather in terms of the need for societal protection against genetic deterioration. The genetic information which made such an analysis valid thirty or even ten years ago has been substantially amended today.

In the recent past, the chief proponent of the need for eugenic practice was Hermann Muller. In 1959 he stated: "If we fail to act now to eradicate genetic defects, the job of ministering to infirmities would come to consume all the energy that society could muster for it, leaving no surplus for general, cultural purposes."[18] Other, more contemporary authors have voiced similarly concerned if not alarmist views.[19]

While no one can conclusively refute the contention that *sometime* in the future we may have to come to grips with an increased incidence of genetically disabling disorders, it would have been extremely difficult to have made the case, even in 1959, for our moral obligations to act to anticipate them. As Martin Golding, in a review of genetic responsibility to future generations, concluded: "We are thus raising a question about our moral obligation to the community of the remote future. I submit that this relationship is far from clear, certainly less clear than our moral obligations to communities of the present? . . ."[20]

What actually is the "threat" posed

to future generations (or, for that matter, to our very own children) by the specter of genetic deterioration? Golding and others appear to believe that current trends in medical treatment and protection of the "genetically unfit" condemn the future to suffer the weight of our omissions. He states, for example, that "the tragedy of the situation may be that we will have to reckon with the fact that the amelioration of short-term evils . . . and the promotion of good for the remote future are mutually exclusive alternatives."[21]

Part of the fallacy of this form of pessimisim is the assumption that genes and genes alone are the only means by which we project ourselves into the future. Certainly, most anthropologists, when faced with the question of the most important way in which we influence the future, would emphasize the primacy of *cultural* factors in establishing human societies through time, because purely genetic trends are highly uncertain in fluctuating and migrating human populations.

The Fallacy of a Genetic Apocalypse

The other part of the fallacy is the assumption that we actually do face a genetically deteriorating situation. In the ten years since Dobzhansky originally posed the dilemma of a "genetic twilight," we have acquired enough information to enable us to draw back from the vision of a genetic apocalypse. Imminent "genetic deterioration" of the species is, for all intents and purposes, a red herring. The officers of the American Eugenics Society acknowledged this in a six-year report ending in 1970. In spite of the fact that they reaffirmed the long-range objective of the society to pursue the goal of maintaining or improving genetic potentialities of the human species, they stated that "neither present scientific knowledge, current genetic trends, nor social value justify coercive measures as applied to human reproduction." In fact, the officers wrote, "at this stage the need is for better identification of present and potential directions of changes rather than action to alter these trends in any major way."[22]

Our contemporary population is in a unique situation. The "gene pool" is in fact undergoing a period of stabilization, not change. In an analysis of the

demographic trends characterizing the current population in the United States, Dudley Kirk observed that while the tremendous relaxation in the intensity of selection accomplished by modern medical achievements may be inexorably increasing the load of mutations the population carries, the overall demographic trends are such as to reduce the number of children born with serious congenital abnormalities. He summarized his paper in the following way:

A relaxation of selection intensity of the degree and durability now existing among Western and American peoples has surely never before been experienced by man. . . . In the short run, demographic trends (in and of themselves) are reducing the incidence of serious congenital anomalies. . . . In the foreseeable future, the possibility of medical and environmental correction of genetic defects will far outrun the effects of the growing genetic load.[23]

Demographic trends such as lowered average age of childbearing, smaller number of children, and the reduction of consanguineous marriages, *themselves* effect dramatic changes in the quality of life experienced by the next generation. In the thirteen years between 1947 and 1960 when Japan instituted a revolutionary (if misleadingly termed) "Eugenic Protection Law," there was a ⅓ reduction in the number of children born with Mongolism and a ⅒ reduction in aggregate of all of the other major congenital abnormalities. This startling statistic was accomplished simply as a result of introducing legal abortion and encouraging smaller and earlier families.[24] A similar trend may well be expected in Western countries if we act to encourage the same *non*genetic changes in our population. The data on the close relationship between higher maternal ages at birth, number of previous offspring, and the high incidence of such devastating congenital defects as anencephaly[25] and Mongolism make the moral imperative of recommending basic changes in childbearing patterns obvious. It is important to note that this kind of recommendation (for example, proscribing childbearing in women over thirty-five) has a universal basis, unlike proscriptions on individual childbearing for genetic reasons.

Societal vs. Individual Costs of Genetic Disease

Statistics such as these do not, however, tell us what specific moral questions are at stake for the future childbearing of individuals who themselves are born with a genetically determined disorder. Society's interest in this question acquires legitimacy only if it is true that society is paying an increasing social (not just monetary) cost for the offspring of the genetically unfit.

The origin of the notion of "societal cost" is rooted in the assumption that the care extended by society to the "unfit," while morally desirable, cannot be accomplished without heavy burden. It is widely accepted, for example, that medical advances have contributed to our genetic load by permitting individuals who are born with genetically determined disorders to survive to childbearing age. Is this in fact the case? The answer appears to be that *some* advances in medicine may have this effect, but that on the whole medical practice is neither generating a race of Orwellian invalids requiring daily injections of insulin, enzymes, and other crucial but absent substances *nor* is it permitting a critical number of the truly "unfit" to procreate.[26] A key but unique case in point would be retinoblastoma, a treatable eye tumor which until recently was fatal. "Treatment" here is understood to entail enucleation of the eye, with an increased residual risk of cancer elsewhere in the body even if initial surgery is successful. It is undeniable that the survival of individuals who can transmit the dominant mutant gene to their children poses grave moral problems to both the parents and society as a whole. Between 1930 and 1960 in the Netherlands, for example, the frequency of this dread cancer *doubled*, probably as a result of the procreation of survivors carrying the gene.[27] Another cogent example would be the legitimate societal interest in counseling or even in regulating childbearing in mothers with phenylketonuria, where there is grave danger of fetal damage and retardation. The moral issue becomes whether or not such statistics establish society's right to intervene in childbearing decisions by parents known to carry genes directly or indirectly causing grave disability in offspring.

With rare exception there is, in my opinion, no compelling case for societal restrictions on childbearing. I am profoundly disturbed by the advocacy of societal intervention in childbearing decisions for genetic reasons, denial of medical care to the congenitally damaged, or sterilization of those identified as likely to pass on the genetic basis for a constitutional disability. Such an advocacy is implicit in the tone of the following exerpt from a letter in *Science:* "Even elementary biology tells us that hereditary disease or susceptibility to disease which leads to death or diminished reproduction rids a population of genes which perpetuate these maladies. Yet modern medical practice is leading to the accumulation of such genes in the most highly advanced society of man."[28]

This statement, like the one of Darwin's one hundred years ago, miscasts the facts of natural selection in human populations. *The consensus of the best medical and genetic opinion is that whatever genetic deterioration is occurring as a result of decreased natural selection is so slow as to be insignificant when contrasted to "environmental" changes, including those produced by medical innovation.*[29] Even where we have identified a disease in which medical advances can be *shown* to have increased the overall population incidence, as in schizophrenia,[30] few if any competent geneticists would advocate reducing the number of offspring schizophrenic individuals would be permitted to bear. The principal reason is ignorance. We simply do not know what (if any) intellectually desirable attributes are also transmitted with the complex of genes responsible for schizophrenia. Bodmer notes that the conditions which have led to an increase in the frequency of schizophrenia "may also conceivably increase the frequency of some desirable genetic attributes in other individuals."[31]

The variability that we (and geneticists with considerably more perceptivity) "see" in people represents the top of an iceberg of genetic diversity in human populations. Most of the variability which can be found at the genetic level is the result of spontaneous mutations which become fixed in the population. The traditional attitude of

geneticists was that these mutations were in the main "undesirable," and the number of mutations and the extent to which a population as a whole was subjected to them constituted society's genetic load. Dobzhansky has been diligent in pointing out that the original definitions of "genetic load" tended to be spurious because they hypothesized a single "best" genotype, specifically one which was "homozygous" (i.e., having the same genes on each chromosome pair) for all of its genes. In Dobzhansky's estimation, this notion was inconsistent with the fact that the nature of human populations is to have a tremendous proportion of their genomes (perhaps as much as 30%) made up of "heterozygous" genes, and thus, to be consistent, geneticists would have to regard genetic uniformity beneficial and genetic heterogeneity inimical to the fitness of the population.[32]

It now appears that the term "genetic load" must be considered as almost synonymous with "genetic variability" and to be similarly bereft of utility. An appreciable portion of the expressed and even greater portion of the concealed variability that we can recognize in man consists of variants that—in most environments—are to some degree unfavorable to the organism.[33] In spite of the tendency to term this unfavorable, deleterious, ostensibly unadaptive part of the genetic "load" or "burden" of the population, there is little evidence that it is deleterious to the population as a whole to carry so many variant genes. In fact, the opposite appears true. To be consistent, those who favor this definition must regard genetic uniformity as the *summum bonum*, an attitude incompatible with the adaptive value of genetic diversity in nature. (A sophisticated analysis of the concept of genetic load is available.)[34]

While many would concur that the "load" imposed by novel or recurrent mutations should be minimized, the natural load of variant genes carried by a population is the result of forces exerted by natural selection. The "burden" of variant genes is a "load," according to Dobzhansky, only in the sense in which the expenditures a community makes to bring up and to educate its younger members are a "load" on that community. Genetic diversity is in one sense capital for investment in future adaptations. Since genetic variability represents evolutionary capability, it is a load we should be ready and willing to bear.

It is indeed ironic that just as man is coming to realize the value of the immense genetic diversity of his species,[35] he has embarked in a direction which threatens to restrict or curtail that diversity. For example, it would be unfortunate if the move to reduce the frequencies of specific "deleterious" genes through identification of heterozygotes by carrier detection screening resulted in broad sanctions on the very mating combinations (heterozygous x normal) which tend to perpetuate genetic diversity. Even where the deleteriousness of a *specific* gene is unquestionable, as in the case of the Hemoglobin S gene responsible for sickle-cell anemia, and the "diversity value" of maintaining high frequencies of the gene largely unsubstantiated, I believe that it would *still* be morally unacceptable to restrict childbearing by those heterozygotes married to normals. Part of the conceptual problem underlying the focus on heterozygous individuals as those responsible for ladening us with our "genetic load" is the false assumption that this load is in fact imposed on society only by a select few individuals. Hermann Muller professed this view when he stated:

A conscience that is socially oriented in regard to reproduction will lead many of the persons who are loaded with more than the average share of defects . . . to refrain voluntarily from engaging in reproduction to the average extent, while vice versa it will be considered a social service for those more fortunately endowed to reproduce to more than the average extent.[36]

Such a statement raises but fails to answer the profound moral question of how one identifies the "unfortunately" or "fortunately" genetically endowed. Today we realize that *each* individual bears a small but statistically significant number (variously estimated at 3–8) of deleterious genes. The moral attitude best fitted by our knowledge is that *a genetic burden is not something that a population is laden with, it is what a family is laden with*.

We now know that the very definition of the phrase "genetic load" is

fraught with difficulty. As an alternative, Muller would ultimately have preferred to evaluate genetic load in man, as Sewall Wright did, in terms of the balance between the contribution that a carrier of a particular genotype makes to society and his "social cost."[37] Yet even this seemingly enlightened view suffers from the assumption that the worth of a man lies exclusively in his social utility. One quickly gets into the moral dilemma that Robert Gorney proposes when he attempts to assess the relative social worth of mentally defective people on the basis of their mother instincts, or dwarfs on the basis of their "court jestering."[38] Do not individuals have value unto themselves and their own families?

Protecting the Gene Pool or Supporting General Well-Being?

What then are the positions of geneticists themselves on the issue of how genetic knowledge should be used to guide human actions? Virtually all geneticists agree with James Crow that the principal hazard facing the human population stems from the introduction of new mutations through environmental agencies. Thus both James Neel and Joshua Lederberg feel that it is the geneticists' primary obligation to "protect the gene pool against damage." (Presumably, this would mean principally reducing the background levels of radiation and population exposure to mutagens.) However, they differ dramatically in their secondary concerns. Neel emphasizes the importance of stabilizing the gene pool through population control, realizing the genetic potential of the individual, and improving the quality of life through parental choice based on genetic counseling and prenatal diagnosis.[39] In contrast, Lederberg speaks of the crucial need for the detection and "humane containment" of the DNA lesions (sic, mutations) once they are introduced into the gene pool.[40]

There is a profound danger in discussing the need for "containment" or "quarantine," for purportedly genetically "hygienic" reasons, of individuals who by no fault of their own carry genes which place their offspring in jeopardy.[41] The case for society's concern for the genetic welfare of the population and its rights in opposing

sanctions on individuals hinges on the demonstration of a clear and present danger of genetic deterioration, which, as I have indicated, is still forthcoming. Yet, a letter I received from a government official rhetorically equated the potential societal threat of genetic disease with that of a highly contagious bacterial one. An individual carrying a deleterious gene was, according to this analysis, analogous to a "Typhoid Mary." Such an attitude is at best naive, and at worst ominously coercive. To equate a genetic disease with one which can be transmitted from person to person is to fail to recognize the salient different between the two: genetic diseases are transmissible only to offspring of the same family. Contagious diseases not only enjoy a much wider and rapid currency, but also an often fateful degree of anonymity, as in the faceless patrons of Typhoid Mary's restaurant. Only in the case of *genetic* disease do affected siblings and relatives serve as constant reminders of the fate of a subsequent affected child. Those who would argue that legal sanctions are necessary to protect society against genetic disease fail to recognize the basic reality of the deep and enduring bonds that draw a parent to his child. As Montaigne put it, "I have never seen a father who has failed to claim his child, however mangy or hunchbacked he might be. Not that he does not perceive his defect . . . but the fact remains the child is his."[42] A father bearing a heritable disorder himself or having experienced a lifetime of suffering in the genetic disability of his child would be the best judge to make the decision to deny life to his subsequent offspring. I know of no such situation (including retinoblastoma) where the decision to procreate or bear children should be the choice of other than the parents. The moral obligations of parents faced with genetic disease are to conscientiously weigh and act based on the prospects for their *children*, not for society at large. Genetic knowledge does not now justify enjoining any family with the societal obligation to refrain from procreation.

The Peril of a Genetic Imperative

In spite of the weight of evidence which shows that we do not have sufficient information to predict any but the grossest genetic changes following individual or population shifts in childbearing habits, the latent fear remains that to do *nothing* will itself lead to an increase in detrimental genes and thereby compound the genetic problem for future generations.[43] Joshua Lederberg has argued that we are so locked into a genetic double bind that we *should* in fact do nothing. He states:

Our problem is compounded by every humanitarian effort to compensate for a genetic defect, insofar as this shelters the carrier [of the defective gene] from natural selection. So it must be accepted that medicine, even prenatal care which may permit the fragile fetus to survive, already intrudes on the questions of "Who shall live." . . .

It is so difficult to do only good in such matters that we are best off putting our strongest efforts in the prevention of mutation, so as to minimize the heavy moral and other burdens of decision making once the gene pool has been seeded with them.[44]

Certainly, any decision to act or not to act in the face of the dilemmas posed by human genetics is a moral choice. But one does not escape the moral burden of choosing by rationalizing that intrinsic contradictions in relative goods freeze one into inaction.

As Lederberg rightfully observes, the moral contradictions in choices of this sort are never more clearly visible than in the protection of the "fragile" and by inference damaged fetus. In fact, developments in prenatal and postnatal care now make it possible to ensure the survival of infants burdened with spina bifida and meningomyelocoele, spinal abnormalities which were life-limiting before this decade. To the extent that such abnormalities (like cleft palate or harelip) are heritable, there is an ethical question in encouraging the survival and successful procreation of the affected individuals. What is too often ignored in simplistic analyses of this sort is that the increased survival of the defective and deformed is *not* the result of special and sometimes "precious" care of the weak, but rather is usually accomplished as an indirect result of dramatic improvements in health care to *all* infants. As a recent editorial in the British Medical Journal observed, "Indiscriminate lowering of early mortality may impose terrible burdens on the survivors. But for the overwhelming majority of infants, the normal and healthy, there is hope and

increasing evidence that the measures which lower mortality tend to produce a corresponding improvement in the quality of life offered them."[45]

Lederberg's course of nonaction is effectively a course of action, and one which is as morally inacceptable today as bringing newborns to the *Lesch* for sorting and disposal in ancient Sparta. Improvement in prenatal and postnatal care may well encourage the survival of more of those "fragile" and presumably genetically defective fetuses and newborns who would normally succumb, but, as the experience in Britain shows, the cost of that type of action may well be worth paying. Would not mothers in a society which offered the promise of nondiscriminative prenatal and postnatal care feel more secure than one (as in ancient Sparta) in which they knew that their children would be subjected to a test of normalcy? If selective care of only the genetically fit leads to a decrease in the survival of the specific few who are congenitally handicapped, it will be at the cost of a general *increase* in the damage wrought by uterine and early environmental deprivation (e.g., cerebral palsy and mental retardation). That would seem a high price for society to pay for its genetic well-being.

Summary

Our knowledge of genes and genetic systems in man shows them to be too complex to readily lend themselves to controlled manipulation. Deep-seated psychologic needs to reduce uncertainty appear to drive our search for genetic control in spite of this complexity. The need for genetic intervention is today justified on the basis of the same unsubstantiated analysis of "genetic deterioration" that characterized the eugenics movement in the late nineteenth century. The notion of a genetic "burden" imposed on society by individuals carrying deleterious variant genes is a misleading concept: the "burden" of deleterious genes is borne by families, not society. Decisions to have or not have children are best made by parents who have experienced genetic disease in their own families, not by society. Society's obligation is to provide universal maternal and postnatal care, even at the cost of survival of the congenitally handicapped. To do less is both to deprive the healthy of the optimum conditions for their development and to jeopardize the moral tone of society itself.

Notes

1. Letter from Oswald Avery to Roy Avery, May 17, 1943, in *Readings in Heredity*, ed. John A. Moore (New York: Oxford Univ. Press, 1972) pp. 249–51.

2. Hans Jonas. *The Phenomenon of Life* (New York: Harper & Row, 1966) p. 205.

3. See Marc Lappé, "Biological Warfare," in *Social Responsibility of the Scientist*, ed. Martin Brown (Berkeley: Free Press, 1970).

4. A condition resulting from an enzymatic defect in the ability to metabolize phenylalanine which is usually associated with mental retardation.

5. Joseph Fletcher, "Ethical Aspects of Genetic Controls," *New England Journal of Medicine* 285 (1971) 776–83. [Reprinted as Chapter 65 of this volume.]

6. See the discussion by Carl Jung in the Introduction to the *I Ching*, tr. Richard Wilhelm (Princeton: Bollingen Series XIX, 1967) p. xix, where he begins: "An incalculable amount of human effort is directed to combating the nuisance and danger represented by chance. . . ."

7. J. F. Crow, "Rates of Genetic Changes under Selection," *Proc. National Academy of Sciences* 59 (1968) 655–61.

8. J. Lederberg, "Experimental Genetics and Human Evolution," *American Naturalist* 100 (1966) 519–26. (Clonal propagation means using the nucleus of a single cell to propagate a whole organism genetically identical with it.)

9. Carl R. Merril, Mark R. Geier, and John Petricciani, "Bacterial Virus Gene Expression in a Human Cell," *Nature* 233 (1971) 398–400.

10. A. G. Schwartz, P. R. Cook, and Henry Harris, "Correction of a Genetic Defect in a Mammalian Cell," *Nature New Biology* 230 (1971) 5–7.

11. Jacques Ellul, *The Technological Society* (New York: Vintage, 1964) p. 11.

12. See J. Lederberg, "Unpredictable Variety Still Rules Human Reproduction," *Washington Post*, Sept. 30, 1967.

13. Eugenics is defined as "an applied science that seeks to maintain or improve the genetic potentialities of the human species" (Gordon Allen, in *International Encyclopedia of the Social Sciences* 5 [1968] 193).

14. Francis Galton, *Hereditary Genius* (London, 1870).

15. Charles Darwin, *The Descent of Man and Selection in Relation to Sex* (1871; New York: Random House Modern Library Edition) pp. 501–2 (italics mine).

16. See in particular Fletcher, *art. cit.*, and Bentley Glass's letter in reply to Leon R. Kass, *Science*, Jan. 8, 1971, p. 23.

17. Theodosius Dobzhansky, "Man and Natural Selection," *American Scientist* 49 (1961) 285–99.

18. H. J. Muller, "The Guidance of Human Evolution," *Perspectives in Biology and Medicine* 1 (1959) 590.

19. W. T. Vukovich, "The Dawning of the Brave New World—Legal, Ethical and Social Issues of Eugenics," *Univ. of Illinois Law Forum* 2 (1971) 189–231; B. Glass, "Human Heredity and Ethical Problems," *Perspectives in Biology and Medicine* 15 (1972) 237–53: R. Gorney, "The New Biology and the Future of Man," *UCLA Law Review* 15 (1968) 273–356.

20. M. Golding, "Our Obligations to Future Generations," *UCLA Law Review* 15 (1968) 443–79.

21. *Ibid.*, p. 463.

22. T. Dobzhansky, D. Kirk, O. D. Duncan, and C. Bajema, *The American Eugenics Society, Inc. Six Year Report, 1965–1970* (published by the Society, New York).

23. Dudley Kirk, "Patterns of Survival and Reproduction in the United States," *Proc. Nat. Acad. Sci.* 59 (1968) 662–70.

24. *Ibid.*

25. Jean Frederick, "Anencephalus: Variation with Maternal Age, Parity, Social Class and Region in England, Scotland, and Wales," *Ann. Human Genetics* (London) 34 (1970) 31–38.

26. Peter Brian Medawar, "Do Advances in Medicine Lead to Genetic Deterioration?" *Mayo Clinic Proceedings* 40 (1965) 23–33.

27. Anonymous, "The Changing Pattern of Retinoblastoma," *Lancet* 2 (1971) 1016–17.

28. "Biological Unsoundness of Modern Medical Practice," *Science* 165 (1969) 1313.

29. James V. Neel, "Lessons from a 'Primitive' People," *Science* 170 (1970) 815–22. See also John R. G. Turner, "How Does Treating Congenital Disease Affect the Genetic Load?" *Eugenics Quarterly*, 1968, pp. 191–96.

30. Walter F. Bodmer, "Demographic Approaches to the Measurement of Differential Selection in Human Populations," *Proc. Nat. Acad. Sci.* 59 (1968) 690–99.

31. *Ibid.*, p. 699.

32. T. Dobzhansky, *Genetics and the Evolutionary Process* (New York: Columbia Univ. Press, 1970) p. 191.

33. Heterozygotes carrying a single dose of a recessive variant gene which is deleterious in the homozygous form are—contrary to popular belief—on the average *less* fit than the person who has both "normal" genes. The sickle-cell heterozygote, for example, is *only* at an advantage in malarial regions, having statistically less fitness than the normal in nonmalarial regions.

34. Bruce Wallace, *Genetic Load: Its Biological and Conceptual Aspects* (Englewood Cliffs, N.J.: Prentice-Hall, 1970).

35. L. C. Dunn, "The Study of Genetics in Man—Retrospect and Prospect," *Birth Defects Original Article Series* (The National Foundation, 1965).

36. H. J. Muller, "The Guidance of Human Evolution," *Perspectives in Biology and Medicine,* 1959, p. 590.

37. Dobzhansky, *Genetics and the Evolutionary Process,* p. 191.

38. Gorney, "The New Biology," pp. 308–9.

39. Neel, "Lessons from a Primitive People."

40. Joshua Lederberg, "The Amelioration of Genetic Defect—A Case Study in the Application of Biological Technology," *Dimensions* 5 (1971) 13–51.

41. Margery Shaw, "*De jure* and *de facto* Restrictions on Genetic Counseling," *Proceedings of the Airlie House Conference on "Ethical Issues in the Application of Human Genetic Knowledge,"* Oct. 10–14, 1971 (Plenum Press, in preparation).

42. Michel de Montaigne, "On the Education of Children," *Selected Essays,* tr. D. M. Frame (New York: Van Nostrand, 1943) chap. 26, p. 5.

43. Bentley Glass, reply to Leon R. Kass.

44. Lederberg, "The Amelioration of Genetic Defect," p. 15.

45. Anonymous, "Early Deaths," *British Medical Journal,* 1971, pp. 315–16.

63

John Fletcher

The Brink: The Parent-Child Bond in the Genetic Revolution

Reprinted with permission of the editor from *Theological Studies,* vol. 33, 1972, pp. 457–485.

New discoveries in human biology have already begun to affect the way parents, with their physicians and genetic counsellors, make decisions about parenthood and childbearing. While a storm of debate swirls about the morality of futuristic proposals[1] for making "better" babies—in the genetic sense—some members of the first generation of parents in history are already crossing a borderline of decision-making, venturing out to use the knowledge obtainable from prenatal diagnosis of genetic disease in their unborn children. I refer specifically to the parents who enter genetic clinics and receive the technique of amniocentesis, which will be described fully below.[2] The first stage of genetic medicine is already being institutionalized, insofar as amniocentesis for diagnostic purposes is no longer considered as "experimental," and a number of genetic clinics with supporting counselling units have been in operation for several years. James Sorenson has recently published the first results of his exploratory studies of the sociological factors which influence parents and genetic counsellors.[3] The point I want to make in this introduction is that whereas genetic counselling has been primarily a verbal transaction based upon the analysis of pedigrees and the risks following the birth of genetically handicapped children, parents have begun to enlist in significant numbers as patients under the care of physicians who use more precise methods for detecting disease or abnormalities in the unborn fetus. The first installment of genetic medicine is upon us. Very grave ethical questions, made sharper by the availability of reliable knowledge, press in upon these parents and their advisers in ways for which the traditions of parenthood and the morality surrounding it are not totally prepared.

The purpose of this article is an analysis of the ethical issues involved in the relations of parents to their children, born and unborn, when parents are involved in prenatal diagnosis and genetic counselling. I will use as my primary data interviews with twenty-five couples who received this test in a genetic counselling center in Washington, D.C.[4]

The argument which I advance through the article, on the basis of my experience with these couples and in the light of my own moral analysis, is that when prenatal diagnosis reveals a severe and untreatable genetic abnormality, some parents may responsibly (though not necessarily) elect to abort the fetus with the view either to attempt once more to bear a less handicapped child or to cease childbearing altogether. A hypothesis is advanced which needs much more testing, namely, that the experience of parents in prenatal diagnosis and genetic counselling does not lessen the affection they bear for their children, already born or to be born, even though that relationship is permanently altered by the character of the experience of genetic counselling and amniocentesis. The effects of amniocentesis and genetic counselling on public social policy should be held, in the eyes of legislators, physicians, and parents, as an interim and temporary measure, affording them some space in the long-range task of discovering treatment to genetic disease *in utero.* This view, in my opinion, is fundamentally compatible with the central values guiding the way the relation between family life and the progress of biomedical science should be regulated. At the same time, great care should be taken in the counselling of parents and in the public support of biomedical science to assure that treatment, not abortion, of genetically handicapped children is our ultimate goal.

Parents in Genetic Counselling

My primary interest in research is the dependency relationship in all of its forms, especially where the dependent person relates to an "expert" who controls highly significant or risk-laden knowledge, technique, or processes. On the basis of an investigation into the morality of informed consent in human experimentation,[5] and due to the great interest generated by the application of amniocentesis to prenatal genetic diagnosis, it seemed mandatory to initiate an action-research project to investigate the moral problems actually experienced by parents who seek genetic counselling supported by amniocentesis.

Withdrawal of amniotic fluid from a pregnant woman, for therapeutic purposes, has been practiced in medicine for over a century.[6] The use of amniotic fluid for diagnostic purposes relating to Rh-factor was first done by Bevis in 1952.[7] Fuchs was the first physician to withdraw amniotic fluid for purposes of examination of sex chromatin in the nuclei of cells in the fluid.[8] In cases of sex-linked genetic disease, Fuchs and his colleagues were able to identify fetuses at risk and inform the parents. Since 1965, much progress has been made in improving the technique of karyotyping the cells of the fetus which float in amniotic fluid, for the purpose of diagnosis of genetic disease. The cells can be cultured and pictures taken of the arrangement of chromosomes for the inspection of physicians and genetic counsellors. The pregnancies for which amniocentesis is applicable are (1) patients who are definite carriers of a chromosomal translocation which results in repetition of multiple chromosomal anomalies, e.g., Down's Syndrome, (2) carriers of a Mendelian gene for which a reliable heterozygote test is available, (3) patients who have had significant exposure to radiation or virus infections, (4) patients with a poor reproductive history of recurrent fetal anomalies and early abortion.[9] Thus, parents who have had one child with Down's Syndrome, Tay-Sachs disease, or Lesch-Nyhan Syndrome, plus many other genetic diseases, upon becoming pregnant the second or third time, enter genetic counselling and receive amniocentesis. Between the fourteenth and eighteenth week of pregnancy, when a fetal heartbeat is detected, amniotic fluid is extracted by needle-puncture, analyzed, and diagnosed. Parents who, through tests, are determined to be carriers of such genetic diseases can also receive amniocentesis during their first pregnancy.

A study was designed to develop hypotheses about the structure of moral problems of parents in one genetics counselling unit. I interviewed a series of twenty-five couples and the counsellor at crucial points in the counselling process: (1) after their meeting with the counsellor, (2) with the counsellor after the initial counselling session, (3) with the couple after the report on the results of amniocentesis, (4) with the couple following birth or abortion. In addition to these interviews in the immediate process, a follow-up interview was conducted six months to one year after birth or abortion in order to identify their central perceptions and feelings as parents. The results of these latter interviews are most pertinent to the substance of this article, although the previous interviews form an introduction to a discussion of the morality of prenatal diagnosis and its relation to the ethics of parenthood.

For the purposes of this study, a "moral problem" was defined within the framework of two types of human conflicts. The first is when a person or group is perceived by others to be in fundamental violation of responsibilities to the welfare of a significant human community. The important feature of this situation is that the moral problem is defined in collective terms. The collective poses the question of basic loyalty to the decision-maker. "Are you with us or against us on this matter?"[10] A Catholic mother who decided on abortion of a genetically defective fetus would be judged by the norms of a significant segment of the Catholic community, whether she felt guilty or not.

The second situation finds a person confronting sharply conflicting responsibilities, divided within himself, and making a decision which expresses the conflict. This situation has been described as the "conflict of rule situation."[11] For example, some genetic counsellors allow couples to believe that each contributes to a particular genetic disease, when in fact one is the carrier. Robert Murray reported a case involving his response to possible non-paternity in a couple seeking genetic counselling for sickle-cell anemia. He commented that "it was explained to them that an egg from the mother containing a sickle cell gene was fertilized by a sperm in which a fresh mutation also producing a sickle cell gene had occurred. It was *not* pointed out that mutations are extremely rare."[12] Caught between a concern for the marriage and a concern to give accurate information, the counsellor may be untruthful and hence suffer some remorse. The most intense moral suffering may occur when these two situations firmly coalesce into one. Most "everyday" moral problems are situations which have elements of demands of collectively defined loyalty and the individuals who are objects of these demands confronting decisions which express conflicts of loyalty. This definition of a moral problem guided our study of parents in genetic counselling. What the patient, couple, or counsellor said about the experience of violating standing in a significant community or an inner conflict of loyalties was the datum to be studied in collecting data for the moral problems of these parents in genetic counselling. A full discussion of the significance of these problems for the ethics of human parenthood will follow my report.

The results of our study with this small sample of parents showed three major periods or phases of decision-making within which "clusters" of problems collected: (1) motivation to seek genetic counselling and a decision about amniocentesis, (2) decision following amniocentesis and learning the results of the diagnosis, (3) postabortion, sterilization, or postbirth decisions. The diagram (Figure 63-1) outlines these phases. On the first line are listed the major events prior to, in, and after the genetic-counselling relationship. On the second line are listed the major moral problems experienced by parents and the genetic counsellor within the time frame of the events on the first line.

Phase 1: Decision about Amniocentesis

The twenty-five couples' experience confirms many research findings about genetic counselling. At certain important points, however, their experience was divergent. All of the couples interviewed were expecting a new baby. All but one of the couples were from the middle class or above, and the majority had graduated from a four-year college. Twenty-four couples were white (Sorenson, 1971 [see note 3]).

The religious affiliation of the couples broke down as follows:

Protestant (both)	11
Jewish (both)	4
Catholic (both)	2
Mixed religious marriages	5
No religious affiliation	3
	25

Thirteen couples came to the unit due to a previously defective child and were now pregnant again. Ten couples were motivated by the "age factor" and its relation to occurrence of

Figure 63-1.
Structure of Moral Problems of Parents in Genetic Counselling

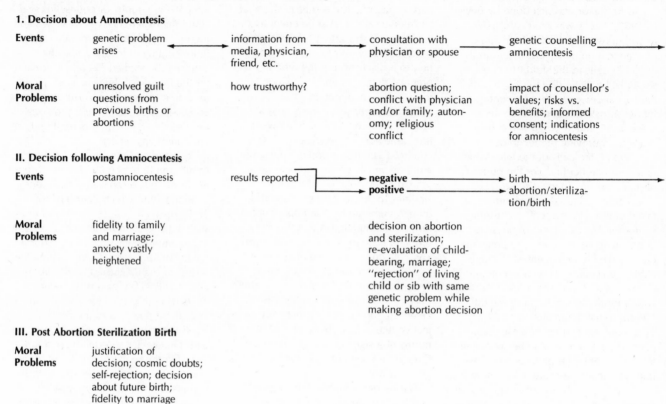

1. Decision about Amniocentesis

Events	genetic problem arises	information from media, physician, friend, etc.	consultation with physician or spouse	genetic counselling amniocentesis
Moral Problems	unresolved guilt questions from previous births or abortions	how trustworthy?	abortion question; conflict with physician and/or family; autonomy; religious conflict	impact of counsellor's values; risks vs. benefits; informed consent; indications for amniocentesis

II. Decision following Amniocentesis

Events	postamniocentesis	results reported	→ negative ——— birth ——— → positive ——— abortion/sterilization/birth
Moral Problems	fidelity to family and marriage; anxiety vastly heightened		decision on abortion and sterilization; re-evaluation of child-bearing, marriage; "rejection" of living child or sib with same genetic problem while making abortion decision

III. Post Abortion Sterilization Birth

Moral Problems	justification of decision; cosmic doubts; self-rejection; decision about future birth; fidelity to marriage

Down's Syndrome. These latter couples discovered the risk ratio largely through reading or the media. One couple sought counselling due to a sibling or twin who had a defective child; one requested counselling because her three brothers had a genetic disease, muscular dystrophy. Recent research done at Princeton on motivation for genetic counselling showed that 80 percent of all cases are parents with a defective child.[13]

More than half of the couples (14) were self-referred to the center. Within this group four couples were "repeaters," having had amniocentesis previously in this center. Three of the four repeating couples had chosen abortion following positive diagnoses of Lesch-Nyhan Syndrome, Patau Syndrome, and sex factor related to muscular dystrophy. Twenty-two fetuses were negatively diagnosed and twenty-two normal babies have now been delivered. Eleven couples had been referred by either a gynecologist or through a program for parents of retarded children.

Unresolved Guilt Parents with one defective child were quick to express their reasons for seeking counselling and amniocentesis when asked. Since the defect had been, for the most part, a shock to them, many acknowledged that though they had learned to live with it, the effect had not worn off. There is often an unusual sense of shame and guilt associated with genetic disease which I came to call a "cosmic guilt." Other investigators have documented this particular form of guilt or sorrow.[14] Having no previous choice over being parents of a defective child, several parents voiced their gratitude at finally being able to do something about the new pregnancy. The sense of being isolated from the community of the "normal," evident in illness generally, is much more in evidence in these particular parents. "I don't know why fate singled me out, but it did," said one mother. The great expense and personal difficulty in adjusting to a defective child was often mentioned. Parents bring their previous problems to the counselling situation in expectation of

the relief of information and the partial freedom that it brings. The relief may stem from a sense of having conquered in part the previously arbitrary fate assigned to them as carriers.

The couples, especially the wives, who were "repeaters" with earlier abortions still bore vivid memories of their disappointment and sense of failure. Later interviews with these couples underlined their need for support and counselling at the time of therapeutic abortion and the deep depression suffered at the time. Each declared an intention to make this "the last time."

Conflicts with Physicians or Family Members In five cases, serious conflicts with obstetrician-gynecologists or with family members had preceded their entering genetic counselling. In the couples' opinion, the physicians had been motivated by either a religious objection to the option of abortion or by a poor opinion of the indication for amniocentesis. One 40-year-old mother of three reported that when she consulted her obstetrician about her intention to seek amniocentesis because of her age, he informed her that her "mental, not physical, health needs attention," and strongly advised her against this course of action. As he had delivered her three children, she felt his words deeply, and she showed considerable ambivalence in counselling. A 26-year-old Catholic mother, carrier of Lesch-Nyhan Syndrome, with one affected child, said that the physician she first consulted "as much as called me a murderer when I said that I wanted a test." Another couple reported opposition from their physician because he thought this an "expensive, unnecessary gimmick which some people are using to build up their reputation."

In twenty-five interviews I detected no substantial disagreement between spouses as to the justifications for seeking help in prenatal diagnosis. Two women told of arguing with family members who strongly disapproved of their actions. One told of her mother-in-law, who herself had given birth to a defective child and kept him at home, attempting to shame her for "taking the easy way out." To the casual observer such conflicts may seem easily dismissed as projection and "sour grapes"; to those who are on the receiving end of them, however, they assume serious proportions. Such is especially true of conflict with physicians.

Prior Consent to Abortion When asked, each of the twenty-five couples answered that they were agreeable to abortion, if indicated by diagnosis, as a morally acceptable means of managing a genetic problem. Judging by content analysis of tapes and notes, the abortion question was the *prevailing moral problem* faced by these parents during the process. More time, energy, and reasoning were expended on explaining their positions on this issue than on their reasons for seeking counselling. Why is this so? My hypothesis is that (a) the structure of the situation calls for a readiness to be committed to abortion as the means of managing a positive diagnosis; (b) being parents strongly motivated to have children and to go to extraordinary lengths to exercise responsible parenthood, these parents are "sensitized" to the abortion

question in considerably more depth than other parents. Therefore, wanting another child (sometimes desperately) and being explicitly committed to abortion constitutes a tension of severely conflicting loyalties and is perceived as a moral problem. Some parents showed signs of what I came to call "moral suffering" of the highest order as they struggled with their conflicts, duties, and changing perception of parenthood. I shall define moral suffering more precisely and discuss it fully in the second major section of this paper.

In this genetics-counselling center the policy was *not* to elicit a firm commitment of the couple to abortion as a prior condition for undergoing amniocentesis. Here we note a difference from what has been reported as the prevailing practice by counsellors and physicians.[15] Such an opinion was emphatically offered by Littlefield when he stated: "Of course amniocentesis should not be undertaken unless the family is committed to subsequent intervention if appropriate."[16] Fuchs, a pioneer in the field, takes the precommitment position because of the risk factor in amniocentesis:

It is virtually impossible to give a reliable estimate of the risks to fetus and mother. The risk of abortion due to infection or trauma may be of the order of one to two percent. It is certainly large enough to contra-indicate amniocentesis in cases where the risk of a particular genetic disorder is less than two percent. In addition, it is certainly large enough to contra-indicate the procedure if the patient and her physician are not prepared to interrupt the pregnancy if a positive diagnosis of a particular disease is made. While it is the experience of several investigators that a patient may change her mind between the amniocentesis and the completion of the fluid analysis, it is imperative that the problems and the risks be thoroughly discussed before the amniocentesis and that a firm decision is made to interrupt the pregnancy if the suspected disorder is proven by the amniotic fluid examination.[17]

As the counselling relationship unfolded, the couples' opinion on the acceptability of abortion was usually revealed, but the counsellor was careful to point out that only the facts were relevant to the decision and deciding on subsequent action should be postponed until after the final report.

The guiding motives for abortion in these parents were largely between the "on demand" and "never" extremes. They explained their own views most often in terms of sufficient reasons for abortion: serious genetic defects, among other reasons (rape, incest, injury to mother), justified abortion. There were many echoes of the theme struck by one mother: "I am nervous about abortion solely for psychiatric or economic reasons, but if my child is seriously affected. I would agree to it."

The parents were almost universally serious about the moral responsibility in being willing to opt for abortion. A father put it: "We have discussed it at length . . . we only want an abortion if we have to for medical reasons . . . it is not an easy decision to make, since you are talking about a life. It is a moral issue." Only one couple approved "abortion on demand." Only one couple gave evidence of coming to genetic counselling on the pretext of having genetic problems but wishing for an abortion of an unwanted child. This couple was not accepted for amniocentesis.

The "moderate" position on abortion held by the great majority of these parents probably stems from their *parental* values as modified by the success of the technique of amniocentesis. They deeply desire children, but they are willing to allow an intervention to test for genetic defects and to act on the consequences. As a mother said, "These days you have a choice about having a healthy baby." While this statement is not exactly true, it reveals a willingness to employ the *technical* utility of prenatal diagnosis while holding firmly to a yearning for children. As the first generation of parents who have had an informed choice about abortion for genetic reasons, as indicated by amniocentesis, they did not consciously suppress affection for the fetus or deny that there was a human life at stake. "When the baby is inside you, you start loving it," said a mother carrying Lesch-Nyhan Syndrome. "When you feel movement, you feel ashamed about contemplating abortion," said another mother. These statements indicate a deep moral problem perceived while in the process of amniocentesis. Follow-up interviews after birth showed even deeper reflections on this problem later. These will be reported in a separate section. Caught between a loyalty to the life of their child and a loyalty to the norm of "healthy" life (as expressed in children with no severe or handicapping genetic defects), there was considerable suffering expressed. It is my hypothesis that the forces assisting these parents in justifying their decision to accept abortions were (1) experience with genetically defective children which led them to believe that the child's life would be unfulfilled, and (2) belief in the values of health and intelligence which their life-style requires for a sense of adequacy and success. Given the choice of accepting a genetically defective child or resorting to abortion, and being informed by their own largely middle-class values, they would choose the latter, even though they suffered from the thought of being responsible for ending the life of their child. Our culture and its preferences tend to reinforce each belief of these parents.

Reasons for Seeking Genetic Counselling In seeking to identify the deeper reasons, a pattern of justification, for the need for genetic counselling, the parents most often offered an argument based on their understanding of parental responsibility to provide for the health of their children and the security of their families. The same mother who spoke of her resistance to abortion for strictly economic or psychiatric reasons said: "It is not fair to it [the child], to the family, to society, or to me to bring another child like the one I have into the world." The concept of "fairness" was often used for justification. Parents with one defective child reasoned from their experiences of psychic and economic loss most often to reflect on their responsibility. The important note in their reasoning was that they included genetic concern as part of parental responsibility. None of these parents could be described as proactive eugenicists, and only a tiny fraction reasoned solely on the basis of individual convenience. In extended conversation about the underlying justification for genetic counselling, it became readily apparent that population problems, genetic responsibility, and parental values were interwoven in the social ethics of the majority of couples. For example, a Catholic father said: "We have an obligation to our children before they are born; you can't turn your back on the future." Another

father said: "I couldn't go through it again . . . it is not doing anything for the child or for society just to be born so sickly . . . it will not make society better for it to happen again."

Several parents, but not a majority, mentioned the concept of a "right to good mental life." In a discussion with one father about this concept, he said that "everyone has a right to live, but each should have a right to a good life, mentally." When I pressed him to try to take the concept to some logical conclusions as applied to society or individual cases, he admitted that he would not want to have rigid standards about "intelligence" or "mental ability" used in screening who would be born. Given the choice, however, between having a child as retarded as his own and abortion, he would choose the latter. He realized that if the majority of people reasoned in a similar manner about all children, a "tyranny of the majority" could develop, aided by an exclusive value on "intelligence" and having little tolerance for weakness or sickness. He made a distinction between those whose mental potential had been drastically destroyed by genetic disease and those who did not have this particular problem, saying that abortion ought only be available on proof of the former. "Medical reasons for genetic betterment are safer than social reasons," he declared.

Parents who sought genetic counselling because of the "age factor" cited social and economic reasons for their inquiry, just as did parents who had defective children. "I have two children and did not intend to get pregnant again," said a 42-year-old mother, "and I must do everything possible to see that my child is healthy. The world has enough problems, I don't want to add to them."

Autonomy Throughout the counselling process, in all three of its phases, these couples showed a consistent reliance on their own authority in decision-making. Only two couples had consulted a nonmedical person for advice, and these advisers were personal friends, not a clergyman, counsellor, or lawyer. Even though the majority perceived moral conflicts in the process of making up their minds, there was no

sufficient cause for official moral "counsel," since they considered their own parental roles the primary source of moral authority for childbearing and family matters. As the previous section illustrated, however, couples freely talked of what "society" had a right to expect, but they did not see society's claims as overriding their own autonomy as parents. They sought medical advice freely, often consulting other physicians. Parents saw no need to consult an authority or helper outside of the medical world for the problems they faced with amniocentesis. Yet there were signs of need for counsel in the moral dimension of their decisions.

At this point I would hypothesize that the time and energy given by the vast majority of the parents to interviews and telephone discussions indicates a need for ventilating their concerns and receiving informed "moral counsel." Parents were extremely diligent in keeping appointments and giving time to the interviews. Several indicated that they enjoyed our discussions, and four relationships of "moral counselling" developed in which the interviewer, on the suggestion of the genetic counsellor, invited couples to discuss their most difficult decisions with him. These discussions suggested to me that alongside an attitude of moral autonomy in these parents may lie a need to establish a sense of moral direction with the larger community. They are not "individualists" and as such found fulfilment in reflecting on their social commitments. I felt that it was striking that the two couples who consulted friends were Catholic, and that the two friends were cited as being very "religious" and knowledgeable about religious matters. Both Catholic couples also asked the genetic counsellor about religious conflicts with their possible course of action. One would normally expect the greatest religious and moral conflict regarding abortion in Catholic couples, or where one spouse is Catholic. In a unique study of parents of retarded children, Zuk found Catholic mothers greatly more accepting of their retarded children than non-Catholic mothers.[18] One Catholic father in a mixed marriage said: "All of my childhood training has suddenly come back to haunt me." He felt that he had achieved a high degree of autonomy in the development of his conscience—until this decision.

Phase 2: Decision Following Amniocentesis

The period following amniocentesis to the report on the results of the tap found the parents in considerable anxiety, and whatever problems existed in their marriage or family relationships were exacerbated. The average time between test and reporting in 25 cases was 20.9 days. The physician told each couple that normally the time lapse was three weeks. Telephone calls to the physician by parents were numerous, and his staff often counselled a spouse over the telephone to tell them of the status of their case.

On looking back at process with the couples, they described "toughest" time as the anxiety in waiting for a report on amniocentesis. "We shouted at each other and fought like tigers," said one husband. Another husband who sought marriage counselling in this period stated that the long wait had made him angrier at his wife for being a carrier, and that he wanted out of the relationship more than ever. Several couples testified to the fact that only their strong marriage relationship sustained them and that without it they would be without support and comfort. "I don't know what I would do without his being with me, since I get so depressed," said a mother carrying Down's Syndrome.

If a marriage is troubled, the strains will most likely break forth in this period, testing to the limits the capacity of the couple to face their problem and make plans. I saw this trouble more often in younger couples than in the older parents. One husband in particular acted out his feeling trapped in a marriage to a carrier partner by making homosexual liaisons. After intensive counselling and some psychotherapy more realistic assessments were made by the parents.

Decisions Following Positive Diagnosis

The most acute personal suffering followed a positive diagnosis. In each of three cases the couples decided for abortion and sterilization by hysterotomy. A great deal of grief and

self-condemnation followed these procedures. Following the report it was as if the whole decision had to be made anew. One might expect that significant preparation had been made which would lessen the burden. Possibly because the couple had so hoped for a normal child, a set of expectations heavily weighted in that direction formed and were shattered.

The reasons offered for the step to be taken were uniformly personal and related to the emotional strain the parents had been under. "I just can't go through this again," said a mother. "If they can't tell me that my child is not normal, I don't want to try again. I have three brothers with muscular dystrophy, and I am not going to take a chance on it." "No one who knows me would say that I don't want children, but I have had enough," said the third mother. The counsellor, sensitive to the profound disappointment of the parents, advised caution in their decision, especially towards sterilization, but none preferred to remain able to bear children.

The three mothers who elected sterilization, and the fathers as well, suffered deeply from guilt and a sense of failure. Added to the guilt associated with being a carrier of genetic disease was their realization that their experiment to get a healthy child had failed, and there would be no more children of their own. I was particularly interested in the plight of the women. One of them stated:

I am just crushed and disappointed. I had so hoped to give my husband a healthy baby, and now I know that I will not. You spend all your life looking at pictures of pretty babies and their mothers and growing up thinking that will be you. It is pretty gruesome when you are the one who is different.

When asked about vasectomy as one option open to them, each mother rejected it vehemently. "It is my fault, why should he have to pay for it?" said one. "He may want to marry again, if anything happens to me, and he should be able to have his own children," said another.

Two mothers electing hysterotomy had living children or family members suffering from genetic disease. They were acutely aware that aborting a fetus affected by the same problem amounted to a type of "rejection" of

the relative. One mother talked of her child:

He knows what's going on. I wonder what he thinks about the baby. He could think . . . they want to put me out of the way, too. And he could think, no one should have to suffer the way I do. I suppose it would be more the second.

Neither mother felt strongly enough about the meaning of abortion to a living person suffering the same disease to choose against it. Several parents with living children remarked that one of the forces driving them against amniocentesis itself was the effect an abortion might have on the security of a child at home with the same problem. One mother gave voice to her sense that an already affected child felt threatened by her visit to the center when she found him hiding in the closet upon returning. Follow-up interviews found parents still concerned about the implied threat to an existing child and finding ways to explain to the new healthier child how it could happen that they once contemplated his destruction if a diagnosis compelled them.

Phase 3: Reflection after Action

An interview was held with parents following childbirth or the termination of pregnancy. No parent regretted using amniocentesis. Parents who could look forward to having a "normal" child said they were greatly eased by the knowledge and that the latter part of pregnancy was easy.

Parents who elected abortion and sterilization were still troubled, but they were also taking other steps to help themselves. Two couples made plans for adoption and a third decided to move to a farm.

Parents electing abortion and sterilization took particular pains to justify their decision and to put the decision into a framework which made sense to them. A Catholic couple alone attempted to place the event in a religious framework, but one which no longer satisfied them morally or intellectually. "Why does God give so many terrible things to children?" queried the mother. She then told of several years of religious doubts due to the birth of a previous child and her rejection by a priest when she earlier sought amniocentesis. "I have a very hard time believing in God any more. I have prayed to God this time for his protection and for a normal baby, and you see nothing has happened." As she talked she cried openly. Feeling that she was reaching for a form of faith which would help interpret suffering without condoning magic, I offered her help in examining the religious views she had been holding. First, she made no distinction between nature and God. "God" was the source of good and bad genes. Secondly, she lived in a universe with a very small margin of moral freedom, if any at all. God determined everything, including one's choices. Thirdly, her anger and cosmic resentment were clearly unacceptable in the eyes of such a God. I reasoned that God was at least as gracious to us as we are to our own children. "Would you always keep your child penned up in the backyard, even when he was older?" I asked. She got the point quickly and began to talk more about her unsatisfactory religious beliefs and fear of the church.

Following Abortion Each mother revealed an element of "cosmic doubt," even though the Catholic mother alone cast her doubt in a strictly religious perspective. "You try to understand how things like this happen," said a Jewish mother, "and there is a scientific explanation . . . but . . . I feel like the fickle finger of fate pointed at me."

"I lie awake nights damning God, even though I don't believe in a God," a third mother with no particular religious persuasions stated. The experience of genetic disease and ending a pregnancy may lead people to the "borderline" question about the meaning of human existence. These questions are of their nature religious questions, since people attempt to come to terms with their fate and a profound sense of isolation from the roles of parenthood. Even if religion is not used as a last line of defense against the arbitrariness of life, parents probably will seek to make some ultimate sense out of these events, and seek some ultimate security in their insecurity.

Following the birth of children, couples who had undergone genetic counselling re-examined their role as parents thoroughly. It was as if the process made them ever more serious about childbearing and parental responsibility. Parents who knew that their children were carriers of a defective gene resolved to instruct them about their problem and to do everything possible to assist them in controlling their marital future. No parent even considered seriously the eugenic possibility of aborting a child who was a carrier. Amniocentesis or another technique would be open to them in the future.

Additional Reflections Discussions with parents at the conclusion of the process provided a good format for inquiry into their attitudes about sex determination and genetic surgery. Only one of the twenty-five couples preferred not to learn the sex of their child. Those who preferred to know gave pragmatic reasons for wanting to know. "It takes some of the mystery out of it, but it helps to prepare us," said a father. Only the parents with sex-linked genetic diseases felt that sex determination was advisable. None of these couples felt that it was wrong to predetermine that a male or female be born if genetic disease could be avoided. Medical indication for sex predetermination was the predominant justification for this step when it becomes feasible. One mother stated: "It wouldn't be a good idea to let everyone select the sex of their children. There would be too many problems. But in our case . . . Fabry's disease . . . it would be a blessing."

In discussing concepts of genetic surgery, these parents were wary of prenatal interventions. None preferred to be the first to allow genetic surgery unless there were good reasons to hope for success. Attitudes of these parents were distinctly conservative in this regard. Yet the same parents had no doubts about the technique they were using. After the birth of a child I asked parents if the possibility of "technical failure" (false negative) had worried them prior to birth. With one exception, a dental surgeon, the answer was "It crossed my mind, but I did not seriously consider it." The exceptional person said that he was not truly at ease until the baby had been examined by a pediatrician. Thus, the power of

technology and the credibility of physicians combine to produce incredible trust in couples using amniocentesis.

None of the mothers who were in a position to discuss "surrogate parenthood" would have chosen this alternative of having a child rather than adoption. Each mother was a carrier of a deleterious gene and would (in surrogate parenthood) have to be the recipient of a donated ovum fertilized by her husband. The husbands preferred to have children either by adoption or when "it is my sperm and her egg."

The Ethics of Parental Care and Prenatal Diagnosis

Will the use of prenatal diagnosis by parents in increasing numbers diminish the sense of care, love, or affection parents must show to their children for the maximal psychic and ethical development of children? More precisely, does the procedure itself, because it inclines the parents to contemplate the abortion of the fetus before they are fully informed as to the results of the test, erode that "basic trust" which is so fundamental as to lead Erik Erikson to assert that "the firm establishment of enduring patterns for the balance of basic trust over basic mistrust is the first task of the budding personality and therefore first of all a task for maternal care"?[19] When evaluated from a Christian ethical perspective, does the use of this technique and its accompanying awareness of elective abortion subvert the deputyship of parents, who as representatives of the love of God for the child are called to represent a love which inspires the confidence that "whatever is, is good," and is no "respecter of persons"?[20]

In preparing answers to these questions, I determined first to interview each of the couples again, more than six months to one year after the birth of a healthier child or after abortion following a positive diagnosis. Four families were not interviewed because of distance and one was unavailable. Twenty couples gladly accepted follow-up interviews.

In my interviews I developed questions around three general areas for the purpose of formulating hypotheses. The areas were: (1) the way they perceived their relationship with a "healthier" or "normal" child born after amniocentesis compared with their perceptions about their relationship with previously born children whether healthy or genetically handicapped; (2) eliciting their feelings about any possible damage to the "trust" dimension of their role as parents caused by the contemplation of abortion; (3) gathering any further moral or ethical reflection they had done as parents at a distance from the birth of the child.

Because the results of the interviews were so uniform, and in the interest of space for further discussion, I shall furnish details of one interview and simply indicate the results of the remainder.

Mr. and Mrs. C. had a Mongoloid daughter, age 4, when Mrs. C. became pregnant the second time. They learned of amniocentesis through a program for parents of the retarded and sought help. She is Protestant, he is Catholic. Following amniocentesis and a negative diagnosis for Down's Syndrome, a son was born over a year ago.

In answer to the first set of questions, the following statements were made by Mrs. C:

It *is* really different, I think, from the experience of parents who do not know if their babies are well before they are born.
I know I feel different about S. [the son] than other mothers do their children. I feel this way about it . . . he is fortunate, it is like adoption, we planned and chose him, we have given him a good gift. Other mothers seem casual about expecting a child, I could never be casual again.
The difference between the way I feel about S. [son] and E. [daughter] is that *we knew him a lot longer* [italics mine].
I feel that there is a "miracle type attitude" around my relationship with S. We worked very hard to get him and went through a lot of terrible worry.

Mr. and Mrs. C. acknowledged having discussed how they would explain later to their son when he was old enough to understand the circumstances of prenatal diagnosis. Both were aware of the possibility of having to answer his questions about "what if you had found that I was like E.?" Mr. C. outlined a future discussion with his son as follows:

We did what we did because of your sister. If she had not been sick, we would not have done what we did with you. We owed it to her not to risk hav-

ing another child like her, since we [the parents] couldn't have survived it. We had a hard enough time taking care of her, and if a second had come along, it would have crushed us for sure. In spite of the risk we ran in having you tested, it was worth it to know that you were really healthy.

Mr. C. acknowledged that he had suffered considerable guilt over the thought that he might have had to decide to abort his own child, "especially since my belief is that the fetus is a life from the earliest stage." He stated that there was "no good way to explain to your own child that you might have had a part in deciding the end of his life." But neither parent felt that the total value of amniocentesis was overshadowed by the possible pain or loss to a son who would one day learn of their decision. They did not think that this knowledge would threaten their son, rather he "will be grateful for being born healthy." They both emphasized the *known* risk involved in their having a healthy child.

In order to stimulate discussion of their later reflection on the morality of elective abortion following amniocentesis, I introduced the facts of the "Baltimore Case"[21] and asked them to compare the morality of what they might have decided with that case. In that case a Mongoloid was born to a couple and needed simple surgery for relief of an internal blockage. They instructed the physician not to operate and to allow the child to die. No food was administered to the child, and it took fifteen days for the child to die.

Mr. and Mrs. C. and each of the other couples interviewed felt strongly that the decision made by the Baltimore parents was "terrible," "wrong," or "immoral." Mrs. C., pointing out the difference between her husband's beliefs and her own, stated: "If a child is born, you must do everything you can to help it. That is different from our decision." When asked *how* it was different, she said:

We would have found out the problem early enough. . . . I do not believe that it would have been wrong in our circumstances to have decided for an abortion . . . especially since we already had E. . . . We had already decided to keep her, no matter what, but we just couldn't risk having another child with the same problem. The difference, though, when you look at it, is

really that we could know so much earlier. We were having such a tough time with E . . . and when we heard that there was a way to find out about the next one, it was the only thing to do. We first were under the impression that we might have twins, which would have made it that much harder. We had to find out the facts in order to save our family. I am thankful that we were able to know. The only difference between the Baltimore people and us is that we knew earlier . . . plus the fact that the doctor supported us.

In order to move into the third area of inquiry, their sense of the ethics of parenthood, I pointed out to them the difference between the arguments they were using, based upon the prediction of certain consequences to them and E. if another Mongoloid child was born, and an "idea of parenthood which accepted the consequences of the birth of children as part of your responsibility." Mrs. C. countered with the assertion:

It would not have been responsible of us not to go to the doctor . . . not to find out . . . if there was a way. . . . If you can know for sure, and the doctor told us there was every chance we could find out . . . then we would have been adding to our troubles to avoid it. We couldn't pretend that we didn't know about the test. We even discussed having the child if we found out it was to be like E. But I was already decided not to do that. If you can be sure that you can have a healthy child, why shouldn't you find out? I can't tell you what a relief it was to know.

Mr. C. added:

I know what you are getting at. I feel it when I am with my own parents and the way they look at me. The fact is that medicine has discovered this test and we needed it. The only other way would have been for us not to have any more children. Given the choice between that and having one normal child . . . I wanted to do what we could. As it happened, we were lucky . . . the worst didn't happen. We love E. very much and are taking care of her ourselves. Having S. gives us everything we ever wanted.

My questions then turned to wider consequences of decisions of parents like them for society, such as the hypothesis that less concern might be shown for Mongoloid or retarded children as a result of widespread use of prenatal diagnosis and elective abortion. Neither parent agreed with this idea, and their answers were supported by most of the other couples questioned. Mrs. C. said that she felt that more people have become aware of the problems of retarded children since amniocentesis has been used. If there are fewer children like E., the ones who are living might have more of a chance to be helped than before. They might get more care when people have more choice. People have told me that what we did might eventually lead to us trying to breed a super-race, but I don't believe that. Maybe it will even lead to a cure for what is wrong with E.

Mr. C. stated:

It is a tremendous thing which we did, when you stop to think about it. I feel good about it now, but I was really worried when it was going on. I was raised Catholic, and all my childhood teachings hit me hard. We went around here screaming at each other. Then, when we sat down and figured out the ways the test would help us and the ways it wouldn't, the first was obvious. For us, with one retarded child at home, it was the right thing. It helped us know and to plan.

I questioned Mr. C. about his concept of the morality of abortion at this stage of his thinking. Was he aware of changing his concept? He answered:

I still *feel* the same way. I was petrified at the thought of having to choose to abort my own child. I would have done it, though, for the sake of saving my family. I am . . . like . . . of two minds on the subject . . . my feelings take me one way and my mind another.

Having concluded that they both felt that this decision was right for them as a family and that the consequences had borne out the fittingness of their decision, I asked about their preferences for social policy on prenatal diagnosis. Should it be required of parents who have one child with Down's Syndrome? Should regulations be passed covering high-risk groups? At this point, one of the most interesting results of the interview emerged. Mrs. C. took a "hard line" and said yes to every social proposal for screening, detection, and prenatal diagnosis. Mr. C. was adamant in the other direction, stressing that only voluntary methods could be used with families in need of genetic counselling. He stated:

I can't see how you can successfully force people to make these decisions. Having the test available and teaching about it was some pressure on me, but I chose to do it. My wife has become a "crusader" about it, but I disagree.

Analysis of the answers of Mr. and Mrs. C. reveals that they do perceive their relation to their second child to be permanently altered due to amniocentesis. It is "different," according to Mrs. C., when parents "know" the child "a lot longer." Descriptions by other couples bore out this perception. Knowing the sex of the child and being reassured of its health bring the couple into a more active relation with the child. "It takes the mystery out of it," said one father, "but it also took the terror out of it." The primary *difference*, in these parents' relation to their tested children, seemed to lie in the fact that active roles as parents began earlier in the course of pregnancy. It was as if the test and its results speeded up activities which most parents begin only after birth. "Most parents may be hoping for a boy, but not knowing," said one mother; "we started to fix up his room as soon as we knew the results of the test." Assurance of the health of the child releases parental care, planning, and symbolic activity usually reserved for birth.

Insofar as Mr. and Mrs. C. already felt enough pressure to begin to construct explanations for later use with their son as to why he was tested, I would make a tentative deduction that they do feel some sense of threat to the type of caring which had characterized the parental roles they had learned. Mr. C.'s remark that "there is no good way" to tell a child that a parent once was partially resigned to its abortion appears to me as evidence of an underlying awareness of threat. When asked, other couples acknowledged having reflected on the task of telling the child about the intervention, though none were as articulate as Mr. C. about an already composed answer. The couples tended to rely on the assurance that the child would be so grateful for being born healthy that no real threat would be perceived. This idea underestimates, in my opinion, the power of the human mind to imagine and enlarge on reasons for rejection. Sidney Callahan, in commenting on the Baltimore case and its possible effect on existing parent-child relations, wrote: "Knowing one's parents let your little brother die because he wasn't 'normal' or was 'sick' would create deep insecurity. 'Will I be done in if I don't measure up? or if I get sick?' "[22] My questions to the parents revolved around their impressions of the feelings of living children where amniocentesis is being used on a fetal sib. Do they worry about their own security? Or did they think that a *tested* child would later grow morbid over the idea that its parents once had him or her tested with a predilection towards abortion? The couples did not know the answers to these questions, nor do I. They showed signs of discomfort at being asked about these possible psychic consequences. Their answers, at this time, revolved around justifications based on the known risk of their having more children and the promise of early knowledge of health in their child. They tended, like the C.'s, to imagine that their tested children would be grateful, not resentful, when they learned the facts with which the parents were faced. Much more study needs to be done of the families of the first generation of parents in amniocentesis to find harder answers to these questions. My conclusions about this small sample of parents would support a hypothesis that parents are aware of some alteration in the formation of trust in their relations to tested and untested children, due to the abortion issue; further, this alteration is seen as justified in the light of known risks about their childbearing.

The moral reasoning of the parents was distinctly along consequentialist lines informed generally by the norm of parental protection. I interviewed no parents who came at their roles from highly conscious norms or principles about parenthood and unconditioned caring. This is not to say that there is not evidence in their discussion of their having internalized such norms, as Mr. C.'s discussion shows. Parents like Mr. C. will show some signs of "moral suffering" as they attempt to come to terms with the impact of genetic counselling on their roles and perceptions of morality. I define moral suffering as the state of being threatened by normlessness, even as one is caught between two forces or principles, both of which are right. Moral suffering is not the direct effect of *anomie*, relative cultural normlessness, on the individual concerned, but rather the opposite, as when a person is caught in a dilemma between two goods. Moral suffering occurs when highly motivated parents who desire children intensely, even desperately, are caught between the rightness of protecting their families from the great strains which genetic disease may place upon them, and the rightness of unconditional caring for the life of their conceived child. In more formal terms, these parents find themselves suffering actively in the process of making society, even as that society and its products "feed back" upon them to introduce new choices into the parent-child relationship. Whether or not this moral suffering will lead to "ethical tragedy," as this term is employed by Henry D. Aiken,[23] depends upon whether the conflict between rights is ethically soluble. It is my position that prenatal diagnosis, taken in the context of the therapeutic goals of genetic medicine and its relation to the circumstances of particular families, does not introduce a permanently insoluble moral conflict in the ethics of parental caring. The remainder of this essay is devoted to this argument.

Amniocentesis and the Morality of Abortion

The most compelling reasons for elective abortion following prenatal diagnosis combine the certain severity of a genetic indication with evidence of potential damaging stress to the family involved. Abortion of a genetically deformed fetus is not "treatment," as Paul Ramsey has so ringingly made clear.[24] When related strictly to the therapeutic goals of genetic medicine, amniocentesis is morally difficult to justify, since there are no basic gene therapies available, and if the medical literature is an indication, genetic therapy will be very difficult to achieve for some time to come.[25] According to Robert Murray, Howard University geneticist, regulating the products of genes will precede any wholesale treatment of defective genes.[26] For example, he predicts that scientists will understand how hemoglobin is synthesized and thus be able to regulate the product of the sickle-cell anemia gene long before they will be able to introduce therapies for the sickling gene itself. Amniocentesis is also difficult to justify morally in relation to studies of the products of genes, unless one wanted to argue that the sacrifice of the genetically deformed fetus is a necessary contribution to the research for a fuller understanding of the genetic problem under consideration. It is not morally right to recruit abortions strictly for research purposes; it is morally

proper to study the remains of an abortus for research into human genetics when that abortus has been obtained legally and without tying the research to the abortion. In genetic counselling centers in which elective abortion also occurs, physicians should be very cautious about the recruitment of their patients and abortuses into research programs. Above all, the physician doing the abortion and the principal investigator doing the research should never be the same person.

Only parents who are definitely at risk for genetically defective children should be admitted to amniocentesis. Not only the risks of the procedure justify this stricture, but more so the ethics of parenthood. Prevention of known and verifiable risk of serious genetic disease may be, in particular families, an acceptable protection of the family. I do not make this as a general principle for all families. Some families cannot survive the addition of one more defective child. In other families, as Daniel Callahan has argued, it is not *inevitable* that the severely handicapped person can expect little or no fulfilment in life.[27] The impressive testimonies of heroic families and their handicapped children, even after the appearance of amniocentesis, are legion.[28] The argument for elective abortion following amniocentesis should only be made related to specifically verified risks in the context of the needs of particular families. At this stage of the development of genetic medicine, *only* if parents are able to tell children, tested or untested, "We made the decision to enter testing because of specific and known risks, and *we* made the decision," will the parent-child bond not be weakened. The more personal and the less coerced a decision, the more opportunity for personally relating to children the reasons why. Nothing could weaken or dissolve the parent-child bond more effectively than children becoming afraid that their parents made such decisions for trivial reasons of personal convenience or because they were forced into it for external societal reasons. The arguments of J. V. Neel, a geneticist, tend, in my view, towards creating a climate of threat to parent-child relations:

. . . I suggest we see the advent and potential applications of prenatal diagnosis as one more of those steps whereby man, consciously, or unconsciously, has grasped the reins of his own genetic destiny. . . .

Early abortion based on prenatal diagnosis can be viewed as the modern counterpart of infanticide based on congenital defect. All over the world, primitive man seems to have recognized the need for curbing his reproduction, and when the limited means at his disposal for so doing failed then practiced infanticide, especially directed towards the defective. I find it difficult to see in our recent and continuing reproductive performance, condemning so many infants to a miserable death and so many of the survivors to marginal diets incompatible with full physical and mental development, any greater respect for the quality of human existence than evinced by our primitive ancestors.[29]

There is nothing in the technique of amniocentesis which "grasps" any gene or inserts any remedial medicine into a child's genetic destiny. No research on the genetic products of the fetus can be done from the fluid withdrawn. The language here is at least inflated and gives the reader an impression that something "genetic" has changed. Nothing could be more destructive of the trust required in parent-child relations than for genetic testing to be understood as motivated by infanticide. The cause of infanticide could never justify prenatal diagnosis within the moral code which presently governs the relation of medicine to the family. The only warrants, at present, which justify abortion following prenatal diagnosis are a positive diagnosis and the undue hardship or misery which would come to a particular family. The portrait of the negotiations in a "condominium" between state, family, physicians, and supporting counsellors drawn by George Williams in an earlier discussion of abortion in this journal presupposes the absolute opposition of the religious communities to the kind of eugenic-abortion policy depicted by Neel.[30] Prenatal diagnosis exists, at this stage, to help particular families gain accurate information about particular at-risk pregnancies. Only in this context can parents exercise the care for the born and the unborn which their roles require. Where parents understand their roles in a religious context, as representative of the love of God to the born and the unborn, and the more personally responsible and accountable the parents are for their decisions, the more adequately they convey the effective meaning of God's love. The more pressure families feel from eugenically inspired groups or "lobbyists" for embryonic transfer or sex determination,[31] the less personal and accountable they can be to their own children for the decisions they make while in genetic counselling.

One could argue, as does Neel, that it is more just and causes least suffering to the fetus to abort it, rather than allowing it to suffer pain and illness, or to endure injustices on the mentally retarded. This argument is vulnerable because of its inherent paternalism. Whenever a strong group argues on behalf of a weaker group that their removal would be better than their survival, we should not be duly impressed.

One could argue, as did H. J. Muller,[32] that it is unjust to society to allow more defective children to be born. This argument is especially vulnerable to the charge of intolerance. By and large the families of genetically defective children must bear the weight of their care and nurture. Consideration of the family's situation and values should be the fulcrum upon which the morality of the uses of genetic knowledge from amniocentesis turns. Daniel Callahan has expressed a view quite similar to mine in his reflection on the Baltimore case:

I am told . . . that we owe it to the fetus to abort it if it has Down's Syndrome. Yet when I read of the actualities of Down's Syndrome it becomes clear that most mongoloids are happy, that many have a minimally adequate intelligence level, that many can be trained for simple jobs, that they are capable of giving and responding to affection.

That does not sound like a life of suffering to me. Perhaps, though, it means a life of suffering for the parents. But, if so, then that is a very different matter; a riddance of the mongoloid serves the parents and not necessarily the child himself. That should be said clearly. . . . Even in the case of Tay-Sachs disease, far more severe than Down's Syndrome, the suffering of the child itself is apparently not great; the course of the disease brings a mercifully quick degeneration of cognitive and affective faculties; the greatest suffering is on the part of the parents. I, myself, would feel that the parents would have a moral right to turn to abortion in that case and for those reasons. But I would hope that no one

would be fooled into thinking we were really acting for the sake of the child, nor that anyone would be fooled into thinking that we were doing anything other than taking the life of the fetus in order to preserve the welfare of the parents.[33]

As Neel himself shows in the same essay cited, as well as in another place,[34] it is highly unlikely that any significant reduction of deleterious genes in the gene pool will be effected through prenatal diagnosis and selective abortion. There is no effective eugenic argument for its wide-scale use. There is an argument for amniocentesis to be used for the relief of certain distressed families. If it can be shown that parental care of the living, in decisions arrived at through accurate information, would be seriously diminished through the birth of a predictable and severely defective child, parents may responsibly elect abortion. In those cases where the existing parent-child or marital bond could be said to be in serious jeopardy, it does not become an ethically insoluble tragedy for the parents to elect abortion. The interest of preservation of the family bond and its resources may, in specific cases, be chosen above the interest of preserving until birth the life of a severely deformed infant for whom no treatment is available.

The Social Consequences of Genetic Intervention

To argue as I have done opens one to the criticism that, if this direction is followed, there will be less tolerance in society for the weak, the imperfect, the unlovely, and the unacceptable. To suggest that we ought to act to reduce the suffering of parents seems to some to deny the good purposes to which pain can be turned. To others, my arguments reinforce the economic and social dominance of the middle and upper classes, since they tend to act upon genetic knowledge much more frequently than minority or lower-class groups. These consequences will be likely if the therapeutic goals of genetic medicine are displaced by eugenic goals. The treatment of the disease is the ultimate goal. Therapy will be a realizable goal in a society where the parent-child bond has not been undercut by well-intentioned scientists.

The avoidance of responsibility in treating genetic disease and acting upon its presence in the unborn undercuts one of the central social values, to reduce suffering in all of its forms. One does not have to hold the position that parents are required to agree to abortion of every defective fetus. I hold that genetic-counselling centers ought not to compel parents to agree to abortion prior to amniocentesis, for this position works against the voluntarism inherent in present practice. Finally, there should be extraordinary efforts to extend genetic medicine to those groups in society who have been discriminated against economically and medically. Unless the benefits of medicine are distributed equally among groups in society, the people will not perceive "benefits" as being in their interest. For practical purposes, medical policy towards genetic treatment should be directed towards those diseases which are catastrophic in their personal and physical consequences. We should beware of those who plan to engineer vast social changes through genetic engineering, such as raising the level of intelligence or reducing aggression in mankind.

New Steps in Genetic Medicine

I chose to follow the progress of couples in amniocentesis because this procedure appears to occupy the center stage of the application of human genetics to practical problems at the present time. It is as if amniocentesis is a "forerunner" of solutions to future problems. I found that the "consumers" of genetic progress (parents) were conservative in their consideration of proposals for sex determination, implantation, and genetic surgery. Their base line for decision on genetic progress was related to serious genetic disease rather than to whole upgrading populations. They realized that they were the first generation of parents to benefit from information gained from prenatal diagnosis, and they were eager that its benefits be extended widely. Their views, on the whole, coincide with mine as to the ethical parameters of progress in genetic medicine. Theological tradition tends to support man's intervention into natural processes to improve his physical and social environment. This is not to say that an unlimited blessing is extended to technical progress. Theologians must beware of providing "cover" for medical progress or codes of behavior which are derived entirely apart from faith. Each proposal in genetics must be evaluated for the benefits and risks to human beings contained in it. Moreover, risks must be assumed by informed human beings who are agreed as to the terms of their experiment. To this theologian, human genetics at present does not violate anything inherently "human," for the most characteristic act of man is to attempt to change himself and his condition. The most authentic Western religious visions prompt interventions into our condition as long as we do not expect to seize eternity or ultimate security through any one or several of these man-made plans. We must not deceive ourselves: human genetics will create as many problems as it solves. Nevertheless, when one has unleashed the full force of ethical self-criticism upon amniocentesis and its effect on parent-child relations, he emerges with no compelling reasons to cry "stop it!" Indeed, one can imagine strictly therapeutic uses for the newest projections for human genetics, including implantation and sex selection. It is the task of the nonmedical professions aligned with physicians to call to them to adhere to their therapeutic calling and resist any attempt to hasten the "kingdom of God" through technical progress.

A New Stage of Life

Others have discussed the development of new "stages of life" in the context of the development of modern culture.[35] It is plausible that the demands of an advanced industrial society create a set of needs plus the means for the appearance of a new stage of life: prenatal. The "discovery" of childhood is a comparatively recent development in the history of the Western family, as Aries shows so convincingly.[36] When Mrs. C. says of her son, "We knew him longer," there is evidence for an intimate involvement of parents, particularly, of the middle class, with their children from conception forward. Given the means to study and monitor the development of the fetus, and given the recognition of the complex demands in the environment the fetus will enter, it stands to reason that some adults in this period will surround the

fetus with whatever supports or interventions they hope will better equip its development. Before this period in history, human beings reckoned that the first stage of life began at birth. Judged by our own actions and inventions, we are assisting in the birth pangs of a new stage of life prior to the birth of the child. One of the consequences of this development emerge will be the assignment of developing human status to the fetus from conception. There is no way to avoid regarding the embryo as human, although the stages of development through which the fetus passes towards birth will carry decisive weight in defining its identity. The more the unknowns of human development prior to birth are exposed to light, possibly the more care can be extended to unborn children. But because care is never "pure" and is mingled with self-interest and ideology, the unprotected fetus is more than ever exposed to the wish fulfilments of adults. One of the primary tasks of ethical inquiry for the generation to come will be defining the limits and possibilities of intervention into the newest human stage of life. The primary task of theological inquiry, as put so well by Gustafson's recent writings, is to frame the ethical inquiry in pondering on two questions: "What do we value about the human?" and "What is the relation of the empirical and descriptive to the ethically normative in our concept of human?"[37] As the family is still a central agent of the experience of being human, no continuing search for the uniquely human can bypass an evaluation of how our changes of ourselves affect our experience of family.

Notes

1. By futuristic proposals I refer to the issues involved in cloning and *in vitro* fertilization of an ovum for eugenic purposes. The issues in the debate emerge clearly by comparing four authors: Leon Kass, "The New Biology: What Price Relieving Man's Estate?" *Science* 174 (1971) 779–88; *id.*, "Making Babies—The New Biology and the 'Old' Morality," *The Public Interest*, no. 26 (1972) 18–56; *id.*, "Babies by Means of In Vitro Fertilization: Unethical Experiments on the Unborn?" *New England Journal of Medicine* 285 (1971) 1174–79; Joseph Fletcher, "Ethical Aspects of Genetic Controls," *New England Journal of Medicine* 285 (1971) 776–83; [reprinted as Chapter 65 of this volume]; Paul Ramsey, *Fabricated Man* (New

Haven: Yale Univ. Press, 1970); Karl Rahner, "Experiment: Man." *Theology Digest* 16 (Feb. 1968) 57–69.

2. The best collection of informed opinion on the technique of amniocentesis is found in Maureen Harris, ed., *Early Diagnosis of Human Genetic Defects: Scientific and Ethical Considerations* (Fogarty International Center Proceedings 6; Washington, D.C.: U.S. Govt. Printing Office, 1972).

3. James R. Sorenson, *Social Aspects of Applied Human Genetics* (*Social Science Frontiers Series;* Russell Sage Foundation, 1971).

4. My thanks go to the Fogarty International Center, NIH, for funding the study, and to Cecil Jacobson, M.D., and the George Washington University Medical School for allowing me to work in the genetics-counselling unit.

5. John Fletcher, "Human Experimentation: Ethics in the Consent Situation," *Law and Contemporary Problems* 32 (1967) 620–49.

6. Fritz Fuchs, "Amniocentesis: Techniques and Complications," in Harris, *op. cit.,* p. 11.

7. D. C. A. Bevis, *Lancet* 1 (1952) 395.

8. P. Riis and F. Fuchs, *Lancet* 2 (1960) 180.

9. Cecil Jacobson and Robert H. Barter, "Intrauterine Diagnosis and Management of Genetic Defects," *American Journal of Obstetrics and Gynecology* 99 (1967) 797.

10. Talcott Parsons, *The Social System* (New York: Free Press, 1951) p. 97.

11. Frederick S. Carney, "Deciding in the Situation: What is Required?" *Norm and Context in Christian Ethics,* ed. Outka and Ramsey (New York: Scribner, 1968) p. 13.

12. Robert F. Murray, Jr., "Problems behind the Promise: Ethical Issues in Mass Genetic Screening," *Hastings Center Report* 2 (April 1972) 12.

13. James R. Sorenson, "Decision Making in Applied Human Genetics: Individual and Societal Perspectives" (Bethesda: Fogarty Center for Advanced Study in the Health Sciences, in press).

14. Among the best studies of this problem are Pauline Cohen, "The Impact of the Handicapped on the Family," *Social Casework* 43 (1962) 137–42; Samuel Olshansky, "Chronic Sorrow: A Response to Having a Mentally Defective Child," *Social Casework* 43 (1962) 190–93; David G. Langsley, "Psychology of a Doomed Family," *American Journal of Psychotherapy* 15 (1961) 531–38.

15. Charles J. Epstein, "Medical Genetics: Recent Advances with Legal Implications," *Hastings Law Journal* 21 (1969) 35–49.

16. John W. Littlefield, "The Pregnancy at Risk for a Genetic Disorder," *New England Journal of Medicine* 282 (1970) 627–28.

17. Fuchs, *op. cit.,* p. 14.

18. G. H. Zuk, "The Religious Factor and the Role of Guilt in Parental Acceptance of the Retarded Child," *American Journal of Mental Deficiency* 64 (1959) 139–47.

19. Erik Erikson, ''Growth and Crises of the Healthy Personality,'' *Psychological Issues* 1 (1959) 63.

20. Others have remarked on the affinity between Erikson's researches into ''basic trust'' and this description of H. R. Neibuhr's of the moral dimension of radical monotheism: *Radical Monotheism and Western Culture* (New York: Harper, 1960) p. 32.

21. This case was the focus of a symposium, ''Choices on Our Conscience,'' sponsored by the Joseph P. Kennedy, Jr. Foundation, Oct. 15–17, 1971, in Washington, D.C. The case was subsequently reported in the press: Harold M. Schmeck, Jr., ''Parley Discusses Life-Death Ethics,'' *New York Times,* Oct. 17, 1971, p. 52; Stuart Auerbach, ''Doctors Ponder Ethics of Letting Mongoloid Die,'' *Washington Post,* Oct. 16, 1971, p. A1.

22. Sidney Callahan, ''Choices on Our Conscience,'' Symposium on Human Rights, Retardation, and Research, *op. cit.,* Morning Plenary Session: ''Who Should Survive: Is Survival a Right?'' p. 20.

23. Henry D. Aiken, *Reason and Conduct* (New York: Knopf, 1962) p. 80.

24. Ramsey, *op. cit.,* pp. 114, 171.

25. Theodore Friedman and Richard Roblin, ''Gene Therapy for Human Genetic Disease?'' *Science* 175 (1972) 949–55.

26. Robert F. Murray, M.D., personal communication.

27. Daniel Callahan, *Abortion: Law, Choice and Morality* (London: Macmillan, 1970) p. 497.

28. One excellent discussion of an afflicted child and his family is found in Robin White, *Be Not Afraid* (New York: Dial, 1972).

29. James V. Neel, ''Ethical Issues Resulting from Pre-Natal Diagnosis,'' in Harris, *op. cit.,* p. 221.

30. George H. Williams, ''Religious Residues and Presuppositions in the American Debate on Abortion,'' *Theological Studies* 31 (1970) 71.

31. The self-understanding of some physicians and lawyers who enter the public debate on crucial ethical matters sometimes resembles that of salesmen or lobbyists. The following quotation should suffice: ''The lobbyists for reform in the laws of drug and alcohol addiction, abortion, and sexual behavior have achieved much public approval in their areas of concern; can biologists in experimental embryology expect so much more by doing any less?'' (Robert G. Edwards and David J. Sharpe, ''Social Values and Research in Human Embryology,'' *Nature* 231 [1971] 90.)

32. H. J. Muller, ''Should We Weaken or Strengthen Our Genetic Heritage,'' in Hudson Hoagland and Ralph W. Burhoe, eds., *Evolution and Man's Progress* (New York: Columbia Univ. Press, 1962) p. 23.

33. Daniel Callahan, ''Who Should Be Born: Is Procreation a Right?'' Symposium on Human Rights, *op. cit.,* Panel no. 1, pp. 7–8.

34. Neel, *op. cit.,* pp. 222, 223; see also Neel, ''Pre-Natal Diagnosis and Therapeutic Abortion,'' *Perspectives in Biology and Medicine* 11 (1967) 129–35.

35. Especially Kenneth Keniston, *Young Radicals* (New York: Harcourt, Brace and World, 1968), and Erik Erikson, *Childhood and Society* (New York: Norton, 1953).

36. Philippe Aries, *Centuries of Childhood* (New York: Vintage, 1962).

37. James M. Gustafson, ''What Is the Normatively Human?'' *American Ecclesiastical Review* 165 (1971) 192–207.

64

Karen A. Lebacqz
Prenatal Diagnosis and Selective Abortion

Reprinted with permission of the editor from *Linacre Quarterly*, vol. 40, 1973, pp. 109–127.

The practice of prenatal diagnosis raises a number of serious ethical dilemmas. I shall focus here on one of these: the selective abortion of defective fetuses. Selective abortion is commonly recognized as the central ethical dilemma in prenatal diagnosis, and it receives new urgency in light of the recent decisions on abortion by the United States Supreme Court.

The questions being raised here are first, what justifications are offered for prenatal diagnosis and selective abortion; and second, what are the implications of the ethical reasoning embodied in these justifications? I shall argue that the current and projected widescale practice of prenatal diagnosis and selective abortion establishes precedents which both violate fundamental principles of justice and threaten the traditional life-preserving orientation of medicine.

I

It may be helpful first to set the entire discussion in the context of two important trends in our changing social ethos. Both these trends have achieved sharp articulation during the time of development of prenatal diagnosis, and both have influenced arguments made on behalf of prenatal diagnosis and selective abortion.

The first trend encompasses a general awareness of "women's rights" and specifically, a movement toward autonomy of women in the reproductive sphere. This trend received significant articulation in the Supreme Court decision in Griswold v. Connecticut (1966), in which a marital right to privacy in reproductive matters was declared to be protected as a constitutional right and its culmination can be seen in the recent declaration by the Supreme Court that "this right of privacy . . . is broad enough to encompass a woman's decision whether or not to terminate her pregnancy."[1]

Current concern for the effects of rapid population growth and the scarcity of resources has contributed to a second trend which influences this discussion: a movement toward a "quality of life" ethic which, according to an editorial in California Medicine, places relative rather than absolute value on human life.[2] This "quality of life" ethic

may be seen generally in the trend toward accepting abortion and specifically in arguments that it is better not to be born than to be born unwanted.

Thus prenatal diagnosis has arisen in a general climate of concern for "population growth, women's rights, the consequences of illegal abortions, the number of 'unwanted' children and the discriminatory aspects of current abortion laws."[3] It is within this general framework and its specific articulation in the recent decisions by the Supreme Court that the practice of prenatal diagnosis and selective abortion must be assessed.

Preliminary Observations

Before considering the morality of selective abortion, some preliminary observations are in order. Prenatal diagnosis itself is an information-gathering procedure. Clearly, the information generated can be used in a variety of ways, and not only as the basis for selective abortion. Indeed, practitioners stress the fact that most diagnoses reveal a normal fetus and hence serve to reassure anxious couples[4] and on occasion to prevent a scheduled abortion.[5] Moreover, a few disorders may be treated prenatally or postnatally on the basis of a prenatal diagnosis,[6] and it is hoped that more treatments will be available in the future.[7] Thus prenatal diagnosis is advocated not only to provide for selective abortions, but because it potentially brings these other benefits as well. Nonetheless, a cursory examination reveals the centrality of selective abortion in the practice of prenatal diagnosis, and hence justifies a focus on this one issue.

To begin with, the importance of the "reassurance" rationale can be tested by asking first, whether any woman could have an amniocentesis just to make sure that the fetus she carries is normal, and second, whether a woman could get amniocentesis if she had no intention of having an abortion in the event of abnormality. The answer to both these questions is "no." First, not all women are considered eligible for amniocentesis, but only those in "high risk" or "moderate risk" groups.[8] Second, even for those women in high risk groups, amniocentesis will not be performed unless abortion is at least an option,[9] and some practitioners would

even say that the woman must be committed to an abortion before diagnosis will be performed.[10] The reason in both cases is simple: the risks associated with the diagnostic procedure are considered sufficiently great so as to preclude the diagnosis in the absence of genuine risk of defect and sufficient benefit—the benefit of reassurance alone does not outweigh the harms of the procedure.[11] No matter how important the reassuring function may be in actual practice, it does not constitute sufficient justification for widescale prenatal diagnosis.

Similarly, the argument that prenatal diagnosis "saves lives" by preventing abortions also depends on the acceptance of selective abortion: the interest here is not in saving the lives of *all* fetuses by preventing *all* abortions, but only in saving the lives of *normal* fetuses by preventing *them* from being aborted. Thus the entire line of reasoning depends on acceptance of the abortion of defective fetuses.

As for treatment, there are currently only a few disorders for which treatments are available and "at the present time, the emphasis is placed on diagnosis of disorders in which there is no treatment."[12] Moreover, even where treatment is available, most practitioners still allow the couple the choice of abortion, and indeed suggest that this is what most parents would prefer.[13] Hence the availability of treatment does not rule out abortion.

Developing Treatments

But even though treatment is not a major possibility now, surely prenatal diagnosis might be justified as a necessary means to gain basic information needed in order to stimulate the development of new treatments.[14] Attractive though this argument might at first seem, however, there are several problems here.

First, if parents would indeed choose abortion over "any but the most trivial treatment,"[15] it is not clear that the impetus to develop treatments will exist. (But even if future fetuses might indeed benefit from information gained through present diagnoses, there remains a serious question: is it justifiable to subject a fetus to risk in an experiment which carries no hope of benefit to *that* fetus but only to future fetuses? The lack of clear legal and ethical guidelines regarding experimentation on the unborn must not obscure the fact that this is a critical question. Should the fetus be protected, for example, by laws that govern experimentation on minors? The answer to this question is beyond the scope of this essay; but the question must be recognized.)

Second, whatever hope there may be for future treatments, such future possibilities do not in fact form sufficient justification for the performance of prenatal diagnosis in the eyes of some practitioners. Dancis states that any attempt previously to diagnose defects prior to birth would have met with the response "why bother?" because no intervention was possible.[16] It is "medical intervention of some sort" that justifies the use of prenatal diagnosis. And, as we have seen, intervention "of some sort" usually means abortion.

It is obvious, then, that whatever other benefits may be claimed for prenatal diagnosis, for the present and for the foreseeable future, its "justifying" or "real" purpose is to provide for selective abortion. Ethically, then, the crux of the matter is whether or not selective abortion of defective fetuses is justifiable.

II

Selective abortion is not, of course, a new issue. While it has rarely been a *central* issue in the "abortion debate," it has received at least sporadic attention following rubella epidemics and the thalidomide scare. A "eugenic abortion" clause has appeared in almost every proposed model code for abortion reform, and a number of states have included such a clause in revised abortion statutes within the last few years.[17] Hence, the issue itself is not new.

What is new in selective abortion following prenatal diagnosis is the certainty of the diagnosis. Previously, a decision for selective or "eugenic" abortion had to be based on statistical probability or "risk" figures; now, an "actual diagnosis" can be made.[18] Thus prenatal diagnosis is hailed as a great advance for "taking the gamble out" of pregnancy and genetic counseling.[19]

The advent of prenatal diagnosis therefore *focuses* the question of selective abortion in a new and dramatic way: for the first time, the problem of selective abortion arises not because of accident or mishap, but because of the deliberate intervention of medical technology. For the first time, selective abortion is not an occasional and regrettable act, but the planned outcome of deliberate programs of medical practice.

Nonetheless, most of the ethical issues raised by prenatal diagnosis and selective abortion are issues that have been implicit or explicit in the "abortion debate" over the past few years. Now this debate has raged so long and hard and covered so much territory that one is well advised to exercise caution when entering the fray. Moreover, the recent decisions by the Supreme Court suggest that the wisest course might be to assume that the legal resolution of the issue also resolves the moral dilemmas.

Arguments Examined

However, I suggest that previous debate and present legal framework notwithstanding, there may yet be a little room for clarification of the issues and moral decision-making with regard to selective abortion. Therefore, I shall examine the arguments offered as justification for selective abortion and place those arguments within a logical framework which will help to ascertain what is really at stake in this practice.

The matter is complicated at the outset by the fact that few practitioners present explicit arguments to justify selective abortion. Most advocates simply refer to the legality of abortion or its acceptance within a significant reference group—for example, "therapeutic abortion may be offered where it is legal,"[20] "most people would probably prefer abortion,"[21] most obstetricians would regard abortion as acceptable,"[22] and so on. Indeed, some practitioners specifically exempt themselves from responsibility for making the ethical decision, on grounds that it is their job to lay the empirical foundations on which legal, ethical, and political decisions will be made by others.[23]

Nonetheless, alongside specific disclaimers and vague references to decision-making groups there emerges from the discussion a constellation of claims for selective abortion.

First, selective abortion is justified on grounds that it procures benefits for individual families: it protects them from the financial and emotional strains associated with bearing and rearing a child with a genetic disease[24] and it minimizes the risks involved in pregnancy. Special pleas are made on behalf of families with a previous history of devastating defect, who may be afraid to "take a chance" with another pregnancy unless they can have prenatal diagnosis.[25]

In addition, there is considerable emphasis on the rights of women and couples and especially on freedom of choice and autonomy in the reproductive sphere. Amniocentesis is seen as a technique which "opens doors"—that is, which expands the options available to women and their spouses, thus enabling them to exercise freedom of choice.[26] It is a cardinal rule in the practice of prenatal diagnosis that the "ultimate" decision for both diagnosis and abortion is to be made by the couple.[27] One practitioner has even suggested that parents have a *right* to healthy children.[28]

First Rationale

Thus the first rationale given for selective abortion is that of the benefits accruing to individual women and their families. As this rationale begins to shade over into questions of women's rights and reproductive freedom, it takes on the character of the first social trend enumerated above, assimilating the trend and contributing to it.

Alongside this concern for the pregnant woman and her family, there emerges another concern: an interest in the impact of genetic disease on society as a whole, and in the public health aspects of prenatal diagnosis. Justification for diagnosis and abortion is therefore also derived from benefits to society gained through wide-scale screening programs.

In the first place, geneticists contend that screening programs could have a eugenic effect in eliminating deleterious genes from the gene pool.[29] In the second place, practitioners argue that screening and abortion would significantly reduce financial burdens to the state, since fewer children would be born needing costly medical or institutional care. Elaborate cost-benefit economic analyses have been made for several disorders.[30] Concern for protection of society at large is thus the second reason given as justification for selective abortion.

Just as arguments regarding benefits to women "shaded over" into arguments about women's rights and procreative freedom, so here the arguments regarding benefits to society shade over into a larger concern, which may be encompassed by the phrase "quality of life." Prenatal diagnosis and selective abortion are justified because they function to preserve a *norm of genetic health* which is a part of the "quality of life."[31]

The concern for a standard of genetic health may be seen to operate, first, in the assumption that prenatal diagnosis and selective abortion function as "preventive medicine." This assumption has been made explicit on several occasions.[32] Moreover, it is implicit in the use of phrases such as "reduce the incidence of disease," "eliminate disease," or "prevent the birth of" rather than "abort." As "preventive medicine," prenatal diagnosis and selective abortion combine to preserve the norm of genetic health which is a part of the quality of life.

Second, concern for the norm of genetic health and the quality of life have been raised explicitly by several advocates. Quality of life questions are most often linked to questions of *quantity*, and it is here that the concern for genetic normalcy becomes most apparent. Prenatal diagnosis is seen as a means of quality control in a quantity-limited system. On the level of the individual family, the quantity-quality link is seen clearly in statements to the effect that with increasing pressure to limit family size, parents will not want to risk any departure from the normal in their offspring.[33] Indeed, under pressures of quantity, quality control becomes a right: "if the size of our families must be limited, surely we are entitled to children who are healthy rather than defective."[34]

Social Needs

The quality problem is seen not only on the individual level, however, but also as a response to societal needs. Thus one practitioner claims: "The world no longer needs all the individuals we are capable of bringing into it," and argues for selective abortion on these grounds.[35] Prenatal diagnosis becomes a tool to ensure that "both the quantity and quality of the human race are kept within reasonable limits."[36] Maintaining the norm of genetic health thus justifies prenatal diagnosis and selective abortion because maintenance of the norm is a necessary step in ensuring quality of life in a time of concern for population growth. The concern here is well summarized by one practitioner reflecting on the work of several pioneers in the field:

Dr. Gerbie and his associates have helped us take still another step down the long road which we must follow if we are going to *improve the quality of human existence while searching for better methods of controlling population density.*[37]

Finally, the norm of genetic health may also be seen in the argument that the fetus has a right to be "well-born."[38] The argument here is that there is a fundamental right to be born "with normal body and mind" and that if this right is not to be fulfilled, then it is better not to be born at all.[39]

In sum, the importance of genetic health is taken as a *given,* which carries its own justification. It is only necessary to know that there is a choice between health and disease: the obvious choice on the part of all parties—family, society, and the individual concerned—will be for health.[40]

These, then, are the justifications for selective abortion: benefits to the woman and family and to society as a whole, both in terms of specific and measurable emotional and economic factors and in terms of the maintenance or restoration of the norm of genetic health.

III

We can now ask how these justifications fit into the context of the "abortion debate," what other assumptions are necessary to explicate them, and what it means to follow out their implications logically.

Several of the justifications offered for selective abortion following prenatal diagnosis are similar to specific arguments used to establish other categories of "indications for abortion."

The concern to protect the woman and family emotionally and financially is not a new concern in the abortion debate, nor is it unique to selective (or eugenic) abortion; rather, it is reminiscent of the "psychiatric" and "socioeconomic" indications for abortion. Thus if these arguments are used to justify selective abortion, the justification becomes similar to that used for the psychiatric and socioeconomic indications. And indeed, it appears to be the practice in some places to require a psychiatric examination and justify the abortion as "therapeutic" on these grounds.[41]

However, some advocates reject the "psychiatric indications" argument: one practitioner calls it "circuitous" and "ridiculous" to require psychiatric examination of the woman following diagnosis of defect in the fetus.[42] They want the presence of defect alone to be sufficient justification for abortion. This argument, therefore, parallels the traditional arguments for a separate category of "eugenic" abortion which has validity independently of other criteria.

The assertion that there should be an independent category of abortion for "eugenic" indications, in which the very presence of defect justifies abortion, is a logical outcome of reasoning on the basis of a norm of genetic health. Thus a psychiatrist commenting on prenatal diagnosis notes that "for some people, abortion of a defective fetus is less unsavory than abortion of a presumably normal fetus," and he explains this fact on the basis that it is "in line with our medical orientation that makes the extirpation of disease a noble act."[43]

If arguments for selective abortion appear at first glance to coincide with various arguments for "indications" for abortion, however, there is also evidence of affinities between arguments used for selective abortion and the so-called "abortion on demand" arguments.[44] Here, the basic claim is that the woman's freedom is an overriding value which dictates the availability of abortion "without reason" (that is, without public or legislative consensus on the reason proffered). Women may thus choose to have a child or not, to have a defective child or not, as they please.

Clearly, then, it is necessary to examine the arguments for selective abortion both within the general context of "abortion on demand" and within the more specific context of special claims made in the case of defect. It will also be necessary to suggest ways in which the recent Supreme Court decision impinges on the various arguments and sets the context for any future action.

IV

I shall begin by examining very briefly the question of "abortion on demand." (Before doing so, however, a brief note is necessary regarding the relation of abortion on demand to the more specialized arguments for abortion in selected categories. This history of the abortion controversy makes it obvious that it is possible to argue for selected categories of justifiable abortion without also condoning abortion on demand. I would argue that it is also *logically* possible to condone abortion on demand without necessarily condoning eugenic abortion. Logically, one can argue that a woman has the right to determine whether or not she is prepared to accept a pregnancy, but that having made that determination the particular status of the fetus should be irrelevant.)

The abortion on demand argument gives primacy to the freedom of choice of the woman. However, it must also deal with the fact that freedom of choice of one human being does not usually extend to the point of killing another human being; that is, there is a *presumption* that a human being has a right to life and that my freedom does not normally extend to the point where it deprives another of his right to life. Thus if the fetus is considered to be a human being, the woman would not normally have the right to kill that human being. To counter this difficulty, advocates of abortion on demand usually take either of two positions: First, they argue that the fetus is not a human being—or not "fully" human —and hence has no right to life. Second, they argue that although the fetus is human and hence has a right to life, there is something in the unique

relationship of the woman and fetus that destroys the "normal" prohibition against killing.

Most advocates have taken the first approach: they assert that the fetus is not (fully) human. Arguments of this sort range from those that assert that the fetus is a mere "tissue" or part of the woman's body[45] to those that recognize the fetus as a "developing" or "potential" human being, but argue that full humanity is not present until a specified time.

Must Set Time

The difficulty with this view is that advocates must then determine a time at which the developing embryo/fetus/neonate is considered to be (fully) human—six weeks? three months? at viability? one year after birth? That is, they are caught in a line-drawing problem: *When* does the individual acquire full human status? The designation of a *time* of attainment of full humanity always presupposes the choice of *criteria* according to which humanity is determined—brain function? lung capacity? personality? speech?

Now these criteria for determining that one has reached full humanity always have to do with functional capacity and personal development. Hence it is always possible to ask whether there would be others besides fetuses who would, logically speaking, be subject to the determination that they are not "fully human" and hence not protectable under the law.

For example, geneticist Joshua Lederberg argues that the moment of conception should not be considered "as the start of human life"; rather, he suggests, "an operationally useful point of divergence of the developing organism would be at approximately the first year of life,"[46] on the basis of development of language and cognitive interaction with others. However, the establishment of this time point on these criteria would obviously allow for the destruction of the newborn child up to one year of age. Logically speaking, Lederberg's criteria would allow for infanticide. At this point, Lederberg draws back from accepting the logical conclusions of his standards and refuses to discuss infanticide, on grounds that our emotional involvement with infants is sufficient to establish "a

pragmatically useful dividing line." He then implies that the "tastes" or emotional involvement of "the majority" determines one's status as a human being to be given full protection under the law: "To discuss the fetus during prenatal life as if he were a human being is merely to reflect the emotional involvement of that observer, according to a set of tastes not now shared by the majority." One must ask, then, whether persons or groups who do not meet the standard of emotional involvement would be considered less than fully human and not protectable—for example, the convicted criminal or any outcast group.[47] Once again, Lederberg draws back from the logical conclusions of his own argument and suggests that the criterion of emotional involvement "should not be confused with any objective biological standard by which we can set up principles of social order."

Lederberg's search for an "objective biological standard" to get him out of the problems he encounters with his own criteria illustrates as well as anything the inherent difficulty in this basic line of approach: any biological point that is chosen will be chosen on the basis of other criteria, and these criteria are all too often the results of our very human weaknesses. (Do we choose "spontaneous lung function" as the determining criterion of humanness because we *really* think it is a decisive criterion, or rather because we would *like* to be able to destroy the fetus prior to viability?) Are we willing to accept the consequences of our choices— what about those who must exist with the help of an iron lung?

Human Standards

In short, there is no "objective biological standard," but only very real *human* standards. To be sure, some choices make more sense than others: Fletcher has suggested, for example, that in order to be consistent with our increasing orientation toward brain activity in defining the *end* of human life, we should also define the *beginning* of human life in terms of brain activity.[48] Certainly, consistency is a desirable trait in both logical thinking and human interaction; indeed, this suggestion makes considerable sense. However, since the presence of brain activity in the fetus has been measured as early as six weeks, considerably before amniocentesis can be performed, Fletcher's criterion would preclude prenatal diagnosis and selective abortion.

In view of the difficulties of drawing a line on the developmental continuum, several advocates of abortion on demand have preferred to take the second route: they argue for abortion on the basis of the special relationship between the woman and the fetus which is deemed to nullify the prohibition against killing. The most intriguing exposition of an argument along this line is that of Judith Jarvis Thomson.[49]

Thomson proposes that we accept, for the sake of argument, the claim that the fetus is human.[50] The question then is, under what circumstances may we justifiably kill a human being? Suppose, says Thomson, that you wake one morning strapped to a famous unconscious violinist who needs your kidneys to survive; "is it morally incumbent on you to accede to this situation? Does the right to life of the violinist require this heroic and self-sacrificing act on the part of another person? Thomson concludes that it does not: "nobody is morally *required* to make large sacrifices, of health, of all other interests and concerns, of all other duties and commitments, for nine years, or even for nine months, in order to keep another person alive." In essence, Thomson's argument rests upon the moral right of the woman to *remove herself* from the violinist—or from the fetus. While separating woman and fetus *in fact* secures the death of the fetus, Thomson is not arguing that a woman has a right to secure the death of the fetus, but only to remove herself. Presumably, if prenatal adoption or an artificial womb were available, either of the options could be used to preserve the fetus while freeing the woman.

This argument is more than intriguing; it has a certain force in its logic. Nonetheless, I think it also admits of some difficulties. Thomson claims that the woman has a right to remove herself from the fetus; the fact that the fetus then dies is perhaps unfortunate, but not central to the moral issue. Perhaps a different scenario will help elucidate the issues.

If one grants, as Thomson does, that the fetus is human, then the issue is whether one human being may remove herself from another when that other is dependent upon her body functions for survival. Surely the closest parallel to pregnancy, then, is the case of siamese twins, in which separation would cause the death of one twin. The moral question then is: could an adult siamese twin choose to "remove" herself from her twin, knowing full well that the twin would die, but claiming that her freedom was the more important value? (The medical practice of involuntarily separating siamese twins at birth, with the resultant death of one, does not change the *moral* argument regarding the rights of adult siamese twins.) If anything, it could be argued that we should feel *more* sympathy toward the plight of the siamese twin than toward the pregnant woman—the twin's predicament is both involuntary and lifelong. Yet I wonder if we would be willing to accept the twin's argument; would we not be inclined to consider the "removal" of one adult twin with the resultant death of the other to be murder, or wrongful killing? It is not clear to me that we are ready to argue *logically* that one human being may "remove" himself from another when that removal causes the other's death.

Other Examples

Indeed, to bring the scenario a little "closer to home" for most of us, let us suppose that a man is responsible for the continued care of his elderly and dependent father, who will die if no one is in attendance at his bedside. Surely this man is morally free to leave his father's bedside if there is someone else to sit and watch over his father. But what if there is no one else? Is he then morally free to walk off, leaving his father to die? Or, suppose a young child needs medication every few hours to survive; is not that child's mother morally (and perhaps legally) culpable if she "removes" herself from the child and it dies?

In short, Thomson's distinction between removing oneself from another and securing the death of another becomes problematic when we consider a variety of cases. In cases where our nurturing function could be served by others, we are perhaps willing to argue that we have a right to remove ourselves provided that we have secured someone else to carry on the nurturing.

But in cases where there is no one else to carry on that function—i.e., in pregnancy today, and in the case of siamese twins—I suggest that a view that really respects the full humanity of the other will not so readily allow us to argue that we may "remove ourselves," causing thereby the death of the other. (Hence, I suspect that Thomson has not really taken the human status of the fetus seriously, that she has not really overcome her own predisposition "that the fetus is not a person from the moment of conception.")

To accept Thomson's argument means to accept what it logically entails: the right of any human being to remove himself from one who is dependent on him, even if that removal results in the other's death—the elderly father, the child in need of medication, and the adult siamese twin. Once again, the argument allows for the destruction of other human beings. If we are not willing to accept these consequences, then we must reject the premises.

V

Thus far, I have dealt with the general question of abortion under the rubric "abortion on demand," locating two basic ways of approaching this issue and suggesting that there are problems in the extension of logic in either of these approaches. It has not been my intention to resolve the issue of whether or not the fetus is entitled to protection of its life, but only to illustrate the difficulties encountered in a position that denies protection to the fetus.

However, the question of selective abortion introduces a new element to the discussion. As Daniel Callahan suggests, with selective abortion we are dealing not with the problem of an unwanted *pregnancy*, but with the problem of an unwanted *child*.[51] A logical exercise will illustrate what is at stake: Suppose that an artificial womb were available. Then, if the purpose of abortion is to free the woman from an unwanted pregnancy, logically the fetus would be placed in the artificial womb. Would a defective fetus also be thus preserved, or would its genetic status somehow "make a difference" in how it is treated?

Since the purpose of selective abortion is not only to protect the woman but also to protect society and preserve the norm of genetic health, it seems logical to assume that simply moving the fetus from one location to another would not be sufficient to fulfill the purposes of selective abortion. To the extent that selective abortion is oriented toward maintenance of the norm of genetic health or the "quality of life," it requires the destruction of those who do not meet this norm.

Now this illustration of the artificial womb is, of course, a hypothetical situation at present. Nonetheless, there are indications in the current practice that demonstrate the centrality of destruction of defective fetuses in this practice.

Determining Sex

First, prenatal diagnosis is used to determine the sex of the fetus in cases at risk for sex-linked disorders such as hemophilia. In such cases, the male fetus which is aborted has a 50 percent chance of being normal. Thus half of the fetuses which are aborted in sex-linked cases will in fact be normal; this destruction of normal fetuses is allowed in order to ensure destruction of defective fetuses.

Now in the case of sex-linked disorders, one does not know whether a *particular* fetus is defective or normal; hence the abortion is done on the supposition that the fetus *might* be defective. A more complicated case, therefore, would be that of a diagnosis of twins which revealed one normal twin and one defective twin. In such a case, in order to "get rid of" the defective fetus, it would be necessary to destroy the normal fetus as well. Would this destruction of normal fetuses be allowed? To date, prenatal diagnosis has missed the presence of twins, but practitioners agree that parents would be allowed the choice.[52] Thus even a known normal fetus could be aborted in order to abort an abnormal fetus.

Finally, since there is always a possibility of error in diagnosis, we can ask whether advocates prefer a false positive which would result in the abortion of a normal fetus, or a false negative which would result in the birth of an affected child. Practitioners

disagree here. One states flatly that the loss of the "rare normal pregnancy" would be "an undefendable catastrophe."[53] Another, however, suggests that it is a "more critical" error if a negative diagnosis is given and the child is born defective than if a positive diagnosis results in abortion of a presumed defective fetus and the defect is not confirmed upon examination of the abortus.[54]

It seems clear that the practice of prenatal diagnosis establishes a distinction between the normal and the defective fetus, and allows for differential treatment of the fetus on this basis. As one concerned practitioner put it: "We are faced with problems of assigning values to individuals with given genetic characteristics and designing programs directed against them."[55]

Serious Problems

What are the implications of adopting this kind of reasoning—of treating fetuses differentially according to their genetic constitution? I suggest that there are a number of serious problems in establishing this kind of precedent, and I shall deal briefly with several of these, illustrating where appropriate with difficulties encountered already in the practice of prenatal diagnosis.[56]

The first problem is that of determining the *categories* of fetuses considered destructible. Where is the line to be drawn on the determination of what constitutes sufficient "quality of life" to enable the fetus to live?

This problem will be encountered in two forms. In the first form, it has to do with the severity of genetic defect. The normative use of prenatal diagnosis is for severe, untreatable disorders (e.g., Tay-Sachs, Down's syndrome). However, even present techniques will diagnose less severe disorders (e.g., XO), and with expanding technology such incidents may be anticipated more frequently. Will abortion be allowed for less severe genetic disorders, or for disorders where treatment is available?

Already this problem is being encountered in the practice of prenatal diagnosis, and advocates appear to be divided in their responses. While some would maintain that "if there is an effective intrauterine treatment, then, of course it should be applied,"[57] probably most would agree that abortion in

the case of a treatable disorder "remains a parental decision based on the informed counsel of their physician."[58]

Second, the determination of destructible fetuses may be extended from clear *genetic* categories to categories of *social desirability* or usefulness. As Kass says, "Once the principle, 'Defectives should not be born,' is established, grounds other than cytological and biochemical may very well be sought."[59] The beginnings of this trend may already be seen in the treatment of fetuses with XYY chromosomes, where the "prognosis" for the child is problematic primarily because of the possibility of socially undesirable behavior. If XYY fetuses are to be aborted, then what about fetuses of women living in undesirable circumstances—for example, women on welfare? Will "quality of life" come to be determined more on the basis of social usefulness than clear genetic disorder? One practitioner has already argued for prenatal diagnosis on grounds that "the world no longer needs all the individuals we are capable of bringing into it—especially those who are unable to compete and an unhappy burden to others."[60] Surely such criteria as "ability to compete" extend the range of destructible fetuses far beyond the severely genetically handicapped.

Indeed, I would stress the fact that *all* categories chosen depend on some social criteria—even those that are most closely tied to genetic anomaly. For example, most practitioners consider Down's syndrome to be a "clear-cut" case calling for abortion.[61] Certainly the genetic component—a trisomy G—is clear enough; and this genetic component is related to certain clinical symptoms such as mental retardation. But to determine therefore that fetuses with trisomy G should be aborted is to make a *social* judgment about the place of retarded individuals in society. It is possible to judge disability or deviation from a norm medically, but to determine that this deviation constitutes a significant handicap is to make a social judgment.[62]

Drawing a Line

The first point, then, is that it is extremely difficult to "draw a line" with regard to the *categories* of fetuses which will be considered destructible, since all determination of such categories includes a social component and will be subject to the vagaries of social opinion. The phrase "quality of life" defines a continuum from the severely disabled through the socially undesirable to the "optimal" child. Where on this continuum will the line be drawn?

The second "line drawing" problem has to do with the *time* continuum. As one practitioner asks: "Are we going to be faced with demands to do away with a child with 21-trisomy whose mother was only 34 years old during her pregnancy and therefore was denied the benefits of prenatal diagnosis."[63] Do not the same arguments that justify abortion of a five month old fetus also justify infanticide?

That this question is not just fanciful is borne out by a recently publicized case at Johns Hopkins Hospital in which a newborn child with Down's syndrome was reportedly starved to death because its parents refused surgery necessary to save its life.[64] It seemed clear that had the child been normal, the surgery would have been performed.

Indeed, some physicians now argue explicitly for a different standard of treatment for newborn children with Down's syndrome. One has said: "Parents of mongoloids have the legal (and I believe the moral) responsibility of determining if their child . . . should live or die," and he suggests that this decision may be seen as a "second chance" for abortion.[65]

Thus it seems that infanticide is simply the logical extension of prenatal diagnosis. Indeed, one practitioner comments: "Early abortion based on prenatal diagnosis can be viewed as the modern counterpart of infanticide based on congenital defect."[66] This, then, is the second serious problem implicit in the reasoning behind prenatal diagnosis and selective abortion.

These first two problems have been line-drawing problems—problems of determining the categories of destructible fetuses, and the time of destruction. The third problem is of a somewhat different nature. It involves the *locus of decision-making* and the possible conflict between "women's rights" on the one hand and the "quality of life"

on the other. I suggest that as increasing value is assigned to the "preventive" function of prenatal diagnosis and selective abortion, the concern to eliminate defectives and preserve the "quality of life" may logically be extended to deprive women and families of decision-making power.

Quality of Life

To be sure, at present advocates assume that the concept of "quality of life" embraces both the familial and the social aspects of prenatal diagnosis, and that there will be a concurrence of benefits to individuals and to society. They assume that if women are given freedom of choice, they will choose to abort defective fetuses and hence their choices will serve the best interests of society as well.

However, it is obvious that the interests of individual families and of society at large will not always coincide—even in the decision to abort the defective fetus. For example, it has been calculated that if all male fetuses at risk for hemophilia were aborted and "replaced" by female children, the result would be a dramatic increase in the number of female carriers of hemophilia—a 50 percent increase in the gene frequency in each generation.[67] Hence, decisions made to benefit individual families might have a dysgenic effect on society as a whole.

On the other hand, at times where it would be beneficial financially to society for a fetus to be aborted, the woman or family might prefer not to abort. Would the woman's freedom of choice be restricted here on grounds of benefiting society or preserving the genetic health? One concerned practitioner has raised the problem by suggesting that the uncertainties could result in an accentuation of the conflict in our society between personal choice and governmental control, which could possibly come in the form of selected programs of compulsory screening and mandatory abortion for some conditions that are deemed socially intolerable.[68]

Indeed, compulsory abortion has already been proposed.[69]

In a situation where the fetus has no inherent rights and genetic health becomes an overriding value, compulsory

amniocentesis and abortion is a logical outcome, as one practitioner rightly anticipates:

The decision to terminate the life of a fetus has traditionally been denied even to the couple at risk, but the more widespread legal acceptance of abortion, the growing awareness of the impending crisis inherent in the population explosion, and increased concern for the social cost of genetic disease lead me to think that attempts to legislate eugenic programs may not be so untimely or even so far in the future as many of us have expected. Individuals in a society which is willing to allow even normal fetuses to be aborted simply at the request of the parents are not likely to be very tolerant of a known abnormal fetus.[70]

To be sure, several practitioners have expressed their alarm and rejection of compulsory programs at the same time as they raise the question. But the point is that the movement toward compulsory abortion of defective fetuses is a logical outcome of elevating the norm of genetic health to override any rights of the fetus.

Further, once a principle has been established that the genetically unequal may be treated unequally in accordance with their genetic potential, other forms of unequal treatment will be encompassed by this principle. One of the first areas to be affected by the application of this principle will be that of procreation: the suggestion has already been made that reproduction be regulated in accordance with genetic inheritance—that "quality control" have a built-in "quality control" component.[71] A practitioner has even claimed that "most of the women screened should not have been pregnant in the first place. All women who would have genetically high-risk pregnancies should be offered sterilization or an effective method of contraception.[72] Thus the way is opened up for other kinds of restrictive programs as well.

Impact on Medicine

Finally, the acceptance of selective abortion and its principle of unequal treatment of unequals will have profound implications for the practice of medicine. On the one hand, if selective abortion is a woman's right, then the physician is *obligated* to provide for it.[73] As with "abortion on demand," the role of the physician is thus radically changed: "For the first time . . . doctors will be expected to do an operation simply because the patient asks that it be done."[74] The physician, then, becomes a technician performing according to the desires of others.

There is evidence already that this dilemma is being encountered in the practice of prenatal diagnosis, and that many practitioners are reluctant to give up entirely their traditional decision-making function. Thus, for example, one suggests that amniocentesis should not be done in cases of LSD ingestion because the physician would be obligated to provide for an abortion if chromosome breaks are found;[75] here, the physician retains his power of making a medical judgment. Another practitioner has suggested that the use of prenatal diagnosis simply to determine the sex of the fetus constitutes an "abuse" of prenatal diagnosis and that information on the sex of the fetus should be withheld "unless it is crucial for management of the case."[76] Prenatal diagnosis, in this view, is not to be a tool for the "frivolous" uses of women; yet if abortion is a woman's right, then it must be performed no matter how "cold-blooded and contrived" it seems to the physician.

On the other hand, if selective abortion is justified not as a woman's right but as a means of maintaining the norm of genetic health and promoting "quality of life," the physician is in danger of becoming a technician for society. Theologian Helmut Thielicke declares that the doctor becomes an "engineer, a technician doing manipulations for a productive society."[77] Thus Friedmann suggests that "it is not difficult to imagine the emergence of pressures to set standards for desirability in genetically determined human characteristics" and we must ask whose standards they might be.[78]

Thus in the long run, this practice threatens the basic orientation of medicine: as geneticist Jerome Lejeune puts it, to "capitulate in the face of our ignorance and propose to eliminate those we cannot help" is to reverse the entire course of medicine. Not only do the principles established here have serious implications for human rights in society, but they also challenge the foundations of medical practice.

VI

Now clearly, many of these same problems have arisen in the general debate on abortion, and are not unique to selective abortion. In a sense, one could say that selective abortion gives a prismatic view of the implications of abortion in general—of the problems of extension of logic, the threats to human rights and to medical practice. Both abortion in general and selective abortion in particular involve the assignment of relative rather than absolute value to human life on the basis of some social criteria; hence both establish precedents which violate fundamental principles of justice as we have understood those principles in Western society.

Nonetheless, if the basic logic of selective abortion does not differ from that of abortion in general, it is focused and reinforced here in a way which makes its implications more striking and perhaps more threatening. As Kass suggests, precisely because the *quality* of the fetus is at stake in the decision for selective abortion, this decision undermines the fundamental moral equality of all human beings.[79]

Further, the practice of prenatal diagnosis adds something to this equation: the deliberate institution of medical programs designed to foster selective treatment of human life. Friedmann captures the truth well in his haunting statement that

Prenatal genetic diagnosis seemed at first no different from most other new diagnostic methods. Now we see that we are faced with problems of assigning values to individuals and designing programs directed against them.[80]

For all these reasons, I submit that the current practice of prenatal diagnosis and selective abortion threatens basic human rights and I urge practitioners to reconsider the implementation of wide-scale programs of diagnosis and abortion. Prenatal diagnosis is indeed a very exciting new technology with many potentially beneficial uses in providing "therapy" for the afflicted fetus and help to anxious parents. These justifiable uses should not be overshadowed by allowing it to become strictly an exercise in selective abortion.

Violate Equality

Even more than abortion on demand, it seems to me, selective abortion embodies principles of unequal treatment which violate the fundamental moral and legal equality of all human beings. In the long run, this violation of fundamental rights of equal treatment is a more serious threat to the "quality of life" of all of us than the birth of numerous children with defects will ever be. I am heartened by the seriousness with which this matter has been taken in general both by parents and by physicians; nonetheless, it is a dangerous move to aid parents by eliminating their children. We must beware of the implications of moving to a "quality of life" ethic in which persons are judged according to their social utility and hence "some are more equal than others."

But perhaps it will be objected that in view of the recent Supreme Court decisions on abortion, physicians really have no choice: Does not the woman now have a right to an abortion, and if so, does the medical practitioner have any choice but to offer prenatal diagnosis and selective abortion?

Admittedly, the Supreme Court's decisions are ambiguous. The Court declares that the "right of privacy" established in the Constitution is "broad enough to encompass a woman's decision whether or not to terminate her pregnancy."[81] At the same time, however, the Court also maintains that "the abortion decision" is "inherently, and primarily, a medical decision," and at all points it appears to give the decision-making power to the physician: "The abortion decision and its effectuation must be left to the medical judgment of the pregnant woman's attending physician."[82] Thus it is not clear that physicians must comply with the demands of the woman; there appears to be room for "medical judgment" in all cases, and especially in cases involving late abortion. Minimally, physicians can choose to make a true "medical judgment" regarding the woman's "life and health" in each case, and not simply to allow the very presence of defect to be considered sufficient justification for abortion without further consideration of the "full setting of the case."[83]

Finally, it seems to me that all of us, physicians and lay persons alike, have a responsibility to women and families to provide the emotional and financial support needed to enable families to care for children born with defects; although I discourage wide-scale prenatal diagnosis and selective abortion because of the serious threats to basic freedoms involved in this practice, I do not think the matter is settled morally by rejecting abortion. The birth of a child with a defect can indeed be a shattering experience for a family; it is the responsibility of all of us to ensure that families are provided with adequate resources. Ironically, as I write this, federal funds for many supportive programs are being curtailed; this we must not allow to happen.

If indeed the strength of a people can be measured by their attitude toward the weak, the defenseless, and the outcast, then selective abortion points to the weaknesses in our society and in ourselves. It seems appropriate, therefore, to close with a word of warning offered by Ralph Potter:

When a fetus is aborted no one asks for whom the bell tolls. No bell is tolled. But do not feel indifferent and secure. The fetus symbolizes you and me and our tenuous hold upon a future here at the mercy of our fellow men.[84]

Notes

1. *Roe* v. *Wade*, 41:4213 at 4225. [Reprinted as Chapter 68 of this volume; see p. 408.]

2. *California Medicine*, September 1970.

3. A. Milunsky, J. W. Littlefield, J. N. Kanfer, E. H. Kolodny, V. E. Smith, and L. Atkins, "Prenatal Genetic Diagnosis," in *New England Journal of Medicine* 283: 1370 and 283: 1498, 1970, at 1501.

4. Ibid., at 1503: "It should be emphasized that for the vast majority of women, these prenatal studies will serve as reassurance that their offspring will be chromosomally normal."

5. See, for example, M. Neil MacIntyre, "Prenatal Chromosome Analysis—A Lifesaving Procedure," *Southern Medical Journal* 64, Supplement 1: 85, 1971.

6. See William Cole, "The Right to Be Well-Born," *Today's Health*, January 1971.

7. Henry Nadler argues repeatedly for the possibility of future treatment; see "Antenatal Detection of Hereditary Disorders," *Pediatrics* 42: 912, 1968.

8. Considerable attention is given to delineating categories of women "at risk." See, for example, John W. Littlefield, "The Pregnancy at Risk for a Genetic Disorder," *New England Journal of Medicine* 282: 627, 1970.

9. MacIntyre expresses the common sentiment when he says: "If I am involved in a situation in which the parents decide that they will continue the pregnancy under any circumstances, I will be opposed to undertaking the amniocentesis." In Maureen Harris (ed.), *Early Diagnosis of Human Genetic Defects*, (Washington, D.C.: D.H.E.W.), 1970, p. 143.

10. For example, T. N. Evans declares: "She must first be committed to an indicated abortion before amniocentesis is justified." In Albert B. Gerbie, Henry L. Nadler, Melvin W. Gerbie, "Amniocentesis in Genetic Counseling," *American Journal of Obstetrics-Gynecology* 109: 765, 1971.

11. Thus MacIntyre declares: "In my judgment, it is wrong to subject a pregnant mother and her fetus to even the slight risk of amniocentesis if the information thus derived will have no effect upon the parents' decision." In Harris, *op. cit.*, p. 143.

12. Henry Nadler, "Human Genetics and Intra-Uterine Diagnosis," in Donald J. Stedman (ed.), *Current Issues in Mental Retardation and Human Development* (The President's Committee on Mental Retardation, 1971.)

13. See, for example, Milunsky et al., *op. cit.* at 1378 and 1502.

14. Nadler argues that "despite the moral, legal and ethical questions" involved in selective abortion, prenatal diagnosis is warranted because it will enable modification of disorders in the future. Nadler, "Antenatal Detection of Hereditary Disorders."

15. A. G. Motulsky, G. R. Fraser, and J. Felsenstein, "Public Health and Long-Term Genetic Implications of Intrauterine Diagnosis and Selective Abortion," in Daniel Bergsma (ed.), *Symposium on Intrauterine Diagnosis* (The National Foundation—March of Dimes, Vol. VII, no. 5, April 1971.)

16. Joseph Dancis, "The Prenatal Detection of Hereditary Defects," *Hospital Practice* 4: 37, 1969.

17. I am indebted to Charles P. Kindregan's excellent discussion, "Eugenic Abortion," *Suffolk University Law Review* 6: 405, 1972.

18. Milunsky et al., *op. cit.*, at 1503. There are, of course, occasional errors in diagnosis: in every publicized instance thus far in which twins were delivered following prenatal diagnosis, the diagnosis failed to reveal this fact.

19. The medical literature is replete with phrases such as "take the gamble out," "reduce the risk," "not take a blind risk," etc.

20. Henry A. Thiede, "Amniocentesis: A New Approach to Some Old Problems in Obstetrics," *Surgery* 67: 383, 1970.

21. Milunsky et al., *op. cit.* at 1504.

22. J. H. Edwards, "Uses of Amniocentesis," *Lancet* 1: 608, 1970.

23. For example, Nadler says: "I do not want to argue the pros and cons of abortion. . . . We are trying to provide a way in which accurate diagnosis can be made in the case of those people with risk factors. Then, *if they wish to,* they can take advantage of that diagnosis." (Nadler, "Human Genetics and Intra-Uterine Diagnosis," emphasis mine.) While Nadler here gives the decision-making power to the individual couple involved, Milunsky et al. suggest that it rests with society: "The medical, moral, legal and economic issues, problems and implications that have been raised will require extensive study over time. . . . Moreover, the challenge of these new responsibilities must be shared with society." Milunsky et al., *op. cit.*, at 1503.

24. "The most obvious purpose of such procedures is to reduce or eliminate the occurrence of genetic diseases that impose a devastating emotional burden on the parents. . . ." Theodore Friedmann, "Prenatal Diagnosis of Genetic Disease," *Scientific American* 225: 34, 1971.

25. See, for example, C. O. Carter, "Practical Aspects of Early Diagnosis," in Harris, *op. cit.*, p. 19.

26. See, for example, MacIntyre, "Prenatal Chromosome Analysis—A Lifesaving Procedure.

27. A statement by Milunsky et al. is typical: "The decision for amniocentesis and subsequent intervention for an affected fetus will be made primarily by the family. . . ." Milunsky et al., *op. cit.*, at 1502.

28. John W. Littlefield, "Prenatal Diagnosis and Therapeutic Abortion," *New England Journal of Medicine* 280: 722, 1969.

29. The most extensive work on the question of *genetic* impact of prenatal diagnosis is the study by Motulsky et al., *op. cit.*; in describing this study, Friedmann concludes: "The directed elimination of genes by selective abortion after prenatal detection is certainly feasible. . . ." Friedmann, *op. cit.*, p. 40.

30. For example, the following calculation of comparative costs was made for Tay-Sachs disease: "The cost of the whole program—of screening the entire Jewish population of the area and monitoring the at-risk pregnancies—is put at somewhere between $100,000 and $200,000, less than the medical costs incurred in caring for just two Tay-Sachs children during their short lives." "Mass Screen for Tay-Sachs Carriers," *Medical World News*, May 14, 1971.

31. I am indebted to Leon Kass for his helpful analysis of "nature as a standard" in "Implications of Prenatal Diagnosis for the Human Right to Life," presented to the Fogarty International Center Symposium at Airlie House on October 12, 1971.

32. In the early stages of development of prenatal genetic diagnosis, J. H. Edwards declared that it had "opened up the possibility of a new field of preventive medicine." Edwards, "Antenatal Detection of Hereditary Disorders," *Lancet* I: 579, 1956.

33. Milunsky et al., op. cit., at 1502. This view is shared by Robert Morison, who suggests that if the "model couple" is to be restricted to 2.1 children, it becomes more important to them that all their children be normal (draft essay: "Implications of Prenatal Diagnosis for the Quality of, and Right to, Human Life," presented to the Fogarty International Center Symposium at Airlie House, October 12, 1971).

34. Littlefield, "Prenatal Diagnosis."

35. Ibid.

36. Morison, op. cit.

37. Dr. T. N. Evans, responding in Gerbie, Nadler, and Gerbie, op. cit. (emphasis mine).

38. Cole, op. cit. The strongest argument of this sort is that of Norman John Berrill: "If a human right exists at all, it is the right to be born with a normal body and mind, with the prospect of developing further to fulfillment. If this is to be denied, then life and conscience are mockery and a chance should be made for another throw of the ovarian dice." The Person in the Womb, p. 153.

39. This line of reasoning has been consistently rejected by the courts.

40. Thus, for example, Irving I. Gottesman and L. Erlenmeyer-Kimling claim: "We accepted as articles of faith that health was better than illness and that normal intelligence was better than mental retardation. Therefore, it is reasonable to maintain that a fetus should not be brought to term when it is known, by amniocentesis, to be a victim of Down's syndrome (mongolism), Tay-Sach's disease, or any of a host of detectable and catastrophic errors of nature." "A Foundation for Informed Eugenics," Social Biology, 24: 54, 1971.

41. Nadler, "Human Genetics and Intra-Uterine Diagnosis."

42. Ibid.

43. E. James Lieberman, "Psychosocial Aspects of Selective Abortion," in Bergsma, op. cit., p. 20.

44. The term "abortion on demand" is problematic. While it focuses attention on the woman's claim to have an abortion, it also implies an obligation to comply with the demand in any and all circumstances, and appears to ignore the physician's right to "conscientious objection."

45. This view is not only medically inaccurate, it is antithetical to the practice of prenatal diagnosis; the separateness of the fetus from the woman enables practitioners to call the fetus the "patient." See Nadler, "Human Genetics and Intra-Uterine Diagnosis."

46. Joshua Lederberg, "A Geneticist Looks at Contraception and Abortion," Annals of Internal Medicine 67: 25, 1967.

47. While our present movement away from capital punishment may indicate a trend to preserve even the lives of those who are most hated in society, we do have a history of treating persons who are "different" as less than human (for example, during the second World War, Japanese Americans were interned in concentration camps without due process of law).

48. Joseph Fletcher, "Ethical Aspects of Genetic Controls," New England Journal of Medicine 285: 776, 1971. [Reprinted as Chapter 65 of this volume.]

49. Judith Jarvis Thomson, "A Defense of Abortion," Philosophy and Public Affairs 1: 1, 1971. [Reprinted as Chapter 70 of this volume.]

50. She says: "I am inclined to agree . . . that the prospects for 'drawing a line' in the development of the fetus look dim. I am inclined to think also that we shall probably have to agree that the fetus has already become a human person well before birth."

51. Daniel Callahan, Abortion: Law, Choice, & Morality (New York: Macmillan, 1970).

52. In one case where a male fetus was detected and the pregnancy terminated, the practitioners comment that "to the surprise of all, non-identical twin male fetuses were delivered." C. J. Epstein, E. L. Schneider, F. A. Conte, and S. Friedman, "Prenatal Detection of Genetic Disorders," American Journal of Human Genetics 24: 214, 1972.

53. Michael Kaback in Harris, op. cit., p. 85. The context for this statement is actually not that of assessing false positives versus false negatives, but of concern for possible complications in widescale use of amniocentesis. Thus it is not certain that Kaback would prefer a false negative to a false positive, although he is clearly concerned about the destruction of normal fetuses.

54. Fritz Fuchs, "Amniocentesis: Techniques and Complications," in Harris, op. cit., p. 15.

55. Friedmann, op. cit., p. 42.

56. There are several critical questions which I ignore here. For example, Leon Kass has suggested that a program to eliminate defective fetuses may have serious implications for our treatment of living persons with defects—undetected by diagnostic mechanisms, who are born with defects in spite of all our efforts (see Kass, op. cit.). This is indeed a serious problem, but will not be dealt with here.

Another serious problem which I ignore is that of experimentation on fetuses—particularly, experimentation with new genetic technologies such as cloning, invitro fertilization, and such. Decisions made with regard to prenatal diagnosis will establish precedents for the treatment of fetal life in and outside the womb, before and after abortion.

57. Carter, op. cit., p. 18.

58. Milunsky et al., op. cit., at 1378.

59. Kass, op. cit., p. 13.

60. Littlefield, "Prenatal Diagnosis," p. 723.

61. Lubs says: ". . . we can approach the prenatal diagnosis of this syndrome with confidence. This is the simplest situation in the spectrum of probabilities with which we and the parents must work." Herbert A. Lubs, "Cytogenetic Problems in Antenatal Diagnosis," in Harris, op. cit., p. 71.

62. The distinction between medical determination of disability and social determination of handicap is forcefully drawn by Beatrice Wright in Physical Disability: A Psychological Approach (New York: Harper, 1960).

63. Orlando J. Miller, "An Overview of Problems Arising from Prenatal Diagnosis," in Harris, op. cit., p. 29.

64. This case has been widely publicized. See, for example, the report in Technology Review, January 1972.

65. Anthony Shaw, "'Doctor, Do We Have a Choice?'" The New York Times Magazine, January 30, 1972.

66. James V. Neel, "Ethical Issues Resulting from Prenatal Diagnosis," in Harris, op. cit., p. 221.

67. Friedmann, op. cit., p. 40.

68. Ibid., p. 42.

69. In "Human Heredity and Ethical Problems," Bentley Glass asks: "Should not the abortion of a seriously defective fetus be obligatory?" Perspectives in Biology and Medicine, 15: 252, 1972.

70. Orlando J. Miller, "An Overview of Problems Arising from Amniocentesis," in Harris, op. cit., p. 28.

71. See William Vukowich, "The Dawning of the Brave New World: Legal, Ethical and Social Issues of Eugenics," 1971 University of Illinois Law Forum 189, for an elaborate system of quality regulation in accordance with genetic endowment. A more generalized statement is the following by Ingle: "I believe that since man must limit his numbers, efforts to control conception should be focused on those who for cultural, genetic, or medical reasons are unable to endow children with a reasonable chance to achieve health, happiness, self-sufficiency, and good citizenship." Dwight J. Ingle, "Ethics of Biomedical Interventions," Perspectives in Biology and Medicine, Spring 1970.

72. Dr. T. N. Evans, responding to Gerbie et al., op. cit. Clearly, Evans's response is not the intent of the current practice of prenatal diagnosis, which can be seen as a means to enable couples at "high risk" to "take a chance" with a pregnancy. Nonetheless, Evans's statement is a logical possibility given acceptance of the basic principle that "some are more equal than others."

73. Nadler and Gerbie state: "The physician who detects a genetic disorder prenatally is committed to providing therapy—if the results indicate an abnormality and the parents wish termination of the pregnancy." Henry Nadler and Albert Gerbie, "Present State of Amniocentesis in Intrauterine Diagnosis of Genetic Defects," Obstetrics-Gynecology 38: 789, 1971. Of course, the physician does not have to perform the abortion.

74. "A Statement on Abortion by One Hundred Professors of Obstetrics," *American Journal of Obstetrics and Gynecology* 112: 992, 1972.

75. Valenti, in Harris, *op. cit.,* p. 179.

76. "An Abuse of Prenatal Diagnosis," letter to the editor, *JAMA* 221: 408, 1972.

77. Helmut Thielicke, "The Doctor as Judge of Who Shall Live and Who Shall Die," in Kenneth Vaux (ed.), *Who Shall Live?* (Philadelphia: Fortress Press, 1970).

78. Friedmann, *op. cit.,* p. 41.

79. Kass, *op. cit.*

80. Friedmann, *op. cit.,* p. 42.

81. *Roe v. Wade,* 41 *Law Week* 4225. [See p. 408 of this volume.]

82. *Ibid.,* 4229.

83. Justice Douglas, concurring opinion in *Doe v. Bolton,* 41 *Law Week* 4244.

84. Ralph B. Potter, "The Abortion Debate," in Donald Cutler (ed.), *Updating Life and Death* (Boston: Beacon Press, 1968).

65

Joseph Fletcher
Ethical Aspects of Genetic Controls: Designed Genetic Changes in Man

Reprinted with permission of the publisher from the *New England Journal of Medicine,* vol. 285, 1971, pp. 776–783.

The essential difference between science and ethics is that science is descriptive and ethics is prescriptive. Science deals with what is, in the indicative mood. Ethics deals with what ought to be, in the imperative mood. Scientific theories and statements depend for their validity upon verification (are they correct?); ethical theories and statements depend upon justification (do they conduce to the good?).

The ethical question, then, is whether we can justify designed genetic changes in man, for the sake of both therapeutic and nontherapeutic benefits. We are able to carry out both negative or corrective eugenics—for example, to obviate gross chromosomal disorders—and positive or constructive eugenics—for example, to specialize an individual's genetic constitution for a special vocation. Like all other problems in ethical analysis, the morality of genetic intervention and engineering comes down to the question of means and ends, or of acts and consequences. Can we justify the goals and the methods of genetic engineering?

Unlike many other problems, however, in this one both the means and the ends are either challenged or actually condemned. This makes it a thornier ethical issue than most others. In bacteriologic warfare, for example, the means or weaponry is sometimes opposed even by those who may morally support a war's goal—i.e., to subjugate an enemy. In education, to take a different kind of case, to have as the end or goal establishing an Orwellian group-think in the populace would be rejected by most of us, even though the means—various mass media—are regarded as morally licit and ordinarily a good thing.

Those who wish to defend or encourage genetic controls are therefore put in the position not only of having to justify such means in embryologic and genetic research as the in vitro fertilization (conception) of human organisms or the vegetative (mitotic) reproduction of human embryos by cloning, but also of having to justify the end—that is, contrived human beings psychophysically improved by biologic design and control.

The relation of means to ends is central to ethical analysis. Does a morally desirable end ever justify a bad means, on the principle of proportionate good? Could a good means ever justify an evil end or consequences—again on the principle of proportionate good? I would answer Yes to both questions, for reasons that will appear as we proceed. The phrase "good end," I shall contend, means only that the end or consequence sought is ordinarily or commonly good, not absolutely good regardless of circumstances. In the same way the phrase "good means" can mean only that this or that method of getting to the goal desired, the act, is ordinarily or commonly right, not absolutely or always right in and of itself. Furthermore, it is obvious that our values, the various elements we hold to make up goodness, must also be identified and declared in this inquiry. Altogether, this poses a complex but important bundle of questions for conscientious people.

A Priori vs. Pragmatic Ethics

Moral judgments differ. Some people fear new and unexplored risks, as we can see (for example) in the debate over construction of nuclear-power plants. They prefer to forget risk-benefit calculations; they like to stay on the safe side. Others distrust any enlargement of potential powers that might give some of us some advantage over others. We are all familiar with C. S. Lewis's observation that each new power won by man is a power over man as well. Certainly, genetic design would be such a power; even though its medical aim were only to gain control over the basic "stuff" of our human constitution it could no doubt also be turned into an instrument of political power, with or without the reinforcement of Huxley's imaginary "soma." Is it possible, some wonder, echoing Henry David Thoreau, that men have become the tools of their tools?

Nobel laureate George Beadle's opinion is that "Man knows enough but is not wise enough to make man."[1] Over against his way of looking at it a Canadian biologist, N. J. Berill, says, "Sooner or later one human society or another will launch out on this adventure, whether the rest of mankind approves or not. If this happens, and a superior race emerges with greater intelligence and longer lives, how will these people look upon those who are lagging behind? One thing is certain: they, not we, will be the heirs to the future, and they will assume control."[2]

Among religionists, Canon Michael Hamilton, of the National Cathedral in Washington, approves of genetic engineering, when and if it is aimed at the personal improvement of humans.[3] At the same time a Jesuit theologian, Richard McCormick, condemns it because, he believes, only monogamously married heterosexual reproduction is morally licit.[4] Wearing his philosopher's hat, J. B. S. Haldane votes for genetic design,[5] but putting on the same hat, another biologist, Theodosius Dobzhansky, votes against it.[6] Disagreement is obviously at work at all levels and in all intellectual camps, from the simplest people to scientific peers.

A careful approach to the issue will avoid what I call the capacity-fallacy—i.e., the notion that because we can do something, such as genetic control, we ought to. It does not follow that because we could, we should. There is an ethical parallel in the necessity-fallacy, the assumption by some culture analysts that because we can do something, we will. Those who are fatalists—a visceral or noncephalic condition that is fairly widespread among us—naturally do not bother to ask policy questions.

Leaving aside technical philosophical conventions, let me suggest that when we tackle right-wrong or good-evil or desirable-undesirable questions there are fundamentally two alternative lines of approach. The first one supposes that whether any act or course of action is right or wrong depends on its consequences. The second approach supposes that our actions are right or wrong according to whether they comply with general moral principles or prefabricated rules of conduct. Kant's formula, "It is always wrong to treat people as means and not as ends," would be an example of decision by moral rules, or the pacifist's use of the fifth of the Ten Commandments, "Thou shalt not kill." The first approach is consequentialist; the second is a priori.

This is the rock-bottom issue, and it is also (I want to suggest) the definitive question in the ethical analysis of genetic control. Are we to reason from general propositions and universals to normative decisions, or are we to reason from empirical data, variable situations and human values to normative decisions? Which? One or the other.

Until modern times the most common form of a priori ethics was religious morality. It usually held in advance of any concrete or actual problem of conscience that certain kinds of acts, such as lying and stealing and fornicating, are always wrong intrinsically, in and of themselves, as such. Their inherent wrongness was believed by faith and by metaphysical opinion to be a matter of "natural" moral law or of divine revelation. They were always negatives, never affirmatives—prohibitions, not obligations. Such "moral laws" were presumably known to the moral agent—the actor or decision maker—through inner guidance or intuition, or by spirit guidance from outside, or by means of some more objective special revelation, like scriptures. In any case, right and wrong were determined by a religious or metaphysical or nonempirical kind of cognition. There is still a widespread disposition to take an ethical posture of this kind, even though it is often unconscious. It is metarational ethics.

Nonconsequentialists would say, therefore, that therapeutic or corrective goals are not enough to justify in vitro fertilization, positive eugenics or designed genetic changes, no matter how desirable they might be. It was this kind of ethics that Daniele Petrucci ran into several years ago in Bologna because of his experiments with artificial fertilization and cell divisions at preblastocyst stages. The Church forced him to stop, in a kind of modern Galileo episode.

The basic moral law here was the religious belief that "only God can make a tree" and only God should make a man. On this basis it would be wrong to use artificial fertilization, insemination or innovulation, or single cell replications in ectogenesis. And this "law" of the divine monopoly is also opposed to any human control of sexually produced conceptuses. In the same way it is believed that fertilization results directly in a "human" being or a "nascent" human being, so that the laboratory sacrifice of such zygotes, or the use of a prostaglandin, being abortifacient, would be intrinsically wrong as such—i.e., "murder."

Good consequences could not, to the a priori moralist, justify such acts or procedures since they are wrong as means, and the a priorist contends that "the end does not justify the means." The principle of proportionate good, or a balance of gains over costs, could not in their ethics make genetic intervention by laboratory reproduction morally permissible. Consequences, as they see it, do not decide what is right. At a recent discussion at Airlie House, Dr. Leon Kass, a molecular biologist working for the National Research Council, put the a priori position succinctly. "Morally," he said, "it is insufficient that your motives are good, that your ends are unobjectionable, that you do the procedure 'lovingly' and even that you may be lucky in the result: you will be engaging in an unethical experiment upon a human subject."[7] This is also the opinion of Paul Ramsey, a Protestant moralist who, like Father McCormick, believes that such procedures as artificial insemination from a donor, artificial innovulation, cloning and other forms of asexual reproduction are wrong—wrong because morally licit reproduction must be done heterosexually by human intercourse within the context of marriage and the family.[8]

However, some a priori moral principles are not based on metaphysical grounds. One school of utilitarians, called "rule utilitarians," make moral choices on the basis of generalizations reached empirically or clinically. They might conclude that in the expectable results of laboratory reproduction and genetic engineering, the good would be outweighed by the evil, or that the attendant risks are unknown or too great, and that therefore such procedures should be disapproved as a class or category.

Here, there is no attempt to assign an intrinsic value or dis-value; it is strictly an extrinsic appraisal. Their reason for resorting to categorical principles is usually like G. E. Moore's: that they are unwilling to trust their own judgment in situations that are apparently exceptions to the general rule. They therefore simply "rule out" some class actions (such as genetic designing) universally and categorically. Outside some theological and philosophical circles, most of the opposition to

designed genetic changes in man, or even to genetic intervention for therapeutic purposes, is based on rule-utilitarianism.

In this connection, by the way, it is only fair to point out that all religionists are not a prioristic; for example, Professor James Gustafson, of the Yale Divinity School, has asked if biomedical changes in man are intrinsically wrong and answered in the negative, but he then added that if its consequences were antihuman it would for that reason be wrong after all.[9] (Later, we shall have cause to return to this matter of the human and nonhuman.)

The more commonly held ethical approach is a different modality, a pragmatic one—sometimes sneered at by a priorists and called a "mere morality of goals." This ethics is my own, and I believe it is implicit in the ethics of all biomedical research and development as well as in medical care. We reason from the data of each actual case or problem and then choose the course that offers an optimum or maximum of desirable consequences.

On this basis we cannot reason deductively from a priori or predetermined rules about the moral justifiability of whole classes of acts, such as the in vitro fertilization of gametes and the experimental sacrifice of test zygotes, or the cloning of animal and human organisms. We agree with Jeremy Bentham: "If any act can with propriety be termed pernicious, it must be so by virtue of some events which are its consequences . . . no act, strictly speaking, can be evil in itself."[10]

For those whom we might call situational or clinical consequentialists results are what counts, and results are good when they contribute to human well-being. On that basis the real issue ethically is whether genetic change in man will, in its foreseeable or predictable results, add to or take away from human welfare. We do not act by a priori categorical rules nor by dogmatic principles, such as the religious-faith proposition that genetic intervention is forbidden to human initiative or the metaphysical claim that every individual has an inalienable right to a unique genotype—presumably according to however chance and the general

gene pool might happen to constitute it. For consequentialists, making decisions empirically is the problem. The question becomes, "When would it be right, and when would it be wrong?"

Genetic Engineering Must Be Selective

What then, might be a situation in which constructive or positive eugenics would be justified because the good to be gained—the proportionate good—would be great enough? Another way of putting it is, "When would its utility justify it?" My ability to futurize, as they say nowadays, is very limited: I am not much of a seer or forecaster, and I feel uncomfortable attempting to predict shocks of the future in long time-spans. But we have to try, even though it raises our anxiety level. We owe a great obligation to the future and to our descendants, and it would be irresponsible to repudiate the problem of genetic control by either a blanket condemnation or an uncritical endorsement. As Kierkegaard said, "To venture causes anxiety, but not to venture is to lose oneself."

Take cloning of humans, for example, as a form of genetic engineering. Although Joshua Lederberg, another Nobelist in microbiology, may be correct when he says that cloning is "merely speculative" until more experimental work with animals is done, it is still possible that such science-fiction scenarios can help value analysis and ethical examination. Diderot, G. B. Shaw, H. G. Wells, Huxley, and Lederberg himself have all foretold genetic engineering. As crystal-ball gazers they have until recently been like Priam's daughter, Cassandra, doubted and pooh-poohed. But now things are different. Now not only the doomsday people but the tut-tut reactors are having a harder time.

And yet, just because cloning is defensible in asparagus or carrot growing, it does not follow that it is all right in human baby making. I respect the ethics of scientists, which is primarily a love for and search for the facts, but some scientists seem to have an almost blind faith that somehow the facts will be used to good purposes, not misused for evil. But this is too complacent as we face the wide margin of personal and social dangers in biomedical research and practice. Therefore, whether and when genetic control could be right would depend on the situation. Let's look at a few cases, both therapeutic and eugenic.

There might be a need in the social order at large for one or more people specially constituted genetically to survive long periods outside bathyspheres at great marine depths, or outside space capsules at great heights. Control of a child's sex by cloning, to avoid any one of 50 sex-linked genetic diseases, or to meet a family's survival need, might be justifiable. I would vote for laboratory fertilization from donors to give a child to an infertile pair of spouses.

It is entirely possible, given our present increasing pollution of the human gene pool through uncontrolled sexual reproduction, that we might have to replicate healthy people to compensate for the spread of genetic diseases and to elevate the plus factors available in ordinary reproduction. It could easily come about that overpopulation would force us to put a stop to general fecundity, and then, to avoid discrimination, to resort to laboratory reproduction from unidentified cell sources. If we had "cell banks" in which the tissue of a species of wild life in danger of extinction could be stored for replication, we could do the same for the sake of endangered humans, such as the Hairy Ainu in northern Japan or certain strains of Romani gypsies.

If the greatest good of the greatest number (i.e., the social good) were served by it, it would be justifiable not only to specialize the capacities of people by cloning or by constructive genetic engineering, but also to bio-engineer or bio-design para-humans or "modified men"—as chimeras (part animal) or cyborg-androids (part prosthetes). I would vote for cloning top-grade soldiers and scientists, or for supplying them through other genetic means, if they were needed to offset an elitist or tyrannical power plot by other cloners—a truly science-fiction situation, but imaginable. I suspect I would favor making and using man-machine hybrids rather than genetically designed people for dull, unrewarding or dangerous roles needed nonetheless for the community's welfare—perhaps the testing of suspected pollution areas or the investigation of threatening volcanos or snow-slides.

Ours is a Promethean situation. We cannot clearly see what the promises and the dangers are. Both are there, in the biomedical potential. Much of the scare-mongering by whole-hog or a priori opponents of genetic control link it with tyranny. This is false and misleading. Their propaganda line supposes, for one thing, that a cloned person would be a "carbon copy" of his single-cell parent because the genotype is repeated, as if such genetically designed individuals would have no individuating personal histories or variable environments. Personalities are not shaped alone by genotypes.

Furthermore, they presume that society will be a dictatorship and that such designed or cloned people would not be allowed to marry or reproduce from the social gene pool, nor be free to choose roles and functions other than the ones for which they had a special constitutional capability. But is this realistic? Is it not, actually, a mood or attitudinal posture rather than a rational or problematic view of the question?

Dr. Lederberg has pointed out that although the scenario of the Brave New World has been widely advertised, emphasizing that a slave state could and probably would use genetic control, still "it could not be so without having instituted slavery in the first place." He adds, "It is indeed true that I might fear the control of my behavior through electrical impulses directed into my brain but . . . I do not accept the implantation of the electrodes except at the point of a gun: the gun is the problem."[11] I agree. The danger of tyranny is a real danger. But genetic controls do not lead to dictatorship—if there is any cause-and-effect relation between them it is the other way around—the reverse. People who appeal to Brave New World and 1984 and Fahrenheit 451 forget this, that the tyranny is set up first and then genetic controls are employed. The problem of misuse is political, not biological.

Reproduction in the Laboratory

The possibility of an ethical justification of genetic control, such as I have indicated, leads at once to the question of an ethical defense of its essential prerequisite—embryologic and genetic research. As I said at the outset, there are serious challenges not only to the end being sought (control) but also to the morality of the means—in vitro fertilizations, bench-made zygotes and embryos, and the entailed practice of their sacrifice in the course of investigation. If we can justify the end, can we justify the means? Does the end justify the means in this particular case? My answer is a positive Yes.

I can see only one possible objection to such research, given a humanistic and situational ethics of the sort I have explained. That objection would be that fertilizations or cloning result directly and instantly in human beings, or in creatures with nascent or proto-human status. Let me say at once that I do not believe this to be true. And that is what such a proposition calls for—belief in a faith assertion, a declaration or confession of faith. It is not in the order of either scientific or rational statements to say that such early cell tissue is human (except in the sense of the biologic specification): it is an a priori metarational opinion. It effectively excludes from its ethics all non-believers.

For example, a Catholic obstetrician in Washington, D.C., has complained that it is "arbitrary" to start regarding a fetus as human at the 20th week or at "viability," and yet the physician himself insists on the even more arbitrary religious doctrine that a fertilized ovum before implantation is human.[12] Granted that it is difficult to check off any specific point on the gestational continuum as the start of a human being, it is obvious that there is much more to be said for viability as that point than for fertilization.

Those who believe such things may be correct. There is no way to know whether they are or not. It follows for them deductively that abortion is wrong in any of its manifold forms, before or after nidation. It would also follow that the experimental sacrifice of zygotes and blastular embryos in the research process is the destruction of innocent human life or the "killing of unborn babies."

This rhetoric is again an instance of how a priori ethics reasons syllogistically from metaphysical and metarational premises to a normative conclusion, rather than consequentially. All the good results in the world, immediately or potentially, could not (they argue) justify what is wrong—in this case "homicide." Indeed, if anybody really believes that a zygote is a human being he or she ought not to terminate a pregnancy or engage in embryologic research, not only for the sake of ethical consistency but for the sake of their own mental and emotional balance.

But most of us do not make that faith assertion. This is precisely and basically what is at stake in the national debate about abortion laws—the fact that they rest on grounds of a private, personal religious conviction and should not therefore be established by government in violation of the Constitution's First Amendment. Obstetricians and gynecologists do not believe this doctrine, nor do surgeons, nor do fetologists, nor do embryologists and geneticists—except for an atypical minority involved in certain religious groups.

There are, be it noted, additional auxiliary arguments used sometimes against the research sacrifice of embryos and other fetal life, such as the claim that "it tends to lower respect for human life." But this begs the question and is not really very convincing as a consequentialist argument (which it is) and is very likely in any case to be a cover-up for the notion that fallopian and uterine cell matter is human. There is also a "feeling" in some discussants that a conceptus somehow has a "right to be born." They would be better advised to follow the reasoning of our common and statutory law, which rejects any idea of "unborn babies" and restricts the status of "baby" to the neonate, denying that any rights at all may be assigned to a fetus.

Nevertheless, these objections to laboratory reproduction uncover two further points I feel obliged to establish. Both points are metaethical in nature or at least prenormative. The first has to do with the idea of "humanness" and the second has to do with the notion of "rights."

What does it mean to say, as Dr. Kass does, that "the laboratory reproduction of human beings is no longer human procreation"?[7] (Indeed, can he reasonably charge that laboratory reproduction is non-human and still call its products "human beings"?) Man is a

maker and a selecter and a designer, and the more rationally contrived and deliberate anything is, the more human it is. Any attempt to set up an antinomy between natural and biologic reproduction, on the one hand, and artificial or designed reproduction, on the other, is absurd. The real difference is between accidental or random reproduction and rationally willed or chosen reproduction. In either case it will be biologic—according to the nature of the biologic process. If it is "unnatural" it can be so only in the sense that all medicine is.

It seems to me that laboratory reproduction is radically human compared to conception by ordinary heterosexual intercourse. It is willed, chosen, purposed and controlled, and surely these are among the traits that distinguish *Homo sapiens* from others in the animal genus, from the primates down. Coital reproduction is, therefore, less human than laboratory reproduction—more fun, to be sure, but with our separation of baby making from lovemaking, both become more human because they are matters of choice, and not chance. This is, of course, essentially the case for planned parenthood. I cannot see how either humanity or morality are served by genetic roulette.

What Is Human?

The fact is that most of our discourse about the ethics of biomedical innovation is a semantic swamp, because what we mean by "human" and ergo by "humanistic" usually remains vague and poorly defined. The question "What is it to be human?" is, however, no longer just an academic exercise for philosophers. Physicians and nurses, as well as geneticists and laboratory technicians, face it every day thousands of times. For them it is literally a life-and-death practical question. It arises in utero or in vitro when sacrifices are indicated, and it arises in terminus when decisions have to made whether to go on prolonging a patient's dying. When does a fetus become human (the better term is "personal"), when is a dying patient no longer so?

Let me suggest a conceptual approach that might be adopted. In the light of medical proposals to redefine death in terms of irreversible coma or a loss of the higher brain function (what some call "cerebral")—it might be due

to a massive hemorrhage, or a neoplasm, or a trauma—if such an excerebral patient is no longer alive in any human sense or personal sense, would it not follow that a pre-cerebral embryo or fetus is not yet alive in any human and personal sense? This would, of course, obviate any further use of such question-begging rhetoric as "killing unborn babies."

In any case, what is called for here, for consequentialists, is a quality-of-life ethics instead of the sanctity-of-life ethics in the classical Western tradition. The metarational premise or a priori that mere life or biologic process is sacrosanct is not only neither verifiable nor falsifiable; by logical inference it is inconsistent with empirical and humanistic medicine, as well as opposed to genetic and embryologic investigation.

The uncomfortable truth is that we have not yet put our heads together in an interdisciplinary way to see if we can find some "common-ground" factors and operational terms for such synthetic concepts as "human" and "personal." Some moralists—for example, Gustafson[9]—doubt if a consensus on "humanness" is possible, but it is worth a try. This may well be the most searching and fundamental problem that faces not only ethicists but society as a whole.

It is already very late. It is urgent that scientists, philosophers, sociologists, lawyers and theologians make the attempt, especially if nondoctrinaire auspices can be found. What makes a creature human? A minimum of cerebrocortical function? Self-awareness and self-control? Memory? A sense of futurity, of time? A capacity for interpersonal relationship? Communication? Love? A minimum I.Q.? Could we add a desire to live? What else? And in what order would we rank them as priorities?

Surely Senator Mondale was on the right track in 1968 when he tried to persuade Congress to propose a National Commission on Health, Science and Society. It was obstructed by people in research medicine objecting to any outside "interference." Another effort, Senate Resolution 98, was also sidetracked, in the 91st Congress of 1969. The alternative to such a thoughtful review of the implications of biomedical pioneering is apt to be hasty, unconsidered legislation. There is a palpable danger of a new Luddism, biologic this time instead of industrial. Little as we should like to be manipulated by what Gerald Leach has called "the biocrats,"[13] neither do we want to be paralyzed by know-nothingism.

Science deals with the possible and the probable, but ethics deals with the preferable—and it is at this level of analysis that the issue of designed genetic changes in man has at last brought us. We cannot any longer sweep it under the rug.

Needs First, Not Rights

My second closing point has to do with what we mean by rights. Reactionaries cannot, of course, "prove" that reproduction is ethical only when it is done heterosexually within the monogamous marriage bond, or that any one set of values or any one preferential order is the correct one, or that particular "rights" alleged by this group or that are sacrosanct. None of them are. For example, we cannot establish a supposed "right to be born," to say nothing of what one theologian has called a "right to be born with a unique genotype."[14] (By this, of course, he can only mean the accidental genotype resulting from random or so-called "natural" conception, and even so, identical twins can and do occur in nature.) All alleged "rights" are at best imperfect and relative. But what is there, then, to appeal to, to validate our humanistic concerns and our person-centered values?

My answer is: Needs are the moral stabilizers, not rights. The legalistic temper gives first place to rights, but the humanistic temper puts needs in the driver's seat. If human rights conflict with human needs, let needs prevail. If medical care can use genetic controls preventively to protect people from disease or deformity, or to ameliorate such things, then let so-called "rights" to be born step aside. If research with embryos and fetal tissue is needed to give us the means to cure and prevent the tragedies of "unique genotypes," even though it involves the sacrifice of some conceptuses, then let rights take a back seat.

Rights are nothing but a formal recognition by society of certain human needs, and as needs change with changing conditions so rights should change too. The right to conceive and bear children has to stop short of knowingly making crippled children—and genetics gives us that knowledge—just as the rights of parents have had to bow to required schooling and the rights of voluntary association have had to bow, in public services, to the human need to be respected regardless of ethnic and racial differences. It is human need that validates rights, not the other way around. I for one am not primarily concerned about any claimed rights to live or to die; I am first of all concerned about human needs, and whether they are met by life or by death will depend on the situation.

To speak of "needs" is to speak of human values. How shall we identify and rank-order them? Here, again, we have to have across-the-board cultural consultation. I agree with Michael Baram, of M.I.T., who says:

I do not think scientific peer groups presently have the objectivity or capability to function as coherent and humane social controls. The members of a peer group share the narrow confines of their discipline, and individual success is measured by the degree to which one plunges more deeply into and more narrowly draws the bounds of his research. There are no peer group rewards for activities or perceptions that extend beyond the discipline or relate it to social problems. Members are therefore neither motivated nor trained to relate their peer group activity to broader social problems.

Self-enclosed peer groups cannot be entrusted with self-control . . . because our educational system does not foster ethical and interdisciplinary values in professional training.[15]

Owing to the work of microbiologists and embryologists we are already able to produce babies born from parents who are separated by space or even by death; women are already able to nourish and gestate other women's children; one man can "father" thousands of children; virgin births or parthenogenesis (for that is what cloning is) are likely soon to be feasible; by genetic intervention we can shape babies, rather than only from the simple seed of our loins; artificial wombs and placentas are projected by biochemists and pharmacologists. All this means that we are going to have to change or alter our old ideas about who or what a father is, or a mother, or a family. Francis Crick, co-describer of DNA, and others are quite right to say that all this is going to destroy to some extent our traditional grounds for ethical beliefs.

But whatsoever new mental images take shape, within new reality situations, as long as they are tailored to a loving concern for human beings we need not be afraid. Fear is at the bottom of this debate—some of it the conventional wisdom's fear of change, some of it a fear of science, and some of it fear of freedom's power and creative control. It is, perhaps, the fear of fear itself that makes for a lot of hangups and cop-outs. But however that may be, the historic moral order has always presupposed heterosexual coital conception as necessary for the continuance of life, and now that is no longer the case. The familiar phrase "the facts of life" is an archaism.

I agree with Roger Shinn that in the sequence or progression from aspirin to insulin to artificial kidneys to brain surgery to genetic engineering there is no point at which we can "change from a clear yes to an absolute no," even though there is a mounting difference in the complexity of the ethical issues posed.[16] We cannot accept the "invisible hand" of blind natural chance or random nature in genetics any more than we could old Professor Jevon's theory of feast and famine in 19th-century laissez-faire economics, based on sun spots and tidal movements. To be men we must be in control. That is the first and last ethical word. For when there is no choice there is no possibility of ethical action. Whatever we are compelled to do is a-moral.

The moral philosopher, sensitive to social ethics, can only echo what the biologist Robert Sinsheimer has said: "As the discoveries accumulate, as new means of biological intervention arise, we can envision such possibilities as the almost indefinite prolongation of life for at least a few, the deliberate predetermination of sex, or the design of human genetic change for varied purposes. With these will come the necessity for multiple social decisions of the most profound consequence."[17]

The pressure of social decision-making is now forcing us to dig deeper than the technical hardware sciences; we now have to grapple with the personal and human software sciences—especially biology and the crossroads it reveals to us, just ahead.

References

1. *Britannica Book of the Year* 1964. Chicago, Encyclopaedia Britannica Inc. 1964, pp. 499–500.

2. Rosenfeld, A. *The Second Genesis: The Coming Control of Life.* Englewood Cliffs, New Jersey, Prentice-Hall, 1969, p. 145.

3. Hamilton M., New life for old: genetic decisions. *Christ Century* 86:741–744, 1969.

4. McCormick, R., Notes on moral theology. *Theologic Studies* 30: 680–692, 1969.

5. Haldane, J. B. S., Biological possibilities for the human species in the next ten thousand years, in *Man and His Future,* ed. G. Wolstenholme. Boston: Little, Brown, 1963, pp. 337–361.

6. Dobzhansky, T. *Heredity and the Nature of Man.* New York: Harcourt, Brace and World, 1964.

7. Kass, L. New beginnings in life, in *Three Medical Futures,* ed. M. Hamilton. Grand Rapids, Michigan: Eerdmans Publishing Company (in press).

8. Ramsey, P., Moral and religious implications of genetic control. *Genetics and the Future of Man,* ed. J. D. Roslansky. Amsterdam: North-Holland Publishing Company, 1966, pp. 107–169.

9. Gustafson, J. Basic ethical issues in the biomedical fields. *Soundings* 52:151–180, 1970.

10. Bentham, J. The influence of time and place in matters of legislation, *The Works of Jeremy Bentham,* Vol. 1, ed. J. Bowring. London, Simpkin, Marshall, and Company, 1843, pp. 169–194.

11. Lederberg, J: Genetic engineering, or the amelioration of genetic defect. *Pharos* 34:9–12, 1971.

12. Helleger, A. Letter to the editor. *Washington Post,* January 9, 1971, p. A21.

13. Leach, G. *The Biocrats,* New York: McGraw-Hill, 1970.

14. Ramsey, P. *Fabricated Man: The Ethics of Genetic Control.* New Haven: Yale University Press, 1970.

15. Baram, M. S., Social control of science and technology. *Science* 172:535–539, 1971.

16. Shinn, R., The ethics of genetic engineering. *N. D. State Univ Bull.,* April 22, 1967, pp. 13–21.

17. Sinsheimer, R., The implications of recent advances in biology for the future of medicine. *Eng. Sci.* 34:6–13, 1970.

Abortion

66

Harold G. Villard

Legalized Elimination of the Unborn in Soviet Russia

Reprinted with permission of the publisher from the *Journal of Social Hygiene*, vol. 12, 1926, pp. 294–298.

By a decree of N. A. Semashko, People's Health Commissary, published in the November 18, 1920, issue of the journal *Isvestija*, expectant mothers in Soviet Russia were granted the right to undergo an operation for the interruption of their pregnancy in the state hospitals of that country whenever they could convince the authorities that they had good reasons, such as poverty or ill-health, for refusing to bring another child into the world. Thus, unlike most other civilized communities where the intentional procuring of a miscarriage is regarded as a crime and is forbidden under severe penalties, the interruption of gestation is legally permissible in Russia in cases where the local Government medical commission is satisfied that a woman has just grounds for wishing to avoid being a mother.

The Russian law only permits physicians on the staff of public hospitals to perform operations for ridding a woman of a coming child and makes it a punishable offense for anyone else to practice such surgery. The statute has run for too short a period as yet to enable one to judge of its ultimate consequences or of its effect in the long run on public morality and the growth of population. According to the latest available advices, however, pregnant Russian women are freely and in increasing numbers availing themselves of the opportunity thus afforded to escape motherhood under the best hygienic conditions and with the least possible risk.

The extent to which this right is being made use of is revealed by certain figures published in the January-March, 1925, issue of the *Bulletin of the Leningrad Province Statistical Office* [pp. 205–207] wherein it is stated that 31,601 infants were born in the district comprising the former Russian capital in 1924. During the same year 6692 legally sanctioned operations, or the equivalent of 21 per cent of the total number of births, were performed in the various municipal hospitals to relieve women with child of their prospective offspring as contrasted with 2983 like operations and 31,906 births in 1923, when only limited facilities existed for disposing of such cases. Only 81 out of every 100 applications for such succor were allowed by the authorities in the last five months of

Table 66-1

Age Categories	Percent of Legal Miscarriages	Percent of All Children Born
16–19	2.5	4.1
20–24	27.5	32.7
25–29	30.7	32.1
30–34	22.6	18.4
35–39	12.6	9.4
40 and over	4.1	3.3
Total	100.0	100.0

1924. Of the rejected petitions 72 per cent were refused on the ground that the parents were possessed of ample means, 8 per cent because pregnancy was too far advanced, 7 per cent because less than a year had elapsed since the last previous miscarriage, and 6 per cent because the health of the mother was held not to be endangered.

On the other hand, in the 3485 instances in which the desired relief was allowed during the five months mentioned the permission was granted in 72 per cent of all cases by reason of the poverty of the parents, and in 17 per cent more because of the mother's state of health. In one out of 24 cases the woman was still nursing her last child and in one out of 45 cases the large size of the family was given as the deciding factor.

As appears from Table 66-1, the average age of the women who were allowed to have miscarriages in Leningrad during 1924 was 29 years.

The above figures show that it is the women over 30 years of age who are most anxious to have a miscarriage. Presumably the majority of these had already been mothers, for from statistics compiled at Jekaterinburg (now known as Sverdlovsk) it was found that those disinclined to undergo another confinement had borne 4.5 children on the average and did not feel able to take care of any more. In these cases of permitted abortions poverty is generally the compelling motive. At Leningrad more than half of the women involved belonged to the working class, a fifth were employees in receipt of a small stipend, while a tenth were without any gainful occupation.

As the public hospitals are not yet fully equipped to handle all cases and as many women are deterred by a feeling of shame or false modesty from presenting themselves at public institutions, the number of illicit abortions in Russia is still very large. It is claimed that women undergoing operations of this character in public hospitals run no greater risk of infection or of injury to their health than in an ordinary case of childbirth. In the Abrikossow maternity hospital, which is the largest establishment of its kind in Moscow, puerperal fever developed in only 2.9 per cent of all the miscarriages treated in 1922, whereas during the same year the corresponding percentage in the city hospitals of Munich was 33 per cent. This bears out the contention of the advocates of legal abortions in Russia that their introduction would cause far less injury to the health of pregnant women than now happens in countries where artificially produced miscarriages are forbidden by law.

For the object of the Russian authorities in sanctioning the destruction of unborn babies under certain safeguards was to lessen as far as possible the harm that is being done to womanhood by deliberately induced abortions. This deplorable evil is prevalent in all countries and is attended by an incalculable amount of bodily and mental anguish on the part of its women victims, of whom from seven to eight thousand are said to die annually in Germany alone. In that country 400,000 cases of such malpractice were estimated to have taken place during 1923, as compared with 1,612,000 births. In the case of France, where less than 800,000 births are now occurring annually, the similar total is given as 300,000, of which 50,000 are attributed to Paris alone. Before the World War a like proportion was reported at Vienna, namely, 14,000 artificially caused miscarriages to 40,000 births. Penal legislation against this social affliction has everywhere proved ineffective and difficult to enforce. Between the years 1881 and 1900 only 277 criminal abortion cases were tried in the whole of France, while elsewhere in Europe it is commonly believed that not one in 1000 of such cases are prosecuted.

Repressive measures have not materially affected the number of premeditated feticides, which in all large centers tend to increase. At Berlin Dr. Vollmann asserts that, instead of ten, as thirty-five years ago, there are now forty miscarriages to every hundred pregnancies. Fully two-thirds of these are deliberately brought on. The laws now in force have not stopped the practice against which they are directed but have made the women resolved on a step of this kind the prey of unscrupulous quacks and degraded midwives. The statutes have failed of their purpose for the reason that they do not touch the cause of the evil which they are supposed to suppress, namely, poverty. Statistics compiled in Austria show, for example, that only one-tenth of 1 per cent of all the transgressing women were well to do, 7.9 per cent possessed small means, while the remaining 92 per cent were extremely poor.

Since the threat of prison has proved a futile corrective the present rulers of Russia feel that the best way of combating this scourge and confining it within the narrowest feasible limits is by their existing system of permissive and medically safeguarded miscarriages. All civilized states exact that enceinte women shall bring children into the world even though the mothers of such infants are often unable to provide them with nourishing food or adequate clothing. This policy the Russians regard as inhumane. In their opinion only where a State obligates itself to look after the babies that see the light of day has it the right to insist on compulsory motherhood. A child is entitled to be happily born and the bestowal of life is no boon to a nonconscious embryo if it is to suffer want and privation from the time of its birth.

The Russian authorities believe further that the doing away with unwanted offsprings will lessen poverty and raise eugenic standards. Where there is barely enough bread to go round the advent of another child means inadequate nourishment for a worker's entire family and operates against the younger members of it growing into strong and healthy adults. It is immoral for parents to have more children than they can provide adequate food for. Measures taken by the State against such an unfortunate contingency are therefore thoroughly justified and would make for the progress of the human race.

So far there is not the least indication of other countries accepting this viewpoint. The teaching of the Christian and in fact of all religions that any interference with the normal course of propagation is sinful still holds the ascendancy.

Not long ago France passed another law with stricter penalties against abortions and the sale of contraceptives. In Germany the doctors have recently opposed any change in the existing statutes on the ground that, while the provisions against artificially induced abortions are disregarded by hundreds of thousands, they are respected by as many more. An overwhelming majority felt that the abolition of the present legal prohibitions would lead to all sorts of evils and corrupt public morals. Until a change occurs in the existing social order it does not seem likely that Russian legislation on the subject of miscarriages passed primarily in the interests of the proletariat will be copied elsewhere.

67

Abortion: Medico-Legal and Ethical Aspects:

A Discussion Held at the Royal Society of Medicine, London, 1927

Reprinted with permission of the publisher from the *British Medical Journal*, vol. 1, 1927, pp. 188–191.

A joint meeting of the Medico-Legal Society and the Section of Obstetrics and Gynaecology of the Royal Society of Medicine was held on January 21st to consider the medico-legal and ethical aspects of abortion. Sir Arthur Claveli Salter (Mr. Justice Salter) presided over a very large attendance.

The Medical View

Dr. J. S. Fairbairn began by outlining, for the benefit of non-medical members of the audience, the medical causes for which abortion might be induced, including diseases peculiar to pregnancy on the one hand, and on the other diseases which pregnancy aggravated or which made it particularly dangerous. In diabetes or kidney or heart disease there was general agreement that if the condition was serious and did not improve in spite of medical treatment, abortion might be induced. With regard to tuberculosis, certain forms of malnutrition, and certain nervous and mental states, there was divergence of opinion as to the advantages of terminating the pregnancy. In the case of women who had been insane in a previous pregnancy, the usual rule was that, if a second pregnancy followed soon, it should be terminated. On the other hand, if there had been some complication not likely to recur, such as excessive bleeding or septic infection, which was clearly the provoking cause of the mental disorder, it was usual to allow the pregnancy to continue. The commonest reason, especially in hospital, for interfering with pregnancy was that some damage had already occurred; in that case the treatment was not the induction of abortion, but the completion of an abortion already started. The original principle that guided the profession was that induction was lawful only if the woman's life was endangered by the pregnancy, but this had been rightly extended to include cases in which serious or permanent damage to health might result. During the last twenty-five years there had been an increasing extension of the practice, and many in the profession acted on the supposition that it was not unlawful to take into consideration other than purely medical factors, including social, economic, and eugenic reasons.

The present meeting arose out of a discussion at the British Medical Association Annual Meeting in Nottingham (*British Medical Journal*, August 7th, 1926, p. 237), and Dr. Fairbairn drew attention to a case cited by the opener of that discussion—the case of a barrister and his wife who took the view that, "the prospective baby being theirs, it was their own affair whether they allowed their work to be completed or not"—as an instance of the casuistical arguments sometimes employed. The pregnancy was terminated in that case, on the ground that rapidly recurring pregnancies affected the mother's health. but within six months pregnancy happened again, and this time interference was refused, but the couple went to another doctor who was more pliable. The rule might be inferred "one abortion per patient," but it did not work, for what happened was "one abortion per patient per doctor"! The effect of the spread of loose views was to produce a vicious circle, for as the public learned that abortion could be easily procured under the guise of medical indications, each individual failed to see why her medical attendant should hesitate in her case, and thus pressure was put upon doctors. The causes of a lowered professional standard were the greater safety and more frequent resort to operative procedure through medicine, the effect of the attitude of the general public on the profession (the ethical standard had been greatly lowered from the same causes which had given an impetus to the conception-control movement), and the changed social conditions which made women more liable to depression and nervous exhaustion under the strain of child-bearing. He advocated that none other than purely medical considerations should be allowed to weigh, and dissented from the "hopelessly inverted" statement of the position by the opener of the discussion at Nottingham that "It is an ethical question of great interest to what extent we as doctors have the right to insist that a woman shall pass through an ordeal which she is unwilling to face, even if we do not think that she will sustain any permanent injury from so doing." It was not a question of "the right to insist," it was a question whether there was any right to interfere with normal pregnancy. This matter should be thought out in terms of hospital rather than of private practice. The private practitioner was more directly under the influence of his patients and their relatives; in hospital factors other than medical did not weigh, and unless her condition was very urgent the patient was kept under observation and treatment until it was seen that all other measures of relief had failed before abortion was induced. Abortion-mongering was but infanticide anticipated by a few months. Perhaps it was too much to expect the populace to think the non-sentient embryo of much account, but medical men knew that the little heart was beating very soon after the patient was aware that she was pregnant. The Soviet Republic of Russia had legalized abortion (*British Medical Journal*, October 30th, 1926, p. 802), and the spread of loose views in the profession regarding its responsibility must tend towards a similar state of affairs in this country. Medical indications alone should be considered in deciding on the induction of abortion; such indications should be defined as those clearly involving danger to life or health of mother or damage to the pregnancy sufficient to interfere with its future development, and the onus of proof should rest on the practitioners concerned. In border-line cases observation of the patient away from home and failure of other methods of treatment should have proved abortion to be the only recourse.

Legal and Ethical Aspects

Lord Riddell summarized the law relating to abortion. The legal position might be stated as follows: if the mother died in consequence of an illegal operation the person performing it might be charged with murder or manslaughter, but these offences could not be committed with respect to a child in the mother's womb, as the child was not *in rerum natura*. If, however, the child was born alive and subsequently died owing to injuries received *en ventre sa mere*, the offender was liable. In Russell on *Crimes* acts were described as lawful which were done in the course of proper treatment and in the interest of the life or health of the mother. *Midwifery by Ten Teachers*

stated that operations of this kind were confined to cases in which the life of the mother would be endangered or her health likely to be permanently damaged by the continuation of the pregnancy. Lord Riddell thought the word "permanent" inaccurate. Induction was not only justifiable, but a duty when the pregnancy indicated grave danger to the mother's health, whether the result was likely to be permanent or not. But it was not justified for the purpose of avoiding the minor risks of pregnancy. The practitioner must not be influenced by the appeals of the patient or her relatives to relieve her of these ordinary risks and discomforts, nor by economic considerations in the case, nor by his compassion for a woman in a distressing situation. He must remember, however, that the mother's life must never be sacrificed for the unborn child, even though she be suffering from incurable disease; on the other hand, the possibility of diseased offspring was no indication for abortion. It could not be denied that there were practitioners ready to seize on any reason to justify abortion when desired by the patient, and offences could not be readily detected in the case of a married woman attended by two medical men. The practitioner dealing with a pregnant unmarried woman was faced with a problem of great difficulty. If he procured abortion his motives were open to question; if he failed to do what was necessary to preserve the life or health of his patient he was liable to grave moral condemnation and possibly legal consequences. The practitioner should always act openly, and seek the support of a second opinion, and if his motives were right he had little to fear. The patient, however, should not be prejudiced by her medical adviser's conscientious scruples. If the practitioner thought abortion necessary, and therefore legally justifiable, but his conscience would not allow him to procure it, the patient should be made to understand that she was being attended by a doctor whose convictions she might or might not share. Lord Riddell sketched the history of abortion from pagan times, and said that the doctrine that the mother was to be sacrificed or risked for the benefit of the unborn child was a relic of the Dark Ages and was biologically unsound. A point to be noted was that even the Roman

Catholic Church discriminated between early and late abortion. The decretal of Gregory IX (1244) defined abortion as homicide if the child had quickened, otherwise not.

Border-line Cases

Dr. H. Russell Andrews, taking the place of Dr. Watts Eden, who was unable to attend, thought that Dr. Fairbairn was going too far when he suggested that the profession in any general way had given up the former definite indications for the induction of abortion. If not, he could only think that Dr. Fairbairn associated with a laxer type of general practitioner than he did himself. Some cases which came to the consultant were easily dealt with, and after investigation a common-sense talk with husband and wife convinced them that the pregnancy ought not to be interrupted. At the other end of the scale were cases in which there could hardly be any difference of opinion that continuation of the pregnancy was fraught with danger to life or possible impairment of health. It was the border-line cases which gave anxiety, and personally he had often had a cowardly wish that the patient's medical adviser had chosen some other consultant. The medical man must sympathize with the tired, exhausted, anxious patient who felt that she could not face the ordeal of many months' disability and ill health, but he realized that he must not allow his judgment to be swayed by sympathy alone, and looked for some definite peg on which to hang his decision one way or the other. The condition was often complicated by what was actually an obsession or fixed idea in the mind of both husband and wife, based on advice given some months or years before, by one or more doctors, that there must not be another pregnancy. On two or three occasions, when he thought that this advice had been given lightly and on insufficient grounds, and remarked that there was a great difference between advising against another pregnancy and destroying life, he was met with the retort that there would not be much difference if only doctors would be more logical. It was impossible to lay down hard and fast rules for the conduct of border-line cases; each case must be judged on its merits. Dr. An-

drews then described in detail two cases in which he had been consulted during the last few months, and in which he had felt justified in advising induction.

Criminal and Non-criminal Abortion

Sir Travers Humphreys said that from his point of view the subject was divided into two parts: criminal and non-criminal abortion. By the latter he meant the steps which were taken by a qualified man to get rid of a condition in his patient which he was satisfied, on medical grounds alone, was dangerous to the patient's life or health. With that the law had no concern whatever. It might be that the patient asked a medical man to induce abortion because, for example, she feared social disgrace or for other non-medical reasons. These might form matters for advice to the patient so long as she was not in the condition of pregnancy, but in considering the induction of abortion he was not entitled to let anything weigh with him except the health of his patient—her medical welfare as distinct from her social or economic welfare. To say that a medical man would fortify his view by obtaining the best opinion he could, and that he would not interfere with the ordinary course of nature except for the gravest reasons, was only to say that he would do what a doctor would do in any case involving grave issues. Criminal abortion in this country was recognized as a very serious crime, and in the United States, France, and Belgium the law was similar to our own. In the Belgian penal code there was a provision that any person who caused abortion, even without desire to do so, by violence, or, as we should say, by ill treatment, was liable to extreme punishment. Those who studied French journals might be disposed to doubt whether in France the practice of abortion was regarded with quite as much distaste as it was by French law, but the mere fact, if it was a fact, that a certain number of people disregarded the law did not alter the law. It must be the law in every civilized country that criminal abortion was regarded in a very serious light, and the fact that abortion was legalized in Soviet Russia

did not alter the case, because he was speaking of civilized countries. The induction of abortion, at all events by any other than the most highly qualified and skilful person, was fraught with the gravest possible danger to the woman. No doubt the increasing prevalence of the crime of abortion in this country was due to the widespread belief that abortion, at least in the early stages of pregnancy, was without risk; but he had heard Sir Bernard Spilsbury combat that idea in the witness-box, and say that there was no such thing as safe procurement, even in the early stage. He hoped medical men would impress that fact upon any of their patients who might be under misapprehensions on the subject.

General Discussion

Dr. Halliday Sutherland referred to the effect of tuberculosis upon pregnancy. It had no constant influence. Women, even in advanced stages of the disease, had brought forth healthy children at full time. There were cases in which the onset of pregnancy was associated with increased severity of the disease, but others in which it was associated with amelioration. He quoted figures from the Stockholm maternity clinic which showed that actually the pregnant tuberculous woman had a rather better expectation of life than the non-pregnant tuberculous woman. He did not doubt that a very early diagnosis of tuberculosis might be of considerable value to those who desired to arrange an "irreproachable" abortion for non-medical reasons, but he hoped that as a result of the present discussion the medical sanctions for abortion, so far from being extended, would be curtailed. Every advance in medical treatment must reduce the occasions on which danger to life or health might be cited in defence of that which was, at best, an act of despair, and at worst a crime akin to murder. If any section of the profession were carried away on the wave of criminal sentimentality passing over the country he would suggest that their activities might be checked by making abortion compulsorily notifiable.

Earl Russell said that, in view of the existing law, it struck him as curious that from some of the cases quoted on the medical side the practice of gynaecologists should have been extended to a degree which went far beyond the narrow consideration of risk to life or health, and amounted in many cases to relieving the patient from a very inconvenient and unpleasant time. It showed how doctors, as he had always maintained, were the high priests of modern civilization and were above the law. The doctors declared in their gynaecological discussions what it was right to do in cases of this sort, and Sir Travers Humphreys said that there was no appeal to a legal tribunal. Sir Travers said that the sole thing they had to consider was the interest of the patient. If that was the case, surely one would apply to the question of removing a foetus the same tests and considerations as one would apply to the removal of any tumour. All operations were dangerous, and Sir Travers had stressed the dangers of abortion. But in these cases of very dangerous operation the choice was generally left to the patient. The ethical view, as stated by Dr. Fairbairn, given the present state of our law, was perfectly correct and unassailable, but the ultimate ethical law was not necessarily that embodied on the statute book, and he was inclined to take the German view which Lord Riddell had quoted, in which it was insisted that the foetus was not yet an independent human being, and that every woman, by virtue of the right over her own body, was entitled to decide whether it should become one. In a matter of this sort the mother, and the mother alone, ought to be the arbiter. What was at present on the statute book was there on religious grounds, and probably could be defended on those grounds, but there was no justification for imposing those grounds on others. Great efforts were being made for the preservation of child life, and he would be the first to recognize the undoubted moral duty of the mother to do the best she could for the child that was to be born, but that did not affect his view that the mother should be mistress of the situation, and the State, unless it said that deliberately it took a certain course for reasons of population and the like, had really no abstract right to deal with the matter. That was not the existing law, but it was his view of the fundamental ethics.

Professor Louise McIlroy agreed with most of what Dr. Fairbairn had said.

She held also that when any abortion took place it ought to be notified to the State, just as was a stillbirth or a live birth. She knew that it was easy for those of them who were specialists in a large city to take a high ethical view, but it was not so easy for the struggling practitioner in his district when perhaps a patient of means and influence wanted him to take this course. He was inclined in such circumstances to look about for some medical excuse for performing abortion, knowing that if he refused she might be the means of greatly injuring his practice. It had been said that this was a woman's question, but the question whether pregnancy should be terminated was a moral question which affected both sexes equally. She greatly resented the assumption of some patients that they could go to the consulting room and lay down to their doctor a line of treatment in much the same spirit as they would approach the bargain counter. She was sure she was speaking for other members of her specialty when she said that none of them looked upon the induction of abortion as anything but homicide. As time went on, and methods of treatment improved, abortion would be regarded as a confession of failure, and would be practised less and less by gynaecologists. In one aspect, however, it was a woman's question—namely, in the cases of pregnancy following rape. There she would like to have legal permission to prevent continuation of the pregnancy, for she saw no reason why the woman should suffer it.

Dr. F. J. McCann said that an extraordinary wave of abortion-mongering had proceeded over Europe since the war. Bills were now tabled in the German, Austrian, and Swiss parliaments seeking to legalize abortion during the first three months. He was one of those who held that there was no ethical reason for procuring abortion. Unless strong opposition were taken to the first ethical loophole being made it would be disastrous to the country. The reason why abortion was spreading was because it was believed that in the early stages there was no life and that abortion in those stages was free from risk. It could not be too widely known by the public that there was life from conception onwards, and that there was grave danger from abortion even in the most skilled hands. He

had seen danger arise from merely dilating the neck of the womb without the necessity of emptying it. He was inclined to criticize the lawyers for certain legal confusions. Thirty years ago the Royal College of Physicians took counsel's opinion, which was that the law did not forbid the procurement of abortion during pregnancy or the destruction of the child during labour where such procurement or destruction was necessary to save the mother's life. It was on that pronouncement that many of them had acted ever since. But there were some peculiarities about the law. One, for example, was that, whether the woman was really pregnant or not, an attempt made by another person with the idea of procuring abortion was a crime, but if the woman made the attempt herself she committed a crime only if she was pregnant.

Dr. Marie Stopes protested against Dr. Fairbairn's statement that the movement for "constructive birth control" tended to produce a slackening of moral fibre. The ethics of abortion had not been touched by any speaker in a fundamental way. Everybody had spoken as if this was an exceptional condition in which a patient came to a medical man, and, if he refused to do what she wanted, there was no more to be said. But abortion was going on all over the country, by other than medical practitioners, in an open and barefaced manner. Thousands of persons assumed that it was the most natural thing, involving no legal or other consequences. She protested strongly against the sale of abortifacients, some of them under her own name, in shops not far from Wimpole Street. She had been to Scotland Yard on the subject, and was told that she could be defied by the participators in this shameless trade, who apparently could use any name they pleased in connexion with their abortifacients, and the person concerned had no redress.

Dr. Beresford Kingsford supported the view taken by Earl Russell that in fundamental ethics the mother should be the mistress of the situation. If depriving the community of potential citizens was really the offence, what about the sale of contraceptive appliances? If abortion prevented the State from having hundreds of future citizens, these appliances—as to which he expressed no opinion—prevented it from having thousands, perhaps hundreds of thousands. But the fact was that the country was getting more children than it needed. It did not need them in peace, because it had more people than it could employ; nor in war, because it had been shown that true reliance in war was not upon a C3 population, but upon the united voluntary effort of the King's dominions.

Sir Bernard Spilsbury said that biologically the individual must be regarded as starting life from the moment of conception. The fact of birth was a mere incident in the life of an individual. Regarded from that point of view, the only sanction for abortion that could be recognized was that the life or health of the mother was seriously endangered by pregnancy. Legally the destruction of the foetus *in utero* was not murder, but morally it certainly was unless there was justification for terminating the pregnancy prematurely owing to danger to the mother from its continuance. There could be no question that abortion was extremely rife. Probably the cases that came into court were only a small proportion of those in which abortion was procured, and the proportion that came into court was lower than it was a quarter of a century ago, partly because the skill of the professional abortionist had increased of recent years.

Dr. Archibald Donald deprecated the view that this was purely a question for the mother—apparently not even for the father. He owed a great deal to the sex, but in these matters he was bound to say that many women seemed to have no moral sense whatever. With regard to medical reasons for inducing abortion, the cases of the kind with which he had been concerned had been, as to the great majority, cases of excessive vomiting of pregnancy; in other cases the patients were seriously ill from heart trouble or uraemia or such conditions. It would be a great disaster if the medical profession departed from its traditions in this matter.

Mr. Justice Salter's Summing Up

The Chairman said that, looking at this question in the precise—he would not say pedantic—manner to which

lawyers were accustomed, it seemed to him to narrow down to this: what was and what ought to be the law with regard to artificially procuring abortion? Every doctor desired to be within the law, and desired the law to be so framed that his duties as a citizen might never conflict with the duties of his profession. Taylor, in his *Medical Jurisprudence,* had a section headed "Justifiable abortion," but laid it down that there was no such thing as abortion justified in law, and the editor of the latest edition of that work had retained that opinion. It seemed to him (the learned judge) to be at least arguable that the Legislature, in forbidding the unlawful use of instruments or drugs, implied that there was such a thing as lawful use. Dr. Fairbairn's position was that either the law allowed, or should be amended to allow, abortion in every case where, after all due examination, delay, and inquiry, it was the considered opinion of the medical man that abortion was absolutely necessary to save the life of the mother or to prevent grave, possibly permanent, injury to her health. The mother's life, certainly; the mother's health, in the grave sense of the word, yes; and there was a third class where it was a question of the future health of the child. Suppose it became clear during the pregnancy that one or other parent was afflicted with some disease very commonly inherited, would there be medical justification for abortion? He would regard that as a very difficult case indeed. Then there were non-medical cases in which it was sought to justify abortion on such grounds as that [pregnancy] would interfere with the mother's social amusements, that abortion would be a means of avoiding disgrace and exposure, or— stronger in its appeal than any of these—that the unfortunate woman had been the victim of rape. Two speakers had urged that the prospective mother was the mistress of the situation. He certainly agreed that she should have more say than anyone else, but if he might put into blunter English the contention of those speakers it was that abortion should be lawful in any case in which the mother desired it or even consented to it. That seemed to him to go rather far. Here was a living thing,

approaching the moment of birth, having in many senses a separate existence already, and the mother was to be at liberty, if she pleased, to have its life ended! After it was born was she still to have that right, and, if not, why not? The ethics of this question could not be considered without bearing in mind the close connexion which there always was between abortion and infanticide. In the later pagan era there was an enormous traffic in the "exposure" of unwanted children, who were taken by speculators and reared as slaves or prostitutes. He had been impressed by a phrase used by Professor McIlroy, that abortion was homicide, and justifiable abortion was justifiable homicide. If abortion were ever sanctioned outside the medical area— in the interest of eugenics, for example, or for economic, social, or personal reasons—he would have great fear that within the medical area there would arise a large class of pliant doctors who would be very easily persuaded that there were sufficient medical reasons in a given case. And in this matter, as in so many others, it would be all to the advantage of the rich, while the poor would find it more difficult to get a favourable "opinion." Some speakers had boggled at the idea of many abortions on the same woman. But if one, why not many? He believed that if it were ever proposed to extend the liberty of abortion outside very strictly recognized and limited medical grounds those who proposed such a change would find themselves up against an enormously powerful body of public opinion—a body rather inarticulate, perhaps, and influenced rather by atavistic ideas, but none the less powerful. One of the most striking features of the early Christian Church was its attitude towards abortion, which in the later pagan era had been practised enormously, and was regarded in the light of a venial wrong, much as sexual excess was regarded. The attitude of the infant Church was from the first uncompromising, and never wavered, and he was certain that if it were ever proposed to extend the liberty of abortion that spirit of unswerving opposition would rise again. The discussion had revealed the great difficulty and delicacy of the question, and certainly its profound importance, and it had been a great satisfaction to him to take the chair.

68

Roe v. *Wade*, Decision on Abortion by the United States Supreme Court

Reprinted from 410 U.S. 116 (1973)

Mr. Justice Blackmun delivered the opinion of the Court.

This Texas federal appeal and its Georgia companion, *Doe* v. *Bolton, post,* p. 179, present constitutional challenges to state criminal abortion legislation. The Texas statutes under attack here are typical of those that have been in effect in many States for approximately a century. The Georgia statutes, in contrast, have a modern cast and are a legislative product that, to an extent at least, obviously reflects the influences of recent attitudinal change, of advancing medical knowledge and techniques, and of new thinking about an old issue.

We forthwith acknowledge our awareness of the sensitive and emotional nature of the abortion controversy, of the vigorous opposing views, even among physicians, and of the deep and seemingly absolute convictions that the subject inspires. One's philosophy, one's experiences, one's exposure to the raw edges of human existence, one's religious training, one's attitudes toward life and family and their values, and the moral standards one establishes and seeks to observe, are all likely to influence and to color one's thinking and conclusions about abortion.

In addition, population growth, pollution, poverty, and racial overtones tend to complicate and not to simplify the problem.

Our task, of course, is to resolve the issue by constitutional measurement, free of emotion and of predilection. We seek earnestly to do this, and, because we do, we have inquired into, and in this opinion place some emphasis upon, medical and medical-legal history and what that history reveals about man's attitudes toward the abortion procedure over the centuries. We bear in mind, too, Mr. Justice Holmes' admonition in his now-vindicated dissent in *Lochner* v. *New York,* 198 U. S. 45, 76 (1905):

[The Constitution] is made for people of fundamentally differing views, and the accident of our finding certain opinions natural and familiar or novel and even shocking ought not to conclude our judgment upon the question whether statutes embodying them conflict with the Constitution of the United States.

I

The Texas statutes that concern us here are Arts. 1191–1194 and 1196 of the State's Penal Code.[1] These make it a crime to "procure an abortion," as therein defined, or to attempt one, except with respect to "an abortion procured or attempted by medical advice for the purpose of saving the life of the mother." Similar statutes are in existence in a majority of the States.[2]

Texas first enacted a criminal abortion statute in 1854. Texas Laws 1854, c. 49, § 1, set forth in 3 H. Gammel, Laws of Texas 1502 (1898). This was soon modified into language that has remained substantially unchanged to the present time. See Texas Penal Code of 1857, c. 7, Arts. 531–536; G. Paschal, Laws of Texas, Arts. 2192–2197 (1866); Texas Rev. Stat., c. 8, Arts. 536–541 (1879); Texas Rev. Crim. Stat., Arts. 1071–1076 (1911). The final article in each of these compilations provided the same exceptions, as does the present Article 1196, for an abortion by "medical advice for the purpose of saving the life of the mother."[3]

II

Jane Roe,[4] a single woman who was residing in Dallas County, Texas, instituted this federal action in March 1970 against the District Attorney of the county. She sought a declaratory judgment that the Texas criminal abortion statutes were unconstitutional on their face, and an injunction restraining the defendant from enforcing the statutes.

Roe alleged that she was unmarried and pregnant; that she wished to terminate her pregnancy by an abortion "performed by a competent, licensed physician, under safe, clinical conditions"; that she was unable to get a "legal" abortion in Texas because her life did not appear to be threatened by the continuation of her pregnancy; and that she could not afford to travel to another jurisdiction in order to secure a legal abortion under safe conditions. She claimed that the Texas statutes were unconstitutionally vague and that they abridged her right of personal privacy, protected by the First, Fourth, Fifth, Ninth, and Fourteenth Amendments. By an amendment to her complaint Roe purported to sue "on behalf of herself and all other women" similarly situated.

James Hubert Hallford, a licensed physician, sought and was granted leave to intervene in Roe's action. In his complaint he alleged that he had been arrested previously for violations of the Texas abortion statutes and that two such prosecutions were pending against him. He described conditions of patients who came to him seeking abortions, and he claimed that for many cases he, as a physician, was unable to determine whether they fell within or outside the exception recognized by Article 1196. He alleged that, as a consequence, the statutes were vague and uncertain, in violation of the Fourteenth Amendment, and that they violated his own and his patients' rights to privacy in the doctor-patient relationship and his own right to practice medicine, rights he claimed were guaranteed by the First, Fourth, Fifth, Ninth, and Fourteenth Amendments.

John and Mary Doe,[5] a married couple, filed a companion complaint to that of Roe. They also named the District Attorney as defendant, claimed like constitutional deprivations, and sought declaratory and injunctive relief. The Does alleged that they were a childless couple; that Mrs. Doe was suffering from a "neural-chemical" disorder; that her physician had "advised her to avoid pregnancy until such time as her condition has materially improved" (although a pregnancy at the present time would not present "a serious risk" to her life); that, pursuant to medical advice, she had discontinued use of birth control pills; and that if she should become pregnant, she would want to terminate the pregnancy by an abortion performed by a competent, licensed physician under safe, clinical conditions. By an amendment to their complaint, the Does purported to sue "on behalf of themselves and all couples similarly situated."

The two actions were consolidated and heard together by a duly convened three-judge district court. The suits thus presented the situations of the pregnant single woman, the childless couple, with the wife not pregnant, and the licensed practicing physician, all joining in the attack on the Texas criminal abortion statutes. Upon the filing of affidavits, motions were made for dismissal and for summary judgment. The court held that Roe and members of her class, and Dr. Hallford, had standing to sue and presented justiciable controversies, but that the Does had failed to allege facts sufficient to state a present controversy and did not have standing. It concluded that, with respect to the requests for a declaratory judgment, abstention was not warranted. On the merits, the District Court held that the "fundamental right of single women and married persons to choose whether to have children is protected by the Ninth Amendment, through the Fourteenth Amendment," and that the Texas criminal abortion statutes were void on their face because they were both unconstitutionally vague and constituted an overbroad infringement of the plaintiffs' Ninth Amendment rights. The court then held that abstention was warranted with respect to the requests for an injunction. It therefore dismissed the Does' complaint, declared the abortion statutes void, and dismissed the application for injunctive relief. 314 F. Supp. 1217, 1225 (ND Tex. 1970).

The plaintiffs Roe and Doe and the intervenor Hallford, pursuant to 28 U. S. C. § 1253, have appealed to this Court from that part of the District Court's judgment denying the injunction. The defendant District Attorney has purported to cross-appeal, pursuant to the same statute, from the court's grant of declaratory relief to Roe and Hallford. Both sides also have taken protective appeals to the United States Court of Appeals for the Fifth Circuit. That court ordered the appeals held in abeyance pending decision here. We postponed decision on jurisdiction to the hearing on the merits. 402 U. S. 941 (1971).

III

It might have been preferable if the defendant, pursuant to our Rule 20, had presented to us a petition for certiorari before judgment in the Court of Appeals with respect to the granting of the plaintiffs' prayer for declaratory relief. Our decisions in *Mitchell* v. *Donovan,* 398 U. S. 427 (1970), and *Gunn* v. *University Committee,* 399 U. S. 383 (1970), are to the effect that § 1253 does not authorize an appeal to this Court from the grant or denial of declaratory relief alone. We conclude, nevertheless, that those decisions do not foreclose our review of both the injunctive and the declaratory aspects of a case of this kind when it is properly here, as this one is, on appeal under § 1253 from specific denial of injunctive relief, and the arguments as to both aspects as necessarily identical. See *Carter* v. *Jury Comm'n,* 396 U. S. 320 (1970); *Florida Lime Growers* v. *Jacobsen,* 362 U. S. 73, 80–81 (1960). It would be destructive of time and energy for all concerned were we to rule otherwise. Cf. *Doe* v. *Bolton, post,* p. 179.

IV

We are next confronted with issues of justiciability, standing, and abstention. Have Roe and the Does established that "personal stake in the outcome of the controversy," *Baker* v. *Carr,* 369 U. S. 186, 204 (1962), that insures that "the dispute sought to be adjudicated will be presented in an adversary context and in a form historically viewed as capable of judicial resolution," *Flast* v. *Cohen,* 392 U. S. 83, 101 (1968), and *Sierra Club* v. *Morton,* 405 U. S. 727, 732 (1972)? And what effect did the pendency of criminal abortion charges against Dr. Hallford in state court have upon the propriety of the federal court's granting relief to him as a plaintiff-intervenor?

A. *Jane Roe.* Despite the use of the pseudonym, no suggestion is made that Roe is a fictitious person. For purposes of her case, we accept as true, and as established, her existence; her pregnant state, as of the inception of her suit in March 1970 and as late as May 21 of that year when she filed an alias affidavit with the District Court; and her inability to obtain a legal abortion in Texas.

Viewing Roe's case as of the time of its filing and thereafter until as late as May, there can be little dispute that it then presented a case or controversy and that, wholly apart from the class aspects, she, as a pregnant single woman thwarted by the Texas criminal abortion laws, had standing to challenge those statutes. *Abele* v. *Markle,* 452 F. 2d 1121, 1125 (CA2 1971); *Crossen* v. *Breckenridge,* 446 F. 2d 833, 838–839 (CA6 1971); *Poe* v. *Menghini,* 339 F. Supp. 986, 990–991 (Kan. 1972). See *Truax* v. *Raich,* 239 U. S. 33 (1915). Indeed, we do not read the appellee's brief as really asserting anything to the contrary. The "logical nexus between the status asserted and the claim sought to be adjudicated," *Flast* v. *Cohen,* 392 U. S., at 102, and the necessary degree of contentiousness, *Golden* v. *Zwickler,* 394 U. S. 103 (1969), are both present.

The appellee notes, however, that the record does not disclose that Roe was pregnant at the time of the District Court hearing on May 22, 1970,[6] or on the following June 17 when the court's opinion and judgment were filed. And he suggests that Roe's case must now be moot because she and all other members of her class are no longer subject to any 1970 pregnancy.

The usual rule in federal cases is that an actual controversy must exist at stages of appellate or certiorari review, and not simply at the date the action is initiated. . . .

But when, as here, pregnancy is a significant fact in the litigation, the normal 266-day human gestation period is so short that the pregnancy will come to term before the usual appellate process is complete. If that termination makes a case moot, pregnancy litigation seldom will survive much beyond the trial stage, and appellate review will be effectively denied. Our law should not be that rigid. Pregnancy often comes more than once to the same woman, and in the general population, if man is to survive, it will always be with us. Pregnancy provides a classic justification for a conclusion of nonmootness. It truly could be "capable of repetition, yet evading review." *Southern Pacific Terminal Co.* v. *ICC,* 219 U. S. 498, 515 (1911).

We, therefore, agree with the District Court that Jane Roe had standing to undertake this litigation, that she presented a justiciable controversy, and that the termination of her 1970 pregnancy has not rendered her case moot.

B. Dr. Hallford. The doctor's position is different. He entered Roe's litigation as a plaintiff-intervenor, alleging in his complaint that he:

[I]n the past has been arrested for violating the Texas Abortion Laws and at the present time stands charged by indictment with violating said laws in the Criminal District Court of Dallas County, Texas to-wit: (1) The State of Texas vs. James H. Hallford, No. C-69-5307-1H, and (2) The State of Texas vs. James H. Hallford, No. C-69-2524-H. In both cases the defendant is charged with abortion. . . .

In his application for leave to intervene, the doctor made like representations as to the abortion charges

pending in the state court. These representations were also repeated in the affidavit he executed and filed in support of his motion for summary judgment.

Dr. Hallford is, therefore, in the position of seeking, in a federal court, declaratory and injunctive relief with respect to the same statutes under which he stands charged in criminal prosecutions simultaneously pending in state court. Although he stated that he has been arrested in the past for violating the State's abortion laws, he makes no allegation of any substantial and immediate threat to any federally protected right that cannot be asserted in his defense against the state prosecutions. Neither is there any allegation of harassment or bad-faith prosecution. In order to escape the rule articulated in the cases cited in the next paragraph of this opinion that, absent harassment and bad faith, a defendant in a pending state criminal case cannot affirmatively challenge in federal court the statutes under which the State is prosecuting him, Dr. Hallford seeks to distinguish his status as a present state defendant from his status as a "potential future defendant" and to assert only the latter for standing purposes here.

We see no merit in that distinction. Our decision in *Samuels* v. *Mackell,* 401 U. S. 66 (1971), compels the conclusion that the District Court erred when it granted declaratory relief to Dr. Hallford instead of refraining from so doing. The court, of course, was correct in refusing to grant injunctive relief to the doctor. . . .

Dr. Hallford's complaint in intervention, therefore, is to be dismissed.[7] He is remitted to his defenses in the state criminal proceedings against him. We reverse the judgment of the District Court insofar as it granted Dr. Hallford relief and failed to dismiss his complaint in intervention. . . .

V

The principal thrust of appellant's attack on the Texas statutes is that they improperly invade a right, said to be possessed by the pregnant woman, to choose to terminate her pregnancy. Appellant would discover this right in the concept of personal "liberty" embodied in the Fourteenth Amendment's

Due Process Clause; or in personal, marital, familial, and sexual privacy said to be protected by the Bill of Rights or its penumbras, see *Griswold* v. *Connecticut,* 381 U. S. 479 (1965); *Eisenstadt* v. *Baird,* 405 U. S. 438 (1972); *id,* at 460 (White, J., concurring in result); or among those rights reserved to the people by the Ninth Amendment, *Griswold* v. *Connecticut,* 381 U. S. at 486 (Goldberg, J., concurring). Before addressing this claim, we feel it desirable briefly to survey, in several aspects, the history of abortion, for such insight as that history may afford us, and then to examine the state purposes and interests behind the criminal abortion laws.

VI

It perhaps is not generally appreciated that the restrictive criminal abortion laws in effect in a majority of States today are of relatively recent vintage. Those laws, generally proscribing abortion or its attempt at any time during pregnancy except when necessary to preserve the pregnant woman's life, are not of ancient or even of common-law origin. Instead, they derive from statutory changes effected, for the most part, in the latter half of the 19th century.

1. *Ancient attitudes.* These are not capable of precise determination. We are told that at the time of the Persian Empire abortifacients were known and that criminal abortions were severely punished.[8] We are also told, however, that abortion was practiced in Greek times as well as in the Roman Era,[9] and that "it was resorted to without scruple."[10] The Ephesian, Soranos, often described as the greatest of the ancient gynecologists, appears to have been generally opposed to Rome's prevailing free-abortion practices. He found it necessary to think first of the life of the mother, and he resorted to abortion when, upon this standard, he felt the procedure advisable.[11] Greek and Roman law afforded little protection to the unborn. If abortion was prosecuted in some places, it seems to have been based on a concept of a violation of the father's right to his offspring. Ancient religion did not bar abortion.[12]

2. *The Hippocratic Oath.* What then of the famous Oath that has stood so long as the ethical guide of the medical

profession and that bears the name of the great Greek (460(?)–377(?) B.C.), who has been described as the Father of Medicine, the "wisest and the greatest practitioner of his art," and the "most important and most complete medical personality of antiquity," who dominated the medical schools of his time, and who typified the sum of the medical knowledge of the past?[13] The Oath varies somewhat according to the particular translation, but in any translation the content is clear: "I will give no deadly medicine to anyone if asked, nor suggest any such counsel; and in like manner I will not give to a woman a pessary to produce abortion,"[14] or "I will neither give a deadly drug to anybody if asked for it, nor will I make a suggestion to this effect. Similarly, I will not give to a woman an abortive remedy."[15]

Although the Oath is not mentioned in any of the principal briefs in this case or in *Doe* v. *Bolton, post,* p. 179, it represents the apex of the development of strict ethical concepts in medicine, and its influence endures to this day. Why did not the authority of Hippocrates dissuade abortion practice in his time and that of Rome? The late Dr. Edelstein provides us with a theory:[16] The Oath was not uncontested even in Hippocrates' day; only the Pythagorean school of philosophers frowned upon the related act of suicide. Most Greek thinkers, on the other hand, commended abortion, at least prior to viability. See Plato, *Republic,* V, 461; Aristotle, *Politics,* VII, 1335b 25. For the Pythagoreans, however, it was a matter of dogma. For them the embryo was animate from the moment of conception, and abortion meant destruction of a living being. The abortion clause of the Oath, therefore, "echoes Pythagorean doctrines," and "[i]n no other stratum of Greek opinion were such views held or proposed in the same spirit of uncompromising austerity."[17]

Dr. Edelstein then concludes that the Oath originated in a group representing only a small segment of Greek opinion and that it certainly was not accepted by all ancient physicians. He points out that medical writings down to Galen (A.D. 130–200) "give evidence of the violation of almost every one of its injunctions."[18] But with the end of antiquity a decided change took place.

Resistance against suicide and against abortion became common. The Oath came to be popular. The emerging teachings of Christianity were in agreement with the Pythagorean ethic. The Oath "became the nucleus of all medical ethics" and "was applauded as the embodiment of truth." Thus, suggests Dr. Edelstein, it is "a Pythagorean manifesto and not the expression of an absolute standard of medical conduct."[19]

This, it seems to us, is a satisfactory and acceptable explanation of the Hippocratic Oath's apparent rigidity. It enables us to understand, in historical context, a long-accepted and revered statement of medical ethics.

3. *The common law.* It is undisputed that at common law, abortion performed *before* "quickening"—the first recognizable movement of the fetus *in utero,* appearing usually from the 16th to the 18th week of pregnancy[20]—was not an indictable offense.[21] The absence of a common-law crime for pre-quickening abortion appears to have developed from a confluence of earlier philosophical, theological, and civil and canon law concepts of when life begins. These disciplines variously approached the question in terms of the point at which the embryo or fetus became "formed" or recognizably human, or in terms of when a "person" came into being, that is, infused with a "soul" or "animated." A loose consensus evolved in early English law that these events occurred at some point between conception and live birth.[22] This was "mediate animation." Although Christian theology and the canon law came to fix the point of animation at 40 days for a male and 80 days for a female, a view that persisted until the 19th century, there was otherwise little agreement about the precise time of formation or animation. There was agreement, however, that prior to this point the fetus was to be regarded as part of the mother, and its destruction, therefore, was not homicide. Due to continued uncertainty about the precise time when animation occurred, to the lack of any empirical basis for the 40–80-day view, and perhaps to Aquinas' definition of movement as one of the two first principles of life, Bracton focused upon

quickening as the critical point. The significance of quickening was echoed by later common-law scholars and found its way into the received common law in this country.

Whether abortion of a *quick* fetus was a felony at common law, or even a lesser crime, is still disputed. Bracton, writing early in the 13th century, thought it homicide.[23] But the later and predominant view, following the great common-law scholars, has been that it was, at most, a lesser offense. In a frequently cited passage, Coke took the position that abortion of a woman "quick with childe" is "a great misprision, and no murder."[24] Blackstone followed, saying that while abortion after quickening had once been considered manslaughter (though not murder), "modern law" took a less severe view.[25] A recent review of the common-law precedents argues, however, that those precedents contradict Coke and that even post-quickening abortion was never established as a common-law crime.[26] This is of some importance because while most American courts ruled, in holding or dictum, that abortion of an unquickened fetus was not criminal under their received common law,[27] others followed Coke in stating that abortion of a quick fetus was a "misprision," a term they translated to mean "misdemeanor."[28] That their reliance on Coke on this aspect of the law was uncritical and, apparently in all the reported cases, dictum (due probably to the paucity of common-law prosecutions for post-quickening abortion), makes it now appear doubtful that abortion was ever firmly established as a common-law crime even with respect to the destruction of a quick fetus.

4. *The English statutory law.* England's first criminal abortion statute, Lord Ellenborough's Act, 43 Geo. 3, c. 58, came in 1803. It made abortion of a quick fetus, § 1, a capital crime, but in § 2 it provided lesser penalties for the felony of abortion before quickening, and thus preserved the "quickening" distinction. This contrast was continued in the general revision of 1828, 9 Geo. 4, c. 31, § 13. It disappeared, however, together with the death penalty, in 1837, 7 Will. 4 & 1 Vict., c. 85, § 6, and did not reappear in the Offenses Against the Person Act

of 1861, 24 & 25 Vict. c. 100, § 59, that formed the core of English anti-abortion law until the liberalizing reforms of 1967. In 1929, the Infant Life (Preservation) Act, 19 & 20 Geo. 5, c. 34, came into being. Its emphasis was upon the destruction of "the life of a child capable of being born alive." It made a willful act performed with the necessary intent a felony. It contained a proviso that one was not to be found guilty of the offense "unless it is proved that the act which caused the death of the child was not done in good faith for the purpose only of preserving the life of the mother."

A seemingly notable development in the English law was the case of *Rex v. Bourne,* [1939] 1 K. B. 687. This case apparently answered in the affirmative the question whether an abortion necessary to preserve the life of the pregnant woman was excepted from the criminal penalties of the 1861 Act. In his instructions to the jury, Judge Macnaghten referred to the 1929 Act, and observed that that Act related to "the case where a child is killed by a wilful act at the time when it is being delivered in the ordinary course of nature." *Id.,* at 691. He concluded that the 1861 Act's use of the word "unlawfully," imported the same meaning expressed by the specific proviso in the 1929 Act, even though there was no mention of preserving the mother's life in the 1861 Act. He then construed the phrase "preserving the life of the mother" broadly, that is, "in a reasonable sense," to include a serious and permanent threat to the mother's *health,* and instructed the jury to acquit Dr. Bourne if it found he had acted in a good-faith belief that the abortion was necessary for this purpose. *Id.,* at 693–694. The jury did acquit.

Recently, Parliament enacted a new abortion law. This is the Abortion Act of 1967, 15 & 16 Eliz. 2, c. 87. The Act permits a licensed physician to perform an abortion where two other licensed physicians agree (a) "that the continuance of the pregnancy would involve risk to the life of the pregnant women, or of injury to the physical or mental health of the pregnant woman or any existing children of her family, greater than if the pregnancy were terminated," or (b) "that there is a substantial risk that if the child were born it would suffer from such physical or mental abnormalities as to be seriously

handicapped." The Act also provides that, in making this determination, "account may be taken of the pregnant woman's actual or reasonably foreseeable environment." It also permits a physician, without the concurrence of others, to terminate a pregnancy where he is of the good-faith opinion that the abortion "is immediately necessary to save the life or to prevent grave permanent injury to the physical or mental health of the pregnant woman."

5. *The American law.* In this country, the law in effect in all but a few States until mid-19th century was the pre-existing English common law. Connecticut, the first State to enact abortion legislation, adopted in 1821 that part of Lord Ellenborough's Act that related to a woman "quick with child."[29] The death penalty was not imposed. Abortion before quickening was made a crime in that State only in 1860.[30] In 1828, New York enacted legislation[31] that, in two respects, was to serve as a model for early anti-abortion statutes. First, while barring destruction of an unquickened fetus as well as a quick fetus, it made the former only a misdemeanor, but the latter second-degree manslaughter. Second, it incorporated a concept of therapeutic abortion by providing that an abortion was excused if it "shall have been necessary to preserve the life of such mother, or shall have been advised by two physicians to be necessary for such purpose." By 1840, when Texas had received the common law,[32] only eight American States had statutes dealing with abortion.[33] It was not until after the War Between the States that legislation began generally to replace the common law. Most of these initial statutes dealt severely with abortion after quickening but were lenient with it before quickening. Most punished attempts equally with completed abortions. While many statutes included the exception for an abortion thought by one or more physicians to be necessary to save the mother's life, that provision soon disappeared and the typical law required that the procedure actually be necessary for that purpose.

Gradually, in the middle and late 19th century the quickening distinction disappeared from the statutory law of most States and the degree of the offense and the penalties were increased.

By the end of the 1950s, a large majority of the jurisdictions banned abortion, however and whenever performed, unless done to save or preserve the life of the mother.[34] The exceptions, Alabama and the District of Columbia, permitted abortion to preserve the mother's health.[35] Three States permitted abortions that were not "unlawfully" performed or that were not "without lawful justification," leaving interpretation of those standards to the courts.[36] In the past several years, however, a trend toward liberalization of abortion statutes has resulted in adoption, by about one-third of the States, of less stringent laws, most of them patterned after the ALI Model Penal Code, § 230.3,[37] set forth as Appendix B to the opinion in *Doe v. Bolton, post,* p. 205.

It is thus apparent that at common law, at the time of the adoption of our Constitution, and throughout the major portion of the 19th century, abortion was viewed with less disfavor than under most American statutes currently in effect. Phrasing it another way, a woman enjoyed a substantially broader right to terminate a pregnancy than she does in most States today. At least with respect to the early stage of pregnancy, and very possibly without such a limitation, the opportunity to make this choice was present in this country well into the 19th century. Even later, the law continued for some time to treat less punitively an abortion procured in early pregnancy.

6. *The position of the American Medical Association.* The anti-abortion mood prevalent in this country in the late 19th century was shared by the medical profession. Indeed, the attitude of the profession may have played a significant role in the enactment of stringent criminal abortion legislation during that period.

An AMA Committee on Criminal Abortion was appointed in May 1857. It presented its report, 12 Trans. of the Am. Med. Assn. 73–78 (1859), to the Twelfth Annual Meeting. That report observed that the Committee had been appointed to investigate criminal abortion "with a view to its general suppression." It deplored abortion and its frequency and it listed three causes of "this general demoralization":

The first of these causes is a widespread popular ignorance of the true character of the crime—a belief, even among mothers themselves, that the foetus is not alive till after the period of quickening.

The second of the agents alluded to is the fact that the profession themselves are frequently supposed careless of foetal life. . . .

The third reason of the frightful extent of this crime is found in the grave defects of our laws, both common and statute, as regards the independent and actual existence of the child before birth, as a living being. These errors, which are sufficient in most instances to prevent conviction, are based, and only based, upon mistaken and exploded medical dogmas. With strange inconsistency, the law fully acknowledges the foetus in utero and its inherent rights, for civil purposes; while personally and as criminally affected, it fails to recognize it, and to its life as yet denies all protection. (Id., at 75–76.)

The Committee then offered, and the Association adopted, resolutions protesting "against such unwarrantable destruction of human life," calling upon state legislatures to revise their abortion laws, and requesting the cooperation of state medical societies "in pressing the subject." Id., at 28, 78.

In 1871 a long and vivid report was submitted by the Committee on Criminal Abortion. It ended with the observation, "We had to deal with human life. In a matter of less importance we could entertain no compromise. An honest judge on the bench would call things by their proper names. We could do no less." 22 Trans. of the Am. Med. Assn. 258 (1871). It proffered resolutions, adopted by the Association, id., at 38–39, recommending, among other things, that it "be unlawful and unprofessional for any physician to induce abortion or premature labor, without the concurrent opinion of at least one respectable consulting physician, and then always with a view to the safety of the child—if that be possible," and calling "the attention of the clergy of all denominations to the perverted views of morality entertained by a large class of females—aye, and men also, on this important question."

Except for periodic condemnation of the criminal abortionist, no further formal AMA action took place until 1967. In that year, the Committee on Human Reproduction urged the adoption of a stated policy of opposition to induced abortion, except when there is "documented medical evidence" of a threat

to the health or life of the mother, or that the child "may be born with incapacitating physical deformity or mental deficiency," or that a pregnancy "resulting from legally established statutory or forcible rape or incest may constitute a threat to the mental or physical health of the patient," two other physicians "chosen because of their recognized professional competence have examined the patient and have concurred in writing," and the procedure "is performed in a hospital accredited by the Joint Commission on Accreditation of Hospitals." The providing of medical information by physicians to state legislatures in their consideration of legislation regarding therapeutic abortion was "to be considered consistent with the principles of ethics of the American Medical Association." This recommendation was adopted by the House of Delegates. Proceedings of the AMA House of Delegates 40–51 (June 1967).

In 1970, after the introduction of a variety of proposed resolutions, and of a report from its Board of Trustees, a reference committee noted "polarization of the medical profession on this controversial issue"; division among those who had testified; a difference of opinion among AMA councils and committees; "the remarkable shift in testimony" in six months, felt to be influenced "by the rapid changes in state laws and by the judicial decisions which tend to make abortion more freely available"; and a feeling "that this trend will continue." On June 25, 1970, the House of Delegates adopted preambles and most of the resolutions proposed by the reference committee. The preambles emphasized "the best interests of the patient," "sound clinical judgment," and "informed patient consent," in contrast to "mere acquiescence to the patient's demand." The resolutions asserted that abortion is a medical procedure that should be performed by a licensed physician in an accredited hospital only after consultation with two other physicians and in conformity with state law, and that no party to the procedure should be required to violate personally held moral principles.[38] Proceedings of the AMA House of Delegates 220 (June 1970). The AMA Judicial Council rendered a complementary opinion.[39]

7. *The position of the American Public Health Association.* In October 1970, the Executive Board of the APHA adopted Standards for Abortion Services. These were five in number:

a. Rapid and simple abortion referral must be readily available through state and local public health departments, medical societies, or other non-profit organizations.

b. An important function of counseling should be to simplify and expedite the provision of abortion services; it should not delay the obtaining of these services.

c. Psychiatric consultation should not be mandatory. As in the case of other specialized medical services, psychiatric consultation should be sought for definite indications and not on a routine basis.

d. A wide range of individuals from appropriately trained, sympathetic volunteers to highly skilled physicians may qualify as abortion counselors.

e. Contraception and/or sterilization should be discussed with each abortion patient. [Recommended Standards for Abortion Services, 61 *Am. J. Pub. Health* 396 (1971).]

Among factors pertinent to life and health risks associated with abortion were three that "are recognized as important":

a. the skill of the physician,
b. the environment in which the abortion is performed, and above all
c. the duration of pregnancy, as determined by uterine size and confirmed by menstrual history. (Id. at 397.)

It was said that "a well-equipped hospital" offers more protection "to cope with unforeseen difficulties than an office or clinic without such resources. . . . The factor of gestational age is of overriding importance." Thus, it was recommended that abortions in the second trimester and early abortions in the presence of existing medical complications be performed in hospitals as inpatient procedures. For pregnancies in the first trimester, abortion in the hospital with or without overnight stay "is probably the safest practice." An abortion in an extramural facility, however, is an acceptable alternative "provided arrangements exist in advance to admit patients promptly if unforeseen complications develop." Standards for an abortion facility were listed. It was said that at present abortions should be performed by physicians or osteopaths who are licensed to practice and who have "adequate training." Id. at 398.

8. *The position of the American Bar Association.* At its meeting in February 1972 the ABA House of Delegates approved, with 17 opposing votes, the Uniform Abortion Act that had been drafted and approved the preceding August by the Conference of Commissioners on Uniform State Laws. 58 *A.B.A.J.* 380 (1972). We set forth the Act in full in the margin.[40] The Conference has appended an enlightening Prefatory Note.[41]

VII

Three reasons have been advanced to explain historically the enactment of criminal abortion laws in the 19th century and to justify their continued existence.

It has been argued occasionally that these laws were the product of a Victorian social concern to discourage illicit sexual conduct. Texas, however, does not advance this justification in the present case, and it appears that no court or commentator has taken the argument seriously.[42] The appellants and *amici* contend, moreover, that this is not a proper state purpose at all and suggest that, if it were, the Texas statutes are overbroad in protecting it since the law fails to distinguish between married and unwed mothers.

A second reason is concerned with abortion as a medical procedure. When most criminal abortion laws were first enacted, the procedure was a hazardous one for the woman.[43] This was particularly true prior to the development of antisepsis. Antiseptic techniques, of course, were based on discoveries by Lister, Pasteur, and others first announced in 1867, but were not generally accepted and employed until about the turn of the century. Abortion mortality was high. Even after 1900, and perhaps until as late as the development of antibiotics in the 1940's, standard modern techniques such as dilation and curettage were not nearly so safe as they are today. Thus, it has been argued that a State's real concern in enacting a criminal abortion law was to protect the pregnant woman, that is, to restrain her from submitting to a procedure that placed her life in serious jeopardy.

Modern medical techniques have altered this situation. Appellants and various *amici* refer to medical data indicating that abortion in early pregnancy, that is, prior to the end of the first trimester, although not without its risk, is now relatively safe. Mortality rates for women undergoing early abortions, where the procedure is legal, appear to be as low as or lower than the rates for normal childbirth.[44] Consequently, any interest of the State in protecting the woman from an inherently hazardous procedure, except when it would be equally dangerous for her to forgo it, has largely disappeared. Of course, important state interests in the areas of health and medical standards do remain. The State has a legitimate interest in seeing to it that abortion, like any other medical procedure, is performed under circumstances that insure maximum safety for the patient. This interest obviously extends at least to the performing physician and his staff, to the facilities involved, to the availability of after-care, and to adequate provision for any complication or emergency that might arise. The prevalence of high mortality rates at illegal "abortion mills" strengthens, rather than weakens, the State's interest in regulating the conditions under which abortions are performed. Moreover, the risk to the woman increases as her pregnancy continues. Thus, the State retains a definite interest in protecting the woman's own health and safety when an abortion is proposed at a late stage of pregnancy.

The third reason is the State's interest—some phrase it in terms of duty—in protecting prenatal life. Some of the argument for this justification rests on the theory that a new human life is present from the moment of conception.[45] The State's interest and general obligation to protect life then extends, it is argued, to prenatal life. Only when the life of the pregnant mother herself is at stake, balanced against the life she carries within her, should the interest of the embryo or fetus not prevail. Logically, of course, a legitimate state interest in this area need not stand or fall on acceptance of the belief that life begins at conception or at some other point prior to live birth. In assessing the State's interest, recognition may be given to the less rigid claim that as long as at least *potential* life is involved, the State may assert interests beyond the protection of the pregnant woman alone.

Parties challenging state abortion laws have sharply disputed in some courts the contention that a purpose of these laws, when enacted, was to protect prenatal life.[46] Pointing to the absence of legislative history to support the contention, they claim that most state laws were designed solely to protect the woman. Because medical advances have lessened this concern, at least with respect to abortion in early pregnancy, they argue that with respect to such abortions the laws can no longer be justified by any state interest. There is some scholarly support for this view of original purpose.[47] The few state courts called upon to interpret their laws in the late 19th and early 20th centuries did focus on the State's interest in protecting the woman's health rather than in preserving the embryo and fetus.[48] Proponents of this view point out that in many States, including Texas,[49] by statute or judicial interpretation, the pregnant woman herself could not be prosecuted for self-abortion or for cooperating in an abortion performed upon her by another.[50] They claim that adoption of the "quickening" distinction through received common law and state statutes tacitly recognizes the greater health hazards inherent in late abortion and impliedly repudiates the theory that life begins at conception.

It is with these interests, and the weight to be attached to them, that this case is concerned.

VIII

The Constitution does not explicitly mention any right of privacy. In a line of decisions, however, going back perhaps as far as *Union Pacific R. Co. v. Botsford,* 141 U. S. 250, 251 (1891), the Court has recognized that a right of personal privacy, or a guarantee of certain areas or zones of privacy, does exist under the Constitution. In varying contexts, the Court or individual Justices have, indeed, found at least the roots of that right in the First Amendment, *Stanley* v. *Georgia,* 394 U. S. 557, 564 (1969); in the Fourth and Fifth Amendments, *Terry* v. *Ohio,* 392 U. S. 1, 8–9 (1968), *Katz* v. *United States,* 389 U. S. 347, 350 (1967), *Boyd* v. *United States,* 116 U. S. 616 (1886), see *Olmstead* v. *United States,* 277 U. S. 438, 478 (1928) (Brandeis, J., dissenting); in the penumbras of the

Bill of Rights, *Griswold* v. *Connecticut,* 381 U. S., at 484–485; in the Ninth Amendment, *id.,* at 486 (Goldberg, J., concurring); or in the concept of liberty guaranteed by the first section of the Fourteenth Amendment, see *Meyer* v. *Nebraska,* 262 U. S. 390, 399 (1923). These decisions make it clear that only personal rights that can be deemed "fundamental" or "implicit in the concept of ordered liberty," *Palko* v. *Connecticut,* 302 U. S. 319, 325 (1937), are included in this guarantee of personal privacy. They also make it clear that the right has some extension to activities relating to marriage, *Loving* v. *Virginia,* 388 U. S. 1, 12 (1967); procreation, *Skinner* v. *Oklahoma,* 316 U. S. 535, 541–542 (1942); contraception, *Eisenstadt* v. *Baird,* 405 U. S., at 453–454, *id.,* at 460, 463–465 (White, J., concurring in result); family relationships, *Prince* v. *Massachusetts,* 321 U. S. 158, 166 (1944); and child rearing and education, *Pierce* v. *Society of Sisters,* 268 U. S. 510, 535 (1925), *Meyer* v. *Nebraska, supra.*

This right of privacy, whether it be founded in the Fourteenth Amendment's concept of personal liberty and restrictions upon state action, as we feel it is, or, as the District Court determined, in the Ninth Amendment's reservation of rights to the people, is broad enough to encompass a woman's decision whether or nor to terminate her pregnancy. The detriment that the State would impose upon the pregnant woman by denying this choice altogether is apparent. Specific and direct harm medically diagnosable even in early pregnancy may be involved. Maternity, or additional offspring, may force upon the woman a distressful life and future. Psychological harm may be imminent. Mental and physical health may be taxed by child care. There is also the distress, for all concerned, associated with the unwanted child, and there is the problem of bringing a child into a family already unable, psychologically and otherwise, to care for it. In other cases, as in this one, the additional difficulties and continuing stigma of unwed motherhood may be involved. All these are factors the woman and her responsible physician necessarily will consider in consultation.

On the basis of elements such as these, appellant and some *amici* argue that the woman's right is absolute and that she is entitled to terminate her pregnancy at whatever time, in whatever way, and for whatever reason she alone chooses. With this we do not agree. Appellant's arguments that Texas either has no valid interest at all in regulating the abortion decision, or no interest strong enough to support any limitation upon the woman's sole determination, are unpersuasive. The Court's decisions recognizing a right of privacy also acknowledge that some state regulation in areas protected by that right is appropriate. As noted above, a State may properly assert important interests in safeguarding health, in maintaining medical standards, and in protecting potential life. At some point in pregnancy, these respective interests become sufficiently compelling to sustain regulation of the factors that govern the abortion decision. The privacy right involved, therefore, cannot be said to be absolute. In fact, it is not clear to us that the claim asserted by some *amici* that one has an unlimited right to do with one's body as one pleases bears a close relationship to the right of privacy previously articulated in the Court's decisions. The Court has refused to recognize an unlimited right of this kind in the past. *Jacobson* v. *Massachusetts,* 197 U. S. 11 (1905) (vaccination); *Buck* v. *Bell,* 274 U. S. 200 (1927) (sterilization).

We, therefore, conclude that the right of personal privacy includes the abortion decision, but that this right is not unqualified and must be considered against important state interests in regulation.

We note that those federal and state courts that have recently considered abortion law challenges have reached the same conclusion. A majority, in addition to the District Court in the present case, have held state laws unconstitutional, at least in part, because of vagueness or because of overbreadth and abridgment of rights. . . . [citations omitted]

Others have sustained state statutes. . . . [citations omitted]

Although the results are divided, most of these courts have agreed that the right of privacy, however based, is broad enough to cover the abortion

decision; that the right, nonetheless, is not absolute and is subject to some limitations; and that at some point the state interests as to protection of health, medical standards, and prenatal life, become dominant. We agree with this approach.

Where certain "fundamental rights" are involved, the Court has held that regulation limiting these rights may be justified only by a "compelling state interest," *Kramer* v. *Union Free School District,* 395 U. S. 621, 627 (1969); *Shapiro* v. *Thompson,* 394 U. S. 618, 634 (1969), *Sherbert* v. *Verner,* 374 U. S. 398, 406 (1963), and that legislative enactments must be narrowly drawn to express only the legitimate state interests at stake. *Griswold* v. *Connecticut,* 381 U. S., at 485; *Aptheker* v. *Secretary of State,* 378 U. S. 500, 508 (1964); *Cantwell* v. *Connecticut,* 310 U. S. 296, 307–308 (1940); see *Eisenstadt* v. *Baird,* 405 U. S., at 460, 463–464 White, J., concurring in result).

In the recent abortion cases, cited above, courts have recognized these principles. Those striking down state laws have generally scrutinized the State's interests in protecting health and potential life, and have concluded that neither interest justified broad limitations on the reasons for which a physician and his pregnant patient might decide that she should have an abortion in the early stages of pregnancy. Courts sustaining state laws have held that the State's determinations to protect health or prenatal life are dominant and constitutionally justifiable.

IX

The District Court held that the appellee failed to meet his burden of demonstrating that the Texas statute's infringement upon Roe's rights was necessary to support a compelling state interest, and that, although the appellee presented "several compelling justifications for state presence in the area of abortions," the statutes outstripped these justifications and swept "far beyond any areas of compelling state interest." 314 F. Supp., at 1222–1223. Appellant and appellee both contest that holding. Appellant, as has been indicated, claims an absolute right that bars any state imposition of criminal penalties in the area. Appellee argues that the State's determination to recognize and protect prenatal life from and after conception constitutes a compelling state interest. As noted above, we do not agree fully with either formulation.

A. The appellee and certain *amici* argue that the fetus is a "person" within the language and meaning of the Fourteenth Amendment. In support of this, they outline at length and in detail the well-known facts of fetal development. If this suggestion of personhood is established, the appellant's case, of course, collapses, for the fetus' right to life would then be guaranteed specifically by the Amendment. The appellant conceded as much on reargument.[51] On the other hand, the appellee conceded on reargument[52] that no case could be cited that holds that a fetus is a person within the meaning of the Fourteenth Amendment.

The Constitution does not define "person" in so many words. Section 1 of the Fourteenth Amendment contains three references to "person." The first, in defining "citizens," speaks of "persons born or naturalized in the United States." The word also appears both in the Due Process Clause and in the Equal Protection Clause. "Person" is used in other places in the Constitution: in the listing of qualifications for Representatives and Senators, Art. I, § 2, cl. 2, and § 3, cl. 3; in the Apportionment Clause, Art. I, § 2, cl. 3;[53] in the Migration and Importation provision, Art. I, § 9, cl. 1; in the Emolument Clause, Art. I, § 9, cl. 8; in the Electors provisions, Art. II, § 1, cl. 2, and the superseded cl. 3; in the provision outlining qualifications for the office of President, Art. II, § 1, cl. 5; in the Extradition provisions, Art. IV, § 2, cl. 2, and the superseded Fugitive Slave Clause 3; and in the Fifth, Twelfth, and Twenty-second Amendments, as well as in §§ 2 and 3 of the Fourteenth Amendment. But in nearly all these instances, the use of the word is such that it has application only postnatally. None indicates, with any assurance, that it has any possible prenatal application.[54]

All this, together with our observation, *supra,* that throughout the major portion of the 19th century prevailing legal abortion practices were far freer than they are today, persuades us that the word "person," as used in the Fourteenth Amendment, does not include the unborn.[55] This is in accord with the results reached in those few cases where the issue has been squarely presented. . . . [citations omitted] Indeed, our decision in *United States* v. *Vuitch,* 402 U. S. 62 (1971), inferentially is to the same effect, for we there would not have indulged in statutory interpretation favorable to abortion in specified circumstances if the necessary consequence was the termination of life entitled to Fourteenth Amendment protection.

This conclusion, however, does not of itself fully answer the contentions raised by Texas, and we pass on to other considerations.

B. The pregnant woman cannot be isolated in her privacy. She carries an embryo and, later, a fetus, if one accepts the medical definitions of the developing young in the human uterus. See *Dorland's Illustrated Medical Dictionary* 478–479, 547 (24th ed. 1965). The situation therefore is inherently different from marital intimacy, or bedroom possession of obscene material, or marriage, or procreation, or education, with which *Eisenstadt* and *Griswold, Stanley, Loving, Skinner,* and *Pierce* and *Meyer* were respectively concerned. As we have intimated above, it is reasonable and appropriate for a State to decide that at some point in time another interest, that of health of the mother or that of potential human life, becomes significantly involved. The women's privacy is no longer sole and any right of privacy she possesses must be measured accordingly.

Texas urges that, apart from the Fourteenth Amendment, life begins at conception and is present throughout pregnancy, and that, therefore, the State has a compelling interest in protecting that life from and after conception. We need not resolve the difficult question of when life begins. When those trained in the respective disciplines of medicine, philosophy, and theology are unable to arrive at any consensus, the judiciary, at this point in the development of man's knowledge, is not in a position to speculate as to the answer.

It should be sufficient to note briefly the wide divergence of thinking on this most sensitive and difficult question. There has always been strong support for the view that life does not begin until live birth. This was the belief of the Stoics.[56] It appears to be the predominant, though not the unanimous, attitude of the Jewish faith.[57] It may be taken to represent also the position of a large segment of the Protestant community, insofar as that can be ascertained; organized groups that have taken a formal position on the abortion issue have generally regarded abortion as a matter for the conscience of the individual and her family.[58] As we have noted, the common law found greater significance in quickening. Physicians and their scientific colleagues have regarded that event with less interest and have tended to focus either upon conception, upon live birth, or upon the interim point at which the fetus becomes "viable," that is, potentially able to live outside the mother's womb, albeit with artificial aid.[59] Viability is usually placed at about seven months (28 weeks) but may occur earlier, even at 24 weeks.[60] The Aristotelian theory of "mediate animation," that held sway throughout the Middle Ages and the Renaissance in Europe, continued to be official Roman Catholic dogma until the 19th century, despite opposition to this "ensoulment" theory from those in the Church who would recognize the existence of life from the moment of conception.[61] The latter is now, of course, the official belief of the Catholic Church. As one brief *amicus* discloses, this is a view strongly held by many non-Catholics as well, and by many physicians. Substantial problems for precise definition of this view are posed, however, by new embryological data that purport to indicate that conception is a "process" over time, rather than an event, and by new medical techniques such as menstrual extraction, the "morning-after" pill, implantation of embryos, artificial insemination, and even artificial wombs.[62]

In areas other than criminal abortion, the law has been reluctant to endorse any theory that life, as we recognize it, begins before live birth or to accord legal rights to the unborn except in narrowly defined situations and except when the rights are contingent upon live birth. For example, the traditional rule of tort law denied recovery for prenatal injuries even though the child was born alive.[63] That rule has been changed in almost every jurisdiction. In most States, recovery is said to be permitted only if the fetus was viable, or at least quick, when the injuries were sustained, though few courts have squarely so held.[64] In a recent development, generally opposed by the commentators, some States permit the parents of a stillborn child to maintain an action for wrongful death because of prenatal injuries.[65] Such an action, however, would appear to be one to vindicate the parents' interest and is thus consistent with the view that the fetus, at most, represents only the potentiality of life. Similarly, unborn children have been recognized as acquiring rights or interests by way of inheritance or other devolution of property, and have been represented by guardians *ad litem*.[66] Perfection of the interests involved, again, has generally been contingent upon live birth. In short, the unborn have never been recognized in the law as persons in the whole sense.

X

In view of all this, we do not agree that, by adopting one theory of life, Texas may override the rights of the pregnant woman that are at stake. We repeat, however, that the State does have an important and legitimate interest in preserving and protecting the health of the pregnant woman, whether she be a resident of the State or a nonresident who seeks medical consultation and treatment there, and that it has still *another* important and legitimate interest in protecting the potentiality of human life. These interests are separate and distinct. Each grows in substantiality as the woman approaches term and, at a point during pregnancy, each becomes "compelling."

With respect to the State's important and legitimate interest in the health of the mother, the "compelling" point, in the light of present medical knowledge, is at approximately the end of the first trimester. This is so because of the now-established medical fact, referred to above [p. 407], that until the end of the first trimester mortality in abortion may be less than mortality in normal childbirth. It follows that, from and after this point, a State may regulate the abortion procedure to the extent that the regulation reasonably relates to the preservation and protection of maternal health. Examples of permissible

state regulation in this area are requirements as to the qualifications of the person who is to perform the abortion; as to the licensure of that person; as to the facility in which the procedure is to be performed, that is, whether it must be a hospital or may be a clinic or some other place of less-than-hospital status; as to the licensing of the facility; and the like.

This means, on the other hand, that, for the period of pregnancy prior to this "compelling" point, the attending physician, in consultation with his patient, is free to determine, without regulation by the State, that, in his medical judgment, the patient's pregnancy should be terminated. If that decision is reached, the judgment may be effectuated by an abortion free of interference by the State.

With respect to the State's important and legitimate interest in potential life, the "compelling" point is at viability. This is so because the fetus then presumably has the capability of meaningful life outside the mother's womb. State regulation protective of fetal life after viability thus has both logical and biological justifications. If the State is interested in protecting fetal life after viability, it may go so far as to proscribe abortion during that period, except when it is necessary to preserve the life or health of the mother.

Measured against these standards, Art. 1196 of the Texas Penal Code, in restricting legal abortions to those "procured or attempted by medical advice for the purpose of saving the life of the mother," sweeps too broadly. The statute makes no distinction between abortions performed early in pregnancy and those performed later, and it limits to a single reason, "saving" the mother's life, the legal justification for the procedure. The statute, therefore, cannot survive the constitutional attack made upon it here.

This conclusion makes it unnecessary for us to consider the additional challenge to the Texas statute asserted on grounds of vagueness. See *United States* v. *Vuitch,* 402 U. S., at 67–72.

XI

To summarize and to repeat:

1. A state criminal abortion statute of the current Texas type, that excepts

from criminality only a *lifesaving* procedure on behalf of the mother, without regard to pregnancy stage and without recognition of the other interests involved, is violative of the Due Process Clause of the Fourteenth Amendment.

a. For the stage prior to approximately the end of the first trimester, the abortion decision and its effectuation must be left to the medical judgment of the pregnant woman's attending physician.

b. For the stage subsequent to approximately the end of the first trimester, the State, in promoting its interest in the health of the mother, may, if it chooses, regulate the abortion procedure in ways that are reasonably related to maternal health.

c. For the stage subsequent to viability, the State in promoting its interest in the potentiality of human life may, if it chooses, regulate, and even proscribe, abortion except where it is necessary, in appropriate medical judgment, for the preservation of the life or health of the mother.

2. The State may define the term "physician," as it has been employed in the preceding paragraphs of this Part XI of this opinion, to mean only a physician currently licensed by the State, and may proscribe any abortion by a person who is not a physician as so defined.

In *Doe* v. *Bolton, post,* p. 179, procedural requirements contained in one of the modern abortion statutes are considered. That opinion and this one, of course, are to be read together.[67]

This holding, we feel, is consistent with the relative weights of the respective interests involved, with the lessons and examples of medical and legal history, with the lenity of the common law, and with the demands of the profound problems of the present day. The decision leaves the State free to place increasing restrictions on abortion as the period of pregnancy lengthens, so long as those restrictions are tailored to the recognized state interests. The decision vindicates the right of the physician to administer medical treatment according to his professional judgment up to the points where important state interests provide compelling justifications for intervention. Up to those points, the abortion decision in all its aspects is inherently, and primarily, a medical decision, and basic responsibility for it must rest with the physician. If an individual practitioner abuses the privilege of exercising proper medical judgment, the usual remedies, judicial and intraprofessional, are available.

XII

Our conclusion that Art. 1196 is unconstitutional means, of course, that the Texas abortion statutes, as a unit, must fall. The exception of Art. 1196 cannot be struck down separately, for then the State would be left with a statute proscribing all abortion procedures no matter how medically urgent the case.

Although the District Court granted appellant Roe declaratory relief, it stopped short of issuing an injunction against enforcement of the Texas statutes. The Court has recognized that different considerations enter into a federal court's decision as to declaratory relief, on the one hand, and injunctive relief, on the other. *Zwickler* v. *Koota,* 389 U. S. 241, 252–255 (1967); *Dombrowski* v. *Pfister,* 380 U. S. 479 (1965). We are not dealing with a statute that, on its face, appears to abridge free expression, an area of particular concern under *Dombrowski* and refined in *Younger* v. *Harris,* 401 U. S., at 50.

We find it unnecessary to decide whether the District Court erred in withholding injunctive relief, for we assume the Texas prosecutorial authorities will give full credence to this decision that the present criminal abortion statutes of that State are unconstitutional.

The judgment of the District Court as to intervenor Hallford is reversed, and Dr. Hallford's complaint in intervention is dismissed. In all other respects, the judgment of the District Court is affirmed. Costs are allowed to the appellee.

It is so ordered.

Mr. Justice Rehnquist, dissenting.

The Court's opinion brings to the decision of this troubling question both extensive historical fact and a wealth of legal scholarship. While the opinion thus commands my respect, I find myself nonetheless in fundamental disagreement with those parts of it that invalidate the Texas statute in question, and therefore dissent.

I

The Court's opinion decides that a State may impose virtually no restriction on the performance of abortions during the first trimester of pregnancy. Our previous decisions indicate that a necessary predicate for such an opinion is a plaintiff who was in her first trimester of pregnancy at some time during the pendency of her lawsuit. While a party may vindicate his own constitutional rights, he may not seek vindication for the rights of others. *Moose Lodge* v. *Irvis,* 407 U. S. 163 (1972); *Sierra Club* v. *Morton,* 405 U.S. 727 (1972). The Court's statement of facts in this case makes clear, however, that the record in no way indicates the presence of such a plaintiff. We know only that plaintiff Roe at the time of filing her complaint was a pregnant woman; for aught that appears in this record, she may have been in her *last* trimester of pregnancy as of the date the complaint was filed.

Nothing in the Court's opinion indicates that Texas might not constitutionally apply its proscription of abortion as written to a woman in that stage of pregnancy. Nonetheless, the Court uses her complaint against the Texas statute as a fulcrum for deciding that States may impose virtually no restrictions on medical abortions performed during the *first* trimester of pregnancy. In deciding such a hypothetical lawsuit, the Court departs from the longstanding admonition that it should never "formulate a rule of constitutional law broader than is required by the precise facts to which it is to be applied." *Liverpool, New York & Philadelphia S. S. Co.* v. *Commissioners of Emigration,* 113 U. S. 33, 39 (1885). See also *Ashwander* v. *TVA,* 297 U. S. 288, 345 (1936) (Brandeis, J., concurring).

II

Even if there were a plaintiff in this case capable of litigating the issue which the Court decides, I would reach a conclusion opposite to that reached by the Court. I have difficulty in concluding, as the Court does, that the right of "privacy" is involved in this case. Texas, by the statute here challenged, bars the performance of a medical abortion by a licensed physician on a plaintiff such as Roe. A transaction resulting in an operation such as this is not "private" in the ordinary usage of that word. Nor is the "privacy" that the Court finds here even a distant relative of the freedom from searches and seizures protected by the Fourth Amendment to the Constitution, which the Court has referred to as embodying a right to privacy. *Katz* v. *United States,* 389 U. S. 347 (1967).

If the Court means by the term "privacy" no more than that the claim of a person to be free from unwanted state regulation of consensual transactions may be a form of "liberty" protected by the Fourteenth Amendment, there is no doubt that similar claims have been upheld in our earlier decisions on the basis of that liberty. I agree with the statement of Mr. Justice Stewart in his concurring opinion that the "liberty," against deprivation, only against deprivation of which without due process the Fourteenth Amendment protects, embraces more than the rights found in the Bill of Rights. But that liberty is not guaranteed absolutely against deprivation, only against deprivation without due process of law. The test traditionally applied in the area of social and economic legislation is whether or not a law such as that challenged has a rational relation to a valid state objective. *Williamson* v. *Lee Optical Co.,* 348 U. S. 483, 491 (1955). The Due Process Clause of the Fourteenth Amendment undoubtedly does place a limit, albeit a broad one, on legislative power to enact laws such as this. If the Texas statute were to prohibit an abortion even where the mother's life is in jeopardy, I have little doubt that such a statute would lack a rational relation to a valid state objective under the test stated in *Williamson, supra.* But the Court's sweeping invalidation of any restrictions on abortion during the first trimester is impossible to justify under that standard, and the conscious weighing of competing factors that the Court's opinion apparently substitutes for the established test is far more appropriate to a legislative judgment than to a judicial one.

The Court eschews the history of the Fourteenth Amendment in its reliance on the "compelling state interest" test. See *Weber* v. *Aetna Casualty & Surety Co.,* 406 U. S. 164, 179 (1972) (dissenting opinion). But the Court adds a new wrinkle to this test by transposing it from the legal considerations associated with the Equal Protection Clause of the Fourteenth Amendment to this case arising under the Due Process Clause of the Fourteenth Amendment. Unless I misapprehend the consequences of this transplanting of the "compelling state interest test," the Court's opinion will accomplish the seemingly impossible feat of leaving this area of the law more confused than it found it.

While the Court's opinion quotes from the dissent of Mr. Justice Holmes in *Lochner* v. *New York,* 198 U. S. 45, 74 (1905), the result it reaches is more closely attuned to the majority opinion of Mr. Justice Peckham in that case. As in *Lochner* and similar cases applying substantive due process standards to economic and social welfare legislation, the adoption of the compelling state interest standard will inevitably require this Court to examine the legislative policies and pass on the wisdom of these policies in the very process of deciding whether a particular state interest put forward may or may not be "compelling." The decision here to break pregnancy into three distinct terms and to outline the permissible restrictions the State may impose in each one, for example, partakes more of judicial legislation than it does of a determination of the intent of the drafters of the Fourteenth Amendment.

The fact that a majority of the States reflecting, after all, the majority sentiment in those States, have had restrictions on abortions for at least a century is a strong indication, it seems to me, that the asserted right to an abortion is not "so rooted in the traditions and conscience of our people as to be ranked as fundamental," *Snyder* v. *Massachusetts,* 291 U. S. 97, 105 (1934). Even today, when society's views on abortion are changing, the very existence of the debate is evidence that the "right" to an abortion is not so universally accepted as the appellant would have us believe.

To reach its result, the Court necessarily has had to find within the scope of the Fourteenth Amendment a right that was apparently completely unknown to the drafters of the Amendment. As early as 1821, the first state law dealing directly with abortion was enacted by the Connecticut Legislature. Conn. Stat., Tit. 22, §§ 14, 16. By the time of the adoption of the Fourteenth Amendment in 1868, there were at least 36 laws enacted by state or territorial legislatures limiting abortion. While many States have amended or updated their laws, 21 of the laws on the books in 1868 remain in effect today. Indeed, the Texas statute struck down today was, as the majority notes, first enacted in 1857 and "has remained substantially unchanged to the present time."

There apparently was no question concerning the validity of this provision or of any of the other state statutes when the Fourteenth Amendment was adopted. The only conclusion possible from this history is that the drafters did not intend to have the Fourteenth Amendment withdraw from the States the power to legislate with respect to this matter.

III

Even if one were to agree that the case that the Court decides were here, and that the enunciation of the substantive constitutional law in the Court's opinion were proper, the actual disposition of the case by the Court is still difficult to justify. The Texas statute is struck down *in toto,* even though the Court apparently concedes that at later periods of pregnancy Texas might impose these selfsame statutory limitations on abortion. My understanding of past practice is that a statute found to be invalid as applied to a particular plaintiff, but not unconstitutional as a whole, is not simply "struck down" but is, instead, declared unconstitutional as applied to the fact situation before the Court. *Yick Wo* v. *Hopkins,* 118 U. S. 356 (1886); *Street* v. *New York,* 394 U. S. 576 (1969).

For all of the foregoing reasons, I respectfully dissent.

Notes

1. Article 1191. Abortion

If any person shall designedly administer to a pregnant woman or knowingly procure to be administered with her consent any drug or medicine, or shall use towards her any violence or means whatever externally or internally applied, and thereby procure an abortion, he shall be confined in the penitentiary not less than two nor more than five years; if it be done without her consent, the punishment shall be doubled. By "abortion" is meant that the life of the fetus or embryo shall be destroyed in the woman's womb or that a premature birth thereof be caused.

Art. 1192. Furnishing the means

Whoever furnishes the means for procuring an abortion knowing the purpose intended is guilty as an accomplice.

Art. 1193. Attempt at abortion

If the means used shall fail to produce an abortion, the offender is nevertheless guilty of an attempt to produce abortion, provided it be shown that such means were calculated to produce that result, and shall be fined not less than one hundred nor more than one thousand dollars.

Art. 1194. Murder in producing abortion

If the death of the mother is occasioned by an abortion so produced or by an attempt to effect the same it is murder.

Art. 1196. By medical advice

Nothing in this chapter applies to an abortion procured or attempted by medical advice for the purpose of saving the life of the mother.

The foregoing Articles, together with Art. 1195, compose Chapter 9 of Title 15 of the Penal Code. Article 1195, not attacked here, reads:

Art. 1195. Destroying unborn child

Whoever shall during parturition of the mother destroy the vitality or life in a child in a state of being born and before actual birth, which child would otherwise have been born alive, shall be confined in the penitentiary for life or for not less than five years.

2. Ariz. Rev. Stat. Ann. § 13–211 (1956); Conn. Pub. Act No. 1 (May 1972 special session) in 4 Conn. Leg. Serv. 677 (1972)), and Conn. Gen. Stat. Rev. §§ 53–29, 53–30 (1968) (or unborn child); Idaho Code § 18–601 (1948); Ill. Rev. Stat., c. 38, § 23–1 (1971); Ind. Code § 35–1–58–1 (1971); Iowa Code § 701.1 (1971); Ky. Rev. Stat. § 436.020 (1962); La. Rev. Stat. § 37:1285 (6) (1964) (loss of medical license) (but see § 14:87 (Supp. 1972) containing no exception for the life of the mother under the criminal statute); Me. Rev. Stat. Ann., Tit. 17, § 51 (1964); Mass. Gen. Laws Ann., c. 272, § 19 (1970) (using the term "unlawfully," construed to exclude an abortion to save the mother's life, *Kudish* v. *Bd. of Registration,* 356 Mass. 98, 248 N. E. 2d 264 (1969)); Mich. Comp. Laws § 750.14 (1948); Minn. Stat. § 617.18 (1971); Mo. Rev. Stat. § 559.100 (1969); Mont. Rev. Codes Ann. § 94–401 (1969); Neb. Rev. Stat. § 28–405 (1964); Nev. Rev. Stat. § 200.220 (1967); N. H. Rev. Stat. Ann. § 585:13 (1955); N. J. Stat. Ann. § 2A:87–1 (1969) ("without lawful justification"); N. D. Cent. Code §§ 12-25–01, 12–25–02 (1960); Ohio Rev. Code Ann. § 2901.16 (1953); Okla. Stat. Ann., Tit. 21, § 861 (1972–1973 Supp.); Pa. Stat. Ann., Tit. 18, §§ 4718, 4719 (1963) ("unlawful"); R. I. Gen. Laws Ann. § 11–3–1 (1969); S. D. Comp. Laws Ann. § 22–17–1 (1967); Tenn. Code Ann. §§ 39–301, 39–302 (1956); Utah Code Ann. §§ 76–2–1, 76–2–2 (1953); Vt. Stat. Ann., Tit. 13, § 101 (1958); W. Va. Code Ann. § 61–2–8 (1966); Wis. Stat. § 940.04 (1969); Wyo. Stat. Ann. §§ 6–77, 6–78 (1957).

3. Long ago, a suggestion was made that the Texas statutes were unconstitutionally vague because of definitional deficiencies. The Texas Court of Criminal Appeals disposed of that suggestion peremptorily, saying only, "It is also insisted in the motion in arrest of judgment that the statute is unconstitutional

and void in that it does not sufficiently define or describe the offense of abortion. We do not concur in respect to this question." *Jackson* v. *State*, 55 Tex. Cr. R. 79, 89, 115 S. W. 262, 268 (1908).

The same court recently has held again that the State's abortion statutes are not unconstitutionally vague or overbroad. *Thompson* v. *State* (Ct. Crim. App. Tex. 1971), appeal docketed, No. 71–1200. The court held that "the State of Texas has a compelling interest to protect fetal life"; that Art. 1191 "is designed to protect fetal life"; that the Texas homicide statutes, particularly Art. 1205 of the Penal Code, are intended to protect a person "in existence by actual birth" and thereby implicitly recognize other human life that is not "in existence by actual birth"; that the definition of human life is for the legislature and not the courts; that Art. 1196 "is more definite than the District of Columbia statute upheld in [*United States* v.] *Vuitch*" (402 U. S. 62); and that the Texas statute "is not vague and indefinite or overbroad." A physician's abortion conviction was affirmed.

In *Thompson*, n. 2, the court observed that any issue as to the burden of proof under the exemption of Art. 1196 "is not before us." But see *Veevers* v. *State*, 172 Tex. Cr. R. 162, 168–169, 354 S. W. 2d 161, 166–167 (1962). Cf. *United States* v. *Vuitch*, 402 U. S. 62, 69–71 (1971).

4. The name is a pseudonym.

5. These names are pseudonyms.

6. The appellee twice states in his brief that the hearing before the District Court was held on July 22, 1970. Brief for Appellee 13. The docket entries, App. 2, and the transcript, App. 76, reveal this to be an error. The July date appears to be the time of the reporter's transcription. See App. 77.

7. We need not consider what different result, if any, would follow if Dr. Hallford's intervention were on behalf of a class. His complaint in intervention does not purport to assert a class suit and makes no reference to any class apart from an allegation that he "and others similarly situated" must necessarily guess at the meaning of Art. 1196. His application for leave to intervene goes somewhat further, for it asserts that plaintiff Roe does not adequately protect the interest of the doctor "and the class of people who are physicians . . . [and] the class of people who are . . . patients. . . ." The leave application, however, is not the complaint. Despite the District Court's statement to the contrary, 314 F. Supp., at 1225, we fail to perceive the essentials of a class suit in the Hallford complaint.

8. A. Castiglioni, *A History of Medicine* 84 (2d ed. 1947), E. Krumbhaar, translator and editor (hereinafter Castiglioni).

9. J. Ricci, *The Genealogy of Gynaecology* 52, 84, 113, 149 (2d Ed. 1950) (hereinafter Ricci); L. Lader, *Abortion* 75–77 (1966) (hereinafter Lader); K. Niswander, Medical Abortion Practices in the United States, in

Abortion and the Law 37, 38–40 (D. Smith ed. 1967); G. Williams, *The Sanctity of Life and the Criminal Law* 148 (1957) (hereinafter Williams); J. Noonan, An Almost Absolute Value in History, in *The Morality of Abortion* 1, 3–7 (J. Noonan ed. 1970) (hereinafter Noonan); Quay, *Justifiable Abortion—Medical and Legal Foundations* (pt. 2), 49 Geo. L. J. 395, 406–422 (1961) (hereinafter Quay).

10. L. Edelstein, *The Hippocratic Oath* 10 (1943) (hereinafter Edelstein). But see Castiglioni 227.

11. Edelstein 12; Ricci 113–114, 118–119; Noonan 5.

12. Edelstein 13–14.

13. Castiglioni 148.

14. *Id.*, at 154.

15. Edelstein 3.

16. *Id.*, at 12, 15–18.

17. *Id.*, at 18; Lader 76.

18. Edelstein 63.

19. *Id.*, at 64.

20. *Dorland's Illustrated Medical Dictionary* 1261 (24th ed. 1965).

21. E. Coke, *Institutes III* *50; 1 W. Hawkins, *Pleas of the Crown*, c. 31, § 16 (4th ed. 1762); 1 W. Blackstone, *Commentaries* *129–130; M. Hale, Pleas of the Crown 433 (1st Amer. ed. 1847). For discussions of the role of the quickening concept in English common law, see Lader 78; Noonan 223–226; Means, *The Law of New York Concerning Abortion and the Status of the Foetus*, 1664–1968: A Case of Cessation of Constitutionality (pt. 1), 14 N. Y. L. F. 411, 418–428 (1968) (hereinafter Means I); Stern, Abortion: Reform and the Law, 59 J. Crim. L. C. & P. S. 84 (1968) (hereinafter Stern); Quay 430–432; Williams 152.

22. Early philosphers believed that the embryo or fetus did not become formed and begin to live until at least 40 days after conception for a male, and 80 to 90 days for a female. See, for example, Aristotle, *Hist. Anim.* 7.3.583b; *Gen. Anim.* 2.3.736, 2.5.741; Hippocrates, *Lib. de Nat. Puer.*, No. 10. Aristotle's thinking derived from his three-stage theory of life: vegetable, animal, rational. The vegetable stage was reached at conception, the animal at "animation," and the rational soon after live birth. This theory, together with the 40/80 day view, came to be accepted by early Christian thinkers.

The theological debate was reflected in the writings of St. Augustine, who made a distinction between *embryo inanimatus*, not yet endowed with a soul, and *embryo animatus*. He may have drawn upon Exodus 21:22. At one point, however, he expressed the view that human powers cannot determine the point during fetal development at which the critical change occurs. See Augustine, *De Origine Animae* 4.4 (Pub. Law 44.527). See also W. Reany, *The Creation of the Human Soul*, c. 2 and 83–86 (1932); Huser. *The Crime of Abortion in Canon Law* 15 (Catholic Univ. of America, Canon Law Studies No. 162, Washington, D.C., 1942).

Galen, in three treatises related to embryology, accepted the thinking of Aristotle and his followers. Quay 426–427. Later, Augustine on abortion was incorporated by Gratian into the Decretum, published about 1140. Decretum Magistri Gratiani 2.32.2.7 to 2.32.2.10, in 1 *Corpus Juris Canonici* 1122, 1123 (A. Friedburg, 2d ed. 1879). This Decretal and the Decretals that followed were recognized as the definitive body of canon law until the new Code of 1917.

For discussions of the canon-law treatment, see Means I, pp. 411–412; Noonan 20–26; Quay 426–430; see also J. Noonan, *Contraception: A History of Its Treatment* by the Catholic Theologians and Canonists 18–29 (1965).

23. Bracton took the position that abortion by blow or poison was homicide "if the foetus by already formed and animated, and particularly if it be animated." 2 H. Bracton, *De Legibus et Consuetudinibus Angliae* 279 (T. Twiss ed. 1879), or, as a later translation puts it, "if the foetus is already formed or quickened, especially if it is quickened," 2 H. Bracton, *On the Laws and Customs of England* 341 (S. Thorne ed. 1968). See Quay 431; see also 2 *Fleta* 60–61 (Book 1, c. 23) (Selden Society ed. 1955).

24. E. Coke, *Institutes III* *50.

25. 1 W. Blackstone, Commentaries *129–130.

26. Means, The Phoenix of Abortional Freedom: Is a Penumbral or Ninth-Amendment Right About to Arise from the Nineteenth-Century Legislative Ashes of a Fourteenth-Century Common-Law Liberty?, 17 *N. Y. L. F.* 335 (1971) (hereinafter Means II). The author examines the two principal precedents cited marginally by Coke, both contrary to his dictum, and traces the treatment of these and other cases by earlier commentators. He concludes that Coke, who himself participated as an advocate in an abortion case in 1601, may have intentionally misstated the law. The author even suggests a reason: Coke's strong feelings against abortion, coupled with his determination to assert common-law (secular) jurisdiction to assess penalties for an offense that traditionally had been an exclusively ecclesiastical or canon-law crime. See also Lader 78–79, who notes that some scholars doubt that the common law ever was applied to abortion; that the English ecclesiastical courts seem to have lost interest in the problem after 1527; and that the preamble to the English legislation of 1803, 43 Geo. 3, c. 58, § 1, referred to in the text, *infra*, at 136 states that "no adequate means have been hitherto provided for the prevention and punishment of such offenses."

27. [Citations omitted.]

28. [Citations omitted.]

29. Conn. Stat., Tit. 20, § 14 (1821).

30. Conn. Pub. Acts, c. 71, § 1 (1860).

31. N. Y. Rev. Stat., pt. 4, c. 1, Tit. 2, Art. 1, § 9, p. 661, and Tit. 6, § 21, p. 694 (1829).

32. Act of Jan. 20, 1840, § 1, set forth in 2 H. Gammel, Laws of Texas 177–178 (1898); see *Grigsby* v. *Reib*, 105 Tex. 597, 600, 153 S. W. 1124, 1125 (1913).

33. The early statutes are discussed in Quay 435–438. See also Lader 85–88; Stern 85–86; and Means II 375–376.

34. Criminal abortion statutes in effect in the States as of 1961, together with historical statutory development and important judicial interpretations of the state statutes, are cited and quoted in Quay 447–520. See Comment, A Survey of the Present Statutory and Case Law on Abortion: The Contradictions and the Problems, 1972 *U. Ill. L. F.* 177, 179, classifying the abortion statutes and listing 25 States as permitting abortion only if necessary to save or preserve the mother's life.

35. Ala. Code, Tit. 14, § 9 (1958); D. C. Code Ann. § 22–201 (1967).

36. Mass. Gen. Laws Ann., c. 272, § 19 (1970); N. J. Stat. Ann. § 2A:87–1 (1969); Pa. Stat. Ann., Tit. 18, §§ 4718, 4719 (1963).

37. Fourteen States have adopted some form of the ALI statute. See Ark. Stat. Ann. §§ 41–303 to 41–310 (Supp. 1971); Calif. Health & Safety Code §§ 25950–25955.5 (Supp. 1972); Colo. Rev. Stat. Ann. §§ 40–2–50 to 40–2–53 (Cum. Supp. 1967); Del. Code Ann., Tit. 24, §§ 1790–1793 (Supp. 1972); Florida Law of Apr. 13, 1972, c. 72–196, 1972 Fla. Sess. Law Serv., pp. 380–382; Ga. Code §§ 26–1201 to 26–1203 (1972); Kan. Stat. Ann. § 21–3407 (Supp. 1971); Md. Ann. Code, Art. 43, §§ 137–139 (1971); Miss. Code Ann. § 2223 (Supp. 1972); N. M. Stat. Ann. §§ 40A–5–1 to 40A–5–3 (1972); N. C. Gen. Stat. § 14–45.1 (Supp. 1971); Ore. Rev. Stat. §§ 435.405 to 435.495 (1971); S. C. Code Ann. §§ 16–82 to 16–89 (1962 and Supp. 1971); Va. Code Ann. §§ 18.1–62 to 18.1–62.3 (Supp. 1972). Mr. Justice Clark described some of these States as having "led the way." Religion, Morality, and Abortion: A Constitutional Appraisal, 2 Loyola U. (L. A.) L. Rev. 1, 11 (1969).

By the end of 1970, four other States had repealed criminal penalties for abortions performed in early pregnancy by a licensed physician, subject to stated procedural and health requirements. Alaska Stat. § 11.15.060 (1970); Haw. Rev. Stat. § 453–16 (Supp. 1971); N. Y. Penal Code § 125.05, subd. 3 (Supp. 1972–1973); Wash. Rev. Code §§ 9.02.060 to 9.02.080 (Supp. 1972). The precise status of criminal abortion laws in some States is made unclear by recent decisions in state and federal courts striking down existing state laws, in whole or in part.

38. Whereas, Abortion, like any other medical procedure, should not be performed when contrary to the best interests of the patient since good medical practice requires due consideration for the patient's welfare and not mere acquiescence to the patient's demand; and

Whereas, The standards of sound clinical judgment, which, together with informed patient consent should be determinative according to the merits of each individual case; therefore be it

Resolved, That abortion is a medical procedure and should be performed only by a duly licensed physician and surgeon in an accredited hospital acting only after consultation with two other physicians chosen because of their professional competency and in conformance with standards of good medical practice and the Medical Practice Act of his state; and be it further

Resolved, That no physician or other professional personnel shall be compelled to perform any act which violates his good medical judgment. Neither physician, hospital, nor hospital personnel shall be required to perform any act violative of personally-held moral principles. In these circumstances good medical practice requires only that the physician or other professional personnel withdraw from the case so long as the withdrawal is consistent with good medical practice. (Proceedings of the AMA House of Delegates 220 [June 1970].)

39. The Principles of Medical Ethics of the AMA do not prohibit a physician from performing an abortion that is performed in accordance with good medical practice and under circumstances that do not violate the laws of the community in which he practices.

In the matter of abortions, as of any other medical procedure, the Judicial Council becomes involved whenever there is alleged violation of the Principles of Medical Ethics as established by the House of Delegates.

40. Uniform Abortion Act
Section 1. [*Abortion Defined; When Authorized.*]
(a) "Abortion" means the termination of human pregnancy with an intention other than to produce a live birth or to remove a dead fetus.
(b) An abortion may be performed in this state only if it is performed:
(1) by a physician licensed to practice medicine [or osteopathy] in this state or by a physician practicing medicine [or osteopathy] in the employ of the government of the United States or of this state, [and the abortion is performed [in the physician's office or in a medical clinic, or] in a hospital approved by the [Department of Health] or operated by the United States, this state, or any department, agency, or political subdivision of either;] or by a female upon herself upon the advice of the physician; and
(2) within [20] weeks after the commencement of the pregnancy [or after [20] weeks only if the physician has reasonable cause to believe (i) there is a substantial risk that continuance of the pregnancy would endanger the life of the mother or would gravely impair the physical or mental health of the mother, (ii) that the child would be born with grave physical or mental defect, or (iii) that the pregnancy resulted from rape or incest, or illicit intercourse with a girl under the age of 16 years].
Section 2. [*Penalty.*] Any person who performs or procures an abortion other than authorized by this Act is guilty of a [felony] and, upon conviction thereof, may be sentenced to pay a fine not exceeding [$1,000] or to imprisonment [in the state penitentiary] not exceeding [5 years], or both.
Section 3. [*Uniformity of Interpretation.*] This Act shall be construed to effectuate its general purpose to make uniform the law

with respect to the subject of this Act among those states which enact it.
Section 4. [*Short Title.*] This Act may be cited as the Uniform Abortion Act.
Section 5. [*Severability.*] If any provision of this Act or the application thereof to any person or circumstance is held invalid, the invalidity does not affect other provisions or applications of this Act which can be given effect without the invalid provision or application, and to this end the provisions of this Act are severable.
Section 6. [*Repeal.*] The following acts and parts of acts are repealed:
(1)
(2)
(3)
Section 7. [*Time of Taking Effect.*] This Act shall take effect ———.

41. This Act is based largely upon the New York abortion act following a review of the more recent laws on abortion in several states and upon recognition of a more liberal trend in laws on this subject. Recognition was given also to the several decisions in state and federal courts which show a further trend toward liberalization of abortion laws, especially during the first trimester of pregnancy.

Recognizing that a number of problems appeared in New York, a shorter time period for "unlimited" abortions was advisable. The time period was bracketed to permit the various states to insert a figure more in keeping with the different conditions that might exist among the states. Likewise, the language limiting the place or places in which abortions may be performed was also bracketed to account for different conditions among the states. In addition, limitations on abortions after the initial 'unlimited' period were placed in brackets so that individual states may adopt all or any of these reasons, or place further restrictions upon abortions after the initial period.

This Act does not contain any provision relating to medical review committees or prohibitions against sanctions imposed upon medical personnel refusing to participate in abortions because of religious or other similar reasons, or the like. Such provisions, while related, do not directly pertain to when, where, or by whom abortions may be performed; however, the Act is not drafted to exclude such a provision by a state wishing to enact the same.

42. See, for example, YWCA v. *Kugler*, 342 F. Supp. 1048, 1074 (N. J. 1972); *Abele* v. *Markle*, 342 F. Supp. 800, 805–806 (Conn. 1972) (Newman, J., concurring in result), appeal docketed, No. 72–56; *Walsingham* v. *State*, 250 So. 2d 857, 863 (Ervin, J., concurring) (Fla. 1971); *State* v. *Gedicke*, 43 N. J. L. 86, 90 (1881); Means II 381–382.

43. See C. Haagensen & W. Lloyd, *A Hundred Years of Medicine* 19 (1943).

44. Potts, Postconceptive Control of Fertility, 8 *Int'l J. of G. & O.* 957, 967 (1970) (England and Wales); Abortion Mortality, 20 *Morbidity and Mortality* 208, 209 (June 12, 1971) (U.S. Dept. of HEW, Public Health Service) (New York City); Tietze, United States: Therapeutic Abortions, 1963–1968, 59 *Studies in Family Planning* 5, 7 (1970); Tietze, Mortality with Contraception and Induced Abortion, 45 *Studies in Family Planning* 6 (1969) (Japan, Czechoslovakia, Hungary); Tietze & Lehfeldt, Legal Abortion in

Eastern Europe, 175 *J.A.M.A.* 1149, 1152 (April 1961). Other sources are discussed in Lader 17–23.

45. See Brief of *Amicus* National Right to Life Committee; R. Drinan, The Inviolability of the Right to Be Born, in *Abortion and the Law* 107 (D. Smith ed. 1967); Louisell, Abortion, The Practice of Medicine and the Due Process of Law, 16 *U. C. L. A. L. Rev.* 233 (1969); Noonan 1.

46. See, *e. g., Abele* v. *Markle,* 342 F. Supp. 800 (Conn. 1972), appeal docketed, No. 72–56.

47. See discussions in Means I and Means II.

48. See, *e. g., State* v. *Murphy,* 27 N. J. L. 112, 114 (1858).

49. *Watson* v. *State,* 9 Tex. App. 237, 244–245 (1880); *Moore* v. *State,* 37 Tex. Cr. R. 552, 561, 40 S. W. 287, 290 (1897); *Shaw* v. *State,* 73 Tex. Cr. R. 337, 339, 165 S. W. 930, 931 (1914); *Fondren* v. *State,* 74 Tex. Cr. R. 552, 557, 169 S. W. 411, 414 (1914); *Gray* v. *State,* 77 Tex. Cr. R. 221, 229, 178 S. W. 337, 341 (1915). There is no immunity in Texas for the father who is not married to the mother. *Hammett* v. *State,* 84 Tex. Cr. R. 635, 209 S. W. 661 (1919); *Thompson* v. *State* (Ct. Crim. App. Tex. 1971), appeal docketed, No. 71–1200.

50. See *Smith* v. *State,* 33 Me., at 55; *In re Vince,* 2 N. J. 443, 450, 67 A. 2d 141, 144 (1949). A short discussion on the modern law on this issue is contained in the Comment to the ALI's Model Penal Code § 207.11, at 158 and nn. 35–37 (Tent. Draft No. 9, 1959).

51. Tr. of Oral Rearg. 20–21.

52. Tr. of Oral Rearg. 24.

53. We are not aware that in the taking of any census under this clause, a fetus has ever been counted.

54. When Texas urges that a fetus is entitled to Fourteenth Amendment protection as a person, it faces a dilemma. Neither in Texas nor in any other State are all abortions prohibited. Despite broad proscription, an exception always exists. The exception contained in Art. 1196, for an abortion procured or attempted by medical advice for the purpose of saving the life of the mother, is typical. But if the fetus is a person who is not to be deprived of life without due process of law, and if the mother's condition is the sole determinant, does not the Texas exception appear to be out of line with the Amendment's command?

There are other inconsistencies between Fourteenth Amendment status and the typical abortion statute. It has already been pointed out, n. 49, *supra,* that in Texas the woman is not a principal or an accomplice with respect to an abortion upon her. If the fetus is a person, why is the woman not a principal or an accomplice? Further, the penalty for criminal abortion specified by Art. 1195 is significantly less than the maximum penalty for murder prescribed by Art. 1257 of the Texas Penal Code. If the fetus is a person, may the penalties be different?

55. Cf. the Wisconsin abortion statute, defining "unborn child" to mean "a human being from the time of conception until it is born alive," Wis. Stat. § 940.04 (6) (1969), and the new Connecticut statute, Pub. Act No. 1 (May 1972 special session), declaring it to be the public policy of the State and the legislative intent "to protect and preserve human life from the moment of conception."

56. Edelstein 16.

57. Lader 97–99; D. Feldman, *Birth Control in Jewish Law* 251–294 (1968). For a stricter view, see I. Jakobovits, Jewish Views on Abortion, in *Abortion and the Law* 124 (D. Smith ed. 1967).

58. Amicus Brief for the American Ethical Union et al. For the position of the National Council of Churches and of other denominations, see Lader 99–101.

59. L. Hellman & J. Pritchard, *Williams Obstetrics* 493 (14th ed. 1971); *Dorland's Illustrated Medical Dictionary* 1689 (24th ed. 1965).

60. Hellman & Pritchard, *supra,* n. 59, at 493.

61. For discussions of the development of the Roman Catholic position, see D. Callahan, *Abortion: Law, Choice, and Morality* 409–447 (1970); Noonan 1.

62. See Brodie, The New Biology and the Prenatal Child, 9 *J. Family L.* 391, 397 (1970); Gorney, The New Biology and the Future of Man, 15 *U. C. L. A. L. Rev.* 273 (1968); Note, Criminal Law—Abortion—The "Morning-After Pill" and Other Pre-Implantation Birth-Control Methods and the Law, 46 *Ore. L. Rev.* 211 (1967); G. Taylor, *The Biological Time Bomb* 32 (1968); A. Rosenfeld, *The Second Genesis* 138–139 (1969); Smith, Through a Test Tube Darkly: Artificial Insemination and the Law, 67 *Mich. L. Rev.* 127 (1968); Note, Artificial Insemination and the Law, 1968 *U. Ill. L. F.* 203.

63. W. Prosser, *The Law of Torts* 335–338 (4th ed. 1971); 2 F. Harper & F. James, *The Law of Torts* 1028–1031 (1956); Note, 63 *Harv. L. Rev.* 173 (1949).

64. See cases cited in Prosser, *supra,* n. 63, at 336–338; Annotation, Action for Death of Unborn Child, 15 *A. L. R. 3d* 992 (1967).

65. Prosser, *supra,* n. 63, at 338; Note, The Law and the Unborn Child: The Legal and Logical Inconsistencies, 46 *Notre Dame Law.* 349, 354–360 (1971).

66. Louisell, Abortion, The Practice of Medicine and the Due Process of Law, 16 *U. C. L. A. L. Rev.* 233, 235–238 (1969); Note, 56 *Iowa Law Rev.* 994, 999–1000 (1971); Note, The Law and the Unborn Child, 46 *Notre Dame Law.* 349, 351–354 (1971).

67. Neither in this opinion nor in *Doe* v. *Bolton, post,* p. 179, do we discuss the father's rights, if any exist in the constitutional context, in the abortion decision. No paternal right has been asserted in either of the cases, and the Texas and the Georgia statutes on their face take no cognizance of the father. We are aware that some statutes recognize the father under certain circumstances. North Carolina, for example, N. C. Gen. Stat. § 14–45.1 (Supp. 1971), requires written permission for the abortion from the husband when the woman is a married minor, that is, when she is less than 18 years of age, 41 N. C. A. G. 489 (1971); if the woman is an unmarried minor, written permission from the parents is required. We need not now decide whether provisions of this kind are constitutional.

69

West German Abortion Decision: A Contrast to *Roe* v. *Wade*?

Translated by Robert E. Jonas and John D. Gorby. Reprinted by permission from the *John Marshall Journal of Practice and Procedure,* vol. 9, spring 1976, pp. 605–684.

[Editors' note: This case came to the Federal Constitutional Court of West Germany. It challenged the constitutionality of a statute, called "the Fifth Statute," which made all abortions performed after the thirteenth day after conception to be criminal violations punishable by fine or imprisonment for up to three years except: (a) abortions performed by a physician with the consent of the mother during the first 12 weeks of pregnancy for any reason; and (b) abortions in later stages of pregnancy performed by a physician with consent of the mother if warranted by specified medical or eugenic reasons. The medical reasons for interruption of pregnancy were considered to be a danger to the mother's life or a serious impairment to her health. The eugenic reasons were related to situations where the child would be defective in regard to its health because of hereditary factors or damage incurred during the pregnancy and as so serious that continuation of the pregnancy could not be demanded of the mother. The statute provided that abortions in the latter category had to be performed in the first 22 weeks of pregnancy. Abortions for medical reasons were not controlled as to time. Furthermore, the statute provided that all pregnant women seeking abortion must receive medical and social counseling at a counseling center or from a physician before a lawful abortion could be performed.

The Constitution of the Federal Republic of Germany, called the Basic Law, contains a provision asserting: "Everyone has the right to life" (article 2, paragraph 2, sentence 1). There is also a provision regarding privacy or personality asserting: "Everyone has the right to the free development of his personality to the extent he does not infringe upon the rights of others and does not violate the constitutional or moral order" (article 2, paragraph 1). The petition to enjoin the effect of the Fifth Statute was brought to the Court by the government of the State, or Land, of Baden-Württemberg.

This is an edited version of the opinion of the Court. The complete opinions of the majority and dissenting judges are published in full in the *John Marshall Journal of Practice and Procedure.*]

Guiding Principles applicable to the judgment of the First Senate of the 25th of February, 1975:

1. The life which is developing itself in the womb of the mother is an independent legal value which enjoys the protection of the constitution (Article 2, Paragraph 2, Sentence 1; Article 1, Paragraph 1 of the Basic Law).

The State's duty to protect forbids not only direct state attacks against life developing itself, but also requires the state to protect and foster this life.

2. The obligation of the state to protect the life developing itself exists, even against the mother.

3. The protection of life of the child *en ventre sa mere* takes precedence as a matter of principle for the entire duration of the pregnancy over the right of the pregnant woman to self-determination and may not be placed in question for any particular time.

4. The legislature may express the legal condemnation of the interruption of pregnancy required by the Basic Law through measures other than the threat of punishment. The decisive factor is whether the totality of the measures serving the protection of the unborn life guarantees an actual protection which in fact corresponds to the importance of the legal value to be guaranteed. In the extreme case, if the protection required by the constitution cannot be realized in any other manner, the legislature is obligated to employ the criminal law to secure the life developing itself.

5. A continuation of the pregnancy is not to be exacted (legally) if the termination is necessary to avert from the pregnant woman a danger to her life or the danger of a serious impairment of her health. Beyond that the legislature is at liberty to designate as non-exactable other extraordinary burdens for the pregnant woman, which are of similar gravity and, in these cases, to leave the interruption of pregnancy free of punishment.

6. The Fifth Statute to Reform the Penal Law of the 18th of June, 1974 (Federal Law Report I, p. 1297) has not in the required extent done justice to the constitutional obligation to protect prenatal life.

Holding

I. Section 218a of the Penal Code in the version of the Fifth Statute to Reform the Penal Law (5 PLRS) of June 18, 1974 (Federal Law Reporter I, p. 1297) is incompatible with Article 2, Paragraph 2, Sentence 1, in conjunction with Article 1, Paragraph 1, of the Basic Law and is null insofar as it excepts the interruption of pregnancy from criminal liability when no reasons are present which, in the sense of the reasons for this decision, have validity in the ordering of values of the Basic Law.

II. Until a new statutory regulation goes into effect the following is ordered under the authority of §35 of the Statute of the Constitutional Court:

1. §218b and §219 of the Penal Code in the version of the Fifth Statute for the Reform of the Penal Law (5 PLRS) of June 18, 1974 (Federal Law Reporter I, p. 1297) are to be applied to interruptions of pregnancy during the first twelve weeks after conception.

2. An abortion performed by a physician with the consent of the pregnant woman within the first twelve weeks after conception is not punishable under §218 of the Penal Code if an illegal act pursuant to §§176–179 of the Penal Code has been committed against the pregnant woman, and compelling reasons demand the assumption that the pregnancy is a result of the act.

3. If the interruption of the pregnancy is performed by a physician within the first twelve weeks after conception with the consent of the pregnant woman to avert from the pregnant woman danger of a serious calamity which cannot be averted in any other way which is exactable from her, the court may forgo a punishment under §218. . . .

The question of the legal treatment of the interruption of pregnancy has been discussed publicly for decades from various points of view. In fact, this phenomenon of social life raises manifold problems of a biological, especially human-genetic, anthropological, medical, psychological, social, social-political, and not least of an ethical and moral-theological nature, which touch upon the fundamental questions of human existence. It is the task of the legislature to evaluate the many sided and often opposing arguments which develop from these various ways of viewing the question, to supplement them through considerations which are specifically legal and political as well as through the practical experiences of the life of the law, and, on this basis, to arrive at a decision as to the manner in which the legal order should respond to this social process. The statutory regulation in the Fifth Statute to Reform the Penal Law which was decided upon after extraordinarily comprehensive preparatory work can be examined by the Constitutional Court only from the viewpoint of whether it is compatible with the Basic Law, which is the highest valid law in the Federal Republic. The gravity and the seriousness of the constitutional question posed becomes clear, if it is considered that what is involved here is the protection of human life, one of the central values of every legal order. The decision regarding the standards and limits of legislative freedom of decision demands a total view of the constitutional norms and the hierarchy of values contained therein.

I

1. Article 2, Paragraph 2, Sentence 1, of the Basic Law also protects the life developing itself in the womb of the mother as an intrinsic legal value.

a) The express incorporation into the Basic Law of the self-evident right to life—in contrast to the Weimar Constitution—may be explained principally as a reaction to the "destruction of life unworthy of life," to the "final solution" and "liquidations," which were carried out by the National Socialistic Regime as measures of state. Article 2, Paragraph 2, Sentence 1, of the Basic Law, just as it contains the abolition of the death penalty in Article 102, includes "a declaration of the fundamental worth of human life and of a concept of the state which stands in emphatic contrast to the philosophies of a political regime to which the individual life meant little and which therefore practiced limitless abuse with its presumed right over life and death of the citizen" (Decisions of the Federal Constitutional Court, 18, 112 117).

b) In construing Article 2, Paragraph 2, Sentence 1, of the Basic Law, one should begin with its language: "Everyone has a right to life. . . ." Life, in the sense of historical existence of a human individual, exists according to definite biological-physiological knowledge, in any case, from the 14th day after conception (nidation, individuation) (cf. on this point the statements of Hinrichsen before the Special Committee for the Reform of the Penal Law, Sixth Election Period, 74th Session, Stenographic Reports, pp. 2142 ff.). The process of development which has begun at that point is a continuing process which exhibits no sharp demarcation and does not allow a precise division of the various steps of development of the human life. The process does not end even with birth; the phenomena of consciousness which are specific to the human personality, for example, appear for the first time a rather long time after birth. Therefore, the protection of Article 2, Paragraph 2, Sentence 1, of the Basic Law cannot be limited either to the "completed" human being after birth or to the child about to be born which is independently capable of living. The right to life is guaranteed to everyone who "lives"; no distinction can be made here between various stages of the life developing itself before birth, or between unborn and born life. "Everyone" in the sense of Article 2, Paragraph 2, Sentence 1, of the Basic Law is "everyone living"; expressed in another way: every life possessing human individuality; "everyone" also includes the yet unborn human being.

c) In opposition to the objection that "everyone" commonly denotes, both in everyday language as well as in legal language, a "completed" person and that a strict interpretation of the language speaks therefore against the inclusion of the unborn life within the effective area of Article 2, Paragraph 2, Sentence 1, of the Basic Law, it should be emphasized that, in any case, the sense and purpose of this provision of the Basic Law require that the protection of life should also be extended to the life developing itself. The security of human existence against encroachments by the state would be incomplete if it did not also embrace the prior step of "completed life," unborn life.

This extensive interpretation corresponds to the principle established in the opinions of the Federal Constitutional Court, "according to which, in doubtful cases, that interpretation is to be selected which develops to the highest degree the judicial effectiveness of the fundamental legal norm" (Decisions of the Federal Constitutional Court. 32, 54 71; 6, 55 72).

d) In support of this result the legislative history of Article 2, Paragraph 2, Sentence 1, of the Basic Law may be adduced here.

After the German Party (DP) had made repeated moves to make explicit reference to "germinating life" in connection with the right to life and bodily inviolability (Federal Council Press 11.48–298 and 12.48–398), the Parliamentary Council deliberated on this circle of problems for the first time in its Committee for Fundamental Questions, the 32nd session, held on January 11, 1949. In the discussion of the question whether a provision should be incorporated into the Basic Law which would forbid medical operations which do not serve health, Representative Dr. Heuss (FDP) explained, without encountering opposition, that compulsory sterilization and abortion in connection with the right to life were at issue. The Main Committee of the Parliamentary Council in its 42nd session on January 18, 1949, thoroughly dealt with, during the second reading on fundamental rights (proceedings of the Chief Committee of the Parliamentary Council, Stenographic Reports, pp. 529 ff.), the question of the inclusion of developing life in the protection of the constitution. Parliamentary Representative Dr. Seebohm (DP) proposed to add both of the following sentences to Article 2, Paragraph 1, of the Basic Law as it existed at that time: "Germinating life is protected" and "the death penalty is abolished." On this point Dr. Seebohm (loc. cit., pp. 533 ff.) commented that the right to life and bodily inviolability possibly does not unconditionally embrace germinating life as well. Therefore, he concluded, it must be specially mentioned in this context. At the least, he continued, one must expressly enter

into the record that germinating life is explicitly included in the right to life and bodily inviolability, if another interpretation is possible.

Parliamentary Representative Dr. Weber explained in the name of the CDU/CSU that her faction, when it intercedes for the right to life, means life simply; and, in the faction's view, germinating life, and above all, the defense of germinating life is contained in the right (loc. cit., p. 534). Dr. Heuss (FDP) agreed with Dr. Weber that the concept of life also embraces developing life; however, matters should not be placed in the constitution which are regulated in the penal law. As a consequence, he considered both the mention of germinating life as well as the death penalty as a special question to be superfluous (loc. cit., p. 535).

"After the unopposed explanations according to which germinating life is embraced in the right to life and bodily inviolability," Dr. Seebohm desired to withdraw his motion (loc. cit., p. 535). However Parliamentary Representative Dr. Greve (SPD) declared: "I must explicitly say here, for the record, that at the least as far as I am concerned, I do not understand the right of germinating life to be within the right to life. I would also like on behalf of my friends, at least for the great majority to them, to deliver a clarification of like content in order to establish for the minutes that the Main Committee of the Parliamentary Council in its entirety does not adopt the standpoint which my colleague Dr. Seebohm just expressed." The motion of Dr. Seebohm was presented once again at that point but was indeed rejected by eleven votes to seven (loc. cit., p. 535). In the written report of the Main Committee (page 7), however, Parliamentary Representative Dr. von Mangoldt (CDU) explained with regard to Article 2 of the Basic Law: "With the guaranteeing of the right to life, germinating life should also be protected. The motions introduced by the German Party in the Main Committee to attach a particular sentence about the protection of germinating life did not attain a majority only because, according to the view prevailing in the Committee, the value to be protected was already secured through the present version."

The plenary Parliamentary Council concurred in Article 2, Paragraph 2, of the Basic Law on May 6, 1949, in the

second reading, there being two votes in opposition. At the third reading on May 8, 1949, both Parliamentary Representatives Dr. Seebohm as well as Dr. Weber stated that, according to their conception, Article 2, Paragraph 2, of the Basic Law would also include germinating life within the protection of this fundamental right (proceedings of the Parliamentary Council, Stenographic Reports, pp. 218, 223). The comments of both speakers stood without opposition.

The history of the origin of Article 2, Paragraph 2, Sentence 1, of the Basic Law suggests that the formulation "everyone has the right to life" should also include "germinating" life. In any case, even less can be concluded from the materials on behalf of the contrary point of view. On the other hand, no evidence is found in the legislative history for answering the question whether unborn life must be protected by the penal law.

e) Furthermore, in the deliberations on the Fifth Statute to Reform the Penal Law there was unity regarding the value of protecting unborn life, although, to be sure, the constitutional structure of the problem has not been treated definitively. In the report of the Special Committee for the Reform of the Penal Law on the statutory draft introduced by the Factions of the SPD and FDP, inter alia, it was stated on this point:

The legal value of unborn life is to be respected in principle equally with that of born life.

This determination is self-evident for the stage in which unborn life would also be capable of independent life outside of the mother's womb. The determination, however, is already justified for the earlier stage of development which begins approximately 14 days after conception, as, among others, Hinrichsen convincingly established in the public hearing (AP, VI, pp. 2142 ff.). . . . That in the entire later development no corresponding point of demarcation may be established in the process is the completely overwhelming view in medical, anthropological, and theological science. . . .

Therefore, it is impermissible to deny the existence of unborn life from the end of nidation on or to contemplate it merely with indifference. The question debated in the literature whether, and if the occasion arises, to what extent the Basic Law should include unborn life in its protection, need not be an-

swered at this point. In any case, if one disregards the extreme ideas of individual groups, the concept of unborn life as a legal value of high rank corresponds to the general public's understanding of the law. This understanding of the law also lies at the basis of this draft.
(Federal Parliamentary Press, 7/1981, new, p. 5)

2. The duty of the state to protect every human life may therefore be directly deduced from Article 2, Paragraph 2, Sentence 1, of the Basic Law. In addition to that, the duty also results from the explicit provision of Article 1, Paragraph 1, Sentence 2, of the Basic Law since developing life participates in the protection which Article 1, Paragraph 1, of the Basic Law guarantees to human dignity. Where human life exists, human dignity is present to it; it is not decisive that the bearer of this dignity himself be conscious of it and know personally how to preserve it. The potential faculties present in the human being from the beginning suffice to establish human dignity.

II

1. The duty of the state to protect is comprehensive. It forbids not only—self-evidently—direct state attacks on the life developing itself but also requires the state to take a position protecting and promoting this life, that is to say, it must, above all, preserve it even against illegal attacks by others. It is for the individual areas of the legal order, each according to its special function, to effectuate this requirement. The degree of seriousness with which the state must take its obligation to protect increases as the rank of the legal value in question increases in importance within the order of values of the Basic Law. Human life represents, within the order of the Basic Law, an ultimate value, the particulars of which need not be established; it is the living foundation of human dignity and the prerequisite for all other fundamental rights.

2. The obligation of the state to take the life developing itself under protection exists, as a matter of principle, even against the mother. Without doubt, the natural connection of unborn life with that of the mother establishes an especially unique relationship, for which there is no parallel in other circumstances of life. Pregnancy belongs to the sphere of intimacy of

the woman, the protection of which is constitutionally guaranteed through Article 2, Paragraph 1, in connection with Article 1, Paragraph 1, of the Basic Law. Were the embryo to be considered only as a part of the maternal organism the interruption of pregnancy would remain in the area of the private structuring of one's life, where the legislature is forbidden to encroach (Decisions of the Federal Constitutional Court, 6, 32 41; 6, 389 433; 27, 344 350; 32, 373 379). Since, however, the one about to be born is an independent human being who stands under the protection of the constitution, there is a social dimension to the interruption of pregnancy which makes it amenable to and in need of regulation by the state. The right of the woman to the free development of her personality, which has as its content the freedom of behavior in a comprehensive sense and accordingly embraces the personal responsibility of the woman to decide against parenthood and the responsibilities flowing from it, can also, it is true, likewise demand recognition and protection. This right, however, is not guaranteed without limits—the rights of others, the constitutional order, and the moral law limit it. A priori, this right can never include the authorization to intrude upon the protected sphere of right of another without justifying reason or much less to destroy that sphere along with the life itself; this is even less so, if, according to the nature of the case, a special responsibility exists precisely for this life.

A compromise which guarantees the protection of the life of the one about to be born and permits the pregnant woman the freedom of abortion is not possible since the interruption of pregnancy always means the destruction of the unborn life. In the required balancing, "both constitutional values are to be viewed in their relationship to human dignity, the center of the value system of the constitution" (Decisions of the Federal Constitutional Court, 35, 202 225). A decision oriented to Article 1, Paragraph 1, of the Basic Law must come down in favor of the precedence of the protection of life for the child en ventre sa mere over the right of the pregnant woman to self-determination. Regarding many opportunities for development of personality,

she can be adversely affected through pregnancy, birth and the education of her children. On the other hand, the unborn life is destroyed through the interruption of pregnancy. According to the principle of the balance which preserves most of competing constitutionally protected positions in view of the fundamental idea of Article 19, Paragraph 2, of the Basic Law;[1] precedence must be given to the protection of the life of the child about to be born. This precedence exists as a matter of principle for the entire duration of pregnancy and may not be placed in question for any particular time. The opinion expressed in the Federal Parliament during the third deliberation on the Statute to Reform the Penal Law, the effect of which is to propose the precedence for a particular time "of the right to self-determination of the woman which flows from human dignity vis-a-vis all others, including the child's right to life" (German Federal Parliament, Seventh Election Period, 96th Session, Stenographic Reports, p. 6492), is not reconcilable with the value ordering of the Basic Law.

3. From this point, the fundamental attitude of the legal order which is required by the constitution with regard to the interruption of pregnancy becomes clear: the legal order may not make the woman's right to self-determination the sole guideline of its rulemaking. The state must proceed, as a matter of principle, from a duty to carry the pregnancy to term and therefore to view, as a matter of principle, its interruption as an injustice. The condemnation of abortion must be clearly expressed in the legal order. The false impression must be avoided that the interruption of pregnancy is the same social process as, for example, approaching a physician for healing an illness or indeed a legally irrelevant alternative for the prevention of conception. The state may not abdicate its responsibility even through the recognition of a "legally free area," by which the state abstains from the value judgment and abandons this judgment to the decision of the individual to be made on the basis of his own sense of responsibility.

III

How the state fulfills its obligation for an effective protection of developing life is, in the first instance, to be decided by the legislature. It determines which measures of protection are required and which serve the purpose of guaranteeing an effective protection of life.

1. In this connection the guiding principle of the precedence of prevention over repression is also valid particularly for the protection of unborn life (Decisions of the Federal Constitutional Court, 30, 336 350). It is therefore the task of the state to employ, in the first instance, social, political, and welfare means for securing developing life. What can happen here and how the assistance measures are to be structured in their particulars is largely left to the legislature and is generally beyond judgment by the Constitutional Court. Moreover, the primary concern is to strengthen readiness of the expectant mother to accept the pregnancy as her own responsibility and to bring the child *en ventre sa mere* to full life. Regardless of how the state fulfills its obligation to protect, it should not be forgotten that developing life itself is entrusted by nature in the first place to the protection of the mother. To reawaken and, if required, to strengthen the maternal duty to protect, where it is lost, should be the principal goal of the endeavours of the state for the protection of life. Of course, the possibilities for the legislature to influence are limited. Measures introduced by the legislature are frequently only indirect and effective only after completion of the time-consuming process of comprehensive education and the alteration in the attitudes and philosophies of society achieved thereby.

2. The question of the extent to which the state is obligated under the constitution to employ, even for the protection of unborn life, the penal law, the sharpest weapon standing at its disposal, cannot be answered by the simplified posing of the question whether the state must punish certain acts. A total consideration is necessary which, on the one hand, takes into account the worth of the injured legal value and the extent of the social harm of the injurious act—in comparison with other acts which socio-ethically are perhaps similarly assessed and which are subject to punishment—and which, on the other hand, takes into account the traditional legal regulation

of this area of life as well as the development of concepts of the role of the penal law in modern society; and, finally, does not leave out of consideration the practical effectiveness of penal sanctions and the possibility of their replacement through other legal sanctions.

The legislature is not obligated, as a matter of principle, to employ the same penal measures for the protection of the unborn life as it considers required and expedient for born life. As a look at legal history shows, this was never the case in the application of penal sanctions and is also true for the situation in the law up to the Fifth Statute to Reform the Penal Law.

a) The task of penal law from the beginning has been to protect the elementary values of community life. That the life of every individual human being is among the most important legal values has been established above. The interruption of pregnancy irrevocably destroys an existing human life. Abortion is an act of killing; this is most clearly shown by the fact that the relevant penal sanction—even in the Fifth Statute to Reform the Penal Law—is contained in the section "Felonies and Misdemeanors against Life" and, in the previous penal law, was designated the "Killing of the Child *en ventre sa mere*." The description now common, "interruption of pregnancy," cannot camouflage this fact. No legal regulation can pass over the fact that this act offends against the fundamental inviolability and indisposability of human life protected by Article 2, Paragraph 2, Sentence 1, of the Basic Law. From this point of view, the employment of penal law for the requital of "acts of abortion" is to be seen as legitimate without a doubt; it is valid law in most cultural states—under prerequisites of various kinds—and especially corresponds to the German legal tradition. Therefore, it follows that the law cannot dispense with clearly labeling this procedure as "unjust." . . .

3. The obligation of the state to protect the developing life exists—as shown—against the mother as well. Here, however, the employment of the penal law may give rise to special problems which result from the unique situation of the pregnant woman. The

incisive effects of a pregnancy on the physical and emotional condition of the woman are immediately evident and need not be set forth in greater detail. They often mean a considerable change of the total conduct of life and a limitation of the possibilities for personal development. This burden is not always and not completely balanced by a woman finding new fulfillment in her task as mother and by the claim a pregnant woman has upon the assistance of the community (Article 6, Paragraph 4, of the Basic Law). In individual cases, difficult, even life-threatening situations of conflict may arise. The right to life of the unborn can lead to a burdening of the woman which essentially goes beyond that normally associated with pregnancy. The result is the question of exactability, or, in other words, the question of whether the state, even in such cases, may compel the bearing of the child to term with the means of the penal law. Respect for the unborn life and the right of the woman not to be compelled to sacrifice the values in her own life in excess of an exactable measure in the interest of respecting this legal value are in conflict with each other. In such a situation of conflict which, in general, does not allow an unequivocal moral judgment and in which the decision for an interruption of pregnancy can attain the rank of a decision of conscience worthy of consideration, the legislature is obligated to exercise special restraint. If, in these cases, it views the conduct of the pregnant woman as not deserving punishment and forgoes the use of penal sanctions, the result, at any rate, is to be constitutionally accepted as a balancing incumbent upon the legislature.

A continuation of the pregnancy appears to be non-exactable especially when it is proven that the interruption is required "to avert" from the pregnant woman "a danger for her life or the danger of a grave impairment of her condition of health" (§218b, No. 1, of the Penal Code in the version of the Fifth Statute to Reform the Penal Law). In this case her own "right to life and bodily inviolability" (Article 2, Paragraph 2, Sentence 1, of the Basic Law) is at stake, the sacrifice of which cannot be expected of her for the unborn life. Beyond that, the legislature has a free hand to leave the interruption of pregnancy free of punishment in the case of other extraordinary burdens for the pregnant woman, which, from the point of view of non-exactability, are as weighty as those referred to in §218b, No. 1. In this category can be counted, especially, the cases of the eugenic (cf. Section 218b, No. 2, of the Penal Code), ethical (criminological), and of the social or emergency indication for abortion which were contained in the draft proposed by the Federal Government in the sixth election period of the Federal Parliament and were discussed both in the public debate as well as in the course of the legislative proceedings. During the deliberations of the Special Committee for the Reform of the Penal Law (Seventh Election Period, 25th Session, Stenographic Reports, pp. 1470 ff.), the representative of the Federal Government explained in detail and with convincing reasons why, in these four cases of indication, the bearing of the child to term does not appear to be exactable. The decisive viewpoint is that in all of these cases another interest equally worthy of protection, from the standpoint of the constitution, asserts its validity with such urgency that the state's legal order cannot require that the pregnant woman must, under all circumstances, concede precedence to the right of the unborn. . . .

In all other cases the interruption of pregnancy remains a wrong deserving punishment since, in these cases, the destruction of a value of the law of the highest rank is subjected to the unrestricted pleasure of another and is not motivated by an emergency. If the legislature wants to dispense (even in this case) with penal law punishment, this would be compatible with the requirement to protect of Article 2, Paragraph 2, Sentence 1, of the Basic Law, only on the condition that another equally effective legal sanction stands at its command which would clearly bring out the unjust character of the act (the condemnation by the legal order) and likewise prevent the interruptions of pregnancy as effectively as a penal provision. . . .

I

The constitutional requirement to protect developing life is directed in the first instance to the legislature. The duty is incumbent on the Federal Constitutional Court, however, to determine, in the exercise of the function allotted to it by the Basic Law, whether the legislature has fulfilled this requirement. Indeed, the Court must carefully observe the discretion of the legislature which belongs to it in evaluating the factual conditions which lie at the basis of its formation of norms, which discretion is fitting for the required prognosis and choice of means. The court may not put itself in the place of the legislature; it is, however, its task to examine carefully whether the legislature, in the framework of the possibilities standing at its disposal, has done what is necessary to avert dangers from the legal value to be protected. This is also fundamentally true for the question whether the legislature is obligated to utilize its sharpest means, the penal law, in which case the examination can extend beyond the individual modalities of punishment.

II

It is generally recognized that the previous §218 of the Penal Code, precisely because it threatened punishment without distinction for nearly all cases of the interruption of pregnancy, has, as a result, only insufficiently protected developing life. The insight that there are cases in which the penal sanction is not appropriate has finally led to the point that cases actually deserving of punishment are no longer prosecuted with the necessary vigor. In addition, with respect to this offense, there is, in the nature of the case, the frequently difficult clarification of the factual situation. Certainly, the statistics on the incidence of illegal abortion differ greatly and it may hardly be possible to ascertain reliable data on this point through empirical investigations. In any case, the number of the illegal interruptions of pregnancy in the Federal Republic was high. The existence of a general penal norm may have contributed to that, since the state had neglected to employ other adequate measures for the protection of developing life. . . .

The weighing in bulk of life against life which leads to the allowance of the destruction of a supposedly smaller number in the interest of the preservation of an allegedly larger number is not reconcilable with the obligation of an individual protection of each single concrete life.

In the judicial opinions of the Federal Constitutional Court the principle has been developed that the unconstitutionality of a statutory provision, which in its structure and actual effect prejudices a definite circle of persons, may not be refuted with the showing that this provision or other regulations of the statute favor another circle of persons. The emphasis of the general tendency of the statute as a whole to favor legal protection is even less adequate for this purpose. This principle (cf. Decisions of the Federal Constitutional Court, 12, 151 168; 15, 328 333; 18, 97 108; 32, 260 269) is valid in special measure for the highest personal legal value, "life." The protection of the individual life may not be abandoned for the reason that a goal of saving other lives, in itself worthy of respect, is pursued. Every human life—the life first developing itself as well—is as such equally valuable and can not therefore be subjected to a discriminatory evaluation, no matter how shaded, or indeed to a balancing on the basis of statistics.

In the basic legal political conception of the Fifth Statute to Reform the Penal Law a concept, which cannot be followed, of the function of a constitutional statute is recognizable. The legal protection for the concrete individual human life required by the constitution is pushed into the background in favor of a more "socio-technical" use of the statute as an intended action of the legislature for the achievement of a definitely desired socio-political goal, the "containing of the abortion epidemic." The legislature may, however, not merely have a goal in view, be it ever so worthy of pursuit; it must be aware that every step on the way to the goal must be justified before the constitution and its indispensable postulates. The fundamental legal protection in individual cases may not be sacrificed to the efficiency of the regulation as a whole. The statute is not only an instrument to steer social processes according to sociological judgments and prognoses but is also the enduring expression of socio-ethical—and as a consequence—legal evaluation of human acts; it should say what is right and wrong for the individual. . . .

The counseling and instruction of the pregnant woman provided under §218c, Par. 1, of the Penal Code cannot, considered by itself, be viewed as suitable to effectuate a continuation of the pregnancy.

The measures proposed in this provision fall short of the concepts of the Alternative Draft of the 16 criminal law scholars, upon which the conception of the Fifth Statute to Reform the Penal Law is, after all, largely based. The counseling centers provided for in §105, Par. 1, No. 2, of the Fifth Statute to Reform the Penal Law should themselves have the means to afford financial, social, and family assistance. Furthermore, they should provide to the pregnant woman and her relatives emotional care through suitable co-workers and work intensively for the continuation of the pregnancy (cf. for particulars, above, pp. 11 ff.).

So to equip the counseling centers, in the sense of this or similar suggestions, so that they are able to arrange direct assistance, would come much nearer the mark, since according to the report of the Special Committee for the Reform of the Penal Law (Printed Materials of the Federal Parliament, 7/1981, new, p. 7, with evidentiary support from the hearings) the unfavorable living situation, the impossibility of caring for a child while pursuing an education or working as well as economic need and special material reasons, and, especially in the case of single mothers, anxiety about social sanctions are supposed to be among the most frequently given causes and motives for the desire for the interruption of pregnancy.

On the other hand, the counseling centers will give instruction about "the public and private assistance available for pregnant women, mothers, and children," "especially regarding assistance which facilitates the continuation of the pregnancy and alleviates the situation of mother and child." This could be interpreted to mean that the counseling centers should only inform, without exerting influence directed to the motivational process. Whether the neutral description of the task of the counseling centers may be attributed to the opinion advocated in the Special

Committee for the Reform of the Penal Law that the pregnant woman should not be influenced in her decision through the counseling (Representative von Schöler, FDP, Seventh Election Period, 25th Session, Stenographic Reports, p. 1473) can remain an open question. If a protective effect in favor of developing life is to accrue to the counseling, it will depend, in any case, decisively upon such an exertion of influence. Section 218c. Par. 1, Nos. 1 and 2, to be sure, allow the interpretation that counseling and instruction should motivate the pregnant woman to carry the pregnancy to term. The report of the Special Committee is probably to be understood in this sense (Printed Materials of the Federal Parliament, 7/1981, new, p. 16); accordingly, the counseling should take into account the total circumstances of life of the pregnant woman and follow up personally and individually, not by telephone or by distributing printed materials (cf. also the previously mentioned resolution of the Federal Parliament, Printed Materials of the Federal Parliament, 7/2042).

Even if one might consider it thinkable that counseling of this kind could exercise a definite effect in the sense of an aversion from the decision for abortion, its structure, in particular, exhibits in any case deficiencies which do not allow the expectation of an effective protection of developing life.

The instruction about the public and private assistance available for pregnant women, mothers and children, according to §218c, Par. 1, No. 1, can also be undertaken by any physician. Social law and social reality are, however, very difficult for the technically trained person to comprehend. A reliable instruction regarding the demands and possibilities in the individual case cannot be expected from a physician, especially since individual inquiries regarding need for frequently required (e.g., for assistance with rent or social assistance). Physicians are neither qualified for such counseling activity by their professional training nor do they generally have the time required for individual counseling.

It is especially questionable that the instruction about social assistance can be undertaken by the same physician who will perform the interruption of pregnancy. Through this provision the medical counseling under §218c,

Par. 1, No. 2, which itself falls within the realm of medical competence will be devalued. The counseling should be structured in conformity with the views of the Special Committee for the Reform of the Penal Law as follows:

Therefore, what is meant is counseling regarding the nature of the operation and its possible consequences for health. That the counseling may however not be limited to this purely medical aspect is emphasized through the conscious choice of the term 'by a physician'. Rather the counseling as far as possible and appropriate must speak to the present and future total situation of the pregnant woman to the extent that she can be affected by the interruption of pregnancy, and, at the same time, correspond to the other task of the physician, which is to work for the protection of the unborn life. The physician must, therefore, make it clear to the pregnant woman that human life is destroyed by the operation and explain its stage of development. Experience shows, as confirmed in the public hearing, for example, by Pross (AP, VI, p. 2255, 2256) and Rolinski (AP, VI, p. 2221) that in this respect many women do not have clear ideas and that this circumstance, if they later learn it, is frequently the occasion for burdening doubts and questionings of conscience. Accordingly, the counseling must be directed to preventing this kind of conflict situation.
(Printed Materials of the Federal Parliament, 7/1981, new, p. 16)

An explanation, in the manner proposed here, which has the required constitutional goal of working for a continuation of the pregnancy cannot be expected from the physician who has been sought out by the pregnant woman precisely for the purpose of performing the interruption of pregnancy. Since, according to the result of the previous inquiries and according to the position statements of representative medical professional panels, it must be assumed that the majority of physicians decline to perform interruptions of pregnancy which are not indicated, only those physicians will make themselves available who either see in the interruption of pregnancy a money-making business or who are inclined to comply with every wish of a woman for interruption of pregnancy because they see in it merely a manifestation of the right to self-determination or a means to the emancipation of women. In both cases, an influence by the physician on the pregnant woman for the continuation of the pregnancy is highly improbable.

The experiences in England show this. There the indication (very broadly conceived) must be determined by any two physicians of the patient's choosing. This has led to the result that almost every desired abortion is carried out by private physicians specializing in such activity. The appearance of professional agents who guide women to these private clinics is an especially unfortunate by-product which is very difficult to avoid (cf. Lane Report, Vol. 1, No. 436 and 452).

Furthermore, the prospects for success are poor since the interruption of pregnancy can immediately follow the instruction and counseling. A serious exchange with the pregnant woman and others involved in which the arguments in the counseling are contrasted with hers is not to be expected under these circumstances. The alternative formulation proposed by the Federal Ministry of Justice to the Special Committee for Penal Law Reform for §218c provided as a consequence that the interruption of pregnancy could first be performed after a minimum of three days had elapsed after the instruction about available assistance (§218, Par. 1, No. 1) (Special Committee, Seventh Election Period, 30th Session, Stenographic Reports, p. 1659). In conformity with a report of the Special Committee, however, "a waiting period, enforced by the penal law, between the counseling and the operation . . . was rejected. This could in individual cases bring with it unreasonable difficulties for the pregnant woman according to her place of residence and her personal situation, with the consequence that the pregnant woman will dispense with the counseling." (Printed Materials of Federal Parliament, 7/1981, new, p. 17). For the woman decided upon an interruption of pregnancy it is only necessary to find an obliging physician. Since he may undertake the social as well as the medical counseling and finally even carry out the operation, a serious attempt to dissuade the pregnant woman from her decision is not to be expected from him.

III

In summary, the following observations should be made on the constitutional adjudication of the regulation of terms encountered in the Fifth Statute to Reform the Penal Law:

That interruptions of pregnancy are neither legally condemned nor subject to punishment is not compatible with the duty incumbent upon the legislature to protect life, if the interruptions are the result of reasons which are not recognized in the value order of the Basic Law. Indeed, the limiting of punishability would not be constitutionally objectionable if it were combined with other measures which would be able to compensate, at least in their effect, for the disappearance of penal protection. That is however—as shown—obviously not the case. The parliamentary discussions about the reform of the abortion law have indeed deepened the insight that it is the principal task of the state to prevent the killing of unborn life through enlightenment about the prevention of pregnancy on the one hand as well as through effective promotional measures in society and through a general alteration of social concepts on the other. Neither the assistance of the kind presently offered and guaranteed nor the counseling provided in the Fifth Statute to Reform the Penal Law are, however, able to replace the individual protection of life which a penal norm fundamentally provides even today in those cases in which no reason for the interruption of pregnancy exists which is worthy of consideration according to the value order of the Basic Law.

If the legislature regards the previously undifferentiated threat of punishment for the interruption of pregnancy as a questionable means for the protection of life, it is not thereby released from the obligation to undertake the attempt to achieve a better protection of life through a differentiated penal regulation by subjecting the same cases to punishment in which the interruption of pregnancy is to be condemned on constitutional grounds. A clear distinction of this group of cases in contrast to other cases in which the continuation of the pregnancy is not exactable from the woman will strengthen the power of the penal norm to develop a legal awareness. He

who generally recognizes the precedence of the protection of life over the claim of the woman for an unrestricted structuring of her life will not be able to dispute the unjust nature of the act in those cases not covered by a particular indication. If the state not only declares that these cases are punishable but also prosecutes and punishes them in legal practice, this will be perceived in the legal consciousness of the community neither as unjust nor as anti-social.

The passionate discussion of the abortion problematic may provide occasion for the fear that in a segment of the population the value of unborn life is no longer fully recognized. This, however, does not give the legislature a right to acquiesce. It rather must make a sincere effort through a differentiation of the penal sanction to achieve a more effective protection of life and formulate a regulation which will be supported by the general legal consciousness.

IV

The regulation encountered in the Fifth Statute to Reform the Penal Law at times is defended with the argument that in other democratic countries of the Western World in recent times the penal provisions regulating the interruption of pregnancy have been "liberalized" or "modernized" in a similar or an even more extensive fashion; this would be, as the argument goes, an indication that the new regulation corresponds, in any case, to the general development of theories in this area and is not inconsistent with fundamental socio-ethical and legal principles.

These considerations cannot influence the decision to be made here. Disregarding the fact that all of these foreign laws in their respective countries are sharply controverted, the legal standards which are applicable there for the acts of the legislature are essentially different from those of the Federal Republic of Germany.

Underlying the Basic Law are principles for the structuring of the state that may be understood only in light of the historical experience and the spiritual-moral confrontation with the previous system of National Socialism. In opposition to the omnipotence of the totalitarian state which claimed for itself limitless dominion over all areas of social life and which, in the prosecution of its goals of state, consideration for the life of the individual fundamentally meant nothing, the Basic Law of the Federal Republic of Germany has erected an order bound together by values which places the individual human being and his dignity at the focal point of all of its ordinances. At its basis lies the concept, as the Federal Constitutional Court previously pronounced (Decisions of the Federal Constitutional Court, 2, 1 12), that human beings possess an inherent worth as individuals in order of creation which uncompromisingly demands unconditional respect for the life of every individual human being, even for the apparently socially "worthless," and which therefore excludes the destruction of such life without legally justifiable grounds. This fundamental constitutional decision determines the structure and the interpretation of the entire legal order. Even the legislature is bound by it; considerations of socio-political expediency, even necessities of state, cannot overcome this constitutional limitation (Decisions of the Federal Constitutional Court, 1, 14 36). Even a general change of the viewpoints dominant in the populace on this subject—if such a change could be established at all—would change nothing. The Federal Constitutional Court, which is charged by the constitution with overseeing the observance of its fundamental principles by all organs of the state and, if necessary, with giving them effect, can orient its decisions only on those principles to the development of which this Court has decisively contributed in its judicial utterances. Therefore, no adverse judgment is being passed about other legal orders "which have not had these experiences with a system of injustice and which, on the basis of an historical development which has taken a different course and other political conditions and fundamental views of the philosophy of state, have not made such a decision for themselves" (Decisions of the Federal Constitutional Court, 18, 112 117).

On the basis of these considerations, §218a of the Penal Code in the version of the Fifth Statute to Reform the Penal

Law is inconsistent with Article 2, Paragraph 2, Sentence 1, in conjunction with Article 1, Paragraph 1, of the Basic Law to the extent that it excepts interruption of pregnancy from punishability if no reasons are present which, according to the present opinion, have standing under the ordering of values of the Basic Law. Within this framework, the nullity of the provision is to be determined. It is a matter for the legislature to distinguish in greater detail the cases of indicated interruption of pregnancy from those not indicated. In the interest of legal clarity, until a valid statutory regulation goes into effect, it appeared necessary, under §35 of the Statute for the Federal Constitutional Court, to issue a directive, the contents of which are obvious from the tenor of this judgment.

There is no occasion to declare further provisions of the Fifth Statute to Reform the Penal Law to be invalid.

Dr. Benda
Rupp von Brünneck
Ritterspach
Dr. Böhmer
Dr. Haager
Dr. Faller
Dr. Brox
Dr. Simon

Dissenting Opinion

Of Justice Rupp von Brünneck and Justice Dr. Simon to the judgment of February 25, 1975, of the First Senate of the Federal Constitutional Court.

The life of each individual human being is self-evidently a central value of the legal order. It is uncontested that the constitutional duty to protect this life also includes its preliminary stages before birth. The debates in Parliament and before the Federal Constitutional Court dealt not with the *whether* but rather only the *how* of this protection. This decision is a matter of legislative responsibility. Under no circumstances can the duty of the state to prescribe punishment for abortion in every stage of pregnancy be derived from the constitution. The legislature should be able to determine the regulations for counseling and the term solution as well as for the indications solution.

A contrary construction of the constitution is not compatible with the liberal character of the fundamental legal

norms and shifts the competence to decide, to a material extent, onto the Federal Constitutional Court (A). In the judgment on the Fifth Statute to Reform the Penal Law, the majority neglects the uniqueness of abortion in relation to other risks of life (B.I.1. = p. 671 *et seq.*). It sufficiently appreciates the social problematic previously found by the legislature as well as the aims of urgent reform (B.I.2. = p. 673 *et seq.*). Because each solution remains patchwork, it is not constitutionally objectionable that the German legislature—in consonance with the reforms in other western civilized states (B.III. = p. 683 *et seq.*)—has given priority to social-political measures over largely ineffective penal sanctions (B.I.3.-5. = p. 675 *et seq.*). The constitution nowhere requires a legal "condemnation" of behavior not morally respectable without consideration of its actual protective effect (B.II. = p. 681 *et seq.*). . . .

Note

1. Article 19, Paragraph 2, of the Basic Law provides: "In no event may a fundamental right be impaired in its essential meaning."

70

Judith Jarvis Thomson
A Defense of Abortion

"A Defense of Abortion," by Judith Jarvis Thomson, *Philosophy and Public Affairs*, vol. 1, no. 1 (copyright © 1971 by Princeton University Press): pp. 47–66. Reprinted by permission of Princeton University Press.

Most opposition to abortion relies on the premise that the fetus is a human being, a person, from the moment of conception. The premise is argued for, but, as I think, not well. Take, for example, the most common argument. We are asked to notice that the development of a human being from conception through birth into childhood is continuous; then it is said that to draw a line, to choose a point in this development and say "before this point the thing is not a person, after this point it is a person" is to make an arbitrary choice, a choice for which in the nature of things no good reason can be given. It is concluded that the fetus is, or anyway that we had better say it is, a person from the moment of conception. But this conclusion does not follow. Similar things might be said about the development of an acorn into an oak tree, and it does not follow that acorns are oak trees, or that we had better say they are. Arguments of this form are sometimes called "slippery slope arguments"—the phrase is perhaps self-explanatory—and it is dismaying that opponents of abortion rely on them so heavily and uncritically.

I am inclined to agree, however, that the prospects for "drawing a line" in the development of the fetus look dim. I am inclined to think also that we shall probably have to agree that the fetus has already become a human person well before birth. Indeed, it comes as a surprise when one first learns how early in its life it begins to acquire human characteristics. By the tenth week, for example, it already has a face, arms and legs, fingers and toes; it has internal organs, and brain activity is detectable.[1] On the other hand, I think that the premise is false, that the fetus is not a person from the moment of conception. A newly fertilized ovum, a newly implanted clump of cells, is no more a person than an acorn is an oak tree. But I shall not discuss any of this. For it seems to me to be of great interest to ask what happens if, for the sake of argument, we allow the premise. How, precisely, are we supposed to get from there to the conclusion that abortion is morally impermissible? Opponents of abortion commonly spend most of their time establishing that the fetus is a person, and hardly any time explaining the step from there to the impermissibility of abortion. Perhaps they think the step too simple and obvious to require much comment. Or perhaps instead they are simply being economical in argument. Many of those who defend abortion rely on the premise that the fetus is not a person, but only a bit of tissue that will become a person at birth; and why pay out more arguments than you have to? Whatever the explanation, I suggest that the step they take is neither easy nor obvious, that it calls for closer examination than it is commonly given, and that when we do give it this closer examination we shall feel inclined to reject it.

I propose, then, that we grant that the fetus is a person from the moment of conception. How does the argument go from here? Something like this, I take it. Every person has a right to life. So the fetus has a right to life. No doubt the mother has a right to decide what shall happen in and to her body; everyone would grant that. But surely a person's right to life is stronger and more stringent than the mother's right to decide what happens in and to her body, and so outweighs it. So the fetus may not be killed; an abortion may not be performed.

It sounds plausible. But now let me ask you to imagine this. You wake up in the morning and find yourself back to back in bed with an unconscious violinist. A famous unconscious violinist. He has been found to have a fatal kidney ailment, and the Society of Music Lovers has canvassed all the available medical records and found that you alone have the right blood type to help. They have therefore kidnapped you, and last night the violinist's circulatory system was plugged into yours, so that your kidneys can be used to extract poisons from his blood as well as your own. The director of the hospital now tells you, "Look, we're sorry the Society of Music Lovers did this to you—we would never have permitted it if we had known. But still, they did it, and the violinist now is plugged into you. To unplug you would be to kill him. But never mind, it's only for nine months. By then he will have recovered from his ailment, and can safely be unplugged from you." Is it morally incumbent on you to accede to this situation? No doubt it would be very nice of you if you did, a great kindness. But do you *have* to accede to it? What if it were not nine months, but nine years? Or longer still? What if the director of the hospital says, "Tough luck, I agree, but you've now got to stay in bed, with the violinist plugged into you, for the rest of your life. Because remember this. All persons have a right to life, and violinists are persons. Granted you have a right to decide what happens in and to your body, but a person's right to life outweighs your right to decide what happens in and to your body. So you cannot ever be unplugged from him." I imagine you would regard this as outrageous, which suggests that something really is wrong with that plausible-sounding argument I mentioned a moment ago.

In this case, of course, you were kidnapped; you didn't volunteer for the operation that plugged the violinist into your kidneys. Can those who oppose abortion on the ground I mentioned make an exception for a pregnancy due to rape? Certainly. They can say that persons have a right to life only if they didn't come into existence because of rape; or they can say that all persons have a right to life, but that some have less of a right to life than others, in particular, that those who came into existence because of rape have less. But these statements have a rather unpleasant sound. Surely the question of whether you have a right to life at all, or how much of it you have, shouldn't turn on the question of whether or not you are the product of a rape. And in fact the people who oppose abortion on the ground I mentioned do not make this distinction, and hence do not make an exception in case of rape.

Nor do they make an exception for a case in which the mother has to spend the nine months of her pregnancy in bed. They would agree that would be a great pity, and hard on the mother; but all the same, all persons have a right to life, the fetus is a person, and so on. I suspect, in fact, that they would not make an exception for a case in which, miraculously enough, the pregnancy went on for nine years, or even the rest of the mother's life.

Some won't even make an exception for a case in which continuation of the pregnancy is likely to shorten the mother's life; they regard abortion as impermissible even to save the mother's life. Such cases are nowadays very rare, and many opponents of abortion do not accept this extreme view. All the same, it is a good place to begin: a number of points of interest come out in respect to it.

1. Let us call the view that abortion is impermissible even to save the mother's life "the extreme view." I want to suggest first that it does not issue from the argument I mentioned earlier without the addition of some fairly powerful premises. Suppose a woman has become pregnant, and now learns that she has a cardiac condition such that she will die if she carries the baby to term. What may be done for her? The fetus, being a person, has a right to life, but as the mother is a person too, so has she a right to life. Presumably that have an equal right to life. How is it supposed to come out that an abortion may not be performed? If mother and child have an equal right to life, shouldn't we perhaps flip a coin? Or should we add to the mother's right to life her right to decide what happens in and to her body, which everybody seems to be ready to grant—the sum of her rights now outweighing the fetus' right to life?

The most familiar argument here is the following. We are told that performing the abortion would be directly killing[2] the child, whereas doing nothing would not be killing the mother, but only letting her die. Moreover, in killing the child, one would be killing an innocent person, for the child has committed no crime, and is not aiming at his mother's death. And then there are a variety of ways in which this might be continued. (1) But as directly killing an innocent person is always and absolutely impermissible, an abortion may not be performed. Or, (2) as directly killing an innocent person is murder, and murder is always and absolutely impermissible, an abortion may not be performed.[3] Or, (3) as one's duty to refrain from directly killing an innocent person is more stringent than one's duty to keep a person from dying, an abortion may not be performed. Or, (4) if one's only options are directly killing an innocent person or letting a person die, one must prefer letting the person die, and thus an abortion may not be performed.[4]

Some people seem to have thought that these are not further premises which must be added if the conclusion is to be reached, but that they follow from the very fact that an innocent person has a right to life.[5] But this seems to me to be a mistake, and perhaps the simplest way to show this is to bring out that while we must certainly grant that innocent persons have a right to life, the theses in (1) through (4) are all false. Take (2), for example. If directly killing an innocent person is murder, and thus is impermissible, then the mother's directly killing the innocent person inside her is murder, and thus is impermissible. But it cannot seriously be thought to be murder if the mother performs an abortion on herself to save her life. It cannot seriously be said that she *must* refrain, that she *must* sit passively by and wait for her death. Let us look again at the case of you and the violinist. There you are, in bed with the violinist, and the director of the hospital says to you, "It's all most distressing, and I deeply sympathize, but you see this is putting an additional strain on your kidneys, and you'll be dead within the month. But you *have* to stay where you are all the same. Because unplugging you would be directly killing an innocent violinist, and that's murder, and that's impermissible." If anything in the world is true, it is that you do not commit murder, you do not do what is impermissible, if you reach around to your back and unplug yourself from that violinist to save your life.

The main focus of attention in writings on abortion has been on what a third party may or may not do in answer to a request from a woman for an abortion. This is in a way understandable. Things being as they are, there isn't much a woman can safely do to abort herself. So the question asked is what a third party may do, and what the mother may do, if it is mentioned at all, is deduced, almost as an afterthought, from what it is concluded that third parties may do. But it seems to me that to treat the matter in this way is to refuse to grant the mother that very status of person which is so firmly insisted on for the fetus. For we cannot simply read off what a person may do from what a third party may do. Suppose you find yourself trapped in a tiny house with a growing child. I mean a very tiny house, and a rapidly growing child—you are already up against the wall of the house and in a few minutes you'll be crushed to death. The child on the other hand won't be crushed to death; if nothing is done to stop him from growing he'll be hurt, but in the end he'll simply burst open the house and walk out a free man. Now I could well understand it if a bystander were to say, "There's nothing we can do for you. We cannot choose between your life and his, we cannot be the ones to decide who is to live, we cannot intervene." But it cannot be concluded that you too can do nothing, that you cannot attack it to save your life. However innocent the child may be, you do not have to wait passively while it crushes you to death. Perhaps a pregnant woman is vaguely felt to have the status of house, to which we don't allow the right of self-defense. But if the woman houses the child, it should be remembered that she is a person who houses it.

I should perhaps stop to say explicitly that I am not claiming that people have a right to do anything whatever to save their lives. I think, rather, that there are drastic limits to the right of self-defense. If someone threatens you with death unless you torture someone else to death, I think you have not the right, even to save your life, to do so. But the case under consideration here is very different. In our case there are only two people involved, one whose life is threatened, and one who threatens it. Both are innocent: the one who is threatened is not threatened because of any fault, the one who threatens does not threaten because of any fault. For this reason we may feel that we bystanders cannot intervene. But the person threatened can.

In sum, a woman surely can defend her life against the threat to it posed by the unborn child, even if doing so involves its death. And this shows not merely that the theses in (1) through (4) are false; it shows also that the extreme view of abortion is false, and so we need not canvass any other possible ways of arriving at it from the argument I mentioned at the outset.

2. The extreme view could of course be weakened to say that while abortion is permissible to save the mother's life,

it may not be performed by a third party, but only by the mother herself. But this cannot be right either. For what we have to keep in mind is that the mother and the unborn child are not like two tenants in a small house which has, by an unfortunate mistake, been rented to both: the mother *owns* the house. The fact that she does adds to the offensiveness of deducing that the mother can do nothing from the supposition that third parties can do nothing. But it does more than this: it casts a bright light on the supposition that third parties can do nothing. Certainly it lets us see that a third party who says "I cannot choose between you" is fooling himself if he thinks this is impartiality. If Jones has found and fastened on a certain coat, which he needs to keep him from freezing, but which Smith also needs to keep him from freezing, then it is not impartiality that says "I cannot choose between you" when Smith owns the coat. Women have said again and again "This body is *my* body!" and they have reason to feel angry, reason to feel that it has been like shouting into the wind. Smith, after all, is hardly likely to bless us if we say to him, "Of course it's your coat, anybody would grant that it is. But no one may choose between you and Jones who is to have it."

We should really ask what it is that says "no one may choose" in the face of the fact that the body that houses the child is the mother's body. It may be simply a failure to appreciate this fact. But it may be something more interesting, namely the sense that one has a right to refuse to lay hands on people, even where it would be just and fair to do so, even where justice seems to require that somebody do so. Thus justice might call for somebody to get Smith's coat back from Jones, and yet you have a right to refuse to be the one to lay hands on Jones, a right to refuse to do physical violence to him. This, I think, must be granted. But then what should be said is not "no one may choose," but only "*I* cannot choose," and indeed not even this, but "*I* will not *act*," leaving it open that somebody else can or should, and in particular that anyone in a position of authority, with the job of securing people's rights, both can and should. So this is no difficulty. I have not been arguing that any given third party must

accede to the mother's request that he perform an abortion to save her life, but only that he may.

I suppose that in some views of human life the mother's body is only on loan to her, the loan not being one which gives her any prior claim to it. One who held this view might well think it impartiality to say "I cannot choose." But I shall simply ignore this possibility. My own view is that if a human being has any just, prior claim to anything at all, he has a just, prior claim to his own body. And perhaps this needn't be argued for here anyway, since, as I mentioned, the arguments against abortion we are looking at do grant that the woman has a right to decide what happens in and to her body.

But although they do grant it, I have tried to show that they do not take seriously what is done in granting it. I suggest the same thing will reappear even more clearly when we turn away from cases in which the mother's life is at stake, and attend, as I propose we now do, to the vastly more common cases in which a woman wants an abortion for some less weighty reason than preserving her own life.

3. Where the mother's life is not at stake, the argument I mentioned at the outset seems to have a much stronger pull. "Everyone has a right to life, so the unborn person has a right to life." And isn't the child's right to life weightier than anything other than the mother's own right to life, which she might put forward as ground for an abortion?

This argument treats the right to life as if it were unproblematic. It is not, and this seems to me to be precisely the source of the mistake.

For we should now, at long last, ask what it comes to, to have a right to life. In some views having a right to life includes having a right to be given at least the bare minimum one needs for continued life. But suppose that what in fact *is* the bare minimum a man needs for continued life is something he has no right at all to be given? If I am sick unto death, and the only thing that will save my life is the touch of Henry Fonda's cool hand on my fevered brow, then all the same, I have no right to be given the touch of Henry Fonda's cool hand on my fevered brow. It would be frightfully nice of him to fly in from the West Coast to provide it. It would be less nice, though no doubt well meant, if my friends flew out to the West Coast and carried Henry Fonda back with them. But I have no right at all against anybody that he should do this for me. Or again, to return to the story I told earlier, the fact that for continued life that violinist needs the continued use of your kidneys does not establish that he has a right to be given the continued use of your kidneys. He certainly has no right against you that *you* should give him continued use of your kidneys. For nobody has any right to use your kidneys unless you give him such a right; and nobody has the right against you that you shall give him this right—if you do allow him to go on using your kidneys, this is a kindness on your part, and not something he can claim from you as his due. Nor has he any right against anybody else that *they* should give him continued use of your kidneys. Certainly he had no right against the Society of Music Lovers that they should plug him into you in the first place. And if you now start to unplug yourself, having learned that you will otherwise have to spend nine years in bed with him, there is nobody in the world who must try to prevent you, in order to see to it that he is given something he has a right to be given.

Some people are rather stricter about the right to life. In their view, it does not include the right to be given anything, but amounts to, and only to, the right not to be killed by anybody. But here a related difficulty arises. If everybody is to refrain from killing that violinist, then everybody must refrain from doing a great many different sorts of things. Everybody must refrain from slitting his throat, everybody must refrain from shooting him—and everybody must refrain from unplugging you from him. But does he have a right against everybody that they shall refrain from unplugging you from him? To refrain from doing this is to allow him to continue to use your kidneys. It could be argued that he has right against us that *we* should allow him to continue to use your kidneys. That is, while he had no right against us that

we should give him the use of your kidneys, it might be argued that he anyway has a right against us that we shall not now intervene and deprive him of the use of your kidneys. I shall come back to third-party interventions later. But certainly the violinist has no right against you that *you* shall allow him to continue to use your kidneys. As I said, if you do allow him to use them, it is a kindness on your part, and not something you owe him.

The difficulty I point to here is not peculiar to the right to life. It reappears in connection with all the other natural rights; and it is something which an adequate account of rights must deal with. For present purposes it is enough just to draw attention to it. But I would stress that I am not arguing that people do not have a right to life—quite to the contrary, it seems to me that the primary control we must place on the acceptability of an account of rights is that it should turn out in that account to be a truth that all persons have a right to life. I am arguing only that having a right to life does not guarantee having either a right to be given the use of or a right to be allowed continued use of another person's body— even if one needs it for life itself. So the right to life will not serve the opponents of abortion in the very simple and clear way in which they seem to have thought it would.

4. There is another way to bring out the difficulty. In the most ordinary sort of case, to deprive someone of what he has a right to is to treat him unjustly. Suppose a boy and his small brother are jointly given a box of chocolates for Christmas. If the older boy takes the box and refuses to give his brother any of the chocolates, he is unjust to him, for the brother has been given a right to half of them. But suppose that, having learned that otherwise it means nine years in bed with that violinist, you unplug yourself from him. You surely are not being unjust to him, for you gave him no right to use your kidney, and no one else can have given him any such right. But we have to notice that in unplugging yourself, you are killing him; and violinists, like everybody else, have a right to life, and thus in the view we were considering just now, the right not to be killed. So here you do what he supposedly has a right you shall not do, but you do not act unjustly to him in doing it.

The emendation which may be made at this point is this: the right to life consists not in the right not to be killed, but rather in the right not to be killed unjustly. This runs a risk of circularity, but never mind: it would enable us to square the fact that the violinist has a right to life with the fact that you do not act unjustly toward him in unplugging yourself, thereby killing him. For if you do not kill him unjustly, you do not violate his right to life, and so it is no wonder you do him no injustice.

But if this emendation is accepted, the gap in the argument against abortion stares us plainly in the face: it is by no means enough to show that the fetus is a person, and to remind us that all persons have a right to life—we need to be shown also that killing the fetus violates its right to life, i.e., that abortion is unjust killing. And is it?

I suppose we may take it as a datum that in a case of pregnancy due to rape the mother has not given the unborn person a right to the use of her body for food and shelter. Indeed, in what pregnancy could it be supposed that the mother has given the unborn person such a right? It is not as if there were unborn persons drifting about the world, to whom a woman who wants a child says "I invite you in."

But it might be argued that there are other ways one can have acquired a right to the use of another person's body than by having been invited to use it by that person. Suppose a woman voluntarily indulges in intercourse, knowing of the chance it will issue in pregnancy, and then she does become pregnant; is she not in part responsible for the presence, in fact the very existence, of the unborn person inside her? No doubt she did not invite it in. But doesn't her partial responsibility for its being there itself give it a right to the use of her body?[6] If so, then her aborting it would be more like the boy's taking away the chocolates, and less like your unplugging yourself from the violinist—doing so would be depriving it of what it does have a right to, and thus would be doing it an injustice.

And then, too, it might be asked whether or not she can kill it even to save her own life: If she voluntarily called it into existence, how can she now kill it, even in self-defense?

The first thing to be said about this is that it is something new. Opponents of abortion have been so concerned to make out the independence of the fetus, in order to establish that it has a right to life, just as its mother does, that they have tended to overlook the possible support they might gain from making out that the fetus is *dependent* on the mother, in order to establish that she has a special kind of responsibility for it, a responsibility that gives it rights against her which are not possessed by any independent person—such as an ailing violinist who is a stranger to her.

On the other hand, this argument would give the unborn person a right to its mother's body only if her pregnancy resulted from a voluntary act, undertaken in full knowledge of the chance a pregnancy might result from it. It would leave out entirely the unborn person whose existence is due to rape. Pending the availability of some further argument, then, we would be left with the conclusion that unborn persons whose existence is due to rape have no right to the use of their mothers' bodies, and thus that aborting them is not depriving them of anything they have a right to and hence is not unjust killing.

And we should also notice that it is not at all plain that this argument really does go even as far as it purports to. For there are cases and cases, and the details make a difference. If the room is stuffy, and I therefore open a window to air it, and a burglar climbs in, it would be absurd to say, "Ah, now he can stay, she's given him a right to the use of her house—for she is partially responsible for his presence there, having voluntarily done what enabled him to get in, in full knowledge that there are such things as burglars, and that burglars burgle." It would be still more absurd to say this if I had had bars installed outside my windows, precisely to prevent burglars from getting in, and a burglar got in only because of a defect in the bars. It remains equally absurd if we imagine it is not a burglar who climbs in, but an innocent person who blunders or falls in. Again, suppose it were like this: people-seeds drift about in the air like pollen, and if you open your windows, one may drift in and take root in your carpets or upholstery. You don't want children, so you fix up your windows with fine

mesh screens, the very best you can buy. As can happen, however, and on very, very rare occasions does happen, one of the screens is defective; and a seed drifts in and takes root. Does the person-plant who now develops have a right to the use of your house? Surely not—despite the fact that you voluntarily opened your windows, you knowingly kept carpets and upholstered furniture, and you knew that screens were sometimes defective. Someone may argue that you are responsible for its rooting, that it does have a right to your house, because after all you *could* have lived out your life with bare floors and furniture, or with sealed windows and doors. But this won't do—for by the same token anyone can avoid a pregnancy due to rape by having a hysterectomy, or anyway by never leaving home without a (reliable!) army.

It seems to me that the argument we are looking at can establish at most that there are *some* cases in which the unborn person has a right to the use of its mother's body, and therefore *some* cases in which abortion is unjust killing. There is room for much discussion and argument as to precisely which, if any. But I think we should sidestep this issue and leave it open, for at any rate the argument certainly does not establish that all abortion is unjust killing.

5. There is room for yet another argument here, however. We surely must all grant that there may be cases in which it would be morally indecent to detach a person from your body at the cost of his life. Suppose you learn that what the violinist needs is not nine years of your life, but only one hour: all you need do to save his life is to spend one hour in that bed with him. Suppose also that letting him use your kidneys for that one hour would not affect your health in the slightest. Admittedly you were kidnapped. Admittedly you did not give anyone permission to plug him into you. Nevertheless it seems to me plain you *ought* to allow him to use your kidneys for that hour—it would be indecent to refuse.

Again, suppose pregnancy lasted only an hour, and constituted no threat to life or health. And suppose that a woman becomes pregnant as a result of rape. Admittedly she did not voluntarily do anything to bring about the

existence of a child. Admittedly she did nothing at all which would give the unborn person a right to the use of her body. All the same it might well be said, as in the newly emended violinist story, that she *ought* to allow it to remain for that hour—that it would be indecent in her to refuse.

Now some people are inclined to use the term "right" in such a way that it follows from the fact that you ought to allow a person to use your body for the hour he needs, that he has a right to use your body for the hour he needs, even though he has not been given that right by any person or act. They may say that it follows also that if you refuse, you act unjustly toward him. This use of the term is perhaps so common that it cannot be called wrong; nevertheless it seems to me to be an unfortunate loosening of what we would do better to keep a tight rein on. Suppose that box of chocolates I mentioned earlier had not been given to both boys jointly, but was given only to the older boy. There he sits, stolidly eating his way through the box, his small brother watching enviously. Here we are likely to say "You ought not to be so mean. You ought to give your brother some of those chocolates." My own view is that it just does not follow from the truth of this that the brother has any right to any of the chocolates. If the boy refuses to give his brother any, he is greedy, stingy, callous—but not unjust. I suppose that the people I have in mind will say it does follow that the brother has a right to some of the chocolates, and thus that the boy does act unjustly if he refuses to give his brother any. But the effect of saying this is to obscure what we should keep distinct, namely the difference between the boy's refusal in this case and the boy's refusal in the earlier case, in which the box was given to both boys jointly, and in which the small brother thus had what was from any point of view clear title to half.

A further objection to so using the term "right" that from the fact that A ought to do a thing for B, it follows that B has a right against A that A do it for him, is that it is going to make the question of whether or not a man has a right to a thing turn on how easy it is to provide him with it; and this seems not merely unfortunate, but morally unacceptable. Take the case of Henry Fonda again. I said earlier that I had no right to the touch of his cool hand on my fevered brow, even though I needed it to save my life. I said it would be frightfully nice of him to fly in from the West Coast to provide me with it, but that I had no right against him that he should do so. But suppose he isn't on the West Coast. Suppose he has only to walk across the room, place a hand briefly on my brow—and lo, my life is saved. Then surely he ought to do it, it would be indecent to refuse. Is it to be said "Ah well, it follows that in this case she has a right to the touch of his hand on her brow, and so it would be an injustice in him to refuse"? So that I have a right to it when it is easy for him to provide it, though no right when it's hard? It's rather a shocking idea that anyone's rights should fade away and disappear as it gets harder and harder to accord them to him.

So my own view is that even though you ought to let the violinist use your kidneys for the one hour he needs, we should not conclude that he has a right to do so—we should say that if you refuse, you are, like the boy who owns all the chocolates and will give none away, self-centered and callous, indecent in fact, but not unjust. And similarly, that even supposing a case in which a woman pregnant due to rape ought to allow the unborn person to use her body for the hour he needs, we should not conclude that he has a right to do so; we should conclude that she is self-centered, callous, indecent, but not unjust, if she refuses. The complaints are no less grave; they are just different. However, there is no need to insist on this point. If anyone does wish to deduce "he has a right" from "you ought," then all the same he must surely grant that there are cases in which it is not morally required of you that you allow that violinist to use your kidneys, and in which he does not have a right to use them, and in which you do not do him an injustice if you refuse. And so also for mother and unborn child. Except in such cases as the unborn person has a right to demand it—and we were leaving open the possibility that there may be such cases—nobody is morally *required* to make large sacrifices, of health, of all other interests and concerns, of all other

duties and commitments, for nine years, or even for nine months, in order to keep another person alive.

6. We have in fact to distinguish between two kinds of Samaritan: the Good Samaritan and what we might call the Minimally Decent Samaritan. The story of the Good Samaritan, you will remember, goes like this:

A certain man went down from Jerusalem to Jericho, and fell among thieves, which stripped him of his raiment, and wounded him, and departed, leaving him half dead.
And by chance there came down a certain priest that way; and when he saw him, he passed by on the other side.
And likewise a Levite, when he was at the place, came and looked on him, and passed by on the other side.
But a certain Samaritan, as he journeyed, came where he was; and when he saw him he had compassion on him.
And went to him, and bound up his wounds, pouring in oil and wine, and set him on his own beast, and brought him to an inn, and took care of him.
And on the morrow, when he departed, he took out two pence, and gave them to the host, and said unto him, "Take care of him; and whatsoever thou spendest more, when I come again, I will repay thee."
(Luke 10:30–35)

The Good Samaritan went out of his way, at some cost to himself, to help one in need of it. We are not told what the options were, that is, whether or not the priest and the Levite could have helped by doing less than the Good Samaritan did, but assuming they could have, then the fact they did nothing at all shows they were not even Minimally Decent Samaritans, not because they were not Samaritans, but because they were not even minimally decent.

These things are a matter of degree, of course, but there is a difference, and it comes out perhaps most clearly in the story of Kitty Genovese, who, as you will remember, was murdered while thirty-eight people watched or listened, and did nothing at all to help her. A Good Samaritan would have rushed out to give direct assistance against the murderer. Or perhaps we had better allow that it would have been a Splendid Samaritan who did this, on the ground that it would have involved a risk of death for himself. But the thirty-eight not only did not do this,

they did not even trouble to pick up a phone to call the police. Minimally Decent Samaritanism would call for doing at least that, and their not having done it was monstrous.

After telling the story of the Good Samaritan, Jesus said "Go, and do thou likewise." Perhaps he meant that we are morally required to act as the Good Samaritan did. Perhaps he was urging people to do more than is morally required of them. At all events it seems plain that it was not morally required of any of the thirty-eight that he rush out to give direct assistance at the risk of his own life, and that it is not morally required of anyone that he give long stretches of his life—nine years or nine months—to sustaining the life of a person who has no special right (we were leaving open the possibility of this) to demand it.

Indeed, with one rather striking class of exceptions, no one in any country in the world is *legally* required to do anywhere near as much as this for anyone else. The class of exceptions is obvious. My main concern here is not the state of the law in respect to abortion, but it is worth drawing attention to the fact that in no state in this country is any man compelled by law to be even a Minimally Decent Samaritan to any person; there is no law under which charges could be brought against the thirty-eight who stood by while Kitty Genovese died. By contrast, in most states in this country women are compelled by law to be not merely Minimally Decent Samaritans, but Good Samaritans to unborn persons inside them. This doesn't by itself settle anything one way or the other, because it may well be argued that there should be laws in this country—as there are in many European countries—compelling at least Minimally Decent Samaritanism.[7] But it does show that there is a gross injustice in the existing state of the law. And it shows also that the groups currently working against liberalization of abortion laws, in fact working toward having it declared unconstitutional for a state to permit abortion, had better start working for the adoption of Good Samaritan laws generally, or earn the charge that they are acting in bad faith.

I should think, myself, that Minimally Decent Samaritan laws would be one thing, Good Samaritan laws quite another, and in fact highly improper.

But we are not here concerned with the law. What we should ask is not whether anybody should be compelled by law to be a Good Samaritan, but whether we must accede to a situation in which somebody is being compelled—by nature, perhaps—to be a Good Samaritan. We have, in other words, to look now at third-party interventions. I have been arguing that no person is morally required to make large sacrifices to sustain the life of another who has no right to demand them, and this even where the sacrifices do not include life itself; we are not morally required to be Good Samaritans or anyway Very Good Samaritans to one another. But what if a man cannot extricate himself from such a situation? What if he appeals to us to extricate him? It seems to me plain that there are cases in which we can, cases in which a Good Samaritan would extricate him. There you are, you were kidnapped, and nine years in bed with that violinist lie ahead of you. You have your own life to lead. You are sorry, but you simply cannot see giving up so much of your life to the sustaining of his. You cannot extricate yourself, and ask us to do so. I should have thought that—in light of his having no right to the use of your body—it was obvious that we do not have to accede to your being forced to give up so much. We can do what you ask. There is no injustice to the violinist in our doing so.

7. Following the lead of the opponents of abortion, I have throughout been speaking of the fetus merely as a person, and what I have been asking is whether or not the argument we began with, which proceeds only from the fetus' being a person, really does establish its conclusion. I have argued that it does not.

But of course there are arguments and arguments, and it may be said that I have simply fastened on the wrong one. It may be said that what is important is not merely the fact that the fetus is a person, but that it is a person for whom the woman has a special kind of responsibility issuing from the fact that she is its mother. And it might be argued that all my analogies are therefore irrelevant—for you do not have that special kind of responsibility for that violinist, Henry Fonda does not have that special kind of responsibility for me. And our attention might be drawn to the fact that men and women both *are* compelled by law to provide support for their children.

I have in effect dealt (briefly) with this argument in section 4 above; but a (still briefer) recapitulation now may be in order. Surely we do not have any such "special responsibility" for a person unless we have assumed it, explicitly or implicitly. If a set of parents do not try to prevent pregnancy, do not obtain an abortion, and then at the time of birth of the child do not put it out for adoption, but rather take it home with them, then they have assumed responsibility for it, they have given it rights, and they cannot *now* withdraw support from it at the cost of its life because they now find it difficult to go on providing for it. But if they have taken all reasonable precautions against having a child, they do not simply by virtue of their biological relationship to the child who comes into existence have a special responsibility for it. They may wish to assume responsibility for it, or they may not wish to. And I am suggesting that if assuming responsibility for it would require large sacrifices, then they may refuse. A Good Samaritan would not refuse—or anyway, a Splendid Samaritan, if the sacrifices that had to be made were enormous. But then so would a Good Samaritan assume responsibility for that violinist; so would Henry Fonda, if he is a Good Samaritan, fly in from the West Coast and assume responsibility for me.

8. My argument will be found unsatisfactory on two counts by many of those who want to regard abortion as morally permissible. First, while I do argue that abortion is not impermissible, I do not argue that it is always permissible. There may well be cases in which carrying the child to term requires only Minimally Decent Samaritanism of the mother, and this is a standard we must not fall below. I am inclined to think it a merit of my account precisely that it does *not* give a general yes or a general no. It allows for and supports our sense that, for example, a sick and desperately frightened fourteen-year-old schoolgirl, pregnant due to rape, may *of course* choose abortion, and that any law which rules this out is an insane law.

And it also allows for and supports our sense that in other cases resort to abortion is even positively indecent. It would be indecent in the woman to request an abortion, and indecent in a doctor to perform it, if she is in her seventh month, and wants the abortion just to avoid the nuisance of postponing a trip abroad. The very fact that the arguments I have been drawing attention to treat all cases of abortion, or even all cases of abortion in which the mother's life is not at stake, as morally on a par ought to have made them suspect at the outset.

Secondly, while I am arguing for the permissibility of abortion in some cases, I am not arguing for the right to secure the death of the unborn child. It is easy to confuse these two things in that up to a certain point in the life of the fetus it is not able to survive outside the mother's body; hence removing it from her body guarantees its death. But they are importantly different. I have argued that you are not morally required to spend nine months in bed, sustaining the life of that violinist; but to say this is by no means to say that if, when you unplug yourself, there is a miracle and he survives, you then have a right to turn round and slit his throat. You may detach yourself even if this costs him his life; you have no right to be guaranteed his death, by some other means, if unplugging yourself does not kill him. There are some people who will feel dissatisfied by this feature of my argument. A woman may be utterly devastated by the thought of a child, a bit of herself, put out for adoption and never seen or heard of again. She may therefore want not merely that the child be detached from her, but more, that it die. Some opponents of abortion are inclined to regard this as beneath contempt—thereby showing insensitivity to what is surely a powerful source of despair. All the same, I agree that the desire for the child's death is not one which anybody may gratify, should it turn out to be possible to detach the child alive.

At this place, however, it should be remembered that we have only been pretending throughout that the fetus is a human being from the moment of conception. A very early abortion is surely not the killing of a person, and so is not dealt with by anything I have said here.

Notes

1. Daniel Callahan, *Abortion: Law, Choice and Morality* (New York, 1970), p. 373. This book gives a fascinating survey of the available information on abortion. The Jewish tradition is surveyed in David M. Feldman, *Birth Control in Jewish Law* (New York, 1968), Part 5, the Catholic tradition in John T. Noonan, Jr., "An Almost Absolute Value in History," in *The Morality of Abortion,* ed. John T. Noonan, Jr. (Cambridge, Mass., 1970).

2. The term "direct" in the arguments I refer to is a technical one. Roughly, what is meant by "direct killing" is either killing as an end in itself, or killing as a means to some end, for example, the end of saving someone else's life. See note 5, below, for an example of its use.

3. Cf. *Encyclical Letter of Pope Pius XI on Christian Marriage,* St. Paul Editions (Boston, n.d.), p. 32: "however much we may pity the mother whose health and even life is gravely imperiled in the performance of the duty allotted to her by nature, nevertheless what could ever be a sufficient reason for excusing in any way the direct murder of the innocent? This is precisely what we are dealing with here." Noonan (*The Morality of Abortion,* p. 43) reads this as follows: "What cause can ever avail to excuse in any way the direct killing of the innocent? For it is a question of that."

4. The thesis in (4) is in an interesting way weaker than those in (1), (2), and (3): they rule out abortion even in cases in which both mother *and* child will die if the abortion is not performed. By contrast, one who held the view expressed in (4) could consistently say that one needn't prefer letting two persons die to killing one.

5. Cf. the following passage from Pius XII, *Address to the Italian Catholic Society of Midwives*: "The baby in the maternal breast has the right to life immediately from God.—Hence there is no man, no human authority, no science, no medical, eugenic, social, economic or moral 'indication' which can establish or grant a valid juridical ground for a direct deliberate disposition of an innocent human life, that is a disposition which looks to its destruction either as an end or as a means to another end perhaps in itself not illicit.—The baby, still not born, is a man in the same degree and for the same reason as the mother" (quoted in Noonan, *The Morality of Abortion,* p. 45).

6. The need for a discussion of this argument was brought home to me by members of the Society for Ethical and Legal Philosophy, to whom this paper was originally presented.

7. For a discussion of the difficulties involved, and a survey of the European experience with such laws, see *The Good Samaritan and the Law,* ed. James M. Ratcliffe (New York, 1966).

71

Sissela Bok
Ethical Problems of Abortion

Reprinted with permission of the author and editors from the *Hastings Center Studies,* vol. 2, no. 1, January 1974, pp. 33–52.

The recent Supreme Court decisions[1] have declared abortions to be lawful in the United States during the first trimester of pregnancy. After the first trimester, the state can restrict them by regulations protecting the pregnant woman's health; and after "viability" the state may regulate or forbid abortions except where the medical judgment is made that an abortion is necessary to safeguard the life or the health of the pregnant woman. But it would be wrong to conclude from these decisions that no *moral* distinctions between abortions can now be made— that what is lawful is always justifiable. These decisions leave the moral issues of abortion open, and it is more important than ever to examine them.

While abortion is frequently rejected for religious reasons,[2] arguments against it are also made on other grounds. The most forceful one holds that if we grant that a fetus possesses humanity, we must accord it human rights, including the right to live. Another argument invokes the danger to *other* unborn humans, should abortion spread and perhaps even become obligatory in certain cases, and the danger to newborns, the retarded, and the senile should society begin to take the lives of those considered expendable. A third argument stresses the danger that physicians and nurses and those associated with the act of abortion might lose their traditional protective attitude toward life if they become involved to taking human lives at the request of mothers.

Among the arguments made in favor of permitting abortion, one upholds the right of the mother to determine her own fertility, and her right to the use of her own body. Another stresses, in cases of genetic defects of a severe variety, a sympathetic understanding of the suffering which might accompany living, should the fetus not be aborted. And a third reflects a number of social concerns, ranging from the problem of overpopulation *per se* to the desire to reduce unwantedness, child abuse, maternal deaths through illegal abortions, poverty and illness.

In discussing the ethical dilemmas of abortion, I shall begin with the basic conflict—that between a pregnant woman and the unborn life she harbors.

Mother and Fetus

Up to very recently, parents had only limited access to birth prevention. Contraception was outlawed or treated with silence. Sterilization was most often unavailable and abortion was left to those desperate enough to seek criminal abortions. Women may well be forgiven now, therefore, if they mistrust the barrage of arguments concerning abortion, and may well suspect that these are rear-guard actions in an effort to tie them still longer to the bearing of unwanted children.

Some advocates for abortion hold that women should have the right to do what they want with their own bodies, and that removing the fetus is comparable to cutting one's hair or removing a disfiguring growth. This view simply ignores the fact that abortion involves more than just one life. The same criticism holds for the vaguer notions which defend abortion on the grounds that a woman should have the right to control her fate, or the right to have an abortion as she has the right to marry. But no one has the clear-cut right to control her fate where others share it, and marriage requires consent by two persons, whereas the consent of the fetus is precisely what cannot be obtained. How, then, can we weigh the rights and the interests of mother and fetus, where they conflict?

The central question is whether the life of the fetus should receive the same protection as other lives—often discussed in terms of whether killing the fetus is to be thought of as killing a human being. But before asking that question, I would like to ask whether abortion can always be thought of as *killing* in the first place. For abortion can be looked upon, also, as the withdrawal of bodily life support on the part of the mother.

Cessation of Bodily Life Support

Would anyone, before or after birth, child or adult, have the right to continue to be dependent upon the bodily processes of another against that person's will? It can happen that a person will require a sacrifice on the part of another in order not to die; does he therefore have the *right* to this sacrifice?

Judith Thomson has argued most cogently that the mother who finds herself pregnant, as a result of rape or in spite of every precaution, does not have the obligation to continue the pregnancy:

I am arguing only that having a right to life does not guarantee having either a right to be given the use of or a right to be allowed the continued use of another person's body—even if one needs it for life itself.[3]

Abortion, according to such a view, can be thought of as the cessation of continued support. It is true that the embryo cannot survive alone, and that it dies. But this is not unjust killing, any more than when Siamese twins are separated surgically and one of them dies as a result. Judith Thomson argues that at least in those cases where the mother is involuntarily pregnant, she can cease her support of the life of the fetus without infringing its right to live. Here, viability—the capability of living independently from the body of the mother—becomes important. Before that point, the unborn life will end when the mother ceases her support. No one else can take over the protection of the unborn life. After the point where viability begins, much depends on what is done by others, and on how much assistance is provided.

It may be, however, that in considering the ethical implications of the right to cease bodily support of the fetus we must distinguish between causing death indirectly through ceasing such support and actively killing the fetus outright. The techniques used in abortion differ significantly in this respect.[4] A method which prevents implantation of the fertilized egg or which brings about menstruation is much more clearly cessation of life support than one which sucks or scrapes out the embryo. Least like cessation of support is abortion by saline solution, which kills and begins to decompose the fetus, thus setting in motion its expulsion by the mother's body. This method is the one most commonly used in the second trimester of pregnancy. The alternative method possible at that time is a hysterotomy, or "small Cesarean," where the fetus is removed intact, and where death very clearly does result from the interruption of bodily support.

If we learn how to provide life support for the fetus outside the natural mother's body, it may happen that parents who wish to adopt a baby may come into a new kind of conflict with those who wish to have an abortion. They may argue that *all* that the aborting mother has a right to is to cease supporting a fetus with her own body. They may insist, if the pregnancy is already in the second trimester, that she has no right to choose a technique which also kills the baby. It would be wrong for the natural parents to insist at that point that the severance must be performed in such a way that others cannot take over the care and support for the fetus. But a conflict could arise if the mother were asked to postpone the abortion in order to improve the chances of survival and well-being of the fetus to be adopted by others.

Are there times where, quite apart from the technique used to abort, a woman has a *special* responsibility to continue bodily support of a fetus? Surely the many pregnancies which are entered upon voluntarily are of such a nature. One might even say that, if anyone ever did have special obligations to continue life support of another, it would be the woman who had *voluntarily undertaken* to become pregnant. For she has then brought about the situation where the fetus has come to require her support, and there is no one else who can take over her responsibility until after the baby is viable.

To use the analogy of a drowning person, one can think of three scenarios influencing the responsibility of a bystander to leap to the rescue. First, someone may be drowning and the bystander arrives at the scene, hesitating between rescue and permitting the person to drown. Secondly, someone may be drowning as a result of the honestly mistaken assurance by the bystander that swimming would be safe. Thirdly, the bystander may have pushed the drowning person out of a boat. In each case the duties of the bystander are different, but surely they are at their most stringent when he has intentionally caused the drowning person to find himself in the water.

These three scenarios bear some resemblance, from the point of view of the mother's responsibility to the fetus, to: first, finding out that she is pregnant against her wishes; second, mistakenly trusting that she was protected against pregnancy; and third, intentionally becoming pregnant.

Every pregnancy which has been intentionally begun creates special responsibilities for the mother.[5] But there is one situation in which these dilemmas are presented in a particularly difficult form. It is where two parents deliberately enter upon a pregnancy, only to find that the baby they are expecting has a genetic disease or has suffered from damage in fetal life, so that it will be permanently malformed or retarded. Here, the parents have consciously brought about the life which now requires support from the body of the mother. Can they now turn about and say that this particular fetus is such that they do not wish to continue their support? This is especially difficult when the fetus is already developed up to the 18th or 20th week. Can they acknowledge that they meant to begin a human life, but not *this* human life? Or, to take a more callous example, suppose, as sometimes happens, that the parents learn that the baby is of a sex they do not wish?[6]

In such cases the justification which derives from wishing to cease life support for a life which had not been intended is absent, since this life *had* been intended. At the same time, an assumption of responsibility which comes with consciously beginning a pregnancy is much weaker than the corresponding assumption between two adults, or the social assumption of responsibility for a child upon birth for reasons which will be discussed in the next section.

To sum up at this point, ceasing bodily life support *of a fetus or of anyone else* cannot be looked at as a breach of duty except where such a duty has been assumed in the first place. Such a duty is closer to existing when the pregnancy has been voluntarily begun. And it does not exist at all in cases of rape. Certain *methods* of abortion, furthermore, are more difficult to think of as cessation of support than others. Finally, pregnancy is perhaps unique in that cessation of support means death for the fetus up to a certain point of its development, so that nearness *to* this point in pregnancy argues against abortion.

I would like now to turn to the larger question of whether the life of the fetus *should* receive the same protection as other lives—whether killing the fetus, by whatever means, and for whatever reason, is to be thought of as killing a human being.

A long tradition of religious and philosophical and legal thought has attempted to answer this question by determining if there is human life before birth, and, if so, when it *becomes* human. If human life is present from conception on, according to this tradition, it must be protected as such from that moment. And if the embryo *becomes* human at some point during a pregnancy, then that is the point at which the protection should set in.

Humanity

The point in a pregnancy at which a human individual can be said to exist is differently assigned. John Noonan generalizes the predominant Catholic view as follows:

If one steps outside the specific categories used by the theologians, the answer they gave can be analyzed as a refusal to discriminate among human beings on the basis of their varying potentialities. Once conceived, the being was recognized as a man because he had man's potential. The criterion for humanity, thus, was simple and all-embracing: If you are conceived by human parents, you are human.[7]

Once conceived, he holds, human life has about an 80% chance to reach the moment of birth and develop further. *Conception,* therefore, represents a point of discontinuity, after which the probabilities for human development are immensely higher than for the sperm or the egg before conception.

Others have held that the moment when *implantation* occurs, 6–7 days after conception, is more significant from the point of view of humanity and individuality than conception itself. This permits them to allow the intrauterine device and the 'morning after pill' as not taking human life, merely interfering with implantation.

Another view is advanced by Jérôme Lejeune, who suggests that unity and uniqueness, "the two headings defining an individual" are not definitely established until between two and four weeks after conception.[8] Up to that time it is possible that two eggs may have collaborated to build together one embryo, known as a "chimera," whereas after that time such a combination is no longer possible. Similarly, up to that time, a fertilized egg from which twins may result may not yet have split in two.

Still another approach to the establishing of humanity is to say that *looking* human is the important factor. A photo of the first cell having divided in half clearly does not depict what most people mean when they use the expression "human being." Even the four-week-old embryo does not look human, whereas the six-week-old one is beginning to. Recent techniques of depicting the embryo and the fetus have remarkably increased our awareness of the "human-ness" at this early stage; this new *seeing* of life before birth may come to increase the psychological recoil from aborting those who already look human—thus adding a powerful psychological factor to the medical and personal factors already influencing the trend to earlier and earlier abortions.

Others reason that the time at which electrical impulses are first detectable from the brain, around the eighth week, marks the line after which human life is present. If brain activity is advocated as the criterion for human life among the dying, they argue, then why not use it also at the very beginning?[9] Such a use of the criterion for human life has been interpreted by some to indicate that abortion would not be killing before electrical impulses are detectable, only afterwards. Such an analogy would seem to possess a symmetry of sorts, but it is only superficially plausible. For the lack of brain response at the end of life has to be shown to be *irreversible* in order to support a conclusion that life is absent. The lack of response from the embryo's brain, on the other hand, is temporary and precisely not irreversible.

Another dividing line, once more having to do with our perception of the fetus, is that achieved when the mother can feel the fetus moving. *Quickening* has traditionally represented an important distinction, and in some legal traditions such as the common law, abortion has been permitted before quickening, but is a misdemeanor, "a great misprision," afterwards, rather than homicide. It is certain that the first felt movements represent an awe-inspiring change for the mother, and perhaps, in some primitive sense, a 'coming to life' of the being she carries.

Yet another distinction occurs when the fetus is considered *viable*. According to this view, once the fetus is capable of living independently of its mother, it must be regarded as a human being and protected as such. The United States Supreme Court decisions on abortion established viability as the "compelling" point for the state's "important and legitimate interest in potential life," while eschewing the question of when "life" or "human life" begins.[10]

A set of later distinctions cluster around the process of birth itself. This is the moment when life begins, according to some religious traditions, and the point at which "persons" are fully recognized in the law, according to the Supreme Court.[11] The first breaths taken by newborn babies have been invested with immense symbolic meaning since the earliest gropings towards understanding what it means to be alive and human. And the rituals of acceptance of babies and children have often served to define humanity to the point where the baby could be killed if it were not named or declared acceptable by the elders of the community or by the head of the household, either at birth or in infancy. Others have mentioned as factors in our concept of humanity the ability to experience, to remember the past and envisage the future, to communicate, even to laugh at oneself.

In the positions here examined, and in the abortion debate generally, a number of concepts are at times used as if they were interchangeable. "Humanity," "human life," "life," are such concepts, as are "man," "person," "human being," or "human individual." In particular, those who hold that humanity begins at conception or at implantation often have the tendency to say that at that time a human being or a person or a man exists as well, whereas others find it impossible to equate them.

Each of these terms can, in addition, be used in different senses which overlap but are not interchangeable. For instance, humanity and human life, in one sense, are possessed by every cell in our bodies. Many cells have the full genetic makeup required for asexual reproduction—so-called cloning—of a human being. Yet clearly this is not the sense of those words intended when the protection of humanity or of human

life is advocated. Such protection would press the reverence for life to the mad extreme of ruling out haircuts and considering mosquito bites murder.

It may be argued, however, that for most cells which have the potential of cloning to form a human being, extraordinarily complex measures would be required which are not as yet sufficiently perfected beyond the animal stage. Is there, then, a difference, from the point of view of human potential, between these cells and egg cells or sperm cells? And is there still another difference in potential between the egg cell before and after conception? While there is a statistical difference in the *likelihood* of their developing into a human being, it does not seem possible to draw a clear line where humanity definitely begins.

The different views as to when humanity begins are not dependent upon factual information. Rather, these views are representative of different worldviews, often of a religious nature, involving deeply held commitments with moral consequences. There is no disagreement as to what we now know about life and its development before and after conception; differences arise only about the names and moral consequences we attach to the changes in this development and the distinctions we consider important. Just as there is no point at which Achilles can be pinpointed as catching up with the tortoise, though everyone knows he does, so too everyone is aware of the distance traveled, in terms of humanity, from before conception to birth, though there is no one point at which humanity can be agreed upon as setting in. Our efforts to pinpoint and to define reflect the urgency with which we reach for abstract labels and absolute certainty in facts and in nature; and the resulting confusion and puzzlement are close to what Wittgenstein described, in *Philosophical Investigations*, as the "bewitchment of our intelligence by means of language."

Even if some see the fertilized egg as possessing humanity and as being "a man" in the words used by Noonan, however, it would be quite unthinkable to act upon all the consequences of such a view. It would be necessary to undertake a monumental struggle against all spontaneous abortions—known as miscarriages—often of severely malformed embryos expelled by

the mother's body. This struggle would appear increasingly misguided as we learn more about how to preserve early prenatal life. Those who could not be saved would have to be buried in the same way as dead infants. Those who engaged in abortion would have to be prosecuted for murder. Extraordinary practical complexities would arise with respect to the detection of early abortion, and to the question of whether the use of abortifacients in the first few days after conception should also count as murder. In view of these inconsistencies, it seems likely that this view of humanity, like so many others, has been adopted for limited purposes having to do with the prohibition of induced abortion, rather than from a real belief in the full human rights of the first few cells after conception.

Purposes for Seeking to Distinguish Human and Non-Human

A related reason why there are so many views and definitions of humanity is that they have been sought for such different *purposes*. I indicated already that many of the views about humanity developed in the abortion dispute seem to have been worked out for one such purpose—that of defending a preconceived position on abortion, with little concern for the other consequences flowing from that particular view. But there have been so many other efforts to define humanity and to arrive at the essence of what it means to be human—to distinguish men from angels and demons, plants and animals, witches and robots. The most powerful one has been the urge to know about the human species and to trace the biological or divine origins and the essential characteristics of mankind. It is magnificently expressed beginning with the very earliest creation myths; in fact, this consciousness of oneself and wonder at one's condition has often been thought one of the essential distinctions between men and animals.

A separate purpose, both giving strength to and flowing from these efforts to describe and to understand humanity, has been that of seeking to define what a *good* human being is—to delineate human aspirations. What ought fully human beings to be like, and how should they differ from and grow beyond their immature, less perfect, sick or criminal fellow men? Who can teach such growth—St. Francis or Nietzsche, Buddha or Erasmus? And what kind of families and societies give support and provide models for growth?

Finally, definitions of humanity have been sought in order to try to set limits to the protection of life. At what level of developing humanity can and ought lives to receive protection? And who, among those many labelled less than human at different times in history—slaves, enemies in war, women, children, the retarded—should be denied such protection?

Of these three purposes for defining "humanity," the first is classificatory and descriptive in the first hand (though it gives rise to normative considerations). It has roots in religious and metaphysical thought, and has branched out into biological and archeological and anthropological research. But the latter two, so often confused with the first, are primarily *normative* or prescriptive. They seek to set norms or guidelines for who is fully human, and who is at least minimally human—so human as to be entitled to the protection of life. For the sake of these normative purposes, definitions of "humanity" established elsewhere have been sought in order to determine action—and all too often the action has been devastating for those excluded.

It is crucial to ask at this point why the descriptive and the normative definitions have been thought to coincide; why it has been taken for granted that the line between human and non-human or not-yet-human is identical with that distinguishing those who may be killed from those who are to be protected.

One or both of two fundamental assumptions are made by those who base the protection of life upon the possession of "humanity." The first is that all human beings are not only different from, but *superior to* all other living matter. This is the assumption which changes the definition of humanity into an evaluative one. It lies at the root of Western religious and social thought, from the Bible and the Aristotelian concept of the 'ladder of life,' all the way to Teilhard de Chardin's view of mankind as close to the intended

summit and consummation of the development of living beings.

The second assumption holds that the superiority of human beings somehow justifies their using what is nonhuman as they see fit, dominating it, even killing it when they wish to. St. Augustine, in *The City of God,*[12] expresses both of these anthropocentric assumptions when he holds that the injunction "Thou shalt not kill" does not apply to killing animals and plants, since, having no faculty of reason, therefore by the altogether righteous ordinance of the Creator both their life and death are a matter subordinate to our needs.

Neither of these assumptions is self-evident. And the results of acting upon them, upon the bidding to subdue the earth, to subordinate its many forms of life to human needs, are no longer seen by all to be beneficial.[13] The very enterprise of *basing* normative conclusions on such assumptions and distinctions can no longer be taken for granted.

Despite these difficulties, many still try to employ definitions of "humanity" to do just that. And herein lies by far the most important reason for abandoning such efforts: the monumental misuse of the concept of "humanity" in so many practices of discrimination and atrocity throughout history. Slavery, witchhunts and wars have all been justified by their perpetrators on the grounds that they held their victims to be less than fully human. The insane and the criminal have for long periods been deprived of the most basic necessities for similar reasons, and excluded from society. A theologian, Dr. Joseph Fletcher, has even suggested recently that someone who has an I.Q. below 40 is "questionably a person" and that those below the 20-mark are not persons at all.[14] He adds that:

This has bearing, obviously, on decion making in gynecology, obstetrics, and pediatrics, as well as in general surgery and medicine.

Here a criterion for "personhood" is taken as a guideline for action which could have sinister and far-reaching effects. Even when entered upon with the best of intentions, and in the most guarded manner, the enterprise of basing the protection of human life upon

such criteria and definitions is dangerous. To question someone's humanity or personhood is a first step to mistreatment and killing.

We must abandon, therefore, this quest for a definition of humanity capable of showing us who has a right to live. To do so must not, however, mean any abandon of concern with the human condition—with the quest for knowledge about human origins and characteristics and with aspirations for human goodness. It is only the use of the concept of 'humanity' as a criterion of *exclusion* which I deplore.

In recent decades, philosophers have devoted much thought to the nature of ethical principles, to the kind of statement they make, and to their internal grammar. Much has been written about the requirement that these principles be universal—that they hold for all mankind, all moral persons, all rational beings. As a rough distinction, such a simple characterization of the *extent* to which ethical principles should hold is undoubtedly natural and relatively unproblematic. It would rule out, for example, the denial of basic rights to some persons while according them to others, whereas it would not prohibit the employment of plant fiber in clothing or lumber in furniture. But I submit that in the many borderline cases where humanity is questioned by some—the so-called "vegetables," the severely retarded, or the embryo—even the seemingly universal yardsticks of "humanity" or rationality are dangerous.

But if we rule out the appeal to a standard of "humanity" in deciding about the protection of life in such difficult cases, may we not have lost the only criterion of objective decisions? Or could there be other criteria less dangerous and vague than that connected with "humanity"?

In order to seek such criteria, it is crucial to arrive at an understanding of the harm that comes from the taking of life. Why do we hold life to be sacred? Why does it require protection beyond that given to anything else? The question seems unnecessary at first—surely most people share what has been called "the elemental sensation of vitality and the elemental fear of its extinction," and what Hume termed "our horrors at annihilation."[15] Many think of this elemental sensation as incapable of further analysis. They view any attempt to say *why* we hold life sacred as an instrumentalist rocking of the boat which may endanger this fundamental and unquestioned respect for life. Yet I believe that such a failure to ask what the respect for life ought to protect lies at the root of the confusion about abortion and many other difficult decisions concerning life and death. I shall try, therefore, to list the most important reasons which underlie the elemental sense of the sacredness of life. Having done so, these reasons can be considered as they apply or do not apply to the embryo and the fetus.

Reasons for Protecting Life

1. Killing is viewed as the greatest of all dangers *for the victim.*

The knowledge that there is a threat to life causes intense anguish and apprehension.

The actual taking of life can cause great suffering.

The continued experience of life, once begun, is considered so valuable, so unique, so absorbing, that no one who has this experience should be unjustly deprived of it. And depriving someone of this experience means that all else of value to him will be lost.

2. Killing is brutalizing and criminalizing *for the killer.* It is a threat to others, and destructive to the person engaged therein.

3. Killing often causes *the family of the victim and others* to experience grief and loss. They may have been tied to the dead person by affection or economic dependence; they may have given of themselves in the relationship, so that its severance causes deep suffering.

4. *All of society,* as a result, has a stake in the protection of life. Permitting killing to take place sets patterns for victims, killers, and survivors, that are threatening and ultimately harmful to all.

These are neutral principles governing the protection of life. They are shared by most human beings reflecting upon the possibility of dying at the hands of others. It is clear that these principles, if applied in the absence of the confusing terminology of 'humanity,' would rule out the kinds of killing perpetrated by conquerors, witch-hunters, slave-holders, and Nazis. Their

victims feared death and suffered; they grieved for their dead; and the societies permitting such killing were brutalized and degraded.

Turning now to abortions once more, how do these principles apply to the taking of the lives of embryos and fetuses?

Reasons to Protect Life in the Prenatal Period

Consider the very earliest cell formations soon after conception. Clearly, most of these *reasons* for protecting human life are absent here.

This group of cells cannot suffer in death, nor can it fear death. Its experiencing of life has not yet begun; it is not yet conscious of the loss of anything it has come to value in life and is not tied by bonds of affection to other human beings. If the abortion is desired by both parents, it will cause no grief such as that which accompanies the death of a child. Almost no human care and emotion and resources have been invested in it. Nor is a very early abortion brutalizing for the person voluntarily performing it, or a threat to other members of the human community.[16] The only factor common to these few cells and, say, a soldier killed in war or a murdered robbery victim is that of the *potential* denied, the interruption of life, the deprivation of the possibility to grow and to experience, to have the joys and sorrows of existence.

For how much should this one factor count? It should count *at least* so much as to eliminate the occasionally voiced notion that pregnancy and its interruption involve only the mother in the privacy of her reproductive life, that to have an abortion is somehow analogous with cutting one's finger nails.

At the same time, I cannot agree that it should count enough so that one can simply equate killing an embryo with murder, even apart from legal considerations or the problems of enforcement. For it *is* important that most of the reasons why we protect lives are absent here. It does matter that the group of cells cannot feel the anguish or pain connected with death, that it is not conscious of the interruption of its life, and that other humans do not mourn it or feel insecure in their own lives if it dies.

But, it could be argued, one can conceive of other deaths with those factors absent, which nevertheless would be murder. Take the killing of a hermit in his sleep, by someone who instantly commits suicide. Here there is no anxiety or fear of the killing on the part of the victim, no pain in dying, no mourning by family or friends (to whom the hermit has, in leaving them for good, already in a sense "died"), no awareness by others that a wrong has been done; and the possible brutalization of the murderer has been made harmless to others through his suicide. Speculate further that the bodies are never found. Yet we would still call the act one of murder. The reason we would do so is inherent in the act itself, and depends on the fact that his life was taken, and that he was denied the chance to continue to experience it.

How does this privation of potential differ from abortion in the first few days of pregnancy? I find that I cannot use words like "deprived," "deny," "take away," and "harm" when it comes to the group of cells, whereas I have no difficulty in using them for the hermit. Do these words require, if not a person conscious of his loss, at least someone who at a prior time has developed enough to be or have been conscious thereof? Because there is no semblance of human form, no conscious life or capability to live independently, no knowledge of death, no sense of pain, one cannot use such words meaningfully to describe early abortion.

In addition, whereas it is possible to frame a rule permitting abortion which causes no anxiety on the part of others covered by the rule—other embryos or fetuses—it is not possible to frame such a rule permitting the killing of hermits without threatening other *hermits.* All hermits would have to fear for their lives if there were a rule saying that hermits can be killed if they are alone and asleep and if the agent commits suicide.

The reasons, then, for the protection of lives are minimal in very early abortions. At the same time, some of them are clearly present with respect to *infanticide,* most important among them the brutalization of those participating in the act and the resultant danger for all who are felt to be undesirable by their families or by others. This is not to say that acts of infanticide have not taken place in our society; indeed, as late as the nineteenth century, newborns were frequently killed, either directly or by giving them into the care of institutions such as foundling hospitals, where the death rate could be as high as 90 percent in the first year of life.[17] A few primitive societies, at the edge of extinction, without other means to limit families, still practice infanticide. But I believe that the *public acceptance* of infanticide in all other societies is unthinkable, given the advent of modern methods of contraception and early abortion, and of institutions to which parents can give their children, assured of their survival and of the high likelihood that they will be adopted and cared for by a family.

Dividing Lines

If, therefore, very early abortion does not violate these principles of protection for life, but infanticide does, we are confronted with a new kind of continuum in the place of that between less human and more human: that of the growth in strength, during the prenatal period, of these principles, these reasons for protecting life. In this second continuum, it would be as difficult as in the first to draw a line based upon objective factors. Since most abortions can be performed earlier or later during pregnancy, it would be preferable to encourage early abortions rather than late ones, and to draw a line before the second half of the pregnancy, permitting later abortions only on a clear showing of need. For this purpose, the two concepts of *quickening* and *viability*—so unsatisfactory in determining when humanity begins—can provide such limits.

Before quickening, the reasons to protect life are, as has been shown, negligible, perhaps absent altogether. During this period, therefore, abortion could be permitted upon request. Alternatively, the end of the first trimester could be employed as such a limit, as is the case in a number of countries.

Between quickening and viability, when the operation is a more difficult one medically and more traumatic for parents and medical personnel, it would not seem unreasonable to hold

that special reasons justifying the abortion should be required in order to counterbalance this resistance; reasons not known earlier, such as the severe malformation of the fetus. After viability, finally, all abortions save the rare ones required to save the life of the mother,[18] should be prohibited, because the reasons to *protect* life may now be thought to be partially present; even though the viable fetus cannot fear death or suffer consciously therefrom, the effects on those participating in the event, and thus on society indirectly, could be serious. This is especially so because of the need, mentioned above, for a protection against infanticide. In the unlikely event, however, that the mother should first come to wish to be separated from the fetus at such a late stage, the procedure ought to be delayed until it can be one of premature birth, not one of harming the fetus in an abortive process.

Medically, however, the definition of "viability" is difficult. It varies from one fetus to another. At one stage in pregnancy, a certain number of babies, if born, will be viable. At a later stage, the percentage will be greater. Viability also depends greatly on the state of our knowledge concerning the support of life after birth, and on the nature of the support itself. Support can be given much earlier in a modern hospital than in a rural village, or in a clinic geared to doing abortions only. It may some day even be the case that almost any human life will be considered viable before birth, once artificial wombs are perfected.

As technological progress pushes back the time when the fetus can be helped to survive independently of the mother, a question will arise as to whether the cutoff point marked by viability ought also be pushed back. Should abortion then be prohibited much earlier than is now the case, because the medical meaning of 'viability' will have changed, or should we continue to rely on the conventional meaning of the word for the distinction between lawful and unlawful abortion?

In order to answer this question it is necessary to look once more at the reasons for which 'viability' was thought to be a good dividing-line in the first place. Is viability important because the baby can survive outside of the mother? Or because this chance of

survival comes at a time in fetal development when the *reasons* to protect life have grown strong enough to prohibit abortion? At present, the two coincide, but in the future, they may come to diverge increasingly.

If the time comes when an embryo *could* be kept alive without its mother and thus be 'viable' in one sense of the word, the reasons for protecting life from the point of view of victims, agents, relatives and society would still be absent; it seems right, therefore, to tie the obligatory protection of life to the present conventional definition of 'viability' and to set a socially agreed upon time in pregnancy after which abortion should be prohibited.

To sum up, the justifications a mother has for not wishing to give birth can operate up to a certain point in pregnancy; after that point, the reasons society has for protecting life become sufficiently weighty so as to prohibit late abortions and infanticide.

Moral Distinctions

But moral distinctions ought nevertheless to be made by the mother considering an abortion even during the period when she may lawfully obtain one. In addition to those having to do with the *method* of abortion and the degree to which the pregnancy was voluntary or involuntary (as discussed previously), the *time* in pregnancy, the weightiness of the *reasons* for wanting the abortion, the desires of the *father*, and the possibility of alternatives such as adoption, must all be considered.

1. The *time* in pregnancy at which the abortion takes place is a very important factor. Very early in pregnancy, the reasons for protecting life are clearly absent. Few will have to face the questions which come with aborting a 4- or 5-month-old fetus when early abortions are generally available. But *in* such late abortions, it is especially important to consider what the reasons are for desiring the abortion.

2. Among all of the reasons why a pregnancy is unwanted, it is possible to perceive a gradation from reasons all would recognize as very compelling, such as a threat to the mother's life, to reasons most would think of as frivolous, such as a determination that only a fetus of a desired sex should be allowed to be born. This gradation

among the reasons for wishing not to have a baby will be part of any judgment concerning the *morality* of acts to prevent births. It is also possible to divide the innumerable reasons for not wanting a pregnancy into two main categories. The first one, sometimes called "selective" unwantedness, refers to those pregnancies which are desired, often planned, by the parents, but during the course of which evidence comes to light concerning a risk, or even a certainty of abnormality in the fetus. If, for example, the mother has Rubella, or German Measles, in the first trimester, there is a probability of fetal abnormality. And it is now possible to learn, through prenatal diagnosis, whether the fetus suffers from a chromosomal abnormality, the most common of which causes mongolism, or from one of a number of genetic diseases which can cause malformation or mental retardation.[19] In all of these cases the parents, while they might ordinarily welcome a pregnancy, may come to the conclusion that they do not wish to give birth in this particular case.

But the determination of such defects through amniocentesis can only be made when the amniotic fluid is present to a sufficient degree, and the final results of the tests may not be available until the fifth month of pregnancy. Only *late* abortions are possible after amniocentesis, and this makes the decision for parents and doctors a much more difficult one.

The reasons for not wanting a malformed baby differ with the capacities of the parents and the severity of the abnormality. Some parents, and families, cope admirably and with great love with children who would prove burdensome and even destructive to other families. A severely disabled fetus, likely to suffer greatly once born and perhaps to die in childhood, could be "unwanted" out of concern for its own welfare, as well as for the welfare of the family. A great deal depends on the help available from the community, in terms of financial assistance, special schooling, medical resources, and general support. Other factors which can be important are the pride of the family, or even parental prejudice, e.g., parents' wish for an abortion after learning that the fetus is of one sex rather than another.

Perhaps most difficult from a moral point of view are the situations where the parents know beforehand that they are carriers of genetic defects, and where they enter upon a pregnancy determined in advance to abort any fetus which is found to exhibit the defect. I say this with the greatest humility, knowing the strength of the urge to have one's own babies. But I see no difference between starting another human life with such plans, and creating "test-tube" fetuses only to throw away those deemed undesirable. In cases such as these, other ways of bringing children into the lives of parents must be worked out. At times artificial insemination may provide an answer,[20] at other times adoption, or working with children in the many capacities where help is needed, may be preferable.

But there are many cases where these distinctions cannot be so clearly made. It may be difficult to know whether there was an intention to have a baby, or to risk becoming pregnant. It might be argued that someone who engaged in sexual activity, even using contraceptives, ought to be willing to take the responsibility for a human life which results. Whereas to abort under such circumstances, or even after a voluntarily begun pregnancy, is not murder, it ought not to be taken lightly. For the same reason, it is insensitive to omit contraceptive measures and to rely on the availability of abortion in the case of pregnancy. (Though the availability of methods making abortions possible in the very earliest days of pregnancy and the hazy line between such abortions and contraception may make such a distinction less pointed.)

Another set of criteria which will be difficult to work out when considering reasons for abortion is that which should govern abortions for the sake of the welfare of the fetus. For while almost all would agree about the extreme cases I have mentioned, there will be disagreement as to what to do in those cases where the affliction is not totally debilitating, or where there is merely a *risk* of disease, not a certainty. What if the risk is small? A recent newspaper article stated that there is one chance out of a hundred that a baby will be born retarded if the mother has had the flu in the first trimester of her pregnancy. Whether or

not this particular concern turns out to be correct, it is going to be increasingly possible to specify odds of this kind, sometimes with a very low probability of danger. It has been suggested that parents will come to want to take very few chances of defects, so long as the choice is open to them of having abortions.

Even if it is possible, however, to work out criteria concerning the welfare of the baby, there are times when the cost at which this welfare is to be purchased must be weighed against the welfare of other human beings. If for example, a fetus is diagnosed as having a disease which can be controlled after birth so as not to cause suffering, but only at staggering costs to the family or the community—say of millions of dollars each day—abortion would clearly be called for in spite of the theoretical possibility of carrying the baby to term and treating it. The other possibility would be not aborting, and permitting the baby to suffer in the absence of such expensive relief, and then once more, the magnitude of the suffering might have argued in favor of abortion.

All these cases, where certain births are unwanted because of the characteristics of the fetus, differ crucially from those in the second category where no children at all are wanted at the time of the pregnancy. In this larger group are the more familiar cases where there is danger to the mother's physical health or her emotional stability, or where there is not enough food, clothing, or shelter to cope with yet another child. Here, too, are cases where there has been rape, or incest, or where a very young girl is pregnant. There are also the frequent cases where the mother feels she is beyond the age best suited for child-caring, or does not want to accept the great change in life—the restriction, the financial pinch, and the feeling of being tied down—which often accompany the birth of a child. These changes affect mothers most powerfully in our society of nuclear families where the burdens of child-rearing often fall on them alone. In all of these cases, contraception could have avoided the pregnancy, and an early abortion is possible as a last resort. Adoption is an alternative resort which should always be considered. It must be remembered, however, that with prevailing attitudes it would be exceedingly difficult for a married woman with existing children to give a baby up for adoption.

The distinction between the two *kinds* of reasons for not wanting a pregnancy is crucial. For while the first group of conceptions—unwanted because of the characteristics of the fetus—often require abortions if births are to be prevented (and often late abortions, since prenatal diagnosis takes time and can rarely begin until the second trimester of pregnancy), the second group can usually be prevented through contraception, sterilization, abstinence, or protection of the mother from sexual assault. Abortion is necessary here only as a last resort, where other methods have failed, and an *early* abortion is possible, presenting fewer medical, ethical, and emotional problems than a later one.

3. At times, there are conflicts between mothers and fathers of the unborn. According to one study,[21] about one-half of the pregnancies unwanted by one or both parents were unwanted by *only one* parent. Very often such disagreements are settled amicably, usually in favor of having the baby. But who should make the decision when the mother wishes to have an abortion, and the father wants to restrain her?[22] In a recent Canadian case,[23] a judge prohibited an abortion desired by a mother. The father had brought suit on his own behalf and on that of the "infant plaintiff."

It is difficult to see how such a disagreement can be anything but disruptive for the relationship between the two parents, as well as very harmful for the child after birth. Whoever "wins" in such a conflict will have won a Pyrrhic victory indeed.

Early in pregnancy, the mother has at her disposal methods of abortion which need not involve the father's knowledge of her condition. The same is true if he does not learn of the pregnancy as it progresses. But barring such eventualities, who would decide in the event of a conflict?

In such a conflict, while it is important to ascertain the father's views when possible, there ought not to be a *requirement* that both parents consent

to an abortion, as is now often the case.[24] The mother has the burden of pregnancy, and most often of caring for the baby she bears. The decision to interrupt her pregnancy should therefore be hers. But into her decision should go the awareness of the heavy price she will have to pay in the relationship with the father, if she aborts their unborn child against his wishes. And the father's reasons for wishing to continue the pregnancy should be given due weight, so as to counterbalance in her judgment all but the most pressing reasons she has for wishing to have the abortion.

The father's wishes should be given great weight, especially if he wants not only to preserve the life of his unborn child, but also to share responsibility and care after birth. At a future time, when it may be possible to remove a fetus relatively early in pregnancy and protect it artifically until "birth," fathers, just as adoptive parents, ought to have the right to declare their intentions to take responsibility for the baby. Mothers at that time, while severing their connections with the fetus, should not be able to demand its death.

Furthermore, if we look back on the reasons for protecting life, one of them concerns the grief felt by family members when someone is killed. If, therefore, a father feels such grief, and if he supports his contention by promising to assume the burdens of child-rearing after birth, this ought to be an important consideration, persuasive to the mother or to her physician or to both. Our society has been moving in the direction of recognizing that men as well as women can provide care and nurturance for children. To permit a father to prevent the abortion of his child on the condition that he bring it up later would seem to be a move in the same direction. If he is unwilling to make such a commitment, however, his grief at the impending death of the fetus is less entitled to respect.

4. The alternatives to abortion differ depending upon whether birth prevention is considered before or after conception. The alternatives open before conception—abstinence, different methods of contraception, and sterilization—do not raise the particular moral problems connected with taking the life of the fetus, or of rejecting the baby after birth.

Once conception *has* occurred, the alternatives to abortion are to accept responsibility for the baby after birth, or to relinquish it to the state or to adoptive parents. It is extremely important to consider these alternatives in the case of each unwanted pregnancy, and only to have recourse to abortion after discarding them. Many pregnant women, whether they are seeking abortions or not, are ambivalent, struggling within themselves in order to reconcile the tenderness normally evoked by the thought of a baby, with fears connected with their pregnancy. The fears may have to do with the future of the baby, or with the future of the family unit into which the baby will come. Sometimes there is no such family unit, and sometimes the relationship with the baby's father is such as to threaten the future of the baby. The decisive point comes when the choice is made to prevent a pregnancy or a birth. And this choice in turn is strongly influenced by social attitudes towards means of birth prevention, and by their availability.

The fact of having children has always been considered "natural," and someone not wishing a child, or any children, has been expected to produce reasons in support of such an attitude. It may be that we are now coming closer to a time when choosing not to have a child will be seen to reflect, not necessarily a hostile and niggardly attitude, a "denial of life," but a respect for the living, and a correct estimate of what kind of life a baby can be given. In that case, reasons will come to be expected *before* giving birth to a new baby, and thoughts for the welfare of the child to be will come to be seen as an important aspect of child-bearing.

In order for such choices to be possible at all, however, *information* is necessary. All those who are physically able to become parents must have wise and full advice regarding family life, sexual life, and birth prevention. From a moral point of view, contraception is greatly preferable to abortion. The *knowledge* about contraceptive alternatives to childbirth, or to abortion, is therefore crucial to all potential parents. Withholding information in order to preserve "innocence" among the young is a self-defeating and unjustifiable exercise of paternalistic power, contributing to the birth of unwanted children and to shattered lives.

I have argued that it may be moral to have an abortion under certain circumstances, but that the range of morally justifiable abortions is more restricted than that of those abortions declared lawful by the Supreme Court. But some argue that such views of morality and legality, if widely followed, could lead to great dangers for society.

Problems of Line-drawing

Can We Allow Abortion Without Risking Infanticide?

Foes of abortion argue that a society which permits abortion may not be able to hold the line against infanticide.[25] Once we admit *reasons* for abortions such as fetal malformation or simply not wanting another child, they say, what is to prevent people from acting upon these very same reasons after birth?[26] A baby just before birth, they argue, is identical to one just after birth. What, then, will provide the discontinuity?

I have argued, on the contrary, that another set of *reasons*—the reasons for protecting human life—gain in strength during pregnancy and are such as to prohibit abortions after a certain point and therefore also to prohibit infanticide. While it is true that no theoretical line can be drawn which distinguishes between a baby just before birth and one just after birth, there is no difficulty in distinguishing an aborted embryo from a newborn baby. A time must therefore be set in pregnancy well before birth for the cutting-off point. The discontinuity will then exist between abortion and infanticide. The argument that the reason *for* aborting may still exist at childbirth does not take into account the reasons *against* killing, and the threat which would be felt by all if infanticide as a parental option were thought to be possible.[27]

How can one *know* whether such a discontinuity can be observed in practice? The only way to know is to consider those societies which have already permitted abortion for considerable lengths of time. These countries do not in fact experience tendencies toward infanticide. The infant mortality statistics in Sweden and Denmark are extremely low, and the protection and care given to all living children, including those born with special problems, is exemplary.

Moreover, Nazi Germany, which is frequently cited as a warning of what is to come once abortion becomes lawful, had *very strict laws prohibiting abortion*. In 1943, Hitler's regime made the existing penalties for women having abortions, and those performing them, even more severe by removing the limit on imprisonment and by including the possibility of "hard labor" for "especially serious cases."[28]

The fear of slipping from abortion towards infanticide, therefore, while understandable, does not seem to be grounded in fact.

Is There a Risk of Compulsory Abortion?

A second type of line-drawing problem is the following: if a beginning is made by permitting amniocentesis and abortion in cases where the mother learns she is expecting a grossly malformed baby, might there not come to be a *requirement* for others to undergo amniocentesis, and to induce abortion if the fetus is found to be defective? And once abortion is no longer reprehensible, might a community not require abortions where expectant mothers are heavily addicted, and where it is not only likely that they will harm or neglect their children after birth, but where they are demonstrably severely harming them even before birth? Might it not be increasingly easy for parents to force their daughters to have abortions should they become pregnant while they are too young, or unmarried?[29] Or even for husbands to require abortions where they judge their wives to be unstable or perhaps ill? And finally, if abortion is permitted for indigent mothers, in part out of sympathy for mother and child, and in part out of a computation of the likely costs to the community of enforcing the births of unwanted children, might there not in the long run be a requirement for abortion where mothers on welfare are concerned, or any others who are judged unable to provide, materially or emotionally or intellectually, for the needs of their children?

One can readily concede that it is important to be vigilant against any

such developments. Any inroads upon a pregnant woman's physical integrity, against her will, are very serious and we need strong protection for the control she should be able to exercise over her own body. Great risks of abuse would obviously accompany any provision for obligatory abortion. But to forbid voluntary abortion because of the danger of involuntary abortion would be like forbidding voluntary adoptions on the grounds that they might lead to involuntary adoption policies. The battle against coercion must be fought at all times, with respect to many social options, but this is no reason to prohibit the options themselves.

Conclusion

There are many reasons which may lead a mother not to wish to give birth, but to have an abortion instead. They range from the most compelling to the most trivial. In early pregnancy, society's reasons for protecting life—the suffering and harm to the victim, to the agent, to the family and friends, and to society as a whole—do not apply, either to the zygote or to the embryo. Abortion, for whatever reasons, should then be available upon request. Preventing birth before conception or just after conception, however, presents fewer ethical conflicts than later abortions.

As pregnancy progresses, the social reasons for preventing killing are more and more applicable to the fetus. At the stage where a fetus is viable—capable of independent life outside the mother's body—these reasons begin to be as substantial as at birth and thereafter. In addition, viability represents the time when cessation of bodily support by the mother need not result in fetal death; as a result a viable fetus is capable of protection by others. For these reasons, I believe that after the established time of possible viability, methods separating fetus and mother so as to kill the fetus should be prohibited. But an earlier time—perhaps 18 rather than 24 weeks—is preferable for all but exceptional cases (such as those occurring after prenatal diagnosis of severe malformation).

Even though abortion may be *lawful* up to this time, however, it is not necessarily an act which an individual may consider right or justifiable. This discrepancy results, I believe, from the fact that the *social* reasons for protecting life may also be looked upon in each case as *individual* reasons. Society may not find that abortion harms either victim or agent, family or social practices. But the individual parent or physician may see risks to himself as a person from such acts and look at them as breaches of personal responsibility toward the unborn. They may then regard abortion as personally distasteful, even though it is lawful.

Some physicians, for example, do feel that they cannot participate in abortions without personal danger of brutalization and without sharing responsibility for killing. This may be especially true when they are called in, as in large hospitals, to perform one abortion after another without any chance to consult with the women involved and to hear their case histories. There should never be a requirement that a physician or nurse must participate in an abortion. Even if women have a right to abortion, they have not therefore the right to force others to perform such acts.

In the same way, a mother or a father may feel personal grief over the death of a fetus, and responsibility for killing it, quite apart from the legality of the act. This grief and this responsibility, which would be present as a matter of course where parents wish for the birth of their baby, may also accompany an unwanted pregnancy. The following factors should then be weighed by the mother before she can be confident that abortion is the right way out of her dilemma, and one she will not come to regret or view with guilt:

Whether or not the pregnancy was voluntarily undertaken

The importance and validity of the *reasons* for wanting the abortion

The technique to be used in the abortion; the extent to which it can be regarded as "cessation of bodily life support," rather than as outright killing

The time of pregnancy

Whether or not the father agrees to the abortion

Whether or not all other alternatives have been considered, such as adoption

Her religious views.

And the father, if he weighs these factors differently, may feel the grief and responsibility differently too, and wish to take over the care of the baby after birth.

Abortion is a last resort, and must remain so. It is much more problematic than contraception, yet it is sometimes the only way out of a great dilemma. Neither individual parents nor society should look at abortion as a policy to be encouraged at the expense of contraception, sterilization, and adoption. At the same time, there are a number of circumstances in which it can justifiably be undertaken, for which public and private facilities must be provided in such a way as to make no distinction between rich and poor.

Notes

1. Roe v. Wade, *United States Law Week* 41, 1973, pp. 4213–33. Doe v. Bolton, *Ibid.,* pp. 4233–40. [Reprinted as Chapter 68 of this volume.]

2. See *The Morality of Abortion,* ed. by John T. Noonan, Jr. (Cambridge: Harvard University Press, 1970), and G. H. Williams, "Religious Residues and Presuppositions in the American Debate on Abortion," *Theological Studies* 31 (1970), 10–75.

3. Judith Thomson, "A Defense of Abortion." [Reprinted as Chapter 70 of this volume.]

4. See Selig Neubardt and Harold Schulman, *Techniques of Abortion* (Boston: Little, Brown and Company, 1972).

5. But lines are hard to draw here. There are many intermediate cases between the pregnancy intentionally begun and, for instance, that resulting from carelessness with contraceptives.

6. See Morton A. Stenchever, "An Abuse of Prenatal Diagnosis," *Journal of the American Medical Association* 221 (July 24, 1972), 408.

7. Noonan, *Morality of Abortion,* p. 51. For a thorough discussion of this and other views concerning the beginning of human life, see Daniel Callahan, *Abortion: Law, Choice and Morality* (New York: Macmillan Company, 1970).

8. Jérôme Lejeune, "On the Nature of Man" (Lecture at the American Society of Human Genetics at San Francisco, October 2–4, 1969).

9. Paul Ramsey, "Feticide/Infanticide upon Request," *Religion in Life* 39 (July, 1970), 170–86. Arthur J. Dyck, "Perplexities for the Would-Be Liberal in Abortion," *Journal of Reproductive Medicine* 8 (June, 1972), 351–54.

10. Roe v. Wade, *United States Law Week 41,* pp. 4227, 4229. [See Chapter 68 of this volume.]

11. *Ibid.,* p. 4227. For further discussion see L. Tribe, "Foreword: Toward a Model of Roles in the Due Process of Life and Law," *Harvard Law Review* 87 (1973), 1–54.

12. Augustine, *The City of God Against the Pagans,* Book I. Ch. XX (Cambridge: Harvard University Press, 1957).

13. C. D. Stone, "Should Trees Have Standing? Toward Legal Rights for Natural Objects," *Southern California Law Review* 45, 450–501, provides an interesting analysis of the extension of rights to those not previously considered persons, such as children, and a discussion of possible future extensions to natural objects.

14. Joseph Fletcher, "Indicators of Humanhood: A Tentative Profile of Man," *The Hastings Center Report* 2 (November, 1972), 1–4.

15. Edward Shils, "The Sanctity of Life," in *Life or Death: Ethics and Options,* ed. by D. H. Labby (Seattle: University of Washington Press, 1968), p. 12. David Hume, "Of the Immortality of the Soul," *Essays: Moral, Political, and Literary* (London: Longmans, Green, and Co., 1882), II, p. 405.

16. This question will be taken up in detail in Part V. It is because all of the reasons for protecting life are *present* when someone considered to be a slave is murdered that the spate of recent sensationalistic comparisons of abortion and slavery do not make sense, even though it is true that in both cases there are denials of the humanity of the victims. Once again, a confusion in the use of the word 'humanity' is at fault.

17. William L. Langer, "Checks on Population Growth: 1750–1850," *Scientific American* 226 (February, 1972).

18. Every effort must be made by physicians and others to construe the Supreme Court's statement "If the State is interested in protecting fetal life after viability, it may go so far as to proscribe abortion during that period except when it is necessary to preserve the life or health of the mother" to concern, in effect, only the life or threat to life of the mother. See Alan Stone, "Abortion and the Supreme Court: What Now?" *Modern Medicine,* April 30, 1973, pp. 33–37, for a discussion of this question and what it means for physicians.

19. Theodore Friedmann, "Prenatal Diagnosis of Genetic Disease," *Scientific American* 225 (November, 1971), 34–42 and A. Milunsky, *et al.,* "Prenatal Genetic Diagnosis," *New England Journal of Medicine* 283 (December 17, 1970), 1370–81; (December 24, 1970), 1441–47; (December 31, 1970), 1498–1504.

20. Especially when genetic evaluation of *donors* becomes a common practice. See Walter Wadlington, "Artificial Insemination: The Dangers of a Poorly Kept Secret," *Northwestern University Law Review* 64 [6] (1970), 777–807.

21. See Edward Pohlman, "Unwanted Conceptions: Research on Undesirable Consequences," *Eugenics Quarterly* 14 [2] (June, 1967), 144.

22. I discuss the reverse situation, where the father wishes to force the mother to have an abortion, on page 441.

23. See *New York Times,* Saturday, January 28, 1972.

24. "When abortion is recommended by a physician, the indications should be stated in the patient's record, and informed consent obtained from the patient and her husband, or herself if she is unmarried, or from her nearest relative or guardian if she is under the age of consent." From *Policy on Abortion,* issued in August, 1970 by the Executive Board of the American College of Obstetricians and Gynecologists. See Tribe, *Harvard Law Review,* 38–41.

25. See for example, Noonan, *Morality of Abortion,* p. 258.

26. Some have used the same argument for the opposite conclusion. Since, or if, we allow abortion, they say, we *should* allow infanticide under certain conditions. See Michael Tooley, "Abortion and Infanticide," *Philosophy and Public Affairs* 2 (Fall, 1972), 37–65, and John M. Freeman and Robert E. Cooke, "Is There a Right to Die— Quickly?," *Journal of Pediatrics* 80 (Spring, 1972), 940–5. Once again, such a conclusion fails to take into account the powerful social reasons against infanticide.

27. It is important to be clear here about the differences between active killing of infants and the fact that the battle for life, in those rare cases where an infant is born with a severe malformation, such as the absence of a brain, is not undertaken or not carried as far as it would otherwise be. There *are* difficult borderline cases, but nothing suggests that killing actively in early pregnancy opens the door to the active killing of infants.

28. See *Reichsgesetzblatt,* 1926, Teil I, Nr. 28, 25 May 1926, § 218, and 1943, Teil I, 9 March 1943, Art. I, "Angriffe auf Ehe, Familie, und Mutterschaft."

29. See the Maryland case *in Re Smith* reported in *41 U.S. Law Week* 2202, 1972, where a 16-year-old girl was jailed at the request of a Circuit Court judge in order to undergo the abortion she refused, but which her mother insisted upon. At the last moment, a higher court freed the girl.

72

John Badertscher
Religious Dimensions of the Abortion Debate

Reprinted with permission of the editor from *Studies in Religion,* vol. 6, no. 2, 1976–1977, pp. 177–183.

The debate over abortion law shows no sign of abating. In 1969, Canada's Parliament amended its law to legalize abortions performed in accredited hospitals when the operation is given prior approval by a three-doctor therapeutic abortion committee according to the criterion that a danger to the life or health of the mother exists. This attempt at reform has met with organized, continuing resistance on both sides. For example, Dr. Henry Morgenthaler was so convinced of the law's arbitrary and unjust character that he launched on a course of classic civil disobedience in 1973. The subsequent judicial proceedings have served to publicize the cause of groups who want abortions restricted as well as those who want the entire abortion statute repealed. As in the case of the 1973 abortion decision of the U.S. Supreme Court, the operation of the judicial process appears to inflame the controversy more than to advance rational discourse.

This inflammation is no doubt due in part to the presence of intemperance and ill-will among the partisans, as evidenced by the invocation of slogans (e.g. "right to life" and "a woman's control over her own body") with whose ostensible meaning no one would want to disagree, but which obviously distort the issue. But perhaps the intractability of the debate might be due as well to factors other than these perennial human weaknesses. Margaret Farley has correctly noted that a major problem in the abortion debate is "an impasse in efforts either to mediate or to join issue between what are fundamentally opposing conscience claims, profoundly different experiences of moral obligation."[1] Professor Farley explores with exceptional clarity the conflict between the "obligation to alleviate situations which are oppressive and harmful to women" and the "obligation to protect the lives of human fetuses."[2]

This paper takes its point of departure from the observation that behind such profound moral conflicts one is likely to find a conflict of religious perspectives. Of course, the conflict over abortion is religious in the superficial sense that some religious communities have been among the most vigorous supporters of anti-abortion law.[3] But this paper will attempt to show that there is a religious dimension behind both of the "experiences of moral obligation" which Margaret Farley has located in the abortion debate. Professor Farley argues that the failure of the contending parties to recognize the moral seriousness of their opponents leads to the presence of "bad faith" in the debate. By elaborating the religious orientations on which that moral seriousness is grounded, I hope to show those interests which, precisely because they are religious or ultimate, will have to be recognized by any public resolution which hopes to be accepted as just by reasonable persons on both sides of the issue. A final purpose of the paper is to outline on the basis of this religious analysis some of the considerations which justice would demand in abortion law.

The contending positions on abortion law are often referred to as "liberal" and "conservative." Since these two labels are often applied in imprecise and misleading ways, it is tempting to discard them and seek others. But, besides their familiarity, there is another good reason for using them, and this paper will do so. The reason is that, at least in the context of the abortion debate, the use of the words can be closely related to their etymology. A liberal is one who values individual freedom, while a conservative is one who seeks to protect and defend some element of the given situation. We can understand a liberal as one who tries to remove impediments to self-fulfillment, while the conservative can perhaps most readily be appreciated on the contemporary scene as a conservationist. We shall see that these characterizations can be applied to the contending positions on abortion law.

My intention is to make the best possible case for each of these positions by tracing them to comprehensive, if contrary, understandings of human good. These terms are not always invoked to such a purpose, so it seems expedient to distinguish two of the most prominent usages which I wish to avoid. The first is their use to characterize positions on social change. The liberal is said to be in favor of change, the conservative opposed. This usage is often accompanied by an evolutionary bias which reads change as the key to reality and interprets the newer as somehow both necessary and better. This usage can be dismissed with the observation that liberals and conservatives on the abortion issue seem equally capable of taking offense at the *status quo* and agitating for change. "Liberal" and "conservative" do not seem to be positions on change *per se*.

The second usage employs the terms to construct a typology. The typology may serve to distinguish between two mutually exclusive positions between which one may choose by a "leap of faith."[4] Another application of the typology serves to locate a mediating position which can serve as a rallying point for those who, while interested in the debate, do not wish to stand with either of the partisans. The typological usage can be distinguished by the tendency to add the adjective "extreme" to the two labels, implying that there is something irrational in a thorough adherence to either position. The use of the labels in this essay, however, will aim at uncovering the rationality inherent in both.

The main problem with using the terms to construct a typology is that, while the terms point to clearly contrary positions on abortion, they do not indicate positions which are necessarily contradictory. There is no reason why one might not be both liberal and conservative in the truest sense of both. For example, I might seek to conserve individual liberties by defending constitutional government. This essay proceeds on the assumption that liberals and conservatives on abortion law can understand and accept each others' basic concerns and commitments, can in that sense inhabit a common world, and therefore can reason toward a just law.

We can now proceed to state the liberal and conservative positions on abortion law. To see the religious dimensions of the positions, the view of human freedom underlying each will be examined. Following that, the criticism of each position by the other will be elaborated, with special attention to their views on the purpose or function of law, on the evaluation of technology, and on God or ultimate reality.

The liberal, understanding freedom as autonomy, will seek to minimize external restraints on human action. This does not imply an ethic of self-indulgence, as conservatives sometimes suppose. On the contrary, the way to autonomy is through the rule of reason. Impulsive gratification of desire is, for the genuine liberal, another and highly subtle form of the loss of autonomy. The liberal understands that the really free act is the one that is chosen on the basis of reason. An act that is not chosen is not free, and an act that is not free cannot be said to be good.

For the pregnant woman, then, the way to good action lies through free, rational decision. The liberal position on abortion law is not fundamentally pro-abortion. Rather, the liberal holds that giving birth, like other human acts, should be freely chosen. A pregnant woman may very well choose that the process which has begun within her body should continue to the end it would reach if no thought were taken, but that choosing has a moral character which is absent if alternatives are not available and considered. In fact, if she chooses the path to maternity the conditions for prenatal development will probably be more auspicious.

The moral decision between abortion or maternity will include consideration of many factors: the woman's health, the network of obligations in which she is presently involved, the life situation into which the child would be born, etc. It is a decision similar to one about the use of contraceptives. The liberal would no doubt agree that the decision about pregnancy should be made beforehand if possible, but since contraceptive techniques fail, occasions for decision about abortion will sometimes arise.

The one point which the liberal would insist we consider is that the nurture which a woman's body gives a fetus is basically involuntary. Of course it can become voluntary, but only when it becomes a matter of free decision. Unless there is opportunity for such decision, pregnancy becomes a form of involuntary servitude. It is this fact, coupled with the observation that only women become pregnant, which makes the abortion debate a legitimate focal point of feminist concern. Seen in this way, an abortion does not primarily intend the cessation of fetal life. Rather, it intends the withdrawal of involuntary support for that life.

The conservative position is sometimes thought to regard the question of freedom as unimportant. In fact, the position is based on a view of human freedom, but one which is different from that of the liberal. Put with dangerous simplicity, the conservative position is that the freedom of the fetus must also be considered in any decision about abortion. The one point on which the conservative position rests is that the fetus is an individuated form of human life.[5] It is human in the basic sense that it has a human mother and father. No talk of potentiality for communication, social life, or reason, should obscure the fact that it is human beings who have such potential. Therefore, the conservative concludes, the fetus is human life and entitled to the protection of law.

The conservative recognizes that there is a difference between fetal and neonate life, and therefore does not expect the fetus to be protected by laws against homicide. Special law is necessary for the special case. But the conservative is unimpressed when notions such as "viability" are introduced, as in Justice Harry Blackmun's 1973 U.S. Supreme Court decision, as a way of determining a point beyond which the law has no legitimate interest. There is no such thing as human freedom apart from biological life, the conservative points out. Further, all human life is dependent upon the sustenance of the natural world. While it is hard to see any person who is not in some sense in need of the nurture of others to gain that sustenance, the less mature are in greater need of this nurture than the more mature, and the fetus in its second trimester is in greater need than a six-month-old baby. But the only real difference that "viability" points to is the difference between a life that can be nurtured by many people and a life that can only be nurtured by one. Pre-viability fetus, post-viability fetus, and neonate alike will die without nurture. Thus the conservative rejects abortion and infanticide on the same grounds, as a culpable refusal to nurture a life which is dependent upon that nurture.

The difference between conservative and liberal views of freedom can be seen in the contrasting interpretation of the significance of the body for moral action, as well as in the contrasting focus on the fetus by the conservative,

and on the pregnant woman by the liberal. The latter, regarding the moral situation of the woman, sees the bodily processes as a potential adversary which the moral agent must subdue by free, rational decision. The conservative looks at the fetus as a potential moral agent and seeks to preserve the physical conditions necessary to the nurture of that potential. When the conservative turns to the moral situation of the pregnant woman, her freedom appears to be something attained in the self-limitation which recognizes and respects the life within her, a life whose claim on freedom would be lost by abortion.

Although these divergent perspectives on freedom suggest alternative religious orientations, the two positions which have been described have not yet been shown to be full-fledged positions consistently applicable to other issues. Further, the religious or ultimate character of these commitments requires elaboration. I propose now to deal with both these problems at once, albeit more by suggestion than by systematic construction. It happens that the abortion question is directly related to at least two other central ethical issues: the function of law and the evaluation of technology. Law is involved since the justice of particular legislation and its impact is being debated. Technological considerations enter into the logic of possible actions and the calculation of their probable results. Finally, we will see that while no positive theological position is necessarily involved in either perspective, the criticism of one by the other can include the charge of idolatry. That is, this criticism imputes a faulty theological position to the other side. Since we will be examining this ultimate dimension of the debate in terms of a mutual criticism, the discussion of law and technology can be readily fitted to the same format of mutual criticism.

While liberal and conservative can agree that law functions rightly when it defends the freedom of a person from the acts of another which would do that person injury or prevent the expression of that person's freedom, the conservative sees abortion law defending the freedom of the fetus, while the

liberal sees that law failing to defend the freedom of the pregnant woman. The liberal believes to be unjust any abortion law which ignores the involuntary character of woman's nurture of the fetus. Both parties suffer from this injustice, the liberal argues. Women are not permitted a free decision about that natural process which many would choose to complete, if they had a real choice. Children who are given nurture under compulsion before birth may well receive far less care than they need later, when the mother has a choice about how she will treat the young child. Even worse, because the law is perceived by women to be arbitrary it is frequently disobeyed and is difficult to enforce. This means that illegal abortions, which are far more dangerous and costly to the woman, take place often enough to bring this law and law in general into disrespect. The liberal, then, criticizes the conservative view of law as arbitrary and finally destructive of the principle of law because it ignores the necessarily voluntary character of moral action.

The conservative, in response, sees the liberal view of law as improperly concerned with convention. The frequency of theft is no argument for repeal of laws against it, and the same is true of the regulation of abortion, the conservative holds. The law serves to defend individual freedom, but it must also embody the best understanding of justice available in a given policy. Law, then, will be educative as well as restrictive. To fail to defend human life at its most defenseless—in its fetal form—would be a betrayal of the very idea of law, and would suggest that law is nothing more than an excuse for the dominance of the weak by the strong. The law should inform freedom, the conservative believes, and this means that the pregnant woman should be led to see that a purpose of her freedom in that particular situation is to nurture the life which is dependent on her alone.

On the question of technology, the conservative many polemically point out the link between the liberal emphasis on freedom as possibility and the emphasis of modern technological society on instrumental domination. Since the liberal values the rational control of natural processes, the appearance of a technological capacity for abortion without great danger to the woman will tend to suggest that the utilization of that capacity is self-evidently good. The conservative will see the abortion issue in the context of other cultural phenomena in which technique is maximized and concern for innocent life is minimized, as in modern warfare. In both, the user of technology never sees his victim. In modern warfare, the killing of civilians takes place "accidentally" and at a distance, in the name of "interdicting supply lines" or some such euphemism. In modern abortion procedure, the fetus is kept hidden and removed quickly from the surgical area, and the operation is euphemistically called "termination of pregnancy." Against the liberal contention that we ought to consider using the possibilities which technology creates, the conservative suggests that the "progress" which is the slogan of technological society is precisely what blinds us to the real ethical issues and makes genuine consideration of alternatives increasingly less likely.

The liberal, however, may also have some things to say about the dangers of overdependence on technique. The conservative, one might reply, has overlooked that modern technique is more a matter of the organization of human action than of the use of machines. The dehumanizing effect of technology, it can be argued, takes place when human action is restricted by participation in the structures and institutions of technological society. In this way persons are not in control of their own lives. The "system" makes their decisions for them. Now the judicial process can be seen as one component of that system. The liberal sees the abortion issue in the context of the technocratically rationalized denial of justice to poor people and minority groups. The judicial process is part of the "system" by which women are oppressed. Both the traditional total proscription of abortion and such recent attempts at reform as the 1969 Canadian legislation subject the decision-making powers of women to the impersonal restriction of judicial technique. The liberal will argue that the person best qualified to know the circumstances of the case and the person

most likely to have the best interests of the fetus at heart should make the decision about abortion, and that person is the pregnant woman.

The two positions, as they have been developed here, need not be advanced on the basis of a commitment to either theism or atheism. The case for the religious nature of these positions could be made simply by showing that their perspectives on human freedom reflect ultimate values. Nevertheless, the religious dimension of these positions can be made clearer by showing how each detects the worship of a false god in the ultimate commitment of the other. Theist and atheist alike can legitimately criticize idolatry.

The liberal wonders at the basis on which the conservative holds that abortion should be a matter determined by law rather than individual choice. Perhaps it is not merely dogma or tradition which guides the conservative, but how can the conservative be so certain that one principle—even one as broad as "the sanctity of life"—can be applied to the variety of situations in which pregnancy is a serious human problem? It appears likely to the liberal that the conservative position is ideological, in that a widely accepted value symbol is invoked to prevent rational consideration of actual cases. The conservative appeals to the importance of the biological basis of life and the essential continuity of the natural process which leads from embryo to mature person. But surely life is more than merely biological existence, and surely not all natural processes are good. To appeal to nature as a basis for law in this way is, the liberal believes, to remove one area of the human situation from decision and thus from responsibility. The god who decrees that nature must take its course, that things must be as they will be, is not a god strange to men. He has been worshipped in many times and places as Fate. The liberal believes that Fate is a false god.

The conservative wonders at the ease with which the liberal excludes a voiceless, defenseless human life from the protection of law, trusting instead to the good will of whoever the pregnant woman may be, or to the guidance of whoever's influence she may be under. Perhaps the liberal is not a mere libertarian, for the liberal may not reject the rule of law in other areas of life. But why is the claim of the fetus

set aside? Is it not because the fetus in a problem pregnancy cannot display any of the powers of reason and decision which in the liberal view distinguishes human life? The liberal recognizes the need for law, the conservative suspects, only when it is necessary to make possible the exercise of the liberal's own powers.

Thus behind the liberal posture the conservative perceives an exaltation of the power of the individual and an emphasis on that which sets mankind apart from creation. When made an ultimate commitment, this too is a familiar form of idolatry—the worship of self. Apart from genuine faith in God, the only defense against the consequence of such pride is respect for law, a law whose validity does not depend on some momentary political consensus, but upon assent to the principle that the will of the individual is not the absolute determinant of the good. The conservative believes that it is the most defenseless who are in greatest danger from the consequences of the self-idolatry of others.

This mutual theological criticism, when not merely implied or imputed but brought explicitly into the debate, can be quite helpful. Whether theist or not, neither liberal nor conservative will want to be open to the charge of idolatry. The conservative will want to state her position in such a way that it cannot be understood as fatalistic. The liberal will want to show that freedom does not mean self-worship of antinomianism. As a result, the liberal can be led to consider whether the cause of freedom might well be advanced by extension of the rule of law to the protection of fetal life, and the conservative can be pressed to take account of the real problems of pregnant women. Seeing the religious dimensions of the abortion debate can thus lead towards the rationalization of that debate, as the two sides begin to incorporate the deepest concerns of the other side into their own position.

From the presence of religious dimensions in this debate we should conclude that no public policy on abortion can be recognized as just unless it shows that the basic commitments of both parties have been taken seriously in the formulation of that policy. The remainder of this essay will be devoted to an outline of a policy which would recognize the validity of both the conservative commitment to the protection of fetal life by the rule of law, and the liberal commitment to the enhancement of the freedom of pregnant women. Such a policy is desirable, not so much because it might bring an end to the controversy as because both parties are arguing on the basis of facts which are true and principles which are right, and such should be embodied in public policy. The conservative is right in arguing that the fetus is human life, and that human life should be protected by law. The liberal is right in arguing that good action is voluntary, and that the sphere of rational decision-making open to pregnant women should be maximized.

To resolve the debate in the direction of public policy, I must take a position on the most basic issue of the debate. Should abortion be regulated by law? Here I conclude that, while both liberal and conservative positions have their validity, the latter has primacy. The conservative can agree that there is more to life than biological existence, and that the liberal is using a more fully elaborated understanding of freedom than the one the conservative applies in this issue. But while the conservative view of freedom as the right to mere life is more elementary than the liberal view, it also deserves prior recognition. Human freedom goes beyond biological existence, but it does not go without it.

So the first step toward a just public policy is the recognition that abortion should be regulated by law. While this commits me to the conservative position, it also forces me to recognize the limits of the conservative claim. I cannot speak of abortion as murder, for I hereby recognize that it needs a special consideration. It cannot be covered by the homicide law. I also recognize that the basic intention of abortion is therapeutic; the end of fetal life is in a real sense accidental to it. This, in turn, compels me to recognize that therapy is not requested unless it is needed, even though the need expressed does not necessarily indicate the most helpful response. The right of the fetus to the conditions of life is not, then, an absolute one. Rather, it must be balanced by the judicial process against the needs of a woman with a problem pregnancy. Thus, the conservative position being developed here is compelled to consider the question of freedom and justice for pregnant women by the logic of its own commitment as well as by the rightness of the liberal's commitment.

Having taken the position that there should be abortion law, the obvious next step is to say what sort of law there should be. This is the point at which liberal interests must be recognized. Just abortion law will be an expression of public policy which is responsive to the just claims and real problems of pregnant women, and is responsive in such a way that women themselves can recognize that this is the case. Just abortion law will be part of a public policy which maximizes the real choices open to women. Just abortion law will be implemented by a judicial process which enhances the dignity and rationality of the participants in it, and recognizes that—in the case of abortion requests as in other areas of law—justice delayed is justice denied.

Since I favor a law which aims at justice for both fetus and pregnant women, it seems proper to consider at this point the Canadian experience with the 1969 amendment which sought to move the law in such a direction. It seems not to have satisfied the requirement that reasonable persons, both liberal and conservative, should be able to regard it as just. In fact, it is widely regarded as unjust. Why has it failed? Two reasons can be given.

First, the judicial process has been foisted upon medical personnel and medical institutions without any terms of reference which would enable them to relate the medical to the judicial approaches. The problems of pregnant women may be medical, and the law can deal with these. But the problems may also be social, moral and political or—more likely—some combination of these with medical problems, and the law does not permit such problems to be dealt with on their own terms. In other words, the law is presently structured so as to exclude consideration of most of the factors which feminists rightly perceive to be related to the question of abortion.

Second, the law can only permit or deny abortion, that is, it either gives unqualified affirmation to the claim of the fetus or unqualified affirmation to the claim of the woman. There may be some cases in which the law must lead to such decision, but abortion does not seem to be one of them. This law, as it stands, serves to close off possibilities for women rather than open them up. If the abortion committee reaches a negative decision on the request of the woman and her physician it must say to her, in effect, "Whatever problems you may have, we deem them to be of no significance."

As a result of this structure and these problems, Canadian abortion law is applied in a highly erratic and apparently arbitrary way. Since the establishment of the therapeutic abortion committee is left to the discretion of the hospital, many hospitals do not have one and therefore do not consider performing abortions. If a woman lives in a community where the only hospital has taken this course, her access to the judicial process is severely limited. Other hospitals which do have such a committee are usually overburdened with applications. Having to pass judgment on a large number of cases on the basis of excessively vague guidelines has led many such committees to invoke the extremely broad definition of health accepted by the World Health Organization, namely, that health is a state of complete physical, mental and social well-being. Obviously, a "danger to life or health" could be found in any problem pregnancy, according to such a definition. Thus, some hospitals limit abortion procedures only by the capacity of their rooms, equipment and personnel. Both sides are correct in regarding a law that produces such arbitrary and capricious results as unjust and undesirable.

Rather than attempt to construct an abortion law which would be universally valid, let me show the implications of this essay for public policy by suggesting some modifications of the law whose shortcomings we have just examined. These modifications are twofold: one concerns abortion law itself, and the other concerns the policies and practices which bear upon problem pregnancies. First, the law

regulating abortion should be unequivocal, and it should be administered
by persons responsible to the public.
Since abortion involves the loss of life,
the procedure should be approved only
when loss of life is deemed likely in
any case.[6] Since the decision is to be
made on medical grounds, the persons
deciding should have the appropriate
medical qualifications, but they should
be recognized as performing a judicial
function.[7] This distinction is especially
important in our present cultural context, in which medical care is understood to be a consumer good rather
than a service in the public interest.
Consequently, those exercising this judicial function would do so independently of any particular health care institution, and the subversion of public
policy by private commitments or institutional incapacity would be less
likely.

The second kind of change needed is
far more complex and costly. In order
that the judicial process on abortion be
able to recognize the legitimacy of
claims of a pregnant woman whose request for an abortion is denied, the
process must be tied directly to institutions which can offer that woman various kinds of compensatory support so
that a "no" to a request for abortion
would lead directly to a "yes" in response to the problems of that pregnancy. Only in this way can the operation of the law be seen as widening the
sphere of free decision. The various
public policies necessary to greater justice in abortion would include intensified research for non-abortifacient
methods of birth control which would
not injure their users' health, further
development of agencies to aid adoption, provision of special facilities for
prenatal and post-natal care, establishment of maternity allowances (perhaps
along the lines of Canada's family al-
lotments), legislation, and labor-union
action to secure greater variability
in work patterns for both men and
women, legislation requiring the provision of maternity leave with pay, and
vastly improved and expanded programs of day care. In short, creation of
the conditions under which abortion
law would not only be just but also respected presupposes realization of
many of the goals of the feminist
movement.

Since I have come to a primarily
conservative conclusion, it seems fitting
that some final words on strategy
should be addressed to those who
share that position. One unhappy aspect of the recent abortion debate has
been the way conservatives have responded to reverses such as the 1973
U.S. Supreme Court decision, as
though we had suddenly been expelled
from the Garden. The struggle to extend the protection of law to the helpless has always been costly and its
victories tenuous. It is not helpful, in
the face of losses, to retreat into the
fortress of aggrieved self-righteousness.
It would, I believe, be far wiser in such
a situation to make common cause
with those who favor the feminist
policies mentioned above, but who do
so from other principles. Such an advocacy would both strengthen the credibility of the conservative concern for
the protection of life, and also help
bring about a situation more auspicious
to the conservative cause.

A hopeful sign from the conservative
camp was the April 1973 statement of
Canadian Council of (Roman Catholic)
Bishops. They said, following an
affirmation of their position against
abortion, "We must take seriously the
rebuke that those who oppose abortion
care too little about the special problems of mothers and the burdens of
rearing children once they are born. If
respect for life seems to end with birth,
our perceptions and values are truncated and incomplete.

"The call of Christ, that we should
bear one another's burdens, demands
that we reach out in practical ways to
share all the burdens of parenthood.
The indicated aid and support will include working to change economic
and social realities in the direction of
justice and respect of life."[8]

Notes

1. Margaret A. Farley, "Liberation, Abortion
and Responsibility," *Reflection* (Yale Divinity School), March 1974, p. 9.

2. Ibid.

3. Some attempts of theological ethicists to
resolve the debate have mistakenly focussed
on this superficially religious aspect and
have consequently suggested that the formula of religious toleration should be
applied. Religious opponents of abortion,
the argument goes, should be content to
regulate the conduct of fellow-believers
through moral suasion and allow persons
with no such religious or moral scruples to

have abortions if they so desire. Such an argument overlooks the point that the arguments advanced by religiously affiliated
anti-abortionists are legal and public rather
than private or religious in any immediate
sense. They seek to protect the fetus because it is a form of human life. The argument for religious tolerance is valid only if
one denies that the fetus has its own body
and life in any significant sense. This is precisely what anti-abortionists are unwilling to
concede.

4. An example is the essay by Roger Wertheimer, "Understanding the Abortion
Debate," *Philosophy and Public Affairs*
1:1, 1971, Princeton University Press,
pp. 67–95. As one might expect, Professor
Wertheimer—having displayed considerable
analytical erudition—is finally unable to
take a constructive position on the basis of
his approach.

5. A remarkably clear and persuasive argument for this position can be found in a letter to the editor of the *Mennonite Medical
Messenger*, vol. 24, no. 3, April–June 1973,
pp. 20–23. The writer is a physician, Dr. H.
Clair Amstutz.

6. This would still leave much room for the
exercise of medical and moral judgment.
However, were the decision to have a judicial as well as a medical character, common law traditions for dealing with doubtful
cases would begin to emerge.

7. I wish to acknowledge the help given by
my students, David Pfau and Ruth Simkin,
in forcing me to clarify my position in this
part of the discussion.

8. As quoted by Gilbert Roxburg, "The Split
on Abortion," *The Globe and Mail*, Toronto,
May 31, 1973, p. W9.

Fetal Experimentation

73

An Act Prohibiting Experimentation on Human Fetuses

Reprinted from The Commonwealth of Massachusetts, "An Act Prohibiting Experimentation on Human Fetuses," Chapter 421, 1974.

Be it enacted by the Senate and House of Representatives in General Court assembled, and by the authority of the same, as follows:

Chapter 112 of the General Laws is hereby amended by inserting after section 12I the following section:

Section 12J No person shall use any live human fetus, whether before or after expulsion from its mother's womb, for scientific, laboratory, research or other kind of experimentation. This section shall not prohibit procedures incident to the study of a human fetus while it is in its mother's womb, provided that in the best medical judgment of the physician, made at the time of the study, said procedures do not substantially jeopardize the life or health of the fetus, and provided said fetus is not the subject of a planned abortion. In any criminal proceeding the fetus shall be conclusively presumed not to be the subject of a planned abortion if the mother signed a written statement at the time of the study, that she was not planning an abortion.

This section shall not prohibit or regulate diagnostic or remedical procedures the purpose of which is to determine the life or health of the fetus involved or to preserve the life or health of the fetus involved or the mother involved.

A fetus is a live fetus for purposes of this section when, in the best medical judgment of a physician, it shows evidence of life as determined by the same medical standards as are used in determining evidence of life in a spontaneously aborted fetus at approximately the same stage of gestational development.

No experimentation may knowingly be performed upon a dead fetus unless the consent of the mother has first been obtained, provided however that such consent shall not be required in the case of a routine pathological study. In any criminal proceeding, consent shall be conclusively presumed to have been granted for the purposes of this section by a written statement, signed by the mother who is at least eighteen years of age, to the effect that she consents to the use of her fetus for scientific, laboratory, research or other kind of experimentation or study; such written consent shall constitute lawful authorization for the transfer of the dead fetus.

No person shall perform or offer to

perform an abortion where part or all of the consideration for said performance is that the fetal remains may be used for experimentation or other kind of research or study.

No person shall knowingly sell, transfer, distribute or give away any fetus for a use which is in violation of the provisions of this section. For purposes of this section, the word "fetus" shall include also an embryo or neonate.

Whoever violates the provisions of this section shall be punished by imprisonment in a jail or house of correction for not less than one year nor more than two and one half years or by imprisonment in the state prison for not more than five years.

74

The National Commission for the Protection of Human Subjects of Biomedical and Behavioral Research, Research on the Fetus: Report and Recommendations

Regulations of the Department of Health, Education, and Welfare Governing Fetal Research

Reprinted from *Federal Register,* vol. 40, no. 154, 1975, pp. 33526–33551.

Report and Recommendations

I. The Mandate

The National Research Act (Pub. L. 93–348) established the National Commission for the Protection of Human Subjects of Biomedical and Behavioral Research and gave the Commission a mandate to investigate and study research involving the living fetus, and to recommend whether and under what circumstances such research should be conducted or supported by the Department of Health, Education, and Welfare. A deadline of four months after the members of the Commission took office was imposed for the Commission to conduct its study and make recommendations to the Secretary, DHEW. The priority assigned by Congress to research involving the fetus indicates the concern that unconscionable acts involving the fetus may have been performed in the name of scientific inquiry, with only proxy consent on behalf of the fetus.

The members of the Commission determined at the outset to undertake a careful study of the nature and extent of research on the fetus, the range of views on the ethical acceptability of such research, and the legal issues involved, prior to formulating their recommendations. To this end, the Commission has accumulated an extensive body of information, held public hearings, questioned a panel of distinguished ethicists, and conducted lengthy deliberations. In the course of these activities, the Commission has given close scrutiny to many important questions that surround research on the fetus, for example: What are the purposes of research on the fetus? What procedures have been employed in such research? Are there alternatives to such research? Can appropriate consent to such research be obtained by proxy? Under what conditions may research be done on a fetus that is to be aborted, or a nonviable delivered fetus? What review of proposed research should be required?

In the remainder of Section I, the background and activities of the Commission are summarized, and the definitions used in this report are set forth. Reports, papers and testimony that were prepared for or presented to the Commission are summarized in Sections II to VII of this report. The Commission's own statement of its deliberations and conclusions appears in Section VIII, and the recommendations themselves are set forth in Section IX, together with a statement by a member of the Commission dissenting in part from the recommendations. Separate views of members of the Commission are set forth in Section X.

The Appendix to the report contains the entire text of the papers and reports that were prepared under contract to the Commission, and certain other materials that were reviewed by the Commission during its deliberations.

Legislative Background

The National Research Act contains two provisions regarding research on the fetus: (1) the mandate to the Commission to conduct studies and make recommendations to the Secretary, DHEW (section 202(b)), and (2) a prohibition, in effect until the Commission has made recommendation, on "research [conducted or supported by DHEW] in the United States or abroad on a living human fetus, before or after the induced abortion of such fetus, unless such research is done for the purpose of assuring the survival of such fetus" (section 213). These two provisions were drafted by a conference committee that resolved the differences between the acts originally passed in 1973 by the House of Representatives and Senate, respectively.

The original House act contained a prohibition against the conduct or support by DHEW of research that would violate any ethical standard adopted by the National Institutes of Health or the National Institute of Mental Heath. This provision was perceived as a prohibition of research on the living fetus, as a result of policy then in force at NIH. In addition, both the House and Senate acts contained floor amendments explicitly prohibiting the conduct or support of research on the fetus by DHEW. The House amendment, adopted by a vote of 354 to 9, proscribed research on a fetus that is outside the uterus and has a beating heart, while the Senate prohibition applied to research in connection with an abortion. Among other differences between the acts, the House prohibitions were

permanent, while the Senate prohibition was temporary. The conference committee applies to research conducted imposing a moratorium until this Commission made recommendations. The moratorium adopted by the conference committee applies to research conducted on a fetus before or after an induced abortion of the fetus (except to assure the survival of the fetus); the mandate for the Commission's study and recommendations applies more generally to research involving the living fetus.

The Commission has reviewed the committee reports (Nos. 93–244, 93–381, and 93–1148), and the record of the floor debate that led to the passage of the National Research Act (Congressional Record, daily eds. May 31, 1973; September 11, 1973; June 27 and 28, 1974). Other legislative materials that have been reviewed include the Hearings on Biomedical Research Ethics and the Protection of Human Subjects, before the House Subcommittee on Public Health and Environment (September 27 and 28, 1973), and the Hearing on Fetal Research before the Senate Subcommittee on Health (July 19, 1974).

It is clear from the legislative history that the National Research Act, as passed by both Houses and signed into law by President Nixon on July 12, 1974, reflects an acknowledgement by the majority of legislators that the issues surrounding research on the fetus require much study and deliberation before policies are established regarding support by the Secretary, DHEW. That assignment was given to the Commission, and this report describes how the assignment was carried out and the conclusions that were reached.

Existing Codes and Other Relevant Material

To assist its deliberations, the Commission referred to the following pre-existing codes and other materials relating to human experimentation:

1. The Nuremberg Code (1946–1949).

2. The Declaration of Helsinki (revised, 1964).

3. The Use of Fetuses and Fetal Material for Research, Report of the Advisory Group, chaired by Sir John Peel (London, 1972).

4. Protection of Human Subjects: Policies and Procedures, draft document of the Department of Health, Education, and Welfare (38 Federal Register No. 221, Part II, November 16, 1973).

5. Protection of Human Subjects: Proposed Policy, Department of Health, Education, and Welfare (39 Federal Register No. 165, Part III, August 23, 1974).

Meetings of the Commission

Secretary Weinberger administered the oath of office to the members of the Commission on December 3, 1974, thereby fixing the deadline for this report. Section 202(b) of the National Research Act requires that recommendations of the Commission with respect to research on the living fetus be transmitted to the Secretary "not later than the expiration of the 4-month period beginning on the first day of the first month that follows the date on which all members of the Commission have taken office." This 4-month period expired April 30, 1975.

The Commission conducted seven meetings devoted primarily to the topic of research on the fetus. These meetings were well attended by the public. One day of the February meeting was devoted to a public hearing of the views of persons interested in research on the fetus; oral testimony was given by 23 witnesses, some representing research, religious or other organizations and some appearing as concerned citizens to express their viewpoints (see Section VI for summaries of the views presented). At the March meeting, three public officials testified about the involvement of their respective agencies or offices in research on the fetus (see Section VI), and the members of the Commission held a roundtable discussion with several ethicists who had prepared papers covering a wide spectrum of secular opinion and religious persuasion (see Section V for summaries of these papers).

Studies and Investigations

The Commission contracted for a number of studies and investigations. These included a study, undertaken primarily through review of the literature, of the nature, extent and purposes of research on the fetus, conducted under contract with Yale University (see Section II); an historical study of the role of research involving living fetuses in certain advances in medical science and practice, conducted under contract with Battelle Columbus Laboratories (see Section III); and a study utilizing available data to establish guidelines for determining fetal viability and death, conducted under contract with Columbia University (see Section VII).

In addition to these studies, papers outlining their views on research on the fetus were prepared by the following ethicists and philosophers: Sissela Bok of Harvard University; Joseph Fletcher of the Institute of Religion and Human Development; Marc Lappé of the Hastings Institute of Society, Ethics, and the Life Sciences; Richard McCormick and LeRoy Walters of the Kennedy Institute for the Study of Human Reproduction and Bioethics; Paul Ramsey of Princeton University; Seymour Siegel of the Jewish Theological Seminary; and Richard Wasserstrom of the University of California at Los Angeles (see Section V). Stephen Toulmin, of the University of Chicago, prepared an analysis of the ethical views that were presented to the Commission, identifying areas of consensus as well as divergence. Leon Kass, of Georgetown University, prepared a philosophical paper on the determination of fetal viability and death (see Section VII). Papers on the legal issues of research on the fetus were prepared by Alexander M. Capron, of the University of Pennsylvania Law School, and John P. Wilson, of Boston University Law School (see Section IV).

Definitions

For the purposes of this report, the Commission has used the following definitions which, in some instances, differ from medical, legal or common usage. These definitions have been adopted in the interest of clarity and to conform to the language used in the legislative mandate.

"Fetus" refers to the human from the time of implantation until a determination is made following delivery that it is viable or possibly viable. If it is viable or possibly viable, it is thereupon designated an infant. (Hereafter, the term "fetus" will refer to a living fetus unless otherwise specified.)

"Viable infant" refers to an infant likely to survive to the point of sustaining life independently, given the support of available medical technology.

This judgment is made by a physician.

"Possibly viable infant" means the fetus ex utero which has not yet been determined to be viable or nonviable. This is a decision to be made by a physician. Operationally, the physician may consider that an infant with a gestational age of 20 to 24 weeks (five to six lunar months; four and one-half to five and one-half calendar months) and a weight between 500 and 600 grams may fall into this indeterminate category. These indices depend upon present technology and should be reviewed periodically.

"Nonviable fetus" refers to the fetus ex utero which, although it is living, cannot possibly survive to the point of sustaining life independently, given the support of available medical technology. Although it may be presumed that a fetus is nonviable at a gestational age less than 20 weeks (five lunar months; four and one-half calendar months) and weight less than 500 grams, a specific determination as to viability must be made by a physician in each instance. The Commission is not aware of any well-documented instances of survival of infants of less than 24 weeks (six lunar months; five and one-half calendar months) gestational age and weighing less than 600 grams; it has chosen lower indices to provide a margin of safety. These indices depend upon present technology and should be reviewed periodically.

"Dead fetus" ex utero refers to a fetus ex utero which exhibits neither heartbeat, spontaneous respiratory activity, spontaneous movement of voluntary muscles, or pulsation of umbilical cord (if still attached). Generally, some organs, tissues and cells (referred to collectively as fetal tissue) remain alive for varying periods of time after the total organism is dead.

"Fetal material" refers to the placenta, amniotic fluid, fetal membranes and the umbilical cord.

"Research" refers to the systematic collection of data or observations in accordance with a designed protocol.

"Therapeutic research" refers to research designed to improve the health condition of the research subject by prophylactic, diagnostic or treatment methods that depart from standard medical practice but hold out a reasonable expectation of success.

"Nontherapeutic research" refers to research not designed to improve the health condition of the research subject by prophylactic, diagnostic or treatment methods.

II. The Nature and Extent of Research Involving the Fetus and the Purposes for Which Such Research Has Been Undertaken

An extensive review of the scientific literature, focusing on a period covering the last 10 years, formed the basis for the Commission's investigation of the nature, extent and purposes of research on the fetus. The review was conducted under contract with Yale University, Maurice J. Mahoney, M.D., Principal Investigator. The investigation included an all-language review of published research, utilizing the MEDLARS computer indexing and search system of the National Library of Medicine, a review of selected bibliographies and abstracts, a survey of departments of pediatrics and obstetrics at medical schools in the United States and Canada to identify current research on the fetus, and a review of NIH grant applications and contracts since 1972 involving research on the fetus. In addition, the Food and Drug Administration provided information on fetal research conducted in fulfillment of its regulations.

For the purpose of summarizing the review, research involving the fetus has been considered in four general categories.

1. *Assessment of fetal growth and development in utero.* Over 600 publications dealing with investigations of fetal development and physiology were identified. In general, the purpose of these investigations was to obtain information on normal developmental processes, as a basis for detecting and understanding abnormal processes and ultimately treating the fetal patient. To this end, numerous experimental approaches were employed.

Studies of normal fetal growth relied primarily on anatomic studies of the dead fetus. Studies of fetal physiology involved both the fetus *in utero* and organs and tissues removed from the dead fetus. In some instances, this research required administration of a substance to the mother prior to an abortion or delivery by caesarean section, followed by analysis to detect the presence of the substance of its metabolic effects in blood from the umbilical cord or in tissues from the dead fetus. Information on the normal volume of amniotic fluid at various stages of pregnancy was obtained by injecting a substance into the fluid and assessing the degree of dilution of that substance; these studies were performed before abortion, during management of disease states (Rh disease), and in normal term pregnancies. Similarly, numerous chemicals were measured in amniotic fluid to establish normal data.

Research also focused on the development of fetal behavior *in utero*. Fetal breathing movements were detected by ultrasound as early as 13 weeks after conception. Fetal hearing was documented by demonstrating changes in fetal heart rate or EEG in response to sound transmitted through the mother's abdomen. Vision was inferred from changes in fetal heart rate in response to light shined transabdominally. Increased rates of fetal swallowing after injection of saccharin into amniotic fluid suggested the presence of fetal taste capability. Observation of the fetus outside the uterus indicated response to touch at 7 weeks and the presence of swallowing movements at 12 weeks of gestation.

2. *Diagnosis of fetal disease or abnormality*. Well over 1000 papers have been published in the last 10 years dealing with intrauterine diagnosis of fetal disease or abnormality. Much of this research involved amniocentesis, a procedure in which a needle is inserted through the mother's abdomen into the uterus and amniotic fluid is removed for analysis. Amniocentesis originally came into extensive use for monitoring the status of the fetus affected by Rh disease in the third trimester of pregnancy. Research related to treating Rh disease indicated that the yellow color of the amniotic fluid correlated with the severity of anemia in the fetus. This color index later was used as an indication of the need for intrauterine transfusion, a procedure subsequently developed to treat severely affected infants.

The knowledge that amniocentesis was safe in the third trimester of pregnancy, coupled with the demonstration that cells shed from the skin of the fetus into the amniotic fluid could be grown in tissue culture, led to application of amniocentesis to detection of genetic disease in the second trimester. The research conducted in developing this procedure focused first on demonstrating in fetal cells from amniotic fluid the normal values for enzymes known to be defective in genetic disease. The research was conducted largely on amniotic fluid samples withdrawn as a routine part of the procedure of inducing abortion. Once it had been demonstrated that the enzyme was expressed in fetal cells and normal values were known, application to diagnosis of the abnormal condition in the fetus at risk was undertaken. The reported research documents a steady progression in development and application of amniocentesis, so that potentially over 60 inborn errors of metabolism (such as Tay-Sachs disease) and virtually all chromosome abnormalities (such as Down's syndrome), as well as the lack of these defects in the fetus at risk, can be diagnosed *in utero*, at a time when the mother can elect therapeutic abortion of an affected fetus.

Research directed at prenatal diagnosis of disease currently focuses on three main objectives. The first involves attempts to extend diagnostic capability to additional diseases, such as cystic fibrosis on the pancreas, which cannot now be detected by amniocentesis. A second approach attempts to detect fetal cells in the maternal circulation and separate these from maternal cells for chemical analysis, thus avoiding any risks and difficulties encountered during amniocentesis. The third direction is the development of fetoscopy, a process by which an instrument is inserted into the uterus and a sample of fetal blood is obtained from the placenta under direct visualization. The blood sample is analyzed to diagnose disorders such as sickle cell disease or thalassemia which cannot be detected by amniocentesis. The time needed for laboratory analysis following fetoscopy is markedly shorter than the four to six weeks required to obtain tissue culture results in amniocentesis. Fetoscopy also permits visual examination of the fetus for external physical defects.

Because of the unknown but theoretically significant risks that remained following animal studies, fetoscopy was developed selectively in women undergoing elective abortion. The first clinical applications have been reported in recent months: three fetuses at risk for beta-thalassemia, whose mothers were seeking abortion to avoid the possibility of having an affected child, were diagnosed as free of disease following fetoscopy. All three have been born and are normal.

Research has also been directed at the identification of physical defects in the developing fetus. The most handicapping defects are those of the neural tube (anencephaly or meningomyelocele). Initial research efforts were devoted to developing X-ray techniques to view the fetus for these defects by injection of radioopaque substances into amniotic fluid (amniography or fetography). These studies primarily involved women having a family history of neural tube defects and whose fetuses were consequently at increased risk. More recently, elevated levels of alpha fetoprotein in amniotic fluid (or maternal blood) were found to be associated with neural tube defects, and may serve as a screening test for these disorders. Ultrasound has come into use to determine internal and external structural detail of the developing fetus and thereby to detect anencephaly, meningomyelocele, and even congenital heart disease.

Amniocentesis also opened another area of fetal research: the assessment of fetal lung maturity. Studies of normal amniotic fluid in the last trimester of pregnancy provided an indication that increased concentrations of lecithin relative to sphingomyelin reflect maturation of the fetal lung; infants with mature lungs did not develop respiratory distress. This predictive test (the L/S ratio) was applied when women went into premature labor, or when induced delivery was indicated due to Rh disease or maternal diabetes, to assess risk that the delivered infant would develop respiratory distress. When the lungs were immature, delivery could be delayed, depending on the relative risks of intrauterine versus extrauterine life. In the last three years, attempts to induce fetal lung maturation by administration of corticosteroids to the mother have added a new dimension to this clinical situation. Following animal studies indicating that this procedure was safe and effective, human studies were undertaken intending to benefit the fetus involved. Results reported to date suggest that the procedure is successful, but studies of possible long-term side effects of this intrauterine therapy are continuing.

Assessment of fetal well-being is another goal of fetal research. Ultrasound has been used to assess fetal size and gestational age, and to monitor fetal respiratory movements, certain types of which have been found to indicate fetal distress. Studies of hormones, metabolic products and chemicals in amniotic fluid (and in maternal blood and urine) identified numerous substances associated with either abnormalities of fetal growth or with fetal distress. In the last decade, monitoring the fetal heart rate and sampling fetal scalp blood during labor developed from research techniques to clinical application for indication of fetal distress.

3. *Fetal pharmacology and therapy.* Over 400 publications in the last 10 years involving fetal pharmacology were identified in the literature search; less than 20 percent of these included research on the living fetus. Of the latter studies, the majority were coincidental studies conducted as an adjunct to clinically accepted procedures. For example, the largest category encompassed studies of transplacental drug movement or effects on the fetus of analgesic or anesthetic agents given to the mother during labor and delivery.

The research techniques employed in investigations of this type included antepartum transfusion of the fetus with blood containing drugs, and administration of drugs or agents to the mother for therapeutic or research reasons. The ensuing studies involved assessment of effects on the fetal electrocardiogram, determination of fetal movements or structures by ultrasound, amniotic fluid sampling, scalp or umbilical cord blood sampling, and studying placental passage and fetal distribution patterns in tissues of the dead fetus. The studies were conducted either prior to abortion or in normal pregnancies, usually at the time of delivery.

In general, studies to determine the effects of a drug on the fetus were retrospective, involved the fetus incidentally or after death, or involved the infant, child or adult. Thus, all studies of the influence of oral contraceptives or

other drugs on multiple births or congenital abnormalities were retrospective. Study of the effects on the fetus of drugs administered to treat maternal illness during pregnancy (including anticonvulsants, antibiotics, hormones and psychopharmacologic agents) in which the fetus was an incidental participant, were also largely retrospective. Studies of effects on the fetus and newborn infant of analgesic and anesthetic agents given at delivery also involved the fetus incidentally, but were conducted prospectively. Recently attempts were made to focus prospective pharmacologic studies of antibiotics intentionally, rather than incidentally, on the fetus. Different antibiotics were administered to pregnant women before abortion to compare quantitative movement of these agents across the placenta, as well as absolute levels achieved in fetal tissues. The results served as a guideline for drug selection to treat intrauterine infections, particularly syphilis. Studies conducted on the dead fetus after abortion showed the clear superiority of one drug over the other.

In addition to assessing effects of drugs on the fetus and measuring placental transfer of drugs, fetal pharmacologic research included attempts to modify drug structures so that they will or will not cross the placenta to affect the fetus. Such research also included study of the effects of certain drugs (such as phenobarbital or corticosteroids) in inducing enzyme activity in the fetus (to prevent hyperbilirubinemia or speed fetal lung maturation and prevent respiratory distress syndrome).

Effects on the fetus of live attenuated virus vaccines administered to the mother were also examined. Preliminary testing of rubella vaccine in monkeys indicated that the vaccine virus did not cross the placenta. In contrast, studies on women requesting therapeutic abortion showed clearly that the vaccine virus did indeed cross the placenta and infect the fetus, indicating the danger of administering the vaccine during pregnancy. Similarly, a study conducted with mumps vaccine virus showed that the virus infected the placenta, but not the fetus.

Attempts at fetal therapy *in utero*, in addition to blood transfusion for Rh

disease and corticosteroid administration to speed fetal lung maturity, were conducted recently as an adjunct to amniocentesis. Examples of this type of fetal therapy include the administration of hydrocortisone to the fetus *in utero* to treat the adrenogenital syndrome, maternal dietary therapy for fetal galactosemia, and administration to the mother of large doses of vitamin B_{12} to treat fetal methylmalonic acidemia.

4. *Research involving the nonviable fetus.* The quantity of research on the nonviable fetus *ex utero* has been small; much of such research included the nonviable fetus only as the extreme end of the spectrum of studies of premature infants. Such studies included measurements of amino acid levels in plasma of infants with intrauterine malnutrition, administration of bromide to measure total body water in low birth weight infants, and the study of hemoglobin in blood from the umbilical cord as an indicator of fetal maturity. The purpose of this research was to gain information that could be of benefit to other fetuses and infants.

Research was also conducted involving the nonviable fetus during abortion by hysterotomy but before the fetus and placenta were physically removed from the uterus. A study conducted in the United States reported the feasibility of delivering a portion of the umbilical cord from the uterus and using it as a site for drug administration and blood sampling. Another study, this one undertaken in Finland, employed the technique to infuse noradrenaline via the umbilical vein; study of metabolites subsequently obtained demonstrated the functional maturity of the fetal sympathetic nervous system. Several studies in Sweden used similar techniques: radiolabeled chemicals were administered to the fetus via the umbilical vessels, and metabolites were then studied in the umbilical vein and, following completion of the abortion, in the fetus. In another Finnish study, arginine and insulin were injected into blood vessels of 8 fetuses (450–600 grams) with the placenta attached to the uterus, and blood samples were taken from the umbilical cord to assess fetal endocrine regulation of glucose metabolism. These studies were conducted solely to gain information on fetal metabolism for the benefit of other fetuses and infants.

The nonviable fetus was the subject of research to develop a life-support system ("artificial placenta") for sustaining very small premature infants, as well as to obtain data on normal fetal physiology. Some of this life support system research was conducted only with larger infants (viable by weight criteria) who had failed on respirators and were tried on experimental systems as an ultimate therapeutic effort to achieve survival. Of the published studies with clearly nonviable fetuses, one was conducted in the United States. Published in 1963, this research involved 15 fetuses, obtained following therapeutic abortion at 9–24 weeks gestational age. The fetuses were immersed in salt solution containing oxygen at extremely high pressure, in an attempt to provide oxygen for the fetus through the skin. The longest survival was 22 hours. In an earlier study in Scandinavia, 7 fetuses weighing 200–375 grams, from both spontaneous and induced abortions, were perfused with oxygenated blood through the umbilical vessels. Longest survival was 12 hours. A third study, conducted in England, utilized a similar method and included 8 fetuses obtained following hysterotomy abortion and weighing 300–980 grams. Longest survival was 5 hours. No other studies of this type involving nonviable fetuses were found in the literature review.

Studies of fetal physiology conducted on the delivered fetus utilized several experimental approaches. In a study conducted in Sweden, the intact fetal-placental unit obtained by hysterotomy abortion was removed and utilized for perfusion studies. A study performed in England involved cannulating the carotid and umbilical arteries of the aborted fetus and measuring fetal glucose levels in response to administration of growth hormone. Four fetuses from hysterotomy abortions at 16–20 weeks gestation were perfused via the umbilical vessels in a study in Scotland which demonstrated that the fetus could synthesize estriol independent of the placenta. A similar study by the same investigators involving six fetuses demonstrated that the 16–20 week fetus could synthesize testosterone from progesterone. To learn whether the human fetal brain could metabolize

ketone bodies as an alternative to glucose, brain metabolism was isolated in 8 human fetuses (12–17 weeks gestation) after hysterotomy abortion by perfusing the head separated from the rest of the body. This study, conducted in Finland, demonstrated that the human fetus, like previously studied animal fetuses, could modify metabolic processes to utilize ketone bodies.

These studies of the nonviable fetus represent the total number reported in the world scientific literature, as well as could be ascertained from review of the most comprehensive bibliographic search ever undertaken of research involving the human fetus. The total number of citations involving fetal research was well in excess of 3000; the reports of research on the nonviable fetus that were found numbered less than 20. Certainly some reports of such research may have been missed even by this thorough review, but it is safe to conclude that the amount of research conducted on the nonviable fetus has been extremely limited. Of the principal investigators conducting this type of research, three were from the United States; two of these investigators conducted their research abroad. The only research conducted in the United States on the nonviable fetus *ex utero* was the study involving attempts to develop an artificial life support system. The literature survey disclosed no reports of research conducted in the United States on the nonviable fetus intended solely to obtain information on normal physiologic function.

In summary, research involving the fetus includes a broad spectrum of studies of the fetus both inside and outside the uterus. The research may be as innocuous as observation, or involve mild manipulation such as weighing or measuring, or more extensive manipulation such as altering the environment, administering a drug or agent, or noninvasive monitoring. Diagnostic studies may involve sampling amniotic fluid, urine, blood, or spinal fluid, or performing biopsies. The most extensive or invasive procedures include perfusion studies and other attempts to maintain function.

The extent of research on the fetus is reflected by the more than 3000 citations included in the literature review of such research. Most involved the

fetus *in utero;* less than 20 articles involved the nonviable fetus.

The purposes for which research on the fetus has been undertaken include obtaining knowledge of normal fetal growth and development as a basis for understanding the abnormal; diagnosing fetal disease or abnormality; studying fetal pharmacology and the effects of chemical and other agents on the fetus, in order to develop fetal therapy; and developing techniques to save the lives of ever smaller premature infants.

III. Alternative Means for Achieving the Purposes for Which Research Involving Living Fetuses Has Been Undertaken

In the development of new medical procedures or drugs to be employed in the treatment of humans, research is usually initiated with animal models, which are used until probable effectiveness and low degree of risk are determined. Ultimately, it becomes necessary to conduct the research on humans, since initial human applications are experimental regardless of the amount of preceding animal research. In some instances, pertinent animal models may not exist or may have certain limitations, so that studies on humans begin at a relatively early stage. In all instances, however, the question may be asked whether studies on humans began at an appropriate time, or whether the information that was required could have been obtained using alternative research means, i.e., studies on animal models.

The broad nature of the survey of the nature and extent of research on the fetus (Section II) did not permit detailed evaluation of alternative means. Therefore, the Commission contracted with Battelle Columbus Laboratories to conduct a more intensive analysis of this issue in connection with four advances in which research on the fetus played a part. The Battelle report to the Commission traces the historical development of (1) rubella vaccine, (2) the use of amniocentesis for prenatal diagnosis of genetic defects, (3) the diagnosis and treatment, as well as prevention, of Rh isoimmunization disease, and (4) the management of respiratory distress syndrome. The study identifies pertinent animal research that was conducted and attempts to assess whether the human research was necessary and appropriate, or whether animal models could have been substituted. Finally, the study evaluates the likelihood that the advance would have been achieved if all research on the fetus, both therapeutic and nontherapeutic, had been prohibited. In preparing the report and analysis, extensive bibliographies on each topic, prepared by staff of the National Library of Medicine, were utilized. In addition, a number of scientists whose research had been of greatest importance to the advances were interviewed.

1. In the case of *congenital rubella syndrome,* descriptions of the condition (which comprises congenital heart disease, cataracts, deafness and mental retardation) and its etiology (maternal rubella infection during pregnancy) were drawn from research on the living child and material from dead fetuses. Attenuation of the rubella virus for vaccine purposes was accomplished in tissue culture using nonhuman cells. Vaccine trials were conducted on adults and children. The vaccine was found safe and effective, and it was licensed in 1969, 28 years after the congenital rubella syndrome was first described.

No research on the living human fetus was required to develop the vaccine. A question remained, however, as to the safety of administering the vaccine during pregnancy or to women in the childbearing years. Should a pregnant woman, without immunity to rubella, be vaccinated to prevent the risk of the fetus that would ensue if she contracted natural rubella? Some experimental animal models for the rubella condition had been developed, the rhesus monkey being the closest one to the human. Accordingly, pregnant monkeys were inoculated with either rubella virus or the vaccine virus. Subsequent study showed that five or six monkey fetuses whose mothers received slightly attenuated rubella virus were infected, but none of the six monkey fetuses whose mothers received vaccine virus was infected. Thus, the animal model suggested that the vaccine virus did not cross the

placenta and was safe to administer during pregnancy, although other vaccine viruses were known to cross the human placenta.

Human studies were then undertaken. Because of the potential risk to the fetus, women requesting therapeutic abortion were employed as subjects. These volunteers received the vaccine and underwent the abortion 11 to 30 days later. Examination of tissues from the dead aborted fetuses showed that, in contrast to the results in monkeys, the vaccine virus did cross the human placenta and infect the fetus. On the basis of this research involving the fetus in anticipation of abortion, as well as subsequent reports of damage to the fetus following accidental rubella vaccination during pregnancy, administration of rubella vaccine to pregnant women or women who might become pregnant within 60 days of vaccination is proscribed.

Two alternatives to the planned testing of rubella vaccine on pregnant women in anticipation of abortion can be considered. First, more extensive animal testing of the vaccine could have been conducted. The usefulness of such a procedure, however, would be questionable. Based on prior experience with the inconsistencies of placental passage of any agent, the human situation would remain unknown after any amount of animal testing. Testing in the human is still required even after negative results in animal models, with the same safeguards as if no animal testing had been conducted.

The second alternative would be to wait for the accidental vaccination of pregnant women and observe the outcome. This in fact occurred in several instances after the planned testing. The women involved, who had wanted pregnancies, elected instead to terminate their pregnancies by abortion due to the risk to the fetus, and studies of tissue from the dead fetuses confirmed that they had been infected by the virus. Thus, the effect in humans could have been learned in this instance by retrospective research. At issue here in the selection of alternatives is the question whether it is preferable to proceed by design with women planning abortions, or to work retrospectively with women who desire pregnancy but were accidentally vaccinated.

2. The use of *amniocentesis* (removal of amniotic fluid via a needle inserted into the uterus through the mother's abdomen) as a clinical procedure dates from 1882, when it was introduced as a treatment for polyhydramnios (excess accumulation of amniotic fluid). There is no evidence that animal studies were conducted prior to that time, and comparatively little research has been done on amniocentesis as a procedure apart from its applications. The Battelle study of amniocentesis thus involved evaluation of the uses to which the procedure has been put, as well as alternative means for developing the procedure. Amniocentesis has found application in three main areas of research: prenatal diagnosis of genetic disease, diagnosis of Rh disease, and assessment of fetal maturity related to respiratory distress syndrome. Its use in the latter two areas will be discussed in parts 3 and 4 of this section.

Two lines of research provided impetus for prenatal diagnosis of genetic disease: development of the technology for tissue culture and identification of the sex chromatin as an indicator of sex in single cells. In 1955 it was shown that fetal sex could be predicted from the sex chromatin pattern of amniotic fluid cells. Application of this technique to prenatal detection of sex-linked disorders was first reported in 1960. Rapid progress in tissue culture research led to success in culturing fetal amniotic fluid cells in 1966, intrauterine diagnosis of a chromosome abnormality in 1967, and the first intrauterine diagnosis of metabolic disorders using cultured amniotic fluid cells in the following year. Research in this area steadily expanded as chromosomal and metabolic disorders were added to the list of conditions diagnosable *in utero.* At present, virtually any chromosomal anomaly and potentially over 60 metabolic disorders can be detected prenatally by amniocentesis. The possibility of diagnosis and selective abortion of abnormal fetuses has enabled the birth of normal children to families that otherwise would not have risked pregnancy, and has permitted families to avoid the impact of the birth of a defective or doomed child.

All research to detect genetic defects involved the living human fetus. Much of it utilized amniotic fluid obtained in the normal course of abortion, in order to ascertain normal values. Such research was obviously nonbeneficial for the fetuses involved. Only research conducted on women at risk for having a fetus with the disorder in question could be considered beneficial, in that many of these women desired an abortion unless it could be shown that the fetus would be normal.

An alternative means to develop the procedure of amniocentesis would have been to conduct more extensive animal research. Animal models have numerous limitations with regard to amniocentesis, however, including shape of the pelvis, size and shape of the uterus, number of fetuses present (which confounds cell analysis), and the marked irritability of the uterus in many species such that even slight manipulation induces abortion, fetal resorption or congenital malformations. Recently some animals have been found in which amniocentesis can be performed, but even in these it is difficult in mid-pregnancy, when it must be done for effective intrauterine diagnosis of genetic defects.

While animal models might have been utilized more extensively in developing the technique of amniocentesis, there is no alternative to human experimentation for the purpose of developing the diagnostic tests for genetic metabolic disorders used with amniocentesis. The conditions are unique to the human species. Only by study of cells in amniotic fluid from pregnant humans, both normal and those at risk for genetic disease in the fetus, was it possible to assess whether the genetic defect was expressed in these cells, and to determine the normal and abnormal values for the responsible enzymes in the cells as the basis for prenatal diagnosis. This research utilized only amniotic fluid and the fetal cells in it, and thus was not invasive of the fetus. In the early stages of developing the technique, however, the possible risks to the fetus were greater than those for many invasive procedures.

3. The history of *Rh isoimmunization disease* encompasses the description of the disorder, determination of its cause, initiation of successful treatment, and development of effective prevention, all

within four decades. Characterization of this disorder, which combines hemolytic anemia, jaundice, and intrauterine death or (if delivered) severe brain damage, was accomplished in the 1930's from study of autopsy material and newborn infants. Research on blood groups, utilizing both human and animal material, led in 1941 to the demonstration from studies of mothers and newborns that Rh sensitization in an Rh negative mother to an Rh positive fetus produced hemolytic anemia in the fetus. In 1945, treatment of affected newborn infants by exchange transfusion was initiated and mortality began to decline.

Use of amniocentesis was introduced in 1956 to obtain amniotic fluid which provided an indicator of how severely the fetus was affected and, late in pregnancy, whether labor should be induced to enable treatment of the fetus outside the uterus. In 1963, treatment of the severely affected fetus by intrauterine blood transfusion was initiated, resulting in a 60 percent reduction of the stillbirth rate for affected infants. Ongoing studies of the etiology of the disease, using pregnant women, provided indications that sensitization of the mother usually occurred at the time of delivery of her first Rh positive infant, when a large volume of fetal Rh positive cells entered the mother's circulation. As the result of research conducted largely with prisoners, a vaccine was developed to prevent this sensitization. Trials of the vaccine, administered to women after delivery, began in 1964. Results indicated virtually complete effectiveness, and the vaccine (RhoGam) became commercial available in 1968.

Research on the fetus played no part in developing the RhoGam vaccine, but such research was essential in demonstrating the basic cause of the disease and in developing methods for prenatal diagnosis and treatment. All significant research on the fetus related to Rh disease was conducted on mothers and fetuses at risk for the disease, and can be categorized as beneficial research. The size of the benefits achieved may be appreciated by reviewing statistics related to the disorder. Approximately 12 percent of couples in the United States are at risk for having an affected infant. Nearly 25,000 infants could be affected yearly.

Since initiation of exchange transfusion, neonatal mortality of affected infants has dropped to about 2.5 percent. Intrauterine transfusion has reduced the annual number of stillbirths due to the disease from 10,000 to less than half that number. The entire amount of money used to support Rh disease research from 1930 through the successful development of the vaccine in 1966 is the equivalent of the present cost to society for lifetime care of six children irreparably brain damaged by the disease.

Limited animal models were available for study of Rh disease and were utilized in some instances. Intrauterine transfusion, for example, was first conducted on animals. Extensive research has been conducted to develop an animal model of the actual disease, but the hamadrayas baboon is the only species that has been found in which the disease is sufficiently similar to the condition in man for the animal to serve as a useful model. The limitations of animal models and the urgency of developing a treatment for fetuses otherwise likely to die led physician researchers to attempt experimental therapy with favorable risk/benefit ratio in human subjects. In these instances, the risk of not doing the research was approximately 50 percent intrauterine death; in the face of such odds, even such a hazardous experimental therapeutic procedure as intrauterine transfusion was considered acceptable.

4. *Respiratory distress syndrome* (RDS) is a major cause of infant mortality. In the United States approximately 40,000 cases occur annually; 95 percent of these cases are premature infants, and overall mortality is in excess of 25 percent. Study of the development of advances related to this condition revealed a picture of frequent interaction of animal model and clinical studies involving the living human fetus in the third trimester. In addition, advances in therapy were achieved from research involving affected premature infants.

The key experimental work elucidating the basic cause of the condition involved study of the lungs of deceased infants who died of RDS or other causes. This research indicated that lungs of infants with RDS lacked a chemical (surfactant) which acted to keep open the smallest air passages in the lung; surfactant was present in the lungs of unaffected infants. Subsequent studies, again relying primarily on autopsy material, delineated the biochemistry of surfactant, and it was suggested that amniotic fluid might provide an indicator of the presence of surfactant. Studies were then conducted of amniotic fluid obtained at various stages in the last trimester of pregnancy, solely to learn the normal values of the phospholipid components of surfactant; this research was non-beneficial for the fetuses involved. Results indicated that a marked increase in the content of lecithin relative to sphingomyelin in amniotic fluid correlated with the appearance of surfactant in the fetal lung, and indicated that the lungs were mature enough that the fetus, if delivered, would probably not develop RDS. The report of these studies in 1971 strongly influenced obstetric management of premature labor and diabetic pregnancy, by providing an index of the time when delivery could proceed with minimum risk of RDS.

Another line of research quickly had an impact on RDS management. Animal studies in the 1950's showed that steroids were capable of inducing enzyme activity in the fetus. Studies involving the pregnant woman and the living fetus in 1961 demonstrated that cortisone crossed the human placenta. Animal studies in the late 1960's and early 1970's indicated that corticosteroids could induce enzymes and thereby increase surfactant in fetal lungs. In the species studied (lambs, rabbits and rats) the steroids did not cross the placenta and had to be administered directly to the fetus. Based on the previous demonstration that steroids crossed the human placenta, and later clinical studies of mothers receiving steroid therapy during pregnancy that had not suggested any ill effects on the fetus, clinical trials were initiated in pregnant women at risk of having infants affected by RDS. The results obtained to date indicate that corticosteroids are highly effective in preventing RDS, without undesirable side effects. Although the treatment remains experimental, it holds promise for markedly reducing the incidence of RDS.

The interplay between animal and human studies was essential in achieving the advances in clinical management and prevention of RDS. Relevant animal models were used when available, and although no extensive search for an animal was evident before the human steroid trials, the research appeared to be a logical and carefully planned step undertaken to provide therapy for a condition of high risk to the fetuses treated.

The following conclusions are drawn from the Battelle study:

A. Animal models were utilized extensively, but adequate and appropriate models were not always available when they were needed. In some instances little or no animal research preceded human studies. In other instances intensive searches for animal models were undertaken (as in Rh disease), but investigators appear to have been reluctant to postpone therapeutic research until an animal model was found.

B. Investigators generally proceeded to clinical trials characterized by very high ratios of benefit to risk.

C. A total ban on all research on the fetus, or postponement of such research until more appropriate and exact animal models were sought and studied, would probably have significantly delayed or halted indefinitely the progress in three of the four areas that were analyzed. Only development of the rubella vaccine could have progressed unimpeded.

A more limited ban would have had less effect, depending on the nature and scope of the prohibitions imposed. For example, a ban only on nontherapeutic research on the fetus would not have affected research on Rh disease, but would have sharply curtailed research with amniocentesis, due to the resulting inability to determine normal values for abnormal enzymes in metabolic disorders. The research which developed L/S ratios, used in RDS diagnosis, might have been possible making use of fluid obtained during caesarean sections or in Rh disease studies. A selective ban on research before or after induced abortion would clearly have permitted the L/S ratio research for RDS diagnosis, but could still have severely curtailed development of amniocentesis for prenatal diagnosis by making ascertainment of normal values extremely difficult. A

ban on invasive research on the fetus would have permitted development of amniocentesis, although the risks to the fetus from this noninvasive procedure were potentially greater than those from many invasive procedures.

IV. Legal Issues

Papers on the legal issues involved in research on the fetus were prepared for the Commission by Professor Alexander M. Capron, University of Pennsylvania Law School, and Assistant Dean John P. Wilson, Boston University School of Law. Both papers are structured, at least in part, according to categories of research, that is, whether the research is therapeutic, or nontherapeutic, whether the fetal subject is viable, nonviable or dead, and whether it is inside or outside the uterus. The interests of the fetus at different stages of development are balanced against the interests of other parties, and the protection of fetal interests is addressed in discussion of appropriate consent requirements. A summary of both papers follows.

The Dead Fetus

The Uniform Anatomical Gift Act (UAGA), which has been adopted in all fifty states and the District of Columbia, permits research on the dead fetus and the products of conception, provided consent has been given by either parent and the other parent has not objected. Professor Capron states that the UAGA should be read in the context of common law requirements on consent; thus, the authorization should be "informed" and "voluntary." In the latter regard, consent should not unnecessarily be sought immediately before or after an abortion. Dean Wilson suggests that it is wise to require the consent of both parents.

Aside from UAGA, Professor Capron points out that the statutes of five states presently impose varying degrees of restriction on research on the dead fetus (Massachusetts, South Dakota, Illinois, Indiana, and Ohio); all of these restrictions apply only to the products of induced and not spontaneous abortions. Other laws that might affect research on the dead fetus are the grave robbing statutes, which would apply only when the consent required by the UAGA has not been obtained. As a matter of medical practice, however, maternal consent is not generally sought for post-abortion examinations. (Both authors note and discuss a pending Massachusetts case.)

Professor Capron states that the various state laws on death certification provide little guidance on the question of defining death with respect to the fetus. Such laws do, however, introduce another complication by recognizing different categories requiring certification. (Other reports prepared for the Commission suggest medical criteria for determining fetal death; see Section VII of this report.)

The Viable Infant

Research on the viable infant is discussed at length by Professor Capron. He states that therapeutic research on a viable infant, whether or not there has been an induced abortion, is generally sanctioned under criminal and civil law. The law is presently unsettled with respect to nontherapeutic research, and, as a practical matter, the exercise of caution in introducing any risk is indicated. The recently enacted fetal research statutes have probably not altered the common law with respect to research on the viable infant after induced abortion, i.e., therapeutic research may be conducted. In the absence of a special statute, the protection afforded the viable infant attaches only after it is in fact ex utero.

Although the interests of the viable infant do not depend on the manner in which it came to be alive ex utero, Professor Capron points out that this might be relevant to the issue of appropriate consent to involvement of the infant in research. The question is whether the decision to abort should disqualify the parents (or at least the mother) from exercising further control after the infant is alive ex utero. The argument for disqualification has an obvious rationale in conflict of interest, but it faces at least three problems: (1) Since the Supreme Court has declared in Roe v. Wade that women have a constitutional right to abortion, basing maternal disqualification on the exercise of that right may be an unconstitutional penalty. (2) Since the abortion itself is legal, the fetus is not thereby deprived of any rights which the parents were obliged to protect. (3) The decision to abort does not necessarily cast the

woman as being irrevocably opposed to the rights of the fetus, since the mother's decision was based on the erroneous assumption that there would be no live issue from the pregnancy. Professor Capron suggests that rather than presumptive disqualification in all cases, judicial proceedings may be an appropriate forum for balancing the rights of all concerned, and that it would be preferable to presume that parents retain control over a viable infant. Certain states, however, have written into their abortion statutes some form of parental forfeiture of rights (Louisiana, Missouri, Montana, Kentucky, Indiana, South Dakota).

Dean Wilson suggests that, at least with respect to therapeutic research, the power of consent should not be removed from a mother and father because they are minors. Also, he expresses the belief that only therapeutic research should be conducted on the viable infant.

The Fetus in Utero

Although the fetus does not achieve the interests of a full person until live birth, it is not entirely without protection while still in utero. Professor Capron points out that the criminal law in various states, with expansions under civil law, recognizes interests of the fetus in utero in two ways of possible relevance to research. First, there are some recent statutes seeking to safeguard the fetus in utero against life threatening intentional injury, and some older statutes that depart from the common law by prohibiting "feticide." It is unlikely that the older statutes would apply to research on the fetus, since the element of intent to do harm would be missing. All of these statutes must, of course, be examined in the light of Roe v. Wade.

Second, interests of the fetus in utero are recognized in the criminal law by protecting the fetus against injuries which cause its death or impairment after it is born alive. The effect of such protection is to put pressure on those involved to assure that the abortion is "effective." Thus, Professor Capron suggests, the law may be recognizing, not fetal interests, but the interests of human beings, after birth, not to suffer because of culpable acts of other persons.

In some jurisdictions, Professor Capron finds out that the civil law recognizes a broader fetal interest in protection against harm in utero. The courts in at least 21 states have recognized a cause of action for injuries to a viable fetus that lead to its stillbirth. Once the fetus is viable, Professor Capron states, the decision in Roe v. Wade does not appear to be an absolute bar to holding that the fetus and its parents have an interest in its potentiality for life.

If the fetus is in fact born alive, the protection under civil law is even broader, with no importance being attached to the question whether the injury that causes impairment or subsequent death occurred before or after viability. (Professor Capron expresses his disagreement with the argument that subsequent live birth is not a necessary element in court decisions regarding the vesting of property interests.)

Finally, if the fetus is both injured and dies before it is viable, recovery for its wrongful death has not been allowed under civil law.

Dean Wilson expresses the opinion that there should be no difference in the rights accorded to the fetus in utero before or after viability, and only therapeutic research or nontherapeutic research that imposes no risk should be permitted in both cases. He would apply the same conditions to research in anticipation of abortion. As grounds for protecting the fetus in utero before viability, he suggests that research on such a fetus might have a brutalizing effect on society as a whole.

With respect to the question of consent to research on the fetus in utero, Professor Capron holds that if the fetus is viable, it is in approximately the same position as a viable infant, i.e., consent by the parents to therapeutic research would be appropriate, but nontherapeutic research that introduces genuine risk should not be undertaken at all. If the fetus is not yet viable, Professor Capron discerns two difficult consent issues: (1) Should there be a separate consent, in addition to that of the mother, when the research is directed at the fetus? A possible answer is that the mother's right of decision to destroy the fetus, recognized by Roe v. Wade, includes a right to permit the fetus to be used in research that is less harmful than total destruction and is done for legitimate scientific reasons. (2) Can the consent of the mother to participate in (nontherapeutic) research directed at the fetus be tied to an agreement to abort? Without such an agreement, parties such as the father and state welfare officials may have grounds to insist that their interests in the potential child be protected. On the other hand, an agreement to abort would probably be unenforceable.

Professor Capron sees no clear answer to the question of appropriate consent to research on the fetus *in utero* before viability. He suggests a partial solution along the lines of the Massachusetts fetal research statute, which provides that research may take place when the fetus is not the subject of a planned abortion and that a statement, signed by the woman, that she is not planning an abortion supplies conclusive evidence on the point. Such an arrangement would not be immune from attack in light of the *Roe* v. *Wade* decision, but it would raise fewer questions, Professor Capron states, if it were a condition of government funding.

In accordance with his views concerning permissible research on the fetus *in utero*, Dean Wilson expresses the belief that the woman should be permitted to consent only to therapeutic research and nontherapeutic research that imposes no risk.

The Nonviable Fetus ex Utero

Professor Capron notes that the law generally does not distinguish between viability and nonviability after birth. Full protection as a person is given, notwithstanding that immaturity may preclude the nonviable fetus from having an independent existence. Professor Capron suggests that legislative consideration of the concept of viability as currently understood might lead to distinctions being made on that basis.

With respect to consent, Professor Capron states that the same rules would apply for therapeutic research on the viable fetus as for such research on the viable infant. For nontherapeutic research on the nonviable fetus, he suggests that judicial review might be appropriate.

V. Ethical Issues

Eight ethicists and philosophers prepared for the Commission papers outlining their views on research on the fetus. Summaries of each of these papers follows:

Sissela Bok, Ph.D.

Dr. Bok identifies two lines of argument opposed to research on the fetus: (1) the fetus is a person and, consequently, research without its consent and not for its benefit is an assault upon its humanity; and (2) research on the fetus will lead society to condone research on other categories of the defenseless. Dr. Bok answers these arguments and concludes that, in order to seek knowledge not otherwise obtainable, research should be permitted at early gestational stages, provided careful safeguards are utilized.

The first argument is countered by a presentation and discussion of four reasons for protecting humans from harm: (1) the victim's anguish, suffering and deprivation of continued experience of life; (2) the brutalization of the agent; (3) the grief of those who care about the victim; and (4) the establishment of a pattern that ultimately will harm all of society. Dr. Bok contends that none of these reasons apply in the early stages of gestational life.

The second argument against research on the fetus advances the last reason for protecting humans from harm as crucial even with respect to research in the first weeks of gestational life. Dr. Bok asserts that no data have been developed to support the applicability of the fourth reason to research on the fetus, and that, in any case, safeguards can be developed to prevent the alleged sequential abuses.

Since the fetus is not a person, consent on its behalf is unnecessary. However, maternal consent should be obtained, even for research following abortion, in deference to the woman's sensitivities.

Dr. Bok concludes that since the means are defensible and the end is desirable, research on the fetus should be permitted during the first 18 weeks of gestational age and when the fetus is under 300 grams in weight. These limits provide a margin of safety to prevent accidental experimentation on a viable fetus. Only therapeutic research on a fetus older than 18 weeks or more than 300 grams in weight should be permitted.

Dr. Bok would permit research on a fetus scheduled for abortion, provided the mother consents and the research is properly reviewed. She would not prohibit experimentation which keeps a nonviable fetus alive for a period of time or which hastens its death.

Joseph Fletcher, D.D.

"Rightness and wrongness are judged according to results, not according to absolute prohibitions or requirements." This statement provides a key to understanding the position taken by Dr. Fletcher regarding the ethics of research on the fetus. The result which justifies such research is the safety of people, especially children, from genetic and congenital disorders, uterine infections and a host of other maladies.

Dr. Fletcher states that the core question is whether the fetus is a person. He contends that although the fetus is a potential person, it does not become an actual person, ethically and legally, until it is born alive and lives entirely outside the mother's body with an independent cardiovascular system. Until the fetus becomes an "actual person" it is an "object," a nonpersonal organism which has value only insofar as it is wanted by its progenitors. It is not entitled to protection as a human subject whether viable or not until it becomes a live-born baby.

Dr. Fletcher states that the following categories of research on the fetus may be justified, depending upon the clinical situation and the design: (1) use of a dead fetus *ex utero* with or without maternal consent; (2) use of a live fetus *ex utero*, nonviable or viable, if survival is not wanted and there is maternal consent; (3) use of a live fetus *in utero* if survival is not wanted and there is maternal consent; and (4) use of a live fetus *in utero*, even if survival is intended, if there is no substantial risk to the fetus and if there is maternal and paternal-spouse consent.

Finally, Dr. Fletcher concludes that regulations by the Executive Branch and legislation by Congress (even though temporary) restricting research on the fetus are unethical if the ethics they are based upon are not fully and frankly disclosed.

Marc Lappé, Ph.D.
Dr. Lappé's essay is developed from a "natural law" perspective. It defends five principles pertaining to research on the fetus and makes five policy recommendations to the Commission.

1. The wanted fetus has a right to protection *in utero*. This principle is based on its unique vulnerability to environmental insult which might interfere with the fulfillment of its genetic potential.

2. Principle (1) is not altered by societal acceptance of abortion. The Supreme Court has allowed a woman to decide that a fetus will no longer receive her protection; it does not follow that others in society are similarly authorized. Further, living fetuses *ex utero* have claims on our duties to afford them protection from experimentation by virtue of our basic medical tenets to preserve life. The Supreme Court offered no guidance on how to treat the fetus once out of the womb.

3. The conditions under which society respects the fetus' right to protection are compromised by the decision and actions taken in the course of an abortion. Moral concern for the fetus dictates a choice of procedures which subject the woman to minimal morbidity risks while expeditiously expelling the fetus and rendering it incapable of survival.

4. The costs of research on the fetus should be balanced by resultant goods. Society should make efforts to endow the abortion process with values it would not otherwise have had. Abortion-related research is therefore justified if and only if it is intended to aid other fetuses.

5. The definition of fetal death and the application of the definition must be made independently from any possible future use of the fetus in experimentation.

Dr. Lappé notes that the problem of consent gives us most difficulty in that even if the fetus were accorded full rights of personhood, it would not do to delegate the parent as proxy since (in the case of abortion) the parent cannot be said to have the interests of the fetus at heart. He offers no solution to the problem, however, except to observe that were the fetus regarded as worthy of all the rights of personhood, we would not sanction nontherapeutic research at all.

Dr. Lappé recommends that the Commission (1) affirm its commitment to protect fetuses *in utero*; (2) provide a statement of concern for abortion-related abuse or neglect, including maternal exposure to harmful agents and insensitive or unethical choice of abortifacients; (3) limit research on the fetus *in utero* which is to be a subject of abortion to cases where no risk to the fetus is involved and the purpose of the research is to aid fetuses as a class; (4) restrict basic nonviable fetal research intended to benefit society generally to dead fetuses; and (5) require that fetal death be ascertained by criteria which separate the purposes of experimentation from the choice of abortion method and from the methodology used to ascertain that death has occurred.

Richard A. McCormick, S.T.D.
Dr. McCormick defends a moral position concerning research on the fetus and distinguishes it from an acceptable public policy concerning such research. Public policy is to be determined, not only by morality, but by feasibility as well. The feasibility test is particularly difficult in a society characterized by moral pluralism and cultural pragmatism.

Dr. McCormick holds that parents may give proxy or vicarious consent for a child to participate in nontherapeutic experimentation where there is "no discernible risk or undue discomfort." Proxy consent is morally legitimate insofar as it is a reasonable construction of what the child *ought* to choose if it were able. This position is rooted in the premise that all humans, including children, have an obligation in social justice to contribute to the benefit of the human community. The same obligation can be extended to the fetus. Research on the fetus is morally permissible if maternal proxy consent is obtained, abortion is not contemplated, the risk or discomfort to the fetus is not discernible, and the results of the experiment cannot be obtained in any other way. Because Dr. McCormick judges most abortions to be immoral, experimental procedures prior to, during, and after abortion (except in the rare instances of legitimate abortion) are morally objectionable because they cooperate with and profit from an immoral system. While Dr. McCormick regards such cooperation as morally

objectionable, he believes that his moral position cannot be fully adopted as public policy, since it cannot pass the feasibility test in a society which allows large-scale abortions.

Dr. McCormick recommends that the measure of proxy consent regarded as valid for subjects of research who are children is suitable to determine acceptable research on the fetus. He makes the following policy proposals which acknowledge both the moral pluralism and the cultural pragmatism characteristic of American society: (1) the research must be necessary; (2) the researcher bears the onus of showing the necessity; (3) there must be no discernible risk for the fetus or the mother or, if the fetus is dying, there must be no added pain or discomfort: (4) the researcher bears the onus of showing that there is no discernible risk; (5) these policy demands must be secured by adequate review and prior approval of all research on the fetus.

Paul Ramsey, Ph.D.
Dr. Ramsey seeks to distinguish between fetal life and fetal viability. Life, he suggests, should be defined for the fetus according to the presence or absence of vital signs which define life and death in other individuals. Viability should not be confused with life, for a fetus may be living yet nonviable. This new human research subject, one which is neither dead nor viable, is the subject of Dr. Ramsey's essay. He is not willing to say it may be entered into research protocols, but he does say that care should be taken not to enter a viable infant by mistake. To this end he recommends that viability be defined for research purposes on the safe side of possibly viable birth weight, crown-rump length or gestational age. He makes the following proposals to the Commission:

1. The Peel Report prohibits procedures carried out with the deliberate intent of ascertaining the harm they might do to the fetus. Such a prohibition should be included in the American policy as well. "Do not harm" encompasses "intend no harm." This principle embraces the intention of the physician and not merely "codes of action."

2. The subjective rule (Peel) must be supplemented by an objective limitation of risks by categorically prohibiting research in anticipation of abortion if that research entails known or uncertain risk.

3. Respect for the dignity of human life must not be compromised whatever the age, circumstances, or expectation of life of the individual. The recent Supreme Court decision on abortion did not nullify the obligation to protect the developing fetus from harm, even if that harm is less than abortion.

4. Vital functions of an individual abortus should not be artificially maintained except where the purpose of the activity is to develop new methods for enabling that abortus to survive to the point of viability.

5. Ethical standards applicable to research on the fetus are the same as would be subscribed to in proposed research on the unconscious, on the dying (in the case of spontaneous abortion), on the (perhaps justly) condemned (in cases of induced abortion), or in experimentation with children.

For the most part, this means that the use of these subjects in nontherapeutic research is an *abuse,* for one ought not to "presume" or "construe" consent for acts of charity. Dr. Ramsey agrees with Dr. McCormick that "one stops and should stop precisely at the point where 'construed' consent does indeed involve self-sacrifice or works of mercy. The dividing line is reached when experiments involve discernible risk, undue discomfort, or inconvenience."

Seymour Siegel, D.H.L.

Dr. Siegel makes the following points:

1. A bias for life is the foundation of the Judeo-Christian world-view and it undergirds medical research. It may be affirmed outside the Judeo-Christian tradition. The bias for life requires individuals to strive to sustain life where it exists, not to terminate or harm life, and in cases of doubt to be on the side of life. A present individual takes precedence over a possible future individual. The bias for life is to be exercised whatever the status of the life before us and whatever the life expectation may be.

2. The indeterminancy of the future requires that utmost caution should be employed in all decisions relating to research on the fetus, since neither the

medical nor the social effects of such research can be predicted with certainty.

3. The fetus is not the same as an infant since it has no independent life system and is tied to the mother.

4. A fetus has real but limited rights, derived from its potential human life. The fetus' right to life is mitigated when the fetus threatens someone else's life; however, unless such a threat is present, the fetus' potential humanity requires that we protect and revere its life.

5. The fetus *in utero* may be the subject of research that (a) helps the mother, (b) is harmless to the fetus, or (c) is designed to help the fetus. Dr. Siegel endorses the Peel Commission dictum that no procedures may be carried out to see what harm they might do the fetus.

6. The fetus *ex utero* has more rights than the fetus *in utero.* Prolongation or early termination of the nonviable fetus should be prohibited.

7. Criteria for death of the fetus should be the same as for other individuals.

8. Consent of the mother or guardian is ordinarily sufficient, but parental consent, when an abortion is contemplated, is dubious. For such cases, consent should be supplemented by a special board. There must be strict separation of attending physician and researcher.

9. Proposed guidelines: (a) fetal research should be limited to cases which present no harm or offer assistance to the life system of the subjects; (b) no procedures should be permitted which are likely to harm the fetus—before, during, or after abortion; (c) a fetus *ex utero* and alive should not be subject to research unless it is intended to enhance the life of that fetus or unless the research involves no risk to the subject; and (d) criteria for determining death of the fetus should be the same as for other human individuals.

Leroy Walters, Ph.D.

Dr. Walters surveys various ways of categorizing research on the fetus: (1) according to the condition of the fetus, (2) according to the chronological age of the fetus, and (3) according to the formal object of the research.

He concludes that research on the fetus is not one but many things, and he focuses on nontherapeutic research on the fetus because it seems to raise serious public policy questions, and on research before, during and after induced abortion since that is a primary concern of the Commission's authorizing legislation. Four possible positions can be developed with respect to such research. Dr. Walters defends the position that nontherapeutic research on the fetus should be permitted only to the extent that such research is permitted on children or on fetuses which will be carried to term.

The essay endorses McCormick's thesis that parents may properly consent to a child's participation in nontherapeutic research which the child should be willing to take part in if the child were able to consent. This position is extended to cover the prenatal period as well. Because of difficulties associated with consent in cases where an abortion decision has been made, nontherapeutic research procedures should be permissible in the case of fetuses before or after abortion to the extent that they are permissible in the case of fetuses which will be brought to term. This position supposes that there is substantial continuity between previable and viable fetal life and postnatal life.

Although public policy making includes an ethical component, it also includes other factors, such as continuity with generally accepted societal principles, accommodation of a variety of belief systems and interests, and clearly understandable formulation. Three public policy propositions are recommended, all of which are based upon a policy of equality of treatment for all categories of human subjects: (1) nontherapeutic research on children should be permitted, if such research involves no risk or only minimal risk to subjects; (2) nontherapeutic research on fetuses which will be carried to term should be permitted, if such research involves no risk or minimal risk to the subjects; (3) nontherapeutic research procedures which are permitted in the case of fetuses which will be carried to term should also be permitted in the case of (a) live fetuses which will be aborted and (b) live fetuses which have been aborted.

Richard Wasserstrom, Ph.D.

Dr. Wasserstrom identifies four views concerning the status of the human fetus. He endorses the view that the fetus is in a unique moral category, closest to that of a newborn infant. The fetus has great value because of its potential to become a fully developed human being. It follows that abortion is morally worrisome because it involves destruction of an entity that possesses the potential to be and to produce things of the highest value. It also follows that if abortion has already taken place and the fetus is nonviable, then research in no way affects the fetus' ability to realize any of its potential.

Dr. Wasserstrom states that the resolution of the problem of consent for research on the fetus depends entirely on how one views the status of the fetus. That is, if one views the fetus as tissue, then consent on behalf of the fetus is meaningless. If one views the fetus as a child, then proxy consent is necessary. Dr. Wasserstrom believes, however, that even if the fetus is considered to be only tissue, consent should be obtained from the parents out of respect for their sensitivities.

Because abortion is a morally worrisome act, the decision to have an abortion should be kept easily revocable until the time of its performance. For this reason, Dr. Wasserstrom recommends that no research on the fetus *in utero* should be permitted if it involves a substantial risk of injury to the fetus.

Dr. Wasserstrom concludes that research on the nonviable fetus *ex utero* is permissible provided that: (1) the mother (if unmarried) or both parents consent before the abortion; (2) a review body has determined that the research may yield important information not otherwise obtainable; (3) the medical counselors of the pregnant woman have in no way been affiliated with the experimentation; and (4) the fetus is not possibly viable. . . .

VI. Views Presented at Public Hearings

Public hearings were held by the Commission to provide interested persons with an opportunity to present their views on research on the fetus. Testimony was given by scientists,

physicians, representatives of various organizations, concerned private citizens, lawyers and public officials. They presented a broad range of views that received careful consideration at the hearings and in the subsequent deliberations of the Commission. Brief summaries of the presentations follow.

1. *C. D. Christian, M.D.* (American College of Obstetricians and Gynecologists). Dr. Christian presented to the Commission a set of guidelines for the conduct of research on the pregnant woman and fetus, as prepared by the Committee on Bioethics of the College. The guidelines include recommendations that animal models be fully explored before human research is initiated, that clinical management of the patient should not be altered by research objectives, that research which would knowingly harm the fetus is not appropriate even in anticipation of abortion, that a fetus of doubtful viability should be treated as a viable infant, and that prolonging or shortening the life of the nonviable fetus only for research purposes is not appropriate.

2. *Robert G. Marshall* (Special Assistant for Congressional Affairs, U.S. Coalition for Life). Mr. Marshall opposed any research that is not directed at preserving the life or restoring the health of the immediate patient. In addition, he suggested adoption of the Golden Rule as a criterion for experimentation; a prohibition on the participation of the medically needy as subjects of research, except in circumstances of immediate danger to life; and a requirement that prospective participants be required to write out their understanding of the purpose of an experiment prior to being accepted as subjects. (During questioning, Mr. Marshall said that he would not object to observational procedures including, for example, fetoscopy.)

3. *Thomas K. Oliver, Jr., M.D.* (Association of American Medical Colleges). Dr. Oliver cited improvement in statistics of infant mortality and morbidity, which may be attributed directly to research on the fetus and newborn infant. He described the research leading to improved care of Rh disease and respiratory distress syndrome, which could have been conducted only on the human fetus and newborn, as specific examples of advances resulting from research on the

fetus. He urged the creation of an Ethical Advisory Board to review those research proposals which raise ethical questions, rather than the imposition of guidelines that would not be responsive to changing circumstances.

4. *Judith Mears* (Reproductive Freedom Project, American Civil Liberties Union). Ms. Mears urged that the Commission not draft protections for the fetus that would undermine the Supreme Court's rulings in *Doe v. Bolton* and *Roe v. Wade* regarding a woman's rights with respect to abortion. In addition, she urged the support of research to improve the safety of abortion procedures. (Ms. Mears agreed, during questioning, that the *Roe* and *Doe* decisions do not speak to the issue of experimentation and would not, therefore, render regulation of such research unconstitutional so long as a woman's access to abortion and other health services is not abridged.)

5. *David G. Nathan, M.D.* (Professor of Pediatrics, Harvard Medical School). Dr. Nathan focused his discussion on fetoscopy. He described this experimental technique for obtaining a sample of fetal blood to enable prenatal detection of disorders such as sickle cell disease and thalassemia, the reasons for conducting initial trials in women about to undergo abortion, and the evolution of the technique to the point where it has had successful clinical application. Dr. Nathan stressed the importance of studies that can be conducted simultaneously with the abortion procedure and consequently avoid any possibility of a change of mind about abortion after the research has begun.

6. *Audrey McMahon* (mother of two developmentally disabled children). Ms. McMahon stressed the need for research into the causes and treatment of developmental disabilities, and urged that such research not be curtailed.

7. *Robert Greenberg, M.D.* (Society for Pediatric Research and the American Pediatric Society). Dr. Greenberg presented statistics on the high rates of infant mortality and abnormal fetal development as indicators that the current health status of the fetus is poor. Dr. Greenberg stated that genuine concern for the fetus requires marked improvement of the health care available to the developing human during intrauterine

life. Such improvements in health care require acquisition of further understanding through increased research.

8. *Sumner Yaffe, M.D.* (American Academy of Pediatrics). Dr. Yaffe cited numerous advances in fetal therapeutics resulting from research on the fetus and emphasized the acute need for more extensive research in fetal clinical pharmacology. He presented the Academy's code of ethics for research involving the fetus and fetal material. The code states that research intended to benefit the mother or fetus *in utero* may be conducted with informed consent; that research on the viable delivered fetus (premature infant) may be carried out as long as nothing is done that is inconsistent with treatment necessary to promote the life of the infant; and that research on the nonviable fetus before or after abortion should be permitted, providing appropriate animal studies have been completed, parental consent is obtained, the researchers have no part in deciding timing or procedures for terminating the pregnancy or in determining viability, the research has been approved by an Institutional Review Board which is satisfied that the information cannot be obtained in any other way, experiments are not done in the delivery room, there is no monetary exchange for fetal material, and full records are kept.

9. *Lois Schiffer* (Women's Equity Action League, Women's Legal Defense Fund, Human Rights for Women). Ms. Schiffer cautioned against developing a policy that would abrogate constitutionally protected interests, such as the preeminence of a pregnant woman's right to health care. She underscored the need for continuing research in order to provide pregnant women with optimum medical advice and treatment (including improved abortion techniques). She suggested, additionally, that a requirement of paternal or spousal consent in conjunction with research on the fetus would contravene the holdings in the *Roe* and *Doe* decisions and that such consent serves no legitimate purpose if no child will be born. Finally, she urged the adequate representation of women on ethical review committees that will be applying policy to specific cases.

10. *Kay Jacobs Katz* (National Capital Tay-Sachs Foundation). Ms. Katz described the illness and death of her daughter, a victim of Tay-Sachs disease, and emphasized that only because of the availability of prenatal diagnosis did she have the courage to risk a further pregnancy that has resulted in the birth of a normal child. She urged the Commission not to restrict research that might develop procedures for prenatal diagnosis of other genetic diseases, nor to curtail research that might lead to the development of effective therapy for inborn errors of metabolism.

11. *Arthur M. Silverstein, Ph.D.* (American Society for Experimental Pathology). Dr. Silverstein pointed out the limitations of animals as models for the human fetus in experimentation. He cited the numerous uses of cells and tissues from the dead fetus in biomedical science, and urged that scientists not be deprived of the opportunity to study such tissues. He urged continued availability of fresh fetal materials for study and for use in transplantation. He concluded by asking the Commission to recognize that society owes to the developing fetus an acknowledgment of its special problems and a determination to attempt to solve these problems and do medical justice to the fetus through research.

12. *Msgr. James T. McHugh* (U.S. Catholic Conference). Msgr. McHugh stated that the fetus is a human being from the earliest stages of development, and that the ethical norms governing research on the fetus derive from those governing research on all human subjects, especially infants and children. Pre-abortion research is inconsistent with human dignity and is therefore unacceptable. Consent by the mother to such research is a mockery, he said, inasmuch as she has already decided to extinguish the life of the fetus; further, such research would eliminate any possibility of a mother's change of mind concerning abortion.

He urged Federal regulation of research on the fetus to permit only projects involving, for example, amniocentesis, fetoscopy, tissue culture, or procedures that would entail no risk to the fetus, and to limit those to circumstances in which their application would serve the purpose of protecting maternal health and assuring safe delivery of the fetus. He urged that animal models be used to the extent possible, even if this would be more expensive and demanding. He stated that the Government should permit research on the fetus only for the purpose of enhancing the survival or well-being of the fetus involved, and only if it can be conducted in a manner that will respect the rights and dignity of the fetus.

13. *Jo Anne Brasel, M.D.* (Endocrine Society). Dr. Brasel cited examples of contributions of fetal endocrinologic research to fetal welfare and survival. Continuation of research on the fetus was urged to permit study of such problems as hormonal deficiency states and care of the fetus of the diabetic mother. She expressed the full support of the Society for efforts to see that ethical considerations are met in the conduct of human research, but asserted that the welfare of future mothers and infants would not be served by wholesale interdiction of research.

14. *Nancy Raymond, R.N.* (Public Relations Director, Maryland Action for Human Life). Ms. Raymond urged that the fetus be treated with fairness and dignity, whether or not an abortion is anticipated or has been conducted. She advocated a prohibition of research on the fetus, but would make the following exceptions from such a prohibition: remedial procedures; procedures to study the fetus within the womb, if they do not substantially jeopardize the fetus and it is not a candidate for planned abortion; diagnostic procedures that do not substantially jeopardize the fetus, even if it is a candidate for planned abortion; and diagnostic procedures that are judged to be in the best interest of the particular fetus and will provide the mother with information about her fetus, even if an abortion is contemplated. She suggested that a panel of medical and nonmedical persons be created to advise scientists on the acceptability of research on the fetus.

15. *Sean O'Reilly, M.D.* (Professor of Neurology at George Washington University). Dr. O'Reilly's testimony (read in his absence) urged protection of the fetus from experimentation without its informed consent. He stated that the fetus obviously cannot give consent, and that parents can consent only to therapeutic research on the fetus. He argued that parents forfeit any right to consent to any other research on the fetus once they have elected to abort it.

16. *Chris Mooney* (President, Pregnancy Aid Centers, Inc.). Ms. Mooney viewed abortion as the worst solution to the problem of unwanted pregnancy, preferring to improve methods and availability of counseling and contraception. She expressed the fear that research on the fetus before and after abortion will further entrench our dependence on this pseudo-solution, by persuading women to abort in order to contribute to the cause of science. If science becomes dependent on abortion for research subjects, scientists and society will be even less inclined to develop viable alternatives to abortion. She urged that no money be offered for the use of an aborted fetus in research. (During questioning, Ms. Mooney said she has no knowledge of cases in which research did, in fact, operate as an inducement to abortion, and agreed that regulations could be devised to avoid that possibility.)

17. *Walter L. Herrmann, M.D.* (Society for Gynecologic Investigation). Dr. Herrmann pointed out that the interrelation of mother and fetus *in utero* requires that they both be considered in research involving either of them. He observed that the attitude of confidence rather than fear of the modern woman contemplating pregnancy is due to improved pregnancy care resulting from maternal and fetal research. Many unanswered questions remain, however, which demand continuation of such research. He urged that, in developing regulations for research on the fetus, the abortion issue be kept separate and emphasis be placed on the pregnant woman as the subject to be protected, so as not to infringe upon her rights or deprive her of the benefits of scientific discovery.

18. *Mary O'Donnell* (Nursing student; member, National Youth Pro-Life Coalition). Ms. O'Donnell argued that fetal life is human life deserving of our respect and protection. She would permit diagnostic procedures when undertaken to promote well-being or survival, and all life-preserving procedures. She would find drug research in anticipation of abortion unacceptable because it deprives a woman of the opportunity to change her mind and violates basic moral values.

19. *Leroy A. Jackson, M.D.* (obstetrician in private practice, Washington, D.C.). Dr. Jackson cited procedures derived from research on the fetus that

have improved his ability as a physician to provide medical care to his patients. He focused his testimony on the need to assure that consent from the mother for research on the fetus is truly informed consent, and that minorities and other groups do not bear a disproportionate share of the research burden. To these ends, he urged that research review committees contain members racially representative of and capable of communicating adequately with individuals on whom the research is conducted, that consent form wording be reviewed in detail, and that non-Government research agencies follow Government guidelines.

20. *Karen Mulhauser* (National Abortion Rights Action League). Ms. Mulhauser urged that the Commission recommend no limitations on research on the nonviable fetus *in utero*, provided informed consent is received from the pregnant woman. She also opposed any limitation of research to develop improved and safer abortion techniques.

21. *Ernest L. Hopkins, M.D.* (Professor of Obstetrics and Gynecology, Howard University). Dr. Hopkins cited statistics indicating that black infants and mothers have markedly higher morbidity and mortality in childbirth and the first year of life than do whites, and thus have a significant stake in research directed toward pregnancy and infancy. It is essential that research be conducted, he stated, as well as mandatory that the rights of the subject be protected. He advised the Commission that a mother often arrives at a decision to terminate pregnancy because she cannot support her present family. These are honorable women with wisdom, he said. They are very emotionally involved with the pregnancy, but they know that the birth of a baby would be catastrophic. They decide, reluctantly, to have an abortion because they see no alternative.

22. *J. V. Klavins, Ph.D.* (Professor of Pathology, State University of New York at Stony Brook). Dr. Klavins suggested that research on the fetus could be conducted with consent of the mother (and father when available). Since abortion is legal, he argued, research that causes no harm or suffering to the fetus-to-be-aborted is certainly

acceptable. He stated that research on the human fetus is no more likely to be dehumanizing than artificial insemination has been, that "do no harm" be used as the guiding principle in research on the fetus, and that society not be allowed to interfere with the parents' right to make decisions concerning the best interests of their offspring.

23. *Myron Winick, M.D.* (American Institute of Nutrition and the American Society for Clinical Nutrition). Dr. Winick reviewed nutrition problems relevant to the fetus and cited research needed to approach solutions to such problems. For example, knowledge is needed of the way the human fetus gets and uses essential nutrients *in utero*. Acquisition of this knowledge may require nonbeneficial research, he stated. The aim of the research, he pointed out, is to improve fetal growth and the quality of life, and, when a malnourished fetus is identified, to assist the fetus, not to terminate the pregnancy.

24. *Aubrey Milunsky, M.D.* (Assistant Professor of Pediatrics, Harvard Medical School). Dr. Milunsky presented written testimony focusing on prenatal diagnosis of genetic disease by amniocentesis. He pointed out that research on the fetus was essential to developing amniocentesis, which is now an accepted clinical procedure. The research aspects of prenatal diagnosis now involve extending diagnostic possibilities to other diseases and developing methods of prenatal treatment of an affected fetus as an alternative to abortion. He argued that to halt such research now would prohibit extending to other populations (such as those affected by sickle cell disease) the option of prenatal diagnosis, and also would prohibit the possible development of treatments for the diagnosed diseases.

25. *Louis Hellman, M.D.* (Deputy Assistant Secretary for Population Affairs, DHEW). Dr. Hellman reviewed the activities of his office in supporting research and providing services in family planning, noting that the objectives directly affected the health of mothers and infants. Enabling women to have fewer children implies that those born should have optimum chances for survival and good health. Thus, the Office of Population Affairs has an interest in all aspects of maternal and fetal research directed at reducing mortality

and morbidity. In the conduct of such research, Dr. Hellman stated, obtaining properly informed consent and review of the research by a committee of peers do not constitute significant barriers. He advocated conducting such reviews locally rather than in Washington. He expressed a personal distaste for non-beneficial research on the aborted fetus, for which an outright prohibition might be considered, but cautioned that such a course would be unlikely to stop the search for new knowledge, perhaps in another country or in another generation. He concluded that knowledge cannot be sequestered nor the course of its attainment blocked, and he suggested that the wiser direction would be adequate regulation of research on the fetus rather than outright prohibition.

26. *Norman Kretchmer, M.D.* (Director, National Institute of Child Health and Human Development, National Institutes of Health). Dr. Kretchmer summarized the policies and procedures presently in effect at NIH for the protection of human subjects studied in research activities. Proposals involving extramural research (which is conducted at institutions other than NIH) undergo a three-stage process of review, including: (1) review by the institution proposing the research, (2) review by scientific peers acting as consultants to NIH, and (3) review by the National Advisory Councils of the Institutes supporting the projects.

The first stage is performed by an Institutional Review Board (IRB), a panel consisting of members with diverse backgrounds and drawn from various disciplines. It is the responsibility of the IRB to review the proposal for scientific merit, community acceptability, the balance of risks and benefits, and any other factors that might bear upon the protection of the rights and welfare of the subjects.

The second stage of review is conducted by scientific peers, to evaluate the soundness of the research design, the relevant professional experience of the investigator, adequacy of facilities, scientific importance of the research, and the like. In addition, the reviewing body may consider the investigator's evaluation of risks and benefits, as well as any procedures suggested to protect the subjects against possible risks.

The final stage of review is conducted by a National Advisory Council,

a panel composed of two-thirds scientists and one-third nonscientists. Their responsibility is to recommend policy for the Institute and to advise the Director, NIH (or, in some cases, the Secretary, DHEW) concerning funding of research proposals, giving consideration to the protection of the rights of human subjects, among other things.

Research conducted within NIH (intramural research) undergoes review by the branch chief and clinical director of the Institute conducting the research. It may also be subject to review and approval by the Clinical Research Committee and the Medical Board of the Clinical Center. The Medical Board includes in its membership clinicians, scientists and laymen. All studies involving normal volunteers must be submitted to the Medical Board. Studies which involve potential benefits to patients who have been admitted to the Clinical Center generally are reviewed by clinical associates, attending physicians and the chief of the branch involved. When such studies represent a significant deviation from accepted practice or are associated with unusual hazards, however, they must be reviewed by the Clinical Research Committee.

For fiscal year 1974, NIH has identified about one hundred projects (with a total support of $3.5 million) which involved research on the fetus. These included monitoring of labor, fetal response to growth promoting substances, development of a "fetal risk index," and others. Under the ban imposed by Pub. L. 93–348, research on the living human fetus, before or after induced abortion, is not supported by NIH unless such research is done with the intention of assisting the survival of the fetus.

27. *John Jennings, M.D.* (Associate Commissioner, Food and Drug Administration [Dr. Jennings was accompanied by Dr. Frances Kelsey, Dr. Carl Leventhal and Mr. William Vodra.]). Dr. Jennings testified that FDA has legislative authority to ensure that research submitted to the agency by industry to show the safety and effectiveness of a drug is conducted under conditions that will protect subjects. In this regard, FDA believes it should act in accord, insofar as feasible, with DHEW

guidelines for protection of human subjects in research conducted or supported by the Department.

Most drugs currently marketed bear a warning on the label that they have not been tested for safety in pregnant women. Nevertheless, Dr. Jennings stated, such drugs, with potentially harmful effects on the fetus, are being used by pregnant women and by women of childbearing age, in spite of the label disclaimers. Therefore, the American Academy of Pediatrics has recommended to FDA that all marketed drugs be evaluated regarding their potential for producing adverse effects in the fetus.

Dr. Jennings expressed confidence that although difficult ethical problems are raised by research on the fetus, the Commission would be able to develop flexible guidelines that would safeguard both consumers and subjects.

In response to questions, representatives from FDA explained that no marketing of a drug is permitted until tests on animal teratology and reproduction have been completed. These tests include: (1) studies of normal and reproductive performance from the beginning of pregnancy through delivery, following administration of the drug to both males and females, (2) studies of teratology, following administration of the drug during pregnancy at the time of organ development, and (3) tests following administration of the drug from the end of pregnancy through lactation. FDA requests additional studies in primates if first studies indicate a need for further investigation.

VII. Fetal Viability and Death

The definitions of fetal viability and death present important issues in the conduct of research on the fetus. Accordingly, the Commission contracted for two studies in this area: the first, a medical study to define fetal viability and death based on present capabilities of medical technology; the second, an analysis of ethical and philosophical as well as scientific considerations in defining fetal viability and death.

The first study was conducted under contract with Columbia University, Richard Behrman, M.D., Principal Investigator. It included (1) a survey of the changes over the last 10 years in survival rates of premature infants and the advances in technology that have contributed to improved survival; (2) an assessment of the present state of medical technology designed to sustain premature infants; and (3) based on the foregoing, a recommendation for guidelines for use by physicians in determining whether a fetus, delivered spontaneously or by induced abortion, is viable, nonviable or dead. Consultation with representatives of professional societies in pediatrics and obstetrics, surveys of selected newborn intensive care units in the United States and Canada, statistical surveys and literature reviews were employed in carrying out this charge.

Assessment of changes in survival of premature infants relied primarily on data from New York City and from geographically dispersed infant intensive care units, as no national or international data broken down by weight group under 2500 grams were available. New York data showed a 4.5 percent increase in survival rate (26 percent reduction in mortality) of all infants under 2500 grams for the period covering the years 1962 to 1971. The improvement was primarily in the lower weight groups 68 percent increase in survival rate under 1000 grams, 20 percent increase from 1001 to 1500 grams, and 6 percent from 1501 to 2000 grams. Infants cared for in intensive care units showed an even greater improvement in survival.

Many innovations in caring for the fetus in utero and the delivered premature infant were introduced in the last decade. The large number of these innovations, and their introduction at different times in different centers, generally made it impossible to establish a direct correlation between a given technologic innovation and a change in infant survival. One exception, where such a correlation may be made, is the effect on survival of monitoring fetal heart rate and acid-base balance during labor. At Los Angeles County USC Medical Center, monitoring was introduced as a routine procedure for high risk obstetrical patients in 1970; low risk patients were unmonitored. Between 1970 and 1973, the intrapartum death rate of infants weighing more than 1500 grams decreased 64 percent, and the fetal death

rate became lower for the monitored high risk women than in the unmonitored low risk women. Comparable results were obtained in New York City at Columbia Presbyterian Medical Center, where over 90 percent of the monitoring was done on high risk ward patients, primarily black, poor or Spanish-speaking; the low risk private patients were unmonitored. Following introduction of monitoring, the high risk monitored patients had 10 percent fewer fetal deaths, 14 percent fewer perinatal deaths, and 37 percent fewer intrapartum fetal deaths than the unmonitored low risk private patients.

Overall improvement in premature survival may be traced more generally to the gradual adoption of other innovations. For example, the improved rates during the years 1967 through 1969 may be related to advances first introduced during the years 1964 through 1966, which included amniocentesis for intrauterine diagnosis of infants severely affected with erythroblastosis; fetal transfusion in utero; reorganization of premature nurseries into intensive care centers; extensive monitoring of gases and other substances in blood, and of vital signs, with more aggressive attention to correction of abnormal values; hand ventilation with ambu bags; regulation of the thermal environment; and greater density of nursing personnel. Increases in survival in the period 1970 to 1973 may be correlated with a constellation of advances in the years 1968 through 1970. These included extensive study of amniotic fluid in managing high risk pregnancies; fetal heart rate and uterine pressure monitoring during labor; improved infant transport systems and referral to intensive care units; major advances in design and techniques for use of infant respirators; total intravenous alimentation; and use of phototherapy for jaundice. Numerous other innovations have been introduced, but these are the major advances that have come into widespread use.

Impact of these changes on survival is reflected in data from University College Hospital in London, where survival rate of infants 1001 to 1500 grams was a steady 45 to 50 percent during the 1950's and early 1960's. During the period 1966 to 1970, the survival rate increased to 70 percent. Equally significant is an indication of decreased

morbidity. During the 1950's and 1960's, the handicap rate for infants weighing less than 1500 grams at birth ranged from 33 percent to 60 percent. A recent study evaluating the outcome of such infants born from 1966 to 1970 indicated that 90.5 percent had no detectable handicap.

Despite these advances in the technology of caring for premature infants, there remain limits beyond which the best care cannot result in survival. To ascertain the present limits, surveys were conducted of vital statistics of the United States (including individual States) and Quebec, the medical literature, and 27 major centers with obstetric services and special intensive care units for premature infants. These centers represent the optimal care that present medical technology can provide. Despite differences in data base from various sources, two facts emerged clearly: probability of survival of infants weighing less than 750 grams was extremely small, and no cases were found from any documentable source of any infant surviving with a birth weight below 600 grams at a gestational age of 24 weeks or less. Some rare cases were documented of infants surviving with birth weights below 600 grams, but in each instance the gestational age exceeded 24 weeks, and the cases thus represented more mature infants who for various reasons were small-for-dates. Other rare cases were documented of infants born before 25 weeks gestational age who survived, but in each instance birth weight exceeded 600 grams. Thus, on an empirical basis the current limits of viability are clear: there is no unambiguous documentation that an infant born weighing less than 601 grams at a gestational age of 24 weeks or less has ever survived.

The concept of viability implies a prediction as to whether a delivered fetus is capable of survival. A prematurely delivered fetus is viable when a minimal number of independently sustained, basic, integrative physiologic functions are present. The sum of these functions must support the inference that the fetus is able to increase in tissue mass (growth) and increase the number, complexity and coordination of basic physiologic functions (development) as a self-sustaining organism. This development must be independent of any connection with the mother and supported only by generally accepted medical treatments. If these coordinated functions are not present, the fetus is nonviable. This may be the case even though some signs of life are apparent.

The following functions, taken together, constitute the minimal number of basic integrative physiologic functions to support an inference of viability: (1) Perfusion of tissues with adequate oxygen and prevention of increasing accumulation of carbon dioxide and/or lactic and other organic acids. This function consists of the following components:

a. inflation of the lungs with oxygen,

b. transfer of oxygen across the alveolar membranes into the circulation and elimination of carbon dioxide from the circulation into the expired gas, and

c. cardiac contractions of sufficient strength and regularity to distribute oxygenated blood to tissues and organs throughout the body, and to eliminate organic acids from those tissues and organs. (2) Neurologic regulation of the components of the cardio-respiratory perfusion function, of the capacity to ingest nutrients, and of spontaneous and reflex muscle movements.

These functions in the prematurely delivered fetus cannot at present be assessed separately in a consistent, reliable and exact manner. The absence of the sum of these functions, however, can be assessed indirectly in a reasonable and reliable manner by measurement of weight and an estimation of gestational age. Thus, organisms of less than 601 grams at delivery and gestational age of 24 weeks or less are at present nonviable; signs of life such as a beating heart, spontaneous respiratory movement, pulsation of the umbilical cord and spontaneous movement of voluntary muscles are not adequate in themselves to be used to determine the existence of basic integrative functions.

A weight of 601 grams or more and gestational age over 24 weeks may indicate that the minimal basic functions necessary for independent growth and development are present.

Such a prematurely delivered fetus may be considered at least possibly viable. At these weights and gestational ages, a sign of life such as a beating heart, spontaneous respiratory movement, pulsation of the umbilical cord or spontaneous movement of voluntary muscles indicates possible viability.

Prediction of extrauterine viability of the fetus while it is still in utero takes on an additional dimension of complexity. The fetus in utero, in the absence of clear signs that death has occurred, is always at least potentially viable as long as it remains in the uterus. However, it cannot be weighed, size assessments based on uterine size are inaccurate, and estimates of gestational age based on menstrual history are often inexact. The best medical technology can provide at present is an index of gestational age based on measurement of head size, using ultrasound. In the best hands, this technique is accurate within ±1 week at 20–26 weeks. Relating gestational age to fetal weight, and taking into account the range of error and normal variation, an estimated gestational age of 22 weeks or less by ultrasound would virtually eliminate the possibility of fetal weight above 600 grams and actual gestational age greater than 24 weeks. Such an estimate would permit the prediction that if such a fetus were outside the uterus, it would be nonviable.

Employing present technology, therefore, research on the fetus in utero, undertaken before an abortion to occur not later than 22 weeks gestational age as estimated by ultrasound, would not impact on a fetus with a chance for survival after the abortion. Any reduction of the 22 week limit would provide an additional safeguard.

Whatever the boundaries are for viability, there is always a chance that a viable infant may be born after a prediction of nonviability by gestational age. When this occurs, the premature infant clearly must be cared for in accord with accepted medical practice. Further, these criteria for viability are based on current technology, which is subject to change. Accordingly, the criteria should be reviewed periodically.

Death of the delivered fetus is judged to have occurred when there is a cessation of the minimal basic integrative physiologic functions which,

considered together, may result in self-sustained extrauterine growth and development. The absence of all of the following signs indicates the cessation of these minimal basic integrative physiologic functions: (1) heart beat, (2) spontaneous respiratory movements, (3) spontaneous movement of voluntary muscles, and (4) pulsation of the umbilical cord.

Approaching the same issues of fetal viability and death from the viewpoint of a physician-scientist and philosopher, Dr. Leon Kass, in an essay prepared for the Commission, came to conclusions similar to those reached by Dr. Behrman on criteria for determining death and defining fetal viability (though Dr. Kass was more conservative on the latter). In clarifying the terminology, Dr. Kass distinguished between the terms "viable" and "nonviable" (which refer to states of a living fetus) and "alive" and "dead" (which refer to mutually exclusive conditions of the organism independent of its stage of development). The terms "viable" and "nonviable" are predictive of future outcome, which is dependent on the fetal stage of development and relation to the environment. Thus, the determination of viability is influenced by whether the fetus is inside or outside the uterus, and by the technology available for sustaining life. A fetus that is alive inside the uterus is always at least potentially viable; the same fetus outside the uterus may be viable or nonviable.

As criteria for determining death, Dr. Kass suggested that a fetus be considered dead if, based on ordinary procedures of medical practice, it has experienced an irreversible cessation of spontaneous circulatory and respiratory functions and an irreversible cessation of spontaneous central nervous functions. These criteria are evidenced on examination of the fetus by absence of the following: (1) spontaneous muscular movement, (2) response to external stimuli, (3) elicitable reflexes, (4) spontaneous respiration, and (5) spontaneous heart function manifested by heartbeat and pulse.

These criteria differ from those suggested by Dr. Behrman only by the addition of (2) and (3). Dr. Kass advised that the presence of any one of these functions is a sign that the fetus is alive (again in agreement with Dr.

Behrman), and he further suggested that use of the EEG is unnecessary in making the diagnosis of death. Finally, he recommended that the fetus *in utero* be considered alive until proved dead, and that the fetus being aborted be presumed alive until examination reveals it to be dead.

A viable fetus was defined by Dr. Kass as one that has reached the stage of development at which it is able to sustain itself outside the mother's body. In suggesting criteria for fetal viability based on present technology, Dr. Kass supported use of essentially the same physiologic criteria as suggested by Dr. Behrman, but would not rely upon weight or gestational age to indicate the presence of these integrated functions in the delivered fetus. He suggested that the delivered fetus should be considered viable in the presence of *all five* of the functions listed above (the absence of which is definitive of death). Of these, respiratory activity is the *sine qua non* of viability. Following delivery of the fetus, adequate time should be allowed to assess the presence of life and determine viability before research involving the fetus can be considered. This evaluation should be made by the delivering obstetrician, and then only if he is not himself likely to be engaged in subsequent research involving the fetus.

It is more difficult to determine whether the fetus *in utero* would be viable, if delivered, and, due to the possibility of error, Dr. Kass advised caution. He suggested that viability of the fetus *in utero* be evaluated according to gestational age. The fetus *in utero* is potentially viable before 20 weeks gestational age, but nonviable if removed from the uterus. It should be considered viable after the age of 28 weeks. Accurate evaluation of the viability of a fetus *in utero* between 20 and 28 weeks gestational age is not possible; such a fetus should be presumed viable if a heartbeat is audible using a stethoscope. The fetus which is to be aborted before the heartbeat is audible should be regarded as potentially viable until the abortion procedure is actually in progress, after which it may be considered nonviable.

VIII. Deliberations and Conclusions

The charge to the Commission is to investigate and study research involving the living fetus and to make recommendations to the Secretary, DHEW, on "policies defining the circumstances (if any) under which such research may be conducted or supported." The Commission has attempted to fulfill that duty by conducting investigations into research on the fetus and by providing a public forum for the presentation and analysis of views on this subject. It must be recognized that the Commission was placed under severe limitations of time by its Congressional mandate. As a result, these considerations on research involving fetuses have necessarily been developed prior to the Commission's larger task of studying the nature of research, the basic ethical principles which should guide it, the problem of informed consent and the review process.

After the Commission identified the information that was required for adequate consideration of the charge, a compendium of pertinent scientific literature and medical experience was prepared by consultants and contractors. In addition, a broad range of views was presented in letters, reports and testimony by theologians, philosophers, physicians, scientists, lawyers, public officials and private citizens. The Commission then undertook critical analysis of the studies and presentations, and conducted public deliberations on the issues involved. Finally, the Commission formulated its Recommendations.

This section of the Commission's report summarizes the reasoning and conclusions that emerged during the deliberations. Section IX of the report sets forth the Commission's Recommendations to the Secretary, DHEW. These Recommendations arise from and are consistent with the Deliberations and Conclusions of the Commission. The Recommendations should be considered only within the context of the Deliberations that precede them.

Preface to Deliberations and Conclusions

Throughout the deliberations of the Commission, the belief has been affirmed that the fetus as a human subject is deserving of care and respect.

Although the Commission has not addressed directly the issues of the personhood and the civil status of the fetus, the members of the Commission are convinced that moral concern should extend to all who share human genetic heritage, and that the fetus, regardless of life prospects, should be treated respectfully and with dignity.

The members of the Commission are also convinced that medical research has resulted in significant improvements in the care of the unborn threatened by death or disease, and they recognize that further progress is anticipated. Within the broad category of medical research, however, public concern has been expressed with regard to the nature and necessity of research on the human fetus. The evidence presented to the Commission was based upon a comprehensive search of the world's literature and a review of more than 3000 communications in scientific periodicals. The preponderance of all research involved experimental procedures designed to benefit directly a fetus threatened by premature delivery, disease or death, or to elucidate normal processes or development. Some research constituted an element in the health care of pregnant women. Other research involved only observation or the use of noninvasive procedures bearing little or no risk. A final class of investigation (falling outside the present mandate of the Commission) has made use of tissues of the dead fetus, in accordance with accepted standards for treatment of the human cadaver. The Commission finds that, to the best of its knowledge, these types of research have not contravened accepted ethical standards.

Nonetheless, the Commission notes that there have been instances of abuse in the area of fetal research. Moreover, differences of opinion exist as to whether desired results could have been attained without the use of the human fetus in nontherapeutic research.

Concern has also been expressed that the poor and minority groups may bear an inequitable burden as research subjects. The Commission believes that those groups which are most vulnerable to inequitable treatment should receive special protection.

The Commission concludes that some information which is in the public interest and which provides significant advances in health care can be attained only through the use of the human fetus as a research subject. The Recommendations which follow express the Commission's belief that, while the exigencies of research and the moral imperatives of fair and respectful treatment may appear to be mutually limiting, they are not incompatible.

Ethical Principles and Requirements Governing Research on Human Subjects with Special Reference to the Fetus and the Pregnant Woman

The Commission has a mandate to develop the ethical principles underlying the conduct of all research involving human subjects. Until it can adequately fulfill this charge, its statement of principles is necessarily limited. In the interim, it proposes the following as basic ethical principles for use of human subjects in general, and research involving the fetus and the pregnant woman in particular.

Scientific inquiry is a distinctly human endeavor. So, too, is the protection of individual integrity. Freedom of inquiry and the social benefits derived therefrom, as well as protection of the individual are valued highly and are to be encouraged. For the most part, they are compatible pursuits. When occasionally they appear to be in conflict, efforts must be made through public deliberation to effect a resolution.

In effecting this resolution, the integrity of the individual is preeminent. It is therefore the duty of the Commission to specify the boundaries that respect for the fetus must impose upon freedom of scientific inquiry. The Commission has considered the principles proposed by ethicists in relation to the exigencies of scientific inquiry, the requirements and present limitations of medical practice, and legal commentary. Among the general principles for research on human subjects judged to be valid and binding are: (1) To avoid harm whenever possible, or at least to minimize harm; (2) to provide for fair treatment by avoiding discrimination between classes or among members of the same class; and (3) to respect the integrity of human subjects by requiring informed consent. An additional

principle pertinent to the issue at hand is to respect the human character of the fetus.

To this end, the Commission concludes that in order to be considered ethically acceptable, research involving the fetus should be determined by adequate review to meet certain general requirements:

1. Appropriate prior investigations using animal models and nonpregnant humans must have been completed.

2. The knowledge to be gained must be important and obtainable by no reasonable alternative means.

3. Risks and benefits to both the mother and the fetus must have been fully evaluated and described.

4. Informed consent must be sought and granted under proper conditions.

5. Subjects must be selected so that risks and benefits will not fall inequitably among economic, racial, ethnic and social classes.

These requirements apply to all research on the human fetus. In the application of these principles, however, the Commission found it helpful to consider the following distinctions: (1) therapeutic and nontherapeutic research; (2) research directed toward the pregnant woman and that directed toward the fetus; (3) research involving the fetus-going-to-term and the fetus-to-be-aborted; (4) research occurring before, during or after an abortion procedure; and (5) research which involves the nonviable fetus ex utero and that which involves the possibly viable infant. The first two distinctions encompass the entire period of the pregnancy through delivery; the latter three refer to different portions of the developmental continuum.

The Commission observes that the fetus is sometimes an unintended subject of research when a woman participating in an investigation is incorrectly presumed not to be pregnant. Care should be taken to minimize this possibility.

Application to Research Involving the Fetus

The application of the general principles enumerated above to the use of the human fetus as a research subject presents problems because the fetus cannot be a willing participant in experimentation. As with children, the

comatose and other subjects unable to consent, difficult questions arise regarding the balance of risk and benefit and the validity of proxy consent.

In particular, some would question whether subjects unable to consent should ever be subjected to risk in scientific research. However, there is general agreement that where the benefits as well as the risks of research accrue to the subject, proxy consent may be presumed adequate to protect the subject's interests. The more difficult case is that where the subject must bear risks without direct benefit.

The Commission has not yet studied the issues surrounding informed consent and the validity of proxy consent for nontherapeutic research (including the difficult issue of consent by a pregnant minor). These problems will be explored under the broader mandate of the Commission. In the interim, the Commission has taken various perspectives into consideration in its deliberations about the use of the fetus as a subject in different research settings. The Deliberations and Conclusions of the Commission regarding the application of general principles to the use of the fetus as a human subject in scientific research are as follows:

1. In therapeutic research directed toward the fetus, the fetal subject is selected on the basis of its health condition, benefits and risks accrue to that fetus, and proxy consent is directed toward that subject's own welfare. Hence, with adequate review to assess scientific merit, prior research, the balance of risks and benefits, and the sufficiency of the consent process, such research conforms with all relevant principles and is both ethically acceptable and laudable. In view of the necessary involvement of the woman in such research, her consent is considered mandatory; in view of the father's possible ongoing responsibility, his objection is considered sufficient to veto.

2. Therapeutic research directed toward the pregnant woman may expose the fetus to risk for the benefit of another subject and thus is at first glance more problematic. Recognizing the woman's priority regarding her own health care, however, the Commission concludes that such research is ethically acceptable provided that the woman has been fully informed of the possible impact on the fetus and that

other general requirements have been met. Protection for the fetus is further provided by requiring that research put the fetus at minimum risk consistent with the provision of health care for the woman. Moreover, therapeutic research directed toward the pregnant woman frequently benefits the fetus, though it need not necessarily do so. In view of the woman's right to privacy regarding her own health care, the Commission concludes that the informed consent of the woman is both necessary and sufficient.

In general, the Commission concludes that therapeutic research directed toward the health condition of either the fetus or the pregnant woman is, in principle, ethical. Such research benefits not only the individual woman or fetus but also women and fetuses as a class, and should therefore be encouraged actively.

The Commission, in making recommendations on therapeutic and nontherapeutic research directed toward the pregnant woman (Recommendations (2) and (3)), in no way intends to preclude research on improving abortion techniques otherwise permitted by law and government regulation.

3. Nontherapeutic research directed toward the fetus *in utero* or toward the pregnant woman poses difficult problems because the fetus may be exposed to risk for the benefit of others.

Here, the Commission concludes that where no additional risks are imposed on the fetus (e.g., where fluid withdrawn during the course of treatment is used additionally for nontherapeutic research), or where risks are so minimal as to be negligible, proxy consent by the parent(s) is sufficient to provide protection. (Hence, the consent of the woman is sufficient provided the father does not object.) The Commission recognizes that the term "minimal" involves a value judgment and acknowledges that medical opinion will differ regarding what constitutes "minimal risk." Determination of acceptable minimal risk is a function of the review process.

When the risks cannot be fully assessed, or are more than minimal, the situation is more problematic. The Commission affirms as a general principle that manifest risks imposed upon

nonconsenting subjects cannot be tolerated. Therefore, the Commission concludes that only minimal risk can be accepted as permissible for nonconsenting subjects in nontherapeutic research.

The Commission affirms that the woman's decision for abortion does not, in itself, change the status of the fetus for purposes of protection. Thus, the same principles apply whether or not abortion is contemplated; in both cases, only minimal risk is acceptable.

Differences of opinion have arisen in the Commission, however, regarding the interpretation of risk to the fetus-to-be-aborted and thus whether some experiments that would not be permissible on a fetus-going-to-term might be permissible on a fetus-to-be-aborted. Some members hold that no procedures should be applied to a fetus-to-be-aborted that would not be applied to a fetus-going-to-term. Indeed, it was also suggested that any research involving fetuses-to-be-aborted must also involve fetuses-going-to-term. Others argue that, while a woman's decision for abortion does not change the status of the fetus *per se*, it does make a significant difference in one respect—namely, in the risk of harm to the fetus. For example, the injection of a drug which crosses the placenta may not injure the fetus which is aborted within two weeks of injection, where it might injure the fetus two months after injection. There is always, of course, the possibility that a woman might change her mind about the abortion. Even taking this into account, however, some members argue that risks to the fetus-to-be-aborted may be considered "minimal" in research which would entail more than minimal risk for a fetus-going-to-term.

There is basic agreement among Commission members as to the validity of the equality principle. There is disagreement as to its application to individual fetuses and classes of fetuses. Anticipating that differences of interpretation will arise over the application of the basic principles of equality and the determination of "minimal risk," the Commission recommends review at the national level. The Commission believes that such review would provide the appropriate forum for determination of the scientific and public merit of such research. In addition, such review would facilitate public discussion of

the sensitive issues surrounding the use of vulnerable nonconsenting subjects in research.

The question of consent is a complicated one in this area of research. The Commission holds that procedures that are part of the research design should be fully disclosed and clearly distinguished from those which are dictated by the health care needs of the pregnant woman or her fetus. Questions have been raised regarding the validity of parental proxy consent where the parent(s) have made a decision for abortion. The Commission recognizes that unresolved problems both of law and of fact surround this question. It is the considered opinion, however, that women who have decided to abort should not be presumed to abandon thereby all interest in and concern for the fetus. In view of the close relationship between the woman and the fetus, therefore, and the necessary involvement of the women in the research process, the woman's consent is considered necessary. The Commission is divided on the question of whether her consent alone is sufficient. Assignment of an advocate for the fetus was proposed as an additional safeguard; this issue will be thoroughly explored in connection with the Commission's review of the consent process. Most of the Commissioners agree that in view of the father's possible responsibility for the child, should it be brought to term, the objection of the father should be sufficient to veto. Several Commissioners, however, hold that for nontherapeutic research directed toward the pregnant woman, the woman's consent alone should be sufficient and the father should have no veto.

4. Research on the fetus during the abortion procedure or on the nonviable fetus *ex utero* raises sensitive problems because such a fetus must be considered a dying subject. By definition, therefore, the research is nontherapeutic in that the benefits will not accrue to the subject. Moreover, the question of consent is complicated because of the special vulnerability of the dying subject.

The Commission considers that the status of the fetus as dying alters the situation in two ways. First, the question of risk becomes less relevant, since the dying fetus cannot be "harmed" in the sense of "injured for life." Once the abortion procedure has begun, or after it is completed, there is no chance of a change of mind on the woman's part which will result in a living, injured subject. Second, however, while questions of risk become less relevant, considerations of respect for the dignity of the fetus continue to be of paramount importance, and require that the fetus be treated with the respect due to dying subjects. While dying subjects may not be "harmed" in the sense of "injured for life," issues of violation of integrity are nonetheless central. The Commission concludes, therefore, that out of respect for the dying subjects, no nontherapeutic interventions are permissible which would alter the duration of life of the nonviable fetus *ex utero*.

Additional protection is provided by requiring that no significant changes are made in the abortion procedure strictly for purposes of research. The Commission was divided on the question of whether a woman has a right to accept modifications in the timing or method of the abortion procedure in the interest of research, and whether the investigator could ethically request her to do so. Some Commission members desired that neither the research nor the investigator in any way influence the abortion procedure; others felt that modifications in timing or method of abortion were acceptable provided no new elements of risk were introduced. Still others held that even if modifications increased the risk, they would be acceptable provided the woman had been fully informed of all risks, and provided such modifications did not postpone the abortion beyond the 20th week of gestational age (5 lunar months, four and one-half calendar months). Despite this division of opinion, the Recommendation of the Commission on this matter is that the design and conduct of a nontherapeutic research protocol should not determine the recommendations by a physician regarding the advisability, timing or method of abortion. No members of the Commission desired less stringent measures.

Furthermore, it is possible that, due to mistaken estimation of gestational age, an abortion may issue in a possibly viable infant. If there is any danger that this might happen, research which would entail more than minimal risk

would be absolutely prohibited. In order to avoid that possibility the Commission recommends that, should research during abortion be approved by national review, it be always on condition that estimated gestational age be below 20 weeks. There is, of course, a moral and legal obligation to attempt to save the life of a possibly viable infant.

Finally, the Commission has been made aware that certain research, particularly that involving the living nonviable fetus, has disturbed the moral sensitivity of many persons. While it believes that its Recommendations would preclude objectionable research by adherence to strict review processes, problems of interpretation or application of the Commission's Recommendations may still arise. In that event, the Commission proposes ethical review at a national level in which informed public disclosure and assessment of the problems, the type of proposed research and the scientific and public importance of the expected results can take place.

Review Procedures

The Commission will conduct comprehensive studies of existing review mechanisms in connection with its broad mandate to develop guidelines and make recommendations concerning ethical issues involved in research on human subjects. Until the Commission has completed these studies, it can offer only tentative conclusions and recommendations regarding review mechanisms.

In the interim, the Commission finds that existing review procedures required by statute (Pub. L. 93–348) and DHEW regulations (45 CFR 46) suffice for all therapeutic research involving the pregnant woman and the fetus, and for all nontherapeutic research which imposes minimal or no risk and which would be acceptable for conduct on a fetus *in utero* to be carried to term or on an infant. Guidelines to be employed under the existing review procedures include: (1) importance of the knowledge to be gained; (2) completion of appropriate studies on animal models and nonpregnant humans and existence of no reasonable alternative; (3) full evaluation and disclosure of the risks and benefits that are involved;

and (4) supervision of the conditions under which consent is sought and granted, and of the information that is disclosed during that process.

The case is different, however, for nontherapeutic research directed toward a pregnant woman or a fetus if it involves more than minimal risk or would not be acceptable for application to an infant. Questions may arise concerning the definition of risk or the assessment of scientific and public importance of the research. In such cases, the Commission considers current review procedures insufficient. It recommends these categories be reviewed by a national review body to determine whether the proposed research could be conducted within the spirit of the Commission's recommendations. It would interpret these recommendations and apply them to the proposed research, and in addition, assess the scientific and public value of the anticipated results of the investigation.

The national review panel should be composed of individuals having diverse backgrounds, experience and interests, and be so constituted as to be able to deal with the legal, ethical, and medical issues involved in research on the human fetus. In addition to the professions of law, medicine, and the research sciences, there should be adequate representation of women, members of minority groups, and individuals conversant with the various ethical persuasions of the general community.

Inasmuch as even such a panel cannot always judge public attitudes, panel meetings should be open to the public, and, in addition, public participation through written and oral submissions should be sought.

Compensation

The Commission expressed a strong conviction that considerable attention be given to the issue of provision of compensation to those who may be injured as a consequence of their participation as research subjects.

Concerns regarding the use of inducements for participation in research are only partially met by the Commission's Recommendation (14) on the prohibition of the procurement of an abortion for research purposes. Compensation not only for injury from research but for participation in research as a normal volunteer or in a therapeutic situation will be part of later Commission deliberations.

Research Conducted Outside the United States
The Commission has considered the advisability of modifying its standards for research which is supported by the Secretary, DHEW, and is conducted outside the United States. It has concluded that its recommendations should apply as a single minimal standard, but that research should also comply with any more stringent limitations imposed by statutes or standards of the country in which the research will be conducted.

The Moratorium on Fetal Research
The Commission notes that the restrictions on fetal research (imposed by section 213 of Pub. L. 93-348) have been construed broadly throughout the research community, with the result that ethically acceptable research, which might yield important biomedical information, has been halted. For this reason, it is considered in the public interest that the moratorium be lifted immediately, that the Secretary take special care thereafter that the Commission's concerns for the protection of the fetus as a research subject are met, and appropriate regulations based upon the Commission's recommendations be implemented within a year from the date of submission of this report to the Secretary, DHEW. Until final regulations are published, the existing review panels at the agency and institutional levels should utilize the Deliberations and Recommendations of the Commission in evaluating the acceptability of all grant and contract proposals submitted for funding.

Synthesis
The Commission concludes that certain prior conditions apply broadly to all research involving the fetus, if ethical considerations are to be met. These requirements include evidence of pertinent investigations in animal models and nonpregnant humans, lack of alternative means to obtain the information, careful assessment of the risks and benefits of the research, and procedures to ensure that informed consent

has been sought and granted under proper conditons. Determinations as to whether these essential requirements have been met may be made under existing review procedures, pending study by the Commission of the entire review process.

In the judgment of the Commission, therapeutic research directed toward the health care of the pregnant woman or the fetus raises little concern, provided it meets the essential requirements for research involving the fetus, and is conducted under appropriate medical and legal safeguards.

For the most part, nontherapeutic research involving the fetus to be carried to term or the fetus before, during or after abortion is acceptable so long as it imposes minimal or no risk to the fetus and, when abortion is involved, imposes no change in the timing or procedure for terminating pregnancy which would add any significant risk. When a research protocol or procedure presents special problems of interpretation or application of these guidelines, it should be subject to national ethical review; and it should be approved only if the knowledge to be gained is of medical importance, can be obtained in no other way, and the research proposal does not offend community sensibilities.

IX. Recommendations

1. Therapeutic research directed toward the fetus may be conducted or supported, and should be encouraged, by the Secretary, DHEW, provided such research (a) conforms to appropriate medical standards, (b) has received the informed consent of the mother, the father not dissenting, and (c) has been approved by existing review procedures with adequate provision for the monitoring of the consent process. (Adopted unanimously.)

2. Therapeutic research directed toward the pregnant woman may be conducted or supported, and should be encouraged, by the Secretary, DHEW, provided such research (a) has been evaluated for possible impact on the fetus, (b) will place the fetus at risk to the minimum extent consistent with meeting the health needs of the pregnant woman, (c) has been approved by existing review procedures with adequate provision for the monitoring

of the consent process, and (d) the pregnant woman has given her informed consent. (Adopted unanimously.)

3. Nontherapeutic research directed toward the pregnant woman may be conducted or supported by the Secretary, DHEW, provided such research (a) has been evaluated for possible impact on the fetus, (b) will impose minimal or no risk to the well-being of the fetus, (c) has been approved by existing review procedures with adequate provision for the monitoring of the consent process, (d) special care has been taken to assure that the woman has been fully informed regarding possible impact on the fetus, and (e) the woman has given informed consent. (Adopted unanimously.)

It is further provided that nontherapeutic research directed at the pregnant woman may be conducted or supported (f) only if the father has not objected, both where abortion is not at issue (adopted by a vote of 8 to 1) and where an abortion is anticipated (adopted by a vote of 5 to 4).

4. Nontherapeutic research directed toward the fetus *in utero* (other than research in anticipation of, or during, abortion) may be conducted or supported by the Secretary, DHEW, provided (a) the purpose of such research is the development of important biomedical knowledge that cannot be obtained by alternative means, (b) investigation on pertinent animal models and nonpregnant humans has preceded such research, (c) minimal or no risk to the well-being of the fetus will be imposed by the research, (d) the research has been approved by existing review procedures with adequate provision for the monitoring of the consent process, (e) the informed consent of the mother has been obtained, and (f) the father has not objected to the research. (Adopted unanimously.)

5. Nontherapeutic research directed toward the fetus in anticipation of abortion may be conducted or supported by the Secretary, DHEW, provided such research is carried out within the guidelines for all other nontherapeutic research directed toward the fetus *in utero*. Such research presenting special problems related to the interpretation or application of these guidelines may be conducted or supported by the Secretary, DHEW, provided such research

has been approved by a national ethical review body. (Adopted by a vote of 8 to 1.)

6. Nontherapeutic research directed toward the fetus during the abortion procedure and nontherapeutic research directed toward the nonviable fetus *ex utero* may be conducted or supported by the Secretary, DHEW, provided (a) the purpose of such research is the development of important biomedical knowledge that cannot be obtained by alternative means, (b) investigation on pertinent animal models and nonpregnant humans (when appropriate) has preceded such research, (c) the research has been approved by existing review procedures with adequate provision for the monitoring of the consent process, (d) the informed consent of the mother has been obtained, and (e) the father has not objected to the research; and provided further that (f) the fetus is less than 20 weeks gestational age, (g) no significant procedural changes are introduced into the abortion procedure in the interest of research alone, and (h) no intrusion into the fetus is made which alters the duration of life. Such research presenting special problems related to the interpretation or application of these guidelines may be conducted or supported by the Secretary, DHEW, provided such research has been approved by a national ethical review body. (Adopted by a vote of 8 to 1.)

7. Nontherapeutic research directed toward the possibly viable infant may be conducted or supported by the Secretary, DHEW, provided (a) the purpose of such research is the development of important biomedical knowledge that cannot be obtained by alternative means, (b) investigation on pertinent animal models and nonpregnant humans (when appropriate) has preceded such research, (c) no additional risk to the well-being of the infant will be imposed by the research, (d) the research has been approved by existing review procedures with adequate provision for the monitoring of the consent process, and (e) informed consent of either parent has been given and neither parent has objected. (Adopted unanimously.)

8. Review procedures. Until the Commission makes its recommendations regarding review and consent procedures, the review procedures mentioned above are to be those presently required by the Department of Health, Education, and Welfare. In addition, provision for monitoring the consent process shall be required in order to ensure adequacy of the consent process and to prevent unfair discrimination in the selection of research subjects, for all categories of research mentioned above. A national ethical review, as required in Recommendations (5) and (6), shall be carried out by an appropriate body designated by the Secretary, DHEW, until the establishment of the National Advisory Council for the Protection of Subjects of Biomedical and Behavioral Research. In order to facilitate public understanding and the presentation of public attitudes toward special problems reviewed by the national review body, appropriate provision should be made for public attendance and public participation in the national review process. (Adopted unanimously, one abstention.)

9. Research on the dead fetus and fetal tissue. The Commission recommends that use of the dead fetus, fetal tissue and fetal material for research purposes be permitted, consistent with local law, the Uniform Anatomical Gift Act and commonly held convictions about respect for the dead. (Adopted unanimously, one abstention.)

10. The design and conduct of a nontherapeutic research protocol should not determine recommendations by a physician regarding the advisability, timing or method of abortion. (Adopted by a vote of 6 to 2.)

11. Decisions made by a personal physician concerning the health care of a pregnant woman or fetus should not be compromised for research purposes, and when a physician of record is involved in a prospective research protocol, independent medical judgment on these isssues is required. In such cases, review panels should assure that procedures for such independent medical judgment are adequate, and all conflict of interest or appearance thereof between appropriate health care and research objectives should be avoided. (Adopted unanimously.)

12. The Commission recommends that research on abortion techniques continue as permitted by law and government regulation. (Adopted by a vote of 6 to 2.)

13. The Commission recommends that attention be drawn to Section 214(d) of the National Research Act (Pub. L. 93–348) which provides that:

No individual shall be required to perform or assist in the performance of any part of a health service program or research activity funded in whole or in part by the Secretary of Health, Education, and Welfare, if his performance or assistance in the performance of such part of such program or activity would be contrary to his religious beliefs or moral convictions.

(Adopted unanimously.)

14. No inducements, monetary or otherwise, should be offered to procure an abortion for research purposes. (Adopted unanimously.)

15. Research which is supported by the Secretary, DHEW, to be conducted outside the United States should at the minimum comply in full with the standards and procedures recommended herein. (Adopted unanimously.)

16. The moratorium which is currently in effect should be lifted immediately, allowing research to proceed under current regulations but with the application of the Commission's Recommendations to the review process. All the foregoing Recommendations of the Commission should be implemented as soon as the Secretary, DHEW, is able to promulgate regulations based upon these Recommendations and the public response to them. (Adopted by a vote of 9 to 1.)

Dissenting Statement of Commissioner David W. Louisell

I am compelled to disagree with the Commission's Recommendations (and the reasoning and definitions on which they are based) insofar as they succumb to the error of sacrificing the interests of innocent human life to a postulated social need. I fear this is the inevitable result of Recommendations (5) and (6). These would permit nontherapeutic research on the fetus in anticipation of abortion and during the abortion procedure, and on a living infant after abortion when the infant is considered nonviable, even though such research is precluded by recognized norms governing human research in general. Although the Commission uses adroit language to minimize the appearance of violating standard norms, no facile verbal formula can avoid the reality that under these Recommendations the fetus and nonviable infant will be subjected to nontherapeutic research from which other humans are protected.

I disagree with regret, not only because of the Commission's zealous efforts but also because there is significant good in its Report especially its showing that much of the research in this area is therapeutic for the individuals involved, both born and unborn, and hence of unquestioned morality when based on prudent medical judgment. The Report also makes clear that some research, even though nontherapeutic, is merely observational or otherwise without significant risk to the subject, and therefore is within standard human research norms and as unexceptional morally as it is useful scientifically.

But the good in much of the Report cannot blind me to its departure from our society's most basic moral commitment: the essential equality of all human beings. For me the lessons of history are too poignant, and those of this century too fresh, to ignore another violation of human integrity and autonomy by subjecting unconsenting human beings, whether or not viable, to harmful research even for laudable scientific purposes.

Admittedly, the Supreme Court's rationale in its abortion decisions of 1973—*Roe v. Wade* and *Doe v. Bolton*, 310 U.S. 113, 179—has given this Commission an all but impossible task. For many see in that rationale a total negation of fetal rights, absolutely so for the first two trimesters and substantially so for the third. The confusion is understandable, rooted as it is in the Court's invocation of the specially constructed legal fiction of "potential" human life, its acceptance of the notion that human life must be "meaningful" in order to be deserving of legal protection, and its resuscitation of the concept of partial human personhood, which has been thought dead in American society since the demise of the *Dred Scott* decision. Little wonder that intelligent people are asking: how can one who has no right to life itself have the lesser right of precluding experimentation on his or her person?

It seems to me that there are at least two compelling answers to the notion that *Roe* and *Doe* have placed fetal experimentation, and experimentation on nonviable infants, altogether outside the established protections for human experimentation. First, while we must abide the Court's mandate in a particular case on the issues actually decided even though the decision is wrong and in fact only an exercise of "raw judicial power" (White, J., dissenting in *Roe* and *Doe*), this does not mean we should extend an erroneous rationale to other situations. To the contrary, while seeking to have the wrong corrected by the Court itself, or by the public, the citizen should resist its extension to other contexts. As Abraham Lincoln, discussing the *Dred Scott* decision, put it:

(T)he candid citizen must confess that if the policy of the government upon vital questions affecting the whole people, is to be irrevocably fixed by decisions of the Supreme Court, the instant that they are made, in ordinary litigation between parties in personal actions, the people will have ceased to be their own rulers, having, to that extent, practically resigned their government, into the hands of that eminent tribunal. (4 Basler, The Collected Works of Abraham Lincoln 262, 268 (1963).)

Thus even if the Court had intended by its *Roe* and *Doe* rationale to exclude the unborn, and newly born nonviable infants, from all legal protection including that against harmful experimentation, I can see no legal principle which would justify, let alone require, passive submission to such a breach of our moral tradition and commitment.

Secondly, the Court in *Roe* and *Doe* did not have before it, and presumably did not intend to pass upon and did not in fact pass upon, the question of experimentation on the fetus or born infant. Certainly that question was not directly involved in those cases. Granting the fullest intendment to those decisions possibly arguable, it seems to me that the woman's new-found constitutional right of privacy is fulfilled upon having the fetus aborted. If an infant survives the abortion, there is hardly an additional right of privacy to then have him or her killed or harmed in any way, including harm by experimentation impermissible under standard norms. At least *Roe* and *Doe*

should not be assumed to recognize such a right. And while the Court's unfortunate language respecting "potential" and "meaningful" life is thought by some to imply a total abandonment of *in utero* life for all legal purposes, at least for the first two trimesters, such a conclusion would so starkly confront our social, legal, and moral traditions that I think we should not assume it. To the contrary we should assume that the language was limited by the abortion context in which used and was not intended to effect a departure from the limits on human experimentation universally recognized at least in principle.

A shorthand way, developed during the Commission's deliberations, of stating the principle that would adhere to recognized human experimentation norms and that should be recommended in place of Recommendation (5) is: No research should be permitted on a fetus-to-be-aborted that would not be permitted on one to go to term. This principle is essential if all of the unborn are to have the protection of recognized limits on human experimentation. Any lesser protection violates the autonomy and integrity of the fetus, and even a decision to have an abortion cannot justify ignoring this fact. There is not only the practical problem of a possible change of mind by the pregnant woman. For me, the chief vice of Recommendation (5) is that it permits an escape hatch from human experimentation principles merely by decision of a national ethical review body. No principled basis for an exception has been, nor in my judgment can be, formulated. The argument that the fetus-to-be-aborted "will die anyway" proves too much. All of us "will die anyway." A woman's decision to have an abortion, however protected by *Roe* and *Doe* in the interests of her privacy or freedom of her own body, does not change the nature or quality of fetal life.

Recommendation (6) concerns what is now called the "nonviable fetus ex utero" but which up to now has been known by the law, and I think by society generally, as an infant, however premature. This Recommendation is unacceptable to me because, on approval of a national review body, it makes certain infants up to five months gestational age potential research material, provided the mother who has of course consented to the abortion, also consents to the experimentation and the father has not objected. In my judgment all infants, however premature or inevitable their death, are within the norms governing human experimentation generally. We do not subject the aged dying to unconsented experimentation, nor should we the youthful dying.

Both Recommendations (5) and (6) have the additional vice of giving the researcher a vested interest in the actual effectuation of a particular abortion, and society a vested interest in permissive abortion in general.

I would, therefore, turn aside any approval, even in science's name, that would by euphemism or other verbal device, subject any unconsenting human being, born or unborn, to harmful research, even that intended to be good for society. Scientific purposes might be served by nontherapeutic research on retarded children, or brain dissection of the old who have ceased to lead "meaningful" lives, but such research is not proposed—at least not yet. As George Bernard Shaw put it in "The Doctor's Dilemma": "No man is allowed to put his mother in the stove because he desires to know how long an adult woman will survive the temperature of 500 degrees Fahrenheit, no matter how important or interesting that particular addition to the store of human knowledge may be." Is it the mere youth of the fetus that is thought to foreclose the full protection of established human experimentation norms? Such reasoning would imply that a child is less deserving of protection than an adult. But reason, our tradition, and the U.N. Declaration of Human Rights all speak to the contrary, emphasizing the need of special protection for the young.

Even if I were to approach my task as a Commissioner from a utilitarian viewpoint only, I would have to say that on the record here I am not convinced that an adequate showing has been made of the necessity for nontherapeutic fetal experimentation in the scientific or social interest. The Commission's reliance is on the Battelle Report and its reliance is misplaced.

The relevant Congressional mandate was to conduct an investigation and study of the alternative means for achieving the purposes of fetal research (Pub. L. 93–348, July 12, 1974, sec. 202 (b); National Research Act.)

As Commissioner Robert E. Cooke, M.D., who is sophisticated in research procedures, pointed out in his Critique of the Battelle Report: "The only true objective approach beyond question, since scientists make [the analysis of the necessity for nontherapeutic fetal research], is to collect information and analyze past research accomplishments with the intention of *disproving, not proving* the hypothesis that research utilizing the living human fetus non-beneficially is necessary" (italics in original). The Battelle Report seems to me not in accord with the Congressional intention in that it proceeds from a viewpoint opposite to that quoted, and is really an effort to prove the indispensability of nontherapeutic research. In any event, if that is its purpose, it fails to achieve it, for most of what it claims to have been necessary could be justified as therapeutic research or at least as non-invasive of the fetus (e.g., probably amniocentesis). In view of haste with which this statement must be prepared if it is to accompany the Commission's report, rather than enlarge upon these views now I refer both to the Cooke Critique and the Battelle Report itself both of which I am informed will be a part of or appended to the Commission's Report.

An emotional plea was made at the Commission's hearings not to acknowledge limitations on experimentation that would inhibit the court-granted permissive abortion. However, until its last meeting, I think the Commission for the most part admirably resisted the temptation to distort its purpose by pro-abortion advocacy. But at the last meeting, without prior preparation or discussion, it adopted Recommendation (12) promotive of research on abortion techniques. This I feel is not germane to our task, is imprudent and certainly was not adequately considered.

Finally, I do not think that the Commission should urge lifting the moratorium on fetal research as stated in Recommendation (16). To the extent that duration of the moratorium is controlled by section 213 of the National Research Act, the subject is beyond our

control and we ought not assume authority that is not ours. This is matter not for us and not, ultimately, for any administrative official, but for Congress. If the American people as a democratic society really intend to withdraw from the fetus and nonviable infant the protection of the established principles governing human experimentation, that action I feel should come from the Congress of the United States, in the absence of a practical way to have a national vote. Assuming that any representative voice is adequate to bespeak so basic and drastic a change in the public philosophy of the United States, it could only be the voice of Congress. Of course there is no reason why the Secretary of DHEW cannot immediately make clear that no researcher need stand in fear of therapeutic research.

As noted at the outset, the Commission's work has achieved some good results in reducing the possibilities of manifest abuses and thereby according a measure of protection to humans at risk by reason of research. That it has not been more successful is in my judgment not due so much to the Commission's failings as to the harsh and pervasive reality that American society is itself at risk—the risk of losing its dedication "to the proposition that all men are created equal." We may have to learn once again that when the bell tolls for the lost rights of any human being, even the politically weakest, it tolls for all.

David W. Louisell
*Elizabeth Josselyn Boalt
Professor of Law
University of California, Berkeley*

Statement of Commissioner Karen Lebacqz, With the Concurrence of Commissioner Albert R. Jonsen on the First Item

The following comments include some points of dissent from the Recommendations of the Commission. For the most part, however, these comments are intended as elaborations on the Report rather than dissent from it.

1. At several points, the Commission established as a criterion for permissible research an acceptable level of risk—e.g. "no risk" or "minimal risk."

I support the Commission's Recommendations regarding such criteria, but I wish to make several interpretative comments.

First, I think it should be stressed that in the first trials on human subjects or on a new class of human subjects, the risks are almost always unknown. The Commission heard compelling evidence that differences in physiology and pharmacology between human and other mammalian fetuses are such that even with substantial trials in animal models it is often not possible to assess the risks for the first trials with human fetuses. For example, evidence from animal trials in the testing of thalidomide provided grounds for an estimation of low risk to human subjects; the initial trials in the human fetus resulted in massive teratogenic effects.

I would therefore urge review boards to exercise caution in the interpretation of "risk" and to avoid the temptation to consider the risks "minimal" when in fact they cannot be fully assessed.

Second, I think it important to emphasize the evaluative nature of judgments of risk. The term "risk" means *chance of harm*. Interpretation of risk involves both an assessment of statistical *chance* of injury and an assessment of the *nature* of the injury. Value judgments about what constitutes a "harm" and what percentage chance of harm is acceptable are both involved in the determination of acceptable risk. A small chance of great harm may be considered unacceptable where a greater chance of a smaller harm would be acceptable. For example, it is commonly accepted that a 1–2% chance of having a child with Down's Syndrome is a "high" risk, where the same chance of minor infection from amniocentesis would be considered a "low" risk. Opinions will differ both about what constitutes "harm" or injury and also about what chance of a particular harm is acceptable.

For all these reasons, the interpretation of risk and the designation of acceptable "minimal risk" merit considerable attention by the scientific community and the lay public. The provision of national review in problematic instances should engender serious deliberation on these critical issues.

Third, the establishment of criteria for "no risk" or "minimal risk" is obviously related to the interpretation of "harm." In general, the Commission has discussed "harm" in terms of two indices (1) injury or diminished faculty, and (2) pain. A third commonly accepted definition of "harm" is "offense against right or morality"; this meaning of harm has been subsumed under the rubric of violation of dignity or integrity of the fetus, and thus is separated out of the Commission's deliberations on acceptable levels of risk. In establishing acceptable levels of risk, therefore, the Commission has been concerned with injury and pain to the fetus.

Several ethicists argued cogently before the Commission that the ability to experience pain is morally relevant to decisions regarding research. Indeed, the argument was advanced that the ability to experience pain is a more appropriate consideration than is viability for purposes of establishing the limits of intervention into fetal life.

However, scientific opinion is divided on the question of whether the fetus can experience pain—and on the appropriate indices on which to measure the experience of pain. Several experts argue that the fetus does not feel pain.

I believe that the Commission has implicitly accepted this view in making Recommendation (6) regarding research on the fetus during the abortion procedure and on the nonviable fetus *ex utero*. Should this view not be correct, and should the fetus indeed be able to experience pain before the 20th week of gestation, I would modify Recommendation (6) in two ways:

First, the Recommendation as it now stands does not specify an acceptable level of risk. The reason for this omission is essentially as follows: in a dying subject prior to viability, "diminution of faculties" does not appear to be a meaningful index of harm since this index refers largely to future life expectations. Therefore, the critical meaning of "harm" for such a subject lies in the possibility of experiencing pain. If the fetus does not feel pain it cannot be "harmed" in this sense, and thus there is no risk of harm for such a fetus. It is for this reason that the Commission has not specified an acceptable level of "risk" for fetuses in this category, although it has been careful to protect the dignity of the fetus.

Clearly, however, if the fetus does indeed feel pain, then it can be "harmed" by the above definition of harm. If so, then I would argue that an acceptable level of risk should be established at the same level as that considered acceptable for fetuses *in utero*—namely, "no risk" or "minimal risk."

Second, the Commission has concluded that out of respect for the dying subject, no interventions are permissible which would alter the duration of life of the subject—i.e., by shortening or lengthening the dying process (item 6h). I find the prohibition against shortening the life of the dying fetus to be acceptable provided the fetus does not feel pain. If the fetus does feel pain, however, then its dying may be painful and respect for the dying subject may require that its pain be minimized even if its life-span is shortened in so doing.

2. The Commission has stated that its provisions regarding therapeutic and nontherapeutic research directed toward the pregnant woman are not intended to limit research on improving abortion techniques. I support this stand and wish to clarify the reasons for my support.

In supporting this statement, I neither condone nor encourage widespread abortion. However, I do believe that some abortions are both legally and morally justifiable. It is therefore consonant with the principle of minimizing harm to develop techniques of abortion that are least harmful. Indeed, under the present climate of legal freedom to abort and widespread practice of abortion, adherence to the principle of not-harming may impose an obligation on us to research abortion technology in order to minimize harm. This obligation arises not only out of consideration of the health and well-being of the woman but also from a concern for possible pain or discomfort of the fetus during the abortion procedure.

3. Evidence presented to the Commission indicates that there is a strong emphasis in the law on avoiding possible injury to a child to be born. This evidence, coupled with the uncertainty of risks in a new class of human subjects, suggests that considerable importance ought to be attached to the question of compensation for injury incurred during research.

The Commission will study this question in depth at a later time, and therefore has not made any recommendations on compensation at this time. As a matter of personal opinion, would like to note that I am reluctant to allow any research on the living human fetus unless provision has been made for adequate compensation of subjects injured during research.

4. The Commission's Recommendation on research during the abortion procedure and on the nonviable fetus *ex utero* prevents prolongation of the dying process for purposes of research. This prohibition may appear to have the effect of preventing research on the development of an artificial placenta.

It is my understanding that such an effect does not necessarily follow. Steps toward the development of an artificial placenta are prohibited only through nontherapeutic research; innovative therapy or therapeutic research on the possibly viable infant is not only condoned but encouraged. Thus the development of an artificial placenta may proceed, but under more restricted circumstances in which it is limited to therapeutic research or to nontherapeutic research which does not alter the duration of life. I do not believe that it was the intention of the Commission to curtail all research toward the development of an artificial placenta, nor do I believe that such will be the effect of the Commission's Recommendations.

Were the Recommendations to have such an effect, however, I would dissent. Indeed, I would argue that a prematurely delivered fetus that is unable to survive, given the support of available medical technology, would have an interest in the development of an artificial placenta that would allow others like it to survive. Thus it would not be contrary to the interests of that fetus for it to be subjected to nontherapeutic research in the development of an artificial placenta.

In making such an argument, I invoke a principle that I call the "principle of proximity": namely, that research is ethically more acceptable the more closely it approximates what the considered interests of the subject would reasonably be. For example, Hans Jonas has argued that dying subjects should not be used in nontherapeutic research, even when they have

consented, unless the research deals directly with the cause from which they are dying; that is, it is presumed that a dying subject has an interest in his/her own disease which legitimates research on that disease where research in general would not be legitimate.

Such a principle is, of course, open to wide interpretation. But I think it not unreasonable to suggest that the dying fetus would have an interest in the cause of its dying or in the development of technology which would allow others like it to survive. On such a principle, one might argue that it is more ethically acceptable to use dying fetuses with Tay-Sachs disease as subjects in nontherapeutic research on Tay-Sachs disease than in nontherapeutic research on general fetal pharmacology. Similarly, one might argue that it is ethically acceptable to use nonviable fetuses *ex utero* as subjects in nontherapeutic research on the development of an artificial placenta. The development of a full rationale for such a position would require an analysis along the lines suggested by McCormick and Toulmin, and I cannot attempt that here. At this point I simply wish to suggest that I believe it is possible to argue for both therapeutic and nontherapeutic research directed to-. ward the development of an artificial placenta.

5. Finally, members of the Commission disagreed about changes in the timing or method of abortion in relation to research. Recommendation (10) states clearly that the recommendations of a physician regarding timing and method of abortion should not be determined by the design or conduct of nontherapeutic research. I am in full agreement with this Recommendation.

The provision in Recommendation (6) (item g), however, is more ambiguous. I would argue that changes in timing or method of abortion are ethically acceptable provided that they are freely chosen by the woman and that she has been fully informed of all possible risks from such changes. I base this argument on the right of any patient to be informed about alternative courses of treatment and to choose between them. It seems to me that the pregnant woman, as a patient, may choose the timing and method of abortion, provided that she has been fully informed

of the following: (1) the relation of alternative methods of abortion to possible research on the fetus; (2) risks to herself and to possible future children of alternative possible methods of abortion; and (3) procedures which would be introduced into the abortion as part of the research design which would not be medically indicated.

Some members of the Commission have argued that a woman might choose such changes provided that they entail no additional risk. While I appreciate the concern to protect the woman's health and well-being, such a restriction seems to me a violation of her right to freedom of choice as a patient. Thus I would allow a woman to choose to delay her abortion until the second trimester for purposes of research, *provided that* she has been fully informed of all risks in so doing. One restriction seems imperative to me, however: in no case, should she be allowed to delay the abortion beyond the 20th week of gestation *for research purposes*. This position is reflected in the Deliberations and Conclusions of the Commission's Report.

Regulations

Protection of Human Subjects: Fetuses, Pregnant Women, in Vitro Fertilization

Basic regulations governing the protection of human subjects involved in research development, and related activities supported or conducted by the Department through grants and contracts were published in the *Federal Register* on May 30, 1974 (39 FR 18914). [These were readopted with minor technical amendments in the *Federal Register* for March 13, 1975 (40 FR 11854).] At that time it was indicated that notices of proposed rulemaking would be developed to provide additional protection for subjects of research who may have diminished capacity to provide informed consent. On August 23, 1974, a notice of proposed rulemaking was published for public comment (39 FR 30648) in which it was proposed to amend 45 CFR Part 46 to provide further protective measures for the fetus, the abortus, prisoners, and the institutionalized mentally disabled as subjects of research activities.

On July 12, 1974, the National Research Act (Pub. L. 93–348) was signed into law, thereby creating the National Commission for the Protection of Human Subjects of Biomedical and Behavioral Research. One of the charges to the Commission was to investigate and study the nature and extent of research involving the living human fetus and to recommend to the Secretary the circumstances (if any) under which such research should be conducted or supported by the Department. Pursuant to section 202(b) of that Act, the Commission has transmitted Recommendations to the Secretary. Pursuant to section 205 of the Act, the Secretary is publishing that Report elsewhere in this issue of the *Federal Register*.

After considering both the public comments to the proposed rulemaking published August 23, 1974, and the Recommendations of the Commission, the Secretary has determined to amend 45 CFR 46 by adding a subpart governing research involving the fetus, the pregnant woman, and products of human *in vitro* fertilization consistent with the public comments and the Recommendations of the Commission. This amendment to the regulations is to be effective immediately. The Secretary, as required by Pub. L. 93–348, section 205, will take into consideration any comments submitted regarding the Recommendations and, if it appears necessary, will propose further rulemaking with respect to any amendments to these regulations which appear warranted.

The Secretary also concludes that the moratorium on fetal research which was imposed by the Department on August 27, 1974 (39 FR 30962) may now be lifted, allowing research to go forward under the regulations issued herewith. The Secretary notes in this regard that the restrictions imposed by section 213 of the National Research Act (Pub. L. 93–348) extended only until the Commission had submitted its Recommendations to the Secretary on May 21, 1975.

Over 125 individuals commented on subpart C (here stated as subpart B) of the proposed rulemaking which pertains to the fetus, the abortus, the pregnant woman, and the products of human *in vitro* fertilization. Those comments, and the Recommendations of the Commission, are summarized as follows:

Applicability

Commenters objected to the applicability of this subpart to "activities involving women who could become pregnant, except where the applicant or offeror shows to the satisfaction of the Secretary that adequate steps will be taken to avoid involvement of women who are pregnant." Concern was expressed that implementation of such a provision might involve numerous pregnancy tests during the course of an investigation, and still not achieve this goal. The Department notes that although the Commission expressed concern that the fetus not be involved unintentionally in research activities, it did not make a specific recommendation with respect to this. The Department concludes that the Institutional Review Boards should determine whether adequate measures will be taken to avoid unintentional involvement of pregnant women in research activities which are not designed to include pregnant women or the fetus and which might present a risk to a fetus if such existed. Section 46.102(b) (5) of subpart A is therefore amended to add such determinations as one of the duties of the Institutional Review Board.

The notice published August 23, 1974, was limited to biomedical research. That limitation has been removed because, while the Department believes that this subpart applies primarily to biomedical research, other research may be proposed which might fall under the scope of this subpart.

Definitions

The Department has reviewed with care the definitions adopted by the Commission, and determined that those definitions should be incorporated substantially as drafted into the regulations. It should be noted that in so doing, the Department has extended the meaning of the term "fetus" to include the fetus *ex utero* until such time as such a fetus is determined to be viable. The effect of this change is to delete the term "abortus" which appeared in the proposed rulemaking, and refer instead to a fetus *ex utero*. The Department agrees with the Commission that such usage serves the interests of both consistency and clarity, although it may vary at times from legal, medical, or common usage. Also, consistent with the determination discussed above, the definition of "biomedical research" has been dropped.

Ethical Advisory Boards

A number of respondents expressed concern that an Ethical Advisory Board, as proposed, would be overburdened and would add an unnecessary layer to a review process which is already time consuming. It was also suggested that the Institutional Review Boards can, and in many instances already do, perform at the local level many of the tasks suggested for the Board. On the other hand, some respondents endorsed the proposal as a welcome measure to insure that projects would be stringently reviewed at a national level for ethical considerations prior to receiving support with public monies.

The Commission recommended that a national review body (similar to that proposed by the Department) consider the ethical problems raised by research proposals to which the application of standards enumerated in their recommendations proves difficult.

The Department has considered these suggestions and agrees that whereas the Institutional Review Boards may be able to assume a large share of the ethical review of proposals, it is also true that there will be instances in which the application of standards to specific cases will be difficult or in which review at the national level is desirable. The Department therefore has determined that such an Ethical Advisory Board is necessary to assure that projects supported or conducted by the Department meet ethical standards acceptable to the general community. However, because the nature of the activities may be different and the number of activities requiring review may be large, one Board will be established to provide advice to the Public Health Service and one Board will be established to provide advice to other components of the Department, with respect to policy governing certain kinds of research, and also with respect to the funding of individual proposals which raise ethical problems. While the Boards will propose to the Secretary categories of research which the Board believes either require or do not require their review, research protocols and procedures which involve minimal or no risk, and which clearly conform to the requirements of this subpart, generally need not be reviewed by the Ethical Advisory Board. Research proposals which are judged by agency advisors or staff to require further evaluation of risk or the interpretation of the requirements or which raise ethical problems, may not be conducted or supported by the Secretary unless the Ethical Advisory Board has reviewed and rendered its advice concerning the research activity. It is intended, ultimately, that a similar requirement for Board review be extended to other classes of research subjects.

A number of comments were received regarding the composition of the Ethical Advisory Board, its duties, or the manner in which it should conduct its meetings. Specifically, the Commission recommended that women and minorities be adequately represented on the Board, and that its deliberations be conducted with full public participation. Many of the suggestions are currently incorporated in regulations governing Federal committee membership and activities. Others will be addressed in the Charter of the Board which the Secretary will publish in the *Federal Register* at a later date.

Establishment of a Consent Committee
Although there was general agreement among commenters that provisions should be made to monitor conditions surrounding the consent process, there was criticism of the proposal to create separate committees to perform this function. For the most part, it was felt that the Institutional Review Boards could and should perform this function as part of continuing responsibility for the protection of human subjects. It was further suggested that additional panels should not be created unless the Department has evidence that the necessary functions could not be performed by the Institutional Review Boards or other existing committees.

The Commission noted that it will be undertaking a study, as part of its mandate under Pub. L. 93–348, of the effectiveness of Institutional Review

Boards in implementing DHEW regulations for the protection of human subjects. It recommended that until the study is completed, the responsibility for monitoring the consent process should be assumed by the Institutional Review Boards. The Department agrees. The provisions for creating Consent Committees have therefore been deleted, and the duties delegated to them in the proposed rulemaking have been given to the Institutional Review Boards. This is reflected in § 46.205, titled "Additional duties of the Institutional Review Boards in connection with activities involving fetuses, pregnant women, or human *in vitro* fertilization."

The Department received a number of criticisms regarding the provision that the Consent Committee be authorized to terminate the participation of subjects without their consent (§ 46.305(a) (2) of the proposed rulemaking). It was argued that this would be an unwarranted infringement of an individual's right to consent. The Department agrees, and such authority has been deleted.

Research Involving in Vitro Fertilization
Commenters generally endorsed the Department's proposal not to regulate research involving human *in vitro* fertilization other than to require that all proposals involving such research be reviewed for approval by the Ethical Advisory Board. The Commission did not make any recommendation concerning this category of research in the report submitted on May 21. The Department therefore makes no change from the proposed rulemaking with respect to research involving *in vitro* fertilization. The requirement that all such proposals be reviewed by the Ethical Advisory Board, as well as by the Institutional Review Board, appears in §§ 46.204(c) and 46.205 respectively.

Because biomedical research is not yet near the point of being able to maintain for a substantial period the non-implanted product of *in vitro* fertilization, these regulations do not address this point. Given the state of the research, we believe that regulations would be premature. However, the Department anticipates that such a regulation will be prepared when the state of biomedical science so warrants.

Activities Involving Fetuses in Utero or Pregnant Women
A number of commenters suggested that the rulemaking, as proposed, would hamper research necessary to meet the health needs of pregnant women, fetuses, and neonates. The most frequent references were to studies on placental transfer, the normal course of pregnancy, and the delivery process. Some individuals objected to the prohibition of research prior to the commencement of a procedure to terminate pregnancy, while others objected to any conduct of research even during the process of abortion.

The Commission, in its Recommendations, separated that category of research directed toward the pregnant woman from that directed toward the fetus *in utero*. It further distinguished between therapeutic research and nontherapeutic research, finding therapeutic research to be generally acceptable and desirable, whether directed toward the fetus or the pregnant woman, provided certain specified preconditions are met. The Department agrees that it is useful to distinguish between the fetus *in utero* and the pregnant woman as the primary subject of a research activity and also that research directed at meeting the health needs of the subject is generally acceptable provided certain conditions are met. The regulations therefore address these topics in separate sections.

General Limitations
There were no substantive objections to the intent of restrictions which appeared in various parts of the proposed rulemaking pertaining to: (1) the necessary completion of appropriate animal studies; or (2) the separation of research personnel from decisions regarding the timing or method of terminating pregnancy or regarding the viability of a delivered fetus. Some commenters, and the Commission, recommended the addition of appropriate studies on nonpregnant humans as a prerequisite for research activities covered by this subpart. The Commission further recommended that there should be no significant changes introduced into a delivery procedure solely in the interests of research. The Department

has incorporated these provisions in a section titled "General limitations" (§ 46.206) which governs all research activities covered by this subpart.

Activities Directed toward Pregnant Women as Subjects

As noted above, there was little objection from commenters or from the Commission regarding research directed toward the health needs of the pregnant woman. In fact, some respondents urged that care be taken not to infringe the woman's right to privacy and her access to health care. With respect to women's rights, a number of individuals objected to the provision requiring consent other than that of the pregnant woman for research directed toward the health needs of the pregnant woman, and some objected to such consent provisions even when the woman would be participating in nontherapeutic research activities.

The Commission considered that the woman's right to health care is preeminent, and recommended essentially no restrictions on research directed toward the health care of the pregnant woman, so long as the risks to her fetus are minimized as much as possible consistent with meeting her health needs, and provided that she is fully advised of the risks to herself and her fetus. In addition, the general provisions for prerequisite research and for adequate review and supervision of the consent process should be met. The Department agrees.

With respect to research directed toward the pregnant woman but which is not directed toward her health care, there seems to be general agreement that such research should be permitted only if it imposes minimal or no risk to the fetus. There is disagreement among the commenters with respect to paternal consent for this category of research. The Department has considered with care the various arguments with respect to consent other than the pregnant woman's for nontherapeutic research involving the pregnant woman, and concludes that such consent should be obtained except where such research involves the health needs of the woman.

In general, women who are victims of rape are not appropriate subjects for nontherapeutic research. There are some instances, however, in which

their participation may be sought (as in studies concerning the effects of rape.) Consent other than hers is not necessary in such cases.

It should be noted in this regard that the Commission, in a number of instances, recommended that research be permitted if the mother has consented and the father has not objected. The Department has concluded that implementation of a provision for absence of objection might present serious problems. Since the absence of objection can best be verified by requesting consent, the Department has retained the requirement for paternal consent when the father's identity and whereabouts can reasonably be ascertained, and if he is reasonably available.

Activities Directed towards Fetuses in Utero as Subjects

No comments were received which expressed objections to the conduct of research activities directed toward the health care of the fetus *in utero.* Rather, the Department was urged not to restrict, and even to encourage, such research.

On the other hand there was considerable division of opinion regarding research directed toward the fetus which is not related to its health care. Concern was expressed that the fetus might be used as an experimental "object," in a manner inconsistent with its human genetic heritage. This is particularly true when termination of pregnancy is a factor in the research, as in protocols designed to determine the effect on the fetus of drugs administered to a pregnant woman. Questions were raised regarding the ethical validity of consent by a pregnant woman on behalf of a fetus, for its inclusion in a research activity of no benefit to that fetus, especially if the woman has already decided to terminate her pregnancy.

The Department is sensitive to these concerns. It has reviewed the Recommendations of the Commission regarding this category of research, and is persuaded that those recommendations are sound; namely, that no research be conducted or supported which fails to treat the fetus with proper care and dignity. In addition, the Department agrees that a pregnant woman need not

be presumed to lack interest in her fetus even when she has decided to terminate her pregnancy; thus, she may validly be asked for consent for research involving the fetus.

The Department notes that the Commission was created to represent the best judgment of the community, and to make recommendations following an intensive study of the issues. All of the arguments which were submitted to the Department were considered by the Commission in its deliberations, and it is therefore reasonable to accept the findings of the Commission as the best possible judgment on the matter. The Department concludes that the Recommendations of the Commission with respect to research involving the fetus *in utero* should be adopted. These are incorporated in the regulations in § 46.208, with modifications, as noted above, in the provisions for paternal consent.

Activities Directed toward Fetuses ex Utero as Subjects

Although some commenters suggested that no research be permitted on the fetus ex *utero,* others were concerned that the proposed rulemaking was too restrictive, and would preclude the development of technology for sustaining premature infants. The Commission recommended that no procedures be applied to a nonviable fetus *ex utero* which would alter its duration of life. It further recommended that if the fetus might possibly be viable, but has not yet been determined to be so, no additional risk to the well-being of that fetus should be imposed by research. It is expected that no procedures will be undertaken which fail to treat the fetus with due care and dignity, or which affront community sensibilities. Further, it is required that if a delivered fetus is determined to be viable, it will be treated as a premature infant, and may be included in research activities according to the regulations to be proposed governing the participation of children in research.

For the reasons stated above, the Department has concluded that the Recommendations of the Commission regarding research on the fetus *ex utero* should be adopted, for the most part. These are incorporated in § 46.209 of the regulations with modifications, as noted above, in the provisions for paternal consent. However, the Secretary is persuaded by the weight of scientific evidence that research performed on the nonviable fetus ex *utero* has contributed substantially to the ability of physicians to bring to viability increasingly small fetuses. The Secretary perceives that it is in the public interest to continue this successful research and accordingly an exception is made to the Recommendations of the Commission to permit research to develop new methods for enabling fetuses to survive to the point of viability.

Activities Involving the Dead Fetus, Fetal Material, or the Placenta

The Department notes, as did the Commission, that research involving the dead fetus and fetal material is governed in part by the Uniform Anatomical Gift Act which has been adopted by 49 States, the District of Columbia and Puerto Rico. There were no substantive recommendations concerning this section, and the regulation therefore differs from the proposed rulemaking only with respect to minor additions for clarification. Any applicable State or local laws regarding such activities are, of course, controlling.

Activities to Be Performed Outside the United States

Consistent with the Commission's Recommendations, § 46.210 of the proposed rulemaking has been deleted, thereby making these regulations applicable to all research conducted or supported by the Department within the United States or abroad.

Modification or Waiver of Specific Requirements

Recognizing the difficulty of applying a specific set of regulations to all situations that may arise in the future, the Department has elected to provide a mechanism for waiver or modification of specific provisions under certain circumstances. Requests from an applicant or offeror for such a waiver or modification must be reviewed by the appropriate Ethical Advisory Board, which after opportunity for public input, shall advise the Secretary as to whether or not the request should be approved. These Boards will conform to the operating procedures required by the Federal Advisory Committee Act.

Activities Conducted by Departmental Employees

In order to make it clear that the requirements of these regulations (Part 46) apply to activities conducted by its own employees, the Department is adding subpart C titled "Activities Conducted by Departmental Employees" as § 46.301.

The moratorium on fetal research imposed on August 27, 1974, is hereby lifted, but such research will be conducted or supported by the Department only in accordance with the following regulations.

Written comments concerning the Recommendations of the Commission may be sent to the Office of Protection from Research Risks, National Institutes of Health, 9000 Rockville Pike, Bethesda, Maryland 20014. All comments received will be available for inspection at the National Institutes of Health, Room 303, Westwood Building, 5333 Westbard Avenue, Bethesda, Maryland, weekdays (Federal holidays excepted) between the hours of 9 a.m. and 4:30.

These regulations shall become effective on August 8, 1975.

Date: July 17, 1975

Theodore Cooper
Assistant Secretary for Health

Approved: July 29, 1975

Caspar W. Weinberger
Secretary

Accordingly Part 46 of 45 CFR Subtitle A is amended by:

46.101–46.122 [Redesignated]

1. Designating §§ 46.1 through 46.22 as Subpart A, renumbering these as §§ 46.101 through 46.122, and modifying all references thereto accordingly.

46.102 [Amended]

2. Adding the word "and" at the end of § 46.102(b) (2), changing the semicolon at the end of § 46.102(b) (3) to a period, and deleting § 46.102(b) (4).

3. Redesignating § 46.102(c) as § 46.102(e) and inserting the following new §§ 46.102(c) and 46.102(d).

46.102 Policy

(c) Unless the activity is covered by Subpart B of this Part, if it involves as subjects women who could become

pregnant, the Board shall also determine as part of its review that adequate steps will be taken in the conduct of the activity to avoid involvement of women who are in fact pregnant, when such activity would involve risk to a fetus.

(d) Where the Board finds risk is involved under paragraph (b) of this section, it shall review the conduct of the activity at timely intervals.

4. Adding the following new Subparts B and C.

Subpart B—Additional Protections Pertaining to Research, Development, and Related Activities Involving Fetuses, Pregnant Women, and Human In Vitro Fertilization

46.201 Applicability a. The regulations in this subpart are applicable to all Department of Health, Education, and Welfare grants and contracts supporting research, development, and related activities involving: (1) The fetus, (2) pregnant women, and (3) human *in vitro* fertilization.

b. Nothing in this subpart shall be construed as indicating that compliance with the procedures set forth herein will in any way render inapplicable pertinent State or local laws bearing upon activities covered by this subpart.

c. The requirements of this subpart are in addition to those imposed under the other subparts of this part.

46.202 Purpose It is the purpose of this subpart to provide additional safeguards in reviewing activities to which this subpart is applicable to assure that they conform to appropriate ethical standards and relate to important societal needs.

46.203 Definitions As used in this subpart:

a. "Secretary" means the Secretary of Health, Education, and Welfare and any other officer or employee of the Department of Health, Education, and Welfare to whom authority has been delegated.

b. "Pregnancy" encompasses the period of time from confirmation of implantation until expulsion or extraction of the fetus.

c. "Fetus" means the product of conception from the time of implantation until a determination is made, following expulsion or extraction of the fetus, that it is viable.

d. "Viable" as it pertains to the fetus means being able, after either spontaneous or induced delivery, to survive (given the benefit of available medical therapy) to the point of independently maintaining heart beat and respiration. The Secretary may from time to time, taking into account medical advances, publish in the *Federal Register* guidelines to assist in determining whether a fetus is viable for purposes of this subpart. If a fetus is viable after delivery, it is a premature infant.

e. "Nonviable fetus" means a fetus *ex utero* which, although living, is not viable.

f. "Dead fetus" means a fetus *ex utero* which exhibits neither heartbeat, spontaneous respiratory activity, spontaneous movement of voluntary muscles, nor pulsation of the umbilical cord (if still attached).

g. *"In vitro* fertilization" means any fertilization of human ova which occurs outside the body of a female, either through admixture of donor human sperm and ova or by any other means.

46.204 Ethical Advisory Boards a.
Two Ethical Advisory Boards shall be established by the Secretary. Members of these Boards shall be so selected that the Boards will be competent to deal with medical, legal, social, ethical, and related issues and may include, for example, research scientists, physicians, psychologists, sociologists, educators, lawyers, and ethicists, as well as representatives of the general public. No board member may be a regular, full-time employee of the Federal Government.

b. One Board shall be advisory to the Public Health Service and its components. One Board shall be advisory to all other agencies and components within the Department of Health, Education, and Welfare.

c. At the request of the Secretary, the appropriate Ethical Advisory Board shall render advice consistent with the policies and requirements of this Part as to ethical issues, involving activities covered by this subpart, raised by individual applications or proposals. In addition, upon request by the Secretary, the appropriate Board shall render advice as to classes of applications or proposals and general policies, guidelines, and procedures.

d. A Board may establish, with the approval of the Secretary, classes of applications or proposals which: (1) Must be submitted to the Board, or (2) need not be submitted to the Board. Where the Board so establishes a class of applications or proposals which must be submitted, no application or proposal within the class may be funded by the Department or any component thereof until the application or proposal has been reviewed by the Board and the Board has rendered advice as to its acceptability from an ethical standpoint.

e. No application or proposal involving human *in vitro* fertilization may be funded by the Department or any component thereof until the application or proposal has been reviewed by the Ethical Advisory Board and the Board has rendered advice as to its acceptability from an ethical standpoint.

46.205 Additional Duties of the Institutional Review Boards in Connection with Activities Involving Fetuses, Pregnant Women, or Human in Vitro Fertilization a.
In addition to the responsibilities prescribed for Institutional Review Boards under Subpart A of this part, the applicant's or offeror's Board shall, with respect to activities covered by this subpart, carry out the following additional duties:

(1) Determine that all aspects of the activity meet the requirements of this subpart;

(2) Determine that adequate consideration has been given to the manner in which potential subjects will be selected, and adequate provision has been made by the applicant or offeror for monitoring the actual informed consent process (e.g., through such mechanisms, when appropriate, as participation by the Institutional Review Board or subject advocates in: (i) Overseeing the actual process by which individual consents required by this subpart are secured either by approving induction of each individual into the activity or verifying, perhaps through sampling, that approved procedures for induction of individuals into the activity are being followed, and (ii) monitoring the progress of the activity and intervening as necessary through such steps as visits to the activity site and continuing evaluation to determine if any unanticipated risks have arisen);

(3) Carry out such other responsibilities as may be assigned by the Secretary.

b. No award may be issued until the applicant or offeror has certified to the Secretary that the Institutional Review Board has made the determinations required under paragraph (a) of this section and the Secretary has approved these determinations, as provided in § 46.115 of Subpart A of this part.

(c) Applicants or offerors seeking support for activities covered by this subpart must provide for the designation of an Institutional Review Board, subject to approval by the Secretary, where no such Board has been established under Subpart A of this part.

46.206 General Limitations a.
No activity to which this subpart is applicable may be undertaken unless:

(1) Appropriate studies on animals and nonpregnant individuals have been completed;

(2) Except where the purpose of the activity is to meet the health needs of the particular fetus, the risk to the fetus is minimal and, in all cases, is the least possible risk for achieving the objectives of the activity;

(3) Individuals engaged in the activity will have no part in: (i) Any decisions as to the timing, method, and procedures used to terminate the pregnancy, and (ii) determining the viability of the fetus at the termination of the pregnancy; and

(4) No procedural changes which may cause greater than minimal risk to the fetus or the pregnant woman will be introduced into the procedure for terminating the pregnancy solely in the interest of the activity.

b. No inducements, monetary or otherwise, may be offered to terminate pregnancy for purposes of the activity.

46.207 Activities Directed toward Pregnant Women as Subjects a.
No pregnant woman may be involved as a subject in an activity covered by this subpart unless: (1) The purpose of the activity is to meet the health needs of

the mother and the fetus will be placed at risk only to the minimum extent necessary to meet such needs, or (2) the risk to the fetus is minimal.

b. An activity permitted under paragraph (a) of this section may be conducted only if the mother and father are legally competent and have given their informed consent after having been fully informed regarding possible impact on the fetus, except that the father's informed consent need not be secured if: (1) The purpose of the activity is to meet the health needs of the mother; (2) his identity or whereabouts cannot reasonably be ascertained; (3) he is not reasonably available; or (4) the pregnancy resulted from rape.

46.208 Activities Directed toward Fetuses in Utero as Subjects a. No fetus in utero may be involved as a subject in any activity covered by this subpart unless: (1) The purpose of the activity is to meet the health needs of the particular fetus and the fetus will be placed at risk only to the minimum extent necessary to meet such needs, or (2) the risk to the fetus imposed by the research is minimal and the purpose of the activity is the development of important biomedical knowledge which cannot be obtained by other means.

b. An activity permitted under paragraph (a) of this section may be conducted only if the mother and father are legally competent and have given their informed consent, except that the father's consent need not be secured if: (1) His identity or whereabouts cannot reasonably be ascertained, (2) he is not reasonably available, or (3) the pregnancy resulted from rape.

46.209 Activities Directed toward Fetuses ex Utero, Including Nonviable Fetuses, as Subjects a. No fetus ex utero may be involved as a subject in an activity covered by this subpart until it has been ascertained whether the particular fetus is viable, unless: (1) There will be no added risk to the fetus resulting from the activity, and (2) the purpose of the activity is the development of important biomedical knowledge which cannot be obtained by other means.

b. No nonviable fetus may be involved as a subject in an activity covered by this subpart unless: (1) Vital functions of the fetus will not be artificially maintained except where the purpose of the activity is to develop new methods for enabling fetuses to survive to the point of viability, (2) experimental activities which of themselves would terminate the heartbeat or respiration of the fetus will not be employed, and (3) the purpose of the activity is the development of important biomedical knowledge which cannot be obtained by other means.

c. In the event the fetus ex utero is found to be viable, it may be included as a subject in the activity only to the extent permitted by and in accordance with the requirements of other subparts of this part.

d. An activity permitted under paragraph (a) or (b) of this section may be conducted only if the mother and father are legally competent and have given their informed consent, except that the father's informed consent need not be secured if: (1) his identity or whereabouts cannot reasonably be ascertained, (2) he is not reasonably available, or (3) the pregnancy resulted from rape.

46.210 Activities Involving the Dead Fetus, Fetal Material, or the Placenta Activities involving the dead fetus, mascerated fetal material, or cells, tissue, or organs excised from a dead fetus shall be conducted only in accordance with any applicable State or local laws regarding such activities.

46.211 Modification or Waiver of Specific Requirements Upon the request of an applicant or offeror (with the approval of its Institutional Review Board), the Secretary may modify or waive specific requirements of this subpart, with the approval of the Ethical Advisory Board after such opportunity for public comment as the Ethical Advisory Board considers appropriate in the particular instance. In making such decisions, the Secretary will consider whether the risks to the subject are so outweighed by the sum of the benefit to the subject and the importance of the knowledge to be gained as to warrant such modification or waiver and that such benefits cannot be gained except through a modification or waiver. Any such modifications or waivers will be published as notices in the Federal Register.

Subpart C—General Provisions

46.301 Activities Conducted by Department Employees The regulations of this part are applicable as well to all research, development, and related activities conducted by employees of the Department of Health, Education, and Welfare, except that each Principal Operating Component head may adopt such nonsubstantive procedural modifications as may be appropriate from an administrative standpoint.

Illustrative Cases

A 35-year-old married woman, sixteen weeks pregnant, undergoes amniocentesis to determine the presence of fetal defects. The procedure, which takes about three weeks to complete, involves removing fetal cells from the fluid surrounding the fetus in the uterus, growing, and then analyzing the cells. The procedure carries little risk for either mother or child. Her physician reports that the fetus shows no signs of abnormality and that the woman can expect to give birth to a girl. Several days later the woman requests an abortion. The reason she gives the doctor is that she does not want to have another daughter. She has two children, 3 and 5 years old—both girls. Her husband is opposed to the abortion and would prefer to have the additional child. The marriage appears to be stable and happy, and the couple are well-to-do. The physician did not know that the information regarding the sex of the fetus would lead to a request for an abortion.

1. Assume that you are the physician. What justification would you have for doing the abortion? For not doing the abortion? If a serious defect had been detected in the fetus, would this alter your actions?

A young couple has decided to be married. They learn from their physician that the woman carries a gene with a 50 percent chance of blindness in the male offspring of the marriage and that could cause half of the female offspring to be carriers of the defect. Through amniocentesis, physicians can detect both the fetus who will be blind and the fetus who will be a carrier of the defect. Yet both the prospective husband and wife are opposed to abortion and willing to risk transmitting this disorder to the children they hope to bear.

1. If you were the physician, what counsel would you give this couple?
2. Should government take steps to deal with the social interests at stake in this case or in cases like it?

VII

Suffering and Dying

Introduction to Part VII

Modern medicine wins many accolades for its conquests over disease and its increasing sophistication in saving lives from the very brink of death. Yet some of the very skills and technologies that heighten the ability to save lives that would have been lost in a former era are contributing to increased frustrations for health professionals and patients. People who are comatose or in the very debilitated end states of fatal illnesses can have their lives sustained for longer periods than ever before. Thus, ironically enough, medical advances in pain relief and life-sustaining techniques may either alleviate or heighten the suffering that often accompanies dying and irreversible handicapping injuries or diseases. The task of medicine throughout its long history has included relief of pain and suffering and care for the dying, as well as the cure and management of diseases and saving lives. How best to deal with suffering and dying?

The article by Stanley J. Reiser provides a perspective on the range of responses to suffering and dying on the part of English and American physicians during the past century. Reiser shows that the types of responses involve more than the usual alternatives discussed in the overly polarized presentations typical of the media. Carl F. H. Marx, writing in the nineteenth century, further documents the thinking and attitudes of physicians confronted by suffering and dying patients. To round out the background for understanding the moral issues that are raised by caring for suffering and dying patients, the next five selections are among historically significant attempts to cope with the contemporary situation. In these documents, legislators, religious leaders, and prestigious physicians represent forces at work within medicine, as well as forces emanating from a concerned public.

The essays by Cicely Saunders and Diana Crane indicate how adults who are suffering and dying can be cared for and also provide a contemporary view of medical attitudes toward those who are critically ill.

The Karen Quinlan case is an unprecedented and rather agonizing attempt of the Supreme Court in New Jersey to try to say what is legally required of health professionals and relatives in a case where a comatose person does not meet the criteria of brain death (as specified in the document that precedes it), yet is given no prospect of living in anything but a comatose state. What does mercy require of us in instances like this?

Arthur J. Dyck critically analyzes two different philosophies regarding how we are to see the value of human life and how we are to continue to protect our positive affirmations of its value while still providing relief for those who are suffering.

The question of mercy killing is sharply pressing on us in the context of caring for desperately ill and handicapped infants. The Joseph P. Kennedy, Jr. Foundation had a film made of a case of failing to provide lifesaving intervention for a child diagnosed as having Down's syndrome (mongolism). Paul Freund's essay, "Mongoloids and 'Mercy Killing,' " was written in response to this case and presented at a conference sponsored by the Kennedy Foundation in 1971. Drs. Raymond S. Duff and A. G. M. Campbell take issue with Freund's attitude toward the law and its protection of handicapped infants. Indeed, the article by Duff and Campbell has sparked a continuing debate regarding the care of infants whose life prospects and prognoses are extremely poor. Religious ethicist Richard A. McCormick has responded to the kinds of practices Duff and Campbell are condoning. McCormick takes up the difficult task of trying to sort out some of the circumstances when it may be less than compassionate to try to prolong life and others when the obligation to save life should persist.

75

Stanley Joel Reiser

The Dilemma of Euthanasia in Modern Medical History: The English and American Experience

Reprinted with minor revision by permission of author and editors from John A. Behnke and Sissela Bok, eds., *The Dilemmas of Euthanasia* (New York: Anchor Press, 1975), pp. 27–49.

During most of the nineteenth century, Western physicians usually rejected suggestions to shorten the lives of incurable or dying patients to mitigate their suffering. When Napoleon proposed that his physician Desgenettes fatally drug several plague-stricken, mortally ill soldiers unable to march and likely to fall into enemy hands, the doctor refused. He declared that his obligation was to cure people, not to kill them (Wilson 1896: 633–34, quoting Napoleon). John Keats, the poet, hoping to end his torment from the last stages of tuberculosis, and spare his friend Joseph Severn the miseries of attending and beholding him, could not induce either Severn or his physician to give him a lethal dose of laudanum. And the composer Hector Berlioz recalled bitterly, in his memoirs, the despair he felt when physicians refused to end the life of his dying sister:

I have lost my eldest sister; she died of a cancer of the breast after six months of horrible suffering which drew heart rending screams from her day and night. My other sister, who went to Grenoble to nurse her, and who did not leave her till the end, all but died from the fatigue and the painful impressions caused by this slow agony. And not a doctor dared to have the humanity to put an end to this martyrdom by making my sister inhale a bottle of chloroform. This is done to save a patient the pain of a surgical operation which lasts a quarter of a minute, and it is not had recourse to in order to deliver one from a torture lasting six months. [*sic*] When it is proved certain that no remedy, nothing, not even time, can cure a dreadful disease; when death is evidently the supreme good, deliverance, joy, happiness!
. . . The most horrible thing in the world for us, living and sentient beings, is inexorable suffering, pain without any possible compensation when it has reached this degree of intensity; and one must be barbarous, or stupid, or both at once, not to use the sure and easy means now at our disposal to bring it to an end. Savages are more intelligent and more humane. (Wilson 1896: 633–34; see also Ferriar 1816: 392)

Beginnings of the Euthanasia Debate in England and the United States

At the start of the 1870s, essays appeared by two laymen that stirred public and medical consideration of euthanasia (or painless death) in England and the United States. In the first

paper, S. D. Williams proposed that when patients stricken with a hopeless and agonizing sickness requested that their lives be ended, the physician should have the legal right to assist them. Lionel Tollemache followed shortly with an essay supporting this viewpoint and focusing, like Williams, on the excessive burden, suffering, and anxiety borne by unhealable patients.

Any of us may one day have to bear—many of us will certainly have to witness—either cancer, creeping paralysis, or something equally unpleasant; some may even have to endure the hardest fate of all—the fate of a mortally-wounded soldier, who wishes to die, but whose wounds are laboriously tended; so that, by an ingenious cruelty, he is kept suffering, against nature, and against his own will. Hence, even from the most selfish point of view, we all have an interest that this question should be speedily discussed; so that, in case any change should be thought possible and right, that change may occur in our lifetime. (Tollemache 1873: 218–19)

Although no modification in laws or codes of medical ethics occurred, these essays moved people to consider the issues raised by euthanasia.

By the beginning of the twentieth century, advances in medicine had given physicians increasingly potent weapons to keep alive the patient who would quickly die if natural biological forces could prevail. As Judge Simeon Baldwin noted in 1904:

The family ask the doctor if there is no hope, and he responds with some sharp stimulant; some hypodermic injection; some transfusion or infusion to fill out for a few hours the bloodless veins. . . . The sufferer wakes to pain and gasps back to a few more days or weeks of life. Were they worth the having? Do they bring life or a parody of life? . . . Has nature—that is, the divine order of things—been helped or thwarted? For the time thwarted; but not for long. The suffering, or at best lethargic existence, has been successfully protracted, but the body will soon falter and fail in the unwonted functions forced upon parts of it made for other uses, and death come, to the relief of the dying and living, alike. (Baldwin 1904: 4)

Baldwin's reservations about the benefits of medical advances are strikingly similar to those expressed more than a half century later by Dr. William Williamson. By this time, powerful drugs, efficient respirators, pacemakers, and artificial organs, in concert with aggressive nursing care, saved many lives. Although the physician had acquired substantial technical ability to prolong lives, he had developed no moral principles that told him when to apply or withhold his remedies in the new kinds of medical situations he confronted. For example, prior to the 1960s, a mortally ill patient who stopped breathing was pronounced dead. But modern respirators gave physicians the ability to treat the condition. As Williamson recounted:

I have seen patients with brain-stem failure, with dilated, fixed pupils, decerebrate rigidity, and cessation of spontaneous respiration, who have had a tracheostomy and were assisted with a mechanical respirator. With fluids, electrolytes, and good nursing care, the essentially isolated heart in such a patient can sometimes be kept beating for a week. I have never seen such a patient begin to breathe spontaneously and survive, and autopsy always shows advanced liquefaction necrosis of the brain, for it "died" several days before the heart did. (Williamson 1966: 793)

Laymen and physicians had warned that the temptation to hold back such patients from the grave for days or years threatened the sensibilities and humanity of the patient and the doctor. They declared that the power to detain death was not a warrant for its use, when the result might be only a short postponement of death, purchased at the cost of pain, and barren of real opportunities for good.[1] Yet most twentieth-century physicians seemed disposed to sustain life at the expense of great anguish:

Of all that modern science has achieved in the alleviation of human suffering, the fact remains that vast numbers of human beings are doomed to end their earthly existence by a lingering, painful and often agonizing form of death. (Millard 1931: 39; see also The Right to Die 1935: 1616)

By the twentieth century, cancer had become a highly prevalent incurable disease. For example, the 60,000 deaths caused by cancer in England during 1940 represented a doubling since the dawn of the century. The application of twentieth-century medical discoveries also had lengthened the expectancy of life. The number of people over sixty years old in England increased from fewer than 2,500,000 in 1901 to 6,250,000 in 1944. The aged were susceptible not only to cancer but other debilitating chronic disorders that resisted medical therapy. Physicians treating elderly, terminally ill people

were often discouraged; one medical journal characterized such patients as dull, apathetic, helpless, and hopeless individuals who lingered on while those around them whispered hopes for their death. (Editorial 1946: 343) The growth of the elderly population led some physicians to advocate the development of strategies to deal with the threat they posed to the public purse, and the aggregate increase of societal suffering that they brought with their augmented years. Euthanasia was one of the options suggested.[2]

Policies for Euthanasia

The controversies generated by the subject of euthanasia during the nineteenth and twentieth centuries have been provoked, in part, by the two senses in which the word has been used by physicians and laymen, and by the four different courses of medical action that these definitions prompted. Some have meant by euthanasia giving a painless death to people suffering from incurable disease who were not close to death; others have applied it to helping people who were dying to exit from life with as little anguish as possible, the sense in which it was used most often. Based upon these meanings of euthanasia, four therapeutic policies evolved. In the first policy (1) the physician consciously endeavored to make the period of terminal illness as happy and free from pain as possible, consistent with doing nothing that would hasten death. A second approach (2) also specified efforts to moderate discomfort, but condoned jeopardizing the patient's life in the process. In the third approach (3) the physician acknowledged his inability to heal the patient, ceased his therapy, and surrendered to the superior biological forces. A fourth policy (4) suggested that the physician actively participate in ending the life of a patient who pleaded for release from the tribulations of incurable disease or the throes of dying. Physicians applied the first and second measures mainly to patients near death; they applied the third and fourth measures to patients near death as well as to patients having painful, unhealable disease with no prospect of imminent death.

1. The first policy was euthanasia in the sense of making dying gentle and

easy. It was reflected in John Ferriar's 1816 observation: "When all hopes of revival are lost, it is still the duty of the physician to soothe the last moments of existence" (p. 392). A crucial requirement for the physician subscribing to this viewpoint was developing skills to ameliorate the oppressive features of terminal illness, so that the time remaining might be lived with as little pain and distress as possible. The patient received food and wine that comforted and pleased him. Attendants made his bedchamber bright and cheerful, and administered powerful pain-killing drugs when the patient requested them. The patient was encouraged to think of his past and dwell on his accomplishments. Religion was invoked, when appropriate, to give him hope of future salvation. Advocates believed it was the

sacred duty of every physician to make this subject a part of his studies. . . . It should be a grateful and sacred duty, nay, it should be the highest triumph of the physician to minister unto the wants of a dying fellow creature by effecting the Euthanasia. (Williams 1894: 909; see also Hammond 1934: 486)

But the physician could prescribe only to relieve the suffering and not to hasten death. He could comfort patients, but not diminish their vital powers. (Euphoria vs. Euthanasia 1899: 674; Euthanasia 1903: 1094)

2. The second policy declared that patients with terminal illness must have their ordeal moderated, even if it involved shortening their lives. Supporters of this position believed that the quality was more important than the length of life. The physician's first thought was to assuage pain. Lionel Tollemache noted in 1873:

I am told on medical authority that in the last stages of cancer (perhaps also in hydrophobia) it is now not uncommon to give strong narcotics, which no one would have dreamt of giving half a century ago, and which, while they much mitigate the final agony, by no means tend to prolong it. (Tollemache 1873: 222)

The thoughtful doctor distinguished between extending life and lengthening dying; he constantly judged how the patient tolerated the difficult fight for life:

The two extremes of dying in pain and being killed do not exhaust the possibilities of the stricken patient, because there is a middle course created by a kindly and skilful doctor who gives assistance in an equally kindly nature, and that is what is implicit in the patient's question: "You will stand by me, won't you?" and the doctor's assurance: "Yes, I will."[3]

These physicians dealt with the anguish of the patient by prescribing operative or pharmacological measures in whatever amount necessary to reduce it. If such actions abbreviated existence, the justification was deemed adequate that they were initiated with the objective to prevent pain and not to curtail life:

They undertake the operation or the administration of the drug which they *know* will bring relief to pain, which they *hope* will prolong life a little, but which both patient and surgeon *know* may bring death sooner than it would otherwise come. It is their duty to do it. (Euthanasia—Degenerated Sympathy 1906: 331)

In 1949, the Academy of Moral and Political Sciences, in the United States, passed a resolution telling doctors that the threat of death from measures taken to relieve suffering should not inhibit their therapeutic actions, as long as physicians did not deliberately seek to provoke death.[4]

Accordingly, the approach under discussion entailed a commitment to the use of powerful remedies to reduce suffering, as opposed to the previous policy of comprehensive concern for the physical, psychological, and spiritual needs of the dying or incurable patient.

3. The *Boston Medical and Surgical Journal* endorsed the third approach in an 1884 editorial:

We suspect few physicians have escaped the suggestion in a hopeless case of protracted suffering to adopt the policy of *laisser-aller*, to stand aside passively and give over any further attempt to prolong a life which has become a torment to its owner. . . . Shall not a man under such circumstances give up the fight, take off the spur of the stimulant, and let exhausted nature sink to rest? . . . Perhaps logically it is difficult to justify a passive more than active attempt to euthanasia; but certainly it is much less abhorrent to our feelings. . . . May there not come a time when it is a duty in the interest of the survivors to stop a fight which is only prolonging a useless and hopeless struggle? (Permissive Euthanasia 1884: 20)

Euthanasia, in this usage, is the outcome of negative acts—the doctor halts active therapy, he suspends tormenting the human frame with strong remedies directed at cure (Munk 1888: 473).

However, sometimes this approach amounted to abandonment of the patient by his doctor, and received sharp criticism. Answering the assertion of Sir William Temple that "an honest physician is excused for leaving his patient, when he finds the disease growing desperate, and can, by his attendance, expect only to receive his fees, without any hopes or appearance of deserving them," the English doctor Thomas Percival admonished physicians not to desert the incurable patient. In his 1803 treatise on medical ethics, the most extensive commentary on the subject written to that date, he claimed physicians could soothe the mental anguish of the patient and his family, even in the last stages of fatal disease:

To decline attendance, under such circumstances, would be sacrificing, to fanciful delicacy and mistaken liberality, that moral duty which is independent of, and far superior to, all pecuniary appreciation. (Percival 1803: 38–39)

The Code of Ethics of the American Medical Association, adopted in 1847 and heavily drawn from Percival's work, repeated his injunction against abandoning patients (Leake 1927: 221).

4. A fourth course of action suggested that physicians had the moral right to purposely terminate a patient's life when he suffered from an incurable and agonizing disease, and wanted to die (Rosenberg and Aronstam 1901: 109). Defenders of this form of euthanasia labeled as irrational the reverence for human life without regard to its character, or the maintenance of body function in a patient whose intelligence and consciousness had fundamentally eroded, leaving nothing but the external form with its associations of memory to show that it has been the abiding place of a soul now evicted. Would it not be a more respectful treatment of the loved ones, a more dignified ending of a worthy life, if respiration were allowed to cease when all higher functions have irrevocably departed? Would not memories associated with a previous life of usefulness and beauty be more precious than those dependent upon the prolongation of the lowest animal existence? (Euthanasia—Degenerated Sympathy 1906: 331)

One physician described a case in which his patient continually cried in agony, "Oh, God, take me." The imminence of death, in addition to the

suffering, led the physician to administer large doses of morphine until the patient died. He defended his act:

Would you, Sir, rather be attended at your latter end by a man who thought of you first and last, or by one who was determined at all cost to your feelings to keep you alive a few hours or days longer in order to satisfy some legal or ethical fetish? (Richards 1936: 557)

On several occasions during the twentieth century, advocates of this form of euthanasia sought legislation to liberate physicians from the need to maintain life in patients who desired a speedy and painless death as a matter of right. Dr. R. H. Gregory introduced a bill into the legislature of Iowa, and Miss Anne Hall presented one to the legislature of Ohio to give legal sanction to the participation of physicians in euthanasia. Gregory claimed that many doctors defied the law and commonly practiced euthanasia on their suffering and incurable patients. The *British Medical Journal* labeled Gregory "a liar of the basest kind," and Anne Hall was criticized in a similar manner by physicians. The lawmakers rejected both bills, but the proposals created a sufficient alarm for a New York State legislator to offer a law that anyone suggesting such euthanasia, verbally or through a written document, be guilty of a felony. That bill was also set aside.[5]

The second major flurry of legislative debate occurred in England during the 1930s. Dr. Killick Millard initiated the activity with a proposal to legalize termination of life by physicians, if requested by a patient suffering from a painful, irreparable disease. Millard's recommendation drew support from many people in England, who believed they had a right to die painlessly without being in defiance of the law. Even when incurably ill, existing statutes made ending one's life a felony. The felony not only tarnished the family name, but opened the abetting doctor, nurse, friend, or relative to a charge of manslaughter, or possibly murder (Voluntary Euthanasia 1932: 321; Wanner 1933: 71). To promote legalization of painless death, and to educate public opinion concerning it, the Voluntary Euthanasia Legalization Society was formed in England. Drawing support from a number of distinguished physicians and laymen who had become members, the society redrafted Millard's proposal and presented it to Parliament. The bill specified the candidate for euthanasia must be over twenty-one, suffering from a disorder involving severe pain, and incurable. To initiate action required a formal written application, certified by two witnesses, which was sent to a referee who reviewed the request and interviewed the candidate. Permission granted, someone other than the patient's doctor carried out the euthanasia.[6]

Proponents of legalizing this form of euthanasia believed that the tradition requiring doctors to maintain life to the limit of their medical powers, irrespective of the patient's suffering, should be replaced by a tradition making reduction of suffering more urgent, even if it involved abbreviating life. They argued that civilized man must exert greater control over his existence. Wrote Lord Moynihan, president of the Voluntary Euthanasia Legalization Society:

Many people insist that God sent suffering into the world. But they seem to forget that God also sent the means of relief. Our duty at present seems to be to keep people alive, even when their lives are useless, at the expense of great suffering. Some of us in the medical profession are unhappy when this necessity is inflicted on us. We feel that under the strictest supervision power should be given to end life that is a curse to itself and a torture to all who love the afflicted individual. There is nothing compulsory about our proposals. The patient would decide for himself or herself whether the right to die should be exercised.[7]

These physicians disparaged the effectiveness of therapy to reduce suffering. They pointed to cases where drugs provided no relief, where patients received an immediate benefit from a drug only to acquire subsequent tolerance of it, or where the continued administration of a remedy such as morphine could debase the character of the patient and from its side effects, cause him great suffering (Cockshut 1941: 65; Voluntary Euthanasia: The New Society States Its Case 1935: 1168).

Supporters of the bill also argued that the widespread, secret, criminal, and often ineffective attempts at euthanasia made open and lawful conduct of the procedure preferable. The physician asked to administer euthanasia had to choose between helping his patient or chancing a prison sentence. Legal sanction of euthanasia would end the risk of criminal prosecution, and make the act and the participation of the doctor in it socially acceptable (see Chap. 3, Meyers, and Chap. 4, Cantor). The physician would cease to bear the total responsibility for euthanasia, but would be joined in the decision by legal, religious, and other agents of society. Further, under legalized euthanasia, the patient's chance of escaping a lingering death would no longer depend fortuitously on the character of the physician. Finally, not only would patient and doctor benefit from such legislation, but so would relatives of the patient by escaping the financial and emotional strain of a prolonged illness. In spite of these arguments, the English Parliament rejected the euthanasia bill (Notes on the Debate in the House of Lords in 1936: 1232–34).

Opposition to the Deliberate Ending of Life

During the nineteenth and twentieth centuries, efforts to relieve suffering, as proposed in the first three policies for euthanasia, did not arouse strong medical antagonism. Yet the defeat of the euthanasia bills revealed the great opposition within society and the medical profession to all suggestions favoring the fourth policy for euthanasia—that physicians explicitly act to end the lives of unhealable, pain-burdened patients. "If a life is worth living at all, it is certainly worth living to the very end, a position from which the conscientious physician has no possible escape in the care of the cases which he is called upon to treat," wrote a doctor summing up the attitudes of many colleagues (Our Attitude Toward Incurable Disease 1899: 531; May the Physician Ever End Life? 1897: 934). The most important aspect of the Hippocratic Oath was declared the passage forbidding the physicians to give "deadly medicine to anyone, even if asked, nor [to] suggest such counsel."[8] Many doctors believed it would be dangerous and dishonorable to profession and public if any departure from this clear principle were sanctioned.

Of great concern to these antagonists was the threat to the relation between doctor and patient posed by acts directed at producing death. The patient's trust of doctors might decline if they assumed the role of executioners. "Euthanasia is a rather euphemistic term for what may be called professional murder," the Journal of the American Medical Association bluntly put it (Editorial, The Moral Side of Euthanasia 1885: 382). "To suggest that physicians, in the secrecy of the bed chamber, are to hold themselves ready to practise thugee on their patients, either on the patient's own suggestion or to please distraught or designing by-standers, would be absurd if it were not so horrible," declared the British Medical Journal.[9] Doctors feared patients would lose faith in them as guardians of life. If a part of the doctor's duty was to hasten his patient's passage into the other world,

his very presence would necessarily be associated with the idea of death. He would enter the sick-room, into which he should bring life and hope, with the dark shadow of death behind him. (The Right to Die 1911: 1217; see also Euthanasia Again Debated 1939: 608)

Physicians also were apprehensive that all medical practice would become more difficult if they condoned such euthanasia. The treatment even of non-fatal illness required the physician to strengthen the will of the sufferer to endure. How could will be summoned if the patient knew euthanasia was a legally and medically acceptable option for him? (Euphoria vs. Euthanasia 1899: 674; Fleming 1936: 86) As for the doctor himself, unless he learned to stretch the techniques of his craft to its limits, he too might develop a defeatist attitude when facing illness. To carry out the mercy killing implied the physician had failed to fully utilize his personal and scientific resources for the patient. Some physicians even thought that it might threaten the development of new drugs to relieve pain (Voluntary Euthanasia 1932: 321; Fleming 1935: 1181).

Crucial also to the argument against deliberate actions to produce death was the belief that natural dying was not an ordeal:

The nearer we approach the dying state, the more we throw upon it the light of science, the less we find of the bodily sufferings which in the popular belief are all but inseparable from it, and are emphasized in the terms "mortal agony and death struggle."

The medical profession, the clergy, intelligent nurses, all who have frequently witnessed the phenomena of dying, testify that they do not see signs of pain or fear of death. Natural anaesthesia is bestowed by the hand of the "Great Physician."[10]

Dr. William Osler kept careful records of 500 patients, in which he recorded the causes of their death and their sensations during the act of dying. He found ninety experienced bodily pain, eleven mental apprehension, two positive terror, one spiritual exaltation, and one bitter remorse. The great majority gave no sign either way: "like their birth, their death was a sleep and a forgetting."[11]

Studies and observations of patients in hospitals for the incurable related that patients roused their courage to face the ordeal of pain and death; that it was rare for them to express the wish to die. The *British Medical Journal* editorialized:

We have no recollection of any case in which the patient himself, unless he were in the very grasp of death, said plainly that the moment for the sundering the bond of life had actually arrived. The protests are conditional. To-morrow if things be no better; but let to-morrow dawn; I may have a better night.[12]

Some doctors believed it was the neurotic patient suffering mental, not physical pain, who usually asked to die. Moreover, even lengthening life by a day might ease the final hours by allowing the person to soothe a guilty conscience, to sign a will, to heal a breach of friendship, or to say farewell to someone.

Several adversaries of deliberate euthanasia pointed out that the meaning of suffering and dying eluded people; that the Bible said man must endure the pain of death as the penalty for sin: "Providence ordains the day of our death. . . . To hasten that day is an act of rebellion against the Divine Will."[13] The doctor could not decide what the value of life was for his most tormented and hopeless patient, and so could have no part in actively causing death. Opponents believed that calls for euthanasia often indicated moral deficiency and weakness, not in the dying patient, but in beholders unable to bear his torment: "The sight of pain is distressing; therefore let the suffering person be got rid of. That is really what the whole thing comes to."[14] Some

even feared that the patient might decide to sacrifice himself to mitigate the tribulation that he caused his relatives (Earengey 1940: 97).

But even those inclined to purposely shorten a life of suffering expressed apprehension that medical diagnosis and prognosis were unequal to the task. The chance of error in predicting the nature or course of a disorder made the judgment to administer euthanasia weighty and perilous:

Who is to decide whether an illness is certain to prove fatal? Medicine is not an exact science and patients who have been deemed incurable by some physicians have not infrequently recovered, even patients with cancer who seemed to be dying. (Euthanasia Again 1926: 1491)

Physicians knew that apparently unhealable patients sometimes got well, and hesitated to bear the responsibility of deciding whether to use extreme measures to hasten death. One miraculous cure given a great deal of publicity was that of a clergyman's wife who, in a widely circulated letter, had begged for "scientific kindness" by her physicians to terminate her suffering and give her painless death. Many laymen supported her arguments, but the physicians ignored them and succeeded in restoring her health. She rejoiced that her pleas were disregarded.[15] Equally disturbing were studies conducted during the twentieth century that demonstrated considerable flaws in medical judgments. A pioneer analysis by Richard Cabot in 1910 found widespread diagnostic errors occurred among cases in which autopsy evidence was available for verification (Cabot 1910: 1343–50; see also V. Robinson 1913: 146).

The possibilities of future therapeutic discoveries also raised imponderable questions. Who knew if a cure for a given disease might not be found tomorrow? Moreover, the duty of the physician was to maintain an encouraging attitude in the patient: "Where there is life there is hope, and it is the duty of the doctor to hope until the final breath." (Wolbarst 1939: 681; see also V. Robinson 1913: 146) Patients tenaciously clung to hope. Sentiment aside, skepticism about the fallibility of human judgment fed the spirits of the dying.

Some physicians feared that social approval of medical actions to hasten death would contribute to undermine civilization by reviving repressed sadism. The "Thou Shalt Not Kill" rule held society together. The homicide instinct in man, part of his natural aggressive component, had to be repressed. Once let loose, as in war, it became difficult to control. These physicians believed that mercy killing, even if humanely applied, could demoralize medicine and society. Physicians under the pretense of mercy might commit a felony, if promised large sums of money by greedy in-laws of the patient. Or perhaps, if a person were encouraged to take his own life when ill, people burdened with unfortunate love affairs, financial loss, or other serious problems would be inclined to do the same. The principle might be widened to incurably insane persons, who could not express valid consent, to aged people, or to any individual whom a majority of interested persons considered better dead than alive.[16] Physicians might seize upon the alternative of euthanasia to relieve society, hospitals, families, and themselves from the burdens of caring for patients whom they could not rehabilitate, and who threatened the physician's belief in his medical omnipotence. As the public contributed growing amounts of tax money to medical care, the question would inevitably arise whether public funds should be allocated first to people considered more valuable to society than others. At this point, the euthanasia alternative for unproductive or burdensome patients might become a tempting social solution (Alexander 1949: 45–46).

These were not empty misgivings. Suggestions to make the incurable mental patient an object of euthanasia arose from several quarters in England and the United States during the twentieth century, such as the proposal written by a San Francisco physician in 1944:

To end a life that is useless, helpless and hopeless seems merciful. The end should be welcome. The act then is kind rather than ruthless and the result could not but benefit the living. In this sense, domestic animals receive better treatment than human beings. The useless, helpless and hopeless are of many kinds. They either always have been or have become unfit in the struggle of life. The opinion of many would include in this classification idiots and the insane, imbeciles and morons, psychopaths both mild and severe, criminals and delinquents, monsters and defectives, incurables and the worn-out senile. Most of these unfits are of no apparent use in the world. They require care and many are without hope of betterment. Not only are they a great burden upon society but, supported and protected, they are fast increasing their dead weight by reproducing their kind.[17]

In Germany, such proposals became social policy. Before the Nazi takeover, in the early 1930s, German physicians discussed the conduct of euthanasia on people with chronic mental illness. In 1939, after Hitler came to power, all state institutions submitted reports on patients who were ill and were unable to work the previous five years to a central bureau, which selected patients for euthanasia. An organization devoted to determining appropriate children for euthanasia also existed, having the title: Realms Committee for Scientific Approach to Severe Illness Due to Heredity and Constitution. The hundreds of thousands of people killed through these organizations included mentally ill, epileptics, the aged sick, and sufferers from neurological diseases such as infantile paralysis and brain tumors.[18]

Concluding Remarks

Despite the literature examined in this essay, discussion by doctors of the suffering of the incurable and care for the dying is appallingly meager in American and English medical journals from the nineteenth to mid-twentieth century. Most commentary deals with the management of the dying, but even this is scant. John Ferriar wrote in 1816 that there was no subject less studied in its fine details than the terminally ill patient: "The wise look beyond it, and the inconsiderate escape from [it]" (p. 392).[19] By the end of the nineteenth century, educators and practitioners continued to ignore the problems of the dying patient. The subject was not examined in medical schools; the young physician had to "learn for himself what to do and what not to do, in the most solemn and delicate position in which he can be placed" (Hitchcock 1889: 40). It still remained a tenet of practice that when no more could be

done to arrest the progress of disease, both the laity and medical profession assumed that the physician had no further duty to the patient (Munk 1888: 473). This attitude persisted during the twentieth century. Dr. T. E. Hammond in 1934 noted a

tendency for many in the profession to concentrate on the prevention of disease and the maintenance of health and to forget that one of its aims should be the endeavor to make the living of life and the passing out from life as easy as possible for the patient and his friends.[20]

Public and professional discussion of euthanasia continued to be sparse up to the mid-1960s. Then, the subject was given much attention as a consequence of the moral problems raised by the growing medical use of machines which sustained the physical functioning of dying patients but usually could not alter their grave prognosis. Until this time, incurable disease and death meant defeat for the physician as well as for the patient: both appeared to prefer the remedy of silence.

Notes

1. Baldwin 1904: 8–9; Ferriar 1816: 392–96; Euthanasia, *St. Louis Medical Review* 1906: 66.

2. Lund 1949: 758; Hickey 1949: 759; Voluntary Euthanasia: The New Society States Its Case 1935:1168; Davis 1950: 311; Millard 1940: 881; Millard 1931: 39.

3. Earengey 1940: 99, citing Dawson; also see Millard 1931: 39; Earengey 1940: 99, citing FitzAlan.

4. Euthanasia 1950: 744; Hammond 1934: 487–88; Kelleher 1940: 880–81; Richards 1936: 556–57.

5. Euthanasia (editorial) 1906: 638–39; Euthanasia—Degenerated Sympathy 1906: 330; Euthanasia, *St. Louis Medical Review* 1906: 66–69.

6. Notes on the Debate in the House of Lords 1936: 1232–34; Millard 1931: 39–47; Voluntary Euthanasia: Propaganda for Legislation 1935: 850; Rejection of the Bill to Legalize Voluntary Euthanasia 1937: 215–16.

7. The Right to Die 1935: 1616; also see Voluntary Euthanasia: The New Society States Its Case 1935: 1168; Notes on the Debate in the House of Lords 1936: 1232–33.

8. The Right to Die 1911: 1217; also see Roche 1935: 926; Euthanasia 1904: 1385; Euthanasia, *B.M.J.* 1906: 539.

9. Sufferers Who Long to Die 1895: 941; also see The Right to Die 1911: 1217; Euthanasia (letter) 1919: 1557; Shaker Held for Murder 1911: 681.

10. Hitchcock 1889: 32; The Problem of Euthanasia 1913: 1897; also see Euthanasia Again 1926: 1491; The Scientific Argument Against Euthanasia 1914: 882.

11. Osler 1905: 19; also see Ferriar 1816: 394; Hawkins 1865: 181–85.

12. May the Physician Ever End Life? 1897: 934; also see Banks 1950: 297–305; V. Robinson 1913: 147–48; Walsh 1935: 333–34.

13. Tollemache 1873: 219; The Right to Die 1911: 1217; also see Walsh 1935: 333–34.

14. Roche 1935: 926; The Right to Die 1911: 1217; V. Robinson 1913: 147.

15. Supplicant for Euthanasia Recovers 1914: 700; The Tonic Effect of Sympathy With Others 1914: 327–28; Wolbarst 1935: 331; The Problem of Euthanasia 1913: 1897; Jacobi 1912: 363; Brill 1936: 2–3.

16. Brill 1936: 9–12; Rosenberg and Aronstam 1901: 110; The Right to Die 1911: 1217; Voluntary Euthanasia 1935: 1053; Tredgold 1936: 33.

17. Hinman 1944: 640; also see W. Robinson 1913: 86–90; Euthanasia Again 1955: 65; Euthanasia Trial Opens 1964: 945.

18. Alexander 1949: 45–46; Ivy 1947: 133–46; Kamisar 1958: 969–1042.

19. A similar viewpoint was held by German physicians; *see* Marx 1826: 404–5.

20. Hammond 1934: 487; also see Bowman 1939: 727; Millard 1931: 39.

References

[The following journals appear in abbreviated form after the first citation to each: *Boston Medical and Surgical Journal* (*B.M.S.J.*); *British Medical Journal* (*B.M.J.*); *Journal of the American Medical Association* (*J.A.M.A.*); *Journal of Nervous and Mental Disease* (*J.N.M.D.*); *Medical Review of Reviews* (*M.R.R.*) and *New England Journal of Medicine* (*N.E.J.M.*)].

Alexander, Leo. 1949. Medical Science Under Dictatorship. *New England Journal of Medicine* 241: 39–47.

Baldwin, Simeon E. 1904. *The Natural Right to a Natural Death.* Cincinnati: Frank H. Vehr.

Banks, Leslie A. 1950. Euthanasia. *Bulletin of the New York Academy of Medicine* 26: 297–305.

Bowman, W. M. 1939. Euthanasia. *Virginia Medical Monthly* 66: 723–29.

Brill, A. A. 1936. Reflections on Euthanasia. *Journal of Nervous and Mental Disease* 84: 1–12.

Cabot, Richard. 1910. A Study of Mistaken Diagnoses. *Journal of the American Medical Association* 55: 1343–50.

Cockshut, R. W. 1941. Euthanasia (letter). *British Medical Journal* 1: 65.

Davis, Edwin. 1950. Should We Prolong Suffering? *Nebraska Medical Journal* 35: 310–12.

Earengey, W. G. 1940. Voluntary Euthanasia. *Medico-Legal Review* 8: 91–110.

Editorial. 1946. *N.E.J.M.* 235: 343.

Euphoria vs. Euthanasia. 1899. *J.A.M.A.* 32: 674.

Euthanasia. 1903. *J.A.M.A.* 41: 1094.

Euthanasia. 1904. *B.M.J.* 1: 1384–86.

Euthanasia. 1906. (editorial) *B.M.J.* 1: 638–39.

Euthanasia. 1906. *B.M.J.* 1: 539.

Euthanasia. 1906. *St. Louis Medical Review* 2: 66–69.

Euthanasia. 1919. (letter) *J.A.M.A.* 72: 1557.

Euthanasia. 1950. (letter) *J.A.M.A.* 142: 744–45.

Euthanasia Again. 1926. *J.A.M.A.* 87: 1491.

Euthanasia Again. 1955. *J.A.M.A.* 159: 65.

Euthanasia Again Debated. 1939. *J.A.M.A.* 113: 608.

Euthanasia —Degenerated Sympathy. 1906. *Boston Medical and Surgical Journal* 154: 330–31.

Euthanasia Trial Opens. 1964. *J.A.M.A.* 188: 945.

Ferriar, John. 1816. Medical Histories and Reflections. Philadelphia: Thomas Dobson.

Fleming, Robert A. 1935. Voluntary Euthanasia (letter). *B.M.J.* 2: 1181.

———. 1936. Voluntary Euthanasia (letter). *B.M.J.* 2: 86.

Hammond, T. E. 1934. Euthanasia *Practitioner* 132: 485–94.

Hawkins, Charles, ed. 1865, *The Works of Sir Benjamin Collins Brodie*. London: Longmans Green.

Hickey, E. M. 1949. Reply to Lund. *B.M.J.* 2: 759.

Hinman, Frank. 1944. Euthanasia. *J.N.M.D.* 99: 640.

Hitchcock, Frank E. 1889. Annual Oration, Euthanasia. *Transactions of the Maine Medical Association* 10: 30–43.

Ivy, Andrew. 1947. Nazi Crimes of a Medical Nature. *Federation Bulletin* 33: 133–46. [Reprinted as Chapter 46 of this volume.]

Jacobi, Abraham. 1912. Euthanasia. *Medical Review of Reviews* 18: 362–63.

Kamisar, Yale. 1958. Some Non-religious Views Against Proposed "Mercy Killing" Legislation. *Minnesota Law Review* 42: 969–1042.

Kelleher, D. 1940. Euthanasia (letter). *B.M.J.* 2: 880–81.

Leake, Chauncey, 1927. *Percival's Medical Ethics*. Baltimore: Williams & Wilkins.

Lund, J. Ruthworth. 1949. Old Age. *B.M.J.* 2: 758.

Marx, C. F. H. 1826. Medical Euthanasia, Translated by Walter Cane, 1952, in *Journal of History of Medical and Allied Sciences* 7:401–16. [Reprinted as Chapter 76 of this volume.]

May the Physician Ever End Life? 1897. *B.M.J.* 1: 934.

Millard, Killick. 1931. The Legalization of Voluntary Euthanasia. *Public Health* 45: 39–47.

———. 1940. (Euthanasia. *B.M.J.* 2: 880–81. Moral Side of) Euthanasia, The. 1885. (editorial) *J.A.M.A.* 5: 382–83.

Munk, William. 1888. Review of Euthanasia, A Medical Treatment in Aid of an Early Death. *B.M.J.* 1: 473.

Notes on the Debate in the House of Lords. 1936. *B.M.J.* 2: 1232–34. [Reprinted as Chapter 77 of this volume.]

Osler, William. 1905. *Science and Immortality*. Boston: Houghton.

Our Attitude Toward Incurable Disease. 1899. *B.M.S.J.* 141: 531.

Percival, Thomas. 1803. *Medical Ethics*. London: W. Jackson. [Reprinted as Chapter 7 of this volume.]

Permissive Euthanasia. 1884. *B.M.S.J.* 110: 19–20.

Problem of Euthanasia, The. 1913. *J.A.M.A.* 60: 1897.

Rejection of the Bill to Legalize Voluntary Euthanasia. 1937. *J.A.M.A.* 108: 215–16.

Richards, W. Guyon. 1936. Euthanasia (letter). *B.M.J.* 1: 556–57.

Right to Die, The. 1911. *B.M.J.* 2: 1215–17.

Right to Die, The. 1935. *J.A.M.A.* 105: 1616–17.

Robinson, Victor, ed. 1913. A Symposium on Euthanasia. *M.R.R.* 20, Pp. 143–155.

Robinson, William J. 1913. Euthanasia. *Medical Pharmacology Critic and Guide* 6: 85–90.

Roche, Redmond. 1935. Voluntary Euthanasia (letter). *B.M.J.* 2: 926.

Rosenberg, Louis J., and Aronstam, N. E. 1901. Euthanasia—A Medicolegal Study. *J.A.M.A.* 36: 108–10.

Scientific Argument Against Euthanasia, The. 1914. (editorial) *B.M.J.* 2: 881–82.

Shaker Held for Murder. 1911. *Medical Record* 1: 681.

Suffers Who Long to Die. 1895. *B.M.J.* 1: 940–41

Supplicant for Euthanasia Recovers. 1914. *J.A.M.A.* 62: 705–6.

Tollemache, Lionel. 1873. The New Cure for Incurables. *Fortnightly Review*, pp. 218–30.

Tonic Effect of Sympathy With Others, The. 1914. *J.A.M.A.* 63: 327–28.

Tredgold, A. F. 1936. Voluntary Euthanasia. *B.M.J.* 1: 33.

Voluntary Euthanasia. 1932. *B.M.J.* 2: 321–22.

Voluntary Euthanasia. 1935. *B.M.J.* 2: 1052–53.

Voluntary Euthanasia: Propaganda for Legislation. 1935. *B.M.J.* 2: 856.

Voluntary Euthanasia: The New Society States Its Case. 1935. *B.M.J.* 2: 1168.

Walsh, James J. 1935. Life Is Sacred. *Forum and Century Magazine* 1: 333–34.

Wanner, Jay G. 1933. The Privilege of Death. *Colorado Medicine* 30: 71–72.

Williams, Charles B. 1894. Euthanasia. *Medical and Surgical Report* 70: 909–11.

Williamson, William P. 1966. Life or Death—Whose Decision? *J.A.M.A.* 197: 793–95.

Wilson, Sir Robert. 1896. A Medico-Literary Causerie Euthanasia. *Practitioner* 56: 631–35.

Wolbarst, Abraham L. 1935. The Right to Die, A Debate: Part I, Legalize Euthanasia. *Forum and Century Magazine* 1: 330–32.

———. 1939. The Doctor Looks at Euthanasia. *Medical Record* 1: 681.

76

Carl F. H. Marx

From "Medical Euthanasia," trans. Walter Cane

Reprinted in abridged form with permission of the editor from Carl F. H. Marx, "Medical Euthanasia" (1826), translated from the German by Walter Cane, *Journal of the History of Medicine and Allied Sciences,* vol. 7, 1952, pp. 404–407, 410–413, 416.

Since death, which cannot be exorcised by any means, does not befall us in one assault but proceeds gradually and by certain steps, one following the other, it may be asked what can be done so the passing from life may be gentle and bearable. Why should not man, with his intellect mastering so many problems, find and produce some skilful contrivance for the care of the dying? Indeed the philosophers and the priests have much to offer, both in teaching and in comforting, with which to remove fear of future death from the living and to stretch out and to strengthen hope for a life beyond to the dying; the physician, on the other hand, who is present at the greatest peril to, and crisis of, life is the best judge as to when illness turns for the worse, and he is a continuous observer of his patient's ailment. He is not expected to have a remedy for death but for skilful alleviation of suffering, and he should know how to apply it where any hope has departed. This is that science, called euthanasia, which checks oppressing features of illness, relieves pain, and renders the supreme and inescapable hour a most peaceful one. To this aim our greatest efforts should be devoted, as was urged by that great Englishman who said:

Again, to go a little further; I esteem it likewise to be clearly the office of a physician, not only to restore health, but also to mitigate the pains and torments of diseases; and not only when such mitigation of pain, as of a dangerous symptom, helps and conduces to recovery; but also when, all hope of recovery being gone, it serves only to make a fair and easy passage from life. For it is no small felicity which Augustus Caesar was wont so earnestly to pray for, that same Euthanasia; which likewise was observed in the death of Antoninus Pius, which was not so much like death as like falling into a deep and pleasant sleep. . . . But in our times, the physicians make a kind of scruple and religion to stay with the patient after he is given up. Whereas in my judgment, if they would not be wanting to their office, and indeed to humanity, they ought both to acquire the skill and to bestow the attention whereby the dying may pass more easily and quietly out of life. This part I call the inquiry concerning *"outward euthanasia,"* or the easy dying of the body (to distinguish it from that Euthanasia which regards the preparation of the soul); and set it down among the desiderata.[1]

This subject does not seem to have been thoroughly studied at all up to the present time. Most physicians, once they see the expected result of their treatment to be wanting, and once they are convinced of the hopelessness of the patient's case, start to lose interest themselves, thinking they have all but discharged their duties if they have made ample use of the therapeutic means, believing they are dealing with a disease, not with a human being. Those very few, indeed, whom God has given a nobler heart will just then, with no shining ray of hope remaining, consider it their more lofty duty to lay to peaceful rest a life they can no longer save. Accordingly they will extend their energy and their affection, they will follow each successive turn of events, they will apply palliatives wherever they can, and with an all-caring heart they will put themselves in readiness for the great event, so that the last breath of passing may be light and not dreadful to those left behind.

There are three points on which the doctor's efforts to discharge this sacred duty can be observed: first, that he by every means possible alleviates the patient's condition through foresight and guidance; second, that he avoids and removes everything that might increase the patient's pain and suffering; third, that he cheers the patient's soul and mind with gracious and convincing comfort. In the fourth place may be added consideration of objects and of persons that such care embraces. To follow this too literally and to write down just what should be done in any particular case would be unending and fruitless labor. Nor will such a thing be expected from this paper, limited in its scope as it is. However, points of general interest and those constituting in a way the main subject of this treatise, those to develop in a comprehensive manner seems to be the guiding principle of this study. May the reading of this paper fall on fertile ground.

For aiding the condition of a hopelessly afflicted patient, whatever can possibly be done through the doctor's foresight is best of all carried out by attendants and by properly trained nurses if they are considerate, watchful, quiet, clean, free of prejudice toward people, and if they follow, and adhere to, the doctor's orders with greatest obedience. (For training and obtaining such kind of people an institution with funds providing them with old-age insurance is needed. If only Professor

Mai of Heidelberg could find followers of his example! A few years ago he gave free courses for married and unmarried women in which he taught clearly how those to whom the care of the sick is entrusted should deport themselves, and the expenditures for the undertaking were met by Amalia, Duchess of Baden. But the whole project died later on, together with the venerable old gentleman.) Indeed any people who move about the patient and give him a helping hand at his bedside, friends, domestic help, and relatives, should be required to be quiet and silent. Furthermore, care should be taken that no news is told him about any misfortune, danger, or death; not many people should be admitted just to see him lest those persons in their obtrusiveness cause noise and stir. For this reason even the doctor will not enter too often: but all should deport themselves in such a manner that the patient feels affectionate attention from human beings, and that he gains the conviction of being best cared for by them.

What would be more desirable than pure and fresh air in a secluded room? Therefore as often as is possible in view of the kind of illness, site of sickroom, and position of bed as to doors and windows, the air should be purified and renewed or, if this is less permissible, refreshed with fumigating agents obtained through the doctor's prescription. Whatever can contaminate or deteriorate the air should be moved far out of the sickroom, and the greatest cleanliness should be observed within and around the bed. Who does not see the importance of this in cases of stool incontinence, excessive diarrhea, of ample secretion of pus or of purulent matter? For that purpose much is accomplished with beds whose mattresses consist of small sections which can be easily pulled out and others put in their places.

A suitable and comfortable position of the patient in bed will offer greatest relief, particularly where parts are swollen and painful, such as in hydrops, especially in hydrothorax, after serious amputations, or when bedsores tend to deepen. Among the many beds designed for this purpose which have been recommended here and there, like recently in England,[2] one is worth

remembering that is in use for hydrothorax in the Karlsruhe Military Hospital. This can be raised and lowered at its head and foot ends by straps attached to a bedtable.

Bedsores, often the most vicious and almost unbearable affliction of these patients, will be obviated without much difficulty if greatest cleanliness is observed and if bedsheet folds are avoided which is customarily done by the use of thin bedsheets made of buckskin. The physician's alertness must be directed toward suspecting such afflictions in any protracted illness. For those patients may be already deprived of their sense of feeling, may suffer from numbness and stupor, may be seized by paralysis of their limbs, may rarely raise their voice, rarely complain. The doctor will with his own eyes repeatedly search for bedsores. For the same reason he will, as a matter of routine, also go over the patient's dry tongue and pharynx and will moisten them.

It is easily apparent what can be accomplished by administration of medicines where there is no room for the preservation of life or for the restitution of health. What good will it do the incurable patient to apply dangerous and dubious therapeutic measures? The entire plan of treatment will here confine itself within "symptomatic and palliative indication." . . .

In the second place the serious and important question arises: Where it appears that a slight chance to save a life depends on the surgical knife, should the patient undergo the hazards of a questionable "operation"? By no means can it be denied, and every day's experience proves it, that occasionally, under most unfavorable conditions of physical strength, a life has been saved and extended only by performing a paracentesis, a lithotomy, herniotomy, amputation, or trepanation. But on the other hand, just as many, who with equanimity and with greatest patience submitted to the surgeon's incision, died under excruciating pain either right under his eyes or a few days later. Who on earth whose mind is open to any sense of mercy does not shrink from such a sight where the most cruel operation is performed even when one may recognize approaching death from the limbs and from the face? Indeed those surgeons

who for mankind's and for science's sake, without any thought of themselves, hesitatingly enter the uncertain path of experimentation should imprint into their minds the words of Bichat: "Those operations are dreadful therapeutic measures where assurance of retarding fatal outcome can be bought only at the risk of precipitating it. Successes are interspersed with failures, and the real results are at times only cruel surgical exploits. The virtue to stay away from those operations should be rated higher than the virtue to perform them well; and if there is any doubt as to their indication it is a wise move not to go ahead."[3] Particularly where a local lesion is the result of generalized humoral disintegration, and where even by undertaking surgery little hope remains as to recovery, the experienced physician should apply himself much rather to euthanasia than to surgery.

Now, however, let us approach that task of the physician which is less concerned with dispensing medicines than with administering some kind of higher comfort. Whoever refuses his part in this duty and assigns it solely to priests deprives himself of the most noble and rewarding aspect of his work. Where the priest, administering the sacraments, comes to the bedside to soothe the longing soul with the last solace of religion and of comfort, who will not see the patient's deep shock when he faces this quasi-harbinger of death? The physician, on the other hand, to whose sight the patient's eyes are accustomed, from whose hand he is used to receive relief in his misery, from whose lips he is used to derive hope for the future, whose entrance is always expected and desired, can even in utter despair speak out freely what no one else may be permitted to mention. Take, for instance, the writing of a will, often desired by the family who yet do not dare to ask this of the patient for fear of upsetting him with thoughts about his estate. Every single person should be aware of this duty while enjoying good health and full strength so he can at all times say: "I am ready for death, hence I may enjoy life."[4] But where a will has been neglected, no one is more fitted than the doctor to remind his patient of this fact. For with encouragement and with promise he will bring spirit to the dejected, hope to the fearful, confidence to the despairing. Likewise he may tell him how often other people have recovered from more serious illness, or how many effective medicines for aid and support are still available, or he may cheer up his patient's mind in many ways, holding out the prospect of a bluer sky, of fairer weather, and even of a trip to hot and medicinal springs.

Furthermore, when all hope is gone for the patient and when death draws nearer and nearer, the doctor will not desist from his efforts to help. As he knows from experience how to alleviate the supreme anguish of the patient's mind by conferring confidence to the dying about the safe and secure future of those to be left behind, his wife, his children, his dearest stakes in life, he will now put forth his best efforts in this kind of comforting. Likewise, he will assure the doubtful and agitated of an honorable funeral and of a not-too-hasty interment. Finally, as a truthful interpreter of nature, he will relieve the troubled from his fear of complete extinction by giving him hope of immortality and of everlasting life of the souls. "Don't shrink away from that day as if it were the last one, for it is the birthday of eternity."[5] Since nothing of earthly matter is destroyed, why assume extinction of the mind, partaker of the divine spirit? This theory is not only compatible with our inborn desire for fairness and truthfulness, it is based also on the unshakably firm conviction of the wisest men. The more he who administers this comfort is a noble-minded man himself and irreproachable and blameless in life and esteemed by his patient for his skill, his devotion, and his effort, the more likely he will succeed in reassuring his patient's mind.

At the approach of the last moments care should be taken that more and more silence and quietness is maintained around the bedside and that anything unpleasant is removed from the eyes of the departing. All of the dearest ones, if they can bear staying with him, should with poise, their grief concealed, endure the final sigh. Wrong indeed is the opinion of those who claim that the presence of the dearest ones makes the passing harder. Where there is love, life is sweet and death is not bitter. Thus it is related that Caesar Augustus passed away calmly under Livia's kisses. The hearing in particular, last of the senses to abandon the dying, should not be blotted out with noise, nor with lamentation, nor with the mournful sound of funeral songs. It should much rather be soothed and lulled to sleep with sweet chords from harps and flutes, unless deep silence is preferred. There is a custom of cruel people who deafen the ears of the departing even with howling and with the shrill din of trumpets and of metal tools.

Now, when on first inspection death has apparently arrived, as shown by the cooling off of the body, cessation of respiration and of the heart beat, the duty toward the deceased is not yet fulfilled. Instances are known where individuals at that stage, after cessation of all motor function, have perceived over a number of hours everything that took place around them. "For this is peculiar to all of us mortals, born to live through the strangest adversities, that we must not take anything for granted about man, not even his death."[6]

It is wise, therefore, to see to it that the deceased is not taken out of the natural warmth of his bed, that his nose, his mouth, or eyes are not closed as is indiscriminately being done, nor should his face be turned upward, nor should he be placed on a straw tick, nor on the bare floor. He should much rather quietly remain either in his house or in a public building designed for this purpose, and he should be guarded by attentive and watchful persons until it becomes evident that the abdomen is swollen, the intercostal muscles greenish, the privates dark, the cornea cloudy and full of phlegm, the lips and the tips of fingers and toes dry and blackish, the nails bluish, the skin loose, the expression of face and mouth changed and distorted. Then it will be clear that, with all ties to any spiritual life finally severed, there is no room for hope or, for that matter, for fear.

In the fourth and last place the doctor's task in providing euthanasia concerns his duty to pay attention to the speed of progression of the disease process, to the kind of illness, and to the patient with regard to temperament and age group.

The speed of progression of the disease process is certainly of great importance, in order to find out, if at all, just when the task should be fulfilled. This will generally be the case when there is no definite trace left of nature's own healing power or of the value of therapeutic agents, or when neither of them seems to promise any help. It behooves the intelligent and foreseeing neither to come to any rash conclusion in this matter nor to divulge such to the family or to those who remain at the patient's bedside. For we are subject to human nature, and we don't know yet the whole medical armamentarium, and it is altogether better to wait for future developments in such a case and to think of remedies against them than to pronounce something for certain that also may take a different course of events. "As for the patient, as long as there is life, there is hope."[7]

It is therefore the physician's duty to make an effort to extend the span of life in every way, and least of all should he be permitted, prompted either by other people's requests or by his own sense of mercy, to end the patient's pitiful condition by purposely and deliberately hastening death. How can it be permitted that he who is by law required to preserve life be the originator of, or partner in, its destruction? This would be both against religion and against utterances of the wisest men. "Pythagoras forbids that you desert your stand and post in life without orders from the supreme commander which means God."[8] . . .

When the physician has thus become adept in the whole knowledge of this art in medicine, he may be in good and cheerful mood for he may some day expect a life service from others. To the best of his ability he has undertaken to administer euthanasia; athanasia[9] he is unable to give.

Notes

1. Bacon. *Advancement of Science,* IV, 2.

2. *Edinburgh Med. Surg. J.,* 1820, *16,* 296.

3. Bichat. *Oeuvres Chirurgicales.* Paris, 1798, I:8, p. 28.

4. Seneca. *Letters to Lucilius,* LXI.

5. *Ibid.,* CII.

6. Pliny. *Natural History,* Book VII, Chap. LII.

7. Cicero. *Letters to Atticus,* IX, 10.

8. Cicero. *Cato Major, An Essay on Old Age,* XX.

9. Greek, meaning "immortality." (W.C.)

77

Voluntary Euthanasia: Debate in the House of Lords (1936)

Reprinted with permission of the publisher from the *British Medical Journal*, vol. 2, 1936, pp. 1232–1234.

[Editors' Note: On November 4, 1936, Lord Ponsonby introduced a bill into the House of Lords to legalize, under certain conditions, the administration of euthanasia to patients requesting it who suffered from an illness that was fatal, incurable, and the cause of great pain. The bill specified that such a patient must be over 21, must be of sound mind, must have his petition witnessed by two people, and must submit the petition to a euthanasia referee appointed by the minister of health together with certificates signed by two physicians, one of whom must be the patient's doctor. Before the euthanasia petition can be acted on the patient must be interviewed by the referee, who makes sure that the patient understands his request and reviews the entire application. These conditions satisfied, a physician must administer the euthanasia.]

The House of Lords declined on December 1st, by 35 votes to 14, to give a second reading to the Voluntary Euthanasia (Legalization) Bill.

Lord Ponsonby, in moving the second reading of the Bill, first expressed regret that his place was not more worthily filled by the late Lord Moynihan. The latter's untimely death had not only deprived the medical profession and those who were his patients of a great friend and a notable figure, but also many, like himself, who had no professional contact with him but enjoyed his charming intercourse, which he was ever ready to extend to those to whose sympathy he responded. His absence that day was nothing short of a calamity for those who wished the promotion of the measure.

Continuing, Lord Ponsonby said that this was not a measure which was supported by a few cranks, but it had the strong support of a good many notable men and women of different professions and callings in our community. He knew that the medical profession was not in full agreement with the provisions of this Bill. But this was not exclusively a medical question; it was an ethical, social, and legal one, and he hoped that the House would not be swept away by the eloquence of Lord Horder and Lord Dawson if they opposed the Bill. It sought to legalize, under certain conditions, the administration of euthanasia to persons desiring it and who were suffering from illness of a fatal and incurable character involving severe pain.

Change in Public Opinion

There had in the last generation been a great change in public opinion in regard to suicide. The law still remained, however, and suicide was legally regarded as a common law misdemeanour. However, a more lenient view was taken, and coroners' juries brought in verdicts of "Suicide while of unsound mind," which might be true in a few cases, but in many more were not grounded on a certificate of insanity, and were not, strictly speaking, justified by the evidence. By some throughout the ages suicide had not been regarded as a criminal offence. When Father Damien went out to attend the lepers he knew that he was going to kill himself. Another striking example was Captain Oates in the Antarctic. Scott said that his act was the act of a brave man and an English gentleman. Lord Ponsonby, in conclusion, hoped their lordships would give the Bill a second reading.

Lord Denman, who seconded the motion, said he wished to remove misapprehension that might be felt outside the House, and to say that it was not proposed, for example, that imbeciles and mental defectives should be deprived of life, or that old people who had become a burden to their relatives should be done away with, and it was not proposed that any person who wished to do so should be allowed—still less encouraged—to commit suicide. It was proposed that persons who were suffering from an incurable and fatal disease should be allowed by law, if they so desired, to substitute for a slow and painful death a quick and painless one. In that respect we were more merciful in our treatment of animals than we were of human beings. It had been said that euthanasia was practised to-day. Doctors, with a dose of morphine or other powerful drug, eased their patient's death. As the law stood, if a doctor practised euthanasia he did so at the risk of criminal prosecution or of professional ruin. It was unfair and unjust that a doctor should be put in that invidious position for performing what was really an act of mercy.

Rejection Moved

Viscount Fitzalan moved the rejection of the Bill. He said that it contained complicated provisions for its administration. Notwithstanding the voluntary character of the Bill, if it became an Act he should be indeed sorry for the relatives of the patient, who would have a great responsibility thrust upon them. He should be still more sorry for the doctors who would have the responsibility of perpetrating the act, and he should be most sorry of all for the unfortunate patient, who would be exposed to a great mental anxiety while all the formalities laid down by the Bill were being prepared. Might he point out to the two noble lords in the House who were members of the medical profession that their duty was to cure and not to kill? He could not congratulate Lord Ponsonby on the title of his Bill. Instead of giving it a classical title he should have given it a good plain English one, understandable by the people, and called it what it was, a Bill to legalize murder and suicide.

Viscount Dawson's View

Viscount Dawson, who was heard with difficulty, said that compassion was not likely to be lost sight of among those who constantly witnessed human suffering. But he would not like an impression to go out that agonizing pain was a more frequent characteristic of disease than it really was. It would not be correct to say that most cases of cancer were characterized by agonizing pain. There was much more control of pain to-day than existed years ago. He agreed with Lord Fitzalan that the first thought and duty of the medical profession was not only to study the causes of disease, but to give the best of their minds—and they did give the best of their minds—to cure, and in the process of curing to assuage suffering in so far as it was compatible with that end. That was their main purpose. But they had to face the fact that there were diseases which were by their nature incurable. That did not mean that a disease was incurable at the outset, but diseases reached stages when the profession knew that a cure was not

possible. It was their duty and privilege, not being able to cure, to do what they could to make the passage between painful illness and inevitable end as gentle and soft as they could.

Medical opinion had changed on this question. Fifty years ago the profession concentrated on the maintenance of life, in spite of the nature of the illness and even sometimes the imminence of death. It was an accepted tradition that it was the duty of the medical man to continue the struggle for life right up to the end. That had changed. There had gradually crept into medical opinion, as there had into lay opinion, the feeling that one should make the act of dying more gentle and peaceful, even if it did involve curtailment of the length of life. That had become increasingly the custom; it was taken almost as something that was accepted. If they once admitted that they were going to curtail life by a single day they were granting the principle that they must look at life from the point of view of its quality rather than its quantity in such circumstances.

Steady Growth in the Idea of Mercy

There was no disharmony in this matter between the thoughts of the laity and the thoughts of the doctors. They saw a steady growth in the idea of mercy. They should leave thought to grow. There was a cautious but irresistible move to look at life and suffering from a more humane point of view. When a disease was incurable and the patient was carrying a great load of suffering their first course should be assuagement of pain, even if it did involve curtailment of life. The medical profession was a conservative profession, and had within it a tradition long established. This matter should be left to the gentle and slow growth of opinion among both the laity and the medical profession. A woman had an incurable disease and incomparable suffering for nine years, but throughout that time she continued to work and to maintain her family. Eventually, crushed by pain, she asked for kindly timely death to ease her. Was the submerging of her sufferings to be denied her because death might be accelerated by three or

four months? His own view would be that it should not. But there were no two people alike, and only her own doctor should decide whether her desire for death was something more than a passing effect of suffering.

Considerable changes in moral standards had taken place in the course of the years without any change in the statute law, and that was all to the good. There were many things which were much better evolved before the statute law tried to give them expression. He could not conceive a more intimate relation than that which existed between a patient mortally ill and the doctor. If the Act were passed this relationship would be destroyed. The very idea of the sick chamber being visited by officials, and the patient, struggling with a dire and tragic malady, being treated as if he were a case of insanity, was something so opposite from the attitude of the doctor that, far from permitting the general growth of euthanasia in cases of incurable illness, it would have the opposite effect. Doctors would hesitate to touch it. They would not like to introduce such an atmosphere into the sick chamber, and the law would not only remain nugatory, but would deter those who were carrying out a mission of mercy.

Principle and Compassion in Contention

The Archbishop of Canterbury said that to him this was a most difficult question, in which principle and compassion contended. It must be approached on the broad basis of the clear moral principle that no man was entitled voluntarily to take his own life. There must be some exceptions to even that principle, but it was one thing to admit exceptions to that principle and another to give public statutory authority to it. They could not dismiss from their minds the possibly unforeseen effects upon the public conscience of for the first time giving definite legal enactment to the principle that there were circumstances in which a man might for his own sake end his life. He doubted whether a man who was professedly wracked with pain was capable of making a sound moral judgment; and would not the procedure contemplated by the Bill inflict an almost intolerable strain, where the strain was sufficient already, when a man had to ask himself, for his own sake or that of those dear to him, whether he should avail himself of this legal provision? Moreover, they could not dismiss from their minds the possibility of pressure brought by relations from other than motives of compassion.

He could not accept the view of those who contended that the duration of pain must needs be accepted as a divine appointment or means of moral discipline that no man may rightly decline. The whole, increasing, marvellous, and far-reaching use of anaesthetics pointed entirely the other way. But if there were extreme cases where it was morally legitimate to shorten a life of pain it should be left to the medical profession, exercising its intimate and responsible judgement rather than be dragged into the open and regulated by elaborate legal procedure. He would trust the honour and judgement of the medical profession, and would support the rejection of the Bill.

Lord Horder on the Doctor's Reference

Lord Horder, who spoke from the cross benches, said he did not think this was a matter on which the medical profession should be asked to give a definite lead. Indeed, he was sorry that medical men had joined in this movement and had associated themselves with propaganda before the Bill came before the House. Most doctors were very sympathetic towards the modern efforts to secure biological control before life began and while life lasted. But in the matter of putting an end to life, surely a new principle entered, and he submitted that that principle was outside the doctor's reference. If he might use the word, the doctor's reference was clear and generally accepted: it was to cure disease safely and quickly, and, if that ideal could not be achieved, then the doctor's duty must be to prolong life as long as might be, and to relieve pain both bodily and mental. The good doctor was quite aware of the distinction between prolonging life and prolonging the act of dying. The former came within his reference; the latter did not. He should regard with great concern any sanction which led to a different orientation with respect to the

doctor's function, and yet it was difficult to see how such a reorientation could be avoided if the Bill became law.

It was true that the Bill provided that the act of euthanasia should be administered by other than the customary practitioner attending the patient; but was not that very fact a serious one in itself? If it was intended to replace the intimate relationship that existed in the majority of cases between doctor and patient, especially towards the close of life, by the introduction of two, or it might be more, strangers from Whitehall, was that substitution going to be in the patient's interest? The relationship between doctor and patient, when the patient was once assured of it, kept his moral intact. Noble lords had said in a general sense what were the cases in which legalized euthanasia might be sought. He (Lord Horder) suggested that the criteria which justified a decision to terminate life would be found to be extremely difficult to establish for particular patients, so difficult indeed that he should himself hesitate to undertake such great responsibilities as were placed upon the referee.

"Incurability" of Disease

The incurability of a disease was never more than an estimate based upon experience. If the Bill became law it would be in the main to cases of cancer that it would apply, for it was almost only in cancer cases that the criteria laid down could be thought to be fully established. Although it was common knowledge that the essential causes of cancer still eluded them, there were cases to-day of persons suffering from that disease who were living free from pain and who would not have been living ten years ago, and this was the result of advances made in treatment. That being so, and with the prospect of further advances in the near future, the criteria of fatality, if not of curability, would become more and not less difficult to establish as time went on. We never had so many means of relieving pain as we had to-day, and those means might be expected to increase. The Bill made soundness of mind essential to the administration of euthanasia. It was not that the mind of the patient suffering from a lethal illness was unsound—in

the legal sense—but that the patient's mind was variable, with no certainty of purpose. The mental clarity with which those who supported this Bill viewed the situation had no counterpart in the alternating moods and confused judgement of the sick man.

Another possibility must be envisaged if the Bill became law, one which, he supposed, was quite unintended. Would not some persons who were afflicted with illness misinterpret the feelings of their friends and consider that they should avail themselves of the permission to end their lives? The two extremes of dying and being killed did not exhaust the possibilities for the stricken patient, because there was a middle course created by a kindly and skilful doctor who gave assistance to an equally kindly Nature, and that was what was at present implicit in the patient's question: "You'll stand by me, won't you?" and the doctor's assurance: "Yes; trust me."

The Marquess of Crewe said that the Bill before them would throw severe responsibilities on medical men. He could not vote in favour of the Bill. The Bishop of Norwich said that the elaborate safeguards which occupied so great a portion of the Bill showed a certain hesitation on the part of its supporters as to whether they had a right solution to the question. As Lord Dawson had said, this matter should be left to the growth of opinion within the medical profession. Members of the profession always shared with one another all that they had discovered, and there was no profession in which public opinion grew more securely.

The Earl of Listowel said that it was an interesting fact that both Lord Dawson and the Archbishop of Canterbury were in favour of taking human life in certain circumstances, while Lord Horder expressed the view that in certain cases the doctor must act on his own initiative in terminating suffering. That, however, would put upon the doctor a far heavier responsibility than the Bill would place upon him. He was being asked to use his own initiative in performing an action which was at present contrary to law, and to risk being turned out of his profession, in order to satisfy his moral conscience. That was the gravest responsibility that could be imposed upon him.

Bill Psychologically Misconceived

The Earl of Crawford said that the Bill was so misconceived from the psychological point of view that it would cause more suffering than it would ease. He contemplated with horror the strife and dissention its provisions would bring into family life, and with profound distress the unconscious pressure that would be placed on a sick man.

Viscount Gage said that so far as the main principle of the Bill was concerned the Government would leave it to the free vote of the House. If, however, it received a second reading with the present congested state of business the Government could not give any definite guarantee of what facilities could be afforded the measure in the House of Commons.

The House divided, and, as stated above, the Bill was rejected by 35 votes to 14.

78

Pope Pius XII
The Prolongation of Life

Reprinted with permission of the editors from *The Pope Speaks,* vol. 4, 1958, pp. 393–398.

Dr. Bruno Haid, chief of the anesthesia section at the surgery clinic of the University of Innsbruck, has submitted to Us three questions on medical morals treating the subject known as "resuscitation" [*la réanimation*].

We are pleased, gentlemen, to grant this request, which shows your great awareness of professional duties, and your will to solve in the light of the principles of the Gospel the delicate problems that confront you.

Problems of Anesthesiology

According to Dr. Haid's statement, modern anesthesiology deals not only with problems of analgesia and anesthesia properly so-called, but also with those of "resuscitation." This is the name given in medicine, and especially in anesthesiology, to the technique which makes possible the remedying of certain occurrences, which seriously threaten human life, especially asphyxia, which formerly, when modern anesthetizing equipment was not yet available, would stop the heart-beat and bring about death in a few minutes. The task of the anesthesiologist has therefore extended to acute respiratory difficulties, provoked by strangulation or by open wounds of the chest. The anesthesiologist intervenes to prevent asphyxia resulting from the internal obstruction of breathing passages by the contents of the stomach or by drowning, to remedy total or partial respiratory paralysis in cases of serious tetanus, of poliomyelitis, of poisoning by gas, sedatives, or alcoholic intoxication, or even in cases of paralysis of the central respiratory apparatus caused by serious trauma of the brain.

The Practice of "Resuscitation"

In the practice of resuscitation and in the treatment of persons who have suffered headwounds, and sometimes in the case of persons who have undergone brain surgery or of those who have suffered trauma of the brain through anoxia and remain in a state of deep unconsciousness, there arise a number of questions that concern medical morality and involve the principles of the philosophy of nature even more than those of analgesia.

It happens at times—as in the aforementioned cases of accidents and illnesses, the treatment of which offers reasonable hope of success—that the anesthesiologist can improve the general condition of patients who suffer from a serious lesion of the brain and whose situation at first might seem desperate. He restores breathing either through manual intervention or with the help of special instruments, clears the breathing passages, and provides for the artificial feeding of the patient.

Thanks to this treatment, and especially through the administration of oxygen by means of artificial respiration, a failing blood circulation picks up again and the appearance of the patient improves, sometimes very quickly, to such an extent that the anesthesiologist himself, or any other doctor who, trusting his experience, would have given up all hope, maintains a slight hope that spontaneous breathing will be restored. The family usually considers this improvement an astonishing result and is grateful to the doctor.

If the lesion of the brain is so serious that the patient will very probably, and even most certainly, not survive, the anesthesiologist is then led to ask himself the distressing question as to the value and meaning of the resuscitation processes. As an immediate measure he will apply artificial respiration by intubation and by aspiration of the respiratory tract; he is then in a safer position and has more time to decide what further must be done. But he can find himself in a delicate position, if the family considers that the efforts he has taken are improper and opposes them. In most cases this situation arises, not at the beginning of resuscitation attempts, but when the patient's condition, after a slight improvement at first, remains stationary and it becomes clear that only automatic artificial respiration is keeping him alive. The question then arises if one must, or if one can, continue the resuscitation process despite the fact that the soul may already have left the body.

The solution to this problem, already difficult in itself, becomes even more difficult when the family—themselves Catholic perhaps—insist that the doctor in charge, especially the anesthesiologist, remove the artificial respiration apparatus in order to allow the patient, who is already virtually dead, to pass away in peace.

A Fundamental Problem

Out of this situation there arises a question that is fundamental from the point of view of religion and the philosophy of nature. When, according to Christian faith, has death occurred in patients on whom modern methods of resuscitation have been used? Is Extreme Unction valid, at least as long as one can perceive heartbeats, even if the vital functions properly so-called have already disappeared, and if life depends only on the functioning of the artificial-respiration apparatus?

Three Questions

The problems that arise in the modern practice of resuscitation can therefore be formulated in three questions:

First, does one have the right, or is one even under the obligation, to use modern artificial-respiration equipment in all cases, even those which, in the doctor's judgment, are completely hopeless?

Second, does one have the right, or is one under obligation, to remove the artificial-respiration apparatus when, after several days, the state of deep unconsciousness does not improve if, when it is removed, blood circulation will stop within a few minutes? What must be done in this case if the family of the patient, who has already received the last sacraments, urges the doctor to remove the apparatus? Is Extreme Unction still valid at this time?

Third, must a patient plunged into unconsciousness through central paralysis, but whose life—that is to say, blood circulation—is maintained through artificial respiration, and in whom there is no improvement after several days, be considered "de facto" or even "de jure" dead? Must one not wait for blood circulation to stop, in spite of the artificial respiration, before considering him dead?

Basic Principles

We shall willingly answer these three questions. But before examining them We would like to set forth the principles that will allow formulation of the answer.

Natural reason and Christian morals say that man (and whoever is entrusted with the task of taking care of his fellowman) has the right and the duty in case of serious illness to take the necessary treatment for the preservation of life and health. This duty that one has toward himself, toward God, toward the human community, and in most cases toward certain determined persons, derives from well ordered charity, from submission to the Creator, from social justice and even from strict justice, as well as from devotion toward one's family.

But normally one is held to use only ordinary means—according to circumstances of persons, places, times and culture—that is to say, means that do not involve any grave burden for oneself or another. A more strict obligation would be too burdensome for most men and would render the attainment of the higher, more important good too difficult. Life, health, all temporal activities are in fact subordinated to spiritual ends. On the other hand, one is not forbidden to take more than the strictly necessary steps to preserve life and health, as long as he does not fail in some more serious duty.

Administration of the Sacraments

Where the administration of sacraments to an unconscious man is concerned, the answer is drawn from the doctrine and practice of the Church which, for its part, follows the Lord's will as its rule of action. Sacraments are meant, by virtue of divine institution, for men of this world who are in the course of their earthly life, and, except for baptism itself, presuppose prior baptism of the recipient. He who is not a man, who is not yet a man, or is no longer a man, cannot receive the sacraments. Furthermore, if someone expresses his refusal, the sacraments cannot be administered to him against his will. God compels no one to accept sacramental grace.

When it is not known whether a person fulfills the necessary conditions for valid reception of the sacraments, an effort must be made to solve the doubt. If this effort fails, the sacrament will be conferred under at least a tacit condition (with the phrase "Si capas est," "If you are capable,"—which is the broadest condition). Sacraments are instituted by Christ for men in order to save their souls. Therefore, in cases of extreme necessity, the Church tries extreme solutions in order to give man sacramental grace and assistance.

The Fact of Death

The question of the fact of death and that of verifying the fact itself ("de facto") or its legal authenticity ("de jure") have, because of their consequences, even in the field of morals and of religion, an even greater importance. What We have just said about the presupposed essential elements for the valid reception of a sacrament has shown this. But the importance of the question extends also to effects in matters of inheritance, marriage and matrimonial processes, benefices (vacancy of a benefice), and to many other questions of private and social life.

It remains for the doctor, and especially the anesthesiologist, to give a clear and precise definition of "death" and the "moment of death" of a patient who passes away in a state of unconsciousness. Here one can accept the usual concept of complete and final separation of the soul from the body; but in practice one must take into account the lack of precision of the terms "body" and "separation." One can put aside the possibility of a person being buried alive, for removal of the artificial respiration apparatus must necessarily bring about stoppage of blood circulation and therefore death within a few minutes.

In case of insoluble doubt, one can resort to presumptions of law and of fact. In general, it will be necessary to presume that life remains, because there is involved here a fundamental right received from the Creator, and it is necessary to prove with certainty that it has been lost.

We shall now pass to the solution of the particular questions.

A Doctor's Rights and Duties

1. Does the anesthesiologist have the right, or is he bound, in all cases of deep unconsciousness, even in those that are considered to be completely hopeless in the opinion of the competent doctor, to use modern artificial respiration apparatus even against the will of the family?

In ordinary cases one will grant that the anesthesiologist has the right to act in this manner, but he is not bound to do so, unless this becomes the only way of fulfilling another certain moral duty.

The rights and duties of the doctor are correlative to those of the patient.

The doctor, in fact, has no separate or independent right where the patient is concerned. In general he can take action only if the patient explicitly or implicitly, directly or indirectly, gives him permission. The technique of resuscitation which concerns us here does not contain anything immoral in itself. Therefore the patient, if he were capable of making a personal decision, could lawfully use it and, consequently, give the doctor permission to use it. On the other hand, since these forms of treatment go beyond the ordinary means to which one is bound, it cannot be held that there is an obligation to use them nor, consequently, that one is bound to give the doctor permission to use them.

The rights and duties of the family depend in general upon the presumed will of the unconscious patient if he is of age and "sui juris." Where the proper and independent duty of the family is concerned, they are usually bound only to the use of ordinary means.

Consequently, if it appears that the attempt at resuscitation constitutes in reality such a burden for the family that one cannot in all conscience impose it upon them, they can lawfully insist that the doctor should discontinue these attempts, and the doctor can lawfully comply. There is not involved here a case of direct disposal of the life of the patient, nor of euthanasia in any way: this would never be licit. Even when it causes the arrest of circulation, the interruption of attempts at resuscitation is never more than an indirect cause of the cessation of life, and one must apply in this case the principle of double effect and of "voluntarium in causa."

Extreme Unction

2. We have, therefore, already answered the second question in essence: "Can the doctor remove the artificial respiration apparatus before the blood circulation has come to a complete stop? Can he do this, at least, when the patient has already received Extreme Unction? Is this Extreme Unction valid when it is administered at the moment when circulation ceases, or even after?"

We must give an affirmative answer to the first part of this question, as We have already explained. If Extreme Unction has not yet been administered, one must seek to prolong respiration until this has been done. But as far as concerns the validity of Extreme Unction at the moment when blood circulation stops completely or even after this moment, it is impossible to answer "yes" or "no."

If, as in the opinion of doctors, this complete cessation of circulation means a sure separation of the soul from the body, even if particular organs go on functioning, Extreme Unction would certainly not be valid, for the recipient would certainly not be a man anymore. And this is an indispensable condition for the reception of the sacraments.

If, on the other hand, doctors are of the opinion that the separation of the soul from the body is doubtful, and that this doubt cannot be solved, the validity of Extreme Unction is also doubtful. But, applying her usual rules: "The sacraments are for men" and "In case of extreme necessity one tries extreme measures," the Church allows the sacrament to be administered conditionally in respect to the sacramental sign.

When Is One "Dead"?

3. "When the blood circulation and the life of a patient who is deeply unconscious because of a central paralysis are maintained only through artificial respiration, and no improvement is noted after a few days, at what time does the Catholic Church consider the patient "dead," or when must he be declared dead according to natural law (questions 'de facto' and 'de jure')?"

(Has death already occurred after grave trauma of the brain, which has provoked deep unconsciousness and central breathing paralysis, the fatal consequences of which have nevertheless been retarded by artificial respiration? Or does it occur, according to the present opinion of doctors, only when there is complete arrest of circulation despite prolonged artificial respiration?)

Where the verification of the fact in particular cases is concerned, the answer cannot be deduced from any religious and moral principle and, under this aspect, does not fall within the competence of the Church. Until an answer can be given, the question must remain open. But considerations of a general nature allow us to believe that human life continues for as long as its vital functions—distinguished from the simple life of organs—manifest themselves spontaneously or even with the help of artificial processes. A great number of these cases are the object of insoluble doubt, and must be dealt with according to the presumptions of law and of fact of which We have spoken.

May these explanations guide you and enlighten you when you must solve delicate questions arising in the practice of your profession. As a token of divine favors which We call upon you and all those who are dear to you, We heartily grant you Our Apostolic Blessing.

79

A Definition of Irreversible Coma: Report of the Ad Hoc Committee of the Harvard Medical School to Examine the Definition of Brain Death

Reprinted with permission of the editors from the *Journal of the American Medical Association*, vol. 205, 1968, pp. 337–340. Copyright © 1968, American Medical Association.

Our primary purpose is to define irreversible coma as a new criterion for death. There are two reasons why there is need for a definition: (1) Improvements in resuscitative and supportive measures have led to increased efforts to save those who are desperately injured. Sometimes these efforts have only partial success so that the result is an individual whose heart continues to beat but whose brain is irreversibly damaged. The burden is great on patients who suffer permanent loss of intellect, on their families, on the hospitals, and on those in need of hospital beds already occupied by these comatose patients. (2) Obsolete criteria for the definition of death can lead to controversy in obtaining organs for transplantation.

Irreversible coma has many causes, but *we are concerned here only with those comatose individuals who have no discernible central nervous system activity.* If the characteristics can be defined in satisfactory terms, translatable into action—and we believe this is possible—then several problems will either disappear or will become more readily soluble.

More than medical problems are present. There are moral, ethical, religious, and legal issues. Adequate definition here will prepare the way for better insight into all of these matters as well as for better law than is currently applicable.

Characteristics of Irreversible Coma

An organ, brain or other, that no longer functions and has no possibility of functioning again is for all practical purposes dead. Our first problem is to determine the characteristics of a *permanently* nonfunctioning brain.

A patient in this state appears to be in deep coma. The condition can be satisfactorily diagnosed by points 1, 2, and 3 to follow. The electroencephalogram (point 4) provides confirmatory data, and when available it should be utilized. In situations where for one reason or another electroencephalographic monitoring is not available, the absence of cerebral function has to be determined by purely clinical signs, to be described, or by absence of circulation as judged by standstill of blood in the retinal vessels, or by absence of cardiac activity.

Unreceptivity and Unresponsitivity

There is a total unawareness to externally applied stimuli and inner need and complete unresponsiveness—our definition of irreversible coma. Even the most intensely painful stimuli evoke no vocal or other response, not even a groan, withdrawal of a limb, or quickening of respiration.

No Movements or Breathing

Observations covering a period of at least one hour by physicians is adequate to satisfy the criteria of no spontaneous muscular movements or spontaneous respiration or response to stimuli such as pain, touch, sound, or light. After the patient is on a mechanical respirator, the total absence of spontaneous breathing may be established by turning off the respirator for three minutes and observing whether there is any effort on the part of the subject to breathe spontaneously. (The respirator may be turned off for this time provided that at the start of the trial period the patient's carbon dioxide tension is within the normal range, and provided also that the patient had been breathing room air for at least 10 minutes prior to the trial.)

No Reflexes

Irreversible coma with abolition of central nervous system activity is evidenced in part by the absence of elicitable reflexes. The pupil will be fixed and dilated and will not respond to a direct source of bright light. Since the establishment of a fixed, dilated pupil is clear-cut in clinical practice, there should be no uncertainty as to its presence. Ocular movement (to head turning and to irrigation of the ears with ice water) and blinking are absent. There is no evidence of postural activity (decerebrate or other). Swallowing, yawning, vocalization are in abeyance. Corneal and pharyngeal reflexes are absent.

As a rule the stretch of tendon reflexes cannot be elicited: ie, tapping the tendons of the biceps, triceps, and pronator muscles, quadriceps and gastrocnemius muscles with the reflex hammer elicits no contraction of the respective muscles. Plantar or noxious stimulation gives no response.

Flat Electroencephalogram

Of great confirmatory value is the flat or isoelectric EEG. We must assume that the electrodes have been properly applied, that the apparatus is functioning normally, and that the personnel in charge is competent. We consider it prudent to have one channel of the apparatus used for an electrocardiogram. This channel will monitor the ECG so that, if it appears in the electroencephalographic leads because of high resistance, it can be readily identified. It also establishes the presence of the active heart in the absence of the EEG. We recommend that another channel be used for a noncephalic lead. This will pick up space-borne or vibration-borne artifacts and identify them. The simplest form of such a monitoring noncephalic electrode has two leads over the dorsum of the hand, preferably the right hand, so the ECG will be minimal or absent. Since one of the requirements of this state is that there be no muscle activity, these two dorsal hand electrodes will not be bothered by muscle artifact. The apparatus should be run at standard gains $10\mu v/mm$, $50\mu v/5$ mm. Also it should be isoelectric at double this standard gain which is $5\mu v/mm$ or $25\mu v/5$ mm. At least ten full minutes of recording are desirable, but twice that would be better.

It is also suggested that the gains at some point be opened to their full amplitude for a brief period (5 to 100 seconds) to see what is going on. Usually in an intensive care unit artifacts will dominate the picture, but these are readily identifiable. There shall be no electroencephalographic response to noise or to pinch.

All of the above tests shall be repeated at least 24 hours later with no change.

The validity of such data as indications of irreversible cerebral damage depends on the exclusion of two conditions: hypothermia (temperature below 90 F [32.2 C] or central nervous system depressants, such as barbiturates.

Other Procedures

The patient's condition can be determined only by a physician. When the patient is hopelessly damaged as defined above, the family and all colleagues who have participated in major decisions concerning the patient, and all nurses involved, should be so informed. Death is to be declared and *then* the respirator turned off. The decision to do this and the responsibility for it are to be taken by the physician-in-charge, in consultation with one or more physicians who have been directly involved in the case. It is unsound and undesirable to force the family to make the decision.

Legal Commentary

The legal system of the United States is greatly in need of the kind of analysis and recommendations for medical procedures in cases of irreversible brain damage as described. At present, the law of the United States, in all 50 states and in the federal courts, treats the question of human death as a question of fact to be decided in every case. When any doubt exists, the courts seek medical expert testimony concerning the time of death of the particular individual involved. However, the law makes the assumption that the medical criteria for determining death are settled and not in doubt among physicians. Furthermore, the law assumes that the traditional method among physicians for determination of death is to ascertain the absence of all vital signs. To this extent, *Black's Law Dictionary* (fourth edition, 1951) defines death as

The cessation of life; the ceasing to exist; *defined by physicians* as a total stoppage of the circulation of the blood, and a cessation of the animal and vital functions consequent thereupon, such as respiration, pulsation, etc. [italics added].

In the few modern court decisions involving a definition of death, the courts have used the concept of the total cessation of all vital signs. Two cases are worthy of examination. Both involved the issue of which one of two persons died first.

In *Thomas vs. Anderson*, (96 Cal. App. 2d 371, 211 P 2d 478) a California District Court of Appeal in 1950 said, "In the instant case the question as to which of the two men died first was a question of fact for the determination of the trial court. . . ."

The appellate court cited and quoted in full the definition of death from *Black's Law Dictionary* and concluded,

". . . death occurs precisely when life ceases and does not occur until the heart stops beating and respiration ends. Death is not a continuous event and is an event that takes place at a precise time."

The other case is *Smith vs. Smith* (229 Ark, 579, 317 SW 2d 275) decided in 1958 by the Supreme Court of Arkansas. In this case the two people were husband and wife involved in an auto accident. The husband was found dead at the scene of the accident. The wife was taken to the hospital unconscious. It is alleged that she "remained in coma due to brain injury" and died at the hospital 17 days later. The petitioner in court tried to argue that the two people died simultaneously. The judge writing the opinion said the petition contained a "quite unusual and unique allegation." It was quoted as follows:

That the said Hugh Smith and his wife, Lucy Coleman Smith, were in an automobile accident on the 19th day of April, 1957, said accident being instantly fatal to each of them at the same time, although the doctors maintained every effort to revive and resuscitate said Lucy Coleman Smith until May 6th, 1957, when it was finally determined by the attending physicians that their hope of resuscitation and possible restoration of human life to the said Lucy Coleman Smith was entirely vain, and

That as a matter of modern medical science, your petitioner alleges and states, and will offer the Court competent proof that the said Hugh Smith, deceased, and said Lucy Coleman Smith, deceased, lost their power to will at the same instant, and that their demise as earthly human beings occurred at the same time in said automobile accident, neither of them ever regaining any consciousness whatsoever.

The court dismissed the petition as a *matter of law*. The court quoted *Black's* definition of death and concluded,

Admittedly, this condition did not exist, and as a matter of fact, it would be too much of a strain of credulity for us to believe any evidence offered to the effect that Mrs. Smith was dead, scientifically or otherwise, unless the conditions set out in the definition existed.

Later in the opinion the court said, "Likewise, we take judicial notice that one breathing, though unconscious, is not dead."

"Judicial notice" of this definition of death means that the court did not consider that definition open to serious controversy; it considered the question as settled in responsible scientific and medical circles. The judge thus makes proof of uncontroverted facts unnecessary so as to prevent prolonging the trial with unnecessary proof and also to prevent fraud being committed upon the court by quasi "scientists" being called into court to controvert settled scientific principles at a price. Here, the Arkansas Supreme Court considered the definition of death to be a settled, scientific, biological fact. It refused to consider the plaintiff's offer of evidence that "modern medical science" might say otherwise. In simplified form, the above is the state of the law in the United States concerning the definition of death.

In this report, however, we suggest that responsible medical opinion is ready to adopt new criteria for pronouncing death to have occurred in an individual sustaining irreversible coma as a result of permanent brain damage. If this position is adopted by the medical community, it can form the basis for change in the current legal concept of death. No statutory change in the law should be necessary since the law treats this question essentially as one of fact to be determined by physicians. The only circumstance in which it would be necessary that legislation be offered in the various states to define "death" by law would be in the event that great controversy were engendered surrounding the subject and physicians were unable to agree on the new medical criteria.

It is recommended as a part of these procedures that judgment of the existence of these criteria is solely a medical issue. It is suggested that the physician in charge of the patient consult with one or more other physicians directly involved in the case before the patient is declared dead on the basis of these criteria. In this way, the responsibility is shared over a wider range of medical opinion, thus providing an important degree of protection against later questions which might be raised about the particular case. It is further suggested that the decision to declare the person dead, and then to turn off the respirator, be made by physicians not involved in any later effort to transplant organs or tissue from the deceased individual. This is advisable in order to avoid any appearance of self-interest by the physicians involved.

It should be emphasized that we recommend the patient be declared dead before any effort is made to take him off a respirator, if he is then on a respirator. This declaration should not be delayed until he has been taken off the respirator and all artificially stimulated signs have ceased. The reason for this recommendation is that in our judgment it will provide a greater degree of legal protection to those involved. Otherwise, the physicians would be turning off the respirator on a person who is, under the present strict, technical application of the law, still alive.

Comment

Irreversible coma can have various causes: cardiac arrest; asphyxia with respiratory arrest; massive brain damage; intracranial lesions, neoplastic or vascular. It can be produced by other encephalographic states such as the metabolic derangements associated, for example, with uremia. Respiratory failure and impaired circulation underlie all of these conditions. They result in hypoxia and ischemia of the brain.

From ancient times down to the recent past it was clear that, when the respiration and heart stopped, the brain would die in a few minutes; so the obvious criterion of no heart beat as synonymous with death was sufficiently accurate. In those times the heart was considered to be the central organ of the body; it is not surprising that its failure marked the onset of death. This is no longer valid when modern resuscitative and supportive measures are used. These improved activities can now restore "life" as judged by the ancient standards of persistent respiration and continuing heart beat. This can be the case even when there is not the remotest possibility of an individual recovering consciousness following massive brain damage. In other situations "life" can be maintained only by means of artificial respiration and electrical stimulation of the heart beat, or in temporarily by-passing the heart, or, in conjunction with these things, reducing with cold the body's oxygen requirement.

In an address, "The Prolongation of Life," (1957),[1] Pope Pius XII raised many questions; some conclusions stand out: (1) In a deeply unconscious individual vital functions may be maintained over a prolonged period only by extraordinary means. Verification of the moment of death can be determined, if at all, only by a physician. Some have suggested that the moment of death is the moment when irreparable and overwhelming brain damage occurs. Pius XII acknowledged that it is not "within the competence of the Church" to determine this. (2) It is incumbent on the physician to take all reasonable, ordinary means of restoring the spontaneous vital functions and consciousness, and to employ such extraordinary means as are available to him to this end. It is not obligatory, however, to continue to use extraordinary means indefinitely in hopeless cases. "But normally one is held to use only ordinary means—according to circumstances of persons, places, times, and cultures—that is to say, means that do not involve any grave burden for oneself or another." It is the church's view that a time comes when resuscitative efforts should stop and death be unopposed.

Summary

The neurological impairment to which the terms "brain death syndrome" and "irreversible coma" have become attached indicates diffuse disease. Function is abolished at cerebral, brain-stem, and often spinal levels. This should be evident in all cases from clinical examination alone. Cerebral, cortical, and thalamic involvement are indicated by a complete absence of receptivity of all forms of sensory stimulation and a lack of response to stimuli and to inner need. The term "coma" is used to designate this state of unreceptivity and unresponsivity. But there is always coincident paralysis of brain-stem and basal ganglionic mechanisms as manifested by an abolition of all postural reflexes, including induced decerebrate postures; a complete paralysis of respiration; widely dilated, fixed pupils; paralysis of ocular movements; swallowing; phonation; face and tongue muscles. Involvement of spinal cord, which is less constant, is reflected usually in loss of tendon reflex and all flexor withdrawal or nocifensive reflexes. Of the brain-stem-spinal mechanisms which are conserved for a time, the vasomotor reflexes are the most persistent, and they are responsible in part for the paradoxical state of retained cardiovascular function, which is to some extent independent of nervous control, in the face of widespread disorder of cerebrum, brain stem, and spinal cord.

Neurological assessment gains in reliability if the aforementioned neurological signs persist over a period of time, with the additional safeguards that there is no accompanying hypothermia or evidence of drug intoxication. If either of the latter two conditions exist, interpretation of the neurological state should await the return of body temperature to normal level and elimination of the intoxicating agent. Under any other circumstances, repeated examinations over a period of 24 hours or longer should be required in order to obtain evidence of the irreversibility of the condition.

Notes

The Ad Hoc Committee includes Henry K. Beecher, MD, *chairman*; Raymond D. Adams, MD; A. Clifford Barger, MD; William J. Curran, LLM, SMHyg; Derek Denny-Brown, MD; Dana L. Farnsworth, MD; Jordi Folch-Pi, MD; Everett I. Mendelsohn, PhD; John P. Merrill, MD; Joseph Murray, MD; Ralph Potter, ThD; Robert Schwab, MD; and William Sweet, MD.
Reprint requests to Massachusetts General Hospital, Boston 02114 (Dr. Henry K. Beecher).

Reference

1. Pius XII: The Prolongation of Life, *Pope Speaks* 4:393–398 (No. 4) 1958 [Reprinted as Chapter 78 of this volume.]

80

John S. Ames III
An Act Relating to Certain Medical Treatment

Reprint of a Legislative Proposal in the Commonwealth of Massachusetts (1974).

[Editors' note: As this volume was in press, the California Natural Death Act was passed by the California legislature. We have included this unprecedented law in its entirety as an appendix (p. 665). Readers will note that the California legislation makes the living will binding; the Ames bill, if it had been approved, would not have had this effect.]

Be it enacted by the Senate and House of Representatives in General Court assembled, and by the authority of the same, as follows:

Section 1 The availability of medical technology does not eliminate the need for human choices regarding its use. This is especially true when a patient is irreversibly ill. The decision to cease employment of artificial means or heroic measures to prolong the life of the body belongs to the patient and/or the immediate family with the approval of the family physician. Such a decision is always in some respects unique, for even the determination of what constitutes "heroic measures," or "extraordinary means," is relative to the available medical resources, the condition of the patient, and the consequences of the treatment for both the patient and other affected persons. In order that the rights of patients may be respected even after they are no longer able to participate actively in decisions about themselves, they may choose to indicate their wishes regarding refusal of treatment in a written statement as contained in section 2 of this act.

Section 2 As used in this act, unless the text indicates otherwise:

1. "Terminal illness" or "injury" means any illness or injury that will result in the expiration of life, regardless of the use or discontinuance of medical treatment to sustain the life processes,

2. "Physician" means any person licensed to practice medicine under chapter 112 of the general laws and who is a member of the staff of a hospital licensed under chapter 111 of the general laws,

3. "Maintenance medical treatment" means artificial means or heroic measures administered as medical treatment designed solely to sustain the life processes where there is no reasonable chance for recovery,

4. "Document" means an executed instrument, as hereinafter contained, which requests that the individual be allowed to die and not be kept alive by maintenance medical treatment or other extraordinary measures. Said document is designed to provide an opportunity to indicate a present desire on the part of said individual, if at some point in the future said individual is unable to indicate his desires, to have his physician and family carefully consider whether the administration of maintenance medical treatment is in the best interest of the patient.

The document shall read substantially as follows [material restating Section 1 omitted]:

To My Family, My Physician, My Clergyman, My Lawyer—

If the time comes when I am no longer able to indicate my desires, I wish this statement to stand as the testament of my wishes.

If there is no reasonable expectation of my recovery from physical or mental disability, as certified by two physicians, I, ———, request that I be allowed to die and not be kept alive by artificial means or heroic measures. I value life and the dignity of life, so that I am not asking that my life be directly taken, but that my dying not be unreasonably prolonged, nor the dignity of life destroyed.

This request is made, after careful reflection, while I am in good health and spirits. I recognize that it places a heavy burden of responsibility upon you, and it is with the intention of sharing this responsibility that this statement is made.

Date:
Signed:
Notarized by:

5. "Family" means a spouse and persons of the first degree of kinship.

Section 3 Any individual of sound mind, eighteen years of age or older, may in the presence of a notary public, execute a document requesting that no maintenance medical treatment be utilized for the prolongation of his life at such time as he suffers a terminal injury or illness. Said document shall become a permanent part of the individual's medical record and shall serve as an indication of the patient's wishes regarding further medical care, when said individual is certified as terminally ill by two physicians; and when said individual is unable to indicate his present desires.

An individual who has executed such a document, may, at any time thereafter, revoke such document by destruction or by oral or written statement provided however that such revocation be witnessed by one person.

Section 4 A physician who acts in reliance on a document executed under this act, where such physician has no actual notice of revocation or contrary indication, by withholding maintenance medical treatment from an individual who executed such document is presumed to be acting in good faith, and unless negligent shall be immune from civil or criminal liability.

For the purposes of this act, a physician may presume in the absence of actual notice to the contrary that an individual who executed a document under section 2 of this act was of sound mind when it was executed.

Section 5 Nothing in this act shall be construed to impose any limitation on the medical judgment of any physician in the treatment and care of any patient.

81

On the Rights of the Sick and Dying

Reprinted from text of Recommendation 779 adopted by the Parliamentary Assembly of the Council of Europe, January 29, 1976.

The Assembly,

1. Considering that the rapid and continuing progress of medical science creates problems, and may even pose certain threats, with respect to the fundamental human rights and the integrity of sick people;

2. Noting the tendency for improved medical technology to lead to an increasingly technical—sometimes less humane—treatment of patients;

3. Observing that sick persons may find it difficult to defend their own interests, especially when undergoing treatment in large hospitals;

4. Considering that recently it has become generally agreed that doctors should in the first place respect the will of the sick person with respect to the treatment he or she has to undergo;

5. Being of the opinion that the right to personal dignity and integrity, to information and proper care, should be clearly defined and granted to every person;

6. Convinced that the duty of the medical profession is to serve mankind, to protect health, to treat sickness and injury, and to relieve suffering, with respect for human lfe and the human person, and convinced that the prolongation of life should not in itself constitute the exclusive aim of medical practice, which must be concerned equally with the relief of suffering;

7. Considering that the doctor must make every effort to alleviate suffering, and that he has no right, even in cases which appear to him to be desperate, intentionally to hasten the natural course of death;

8. Emphasising that the prolongation of life by artificial means depends to a large extent on factors such as the availability of efficient equipment, and that doctors working in hospitals where the technical equipment permits a particularly long prolongation of life are often in a delicate position as far as the continuation of the treatment is concerned, especially in cases where all cerebral functions of a person have irreversibly ceased;

9. Insisting that doctors shall act in accordance with science and approved medical experience, and that no doctor or other member of the medical profession may be compelled to act contrary to the dictates of his own conscience in relation to the right of the sick not to suffer unduly.

10. Recommends that the Committeee of Ministers invite the governments of the member states:

I. a. to take all necessary action, particularly with respect to the training of medical personnel and the organisation of medical services, to ensure that all sick persons, whether in hospital or in their own homes, receive relief of their suffering as effective as the current state of medical knowledge permits;

   b. to impress upon doctors that the sick have a right to full information, if they request it, on their illness and the proposed treatment, and to take action to see that special information is given when entering hospital as regards the routine, procedures and medical equipment of the institution;

   c. to ensure that all persons have the opportunity to prepare themselves psychologically to face the fact of death, and to provide the necessary assistance to this end both through the treating personnel—doctors, nurses, and aids—who should be given the basic training to enable them to discuss these problems with persons approaching the end of life, and through psychiatrists, clergymen or specialised social workers attached to hospitals;

II. to establish national commissions of enquiry, composed of representatives of all levels of the medical profession, lawyers, moral theologians, psychologists and sociologists, to establish ethical rules for the treatment of persons approaching the end of life, and to determine the medical guiding principles for the application of extraordinary measures to prolong life, thereby considering inter alia the situation which may confront members of the medical profession, such as legal sanctions, whether civil or penal, when they have refrained from effecting artificial measures to prolong the death process in the case of terminal patients whose lives cannot be saved by present-day medicine, or have taken positive measures whose primary intention was to relieve suffering in such patients and which could have a subsidiary effect on the process of dying, and to examine the question of written declarations made by legally competent persons, authorising doctors to abstain from life-prolonging measures, in particular in the case of irreversible cessation of brain function;

III. to establish, if no comparable organisations already exist, national commissions to consider complaints against medical personnel for errors or negligence in the practice of their profession, and this without prejudice to the jurisdiction of the ordinary courts;

IV. to inform the Council of Europe of their analytical findings and conclusions for the purpose of harmonising criteria regarding the rights of the sick and dying and the legal and technical means of guaranteeing their application.

82

Cicely M. S. Saunders
The Care of the Dying Patient and His Family

Reprinted with permission of the author and editor from *Contact,* supplement 38, Summer 1972, pp. 12–18.

The care of dying patients or terminal care, as it has come to be called, is no new thing. Few of us do more than learn from other people, and St. Christopher's has joined St. Joseph's Hospice, the Hostel of God, St. Luke's Hospital, and Marie Curie Foundation and others in trying to fill what has been a gap in the general medical services. The teaching which is represented here is based on their long experience. You are asked to forget one special place and to put the patients we discuss into your own setting, translating general principles into particular situations. All those who work with dying people are anxious that what is known already should be developed and extended and that terminal care everywhere should become so good that no one need ever ask for voluntary euthanasia.

The Family the Unit of Care

Nothing that we do should serve to separate someone who is dying from his family. There may be moments of difficulty or even despair but it is of first importance that they should come through to the end together. The journey itself may ease the next stages for those who have to go on living afterwards.

The first meeting with more than half of our patients takes place in their own homes. This is sometimes a visit to assess the need for admission which may be arranged immediately. At other times most of the care given by the Hospice consists of visits by our Out-Patient Sister and her staff over many weeks or even months. Patients may never need admission at any time but remain at home under the care of their own doctors and district nurses.

A family doctor asked our clinic staff to visit one young woman in her forties whose pain and vomiting had become uncontrollable. We discovered later that by this time her distress was so great that not only had she attempted suicide but when she failed the family had discussed whether they should not add together all the pills in the house and try to end her life. We were not told this until a year later. Instead, she spent most of that year at home with her family, able once again to enjoy life, to cook and even to shop and to

care for the three children. She overcame her fear of hospitals, attended our Out-Patients, came for one short stay to re-establish control of her vomiting and finally came in peacefully for her last few weeks. One of the things she said to us at the stage was, "The children are a year older." It was when she was dying that we were told of the despairing attempts of a year before. We asked if she had ever again demanded for her life to be ended. We were told, "Never. Not after the Sister came, because she never had any more pain." We know that this family has really begun to live once more, as her husband calls frequently at a social club at the Hospice designed for such informal "follow-up." How different it would have been if they had remembered only the bewilderment and guilt that follow a suicide or the course they had discussed. And they all needed that extra year.

We should aim to involve the family from the beginning. For example, we may be able to ask for their help in getting a patient comfortable in the bed as he first arrives, thus symbolising their inclusion in all that happens. At other times we have to go more slowly. The fear of seeing physical distress and being able to do nothing about it, coupled with the other demands which can seem too great to meet, may often make a family withdraw from real communication with a dying patient. When one sees tensions relax, children really listening to what their father says, a wife sitting quietly reading her paper beside her husband in bed, we believe that isolation has been overcome and that this is, perhaps, the most important result of all our efforts. This may stem as much from the informal atmosphere of a community planned for such care with the minimum of hierarchy as from the skills which relieve pain, fits, confusion or other distress. After such a coming together the final parting is far more peaceful. We see desperation fade and people come to the place where they are able to let go quietly.

We are finding in our research among bereaved families that just as most patients wish to remain in their own homes as long as they can, so families also wish to manage if only they have enough medical, nursing, and social support. The pattern of care

which appears to leave the least stress and feeling of guilt in bereavement is that in which a patient is cared for at home as long as possible and admitted to hospital within a week or two of his death.

The Control of Physical Distress

Terminal pain can be a kind of "total" pain which obliterates almost everything else from consciousness. Some of our patients have illustrated feelings of their imprisonment in pain in drawings. They portray a situation completely different in character from the temporary events of acute pain with which we are too apt to compare it. Even such total pain can be relieved and forgotten.

Treatment for such pain should begin with the use of any specific treatments which may be relevant. Painful infections must be treated, fractures immobilized by fixation or traction; radiotherapy and chemotherapy may still be of value. The use of steroids may also help greatly towards the relief of pain as well as of anorexia (often a particularly depressing symptom). We must also remember that such complaints as haemorrhoids and toothache hurt just as much or more when one is dying and that distractions and pleasures still give temporary forgetfulness.

There are many drugs that may be useful for moderate pain and they should be used concurrently with such treatments as are mentioned above and certainly as soon as pain becomes part of a patient's life. Relief is self perpetuating and the expectation that something will help is an important factor in pain control at a later stage. It is, however, the experience of all those who care for numbers of such patients that narcotic drugs are at present irreplaceable and can be used effectively for weeks or months. They can also be withdrawn if the need for them ceases. There will always be the small number of patients who confound the prognostications of all the doctors and enter a period of unexpected remission. Sometimes this seems to be induced by the very relief of pain itself; more often it seems to be linked with the renewed appetite and the other effects of steroid therapy. It is certainly helped by the stimulation of occupation, interest, and

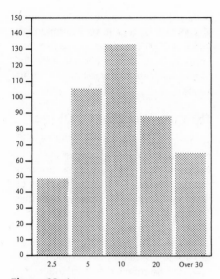

Figure 82–1

pleasure. Parties are an important factor in terminal care.

Constant pain, typical of terminal malignant disease, calls for constant control. Constant control calls for drugs given regularly on a schedule and at a dose level which will prevent pain from occurring at all or at least from becoming severe enough for a patient to add to it by fear and tension. Pain is the strongest antagonist to any analgesic. Once pain has been permitted to take any kind of hold it will call for a larger dose for its control. If a drug is balanced or "titrated" against a patient's need for it in such a way that it covers slightly longer than the chosen routine time it will arrive automatically before the pain has begun to move into the vicious spiral of self-perpetuation and dose increase. The patient who does not receive his analgesics regularly and who is continually having to ask for them is reminded each time of his dependence upon the drug and upon the people who give it to him. Most pain can be controlled on such a regime by narcotics given orally. We do not find that we have to increase doses continually or to push them up to high levels, except in a minority of patients, and never have we lost control. Many of our patients receive narcotics for weeks and months, at home or in the Hospice, and we have not found that the drugs become ineffective nor that patients become psychologically dependent. The majority of doses are given by mouth. Figure 82–1 shows the

maximum levels ever needed by all the patients among a group of 500 at the Hospice. The number needing more than a 30 mgm. dose at a time included a few who reached levels of 60 or even 90 mgm. Occasionally we need to be bold in the relief of pain and the fact that most patients do not need this should never lead to one of them failing to receive what for him is the only adequate dose. Even with these patients we may find then no further increase in dose for a period of weeks while relief remains good.

Dyspnoea, with its almost inevitable accompaniment of anxiety and nausea and vomiting, which are so often coupled with a most understandable depression, may demand more skill and confidence for their control than pain itself. Again, we may need to use heavy sedation with a small minority of patients, usually for a short time only.

Relief of Mental Distress

This includes all that we can learn of what it feels like to be so ill and of the stages of emotion which many seem to pass through.[1] We need to learn to recognize the difference between clinical depression (surprisingly rare in this situation) and sorrow or what has been called "the bereavement of the dying." Drugs may help the first but only the real listener will reach through to the second. We see anxiety and have to learn not to pass by. Patients, too, often come in with some such remark as "It seemed so strange, no one wanted to look at me." Those who come to terms with what is happening have so much to teach us if we will only come close enough to learn.

The very old suffer deeply from weariness and the feeling that their years are a burden to others as well as to themselves. Confusion is sometimes a retreat from reality and whereas drugs may help here it is again the listener who will reach through more positively. But just as isolation is a "state inaccessible to drugs"[2] so words may not reach and some needs can only be met by touch and silent communication.

Care for the Spirit

There are many different ways in which people illustrate their fear of the future—the kind of dread which may be expressed as "I cannot die in

meaninglessness." Spiritual care includes the personal and the informal but more often than might be expected people are helped by long-forgotten sacraments. This is not the province of the Chaplain only, any member of staff may be called on to remain, often without words, with a family or a lonely patient. Spiritual care includes all that we can do to bring a sense of security into the situation. Our own philosophy must never be imposed upon another person but an unspoken conviction that there is still purpose and meaning in his life may create a climate in which he can find his own answer.

How do the staff of such units involve themselves so deeply in the needs of their patients and still carry on? We have found that we need to meet constantly in small groups for discussion so that we share the work fully. A social psychiatrist visits weekly and sees about 15% of the patients but spends much of his time in such groups. The volunteers and visiting students, part-time staff, the elderly residents in their own Wing, and the children of the staff in their Playgroup, form a mixed community which gives mutual support.

Decisions

Terminal care includes the making of decisions concerning the correct treatment for an individual patient. There is a time for giving dexamethazone to a patient with a cerebral tumour but there is also a time to withdraw it. We have to concern ourselves with the quality of life as well as with its length and with the pressures imposed upon a family when we are maintaining what has become only a travesty of life. There are patients for whom chemotherapy gives great benefits but there are others for whom it becomes increasingly irrelevant, producing more side effects with diminishing returns. We must learn when to withdraw such treatment.

There are other manoeuvres which should never be undertaken. There are times when the treatment for a haemorrhage is not a blood transfusion with its attendant alarms but instead an injection and someone who stays there. There are infusions which should never have been put up, feelings of thirst can be relieved by the right use of narcotics. It is far better to have a cup of tea given slowly on your last afternoon than to have drips and tubes in all directions. This is not ineffectual sentimentality but proper care with all the compassionate matter-of-factness that the nuns of St. Joseph's Hospice and many other experienced nurses have shown us over the years. Again, we sometimes need to make decisions concerning the use of antibiotics and other measures for the very old or the very ill who develop pneumonia. There are ways of relieving the dyspnoea, cough and any other distress which do not prolong further a life which has come to its close. These are not "untreated" patients but rather those who have received the treatment relevant to their condition and so often to their wishes.

All the above would, we believe, be included in the "good medical care" as referrred to by the President of this College in his opening speech. This kind of terminal care, which needs to be developed and shared between the general and the special hospital, the patient's own home and units of various kinds, is the answer to most of the fears which lead to support for the principle of voluntary euthanasia.

Requests?

A very small number of patients have wanted to discuss euthanasia with us. No one has come back to make a considered request for us to carry it out. Once pain and the feeling of isolation had been relieved they never asked again.

We had such discussions with two young men, both with motor neurone disease. One said, "If it were available I would ask." Yet he always demanded antibiotics if he had an incipient chest infection and he well knew how inconsistent were his feelings and wishes. Finally he said, "Yes, I would have asked, but now I see the snags." Weighed against all his problems were his deepening relationship with his wife and his growing confidence that we would never let him choke. He died quietly in his sleep after a massive pulmonary embolus. The two of them had shared the hardness throughout and there were no guilts or hang-ups as his wife began her new life.

The other man died later. He found that the stage of physical helplessness in the first, which he had watched with apprehension, was totally different when he reached it himself. He maintained his essential independence, never giving in to anything and fought his way into a peace in which he could say, "I can't see round the next bend but I know it will be all right."

A young man said to me, as he faced leaving life and his strong family ties and responsibilities, "I've fought and I've fought—but now I've accepted." We, too, have to learn to accept as well as to fight and to realize that part of our work can have nothing to do with cure but only with the giving of relief and comfort. We will learn by looking at patients, by listening to what they want to say and by meeting their needs as far as we can both practically and philosophically. His readiness finally to say "yes" to death was in itself an affirmation of life. We need him as much and more than he needs us. Anything which says to the very ill or the very old that there is no longer anything that matters in their life would be a deep impoverishment to the whole of society.

References

1. Kubler-Ross, Elisabeth (1970), *On Death and Dying*. Tavistock Publications, London.

2. Hackett, T. P., Weissmann, A. D. (1962), The Treatment of the Dying. *Curr. Psychiat. Ther.* 2 121.

83

Diana Crane
Physicians' Attitudes toward the Treatment of Critically Ill Patients

Reprinted with deletion of pictures by permission of the author and the editor from the *Radcliffe Quarterly,* vol. 62, March 1976, pp. 18–21.

In recent years, because of advances in medical knowledge and technology, chronic rather than acute diseases have become the most prevalent causes of death in industrial societies. Difficult decisions concerning the prolongation of life are more common during the course of chronic disease than during the course of acute disease. As these problems occur more frequently, popular pressure to resolve the contradictions inherent in these situations increases.

Sissela Bok . . . defines euthanasia as causing death painlessly to end suffering. This definition is generally considered to apply to cases of direct killing with the consent of the patient. Cases where treatment is withdrawn or omitted from the care of conscious patients are considered by some, but not all, writers to fall within the category of euthanasia (often called passive or negative euthanasia). It is understood that this type of action is taken by the physician in accord with the wishes of the patient. A few writers include under the category of euthanasia direct killing or withdrawal of treatment from brain-damaged or unconscious patients. The rationale for including this behavior under the rubric of euthanasia is presumably that the patient would not have wished to have his life maintained or prolonged under such circumstances, so that his consent can be assumed. In other words, it is only by considerably extending the usual definition of euthanasia that it is possible to include the full range of medical problems that create anxiety and concern to doctors and public alike at the present time.

Information concerning doctors' attitudes toward the treatment of critically ill patients was obtained through questionnaires which were sent by the author to physicians in 1970–71 in four medical specialties: internal medicine, neurosurgery, pediatrics, and pediatric heart surgery. The samples were large. The proportion of respondents returning the questionnaire was over 70 percent in all samples. There were 1,410 internists, 650 neurosurgeons, 922 pediatricians, and 207 pediatric heart surgeons.

Samples of neurosurgeons and pediatric heart surgeons were drawn from lists of members of these specialties. Because hospital environment is an important influence upon the behavior of physicians, it was decided to select pediatricians and internists from staffs of hospitals which represent different types of hospital environments. Since residents participate in these decisions, they were also included.

Case Histories

The physicians were presented with case histories of patients which were different for each specialty. Surgeons were asked to indicate whether or not they would usually operate in such cases. Physicians were asked to check items on an accompanying list of medical procedures to indicate how actively they would treat such patients. There were three versions of the questionnaire for internal medicine and two versions for pediatrics. Each version included the same case histories, but social characteristics such as family attitude, patient attitude, or social class were varied.

Sample cases may prove illuminating: A 65-year-old woman with severe cerebral atrophy cannot walk, feed herself, or communicate meaningfully with others. She is admitted to the ward service dehydrated and septic. Her family is unwilling to care for her at home if discharged from the hospital following treatment. Which of the following would you be likely to perform? *(Check yes, maybe, or no for each of the following.)* The list of ten items with squares to be checked for the three responses were: 1. Intravenous feeding for dehydration. 2. Lumbar puncture for stiff neck and fever. 3. Urine culture for pyuria. 4. Six blood cultures for fever and murmur. 5. Appendectomy for incidental suspected appendicitis. 6. Small bowel resection for suspected infarcted bowel. 7. If respiratory insufficiency due to pneumonia became severe, would you use endotrachial tube and respirator? 8. If respiratory distress lasted two days, would you perform tracheostomy? 9. If cardiac arrest occurred, would you begin resuscitation? 10. If resuscitation was unsuccessful after 15 minutes, would you continue?

A 45-year-old, 140-pound man in the last stages of terminal cancer has been receiving 40 mg. of morphine p.r.n. Later 40 mg. of morphine no longer gives him relief from pain.

Which of the following would you be likely to prescribe? *(Check one of the following.)* The items physicians were asked to check included: 1. No increase in dosage. 2. Increased dosage but not to the extent that there is danger of producing respiratory arrest. 3. Increased dosage to the point where pain is relieved even if it might risk respiratory arrest. 4. If dosage described in (3) was not effective, increased dosage to the point where pain is relieved even if it will probably lead to respiratory arrest.

The Affirmative Act Causing Death

An affirmative act designed to cause death to a patient would be considered as criminal homicide in terms of the law. Data obtained from the questionnaires suggest that physicians in at least one medical specialty quite frequently perform acts which have the effect of hastening the deaths of their patients. Specialists in internal medicine were asked to indicate whether or not they would increase the dosage of narcotics for a terminal cancer patient to the point where it might risk or would probably lead to respiratory arrest. Forty-three percent of the physicians and 29 percent of the residents in the sample were willing to incur high risk of inducing respiratory arrest in such a patient by increasing his dosage of narcotics.

On the other hand, response to a question addressed to pediatricians concerning direct killing of an anencephalic infant (one born without a brain) was overwhelmingly negative. Among the respondents (both residents and physicians), only one percent said that they would be likely to give an "intravenous injection of a lethal dose of potassium chloride or a sedative drug" to an anencephalic infant; three percent said that they might do so. These low figures are not due to the fact that the case involves an infant, which might be expected to have special significance for physicians. Seventy-six percent of the pediatricians indicated that they would turn off the respirator after brain death had occurred in an infant.

The apparent contradiction between these two sets of findings can probably be explained in terms of differences in the ways in which physicians perceive these two acts. Administration of a lethal drug dose to an anencephalic child is perceived as an instance of direct killing. Ethicist Paul Ramsey has argued that large doses of narcotics which both suppress pain and hasten death are not true examples of euthanasia since the physician's intention is to suppress pain and not to cause death. Comments made to the author during interviews suggested that some physicians defined this type of treatment as euthanasia while others made the same type of distinction between intent and consequence that Ramsey does. Presumably those who use this type of treatment are motivated by their desire to alleviate pain rather than to kill the patient. As a result, the act is apparently not perceived as euthanasia.

Withholding or Terminating Ordinary Medical Treatment

Once a physician has undertaken a particular course of treatment for a patient, the physician may be legally obligated to continue to treat the patient. On the other hand, the patient has the legal right to refuse life-sustaining procedures, such as surgery or blood transfusions. Thus, with the patient's consent, the physician is on safe legal ground in withdrawing treatment. However, if the patient's mental faculties have deteriorated to the point where he is unable to give his consent to withdrawal of treatment, the physician may be legally obligated to continue to treat him.

From a legal point of view, the physician would be expected to continue to treat the brain damaged patient who is incapable of consent and to withdraw treatment from the alert terminal patient who does not wish to be treated actively. In fact, data from the questionnaires obtained from internists and neurosurgeons suggest that the consent of the patient or his agent is only one factor which influences the physician's decision to treat. What criteria is the physician using in making decisions of this kind? To the physician, two considerations are of great importance. First, is the patient salvageable? In other words, if he survives an acute crisis, can he be maintained at a reasonable level of functioning for a considerable period of time?

Second, has the patient's condition affected his physical functioning only or his mental functioning as well? According to the survey, it appears that physicians would rank patients in the following order in terms of how actively they would treat them: (1) the salvageable patient with physical damage only; (2) the salvageable patient with severe mental damage; (3) the unsalvageable patient with physical damage only; and (4) the unsalvageable patient with mental damage.

For example, 67 percent of the physicians in internal medicine indicated that they would treat very actively a patient in the first category, a severely debilitated, semicomatose patient suffering from chronic pulmonary fibrosis whose wife was described as being reluctant to authorize an essential, lifesaving procedure (a tracheostomy). However, 16 percent of the physicians in internal medicine indicated that they would treat very actively a severely brain damaged patient who could not communicate meaningfully with others and whose family had indicated that they were unwilling to care for her at home after discharge from the hospital (case described above).

The Prognosis

The dimension of consent was not included in the neurosurgeons' questionnaire, since the patient's consent is required before surgery can be performed. It was clear that neurosurgeons were using the criteria of prognosis and type of damage in making their decisions about patients. Given two cases of patients who had suffered cerebral hematomas (i.e., a salvageable prognosis), 89 percent of the neurosurgeons indicated that they would operate upon the patient whose physical functioning only was affected by the hematoma while 55 percent indicated that they would operate upon the patient whose mental functioning was affected. Among terminal patients suffering from solitary metastatic brain tumor, 50 percent indicated that they would operate upon the patient whose physical functioning was affected by the tumor while 22 percent indicated that they would operate upon the patient whose mental functioning was affected by it.

The attitude of the adult patient appeared to be more important than the attitude of the adult patient's family. (The family's attitude is, however, very important in the decision to treat children and newborn infants.) In the case of a moderately brain damaged stroke patient, the family's willingness or unwillingness to care for the patient at home upon her discharge from the hospital had a negligible effect upon the physicians' attitudes toward treating her. A terminal cancer patient with physical damage only who was described as requesting that treatment be withdrawn would have been treated by 22 percent of the physicians. On the other hand, when the same patient was described as wanting to be treated vigorously, 51 percent of the physicians indicated that they would do so.

These findings suggest that the dimensions of prognosis and type of damage are of primary importance in the physician's decision to use or withdraw treatment. Within this framework, the patient who wants active treatment is likely to receive it but withdrawal of treatment by the physician depends less upon the consent of the patient or his agent than on the physician's assessment of the patient's prognosis and type of damage.

Withholding or Terminating "Extraordinary" Medical Treatment

One of the most difficult decisions for the physician to make is whether to turn off the respirator which is supporting the respiratory function of a patient who has suffered irreversible cessation of spontaneous brain function. In the absence of legal precedent in this area, it has been argued that the physician who turns off the respirator in such a situation is not committing euthanasia in the legal sense. In other words, the respirator is prolonging the patient's life without any possibility of returning him to health. Withdrawing the machine cannot be said to have caused the patient's death.

When presented with a case which met the criteria for brain death as defined by an interdisciplinary committee at Harvard in 1968, 71 percent of the neurosurgeons and 72 percent of the internists indicated that they would

turn off the respirator. However, in this instance, consent of the family is apparently very important. Forty-nine percent of the members of both specialties said that they would do so only after consultation with family or with family and colleagues. Only nine percent of the neurosurgeons and 19 percent of the internists would do so with the consent of colleagues alone and only 13 percent of the neurosurgeons and two percent of the internists would turn off the machine entirely on their own initiative. Twenty-nine percent of the neurosurgeons and 28 percent of the internists would not turn off the respirator under these conditions.

Interviews suggested that turning off the respirator was viewed by some physicians as an act which directly terminated the patient's life. Apparently this decision is one which physicians fear may be interpreted as euthanasia in spite of the fact that from a legal point of view this is probably unlikely. Possibly their attitude results from their awareness of the traditional interpretation of criminal responsibility as ensuing from acts of commission rather than from acts of omission. Turning off the respirator is viewed as an act of commission.

Implications for Social Policy

It appears that the behavior of physicians is directly contrary in some respects to what might be expected on legal grounds. Legally, the physician can be criminally prosecuted if he performs an act which is designed to bring about or causes the death of a patient, but a significant percentage of physicians said that they would be likely to perform an act which would hasten the death of a terminal cancer patient. While the physician is on the safest ground legally when he withdraws treatment from an alert patient who gives his consent to this course of action, the survey indicates he sometimes withdraws treatment when the patient is incapable of giving consent and gives treatment when the patient or his agent has expressed a desire that treatment be discontinued.

Any discussion of policy has to be phrased in terms of three factors which play important roles in the physician's decision—prognosis, type of damage, and the consent of the patient or his

agent. The survey indicates that the patient with severe physical damage whose condition can be maintained for a considerable period of time is likely to be actively treated against his wishes or those of his agent. Public discussion of the situation of such patients might make it easier for them to exert their right to refuse treatment. Policy implications might include strengthening the legal rights of patients or their families to refuse treatment. A recent court case permitted a woman who was mentally competent but unable to speak to refuse further leg amputations. Generally, in such cases the judge declares the patient "incompetent" so that his wishes can be overridden by a court-appointed guardian.

According to the survey, patients in the other three categories (i.e., the salvageable patient with severe mental damage, the unsalvageable patient with physical damage only, and the unsalvageable patient with mental damage) are less likely to be actively treated against their wishes or those of their agents. There are, however, difficulties in each of these kinds of situations. While the survey suggests that the terminal patient who indicates that he does not want vigorous treatment will not receive such treatment, not all patients are aware of their rights to refuse treatment. Numerous studies show that certain types of patients, particularly those whose ethnic and educational backgrounds are different from those of their physician, find it difficult to communicate with physicians and presumably to engage in the delicate type of negotiations required in order to obtain withdrawal of medical treatment.

Patients' Bill of Rights

Additional support for the patient has recently been provided by the American Hospital Association, which has published as a statement of its national policy a "bill of rights" for patients. Among these rights, the bill includes that of refusing treatment "to the extent permitted by law."

Some issues cannot be translated into public policy before public discussion has taken place. For example, my survey shows that the physician is reluctant to accept the family's judgment concerning the treatment of the adult patient. While the family's attitude plays a very important role in the decision to treat pediatric patients, the physician tends to distrust the family's attitude toward an adult patient. This is particularly the case when he has not known the patient and his family prior to the patient's illness. Should the physician rely upon the family's judgment in cases when the patient is incapable of making such decisions? If so, can the rights of the family in making such decisions be strengthened legally?

The survey also suggests that physicians are inclined not to treat actively either salvageable or unsalvageable patients who are severely brain damaged. The sanctity of individuality rather than the sanctity of life *per se* appears to be the norm. Perhaps the implications of the use of this criterion should also be the subject of public discussion. Finally, it would appear that there is a need for greater exchange of information between the physician and the lawyer concerning the legal implications of turning off the respirator when patients have suffered irreversible brain death.

Growing Public Concern

In conclusion, it is possible that growing public concern with these issues reflects an increasing desire by individuals to control their own lives (and deaths) and increasing unwillingness to accept unquestionably the physician's judgment in these matters. If they are to exercise their rights in a meaningful fashion, patients and families alike will have to educate themselves in advance about the complexities of medical technology and the problems which it can create for medical care. By the time they are actually faced with such decisions, they should know what sorts of alternatives they prefer. Should this happen, physicians in the future may find it necessary to treat the chronically ill patient less as a dependent for whom decisions have to be made and more as an equal. The new demand for greater patient autonomy also means that it is imperative to resolve some of the differences which now separate the perspective of the physician on these matters from that of the layman and the lawyer.

84

In the Matter of Karen Quinlan

Supreme Court of New Jersey, 70 N.J. 10, 355 A.2d 647 (argued January 26, 1976; decided March 31, 1976).

The opinion of the Court was delivered by Hughes, C. J.

The Litigation

The central figure in this tragic case is Karen Ann Quinlan, a New Jersey resident. At the age of 22, she lies in a debilitated and allegedly moribund state at Saint Clare's Hospital in Denville, New Jersey. The litigation has to do, in final analysis, with her life,—its continuance or cessation,—and the responsibilities, rights and duties, with regard to any fateful decision concerning it, of her family, her guardian, her doctors, the hospital, the State through its law enforcement authorities, and finally the courts of justice.

The issues are before this Court following its direct certification of the action under the rule, R. 2:12–1, prior to hearing in the Superior Court, Appellate Division, to which the appellant (hereafter "plaintiff") Joseph Quinlan, Karen's father, had appealed the adverse judgment of the Chancery Division.

Due to extensive physical damage fully described in the able opinion of the trial judge, Judge Muir, supporting that judgment, Karen allegedly was incompetent. Joseph Quinlan sought the adjudication of that incompetency. He wished to be appointed guardian of the person and property of his daughter. It was proposed by him that such letters of guardianship, if granted, should contain an express power to him as guardian to authorize the discontinuance of all extraordinary medical procedures now allegedly sustaining Karen's vital processes and hence her life, since these measures, he asserted, present no hope of her eventual recovery. A guardian *ad litem* was appointed by Judge Muir to represent the interest of the alleged incompetent.

By a supplemental complaint, in view of the extraordinary nature of the relief sought by plaintiff and the involvement therein of their several rights and responsibilities, other parties were added. These included the treating physicians and the hospital, the relief sought being that they be restrained from interfering with the carrying out of any such extraordinary authorization in the event it were to be granted by the court. Joined, as well, was the Prosecutor of Morris County (he being charged with responsibility for enforcement of the criminal law), to enjoin him from interfering with, or projecting a criminal prosecution which otherwise might ensue in the event of, cessation of life in Karen resulting from the exercise of such extraordinary authorization were it to be granted to the guardian.

The Attorney General of New Jersey intervened as of right pursuant to R. 4:33–1 on behalf of the State of New Jersey, such intervention being recognized by the court in the pretrial conference order (R. 4:25–1 et seq.) of September 22, 1975. Its basis, of course, was the interest of the State in the preservation of life, which has an undoubted constitutional foundation.[1]

The matter is of transcendent importance, involving questions related to the definition and existence of death, the prolongation of life through artificial means developed by medical technology undreamed of in past generations of the practice of the healing arts;[2] the impact of such durationally indeterminate and artificial life prolongation on the rights of the incompetent, her family and society in general; the bearing of constitutional right and the scope of judicial responsibility, as to the appropriate response of an equity court of justice to the extraordinary prayer for relief of the plaintiff. Involved as well is the right of the plaintiff, Joseph Quinlan, to guardianship of the person of his daughter.

Among his "factual and legal contentions" under such Pretrial Order was the following:

I. Legal and Medical Death
(a) Under the existing legal and medical definitions of death recognized by the State of New Jersey, Karen Ann Quinlan is dead.

This contention, made in the context of Karen's profound and allegedly irreversible coma and physical debility, was discarded during trial by the following stipulated amendment to the Pretrial Order:

Under any legal standard recognized by the State of New Jersey and also under standard medical practice, Karen Ann Quinlan is presently alive.

Other amendments to the Pretrial Order made at the time of trial expanded the issues before the court. The Prosecutor of Morris County sought a declaratory judgment as to the effect any affirmation by the court of a right in a guardian to terminate life-sustaining procedures would have with regard to enforcement of the criminal laws of New Jersey with reference to homicide. Saint Clare's Hospital, in the face of trial testimony on the subject of "brain death," sought declaratory judgment as to:

Whether the use of the criteria developed and enunciated by the Ad Hoc Committee of the Harvard Medical School on or about August 5, 1968, as well as similar criteria, by a physician to assist in determination of the death of a patient, whose cardiopulmonary functions are being artificially sustained, is in accordance with ordinary and standard medical practice.[3]

It was further stipulated during trial that Karen was indeed incompetent and guardianship was necessary, although there exists a dispute as to the determination later reached by the court that such guardianship should be bifurcated, and that Mr. Quinlan should be appointed as guardian of the trivial property but not the person of his daughter.

After certification the Attorney General filed as of right (R 2:3–4) a cross-appeal[4] challenging the action of the trial court in admitting evidence of prior statements made by Karen while competent as to her distaste for continuance of life by extraordinary medical procedures, under circumstances not unlike those of the present case. These quoted statements were made in the context of several conversations with regard to others terminally ill and being subjected to like heroic measures. The statements were advanced as evidence of what she would want done in such a contingency as now exists. She was said to have firmly evinced her wish, in like circumstances, not to have her life prolonged by the otherwise futile use of extraordinary means. Because we agree with the conception of the trial court that such statements, since they were remote and impersonal, lacked significant probative weight, it is not of consequence to our opinion that we decide whether or not they were admissible hearsay. Again, after certification, the guardian of the person of the incompetent (who had been appointed as a part of the judgment appealed from) resigned and was succeeded by another, but that too seems irrelevant to decision. It is, however, of interest to note the trial court's delineation (in its supplemental opinion of November 12, 1975) of the extent of the personal guardian's authority with respect to medical care of his ward:

Mr. Coburn's appointment is designed to deal with those instances wherein Dr. Morse,[5] in the process of administering care and treatment to Karen Quinlan, feels there should be concurrence on the extent or nature of the care or treatment. If Mr. and Mrs. Quinlan are unable to give concurrence, then Mr. Coburn will be consulted for his concurrence.

Essentially then, appealing to the power of equity, and relying on claimed constitutional rights of free exercise of religion, of privacy and of protection against cruel and unusual punishment, Karen Quinlan's father sought judicial authority to withdraw the life-sustaining mechanisms temporarily preserving his daughter's life, and his appointment as guardian of her person to that end. His request was opposed by her doctors, the hospital, the Morris County Prosecutor, the State of New Jersey, and her guardian ad litem.

The Factual Base

An understanding of the issues in their basic perspective suggests a brief review of the factual base developed in the testimony and documented in greater detail in the opinion of the trial judge. In re Quinlan, 137 N.J.Super. 227, 348 A.2d 801 (Ch.Div.1975).

On the night of April 15, 1975, for reasons still unclear, Karen Quinlan ceased breathing for at least two 15 minute periods. She received some ineffectual mouth-to-mouth resuscitation from friends. She was taken by ambulance to Newton Memorial Hospital. There she had a temperature of 100 degrees, her pupils were unreactive and she was unresponsive even to deep pain. The history at the time of her admission to that hospital was essentially incomplete and uninformative.

Three days later, Dr. Morse examined Karen at the request of the Newton admitting physician, Dr. McGee. He found her comatose with evidence of decortication, a condition relating to derangement of the cortex of the brain causing a physical posture in which the upper extremities are flexed and the lower extremities are extended. She required a respirator to assist her breathing. Dr. Morse was unable to obtain an adequate account of the circumstances and events leading up to Karen's admission to the Newton Hospital. Such initial history or etiology is crucial in neurological diagnosis. Relying as he did upon the Newton Memorial records and his own examination, he concluded that prolonged lack of oxygen in the bloodstream, anoxia, was identified with her condition as he saw it upon first observation. When she was later transferred to Saint Clare's Hospital she was still unconscious, still on a respirator and a tracheotomy had been performed. On her arrival Dr. Morse conducted extensive and detailed examinations. An electroencephalogram (EEG) measuring electrical rhythm of the brain was performed and Dr. Morse characterized the result as "abnormal but it showed some activity and was consistent with her clinical state." Other significant neurological tests, including a brain scan, an angiogram, and a lumbar puncture were normal in result. Dr. Morse testified that Karen has been in a state of coma, lack of consciousness, since he began treating her. He explained that there are basically two types of coma, sleep-like unresponsiveness and awake unresponsiveness. Karen was originally in a sleep-like unresponsive condition but soon developed "sleep-wake" cycles, apparently a normal improvement for comatose patients occurring within three to four weeks. In the awake cycle she blinks, cries out and does things of that sort but is still totally unaware of anyone or anything around her.

Dr. Morse and other expert physicians who examined her characterized Karen as being in a "chronic persistent vegetative state." Dr. Fred Plum, one of such expert witnesses, defined this as a "subject who remains with the capacity to maintain the vegetative parts of neurological function but who . . . no longer has any cognitive function."

Dr. Morse, as well as the several other medical and neurological experts who testified in this case, believed with certainty that Karen Quinlan is not "brain dead." They identified the Ad Hoc Committee of Harvard Medical School report (*infra*) as the ordinary medical standard for determining brain death, and all of them were satisfied

that Karen met none of the criteria specified in that report and was therefore not "brain dead" within its contemplation.

In this respect it was indicated by Dr. Plum that the brain works in essentially two ways, the vegetative and the sapient. He testified:

We have an internal vegetative regulation which controls body temperature which controls breathing, which controls to a considerable degree blood pressure, which controls to some degree heart rate, which controls chewing, swallowing and which controls sleeping and waking. We have a more highly developed brain which is uniquely human which controls our relation to the outside world, our capacity to talk, to see, to feel, to sing, to think. Brain death necessarily must mean the death of both of these functions of the brain, vegetative and the sapient. Therefore, the presence of any function which is regulated or governed or controlled by the deeper parts of the brain which in laymen's terms might be considered purely vegetative would mean that the brain is not biologically dead.

Because Karen's neurological condition affects her respiratory ability (the respiratory system being a brain stem function) she requires a respirator to assist her breathing. From the time of her admission to Saint Clare's Hospital Karen has been assisted by an MA–1 respirator, a sophisticated machine which delivers a given volume of air at a certain rate and periodically provides a "sigh" volume, a relatively large measured volume of air designed to purge the lungs of excretions. Attempts to "wean" her from the respirator were unsuccessful and have been abandoned.

The experts believe that Karen cannot now survive without the assistance of the respirator; that exactly how long she would live without it is unknown; that the strong likelihood is that death would follow soon after its removal, and that removal would also risk further brain damage and would curtail the assistance the respirator presently provides in warding off infection.

It seemed to be the consensus not only of the treating physicians but also of the several qualified experts who testified in the case, that removal from the respirator would not conform to medical practices, standards and traditions.

The further medical consensus was that Karen in addition to being comatose is in a chronic and persistent "vegetative" state, having no awareness of anything or anyone around her and existing at a primitive reflex level. Although she does have some brain stem function (ineffective for respiration) and has other reactions one normally associates with being alive, such as moving, reacting to light, sound and noxious stimuli, blinking her eyes, and the like, the quality of her feeling impulses is unknown. She grimaces, makes stereotyped cries and sounds and has chewing motions. Her blood pressure is normal.

Karen remains in the intensive care unit at Saint Clare's Hospital, receiving 24-hour care, by a team of four nurses characterized, as was the medical attention, as "excellent." She is nourished by feeding by way of a nasal-gastro tube and is routinely examined for infection, which under these circumstances is a serious life threat. The result is that her condition is considered remarkable under the unhappy circumstances involved.

Karen is described as emaciated, having suffered a weight loss of at least 40 pounds, and undergoing a continuing deteriorative process. Her posture is described as fetal-like and grotesque; there is extreme flexion-rigidity of the arms, legs and related muscles and her joints are severely rigid and deformed.

From all of this evidence, and including the whole testimonial record, several basic findings in the physical area are mandated. Severe brain and associated damage, albeit of uncertain etiology, has left Karen in a chronic and persistent vegetative state. No form of treatment which can cure or improve that condition is known or available. As nearly as may be determined, considering the guarded area of remote uncertainties characteristic of most medical science predictions, she can *never* be restored to cognitive or sapient life. Even with regard to the vegetative level and improvement therein (if such it may be called) the prognosis is extremely poor and the extent unknown if it should in fact occur.

She is debilitated and moribund and although fairly stable at the time of argument before us (no new information having been filed in the meanwhile in expansion of the record), no physician risked the opinion that she could live more than a year and indeed she may die much earlier. Excellent medical and nursing care so far has been able to ward off the constant threat of infection, to which she is peculiarly susceptible because of the respirator, the tracheal tube and other incidents of care in her vulnerable condition. Her life accordingly is sustained by the respirator and tubal feeding, and removal from the respirator would cause her death soon, although the time cannot be stated with more precision.

The determination of the fact and time of death in past years of medical science was keyed to the action of the heart and blood circulation, in turn dependent upon pulmonary activity, and hence cessation of these functions spelled out the reality of death.[6]

Developments in medical technology have obfuscated the use of the traditional definition of death. Efforts have been made to define irreversible coma as a new criterion for death, such as by the 1968 report of the Ad Hoc Committee of the Harvard Medical School (the Committee comprising ten physicians, an historian, a lawyer and a theologian), which asserted that:

From ancient times down to the recent past it was clear that, when the respiration and heart stopped, the brain would die in a few minutes; so the obvious criterion of no heart beat as synonymous with death was sufficiently accurate. In those times the heart was considered to be the central organ of the body; it is not surprising that its failure marked the onset of death. This is no longer valid when modern resuscitative and supportive measures are used. These improved activities can now restore "life" as judged by the ancient standards of persistent respiration and continuing heart beat. This can be the case even when there is not the remotest possibility of an individual recovering consciousness following massive brain damage. ["A Definition of Irreversible Coma," 205 J.A.M.A. 337, 339 (1968)].

The Ad Hoc standards, carefully delineated, included absence of response to pain or other stimuli, pupilary reflexes, corneal, pharyngeal and other reflexes, blood pressure, spontaneous respiration, as well as "flat" or isoelectric electroencephalograms and the like, with all tests repeated "at least 24 hours later with no change." In such circumstances, where all of such criteria have been met as showing

"brain death," the Committee recommends with regard to the respirator:

The patient's condition can be determined only by a physician. When the patient is hopelessly damaged as defined above, the family and all colleagues who have participated in major decisions concerning the patient, and all nurses involved, should be so informed. Death is to be declared and *then* the respirator turned off. The decision to do this and the responsibility for it are to be taken by the physician-in-charge, in consultation with one or more physicians who have been directly involved in the case. It is unsound and undesirable to force the family to make the decision. [205 J.A.M.A., *supra* at 338 [emphasis in original].

But, as indicated, it was the consensus of medical testimony in the instant case that Karen, for all her disability, met none of these criteria, nor indeed any comparable criteria extant in the medical world and representing, as does the Ad Hoc Committee report, according to the testimony in this case, prevailing and accepted medical standards.

We have adverted to the "brain death" concept and Karen's disassociation with any of its criteria, to emphasize the basis of the medical decision made by Dr. Morse. When plaintiff and his family, finally reconciled to the certainty of Karen's impending death, requested the withdrawal of life support mechanisms, he demurred. His refusal was based upon his conception of medical standards, practice and ethics described in the medical testimony, such as in the evidence given by another neurologist, Dr. Sidney Diamond, a witness for the State. Dr. Diamond asserted that no physician would have failed to provide respirator support at the outset, and none would interrupt its life-saving course thereafter, except in the case of cerebral death. In the latter case, he thought the respirator would in effect be disconnected from one already dead, entitling the physician under medical standards and, he thought, legal concepts, to terminate the supportive measures. We note Dr. Diamond's distinction of major surgical or transfusion procedures in a terminal case not involving cerebral death, such as here:

The subject has lost human qualities. It would be incredible, and I think unlikely, that any physician would re-

spond to a sudden hemorrhage, massive hemorrhage or a loss of all her defensive blood cells, by giving her large quantities of blood. I think that . . . major surgical procedures would be out of the question even if they were known to be essential for continued physical existence.

This distinction is adverted to also in the testimony of Dr. Julius Korein, a neurologist called by plaintiff. Dr. Korein described a medical practice concept of "judicious neglect" under which the physician will say:

Don't treat this patient anymore, . . . it does not serve either the patient, the family, or society in any meaningful way to continue treatment with this patient.

Dr. Korein also told of the unwritten and unspoken standard of medical practice implied in the foreboding initials DNR (do not resuscitate), as applied to the extraordinary terminal case:

Cancer, metastatic cancer, involving the lungs, the liver, the brain, multiple involvements, the physician may or may not write: Do not resuscitate. . . . [I]t could be said to the nurse: if this man stops breathing don't resuscitate him. . . . No physician that I know personally is going to try and resuscitate a man riddled with cancer and in agony and he stops breathing. They are not going to put him on a respirator. . . . I think that would be the height of misuse of technology.

While the thread of logic in such distinctions may be elusive to the nonmedical lay mind, in relation to the supposed imperative to sustain life at all costs, they nevertheless relate to medical decisions, such as the decision of Dr. Morse in the present case. We agree with the trial court that that decision was in accord with Dr. Morse's conception of medical standards and practice.

We turn to that branch of the factual case pertaining to the application for guardianship, as distinguished from the nature of the authorization sought by the applicant. The character and general suitability of Joseph Quinlan as guardian for his daughter, in ordinary circumstances, could not be doubted. The record bespeaks the high degree of familial love which pervaded the home of Joseph Quinlan and reached out fully to embrace Karen, although she was living elsewhere at the time of her collapse. The proofs showed him to be deeply religious, imbued with a morality so sensitive that months of tortured indecision preceded his belated conclusion (despite earlier moral judgments reached by the other family members, but unexpressed to him in order not to influence him) to seek the termination of life-supportive measures sustaining Karen. A communicant of the Roman Catholic Church, as were other family members, he first sought solace in private prayer looking with confidence, as he says, to the Creator, first for the recovery of Karen and then, if that were not possible, for guidance with respect to the awesome decision confronting him.

To confirm the moral rightness of the decision he was about to make he consulted with his parish priest and later with the Catholic chaplain of Saint Clare's Hospital. He would not, he testified, have sought termination if that act were to be morally wrong or in conflict with the tenets of the religion he so profoundly respects. He was disabused of doubt, however, when the position of the Roman Catholic Church was made known to him as it is reflected in the record in this case. While it is not usual for matters of religious dogma or concepts to enter a civil litigation (except as they may bear upon constitutional right, or sometimes, familial matters; cf. In re Adoption of E, 59 N.J. 36, 279 A.2d 785 (1971)), they were rightly admitted in evidence here. The judge was bound to measure the character and motivations in all respects of Joseph Quinlan as prospective guardian; and insofar as these religious matters bore upon them, they were properly scrutinized and considered by the court.

Thus germane, we note the position of that Church as illuminated by the record before us. We have no reason to believe that it would be at all discordant with the whole of Judeo-Christian tradition, considering its central respect and reverence for the sanctity of human life. It was in this sense of relevance that we admitted as amicus curiae the New Jersey Catholic Conference, essentially the spokesman for the various Catholic bishops of New Jersey, organized to give witness to spiritual values in public affairs in the statewide community. The position statement of Bishop Lawrence B. Casey, reproduced in the amicus brief, projects these views:

(a) The verification of the fact of death in a particular case cannot be deduced from any religious or moral principle and, under this aspect, does not fall within the competence of the church;—that dependence must be had upon traditional and medical standards, and by these standards Karen Ann Quinlan is assumed to be alive.

(b) The request of plaintiff for authority to terminate a medical procedure characterized as "an extraordinary means of treatment" would not involve euthanasia. This upon the reasoning expressed by Pope Pius XII in his "allocutio" (address) to anesthesiologists on November 24, 1957, when he dealt with the question:

Does the anesthesiologist have the right, or is he bound, in all cases of deep unconsciousness, even in those that are completely hopeless in the opinion of the competent doctor, to use modern artificial respiration apparatus, even against the will of the family?

His answer made the following points:

1. In ordinary cases the doctor has the right to act in this manner, but is not bound to do so unless this is the only way of fulfilling another certain moral duty.
2. The doctor, however, has no right independent of the patient. He can act only if the patient explicitly or implicitly, directly or indirectly gives him the permission.
3. The treatment as described in the question constitutes extraordinary means of preserving life and so there is no obligation to use them nor to give the doctor permission to use them.
4. The rights and the duties of the family depend on the presumed will of the unconscious patient if he or she is of legal age, and the family, too, is bound to use only ordinary means.
5. This case is not be considered euthanasia in any way; that would never be licit. The interruption of attempts at resuscitation, even when it causes the arrest of circulation, is not more than an indirect cause of the cessation of life, and we must apply in this case the principle of double effect.

So it was that the Bishop Casey statement validated the decision of Joseph Quinlan:

Competent medical testimony has established that Karen Ann Quinlan has no reasonable hope of recovery from her comatose state by the use of any available medical procedures. The continuance of mechanical (cardiorespiratory) supportive measures to sustain continuation of her body functions and her life constitute extraordinary means of treatment. *Therefore, the decision of Joseph . . . Quinlan to request the discontinuance of this treatment is, according to the teachings of the Catholic Church, a morally correct decision.* (emphasis in original)

And the mind and purpose of the intending guardian were undoubtedly influenced by factors included in the following reference to the interrelationship of the three disciplines of theology, law and medicine as exposed in the Casey statement:

The right to a natural death is one outstanding area in which the disciplines of theology, medicine and law overlap; or, to put it another way, it is an area in which these three disciplines convene.

Medicine with its combination of advanced technology and professional ethics is both able and inclined to prolong biological life. Law with its felt obligation to protect the life and freedom of the individual seeks to assure each person's right to live out his human life until its natural and inevitable conclusion. Theology with its acknowledgment of man's dissatisfaction with biological life as the ultimate source of joy . . . defends the sacredness of human life and defends it from all direct attacks.

These disciplines do not conflict with one another, but are necessarily conjoined in the application of their principles in a particular instance such as that of Karen Ann Quinlan. Each must in some way acknowledge the other without denying it own competence. The civil law is not expected to assert a belief in eternal life; nor, on the other hand, is it expected to ignore the right of the individual to profess it, and to form and pursue his conscience in accord with that belief. Medical science is not authorized to directly cause natural death; nor, however, is it expected to prevent it when it is inevitable and all hope of a return to an even partial exercise of human life is irreparably lost. Religion is not expected to define biological death; nor, on its part, is it expected to relinquish its responsibility to assist man in the formation and pursuit of a correct conscience as the acceptance of natural death when science has confirmed its inevitability beyond any hope other than that of preserving biological life in a merely vegetative state.

And the gap in the law is aptly described in the Bishop Casey statement:

In the present public discussion of the case of Karen Ann Quinlan it has been brought out that responsible people involved in medical care, patients and families have exercised the freedom to terminate or withhold certain treatments as extraordinary means in cases judged to be terminal, i.e., cases which hold no realistic hope for some recovery, in accord with the expressed or implied intentions of the patients themselves. To whatever extent this has been happening it has been without sanction in civil law. Those involved in such actions, however, have ethical and theological literature to guide them in the judgments and actions. Furthermore, such actions have not in themselves undermined society's reverence for the lives of sick and dying people.

It is both possible and necessary for society to have laws and ethical standards which provide freedom for decisions, in accord with the expressed or implied intentions of the patient, to terminate or withhold extraordinary treatment in cases which are judged to be hopeless by competent medical authorities, without at the same time leaving an opening for euthanasia. Indeed, to accomplish this, it may simply be required that courts and legislative bodies recognize the present standards and practices of many people engaged in medical care who have been doing what the parents of Karen Ann Quinlan are requesting authorization to have done for their beloved daughter.

Before turning to the legal and constitutional issues involved, we feel it essential to reiterate that the "Catholic view" of religious neutrality in the circumstances of this case is considered by the Court only in the aspect of its impact upon the conscience, motivation and purpose of the intending guardian, Joseph Quinlan, and not as a precedent in terms of the civil law.

If Joseph Quinlan, for instance, were a follower and strongly influenced by the teachings of Buddha, or if, as an agnostic or atheist, his moral judgments were formed without reference to religious feelings, but were nevertheless formed and viable, we would with equal attention and high respect consider these elements, as bearing upon his character, motivations and purposes as relevant to his qualification and suitability as guardian.

It is from this factual base that the Court confronts and responds to three basic issues:

1. Was the trial court correct in denying the specific relief requested by plaintiff, i.e., authorization for termination of the life-supporting apparatus, on the case presented to him? Our determination on that question is in the affirmative.

2. Was the court correct in withholding letters of guardianship from the plaintiff and appointing in his stead a stranger? On that issue our determination is in the negative.

3. Should this Court, in the light of the foregoing conclusions, grant declaratory relief to the plaintiff? On that question our Court's determination is in the affirmative.

This brings us to a consideration of the constitutional and legal issues underlying the foregoing determinations.

Constitutional and Legal Issues

At the outset we note the dual role in which plaintiff comes before the Court. He not only raises, derivatively, what he perceives to be the constitutional and legal rights of his daughter Karen, but he also claims certain rights independently as parent.

Although generally litigant may assert only his own constitutional rights, we have no doubt that plaintiff has sufficient standing to advance both positions.

While no express constitutional language limits judicial activity to cases and controversies, New Jersey courts will not render advisory opinions or entertain proceedings by plaintiffs who do not have sufficient legal standing to maintain their actions. Walker v. Stanhope, 23 N.J. 657, 660, 130 A.2d 372 (1957). However, as in this case, New Jersey courts commonly grant declaratory relief. Declaratory Judgments Act, N.J.S.A. 2A:16–50 et seq. And our courts hold that where the plaintiff is not simply an interloper and the proceeding serves the public interest, standing will be found. Walker v. Stanhope, supra, 23 N.J. at 661–66, 130 A.2d 372; Koons v. Atlantic City Bd. of Comm'rs, 134 N.J.L. 329, 338–39, 47 A.2d 589 (Sup.Ct.1946), aff'd, 135 N.J.L. 204, 50 A.2d 869 (E. & A. 1947). In Crescent Park Tenants Ass'n v. Realty Equities Corp., 58 N.J. 98, 275 A.2d 433 (1971), Justice Jacobs said:

... [W]e have appropriately confined litigation to those situations where the litigant's concern with the subject matter evidenced a sufficient stake and real adverseness. In the overall we have given due weight to the interests of individual justice, along with the public interest, always bearing in mind that throughout our law we have been

sweepingly rejecting procedural frustrations in favor of "just and expeditious determinations on the ultimate merits." [58 N.J. at 107–08, 275 A.2d at 438 (quoting from Tumarkin v. Friedman, 17 N.J.Super. 20, 21, 85 A.2d 304 (App.Div.1951), certif. den., 9 N.J. 287, 88 A.2d 39 (1952))].

The father of Karen Quinlan is certainly no stranger to the present controversy. His interests are real and adverse and he raises questions of surpassing importance. Manifestly, he has standing to assert his daughter's constitutional rights, she being incompetent to do so.

I. The Free Exercise of Religion

We think the contention as to interference with religious beliefs or rights may be considered and dealt with without extended discussion, given the acceptance of distinctions so clear and simple in their precedential definition as to be dispositive on their face.

Simply stated, the right to religious beliefs is absolute but conduct in pursuance thereof is not wholly immune from governmental restraint. John F. Kennedy Memorial Hosp. v. Heston, 58 N.J. 576, 580–81, 279 A.2d 670 (1971). So it is that, for the sake of life, courts sometimes (but not always) order blood transfusions for Jehovah's Witnesses (whose religious beliefs abhor such procedure), Application of President & Directors of Georgetown College, Inc., 118 U.S.App.D.C. 80, 331 F.2d 1000 (D.C.Cir.), cert. den., 337 U.S. 978, 84 S.Ct. 1883, 12 L.Ed.2d 746 (1964); United States v. George, 239 F.Supp. 752 (D.Conn. 1965); John F. Kennedy Memorial Hosp. v. Heston, supra; Powell v. Columbia Presbyterian Medical Center, 49 Misc.2d 215, 267 N.Y.S.2d 450 (Sup.Ct.1965); but see In re Osborne, 294 A.2d 372 (D.C.Ct.App.1972); In re Estate of Brooks, 32 Ill.2d 361, 205 N.E.2d 435 (Sup.Ct.1965); Erickson v. Dilgard, 44 Misc.2d 27, 252 N.Y.S.2d 705 (Sup.Ct.1962); see generally Annot., "Power Of Courts Or Other Public Agencies, In The Absence Of Statutory Authority, To Order Compulsory Medical Care for Adult," 9 A.L.R.3d 1391 (1966); forbid exposure to death from handling virulent snakes or ingesting poison (interfering with deeply held religious sentiments in such regard), e.g., Hill v. State, 38 Aa.App. 404, 88

So.2d 880 (Ct.App.), *cert. den.,* 264 Ala. 697, 88 So.2d 887 (Sup.Ct.1956); *State v. Massey,* 229 N.C. 734, 51 S.E.2d 179 (Sup.Ct.), appeal dismissed *sub nom., Bunn v. North Carolina,* 336 U.S. 942, 69 S.Ct. 813, 93 L.Ed. 1099 (1949); *State ex rel. Swann v. Pack,* Tenn., 527 S.W.2d 99 (Sup.Ct.1975), *cert. den.,* —— U.S. ——, 96 S.Ct.1429, 46 L.Ed.2d 360, 44 U.S.L.W. 3498, No. 75–956 (March 8, 1976); and protect the public health as in the case of compulsory vaccination (over the strongest of religious objections), *e.g., Wright v. DeWitt School Dist. 1,* 238 Ark. 906, 385 S.W.2d 644 (Sup.Ct.1965); *Mountain Lakes Bd. of Educ. v. Maas,* 56 N.J.Super. 245, 152 A.2d 394 (App.Div.1959), aff'd o. b., 31 N.J. 537, 158 A.2d 330 (1960), *cert. den.,* 363 U.S. 843, 80 S.Ct. 1613, 4 L.Ed.2d 1727 (1960); *McCartney v. Austin,* 57 Misc.2d 525, 293 N.Y.S.2d 188 (Sup.Ct.1968). The public interest is thus considered paramount, without essential dissolution of respect for religious beliefs.

We think, without further examples, that, ranged against the State's interest in the preservation of life, the impingement of religious belief, much less religious "neutrality" as here, does not reflect a constitutional question, in the circumstances at least of the case presently before the Court. Moreover, like the trial court, we do not recognize an independent parental right of religious freedom to support the relief requested. 137 N.J.Super. at 267–68, 348 A.2d 801.

II. Cruel and Unusual Punishment

Similarly inapplicable to the case before us is the Constitution's Eighth Amendment protection against cruel and unusual punishment which, as held by the trial court, is not relevant to situations other than the imposition of penal sanctions. Historic in nature, it stemmed from punitive excesses in the infliction of criminal penalties.[7] We find no precedent in law which would justify its extension to the correction of social injustice or hardship such as, for instance, in the case of poverty. The latter often condemns the poor and deprived to horrendous living conditions which could certainly be described in the abstract as "cruel and unusual

punishment." Yet the constitutional base of protection from "cruel and unusual punishment" is plainly irrelevant to such societal ills which must be remedied, if at all, under other concepts of constitutional and civil right.

So it is in the case of the unfortunate Karen Quinlan. Neither the State, nor the law, but the accident of fate and nature, has inflicted upon her conditions which though in essence cruel and most unusual, yet do not amount to "punishment" in any constitutional sense.

Neither the judgment of the court below, nor the medical decision which confronted it, nor the law and equity perceptions which impelled its action, nor the whole factual base upon which it was predicated, inflicted "cruel and unusual punishment" in the constitutional sense.

III. The Right of Privacy[8]

It is the issue of the constitutional right of privacy that has given us most concern, in the exceptional circumstances of this case. Here a loving parent, *qua* parent and raising the rights of his incompetent and profoundly damaged daughter, probably irreversibly doomed to no more than a biologically vegetative remnant of life, is before the court. He seeks authorization to abandon specialized technological procedures which can only maintain for a time a body having no potential for resumption or continuance of other than a "vegetative" existence.

We have no doubt, in these unhappy circumstances, that if Karen were herself miraculously lucid for an interval (not altering the existing prognosis of the condition to which she would soon return) and perceptive of her irreversible condition, she could effectively decide upon discontinuance of the life-support apparatus, even if it meant the prospect of natural death. To this extent we may distinguish *Heston, supra,* which concerned a severely injured young woman (Delores Heston), whose life depended on surgery and blood transfusion; and who was in such extreme shock that she was unable to express an informed choice (although the Court apparently considered the case as if the patient's own religious decision to resist transfusion were at stake), but most importantly a patient apparently salvable to long life and vibrant

health;—a situation not at all like the present case.

We have no hesitancy in deciding, in the instant diametrically opposite case, that no external compelling interest of the State could compel Karen to endure the unendurable, only to vegetate a few measurable months with no realistic possibility of returning to any semblance of cognitive or sapient life. We perceive no thread of logic distinguishing between such a choice on Karen's part and a similar choice which, under the evidence in this case, could be made by a competent patient terminally ill, riddled by cancer and suffering great pain; such a patient would not be resuscitated or put on a respirator in the example described by Dr. Korein, and *a fortiori* would not be kept *against his will* on a respirator.

Although the Constitution does not explicitly mention a right of privacy, Supreme Court decisions have recognized that a right of personal privacy exists and that certain areas of privacy are guaranteed under the Constitution. *Eisenstadt v. Baird,* 405 U.S. 438, 92 S.Ct. 1029, 31 L.Ed.2d 349 (1972); *Stanley v. Georgia,* 394 U.S. 557, 89 S.Ct. 1243, 22 L.Ed.2d 542 (1969). The Court has interdicted judicial intrusion into many aspects of personal decision, sometimes basing this restraint upon the conception of a limitation of judicial interest and responsibility, such as with regard to contraception and its relationship to family life and decision. *Griswold v. Connecticut,* 381 U.S. 479, 85 S.Ct. 1678, 14 L.Ed.2d 510 (1965).

The Court in *Griswold* found the unwritten constitutional right of privacy to exist in the penumbra of specific guarantees of the Bill of Rights "formed by emanations from those guarantees that help give them life and substance." 381 U.S. at 484, 85 S.Ct. at 1681, 14 L.Ed.2d at 514. Presumably this right is broad enough to encompass a patient's decision to decline medical treatment under certain circumstances, in much the same way as it is broad enough to encompass a woman's decision to terminate pregnancy under certain conditions. *Roe v. Wade,* 410 U.S. 113, 153, 93 S.Ct. 705, 727, 35 L.Ed.2d 147, 177 (1973).

Nor is such right of privacy forgotten in the New Jersey Constitution. N.J.Const. (1947), Art. I, par. 1.

The claimed interests of the State in this case are essentially the preservation and sanctity of human life and defense of the right of the physician to administer medical treatment according to his best judgment. In this case the doctors say that removing Karen from the respirator will conflict with their professional judgment. The plaintiff answers that Karen's present treatment serves only a maintenance function; that the respirator cannot cure or improve her condition but at best can only prolong her inevitable slow deterioration and death; and that the interests of the patient, as seen by her surrogate, the guardian, must be evaluated by the court as predominant, even in the face of an opinion *contra* by the present attending physicians. Plaintiff's distinction is significant. The nature of Karen's care and the realistic chances of her recovery are quite unlike those of the patients discussed in many of the cases where treatments were ordered. In many of those cases the medical procedure required (usually a transfusion) constituted a minimal bodily invasion and the chances of recovery and return to functioning life were very good. We think that the State's interest *contra* weakens and the individual's right to privacy grows as the degree of bodily invasion increases and the prognosis dims. Ultimately there comes a point at which the individual's rights overcome the State interest. It is for that reason that we believe Karen's choice, if she were competent to make it, would be vindicated by the law. Her prognosis is extremely poor,—she will never resume cognitive life. And the bodily invasion is very great,—she requires 24 hour intensive nursing care, antibiotics, the assistance of a respirator, a catheter and feeding tube.

Our affirmation of Karen's independent right of choice, however, would ordinarily be based upon her competency to assert it. The sad truth, however, is that she is grossly incompetent and we cannot discern her supposed choice based on the testimony of her previous conversations with friends, where such testimony is without sufficient probative weight. 137 N.J.Super. at 260, 348 A.2d 801. Nevertheless we have concluded that

Karen's right of privacy may be asserted on her behalf by her guardian under the peculiar circumstances here present.

If a putative decision by Karen to permit this non-cognitive, vegetative existence to terminate by natural forces is regarded as a valuable incident of her right of privacy, as we believe it to be, then it should not be discarded solely on the basis that her condition prevents her conscious exercise of the choice. The only practical way to prevent destruction of the right is to permit the guardian and family of Karen to render their best judgment, subject to the qualifications hereinafter stated, as to whether she would exercise it in these circumstances. If their conclusion is in the affirmative this decision should be accepted by a society the overwhelming majority of whose members would, we think, in similar circumstances, exercise such a choice in the same way for themselves or for those closest to them. It is for this reason that we determine that Karen's right of privacy may be asserted in her behalf, in this respect, by her guardian and family under the particular circumstances presented by this record.

Regarding Mr. Quinlan's right of privacy, we agree with Judge Muir's conclusion that there is no parental constitutional right that would entitle him to a grant of relief *in propria persona*. *Id.* at 266, 348 A.2d 801. Insofar as a parental right of privacy has been recognized, it has been in the context of determining the rearing of infants and, as Judge Muir put it, involved "continuing life styles." *See Wisconsin v. Yoder*, 406 U.S. 205, 92 S.Ct. 1526, 32 L.Ed.2d 15 (1972); *Pierce v. Society of Sisters*, 268 U.S. 510, 45 S.Ct. 571, 69 L.Ed. 1070 (1925); *Meyer v. Nebraska*, 262 U.S. 390, 43 S.Ct. 625, 67 L.Ed. 1042 (1923). Karen Quinlan is a 22 year old adult. Her right of privacy in respect of the matter before the Court is to be vindicated by Mr. Quinlan as guardian, as hereinabove determined.

IV. The Medical Factor

Having declared the substantive legal basis upon which plaintiff's rights as representative of Karen must be deemed predicated, we face and respond to the assertion on behalf of defendants that our premise unwarranta-

bly offends prevailing medical standards. We thus turn to consideration of the medical decision supporting the determination made below, conscious of the paucity of pre-existing legislative and judicial guidance as to the rights and liabilities therein involved.

A significant problem in any discussion of sensitive medical-legal issues is the marked, perhaps unconscious, tendency of many to distort what the law is, in pursuit of an exposition of what they would like the law to be. Nowhere is this barrier to the intelligent resolution of legal controversies more obstructive than in the debate over patient rights at the end of life. Judicial refusals to order lifesaving treatment in the face of contrary claims of bodily self-determination or free religious exercise are too often cited in support of a preconceived "right to die," even though the patients, wanting to live, have claimed no such right. Conversely, the assertion of a religious or other objection to lifesaving treatment is at times condemned as attempted suicide, even though suicide means something quite different in the law. [Byrn, "Compulsory Lifesaving Treatment For The Competent Adult," 44 Fordham L. Rev. 1 (1975)].

Perhaps the confusion there adverted to stems from mention by some courts of statutory or common law condemnation of suicide as demonstrating the state's interest in the preservation of life. We would see, however, a real distinction between the self-infliction of deadly harm and a self-determination against artificial life support or radical surgery, for instance, in the face of irreversible, painful and certain imminent death. The contrasting situations mentioned are analogous to those continually faced by the medical profession. When does the institution of life-sustaining procedures, ordinarily mandatory, become the subject of medical discretion in the context of administration to persons *in extremis*? And when does the withdrawal of such procedures, from such persons already supported by them, come within the orbit of medical discretion? When does a determination as to either of the foregoing contingencies court the hazard of civil or criminal liability on the part of the physician or institution involved?

The existence and nature of the medical dilemma need hardly be discussed at length, portrayed as it is in the present case and complicated as it has recently come to be in view of the dramatic advance of medical technology. The dilemma is there, it is real, it is constantly resolved in accepted medical practice without attention in the courts, it pervades the issues in the very case we here examine. The branch of the dilemma involving the doctor's responsibility and the relationship of the court's duty was thus conceived by Judge Muir:

Doctors . . . to treat a patient, must deal with medical tradition and past case histories. They must be guided by what they do know. The extent of their training, their experience, consultation with other physicians, must guide their decision-making processes in providing care to their patient. The nature, extent and duration of care by societal standards is the responsibility of a physician. The morality and conscience of our society places this responsibility in the hands of the physician. What justification is there to remove it from the control of the medical profession and place it in the hands of the courts? [137 N.J.Super. at 259, 348 A.2d at 818].

Such notions as to the distribution of responsibility, heretofore generally entertained, should however neither impede this Court in deciding matters clearly justiciable nor preclude a re-examination by the Court as to underlying human values and rights. Determinations as to these must, in the ultimate, be responsive not only to the concepts of medicine but also to the common moral judgment of the community at large. In the latter respect the Court has a nondelegable judicial responsibility.

Put in another way, the law, equity and justice must not themselves quail and be helpless in the face of modern technological marvels presenting questions hitherto unthought of. Where a Karen Quinlan, or a parent, or a doctor, or a hospital, or a State seeks the process and response of a court, it must answer with its most informed conception of justice in the previously unexplored circumstances presented to it. That is its obligation and we are here fulfilling it, for the actors and those having an interest in the matter should not go without remedy.

Courts in the exercise of their *parens patriae* responsibility to protect those under disability have sometimes implemented medical decisions and authorized their carrying out under the doctrine of "substituted judgment." *Hart v. Brown*, 29 Conn.Sup. 368, 289

A.2d 386, 387–88 (Super.Ct.1972); *Strunk v. Strunk*, 445 S.W.2d 145, 147–48 (Ky.1969). For as Judge Muir pointed out:

As part of the inherent power of equity, a Court of Equity has full and complete jurisdiction over the persons of those who labor under any legal disability. . . . The Court's action in such a case is not limited by any narrow bounds, but it is empowered to stretch forth its arm in whatever direction its aid and protection may be needed. While this is indeed a special exercise of equity jurisdiction, it is beyond question that by virtue thereof the Court may pass upon purely personal rights. [137 N.J.Super. at 254, 348 A.2d at 816 (quoting from *Am.Jur.*2d, Equity § 69 (1966))].

But insofar as a court, having no inherent medical expertise, is called upon to overrule a professional decision made according to prevailing medical practice and standards, a different question is presented. As mentioned below, a doctor is required

"to exercise in the treatment of his patient the degree of care, knowledge and skill ordinarily possessed and exercised in similar situations by the average member of the profession practicing in his field." *Schueler v. Strelinger*, 43 N.J. 330, 344, 204 A.2d 577, 584 (1964). If he is a specialist he "must employ not merely the skill of a general practitioner, but also that special degree of skill normally possessed by the average physician who devotes special study and attention to the particular organ or disease or injury involved, having regard to the present state of scientific knowledge". *Clark v. Wichman*, 72 N.J.Super. 486, 493, 179 A.2d 38, 42 (App.Div.1962). This is the duty that establishes his legal obligations to his patients. [137 N.J.Super. at 257–58, 348 A.2d at 818].

The medical obligation is related to standards and practice prevailing in the profession. The physicians in charge of the case, as noted above, declined to withdraw the respirator. That decision was consistent with the proofs below as to the then existing medical standards and practices.

Under the law as it then stood, Judge Muir was correct in declining to authorize withdrawal of the respirator.

However, in relation to the matter of the declaratory relief sought by plaintiff as representative of Karen's interests, we are required to reevaluate the applicability of the medical standards

projected in the court below. The question is whether there is such internal consistency and rationality in the application of such standards as should warrant their constituting an ineluctable bar to the effectuation of substantive relief for plaintiff at the hands of the court. We have concluded not.

In regard to the foregoing it is pertinent that we consider the impact on the standards both of the civil and criminal law as to medical liability and the new technological means of sustaining life irreversibly damaged.

The modern proliferation of substantial malpractice litigation and the less frequent but even more unnerving possibility of criminal sanctions would seem, for it is beyond human nature to suppose otherwise, to have bearing on the practice and standards as they exist. The brooding presence of such possible liability, it was testified here, had no part in the decision of the treating physicians. As did Judge Muir, we afford this testimony full credence. But we cannot believe that the stated factor has not had a strong influence on the standards, as the literature on the subject plainly reveals. (See footnote 9, *infra*). Moreover our attention is drawn not so much to the recognition by Drs. Morse and Javed of the extant practice and standards but to the widening ambiguity of those standards themselves in their application to the medical problems we are discussing.

The agitation of the medical community in the face of modern life prolongation technology and its search for definitive policy are demonstrated in the large volume of relevant professional commentary.[9]

The wide debate thus reflected contrasts with the relative paucity of legislative and judicial guides and standards in the same field. The medical profession has sought to devise guidelines such as the "brain death" concept of the Harvard Ad Hoc Committee mentioned above. But it is perfectly apparent from the testimony we have quoted of Dr. Korein, and indeed so clear as almost to be judicially noticeable, that humane decisions against resuscitative or maintenance therapy are frequently a recognized *de facto* response in the medical world to the irreversible, terminal, pain-ridden patient, especially with familial consent. And these cases, of course, are far short of "brain death."

We glean from the record here that physicians distinguish between curing the ill and comforting and easing the dying; that they refuse to treat the curable as if they were dying or ought to die, and that they have sometimes refused to treat the hopeless and dying as if they were curable. In this sense, as we were reminded by the testimony of Drs. Korein and Diamond, many of them have refused to inflict an undesired prolongation of the process of dying on a patient in irreversible condition when it is clear that such "therapy" offers neither human nor humane benefit. We think these attitudes represent a balanced implementation of a profoundly realistic perspective on the meaning of life and death and that they respect the whole Judeo-Christian tradition of regard for human life. No less would they seem consistent with the moral matrix of medicine, "to heal," very much in the sense of the endless mission of the law, "to do justice."

Yet this balance, we feel, is particularly difficult to perceive and apply in the context of the development by advanced technology of sophisticated and artificial life-sustaining devices. For those possibly curable, such devices are of great value, and, as ordinary medical procedures, are essential. Consequently, as pointed out by Dr. Diamond, they are necessary because of the ethic of medical practice. But in light of the situation in the present case (while the record here is somewhat hazy in distinguishing between "ordinary" and "extraordinary" measures), one would have to think that the use of the same respirator or like support could be considered "ordinary" in the context of the possibly curable patient but "extraordinary" in the context of the forced sustaining by cardiorespiratory processes of an irreversibly doomed patient. And this dilemma is sharpened in the face of the malpractice and criminal action threat which we have mentioned.

We would hesitate, in this imperfect world, to propose as to physicians that type of immunity which from the early common law has surrounded judges and grand jurors, see e.g., Grove v. Van Duyn, 44 N.J.L. 654, 656–57 (E & A.1882); O'Regan v. Schermerhorn, 25 N.J.Misc. 1, 19–20, 50 A.2d 10 (Sup.Ct.1940), so that they might without fear of personal retaliation perform

their judicial duties with independent objectivity. In Bradley v. Fisher, 80 U.S. (13 Wall.) 335, 347, 20 L.Ed. 646, 649 (1872), the Supreme Court held:

[I]t is a general principle of the highest importance to the proper administration of justice that a judicial officer, in exercising the authority vested in him, shall be free to act upon his own convictions, without apprehension of personal consequences to himself.

Lord Coke said of judges that "they are only to make an account to God and the King [the State]." 12 Coke Rep. 23, 25, 77 Eng.Rep. 1305, 1307 (S.C.1608).

Nevertheless, there must be a way to free physicians, in the pursuit of their healing vocation, from possible contamination by self-interest or self-protection concerns which would inhibit their independent medical judgments for the well-being of their dying patients. We would hope that this opinion might be serviceable to some degree in ameliorating the professional problems under discussion.

A technique aimed at the underlying difficulty (though in a somewhat broader context) is described by Dr. Karen Teel, a pediatrician and a director of Pediatric Education, who writes in the Baylor Law Review under the title "The Physician's Dilemma: A Doctor's View: What The Law Should Be." Dr. Teel recalls:

Physicians, by virtue of their responsibility for medical judgments are, partly by choice and partly by default, charged with the responsibility of making ethical judgments which we are sometimes ill-equipped to make. We are not always morally and legally authorized to make them. The physician is thereby assuming a civil and criminal liability that, as often as not, he does not even realize as a factor in his decision. There is little or no dialogue in this whole process. The physician assumes that his judgment is called for and, in good faith, he acts. Someone must and it has been the physician who has assumed the responsibility and the risk.

I suggest that it would be more appropriate to provide a regular forum for more input and dialogue in individual situations and to allow the responsibility of these judgments to be shared. Many hospitals have established an Ethics Committee composed of physicians, social workers, attorneys, and theologians, . . . which serves to review the individual circumstances of ethical dilemma and which has provided

much in the way of assistance and safeguards for patients and their medical caretakers. Generally, the authority of these committees is primarily restricted to the hospital setting and their official status is more that of an advisory body than of an enforcing body.

The concept of an Ethics Committee which has this kind of organization and is readily accessible to those persons rendering medical care to patients, would be, I think, the most promising direction for further study at this point. . . . [This would allow] some much needed dialogue regarding these issues and [force] the point of exploring all of the options for a particular patient. It diffuses the responsibility for making these judgments. Many physicians, in many circumstances, would welcome this sharing of responsibility. I believe that such an entity could lend itself well to an assumption of a legal status which would allow courses of action not now undertaken because of the concern for liability. [27 Baylor L.Rev. 6, 8–9 (1975)].

The most appealing factor in the technique suggested by Dr. Teel seems to us to be the diffusion of professional responsibility for decision, comparable in a way to the value of multi-judge courts in finally resolving on appeal difficult questions of law. Moreover, such a system would be protective to the hospital as well as the doctor in screening out, so to speak, a case which might be contaminated by less than worthy motivations of family or physician. In the real world and in relationship to the momentous decision contemplated, the value of additional views and diverse knowledge is apparent.

We consider that a practice of applying to a court to confirm such decisions would generally be inappropriate, not only because that would be a gratuitous encroachment upon the medical profession's field of competence, but because it would be impossibly cumbersome. Such a requirement is distinguishable from the judicial overview traditionally required in other matters such as the adjudication and commitment of mental incompetents. This is not to say that in the case of an otherwise justiciable controversy access to the courts would be foreclosed; we speak rather of a general practice and procedure.

And although the deliberations and decisions which we describe would be professional in nature they should obviously include at some stage the feelings of the family of an incompetent relative. Decision-making within health care if it is considered as an expression of a primary obligation of the physician, *primum non nocere,* should be controlled primarily within the patient-doctor-family relationship, as indeed was recognized by Judge Muir in his supplemental opinion of November 12, 1975.

If there could be created not necessarily this particular system but some reasonable counterpart, we would have no doubt that such decisions, thus determined to be in accordance with medical practice and prevailing standards, would be accepted by society and by the courts, at least in cases comparable to that of Karen Quinlan.

The evidence in this case convinces us that the focal point of decision should be the prognosis as to the reasonable possibility of return to cognitive and sapient life, as distinguished from the forced continuance of that biological vegetative existence to which Karen seems to be doomed.

In summary of the present Point of this opinion, we conclude that the state of the pertinent medical standards and practices which guided the attending physicians in this matter is not such as would justify this Court in deeming itself bound or controlled thereby in responding to the case for declaratory relief established by the parties on the record before us.

V. Alleged Criminal Liability
Having concluded that there is a right of privacy that might permit termination of treatment in the circumstances of this case, we turn to consider the relationship of the exercise of that right to the criminal law. We are aware that such termination of treatment would accelerate Karen's death. The County Prosecutor and the Attorney General maintain that there would be criminal liability for such acceleration. Under the statutes of this State, the unlawful killing of another human being is criminal homicide. N.J.S.A. 2A:113-1, 2, 5. We conclude that there would be no criminal homicide in the circumstances of this case. We believe, first, that the ensuing death would not be homicide but rather expiration from existing natural causes. Secondly, even if it were to be regarded as homicide, it would not be unlawful.

These conclusions rest upon definitional and constitutional bases. The termination of treatment pursuant to the right of privacy is, within the limitations of this case, *ipso facto* lawful. Thus, a death resulting from such an act would not come within the scope of the homicide statutes proscribing only the unlawful killing of another. There is a real and in this case determinative distinction between the unlawful taking of the life of another and the ending of artificial life-support systems as a matter of self-determination.

Furthermore, the exercise of a constitutional right such as we have here found is protected from criminal prosecution. *See Stanley v. Georgia, supra,* 394 U.S. at 559, 89 S.Ct. at 1245, 22 L.Ed.2d at 546. We do not question the State's undoubted power to punish the taking of human life, but that power does not encompass individuals terminating medical treatment pursuant to their right of privacy. *See id.* at 568, 89 S.Ct. at 1250, 22 L.Ed.2d at 551. The constitutional protection extends to third parties whose action is necessary to effectuate the exercise of that right where the individuals themselves would not be subject to prosecution or the third parties are charged as accessories to an act which could not be a crime. *Eisenstadt v. Baird, supra,* 405 U.S. at 445-46, 92 S.Ct. at 1034-35, 31 L.Ed.2d at 357-58; *Griswold v. Connecticut, supra,* 381 U.S. at 481, 85 S.Ct. at 1679-80, 14 L.Ed.2d at 512-13. And, under the circumstances of this case, these same principles would apply to and negate a valid prosecution for attempted suicide were there still such a crime in this State.[10]

VI. The Guardianship of the Person
The trial judge bifurcated the guardianship, as we have noted, refusing to appoint Joseph Quinlan to be guardian of the person and limiting his guardianship to that of the property of his daughter. Such occasional division of guardianship, as between responsibility for the person and the property of an incompetent person, has roots deep in the common law and was well within the jurisdictional capacity of the trial judge. *In re Rollins,* 65 A.2d 667, 679-82 (N.J.Cty.Ct.1949).

The statute creates an initial presumption of entitlement to guardianship in the next of kin, for it provides:

In any case where a guardian is to be appointed, letters of guardianship shall be granted . . . to the next of kin, or if . . . it is proven to the court that no appointment from among them will be to the best interest of the incompetent or his estate, then to such other proper person as will accept the same. [N.J.S.A. 3A:6-36. *See In re Roll,* 117 N.J.Super. 122, 124, 283, A.2d 764, 765 (App.Div.1971)].

The trial court was apparently convinced of the high character of Joseph Quinlan and his general suitability as guardian under other circumstances, describing him as "very sincere, moral, ethical and religious." The court felt, however, that the obligation to concur in the medical care and treatment of his daughter would be a source of anguish to him and would distort his "decision-making processes." We disagree, for we sense from the whole record before us that while Mr. Quinlan feels a natural grief, and understandably sorrows because of the tragedy which has befallen his daughter, his strength of purpose and character far outweighs these sentiments and qualifies him eminently for guardianship of the person as well as the property of his daughter. Hence we discern no valid reason to overrule the statutory intendment of preference to the next of kin.

Declaratory Relief

We thus arrive at the formulation of the declaratory relief which we have concluded is appropriate to this case. Some time has passed since Karen's physical and mental condition was described to the Court. At that time her continuing deterioration was plainly projected. Since the record has not been expanded we assume that she is now even more fragile and nearer to death than she was then. Since her present treating physicians may give reconsideration to her present posture in the light of this opinion, and since we are transferring to the plaintiff as guardian the choice of the attending physician and therefore other physicians may be in charge of the case who may take a different view from that of the present attending physicians, we herewith declare the following affirmative relief on behalf of the plaintiff. Upon the concurrence of the guardian and family of Karen, should the responsible attending physicians conclude that there is no reasonable possibility of Karen's ever emerging from her present comatose condition to a cognitive, sapient state and that the life-support apparatus now being administered to Karen should be discontinued, they shall consult with the hospital "Ethics Committee" or like body of the institution in which Karen is then hospitalized. If that consultative body agrees that there is no reasonable possibility of Karen's ever emerging from her present comatose condition to a cognitive, sapient state, the present life-support system may be withdrawn and said action shall be without any civil or criminal liability therefor on the part of any participant, whether guardian, physician, hospital or others.[11] We herewith specifically so hold.

Conclusion

We therefore remand this record to the trial court to implement (without further testimonial hearing) the following decisions:
1. To discharge, with the thanks of the Court for his service, the present guardian of the person of Karen Quinlan, Thomas R. Curtin, Esquire, a member of the Bar and an officer of the court.
2. To appoint Joseph Quinlan as guardian of the person of Karen Quinlan with full power to make decisions with regard to the identity of her treating physicians.

We repeat for the sake of emphasis and clarity that upon the concurrence of the guardian and family of Karen, should the responsible attending physicians conclude that there is no reasonable possibility of Karen's ever emerging from her present comatose condition to a cognitive, sapient state and that the life-support apparatus now being administered to Karen should be discontinued, they shall consult with the hospital "Ethics Committee" or like body of the institution in which Karen is then hospitalized. If that consultative body agrees that there is no reasonable possibility of Karen's ever emerging from her present comatose condition to a cognitive, sapient state, the present life-support system may be withdrawn and said action shall be without any civil or criminal liability therefor on the part of any participant, whether guardian, physician, hospital or others.

By the above ruling we do not intend to be understood as implying that a proceeding for judicial declaratory relief is necessarily required for the implementation of comparable decisions in the field of medical practice.

Modified and remanded.

For modification and remandment: Chief Justice Hughes, Justices Mountain, Sullivan, Pashman, Clifford and Schreiber and Judge Conford—7.

Opposed: None.

Notes

1. The importance of the preservation of life is memorialized in various organic documents. The Declaration of Independence states as self-evident truths "that all men . . . are endowed by their Creator with certain unalienable Rights, that among these are Life, Liberty and the pursuit of Happiness." This ideal is inherent in the Constitution of the United States. It is explicitly recognized in our Constitution of 1947 which provides for "certain natural and unalienable rights, among which are those of enjoying and defending life. . . ." N.J.Const. (1947), Art. I, par. 1. Our State government is established to protect such rights, N.J.Const. (1947), Art. I, par. 2, and, acting through the Attorney General (N.J.S.A. 52:17A–4(h)), it enforces them.

2. Dr. Julius Korein, a neurologist, testified:
A. . . . [Y]ou've got a set of possible lesions that prior to the era of advanced technology and advances in medicine were no problem inasmuch as the patient would expire. They could do nothing for themselves and even external care was limited. It was—I don't know how many years ago they couldn't keep a person alive with intravenous feedings because they couldn't give enough calories. Now they have these high caloric tube feedings that can keep people in excellent nutrition for years so what's happened is these things have occurred all along but the technology has now reached a point where you can in fact start to replace anything outside of the brain to maintain something that is irreversibly damaged.
Q. Doctor, can the art of medicine repair the cerebral damage that was sustained by Karen?
A. In my opinion, no. . . .
Q. Doctor, in your opinion is there any course of treatment that will lead to the improvement of Karen's condition?
A. No.

3. The Harvard Ad Hoc standards, with reference to "brain death," will be discussed *infra*. [Reprinted as Chapter 79 of this volume.]

4. This cross-appeal was later informally withdrawn but in view of the importance of the matter we nevertheless deal with it.

5. Dr. Robert J. Morse, a neurologist, and Karen's treating physician from the time of her admission to Saint Clare's Hospital on April 24, 1975 (reference was made *supra* to "treating physicians" named as

defendants; this term included Dr. Arshad Javed, a highly qualified pulmonary internist, who considers that he manages that phase of Karen's care with primary responsibility to the "attending physician," Dr. Morse).

6. Death. The cessation of life; the ceasing to exist; defined by physicians as a total stoppage of the circulation of the blood, and a cessation of the animal and vital functions consequent thereon, such as respiration, pulsation, etc. *Black's Law Dictionary* 488 (rev. 4th ed. 1968).

7. It is generally agreed that the Eighth Amendment's provision of "[n]or cruel and unusual punishments inflicted" is drawn verbatim from the English Declaration of Rights. *See* 1 Wm. & M., sess. 2, c. 2 (1689). The prohibition arose in the context of excessive punishments for crimes, punishments that were barbarous and savage as well as disproportionate to the offense committed. *See generally* Granucci " 'Nor Cruel and Unusual Punishments Inflicted:' The Original Meaning," 57 Calif.L.Rev. 839, 844–60 (1969); Note, "This Cruel and Unusual Punishment Clause and the Substantive Criminal Law," 79 Harv.L.Rev. 635, 636–39 (1966). The principle against excessiveness in criminal punishments can be traced back to Chapters 20–22 of the *Magna Carta* (1215). The historical background of the Eighth Amendment was examined at some length in various opinions in *Furman v. Georgia*, 408 U.S. 238, 92 S.Ct. 2726, 33 L.Ed.2d 346 (1972).
The Constitution itself is silent as to the meaning of the word "punishment." Whether it refers to the variety of legal and nonlegal penalties that human beings endure or whether it must be in connection with a criminal rather than a civil proceeding is not stated in the document. But the origins of the clause are clear. And the cases construing it have consistently held that the "punishment" contemplated by the Eighth Amendment is the penalty inflicted by a court for the commission of a crime or in the enforcement of what is a criminal law. *See, e.g., Trop v. Dulles,* 356 U.S. 86, 94–99, 78 S.Ct. 590, 594–97, 2 L.Ed.2d 630, 638–41 (1957). *See generally* Note, "The Effectiveness of the Eighth Amendment: An Appraisal of Cruel and Unusual Punishment," 36 N.Y.U.L.Rev. 846, 854–57 (1961). A deprivation, forfeiture or penalty arising out of a civil proceeding or otherwise cannot be "cruel and unusual punishment" within the meaning of the constitutional clause.

8. The right we here discuss is included within the class of what have been called rights of "personality." *See* Pound, "Equitable Relief against Defamation and Injuries to Personality," 29 Harv.L.Rev. 640, 668–76 (1916). Equitable jurisdiction with respect to the recognition and enforcement of such rights has long been recognized in New Jersey. *See, e.g., Vanderbilt v. Mitchell,* 72 N.J.Eq. 910, 919–20, 67 A. 97 (E. & A. 1907).

9. *See, e.g.,* Downing, *Euthanasia and the Right to Death* (1969); St. John-Stevas, *Life, Death and the Law* (1961); Williams, *The Sanctity of Human Life and the Criminal Law* (1957); Appel, "Ethical and Legal Questions Posed by Recent Advances in Medicine," 205 J.A.M.A. 513 (1968); Cantor, "A Patient's Decision To Decline Life-Saving Medical Treatment: Bodily Integrity Versus The Preservation Of Life," 26 Rutgers L.Rev. 228 (1973); Claypool, "The Family Deals with Death," 27 Baylor L.Rev. 34 (1975); Elkington, "The Dying Patient, The Doctor and The Law," 13 Vill.L.Rev. 740 (1968); Fletcher, "Legal Aspects of the Decision Not to Prolong Life," 203 J.A.M.A. 65 (1968); Foreman, "The Physician's Criminal Liability for the Practice of Euthanasia," 27 Baylor L.Rev. 54 (1975); Gurney, "Is There A Right To Die?—A Study of the Law of Euthanasia," 3 Cumb.-Sam.L.Rev. 235 (1972). Mannes, "Euthanasia vs. The Right to Life," 27 Baylor L.Rev. 68 (1975); Sharp & Crofts, "Death with Dignity and The Physician's Civil Liability," 27 Baylor L.Rev. 86 (1975); Sharpe & Hargest, "Lifesaving Treatment for Unwilling Patients," 36 Fordham L.Rev. 695 (1968); Skegg, "Irreversibly Comatose Individuals: 'Alive' or 'Dead'?," 33 Camb.L.J. 130 (1974); Comment, "The Right to Die," 7 Houston L.Rev. 654 (1970); Note, "The Time Of Death—A Legal, Ethical and Medical Dilemma," 18 Catholic Law, 243 (1972); Note, "Compulsory Medical Treatment: The State's Interest Re-evaluated," 51 Minn.L.Rev. 293 (1966).

10. An attempt to commit suicide was an indictable offense at common law and as such was indictable in this State as a common law misdemeanor. 1 Schlosser, *Criminal Laws of New Jersey* § 12.5 (3d ed. 1970); see N.J.S.A. 2A:85–1. The legislature downgraded the offense in 1957 to the status of a disorderly persons offense, which is not a "crime" under our law. N.J.S.A. 2A:170–25.6. And in 1971, the legislature repealed all criminal sanctions for attempted suicide. N.J.S.A. 2A:85–5.1. Provision is now made for temporary hospitalization of persons making such an attempt. N.J.S.A. 30:4–26.3a. We note that under the proposed New Jersey Penal Code (Oct. 1971) there is no provision for criminal punishment of attempted suicide. *See* Commentary, § 2C:11–6. There is, however, an independent offense of "aiding suicide." § 2C:11–6b. This provision, if enacted, would not be incriminatory in circumstances similar to those presented in this case.

11. The declaratory relief we here award is not intended to imply that the principles enunciated in this case might not be applicable in divers other types of terminal medical situations such as those described by Drs. Korein and Diamond, *supra,* not necessarily involving the hopeless loss of cognitive or sapient life.

85

Arthur J. Dyck
An Alternative to the Ethic of Euthanasia

Reprinted with permission of author and publisher from R. H. Williams, ed., *To Live and to Die: When, Why and How?* (New York: Springer-Verlag, 1973), pp. 98–112.

Contemporary society and modern medicine face difficult policy decisions. This is illustrated most recently in the Voluntary Euthanasia Act of 1969, submitted for consideration in the British Parliament. The purpose of that act is to provide for "the administration of euthanasia to persons who request it and who are suffering from an irremediable condition" (Downing, 1971) and to enable such persons to make such a request in advance. For the purposes of that act, euthanasia means "the painless inducement of death" to be administered by a physician, i.e., "a registered medical practitioner."

The declaration that one signs under this act, should one become incurably ill and wish to have euthanasia administered, reads as follows:

If I should at any time suffer from a serious physical illness or impairment reasonably thought in my case to be incurable and expected to cause me severe distress or render me incapable of rational existence, I request the administration of euthanasia at a time or in circumstances to be indicated or specified by me or, if it is apparent that I have become incapable of giving directions, at the discretion of the physician in charge of my case.
In the event of my suffering from any of the conditions specified above, I request that no active steps should be taken . . . to prolong my life or restore me to consciousness.
This declaration is to remain in force unless I revoke it, which I may do at any time. . . .
I wish it to be understood that I have confidence in the good faith of my relatives and physicians, and fear degeneration and indignity far more than I fear premature death.

The ethic by which one justifies making such a declaration has been eloquently expressed by Joseph Fletcher. He speaks of "the right of spiritual beings to use intelligent control over physical nature rather than to submit beastlike to its blind workings." For Fletcher, "Death control, like birth control, is a matter of human dignity. Without it persons become puppets. To perceive this is to grasp the error lurking in the notion—widespread in medical circles—that life as such is the highest good."

Within our society today there are those who agree with the ethic of Joseph Fletcher. They agree also that an ethic that places a supreme value upon life is dominant in the medical profession. In a candid editorial (*Cal. Med.*), the traditional Western ethic with its affirmation of "the intrinsic worth and equal value of every human life regardless of its stage or condition" and with its roots in the Judaic and Christian heritage, is declared to be the basis for most of our laws and much of our social policy. What is more, the editorial says, "the reverence for each and every human life" is "a keystone of Western medicine and is the ethic which has caused physicians to try to preserve, protect, repair, prolong and enhance every human life which comes under their surveillance." Although this medical editor sees this traditional ethic as still clearly dominant, he is convinced that it is being eroded and that it is being replaced by a new ethic that he believes medicine should accept and applaud. This editor sees the beginning of the new ethic in the increasing acceptance of abortion, the general practice of which is in direct defiance of an ethic that affirms the "intrinsic and equal value for every human life regardless of its stage, condition, or status." For, in the opinion of this editor, human life begins at conception, and abortion is killing. Such killing is to be condoned and embraced by the new ethic.

In the above editorial a case is made for what is called "the quality of life." To increase the quality of life, it is assumed that the traditional Western ethic will necessarily have to be revised or even totally replaced. This, it is argued, is because it "will become necessary and acceptable to place relative rather than absolute values on such things as human lives, the use of scarce resources and the various elements which are to make up the quality of life or living which is to be sought." On such a view, the new ethic aids medicine in improving the quality of life; the ethic designated as the old ethic, rooted in Judaism and Christianity, is treated as an impediment to medicine's efforts to improve the quality of life. What kind of ethic should guide contemporary decisions regarding sterilization, abortion, and euthanasia—decisions as to who shall live and who shall die? Given the limits of this chapter, we shall discuss and assess the ethic (moral policy) of those who favor a policy of voluntary euthanasia and the ethic (moral policy) of those who oppose it. (Abortion and sterilization are large topics I have discussed in some detail elsewhere [Dyck,

1971].) The term "euthanasia" is used here, exactly as in the Voluntary Euthanasia Act of 1969, to mean "the painless inducement of death."

The Ethic of Euthanasia

What then is the ethic that guides those who support legislation like the Voluntary Euthanasia Act of 1969 and its Declaration? The arguments for euthanasia focus upon two humane and significant concerns: compassion for those who are painfully and terminally ill; and concern for the human dignity associated with freedom of choice. Compassion and freedom are values that sustain and enhance the common good. The question here, however, is how these values affect our behavior toward the dying.

The argument for compassion usually occurs in the form of attacking the inhumanity of keeping dying people alive when they are in great pain or when they have lost almost all of their usual functions, particularly when they have lost the ability or will to communicate with others. Thus, someone like Joseph Fletcher cites examples of people who are kept alive in a hopelessly debilitated state by means of the latest medical techniques, whether these be respirators, intravenous feeding, or the like. Often when Fletcher and others are arguing for the legalization of decisions not to intervene in these ways, the point is made that physicians already make decisions to turn off respirators or in other ways fail to use every means to prolong life. It is this allegedly compassionate behavior that the law would seek to condone and encourage.

The argument for compassion is supplemented by an argument for greater freedom for a patient to choose how and when he or she will die. For one thing, the patient should not be subjected to medical treatment to which that patient does not consent. Those who argue for voluntary euthanasia extend this notion by arguing that the choice to withhold techniques that would prolong life is a choice to shorten life. Hence, if one can choose to shorten one's life, why cannot one ask a physician by a simple and direct act of intervention to put an end to one's life? Here it is often argued that physicians already curtail life by means

of painkilling drugs, which in the doses administered, will hasten death. Why should not the law recognize and sanction a simple and direct hastening of death, should the patient wish it?

How do the proponents of euthanasia view the general prohibition against killing? First of all, they maintain that we are dealing here with people who will surely die regardless of the intervention of medicine. They advocate the termination of suffering and the lawful foreshortening of the dying process. Secondly, although the patient is committing suicide, and the physician is an accomplice in such a suicide, both acts are morally justifiable to cut short the suffering of one who is dying.

It is important to be very clear about the precise moral reasoning by which advocates of voluntary euthanasia justify suicide and assisting a suicide. They make no moral distinction between those instances when a patient or a physician chooses to have life shortened by failing to accept or use life-prolonging techniques and those instances when a patient or a physician shorten life by employing a death-dealing chemical or instrument. They make no moral distinction between a drug given to kill pain, which also shortens life, and a substance given precisely to shorten life and for no other reason. Presumably these distinctions are not honored, because regardless of the stratagem employed—regardless of whether one is permitting to die or killing directly—the result is the same, the patient's life is shortened. Hence, it is maintained that, if you can justify one kind of act that shortens the life of the dying, you can justify any act that shortens the life of the dying when this act is seen to be willed by the one who is dying. Moral reasoning of this sort is strictly utilitarian; it focuses solely on the consequences of acts, not on their intent.

Even though the reasoning on the issue of compassion is so stictly utilitarian, one is puzzled about the failure to raise certain kinds of questions. A strict utilitarian might inquire about the effect of the medical practice of promoting or even encouraging direct acts on the part of physicians to shorten the lives of their patients. And, in the same vein, a utilitarian might also be very concerned about whether the loosening of constraints on physicians may not loosen the constraints on killing generally. There are two reasons these questions are either not raised or are dealt with rather summarily. First, it is alleged that there is no evidence that untoward consequences would result. And second, the value of freedom is invoked, so that the question of killing becomes a question of suicide and assistance in a suicide.

The appeal to freedom is not strictly a utilitarian argument, at least not for some proponents of voluntary euthanasia. Joseph Fletcher, for example, complains about the foolishness of nature in bringing about situations in which dying is a prolonged process of suffering. He feels strongly that the failure to permit or encourage euthanasia demeans the dignity of persons. Fletcher has two themes here: On the one hand, the more people are able to control the process of nature, the more dignity and freedom they have; on the other hand, people have dignity only insofar as they are able to choose when, how, and why they are to live or to die. For physicians this means also choices as to who is to die, because presumably one cannot assist in the suicide of just any patient who claims to be suffering, or who thinks he or she is dying.

The ethic that defends suicide as a matter of individual conscience and as an expression of human dignity is a very old ethic. Both the Stoics and the Epicureans considered the choice of one's own death as the ultimate expression of human freedom and as an essential component of the dignity that attaches to rational personhood. This willingness to take one's life is an aspect of Stoic courage (Tillich, 1952). A true Stoic could not be manipulated by those who threatened death. When death seemed inevitable, they chose it before someone could inflict it upon them. Human freedom for the Stoics was not complete unless one could also choose death and not compromise oneself for fear of it. All the "heroes" in literature exhibit this kind of Stoic courage in the face of death.

A euthanasia ethic, as exemplified already in ancient Stoicism, contains the following essential presuppositions or beliefs:
1. That an individual's life belongs to that individual to dispose of entirely as he or she wishes;
2. That the dignity that attaches to personhood by reason of the freedom to make moral choices demands also the freedom to take one's own life;
3. That there is such a thing as a life not worth living, whether by reason of distress, illness, physical or mental handicaps, or even sheer despair for whatever reason;
4. That what is sacred or supreme in value is the "human dignity" that resides in man's own rational capacity to choose and control life and death.
This commitment to the free exercise of the human capacity to control life and death takes on a distinct religious aura. Speaking of the death control that amniocentesis makes possible, Robert S. Morrison declares that, "the birth of babies with gross physical and mental handicaps will no longer be left entirely to God, to chance, or to the forces of nature."

An Ethic of Benemortasia

From our account of the ethic of euthanasia, those who oppose voluntary euthanasia would seem to lack compassion for the dying and the courage to affirm human freedom. They appear incompassionate because they oppose what has come to be regarded as synonymous with a good death—namely, a painless and deliberately foreshortened process of dying. The term euthanasia originally meant a painless and happy death with no reference to whether such a death was induced. Although this definition still appears in modern dictionaries, a second meaning of the term has come to prevail: euthanasia now generally means "an act or method of causing death painlessly so as to end suffering" (Webster's New World Dictionary, 1962). In short, it would appear that the advocates of euthanasia, i.e., of causing death, are the advocates of a good death, and the advocates of voluntary euthanasia seek for all of us the freedom to have a good death.

Because of this loss of a merely descriptive term for a happy death, it is necessary to invent a term for a happy or good death—namely, benemortasia. The familiar derivatives for this new term are bene (good) and mors (death). The meaning of "bene" in "benemortasia" is deliberately unspecified so that it does not necessarily imply that a death must be painless and/or induced in order to be good. What constitutes a good or happy death is a disputable matter of moral policy. How then should one view the arguments for voluntary euthanasia? And, if an ethic of euthanasia is unacceptable, what is an acceptable ethic of benemortasia?

An ethic of benemortasia does not stand in opposition to the values of compassion and human freedom. It differs, however, from the ethic of euthanasia in its understanding of how these values are best realized. In particular, certain constraints upon human freedom are recognized and emphasized as enabling human beings to increase compassion and freedom rather than diminish them. For the purposes of this essay, we trace the roots of our ethic of benemortasia to Jewish and Christian sources. This does not mean that such an ethic is confined to those traditions or to persons influenced by them any more than an ethic of euthanasia is confined to its Stoic origins or adherents.

The moral life of Jews and Christians alike is and has been guided by the Decalogue, or Ten Commandments. "Thou shalt not kill" is one of the clear constraints upon human decisions and actions expressed in the Decalogue. It is precisely the nature of this constraint that is at stake in decisions regarding euthanasia.

Modern biblical scholarship has discovered that the Decalogue, or Mosaic Covenant, is in the form of a treaty between a Suzerian and his people (Mendenhall, 1955). The point of such a treaty is to specify the relationship between a ruler and his people, and to set out the conditions necessary to form and sustain community with that ruler. One of the most significant purposes of such a treaty is to specify constraints that members of a community must observe if the community is to be viable at all. Fundamentally, the Decalogue articulates the indispensable prerequisites of the common life.

Viewed in this way the injunction not to kill is part of a total effort to prevent the destruction of the human community. It is an absolute prohibition in the sense that no society can be indifferent about the taking of human life. Any act, insofar as it is an act of taking a human life, is wrong, that is to say, taking a human life is a wrong-making characteristic of actions.

To say, however, that killing is prima facie wrong does not mean that an act of killing may never be justified (Ross, 1930). For example, a person's effort to prevent someone's death may lead to the death of the attacker. However, we can morally justify that act of intervention only because it is an act of saving a life, not because it is an act of taking a life. If it were simply an act of taking a life, it would be wrong.[1]

A further constraint upon human freedom within the Jewish and Christian traditions is articulated in a myth concerning the loss of paradise. The loss of Eden comes at the point where man and woman succumb to the temptation to know good and evil, and to know it in the perfect and ultimate sense in which a perfect and ultimate being would know it (Revised Standard Version of the Bible, 1952). To know who should live and who should die, one would have to know everything about people, including their ultimate destiny. Only God could have such knowledge. Trying to decide who shall live and who shall die is "playing god." It is tragic to "play god" because one does it with such limited and uncertain knowledge of what is good and evil.

This constraint upon freedom has a liberating effect in the practice of medicine. Nothing in Jewish and Christian tradition presumes that a physician has a clear mandate to impose his or her wishes and skills upon patients for the sake of prolonging the length of their dying where those patients are diagnosed as terminally ill and do not wish the interventions of the physician. Thus the freedom of the patient to accept his or her dying and to decide whether he or she is to have any particular kind of medical care is surely enhanced. A patient, who has every reason to believe that he or she is dying, would lose the last vestige of freedom were he or she denied the right to choose the circumstances under which the terminal illness would take its course. Presumably that patient is someone who has not chosen to die, but who does have some choices left as to how the last hours and days will be spent. Intervention, in the form of

drugs, drainage tubes, or feeding by injection or whatever, may or may not be what the patient wishes or would find beneficial for these last hours or days. People who are dying have as much freedom as other living persons to accept or to refuse medical treatment when the treatment provides no cure for their ailment. There is nothing in the Jewish or Christian tradition that provides an exact blueprint as to what is the most compassionate thing to do for someone who is dying. Presumably the most compassionate act is to be a neighbor to such a person and to minister to such a person's needs. Depending upon the circumstances, this may or may not include intervention to prolong the process of dying.

Our ethic of benemortasia acknowledges the freedom of patients who are incurably ill to refuse interventions that prolong dying and the freedom of physicians to honor such wishes. However, these actions are not acts of suicide and assisting in suicide. In our ethic of benemortasia, suicide and assisting in suicide are unjustifiable acts of killing. Unlike the ethic of those who would legalize voluntary euthanasia, our ethic makes a moral distinction between acts that *permit* death and acts that *cause* death. As George P. Fletcher notes, one can make a sharp distinction, one that will stand up in law, between "permitting to die" and "causing death." Jewish and Christian tradition, particularly Roman Catholic thought, have maintained this clear distinction between the failure to use extraordinary measures (permitting to die) and direct intervention to bring about death (causing death).[2] A distinction is also drawn between a drug administered to cause death and a drug administered to ease pain which has the added effect of shortening life (see, for example, Smith, 1970).

Why are these distinctions important in instances where permitting to die or causing death both have the effect of shortening life? In both instances there is a failure to try to prolong the life of one who is dying. It is at this point that one must see why consequential reasoning is in itself too narrow, and why it is important also not to limit the discussion of benemortasia to the immediate relationship between a patient and his or her physician.

Where a person is dying of a terminal illness, it is fair to say that no one, including the dying person and his or her physician, has wittingly chosen this affliction and this manner or time of death. The choices that are left to a dying patient, an attendant physician, others who know the patient, and society concern how the last days of the dying person are to be spent.

From the point of view of the dying person, when could his or her decisions be called a deliberate act to end life, the act we usually designate as suicide? Only, it seems to me, when the dying person commits an act that has the immediate intent of ending life and has no other purpose. That act may be to use, or ask the physician to use, a chemical or an instrument that has no other immediate effect than to end the dying person's life. If, for the sake of relieving pain, a dying person chooses drugs administered in potent doses, the intent of this act is not to shorten life, even though it has that effect. It is a choice as to how to live while dying. Similarly, if a patient chooses to forego medical interventions that would have the effect of prolonging his or her life without in any way promising release from death, this also is a choice as to what is the most meaningful way to spend the remainder of life, however short that may be. The choice to use drugs to relieve pain and the choice not to use medical measures that cannot promise a cure for one's dying are not different in principle from the choices we make throughout our lives as to how much we will rest, how hard we will work, how little and how much medical intervention we will seek or tolerate, and the like. For society or physicians to map out life styles for individuals with respect to such decisions is surely beyond anything that we find in Stoic, Jewish, or Christian ethics. Such intervention in the liberty of individuals is far beyond what is required in any society whose rules are intended to constrain people against harming others.

But human freedom should not be extended to include the taking of one's own life. Causing one's own death cannot generally be justified, even when one is dying. To see why this is so, we have to consider how causing one's death does violence to one's self and harms others.

The person who causes his or her own death repudiates the meaningfulness and worth of his or her own life. To decide to initiate an act that has as its primary purpose to end one's life is to decide that that life has no worth to anyone, especially to oneself. It is an act that ends all choices regarding what one's life and whatever is left of it is to symbolize.

Suicide is the ultimately effective way of shutting out all other people from one's life. Psychologists have observed how hostility for others can be expressed through taking one's own life. People who might want access to the dying one to make restitution, offer reparation, bestow last kindnesses, or clarify misunderstandings are cut off by such an act. Every kind of potentially and actually meaningful contact and relation among persons is irrevocably severed except by means of memories and whatever life beyond death may offer. Certainly for those who are left behind by death, there can remain many years of suffering occasioned by that death. The sequence of dying an inevitable death can be much better accepted than the decision on the part of a dying one that he or she has no worth to anyone. An act that presupposes that final declaration leaves tragic overtones for anyone who participated in even the smallest way in that person's dying.

But the problem is even greater. If in principle a person can take his or her own life whenever he or she no longer finds it meaningful, there is nothing in principle that prevents anyone from taking his or her life, no matter what the circumstances. For if the decision hinges on whether one regards his or her own life as meaningful, anyone can regard his or her own life as meaningless even under circumstances that would appear to be most fortunate and opportune for an abundant life.

What about those who would commit suicide or request euthanasia in order to cease being a "burden" on those who are providing care for them? If it is a choice to accept death by refusing non-curative care that prolongs dying, the freedom to embrace death or give one's life in this way is honored by our ethic of benemortasis. What is rejected is the freedom to cause death

whether by suicide or by assisting in one. (Dyck, 1968, distinguished between *giving* one's life and *taking* one's life.)

How a person dies has a definite meaning for those to whom that person is related. In the first year of bereavement, the rate of death among bereaved relatives of those who die in hospitals is twice that of bereaved relatives of those who die at home; sudden deaths away from hospital and home increase the death rate of the bereaved even more (Lasagna, 1970).

The courage to be, as expressed in Christian and Jewish thought, is more than the overcoming of the fear of death, although it includes that Stoic dimension. It is the courage to accept one's own life as having worth no matter what life may bring, including the threat of death, because that life remains meaningful and is regarded as worthy by God, regardless of what that life may be like.

An ethic of benemortasia stresses what Tillich has called the "courage to be as a part"—namely, the courage to affirm not only oneself, but also one's participation as a self in a universal community of beings. The courage to be as a part recognizes that one is not merely one's own, that one's life is a gift bestowed and protected by the human community and by the ultimate forces that make up the cycle of birth and death. In the cycle of birth and death, there may be suffering, as there is joy, but suffering does not render a life meaningless or worthless. Suffering people need the support of others; suffering people should not be encouraged to commit suicide by their community, or that community ceases to be a community.

This consideration brings us to a further difficulty with voluntary euthanasia and its legalization. Not only does euthanasia involve suicide, but also, if legalized, it sanctions assistance in a suicide by physicians. Legislation like the Voluntary Euthanasia Act of 1969 makes it a duty of the medical profession to take someone else's life for him. Here the principle not to kill is even further eroded and violated by giving the physician the power and the encouragement to decide that someone else's life is no longer worth living. The whole notion that a physician can engage in euthanasia implies acceptance of the principle that another person's

life is no longer meaningful enough to sustain, a principle that does not afford protection for the lives of any of the most defenseless, voiceless, or otherwise dependent members of a community. Everyone in a community is potentially a victim of such a principle, particularly among members of racial minorities, the very young, and the very old.

Those who would argue that these consequences of a policy of voluntary euthanasia cannot be predicted fail to see two things: that we have already had an opportunity to observe what happens when the principle that sanctions euthanasia is accepted by a society; and that regardless of what the consequences may be of such acts, the acts themselves are wrong in principle.

With respect to the first point, Leo Alexander's (1949) very careful analysis of medical practices and attitudes of German physicians before and during the reign of Nazism in Germany should serve as a definite warning against the consequences of making euthanasia a public policy. He notes that the outlook of German physicians that led to their cooperation in what became a policy of mass murders,

started with the acceptance of that attitude, basic in the euthanasia movement, that there is such a thing as life not worthy to be lived. This attitude in its early stages concerned itself merely with the severely and chronically sick. Gradually the sphere of those to be included in this category was enlarged to include the socially unproductive, the racially unwanted, and finally all non-Germans. But it is important to realize that the infinitely small wedged-in lever from which this entire trend of mind received its impetus was the attitude toward the nonrehabilitable sick.

Those who reject out of hand any comparison of what happened in Nazi Germany with what we can expect here in the United States should consider current examples of medical practice in this nation. The treatment of mongoloids is a case in point. Now that the notion is gaining acceptance that a fetus diagnosed in the womb as having Down's syndrome (mongolism) can, at the discretion of a couple or the pregnant woman, be justifiably aborted, instances of infanticide in hospitals are being reported. At Johns Hopkins Hospital, for example, an allegedly mongoloid infant whose parents would not permit an operation for an accompanying constriction of part of the intestine which blocked the child's digestive system, was ordered to have "nothing by mouth," condemning that infant to a death that took 15 days. By any of our existing laws, this was a case of murder, justified on the ground that this particular life was somehow not worth saving. (If one argues that the infant was killed because the parents did not want it, we have in this kind of case an even more radical erosion of our restraints upon killing.)

Someone may argue that the child was permitted to die, not killed. But this is faulty reasoning. In the case of an infant whose future life and development could be reasonably assured through surgery, we are not dealing with someone who is dying and with intervention that has no curative effect. The fact that some physicians refer to this as a case of permitting to die is an ominous portent of the dangers inherent in accepting the principle that a physician or another party can decide for a patient that his or her life is not worth living. Equally ominous is the assumption that this principle, once accepted, can easily be limited to cases of patients for whom no curative intervention is known to exist.

With all the risks that attend changing the physician's role from one who sustains life to one who induces death, one may well ask why physicians should be called upon to assist a suicide?

M. R. Barrington, an advocate of suicide and of voluntary euthanasia, is aware of the difficulty of making this request of physicians and of the necessity for justifying legalization of such requests. She suggests that the role of the physician in assisting suicide is essential, "especially as human frailty requires that it should be open to a patient to ask the doctor to choose a time for the giving of euthanasia that is not known to the patient" (Barrington, 1971). This appeal to "human frailty" is very telling. The hesitation to commit suicide and the ambivalence of the dying about their worth should give one pause before one signs a declaration that empowers a physician to decide that at some point one can no longer be trusted as competent to judge whether or not one wants to die. Physicians are also frail humans, and mistaken diagnoses, research interests, and sometimes errors of judgment that

stem from a desire for organs, are part of the practice of medicine.[3]

Comatose patients being kept alive by machines such as respirators pose special problems for an ethic of benemortasia as they do for the advocates of voluntary euthanasia. Where patients are judged to be irreversibly comatose and where sustained efforts have been made to restore such persons to consciousness, no clear case can be made for permitting to die, even though it seems merciful to do so. It seems that the best we can do is to develop some rough social and medical consensus about a reasonable length of time for maintaining a patient by means of life-sustaining technology. Because of the pressures to do research and to transplant organs, it may also be necessary to employ special patient advocates who are not physicians and nurses. These patient advocates, trained in medical ethics, would function as ombudsmen.

In summary, even if the practice of euthanasia were to be confined to those who voluntarily request an end to their lives, no physician could in good conscience participate in such an act. To decide directly to cause the death of a patient is to abandon a cardinal principle of medical practice—namely, to do no harm to one's patient. The relief of suffering, which is surely a time-honored role for the physician, does not extend to an act that presupposes that the life of a patient who is suffering is not worthy to be lived. As we have argued, not even the patient who is dying can justifiably and unilaterally universalize the principle by which a dying life would be declared to be worthless.

Some readers may remain unconvinced that euthanasia is morally wrong as a general policy. Perhaps what still divides us is what distinguishes a Stoic from a Jewish and Christian way of life. The Stoic heritage declares that my life and my selfhood are my own to dispose of as I see fit and when I see fit. The Jewish and Christian heritage declares that my life and my selfhood are not my own, and are not mine to dispose of as I see fit.

In the words of H. Richard Niebuhr,

I live but do not have the power to live. And further, I may die at any moment but I am powerless to die. It

was not in my power, nor in my parents' power, to elect my *self* into existence. Though they willed a child or consented to it they did not will *me*—this I, thus and so. And so also I now, though I *will* to be no more, cannot elect myself out of existence, if the inscrutable power by which I am, elects otherwise. Though I wish to be mortal, if the power that threw me into being in this mortal destructible body elects me into being again there is nothing I can do about that. I can destroy the life of my body. Can I destroy myself? This remains the haunting question of the literature of suicide and of all the lonely debates of men to whom existence is a burden. Whether they shall wake up again, either here in this life or there in some other mode of being, is beyond their control. We can choose among many alternatives; but the power to choose self-existence or self-extinction is not ours. Men can practice birth-control, not self-creation; they can commit *bio*cide; whether they can commit suicide, self-destruction, remains a question.

Although one has the power to commit biocide, this does not give one the right to do so. Niebuhr views our lives as shaped by our responses to others and their responses to us. All of us are in responsible relations to others. The claim that an act of suicide (biocide) would harm no one else is unrealistic. To try to make that a reality would require an incredibly lonely existence cut off from all ties of friendship, cooperation, and mutual dependence. And in so doing, we would repudiate the value and benefits of altruism.

The other points at which the proponents of euthanasia and the advocates of benemortasia part company concern the perception of the context in which all moral decisions are made. Here again the division has religious overtones. Those who decide for euthanasia seem to accept an ethic which ultimately privatizes and subjectivizes the injunction not to kill. Those who oppose euthanasia see the decision not to kill as one that is in harmony with what is good for everyone, and indeed is an expression of what is required of everyone if goodness is to be pervasive and powerful on earth. Once again, H. Richard Niebuhr has eloquently expressed this latter position:

All my specific and relative evaluations expressed in my interpretations and responses are shaped, guided, and formed by the understanding of good and evil I have *upon the whole*. In distrust of the radical action by which I am, by which my society is, by which this world is, I must find my center of valuation in myself, or in my nation, or in my church, or in my science, or in humanity, or in life. Good and evil in this view mean what is good for me and bad for me; or good and evil for my nation, or good and evil for one of these finite causes, such as mankind, or life or reason. But should it happen that confidence is given to me in the power by which all things are and by which I am; should I learn in the depths of my existence to praise the creative source, . . . all my relative evaluations will be subjected to the continuing and great correction. They will be made to fit into a total process producing good—not what is good for me (though my confidence accepts that as included), nor what is good for man (though that is also included), nor what is good for the development of life (though that also belongs in the picture), but what is good for being, for universal being, or for God, center and source of all existence.

Our ethic of benemortasia has argued for the following beliefs and values:

1. that an individual person's life is not solely at the disposal of that person; every human life is part of the human community that bestows and protects the lives of its members; the possibility of community itself depends upon constraints against taking life;

2. that the dignity that attaches to personhood by reason of the freedom to make moral choices includes the freedom of dying people to refuse noncurative, life-prolonging interventions when one is dying, but does not extend to taking one's life or causing death for someone who is dying;

3. that every life has some worth; there is no such thing as a life not worth living;

4. that the supreme value is goodness itself to which the dying and those who care for the dying are responsible. Religiously expressed the supreme value is God. Less than perfectly good beings, human beings, require constraints upon their decisions regarding those who are dying. No human being or human community can presume to know who deserves to live or to die. At the same time, we have implied throughout that religion and the Jewish and Christian expressions of it are not obstacles to modern medicine and a better life; rather they help foster humanity's ceaseless quest to preserve and enhance human life on this earth.

Notes

1. One may be perplexed that societies with their roots in Jewish and Christian traditions have been able to justify capital punishment. If one believes that capital punishment will have a deterrent effect, i.e., will save lives, its justification is at least understandable. We have raised serious doubts in recent years as to its deterrent effect and hence now have good reason to question this practice.

2. See, for example, an excellent discussion by the Protestant Paul Ramsey, *The Patient as Person*, pp. 113–164, which contains many references also to Roman Catholic literature on the care for the dying. For the Jewish views, see the classic text by Immanuel Jakobovits, *Jewish Medical Ethics*. Whereas Jewish law forbids active euthanasia, Jakobovits makes it clear that "Jewish law sanctions and perhaps even demands the withdrawal of any factor—whether extraneous to the patient himself or not—which may artificially delay the demise of the final phase."

3. See Yale Kamisar, "Euthanasia Legislation: Some Non-Religious Objections" for copious documentation of medical error and other aspects of medical practice that would make euthanasia legislation hazardous.

References

Alexander, L. 1949. Medical science under dictatorship. *New Engl. J. Med.* 241:39–47. For a thorough study of the "edge of the wedge" argument as it applies to legalizing voluntary euthanasia, see Sissela Bok, "Voluntary Euthanasia," unpublished Ph.D. thesis.

Barrington, M. R. Apologia for suicide. In Downing (next reference).

Downing, A. B., ed. 1971. *Euthanasia and the Right to Death*. New York, Humanities Press.

Dyck, A. J. *Religious Views and U.S. Population Policy* (prepared for the Commission on Population Growth and the American Future and available at the Institute of Society, Ethics and the Life Sciences, Hastings-On-Hudson, N.Y.). See also Population policies and ethical acceptability. In *Rapid Population Growth: Consequences and Policy Implications*. Roger Revelle et al., eds. Baltimore, Johns Hopkins Press, 1971. See also 1972. Perplexities for the would-be-liberal in abortion, *J. Rep. Med.* 8(6): 351–4.

Dyck, A. J. 1965. Questions for the global conscience. *Psych. Today.* 2(4): 38–42.

Editorial. 1970. A new ethic for medicine and society. *Cal. Med.* 113: 67–68.

Fletcher, G. P. Prolonging life: some legal considerations. In Downing, *op. cit.*

Fletcher, J. The patient's right to die. In Downing, *op. cit.*

Genesis, Chapter 3, *The Holy Bible*. 1952. Revised Standard Version. New York, Thomas Nelson and Sons.

Jakobovits, I. 1967, *Jewish Medical Ethics*. New York, Bloch Publishing Co.

Kamisar, Y. Euthanasia legislation: some non-religious objections. In Downing, *op. cit.*

Lasagna, L. 1970. The prognosis of death. In *The Dying Patient*. O. G. Brim et al., eds. New York, Russell Sage Foundation. Pages 80–81.

Mendenhall, G. E. 1955. *Law and Covenant in Israel and the Ancient Near East*. Pittsburgh, Biblical Colloquium.

Morison, R. S. 1971. Chairman's introduction. In *Early Diagnosis of Human Genetic Defects*. M. Harris, ed. H. E. W. Publication No. (NIH) 72–25. Page 9.

Niebuhr, H. R. 1963. *The Responsible Self*. New York, Harper & Row.

Ramsey, P. 1970. *The Patient as a Person*. New Haven, Yale University Press.

Ross, W. D. 1930. *The Right and the Good*. Clarendon, Oxford University Press (See pp. 19–21 for an explanation and a list of *prima facie* duties.) [The chapter referred to is reprinted as Chapter 16 of this volume.]

Smith, H. L. 1970. *Ethics and the New Medicine*. New York, Abingdon Press.

Tillich, P. 1952. *The Courage To Be*. New Haven, Yale University Press.

86

Paul A. Freund

Mongoloids and "Mercy Killing"

Reprinted with permission of the author and the Foundation as an unpublished paper presented at "Choices of Our Conscience: International Symposium on Human Rights, Retardation and Research," sponsored by the Joseph P. Kennedy, Jr. Foundation, Washington, D.C., October 16, 1971.

[Editors' note: This essay was written in response to the moral questions raised by a case at the Johns Hopkins Hospital, mentioned in the preceding section. A baby was born there who, shortly after birth, was clinically diagnosed to have Down's syndrome (mongolism), a condition associated with mental retardation. An additional confirmation of the clinical diagnosis through a chromosomal analysis in the laboratory, which takes several weeks to perform, was not carried out. The baby also had duodenal atresia, a constriction of a portion of the intestine that prevents the passage of food. It leads to death if not surgically corrected, and operation for it carries a relatively small risk.

The mother of this baby, a nurse, was so distressed on learning the diagnosis of Down's syndrome that she refused to give consent for the operation to remove the intestinal blockage. Her husband accepted this decision, believing that as a nurse his wife was more knowledgeable about this matter than he.

The physician in the case indicated to the parents that children with Down's syndrome often have IQs of between 50 and 80, can perform simple jobs, are usually happy, and can live a long time. This failed to change their minds.

The doctors at the hospital did not attempt to thwart the parents' decision through a court order. In the hospital, after about two weeks, the child died of starvation.]

Who shall live and who shall die? It is an awesome and tragic experience when a decision on this question, agonizing enough for gods, is undertaken to be given by parents and physicians.

In a sense, of course, society makes such choices in a commonplace, almost unnoticed way, when the odds of survival are altered. By setting a speed limit on highways at 70 rather than 30 miles per hour, we make it certain that a predictably greater number of persons will be killed (even allowing for a certain offsetting life-saving potential of rapid travel). We make a similar choice when we set the levels of safety standards for mining operations or allow the sale of cigarettes.

But these decisions for life or death are in the nature of setting the odds in roulette. Individuals retain a measure of choice within the system; to some extent they can decide whether to play at the odds. The collective decision is, to be sure, a moral decision; but it is a matter of statistical morality. Thus men have not quite arrogated to themselves the supreme prerogative of making the final pronouncement of doom on an innocent fellow-man: scope is left for the working of Chance or—describe it as you will—the Divine Order.

The distinction is suggested in the well-known case of shipwreck, where a lifeboat is overloaded or the supply of food is too low to sustain all the lives on board. To sacrifice the life of one companion, or a few, will save the lives of many. Should all be allowed to perish, or is there a right—based on a utilitarian calculus—to choose those who shall serve as involuntary martyrs? When the choice is made by dooming those who are the weakest, the law has deemed the enforced sacrifice to be murder, though mitigation of punishment has in fact ensued.[1] At the same time, some judges have suggested that the legal position would be different if the selection were made by lot.[2] A similar analysis can be seen in a military context. To rescue prisoners of war through an assault that entails a deadly risk to the rescuers, a commander may call for volunteers and, if necessary, may assign men to the mission by lot; but it would be quite another moral issue, would it not, if the commander were to yield to an offer by the enemy to release the prisoners in return for the execution by the commander of certain of his men.

The allocation of scarce medical resources raises serious enough moral problems, but they are usually of the randomized, statistical sort. When, however, decisions are made that focus irretrievably on an innocent individual's right to live or die, the moral judgment, and therefore the legal judgment, becomes excruciatingly difficult. Of such an order is the issue presented by the Baltimore case [at the Johns Hopkins Hospital].

Let me say at once that I cannot agree with the assumption made in the hospital that if the question had been presented to a court the judge would surely have endorsed the parents' right to decide that the child should die. In the case of a more "normal" child, the parents would clearly have no such right, and this appears to be acknowledged on all sides. Even if parents do not will their child's death but refuse consent to a life-saving operation because of religious objections (the conviction of Jehovah's Witnesses that a blood transfusion is a profanation), courts have overridden the religious scruples of the parents and ordered the operation in the child's best interest.[3] (It is, of course, otherwise in the case of an adult of sound mind refusing consent to an operation on himself.)[4] Parents have an obligation not to mistreat or neglect their children, and the courts will enforce that duty. Moreover, physicians who undertake to care for a patient have an obligation to use all reasonable measures (not forbidden by the patient) to promote the patient's well-being and not do him harm. In the face of parental objection, if the situation is an emergency one the physician and hospital would be well advised to follow the life-saving and not the death-inducing course; if there is time, the judgment of a court can be sought, as has been done in cases of religious objection to surgery.

Thus far, of course, we have omitted the salient feature of the case, the fact that the infant was diagnosed as having Down's syndrome, or mongoloidism, a condition in which the degree of subnormal intelligence is unpredictable but which would allow in time simple tests to be performed and which is characterized by a happy disposition, responsive to loving care. To appraise the significance of this feature—that if a relatively safe abdominal operation were performed the child would live but would be a so-called mongoloid— it may be useful to encircle the problem by making comparisons with some situations that are at least superficially similar.

A comparison may be suggested with mercy killing, or euthanasia. In the present state of the law such killings are deemed criminal homicide, despite the motive of mercy.[5] A particularly poignant case came before a federal court obliquely, on a petition for naturalization. The applicant, within five years prior to his application, had been tried for the "mercy killing" of his son, a boy of thirteen, who, in the words of the court, had suffered from birth a brain injury which destined him to be

an idiot and a physical monstrosity malformed in all four limbs. The child was blind, mute, and deformed, incapable of feeding himself, incontinent, his entire life spent in a small crib. Four normal children were cared for faithfully by the father. At the trial the jury rendered a verdict of manslaughter in the second degree (an illogically mild category for a premeditated killing), and recommended utmost clemency. The judge sentenced the father to imprisonment for five to ten years but suspended the sentence and ordered probation, from which he was later relieved. Against this background the naturalization court had to decide whether the applicant had been "of good moral character" during the five years preceding his application. Judge Learned Hand, recognizing the sympathy shown by the jury and the judge in the criminal case, nevertheless felt, as he said, "reasonably secure in holding that only a minority of virtuous persons would deem the practice morally justifiable, while it remains in private hands, even when the provocation is as overwhelming as it was in this instance."[6] The decision may have been made easier for Judge Hand by reason of the fact that the father would become eligible for citizenship after the five-year period elapsed.

However that may be, the facts of that case presented a much more appealing situation for "mercy killing" than the Baltimore case. The former approaches, if it does not reach, the category traditionally termed "monsters," concerning whom there is a long legal tradition, drawing on canon-law sources, treating them as other than human beings.[7] Moreover, in that case the putting to death could be regarded as a mercy to the child, while in the Baltimore case the motivation appears to have been concern for others in the family. On this aspect of the case, more will be said presently.

Even those critics of the law who have advocated the legalization of euthanasia would hedge it about with a set of strict conditions: That the act be willed by the patient: that the illness be terminal and incurable; and that there be suffering from intractable pain.[8] Even with these nominal safeguards, euthanasia would be a dubious legal

innovation, because of the difficulty of administering such a law in actual practice: The reality of the patient's will may be as feeble as his physical state, the motives of relatives may be less than pure, the prospects of medical relief from pain may improve. And in a matter of this kind, where physicians would be called upon to reverse their role by becoming active agents to terminate life, the risk of mistaken judgment should outweigh the possibility of conforming to the formal criteria, when a general rule must be fixed to govern medical practice.

This excursus on euthanasia, however, is a digression, for in the Baltimore case the suggested criteria of the will of the patient, intractable suffering, irreversible terminal illness, and mercy toward the patient, are all notably wanting.

Still, it may be said, there was no active intervention to cause death in the present case, but only inaction that left the infant to the operation of natural processes. Thus the death was caused, it may be argued, not by human agency but by impersonal, inexorable forces. To this argument two answers can be given. First, on the facts it is somewhat disingenuous to ascribe the death to nonhuman causes. Death occurred from starvation, a condition resulting from the directions given at the hospital. To be sure, death would have occurred in any event from an unrelieved intestinal obstruction, but this does not negate the actual cause of death. If A empties a bottle of poison which would have been fatal to B, and then withholds all liquids from B, who dies of dehydration, it is irrelevant that another kind of death would have occurred in any event. Secondly, as a matter of law, inaction is tantamount to action when there is a duty to act and an omission to do so. Thus we are brought back to the basic question of duty, a question which cannot be avoided by drawing distinctions between action and inaction.

There is, to be sure, a sentiment held by sensitive persons that in the care of a patient there comes a time when extraordinary supportive measures may be withheld and the process of dying allowed to take its course. If a patient in a coma, in the terminal stage of cancer, contracts pneumonia, may not a conscientious physician, with the approval of the patient's family, properly withhold antibiotics, even though active lethal intervention, as by injecting air into the veins, would be repugnant to law and a sense of morality? A brilliant physician in Boston became afflicted with Parkinson's disease and when his condition steadily deteriorated he underwent radical neurosurgery, which was not successful, and which left him in a vegetative state of existence, helpless and hospitalized for several years. At one point in this period he contracted pneumonia and was promptly treated for it, successfully, by an intern, thus prolonging his life. I have heard older doctors lament this almost reflexive action of the intern, suggesting that a wiser attitude would come with more experience. If we accept the point of view of these older physicians, are we repudiating the cardinal obligation of the doctor and abandoning the proposition that inaction in the face of a duty is as culpable as positive action? I think not, for the reason that in caring for a dying patient the duty of humane care may present an honest and painful choice between prolonging life—or the process of dying—and allowing the patient to meet his end in as much quiet, peace and dignity as the circumstances will permit. This was not, it seems clear, the situation facing parents and doctors in the Baltimore case. The cases differ as the glow of a sunset differs from that of a sunrise.

We are brought, finally, to the question that has been lurking in the analysis thus far—if one is, without fault on his part, a threat to the well-being of others, may those others in good conscience remove the threat to enhance their own lives and the lives of others dependent on them? We can put to one side the case where there is an immediate threat to the very survival of the others. If three mountain climbers are tied together by a rope, and one of them slips so that his dangling from a cliff menaces the other two, may they cut the rope to save themselves? Whatever our answer may be to that question, it must be plain that to send the dangling companion to his death simply to avoid the discomfort of bruises or a broken bone for the others would be repugnant to our sense

of justice. There are other flaws in the analogy. Insofar as the trauma anticipated by the parents is a psychological one, it is far from clear that this is inevitable, given a judgment from intimate reality rather than from expectation.

The clearer threat that looms up is the drain on time, energy, and material resources. This is really the crux of the problem. That sensitive, decent individuals can be driven to sacrifice a life in the interest of the well-being of the survivors is a reflection less of private morality than of social failure. The contradiction between a religious tradition of the sanctity of life and equality of worth, on the one hand, and judgments of doom on innocent offspring, on the other, could itself be the cause of intense psychological trauma. In this respect we differ from the Romans, among whom infanticide was common practice. Even for those without a formal religious belief, a philosophy of humanism recognizes essential equality of worth based on equality of ignorance: on the important questions of human existence—whence, whither, why—all are equally in the presence of unfathomable mystery. That is why humility is the indispensable condition of wisdom. That is why, in the law, the standard of due process in fundamental matters extends to all "persons," whether citizen or alien, believer or infidel, saint or sinner. Due process of law, and equality of right to live, are recognized and accorded not merely for the sake of the potential victims, but for the sake of the judges and of society, to save us from the agony and absurdity of making ultimate judgments of worth, of assuming the role of a god on the Day of Final Judgment.

We may be destined for a new morality that will encompass an even wider valuing of life, not only human but animal as well. Particularly among young people, solicitude for the survival of other species, and on a smaller scale an aversion to eating animal flesh, may be seen as the glimmer of a more inclusive ethic of life. But if so, it calls for greater self-restraint, less self-indulgence, not a martyrdom forced upon others.

The ultimate question, then, is one of social responsibility for maintaining conditions under which private morality will not be confronted with harrowing choices that are avoidable.

Concretely, this means that resources have to be applied to the provision of life's necessities, including those of the handicapped. Indeed, if society is to continue to insist in its legal codes on the right of infants to live, it behooves society to share in making the right a meaningful reality. Perhaps the most disturbing observation in the Baltimore tragedy was the comment by a nurse that the baby would be better off dead than in the custody of the Rosewood institution.

Who, then, is to make the decisions on the proper care and custody of the child? On that question the doctors are valuable witnesses but not appropriate decision-makers. They can furnish data on the child's physical prospects, but these estimates are only a part of the relevant empirical evidence upon which to base a social-ethical judgment. The same can be said of the parents. They can provide evidence on the prospects for home care, but again this testimony is but a part of the materials for judgment on the best interests of the child. Its best interests, and the interest of society, must be assessed by a disinterested tribunal when the parents are unable or unwilling to bear the responsibility of care. Resort to a court is indicated, not because lawyers and judges have expertise in mongoloidism, which indeed they do not have, but because there all interests can be caught up and valued, and there a guardian *ad litem* for the child can be appointed as spokesman for the child's needs and claims.

In the end, though, we return to the responsibility of society, remembering that in all likelihood, if proper institutional care had been available, the decision of parents and hospital, in harmony with that of the law itself, would have been in favor of life.

Notes

1. *U.S. v. Holmes*, 26 Fed. Cas. 360 (No. 15, 383) (C.C.E.D. Pa. 1842); *Regina v. Dudley*, 14 Q.B.D. 273 (1884).

2. *U.S. v. Holmes*. See Paul Ramsey, *The Patient as Person* (New Haven and London, 1970), pp. 252 et seq.

3. *Wallace v. Labrenz*, 411 Ill. 618, 104 N.E.2d 769 (1952); *State v. Perricone*, 37 N.J. 462, 181 A.2d 751 (1962); *In re Clark*, 185 N.E.2d 128 (Ohio 1962). Even where life was not at stake, but only a severe facial disfigurement, an operation has been ordered. *In re Sampson*, 317 N.Y.S.2d 641 (1970).

4. *In re Brooks' Estate*, 32 Ill. 2d 361, 205 N.E.2d 435 (1965). But where the adult is a pregnant woman, a blood transfusion has been ordered to save the life of the foetus. *Raleigh Fitkin-Paul Morgan Memorial Hospital v. Anderson* 42 N.J. 421, 201 A.2d 557 (1964). A similar order was issued where the woman was the mother of a young child and her mental state may not have been stable at the time of her refusal. *Application of President and Directors of Georgetown College*, 331 P.2d 1000 (D.C. Cir. 1964).

5. See Yale Kamisar, "Some Non-Religious Views Against Proposed 'Mercy-Killing' Legislation," 42 *Minn. L. Rev.* 969 (1958); Silving, "Euthanasia: A Study in Comparative Criminal Law," 103 *U. of Pa. L. Rev.* 350 (1954); N. St. John Stevas, *Life, Death and the Law* (Cleveland and New York, 1961), Chapter 7.

6. *Repouille v. U.S.*, 165 F.2d 152 (1947).

7. See Glanville Williams, *The Sanctity of Life and the Criminal Law* (London, 1957) 31–35.

8. Ibid., Chapter 8; a draft of a law proposed by the Euthanasia Society is published in St. John Stevas, *Life, Death, and the Law*, 14.

87

Raymond S. Duff and A. G. M. Campbell

Moral and Ethical Dilemmas in the Special-Care Nursery

Reprinted with permission of the publisher from the *New England Journal of Medicine*, vol. 289, 1973, pp. 890–894.

Between 1940 and 1970 there was a 58 per cent decrease in the infant death rate in the United States.[1] This reduction was related in part to the application of new knowledge to the care of infants. Neonatal mortality rates in hospitals having infant intensive-care units have been about ½ those reported in hospitals without such units.[2] There is now evidence that in many conditions of early infancy the long-term morbidity may also be reduced.[3] Survivors of these units may be healthy, and their parents grateful, but some infants continue to suffer from such conditions as chronic cardiopulmonary disease, short-bowel-syndrome or various manifestations of brain damage; others are severely handicapped by a myriad of congenital malformations that in previous times would have resulted in early death. Recently, both lay and professional persons have expressed increasing concern about the quality of life for these severely impaired survivors and their families.[4,5] Many pediatricians and others are distressed with the long-term results of pressing on and on to save life at all costs and in all circumstances. Eliot Slater[6] stated, "If this is one of the consequences of the sanctity-of-life ethic, perhaps our formulation of the principle should be revised."

The experiences described in this communication document some of the grave moral and ethical dilemmas now faced by physicians and families. They indicate some of the problems in a large special-care nursery where medical technology has prolonged life and where "informed" parents influence the management decisions concerning their infants.

Background and Methods

The special-care nursery of the Yale–New Haven Hospital not only serves an obstetric service for over 4000 live births annually but also acts as the principal referral center in Connecticut for infants with major problems of the newborn period. From January 1, 1970, through June 30, 1972, 1615 infants born at the Hospital were admitted, and 556 others were transferred for specialized care from community hospitals. During this interval, the average daily census was 26, with a range of 14 to 37.

For some years the unit has had a liberal policy for parental visiting, with the staff placing particular emphasis on helping parents adjust to and participate in the care of their infants with special problems. By encouraging visiting, attempting to create a relaxed atmosphere within the unit, exploring carefully the special needs of the infants, and familiarizing parents with various aspects of care, it was hoped to remove much of the apprehension—indeed, fear—with which parents at first view an intensive-care nursery.[7] At any time, parents may see and handle their babies. They commonly observe or participate in most routine aspects of care and are often present when some infant is critically ill or moribund. They may attend, as they choose, the death of their own infant. Since an average of two to three deaths occur each week and many infants are critically ill for long periods, it is obvious that the concentrated, intimate social interactions between personnel, infants and parents in an emotionally charged atmosphere often make the work of the staff very difficult and demanding. However, such participation and recognition of parents' rights to information about their infant appear to be the chief foundations of "informed consent" for treatment.

Each staff member must know how to cope with many questions and problems brought up by parents, and if he or she cannot help, they must have access to those who can. These requirements can be met only when staff members work closely with each other in all the varied circumstances from simple to complex, from triumph to tragedy. Formal and informal meetings take place regularly to discuss the technical and family aspects of care. As a given problem may require, some or all of several persons (including families, nurses, social workers, physicians, chaplains and others) may convene to exchange information and reach decisions. Thus, staff and parents function more or less as a small community in which a concerted attempt is made to ensure that each member may participate in and know about the major decisions that concern him or her. However, the physician takes appropriate initiative in final decision

making, so that the family will not have to bear that heavy burden alone.

For several years, the responsibilities of attending pediatrician have been assumed chiefly by ourselves, who, as a result, have become acquainted intimately with the problems of the infants, the staff, and the parents. Our almost constant availability to staff, private pediatricians and parents has resulted in the raising of more and more ethical questions about various aspects of intensive care for critically ill and congenitally deformed infants. The penetrating questions and challenges, particularly of knowledgeable parents (such as physicians, nurses, or lawyers), brought increasing doubts about the wisdom of many of the decisions that seemed to parents to be predicated chiefly on technical considerations. Some thought their child had a right to die since he could not live well or effectively. Others thought that society should pay the costs of care that may be so destructive to the family economy. Often, too, the parents' or siblings' rights to relief from the seemingly pointless, crushing burdens were important considerations. It seemed right to yield to parent wishes in several cases as physicians have done for generations. As a result, some treatments were withheld or stopped with the knowledge that earlier death and relief from suffering would result. Such options were explored with the less knowledgeable parents to ensure that their consent for treatment of their defective children was truly informed. As Eisenberg[8] pointed out regarding the application of technology, "At long last, we are beginning to ask, not can it be done, but should it be done?" In lengthy, frank discussion, the anguish of the parents was shared, and attempts were made to support fully the reasoned choices, whether for active treatment and rehabilitation or for an early death.

To determine the extent to which death resulted from withdrawing or withholding treatment, we examined the hospital records of all children who died from January 1, 1970, through June 30, 1972.

Results

In total, there were 299 deaths; each was classified in one of two categories; deaths in Category 1 resulted from

pathologic conditions in spite of the treatment given; 256 (86 per cent) were in this category. Of these, 66 per cent were the result of respiratory problems or complications associated with extreme prematurity (birth weight under 1000 g). Congenital heart disease and other anomalies accounted for an additional 22 per cent (Table 87-1).

Deaths in Category 2 were associated with severe impairment, usually from congenital disorders (Table 87-2): 43 (14 per cent) were in this group. These deaths or their timing was associated with discontinuance or withdrawal of treatment. The mean duration of life in Category 2 (Table 87-3) was greater than that in Category 1. This was the result of a mean life of 55 days for eight infants who became chronic cardiopulmonary cripples but for whom prolonged and intensive efforts were made in the hope of eventual recovery. They were infants who were dependent on oxygen, digoxin and diuretics, and most of them had been treated for the idiopathic respiratory-distress syndrome with high oxygen concentrations and positive-pressure ventilation.

Some examples of management choices in Category 2 illustrate the problems. An infant with Down's syndrome and intestinal atresia, like the much-publicized one at Johns Hopkins Hospital,[9] was not treated because his parents thought that surgery was wrong for their baby and themselves. He died seven days after birth. Another child had chronic pulmonary disease after positive-pressure ventilation with high oxygen concentrations for treatment of severe idiopathic respiratory-distress syndrome. By five months of age, he still required 40 per cent oxygen to survive, and even then, he was chronically dyspneic and cyanotic. He also suffered from cor pulmonale, which was difficult to control with digoxin and diuretics. The nurses, parents and physicians considered it cruel to continue, and yet difficult to stop. All were attached to this child, whose life they had tried so hard to make worthwhile. The family had endured high expenses (the hospital bill exceeding $15,000), and the strains of the illness were believed to be threatening the marriage

Table 87-1

Problems Causing Death in Category 1

Problem	Deaths	Percentage
Respiratory	108	42.2
Extreme prematurity	60	23.4
Heart disease	42	16.4
Multiple anomalies	14	5.5
Other	32	12.5
Totals	256	100.0

Table 87-2

Problems Associated with Death in Category 2

Problem	Deaths	Percentage
Multiple anomalies	15	34.9
Trisomy	8	18.6
Cardiopulmonary	8	18.6
Meningomyelocele	7	16.3
Other central-nervous-system defects	3	7.0
Short-bowel syndrome	2	4.6
Totals	43	100.0

Table 87-3

Selected Comparisons of 256 Cases in Category 1 and 43 in Category 2

Attribute	Category 1	Category 2
Mean length of life	4.8 days	7.5 days
Standard deviation	8.8	34.3
Range	1–69	1–150
Portion living for < 2 days	50.0%	12.0%

bonds and to be causing sibling behavioral disturbances. Oxygen supplementation was stopped, and the child died in about three hours. The family settled down and 18 months later had another baby, who was healthy.

A third child had meningomyelocele, hydrocephalus and major anomalies of every organ in the pelvis. When the parents understood the limits of medical care and rehabilitation, they believed no treatment should be given. She died at five days of age.

We have maintained contact with most families of children in Category 2. Thus far, these families appear to have experienced a normal mourning for their losses. Although some have exhibited doubts that the choices were correct, all appear to be as effective in their lives as they were before this experience. Some claim that their profoundly moving experience has provided a deeper meaning in life, and from this they believe they have become more effective people.

Members of all religious faiths and atheists were participants as parents and as staff in these experiences. There appeared to be no relation between participation and a person's religion. Repeated participation in these troubling events did not appear to reduce the worry of the staff about the awesome nature of the decisions.

Discussion

That decisions are made not to treat severely defective infants may be no surprise to those familiar with special-care facilities. All laymen and professionals familiar with our nursery appeared to set some limits upon their application of treatment to extend life or to investigate a pathologic process. For example, an experienced nurse said about one child, "We lost him several weeks ago.

Isn't it time to quit?" In another case, a house officer said to a physician investigating an aspect of a child's disease, "For this child, don't you think it's time to turn off your curiosity so you can turn on your kindness?" Like many others, these children eventually acquired the "right to die."

Arguments among staff members and families for and against such decisions were based on varied notions of the rights and interests of defective infants, their families, professionals and society. They were also related to varying ideas about prognosis. Regarding the infants, some contended that individuals should have a right to die in some circumstances such as anencephaly, hydranencephaly, and some severely deforming and incapacitating conditions. Such very defective individuals were considered to have little or no hope of achieving meaningful "humanhood."[10] For example, they have little or no capacity to love or be loved. They are often cared for in facilities that have been characterized as "hardly more than dying bins,"[11] an assessment with which, in our experience, knowledgeable parents (those who visited chronic-care facilities for placement of their children) agreed. With institutionalized well children, social participation may be essentially nonexistent, and maternal deprivation severe; this is known to have an adverse, usually disastrous, effect upon the child.[12] The situation for the defective child is probably worse, for he is restricted socially both by his need for care and by his defects. To escape "wrongful life,"[13] a fate rated as worse than

death, seemed right. In this regard, Lasagna[14] notes, "We may, as a society, scorn the civilizations that slaughtered their infants, but our present treatment of the retarded is in some ways more cruel."

Others considered allowing a child to die wrong for several reasons. The person most involved, the infant, had no voice in the decision. Prognosis was not always exact, and a few children with extensive care might live for months, and occasionlly years. Some might survive and function satisfactorily. To a few persons, withholding treatment and accepting death was condemned as criminal.

Families had strong but mixed feelings about management decisions. Living with the handicapped is clearly a family affair, and families of deformed infants thought there were limits to what they could bear or should be expected to bear. Most of them wanted maximal efforts to sustain life and to rehabilitate the handicapped; in such cases, they were supported fully. However, some families, especially those having children with severe defects, feared that they and their other children would become socially enslaved, economically deprived, and permanently stigmatized, all perhaps for a lost cause. Such a state of "chronic sorrow" until death has been described by Olshansky.[15] In some cases, families considered the death of the child right both for the child and for the family. They asked if that choice could be theirs or their doctors.

As Feifel has reported,[16] physicians on the whole are reluctant to deal with the issues. Some, particularly specialists based in the medical center, gave specific reasons for this disinclination. There was a feeling that to "give up" was disloyal to the cause of the profession. Since major research, teaching and patient-care efforts were being made, professionals expected to discover, transmit and apply knowledge and skills; patients and families were supposed to co-operate fully even if they were not always grateful. Some physicians recognized that the wishes of families went against their own, but they were resolute. They commonly agreed that if they were the parents of very defective children, withholding treatment would be most desirable for them. However, they argued that aggressive management was indicated for others. Some believed that allowing death as a management option was euthanasia and must be stopped for fear of setting a "poor ethical example" or for fear of personal prosecution or damage to their clinical departments or to the medical center as a whole. Alexander's report on Nazi Germany[17] was cited in some cases as providing justification for pressing the effort to combat disease. Some persons were concerned about the loss through death of "teaching material." They feared the training of professionals for the care of defective children in the future and the advancing of the state of the art would be compromised. Some parents who became aware of this concern thought their children should not become experimental subjects.

Practicing pediatricians, general practitioners and obstetricians were often familiar with these families and were usually sympathetic with their views. However, since they were more distant from the special-care nursery than the specialists of the medical center, their influence was often minimal. As a result, families received little support from them, and tension in community-medical relations was a recurring problem.

Infants with severe types of meningomyelocele precipitated the most controversial decisions. Several decades ago, those who survived this condition beyond a few weeks usually became hydrocephalic and retarded, in addition to being crippled and deformed. Without modern treatment, they died earlier.[18] Some may have been killed or at least not resuscitated at birth.[19] From the early 1960's, the tendency has been to treat vigorously all infants with meningomyelocele. As advocated by Zachary[20] and Shurtleff,[21] aggressive

management of these children became the rule in our unit as in many others. Infants were usually referred quickly. Parents routinely signed permits for operation though rarely had they seen their children's defects or had the nature of various management plans and their respective prognoses clearly explained to them. Some physicians believed that parents were too upset to understand the nature of the problems and the options for care. Since they believed informed consent had no meaning in these circumstances, they either ignored the parents or simply told them that the child needed an operation on the back as the first step in correcting several defects. As a result, parents often felt completely left out while the activities of care proceeded at a brisk pace.

Some physicians experienced in the care of these children and familiar with the impact of such conditions upon families had early reservations about this plan of care.[22] More recently, they were influenced by the pessimistic appraisal of vigorous management schemes in some cases.[5] Meningomyelocele, when treated vigorously, is associated with higher survival rates,[21] but the achievement of satisfactory rehabilitation is at best difficult and usually impossible for almost all who are severely affected. Knowing this, some physicians and some families[23] decide against treatment of the most severely affected. If treatment is not carried out, the child's condition will usually deteriorate from further brain damage, urinary-tract infections and orthopedic difficulties, and death can be expected much earlier. Two thirds may be dead by three months, and over 90 per cent by one year of age. However, the quality of life during that time is poor, and the strains on families are great, but not necessarily greater than with treatment.[24] Thus, both treatment and nontreatment constitute unsatisfactory dilemmas for everyone, especially for the child and his family. When maximum treatment was viewed as unacceptable by families and physicians in our unit, there was a growing tendency to seek early death as a management option, to avoid that cruel choice of gradual, often slow, but progessive deterioration

of the child who was required under these circumstances in effect to kill himself. Parents and the staff then asked if his dying needed to be prolonged. If not, what were the most appropriate medical responses?

Is it possible that some physicians and some families may join in a conspiracy to deny the right of a defective child to live or to die? Either could occur. Prolongation of the dying process by resident physicians having a vested interest in their careers has been described by Sudnow.[25] On the other hand, from the fatigue of working long and hard some physicians may give up too soon, assuming that their cause is lost. Families, similarly, may have mixed motives. They may demand death to obtain relief from the high costs and the tensions inherent in suffering, but their sense of guilt in this thought may produce the opposite demand, perhaps in violation of the sick person's rights. Thus, the challenge of deciding what course to take can be most tormenting for the family and the physician. Unquestionably, not facing the issue would appear to be the easier course, at least temporarily; no doubt many patients, families, and physicians decline to join in an effort to solve the problems. They can readily assume that what is being done is right and sufficient and ask no questions. But pretending there is no decision to be made is an arbitrary and potentially devastating decision of default. Since families and patients must live with the problems one way or another in any case, the physician's failure to face the issues may constitute a victimizing abandonment of patients and their families in times of greatest need. As Lasagna[14] pointed out, "There is no place for the physician to hide."

Can families in the shock resulting from the birth of a defective child understand what faces them? Can they give truly "informed consent" for treatment or with-holding treatment? Some of our colleagues answer no to both questions. In our opinion, if families regardless of background are heard sympathetically and at length and are given information and answers to their questions in words they understand, the problems of their children as well as the expected benefits and limits of any proposed care can be understood clearly in practically all instances. Parents *are* able to understand the implications of such things as chronic dyspnea, oxygen dependency, incontinence, paralysis, contractures, sexual handicaps and mental retardation.

Another problem concerns who decides for a child. It may be acceptable for a person to reject treatment and bring about his own death. But it is quite a different situation when others are doing this for him. We do not know how often families and their physicians will make just decisions for severely handicapped children. Clearly, this issue is central in evaluation of the process of decision making that we have described. But we also ask, if these parties cannot make such decisions justly, who can?

We recognize great variability and often much uncertainty in prognoses and in family capacities to deal with defective newborn infants. We also acknowledge that there are limits of support that society can or will give to assist handicapped persons and their families. Severely deforming conditions that are associated with little or no hope of a functional existence pose painful dilemmas for the laymen and professionals who must decide how to cope with severe handicaps. We believe the burdens of decision making must be borne by families and their professional advisers because they are most familiar with the respective situations. Since families primarily must live with and are most affected by the decisions, it therefore appears that society and the health professions should provide only general guidelines for decision making. Moreover, since variations between situations are so great, and the situations themselves so complex, it follows that much latitude in decision making should be expected and tolerated. Otherwise, the rules of society or the policies most convenient for medical technologists may become cruel masters of human beings instead of their servants. Regarding any "allocation of death"[26] policy we readily acknowledge that the extreme excess of Hegelian "rational utility" under dictatorships must be avoided.[17] Perhaps it is less recognized that the uncontrolled application of medical technology may be detrimental to individuals and families. In this regard, our views are similar to those of Waitzkin and Stoeckle.[27] Physicians may hold excessive power over decision making by limiting or controlling the information made available to patients or families. It seems appropriate that the profession be held accountable for presenting fully all management options and their expected consequences. Also, the public should be aware that professionals often face conflicts of interest that may result in decisions against individual preferences.

What are the legal implications of actions like those described in this paper? Some persons may argue that the law has been broken, and others would contend otherwise. Perhaps more than anything else, the public and professional silence on a major social taboo and some common practices has been broken further. That seems appropriate, for out of the ensuing dialogue perhaps better choices for patients and families can be made. If working out these dilemmas in ways such as those we suggest is in violation of the law, we believe the law should be changed.

References

1. Wegman, M. E., Annual summary of vital statistics—1970. *Pediatrics* 48:979–983, 1971.

2. Swyer, P. R., The regional organization of special care for the neonate. *Pediatr. Clin. North. Am.* 17:761–776, 1970.

3. Rawlings, G., Reynold, E. O. R., Stewart, A., et al., Changing prognosis for infants of very low birth weight. *Lancet* 1:516–519, 1971.

4. Freeman, E., The god committee. *New York Times Magazine*, May 21, 1972, pp. 84–90.

5. Lorber, J., Results of treatment of myelomeningocele. *Dev. Med. Child Neurol.* 13:279–303, 1971.

6. Slater, E., Health service or sickness service. *Br. Med. J.* 4:734–736, 1971.

7. Klaus, M. H., Kennell, J. H., Mothers separated from their newborn infants. *Pediatr. Clin. North. Am.* 17:1015–1037, 1970.

8. Eisenberg, L., The human nature of human nature. *Science* 176:123–128, 1972.

9. Report of the Joseph P. Kennedy Foundation International Symposium on Human Rights, Retardation and Research, Washington, D.C.: The John F. Kennedy Center for the Performing Arts, October 16, 1971.

10. Fletcher, J., Indicators of humanhood; a tentative profile of man. *The Hastings Center Report* Vol. 2. No. 5. Hastings-on-Hudson, N.Y.: Institute of Society, Ethics and the Life Sciences, November, 1972, pp. 1–4.

11. Freeman, H. F., Brim, O. G., Jr., Williams, G., New dimensions of dying. *The Dying Patient.* Edited by O. G. Brim, Jr., New York: Russell Sage Foundation, 1970, pp. xiii–xxvi.

12. Spitz, R. A., Hospitalism: an inquiry into the genesis of psychiatric conditions in early childhood. *Psychoanal. Study Child* 1:53–74, 1945.

13. Engelhardt, H. T., Jr., Euthanasia and children: the injury of continued existence. *J. Pediatr.* 83:170–171, 1973.

14. Lasagna, L., *Life, Death and the Doctor.* New York: Alfred A. Knopf, 1968.

15. Olshansky, S., Chronic sorrow: a response to having a mentally defective child. *Soc. Casework* 43:190–193, 1962.

16. Feifel, H., Perception of death. *Ann. N.Y. Acad. Sci.* 164:669–677, 1969.

17. Alexander, L., Medical science under dictatorship. *N. Engl. J. Med.* 241:39–47, 1949.

18. Laurence, K. M., and Tew, B. J., Natural history of spina bifida cystica and cranium bifidum cysticum: major central nervous system malformations in South Wales. Part IV. *Arch. Dis. Child.* 46:127–138, 1971.

19. Forrest, D. M., Modern trends in the treatment of spina bifida: early closure in spina bifida: results and problems. *Proc. R. Soc. Med.* 60:763–767, 1967.

20. Zachary, R. B., Ethical and social aspects of treatment of spina bifida. *Lancet* 2:274–276, 1968.

21. Shurtleff, D. B., Care of the myelodysplastic patient. *Ambulatory Pediatrics.* Edited by M. Green, R. Haggerty, Philadelphia: W. B. Saunders Company, 1968, pp. 726–741.

22. Matson, D. D., Surgical treatment of myelomeningocele. *Pediatrics* 42:225–227, 1968.

23. MacKeith, R. C., A new look at spina bifida aperta. *Dev. Med. Child Neurol.* 13:277–278, 1971.

24. Hide, D. W., Williams, H. P., Ellis, H. L., The outlook for the child with a myelomeningocele for whom early surgery was considered inadvisable. *Dev. Med. Child Neurol.* 14:304–307, 1972.

25. Sudnow, D., *Passing On.* Englewood Cliffs, N.J.: Prentice-Hall, 1967.

26. Manning, B., Legal and policy issues in the allocation of death. *The Dying Patient.* Edited by O. G. Brim, Jr., New York: Russell Sage Foundation, 1970, pp. 253–274.

27. Waitzkin, H., Stoeckle, J. D., The communication of information about illness. *Adv. Psychosom. Med.* 8:180–215, 1972. [Reprinted in part as Chapter 37 of this volume.]

88

Richard A. McCormick

To Save or Let Die: The Dilemma of Modern Medicine

Reprinted with permission of the author and the publisher from the *Journal of the American Medical Association*, vol. 229, 1974, pp. 172–176. Copyright © 1974, American Medical Association.

On Feb. 24, the son of Mr. and Mrs. Robert H. T. Houle died following court-ordered emergency surgery at Maine Medical Center. The child was born Feb. 9, horribly deformed. His entire left side was malformed; he had no left eye, was practically without a left ear, had a deformed left hand; some of his vertebrae were not fused. Furthermore, he was afflicted with a tracheal esophageal fistula and could not be fed by mouth. Air leaked into his stomach instead of going to the lungs, and fluid from the stomach pushed up into the lungs. As Dr. Andre Hellegers recently noted, "It takes little imagination to think there were further internal deformities" (*Obstetrical and Gynecological News,* April 1974).

As the days passed, the condition of the child deteriorated. Pneumonia set in. His reflexes became impaired and because of poor circulation, severe brain damage was suspected. The tracheal esophageal fistula, the immediate threat to his survival, can be corrected with relative ease by surgery. But in view of the associated complications and deformities, the parents refused their consent to surgery on "Baby Boy Houle." Several doctors in the Maine Medical Center felt differently and took the case to court. Maine Superior Court Judge David G. Roberts ordered the surgery to be performed. He ruled: "At the moment of live birth there does exist a human being entitled to the fullest protection of the law. The most basic right enjoyed by every human being is the right to life itself."

"Meaningful Life"

Instances like this happen frequently. In a recent issue of the *New England Journal of Medicine*, Drs. Raymond S. Duff and A. G. M. Campbell[1] reported on 299 deaths in the special-care nursery of the Yale–New Haven Hospital between 1970 and 1972. Of these, 43 (14%) were associated with discontinuance of treatment for children with multiple anomalies, trisomy, cardiopulmonary crippling, meningomyelocele, and other central nervous system defects. After careful consideration of each of these 43 infants, parents and physicians in a group decision concluded that the prognosis for "meaningful life" was extremely poor or hopeless, and therefore rejected further treatment. The abstract of the Duff-Campbell report states: "The awesome finality of these decisions, combined with a potential for error in prognosis, made the choice agonizing for families and health professionals. Nevertheless, the issue has to be faced, for not to decide is an arbitrary and potentially devastating decision of default."

In commenting on this study in the *Washington Post* (Oct. 28, 1973), Dr. Lawrence K. Pickett, chief-of-staff at the Yale–New Haven Hospital, admitted that allowing hopelessly ill patients to die "is accepted medical practice." He continued: "This is nothing new. It's just being talked about now."

It has been talked about, it is safe to say, at least since the publicity associated with the famous "Johns Hopkins Case"[2] some three years ago. In this instance, an infant was born with Down's syndrome and duodenal atresia. The blockage is reparable by relatively easy surgery. However, after consultation with spiritual advisors, the parents refused permission for this corrective surgery, and the child died by starvation in the hospital after 15 days. For to feed him by mouth in this condition would have killed him. Nearly everyone who has commented on this case has disagreed with the decision.

It must be obvious that these instances—and they are frequent—raise the most agonizing and delicate moral problems. The problem is best seen in the ambiguity of the term "hopelessly ill." This used to and still may refer to lives that cannot be saved, that are irretrievably in the dying process. It may also refer to lives that can be saved and sustained, but in a wretched, painful, or deformed condition. With regard to infants, the problem is, which infants, if any, should be allowed to die? On what grounds or according to what criteria, as determined by whom? Or again, is there a point at which a life that can be saved is not "meaningful life," as the medical community so often phrases the question? If our past experience is any hint of the future, it is safe to say that public discussion of such controversial issues will quickly collapse into slogans such as "There is no such thing as a life not worth saving" or "Who is the physician to play God?" We saw and continue to see this far too frequently in the abortion debate. We are experiencing it in the euthanasia discussion. For instance, "death with dignity" translates for many into a death that is fast, clean, painless. The trouble with slogans is that they do not aid in the discovery of truth; they co-opt this discovery and promulgate it rhetorically, often only thinly disguising a good number of questionable value judgments in the process. Slogans are not tools for analysis and enlightenment; they are weapons for ideological battle.

Thus far, the ethical discussion of these truly terrifying decisions has been less than fully satisfactory. Perhaps this is to be expected since the problems have only recently come to public attention. In a companion article to the Duff-Campbell report,[1] Dr. Anthony Shaw[3] of the Pediatric Division of the Department of Surgery, University of Virginia Medical Center, Charlottesville, speaks of solutions "based on the circumstances of each case rather than by means of a dogmatic formula approach." Are these really the only options available to us? Shaw's statement makes it appear that the ethical alternatives are narrowed to dogmatism (which imposes a formula that prescinds from circumstances) and pure concretism (which denies the possibility or usefulness of any guidelines).

Are Guidelines Possible?

Such either-or extremism is understandable. It is easy for the medical profession, in its fully justified concern with the terrible concreteness of these problems and with the issue of who makes these decisions, to trend away from any substantive guidelines. As *Time* remarked in reporting these instances: "Few, if any, doctors are willing to establish guidelines for determining which babies should receive lifesaving surgery or treatment and which should not" (*Time,* March 25, 1974). On the other hand, moral theologians, in their fully justified concern to avoid total normlessness and arbitrariness wherein the right is "discovered," or really "created," only in and by brute decision, can easily be insensitive to the moral relevance of the raw experience, of the conflicting tensions and concerns provoked

through direct cradleside contact with human events and persons.

But is there no middle course between sheer concretism and dogmatism? I believe there is. Dr. Franz J. Ingelfinger,[4] editor of the *New England Journal of Medicine,* in an editorial on the Duff-Campbell-Shaw articles, concluded, even if somewhat reluctantly: "Society, ethics, institutional attitudes and committees can provide the broad guidelines, but the onus of decision-making ultimately falls on the doctor in whose care the child has been put." Similarly, Frederick Carney of Southern Methodist University, Dallas, and the Kennedy Center for Bioethics stated of these cases: "What is obviously needed is the development of substantive standards to inform parents and physicians who must make such decisions" (*Washington Post,* March 20, 1974).

"Broad guidelines," "substantive standards." There is the middle course, and it is the task of a community broader than the medical community. A guideline is not a slide rule that makes the decision. It is far less than that. But it is far more than the concrete decision of the parents and physician, however seriously and conscientiously this is made. It is more like a light in a room, a light that allows the individual objects to be seen in the fullness of their context. Concretely, if there are certain infants that we agree ought to be saved in spite of illness or deformity, and if there are certain infants that we agree should be allowed to die, then there is a line to be drawn. And if there is a line to be drawn, there ought to be some criteria, even if very general, for doing this. Thus, if nearly every commentator has disagreed with the Hopkins decision, should we not be able to distill from such consensus some general wisdom that will inform and guide future decisions? I think so.

This task is not easy. Indeed, it is so harrowing that the really tempting thing is to run from it. The most sensitive, balanced, and penetrating study of the Hopkins case that I have seen is that of the University of Chicago's James Gustafson.[2] Gustafson disagreed with the decision of the Hopkins physicians to deny surgery to the mongoloid infant. In summarizing his dissent, he notes: "Why would I draw the line on a different side of mongolism than the physicians did? While reasons can be

given, one must recognize that there are intuitive elements, grounded in beliefs and profound feelings, that enter into particular judgments of this sort." He goes on to criticize the assessment made of the child's intelligence as too simplistic, and he proposes a much broader perspective on the meaning of suffering than seemed to have operated in the Hopkins decision. I am in full agreement with Gustafson's reflections and conclusions. But ultimately, he does not tell us where he would draw the line or why, only where he would *not,* and why.

This is very helpful already, and perhaps it is all that can be done. Dare we take the next step, the combination and analysis of such negative judgments to extract from them the positive criterion or criteria inescapably operative in them? Or more startlingly, dare we *not* if these decisions are already being made? Gustafson is certainly right in saying that we cannot always establish perfectly rational accounts and norms for our decisions. But I believe we must never cease trying, in fear and trembling to be sure. Otherwise, we have exempted these decisions in principle from the one critique and control that protects against abuse. Exemption of this sort is the root of all exploitation whether personal or political. Briefly, if we must face the frightening task of making quality-of-life judgments—and we must—then we must face the difficult task of building criteria for these judgments.

Facing Responsibility

What has brought us to this position of awesome responsibility? Very simply, the sophistication of modern medicine. Contemporary resuscitation and life-sustaining devices have brought a remarkable change in the state of the question. Our duties toward the care and preservation of life have been traditionally stated in terms of the use of ordinary and extraordinary means. For the moment and for purposes of brevity, we may say that, morally speaking, ordinary means are those whose use does not entail grave hardships to the patient. Those that would involve such hardship are extraordinary. Granted the relativity of these terms and the frequent difficulty of their application, still the distinction has had an honored place in medical ethics and medical practice. Indeed, the distinction was recently reiterated by the House of Delegates of the American Medical Association in a policy statement. After disowning intentional killing (mercy killing), the AMA statement continues: "The cessation of the employment of extraordinary means to prolong the life of the body when there is irrefutable evidence that biological death is imminent is the decision of the patient and/or his immediate family. The advice and judgment of the physician should be freely available to the patient and/or his immediate family" (JAMA 227:728, 1974).

This distinction can take us just so far—and thus the change in the state of the question. The contemporary problem is precisely that the question no longer concerns only those for whom "biological death is imminent" in the sense of the AMA statement. Many infants who would have died a decade ago, whose "biological death was imminent," can be saved. Yesterday's failures are today's successes. Contemporary medicine with its team approaches, staged surgical techniques, monitoring capabilities, ventilatory support systems, and other methods, can keep almost anyone alive. This has tended gradually to shift the problem from the means to reverse the dying process to the quality of the life sustained and preserved. The questions, "Is this means too hazardous or difficult to use" and "Does this measure only prolong the patient's dying," while still useful and valid, now often become "Granted that we can easily save the life, what kind of life are we saving?" This is a quality-of-life judgment. And we fear it. And certainly we should. But with increased power goes increased responsibility. Since we have the power, we must face the responsibility.

A Relative Good

In the past, the Judeo-Christian tradition has attempted to walk a balanced middle path between medical vitalism (that preserves life at any cost) and medical pessimism (that kills when life seems frustrating, burdensome, "useless"). Both of these extremes root in

an identical idolatry of life—an attitude that, at least by inference, views death as an unmitigated, absolute evil, and life as the absolute good. The middle course that has structured Judeo-Christian attitudes is that life is indeed a basic and precious good, but a good to be preserved precisely as the condition of other values. It is these other values and possibilities that found the duty to preserve physical life and also dictate the limits of this duty. In other words, life is a relative good, and the duty to preserve it a limited one. These limits have always been stated in terms of the *means* required to sustain life. But if the implications of this middle position are unpacked a bit, they will allow us, perhaps, to adapt to the type of quality-of-life judgment we are now called on to make without tumbling into vitalism or a utilitarian pessimism.

A beginning can be made with a statement of Pope Pius XII[5] in an allocution to physicians delivered Nov. 24, 1957. After noting that we are normally obliged to use only ordinary means to preserve life, the Pontiff stated: "A more strict obligation would be too burdensome for most men and would render the attainment of the higher, more important good too difficult. Life, death, all temporal activities are in fact subordinated to spiritual ends." Here it would be helpful to ask two questions. First, what are these spiritual ends, this "higher, more important good"? Second, how is its attainment rendered too difficult by insisting on the use of extraordinary means to preserve life?

The first question must be answered in terms of love of God and neighbor. This sums up briefly the meaning, substance, and consummation of life from a Judeo-Christian perspective. What is or can easily be missed is that these two loves are not separable. St. John wrote: "If any man says I love God and hates his brother, he is a liar. For he who loves not his brother, whom he sees, how can he love God whom he does not see?" (1 John 4:20–21). This means that our love of neighbor is in some very real sense our love of God. The good our love wants to do Him and to which He enables us, can be done only for the neighbor, as Karl Rahner has so forcefully argued. It is in others that God demands to be recognized and loved. If this is true, it means that, in Judeo-Christian perspective, the

meaning, substance, and consummation of life is found in human *relationships,* and the qualities of justice, respect, concern, compassion, and support that surround them.

Second, how is the attainment of this "higher, more important (than life) good" rendered "too difficult" by life-supports that are gravely burdensome? One who must support his life with disproportionate effort focuses the time, attention, energy, and resources of himself and others not precisely on relationships, but on maintaining the condition of relationships. Such concentration easily becomes overconcentration and distorts one's view of and weakens one's pursuit of the very relational goods that define our growth and flourishing. The importance of relationships gets lost in the struggle for survival. The very Judeo-Christian meaning of life is seriously jeopardized when undue and unending effort must go into its maintenance.

I believe an analysis similar to this is implied in traditional treatises on preserving life. The illustrations of grave hardship (rendering the means to preserve life extraordinary and nonobligatory) are instructive, even if they are outdated in some of their particulars. Older moralists often referred to the hardship of moving to another climate or country. As the late Gerald Kelly, S.J.,[6] noted of this instance: "They (the classical moral theologians) spoke of other inconveniences, too: e.g., of moving to another climate or another country to preserve one's life. For people whose lives were, so to speak, rooted in the land, and whose native town or village was as dear as life itself, and for whom, moreover, travel was always difficult and often dangerous—for such people, moving to another country or climate was a truly great hardship, and more than God would demand as a 'reasonable' means of preserving one's health and life."

Similarly, if the financial cost of life-preserving care was crushing, that is, if it would create grave hardships for oneself or one's family, it was considered extraordinary and nonobligatory. Or again, the grave inconvenience of living with a badly mutilated body was viewed, along with other factors (such as pain in preanesthetic days, uncertainty of success), as constituting the means extraordinary. Even now, the contemporary moralist, M. Zalba, S.J.,[7] states that no one is obliged to preserve his life when the cost is "a most oppressive convalescence" (*molestissima convalescentia*).

The Quality of Life

In all of these instances—instances where the life could be saved—the discussion is couched in terms of the means necessary to preserve life. But often enough it is the kind of, the quality of the life thus saved (painful, poverty-stricken and deprived, away from home and friends, oppressive) that establishes the means as extraordinary. *That* type of life would be an excessive hardship for the individual. It would distort and jeopardize his grasp on the overall meaning of life. Why? Because, it can be argued, human relationships—which are the very possibility of growth in love of God and neighbor—would be so threatened, strained, or submerged that they would no longer function as the heart and meaning of the individual's life as they should. Something other than the "higher, more important good" would occupy first place. Life, the condition of other values and achievements, would usurp the place of these and become itself the ultimate value. When that happens, the value of human life has been distorted out of context.

In his *Morals in Medicine*, Thomas O'Donnell, S.J.,[8] hinted at an analysis similar to this. Noting that life is a relative, not an absolute good, he asks: Relative to what? His answer moves in two steps. First, he argues that life is the fundamental natural good God has given to man, "the fundamental context in which all other goods which God has given man as means to the end proposed to him, must be exercised." Second, since this is so, the relativity of the good of life consists in the effort required to preserve this fundamental context and "the potentialities of the other goods that still remain to be worked out within that context."

Can these reflections be brought to bear on the grossly malformed infant? I believe so. Obviously there is a difference between having a terribly mutilated body as the result of surgery, and having a terribly mutilated body from birth. There is also a difference between a long, painful, oppressive convalescence resulting from surgery, and a life that is from birth one long, painful, oppressive convalescence. Similarly, there is a difference between being plunged into poverty by medical expenses and being poor without ever incurring such expenses. However, is there not also a similarity? Can not these conditions, whether caused by medical intervention or not, equally absorb attention and energies to the point where the "higher, more important good" is simply too difficult to attain? It would appear so. Indeed, is this not precisely why abject poverty (and the systems that support it) is such an enormous moral challenge to us? It simply dehumanizes.

Life's potentiality for other values is dependent on two factors, those external to the individual, and the very condition of the individual. The former we can and must change to maximize individual potential. That is what social justice is all about. The latter we sometimes cannot alter. It is neither inhuman nor unchristian to say that there comes a point where an individual's condition itself represents the negation of any truly human—i.e., relational—potential. When that point is reached, is not the best treatment no treatment? I believe that the *implications* of the traditional distinction between ordinary and extraordinary means point in this direction.

In this tradition, life is not a value to be preserved in and for itself. To maintain that would commit us to a form of medical vitalism that makes no human or Judeo-Christian sense. It is a value to be preserved precisely as a condition for other values, and therefore insofar as these other values remain attainable. Since these other values cluster around and are rooted in human relationships, it seems to follow that life is a value to be preserved only insofar as it contains some potentiality for human relationships. When in human judgment this potentiality is totally absent or would be, because of the condition of the individual, totally subordinated to the mere effort for survival, that life can be said to have achieved its potential.

Human Relationships

If these reflections are valid, they point in the direction of a guideline that may help in decisions about sustaining the lives of grossly deformed and deprived infants. That guideline is the potential for human relationships associated with the infant's condition. If that potential is simply nonexistent or would be utterly submerged and undeveloped in the mere struggle to survive, that life has achieved its potential. There are those who will want to continue to say that some terribly deformed infants may be allowed to die *because* no extraordinary means need be used. Fair enough. But they should realize that the term "extraordinary" has been so relativized to the condition of the patient that it is this condition that is decisive. The means is extraordinary because the infant's condition is extraordinary. And if that is so, we must face this fact head-on—and discover the substantive standard that allows us to say this of some infants, but not of others.

Here several caveats are in order. First, this guideline is not a detailed rule that preempts decisions; for relational capacity is not subject to mathematical analysis but to human judgment. However, it is the task of physicians to provide some more concrete categories or presumptive biological symptoms for this human judgment. For instance, nearly all would very likely agree that the anencephalic infant is without relational potential. On the other hand, the same cannot be said of the mongoloid infant. The task ahead is to attach relational potential to presumptive biological symptoms for the gray area between such extremes. In other words, individual decisions will remain the anguishing onus of parents in consultation with physicians.

Second, because this guideline is precisely that, mistakes will be made. Some infants will be judged in all sincerity to be devoid of any meaningful relational potential when that is actually not quite the case. This risk of error should not lead to abandonment of decisions; for that is to walk away from the human scene. Risk of error means only that we must proceed with great humility, caution, and tentativeness. Concretely, it means that if err we must at times, it is better to err on the side of life—and therefore to tilt in that direction.

Third, it must be emphasized that allowing some infants to die does not imply that "some lives are valuable, others not" or that "there is such a thing as a life not worth living." Every human being, regardless of age or condition, is of incalculable worth. The point is not, therefore, whether this or that individual has value. Of course he has, or rather *is* a value. The only point is whether this undoubted value has any potential at all, in continuing physical survival, for attaining a share, even if reduced, in the "higher, more important good." This is not a question about the inherent value of the individual. It is a question about whether this worldly existence will offer such a valued individual any hope of sharing those values for which physical life is the fundamental condition. Is not the only alternative an attitude that supports mere physical life as long as possible with every means?

Fourth, this whole matter is further complicated by the fact that this decision is being made for someone else. Should not the decision on whether life is to be supported or not be left to the individual? Obviously, wherever possible. But there is nothing inherently objectionable in the fact that parents with physicians must make this decision at some point for infants. Parents must make many crucial decisions for children. The only concern is that the decision not be shaped out of the utilitarian perspectives so deeply sunk into the consciousness of the contemporary world. In a highly technological culture, an individual is always in danger of being valued for his function, what he can do, rather than for who he is.

It remains, then, only to emphasize that these decisions must be made in terms of the child's good, this alone. But that good, as fundamentally a relational good, has many dimensions. Pius XII,[5] in speaking of the duty to preserve life, noted that this duty "derives from well-ordered charity, from submission to the Creator, from social justice, as well as from devotion towards his family." All of these considerations pertain to that "higher, more important good." If that is the case with the duty to preserve life, then the decision not to preserve life must likewise take all of these into account in determining what is for the child's good.

Any discussion of this problem would be incomplete if it did not repeatedly stress that it is the pride of Judeo-Christian tradition that the weak and defenseless, the powerless and unwanted, those whose grasp on the goods of life is most fragile—that is, those whose potential is real but reduced—are cherished and protected as our neighbor in greatest need. Any application of a general guideline that forgets this is but a racism of the adult world profoundly at odds with the gospel, and eventually corrosive of the humanity of those who ought to be caring and supporting as long as that care and support has human meaning. It has meaning as long as there is hope that the infant will, in relative comfort, be able to experience our caring and love. For when this happens, both we and the child are sharing in that "greater, more important good."

Were not those who disagreed with the Hopkins decision saying, in effect, that for the infant, involved human relationships were still within reach and would not be totally submerged by survival? If that is the case, it is potential for relationships that is at the heart of these agonizing decisions.

References

1. Duff, S., Campbell, A. G. M., Moral and ethical dilemmas in the special-care nursery. *N. Engl. J. Med.* 289:890–894, 1973. [Reprinted as Chapter 87 of this volume.]

2. Gustafson, J. M., Mongolism, parental desires, and the right to life. *Perspect. Biol. Med.* 16:529–559, 1973.

3. Shaw, A., Dilemmas of "informed" consent in children. *N. Engl. J. Med.* 289:885–890, 1973.

4. Ingelfinger, F., Bedside ethics for the hopeless case. *N. Engl. J. Med.* 289:914, 1973.

5. Pope Pius XII, *Acta Apostolicae Sedis.* 49:1031–1032, 1957.

6. Kelly, G., *Medico-Moral Problems.* St. Louis, Catholic Hospital Association of the United States and Canada, 1957, p. 132.

7. Zalba, M., *Theologiae Moralis Summa.* Madrid, La Editorial Catolica, 1957, vol. 2, p. 71.

8. O'Donnell, T., *Morals in Medicine.* Westminster, Md.: Newman Press, 1957, p. 66.

Illustrative Cases

A 75-year-old doctor is admitted to a hospital with symptoms that prove to be far-advanced cancer. He is informed of the findings and understands their meaning. An operation is performed to relieve some of the symptoms of the disease, all hope for a curative operation having passed. Despite the operation, he suffers great pain. While in the hospital he goes into cardiac arrest, which is successfully treated by the staff. He expresses appreciation for the good intentions and skill of his colleagues but asks that if another arrest occurs, no further steps be taken to prolong his life: the pain from his cancer had become very severe and cannot be relieved. He even writes a note stating his wishes in his own hospital record. At the time, his mind is judged sound by his physicians.

Nevertheless, when an arrest occurs two weeks after the first episode, he is revived by the emergency resuscitation team of the hospital but becomes comatose. Intravenous feeding and blood transfusions are required. These procedures are continued for two weeks, when another cardiac arrest ends his life before additional resuscitative measures can be initiated.

Consider all these questions from an ethical point of view, not as issues of physiological decision-making.
1. Should the lifesaving procedure have been performed after the first cardiac arrest?
2. Should the patient have been revived after the second arrest?
3. Should the intravenous nourishment and the blood transfusions have been started?
4. If started, should they have been stopped?
5. Would the case have been different if the patient had not *asked* his doctors to cease struggling to keep him alive?
6. How is the case affected by nearness of death?
7. How is it affected by the fact that the patient's suffering could not be mitigated?

A 25-year-old star outfielder for a major league baseball team is in an automobile accident. He suffers serious damage to his spinal cord, which causes paralysis of his body from the neck down. His thinking, speech, and hearing remain unimpaired, but he has lost all movement of his limbs. He re-

quires the constant assistance of attendants and technology to eat and expel wastes. After fifteen months of hospital care, his physicians conclude he has no discernible chance of recovering lost functions and inform him of their conclusions.

He is an intelligent and thoughtful person and thinks a great deal about his future in the weeks that follow disclosure of this prognosis. During this time, he is visited by social and rehabilitation workers at the hospital who attempt to assure him that because he still possesses his mental facilities, he would eventually accommodate to his injuries and develop some meaningful form of life in the future.

He finally decides on a course of action. He calls in his physicians and requests that they discharge him. All parties, the patient included, understand that without hospital facilities death will ensue in several weeks.

1. What are the ethical issues at stake in this case?
2. From the standpoint of ethics, what courses are open to the physicians and the hospital?
3. Which course would you take as the patient's physician?
4. Why?

A 16-year-old girl has been on a dialysis machine for two years. Before this, she had a kidney transplantation, which failed. She is awaiting the availability of a kidney whose compatibility with her tissues might ensure a successful transplantation. But the girl despairs of her life. She must reduce intake of fluids to about 800 millilitres per day, is restricted from food containing sodium or potassium, and cannot travel far from her machine, because she often requires dialysis two to three times a week, for periods of twelve to eighteen hours each session. The girl is deeply concerned about her prospects for a career and marriage, and worries, further, that even if a new transplant operation were tried, the new kidney might be rejected.

One day, she finally decides not to return to the hospital for dialysis. She is an intelligent, rational person and understands she will probably die without dialysis.

1. From a moral viewpoint, what should her parents and physicians do?

VIII

Rights and Priorities in the Provision of Medical Care

Introduction to Part VIII

We come full circle to the subject of our first pages, the therapeutic relationship. In earlier sections we explored the moral and philosophical supports for physicians' obligations to their patients and to the art and science of medicine. In this last part we examine the twentieth-century concept of a right to health care.

Our first contribution is probably the best known expression of the concept on a worldwide basis. The Preamble to the Constitution of the World Health Organization proclaims that the enjoyment of the highest attainable standard of health is "one of the fundamental rights of every human being." Fulfilling this objective has been designated as the main long-term objective of WHO and its member states.

The rest of the selections in this section analyze the debate within medicine and society over how much medical resources should be allowed each individual, what criteria should be used to allocate them, and how medical services should be organized to distribute such resources. A key aspect of this debate is the claim that medical care is the right of all citizens. A perspective on this assertion is given in the opening essay by Carleton Chapman and John M. Talmadge, who trace the history of the notion in the United States. The implications of this right for the status of the physician and the organization of medical care are examined by Robert Sade. His essay, which argues that the freedom of physicians to practice medicine can be impaired by the full acceptance of a right to health care for all people, is defended and criticized in replies to the article. This exchange has political overtones. The ethical justifications of the notion of a right to health care are examined in essays by Charles Fried and Gene Outka. The unique American concept of a right to psychiatric treatment for patients confined against their wills to mental institutions is explored by Judge David L. Bazelon and the psychiatrist Thomas S. Szasz.

These essays focus on the provision of general medical services.

But an equally perplexing set of problems occurs in formulating procedures to allocate medical resources that are particularly expensive and scarce. This problem has received much publicity in recent years, in connection with providing dialysis machines and care to patients afflicted with severe kidney disease. The essay by David Sanders and Jesse Dukeminier describes the administrative procedures and social and moral criteria used by different hospitals to allocate kidney machines in the 1960s when, unlike today, federal funds were not available to aid patients needing them. Nicholas Rescher and James Childress next discuss different schemes for distributing such scarce resources and the ethical justifications for selecting or rejecting them, and Ralph Potter examines the influence of social labels on resource allocation.

Stanley Hauerwas articulates the very basic and profound concern that underlies any of our preoccupation with resources and their limits, namely, our obligation to build and foster human communities. Meeting this obligation entails having and caring for children and developing an ethos in which they are seen not primarily as individual accomplishments, but as precious gifts to and from our communities. Although the essay has an explicitly Christian cast to it, its theme and arguments are not confined to Judeo-Christian origins.

This section concludes with two essays that analyze the use of economic criteria to value human life and allocate medical resources; these criteria often become the basis for government policy. Rashi Fein presents an historical and critical analysis of such standards, and Robert Grosse writes of his experience in the U.S. Department of Health, Education, and Welfare in applying these criteria to government decisions on health.

These materials further illustrate one of the themes that has run through our collection: individual freedoms weighed in the balance with general public welfare.

Health Care as a Right

89

Preamble to the Constitution of the World Health Organization

Reprinted from *World Health Organization: Basic Documents,* 26th ed. (Geneva: World Health Organization, 1976), p. 1.

The States Parties to this Constitution[1] declare, in conformity with the Charter of the United Nations, that the following principles are basic to the happiness, harmonious relations and security of all peoples:

Health is a state of complete physical, mental and social well-being and not merely the absence of disease or infirmity.

The enjoyment of the highest attainable standard of health is one of the fundamental rights of every human being without distinction of race, religion, political belief, economic or social condition.

The health of all peoples is fundamental to the attainment of peace and security and is dependent upon the fullest co-operation of individuals and States.

The achievement of any State in the promotion and protection of health is of value to all.

Unequal development in different countries in the promotion of health and control of disease, especially communicable disease, is a common danger.

Healthy development of the child is of basic importance; the ability to live harmoniously in a changing total environment is essential to such development.

The extension to all peoples of the benefits of medical, psychological and related knowledge is essential to the fullest attainment of health.

Informed opinion and active co-operation on the part of the public are of the utmost importance in the improvement of the health of the people.

Governments have a responsibility for the health of their peoples which can be fulfilled only by the provision of adequate health and social measures.

Note

1. The Constitution was adopted by the International Health Conference held in New York from 19 June to 22 July 1946, and signed on 22 July 1946 by the representatives of 61 States (*Off. Rec. Wld Hlth Org.* 2, 100). Amendments adopted by the Twentieth World Health Assembly (resolution WHA20.36) came into force on 21 May 1975 and are incorporated in the present text.

90

Carleton B. Chapman and John M. Talmadge

The Evolution of the Right to Health Concept in the United States

Reprinted with the permission of the editor of *Pharos,* vol. 34, 1971, pp. 30–51.

Introduction

"Medicine is at the crossroads," incoming president Milford O. Rouse warned the American Medical Association in 1967. He went on to say:

We are faced with the concept of *health care as a right rather than a privilege.* . . . We face proposals and possibilities of increased government control . . . , emphasis on a non-profit approach to medicine, increasing coercion . . . , and emphasis on the academic and institutional environment.[1] (Italics ours.)

In striking contrast, the AMA's House of Delegates, passed a resolution two years later (17 July, 1969) that said in part:

It is the basic *right* of every citizen to have available to him adequate health care.[2] (Italics ours.)

Dr. Rouse was stating a point of view which was clearly in keeping with policy of the AMA as it was officially laid down nearly half a century ago. But the House of Delegates' action in 1969 represented a modification of official policy that may, depending on the actual meaning the Delegates assigned to the resolution, prove to be a profound one.

In linking the word *right* to the word *health,* Dr. Rouse and the House of Delegates were employing a convention that has gradually received wide acceptance in the United States. *Right to health* appears, in modified form, in the Congressional Record (Annals of Congress) as early as 1796 and reappears, largely by inference, at many points during the nineteenth and early twentieth centuries. It came into full flower in Franklin Roosevelt's Economic Bill of Rights (1944) and has been employed by various groups, in and out of government, with increasing frequency ever since.

The meaning assigned to the phrase in 1796 was a very limited one but, even at that early date, it implied a guarantee of protection from certain health hazards to all citizens, regardless of economic or social status. In this sense, it diverged from the ancient view that health care should be provided by government—as a charity, not as a right—only to the indigent. The question of what level of government should concern itself with the right to health entered the debate from the first. And although the question, like the concept, has evolved down the years, it has not been fully resolved even in our own time.

For well over a century, the meaning of right to health had to do with the health of the millions, not of individual. In the 1870's, leaders of organized medicine specifically excluded curative medicine—treatment of the individual—from their definition of the phrase, leaving preventive medicine, as applied to whole communities and populations, to government. There was no quarrel between government and the then relatively young American Medical Association at the time.

Right to health began to assume a much more comprehensive meaning shortly after the turn of the century and the AMA at first went along. But then came reaction.

Since World War One, and especially since the New Deal, the federal government has intermittently broadened its definition of right to health while the AMA has clung to a conservative view of the matter. But there can be no doubt that when Roosevelt used the phrase ("the right to adequate medical care and the opportunity to achieve and enjoy good health"), he was equating it with the most fundamental social and political rights, guaranteed to every citizen. And while the American electorate has never directly expressed its view of the matter, the broadened definition has almost certainly carried the day. Very few elected officials would, at present, be so rash as to declare publicly for the definition of the eighteen seventies. Right to health in today's usage refers to the health of the individual as well as to that of the millions; to curative as well as to preventive medicine.

Virtually by common agreement, the right to health question is about to become a national political issue of major proportions. Linked as it is with the recognition of a national health crisis, no federal administration, conservative or liberal, can evade the moment of truth that is at hand. Neither can the AMA.

The legislation that actually results will unquestionably be massively influenced by many precedents, some of which are already visible in existing laws but many of which have been largely forgotten.

The paper that follows attempts to display most of those precedents, more or less chronologically, and to put them into some sort of context. It is necessarily a wide-ranging chronicle since it involves some of the most fundamental of American political developments and much of the policy-making activity of the AMA. It ends with the dilemmas faced both by the Nixon Administration, and by the present leadership of the AMA.

Parts of the story have been told before but never in continuous form. The AMA's progressive era has been depicted but its origins and effects seem to have been somewhat slighted. So has the very slow process by which the federal government—all three branches—has laid the groundwork for comprehensive federal health legislation, yet to be achieved. In sum, the present account is part, but only a part, of the background needed by medical and lay observers to comprehend the shape of the battlelines now being formed.

Government and Health, 1796 to 1846

When the United States began life as a nation, most of the states already had in force a considerable body of health legislation. Several of the original colonies had acknowledged the obligation of the community to care for the indigent sick; Rhode Island did so as early as 1662 and Connecticut in 1673.[3] Where the total population was concerned—rich or poor—the only health measures passed by the colonies had to do with quarantine. Massachusetts passed a quarantine law (against yellow fever) in 1647 and repealed it two years later when the threat had passed.[4] New York City enacted a quarantine ordinance in 1755 specifying Bedloe's Island as the quarantine site. The Carolinas and Georgia passed similar laws, also in the mid-eighteenth century.[5]

The menace of summer epidemics of yellow fever plagued the new nation as much as it had the colonies. But the Constitution made no mention of health and Congress found no authority to act in the field of health until it was forced to do so by a crisis precipitated by a new yellow fever epidemic. Virtually by default, it turned to the Commerce Clause (Article I, Section

8),* the inference being that if state quarantine laws interfered with interstate and foreign commerce, federal authority was superior to that of the states. But the right to promulgate quarantine laws belonged to the states.

The precedent was a far-reaching one. For decades it had the effect of denying authority to the federal government in health matters, even those relating to quarantine. It was the continuing threat of yellow fever that finally broke the impasse.

Early Federal Health Laws

On 11 September 1793 the *Gazette of the United States* reported on one of its inner pages that "Yesterday, the President of the United States left town [Philadelphia], on a visit to Mount Vernon."[6] For good reason, the *Gazette* did not tell the whole story. The President was actually fleeing a stricken city as almost his entire cabinet had done earlier. Yellow fever, which had appeared in Philadelphia in July, had paralyzed the city and a week after it reported the President's departure, the *Gazette* itself suspended publication until 11 December. The epidemic, which was at its height when Washington headed south, took 4044 lives before it was brought to a halt by cold weather. The President attempted to keep vital government business going from Mount Vernon, but for practical purposes the new nation had no government until the epidemic had run its course. Sensing the great danger in such a hiatus, Washington wrote to the Attorney General and other cabinet members from Mount Vernon to ascertain whether or not he possessed the power to convene Congress elsewhere if epidemics threatened.[7] Since opinions on the matter differed, he asked Congress early in 1794 for the authority to call meetings outside the Capital, if ". . . the prevalence of contagious sickness, or the existence of other circumstances [would] . . . be hazardous to the lives and health of the members. . . ."[8] An Act to this effect was approved on 3 April 1794.[9] On the surface, Congress appears by its action to have been concerned primarily with its own right to health rather than with that of the citizens of the new Nation.

*"To regulate Commerce with foreign Nations, and among the several States, and with the Indian Tribes."

But the move was a pragmatic one, initiated by an anxious chief executive and designed to keep the Nation's government intact at a critical moment. Beyond this, it had no political or philosophic implications.

The severity of the epidemics of 1793 and 1794, and the paralysis they produced in the new nation's commercial life, were not soon to be forgotten. Congress might move its meetings to locations that were not threatened but the country's great seaports were fixed and the populace itself was less mobile than the Congress. Since nothing was known about the nature or mode of transmission of yellow fever except that it was introduced by ships coming from other countries, the resort was to control by quarantine. The inference of proponents of a national quarantine law was that the national government could administer quarantine action more effectively than the individual states. In the spring of 1796, a quarantine bill was introduced by Representative S. Smith of Maryland, requiring federal revenue officers to assist ". . . in the execution of the health laws of the states . . . in such manner as may . . . appear necessary."[10] But very significantly, the proposal gave the President the power to prescribe the conditions of quarantine, a feature that stimulated lively and fundamental debate in Congress. The debate, which went on for two days, centered primarily on questions relating to state and federal authority, a singularly sensitive issue at the time. The limits and extent of federal authority in general were very much in question, and Hamilton's federalist views were strongly contested by the opponents of strong central government headed up by Jefferson.

In the House debate on the quarantine proposal, seventeen representatives from ten states took part. The principle of national, as opposed to state, quarantine was fought most strongly by representatives from Pennsylvania, New York, and Massachusetts, all of which had their own quarantine laws. Southern representatives favored the proposal on the ground that epidemics affect the whole country and ". . . not only embarrass the commerce but injure the revenues of the United States." Representatives from Connecticut and Rhode Island (which had no quarantine laws) agreed.

Only one Representative seems to

have been concerned as much with the health issue as with the question of state versus federal authority. He was William Lyman, of Massachusetts.* Although opposed to giving quarantine authority to the national government Lyman, a staunch Jeffersonian and antifederalist, acknowledged that government at some level may assume an obligation to protect its citizens from epidemic disease. "*The right to the preservation of health,*" said Lyman, "*is inalienable.*"[12] (Italics ours.)

This was the first mention of the right to health in Congress and the meaning inferred by Lyman was a limited one. But the question of protecting the public's health was overwhelmed by the battle over the authority of the states versus that of the Congress and the antifederalists carried the day. The quarantine measure was voted into law shorn of its provisions that were designed to give the federal government more than a permissive role in the matter of quarantine.[13] Within a few years both New York and Philadelphia, whose Representatives had opposed the first national quarantine proposal, asked Congress for a strong national quarantine law but no action was taken owing to the fact that "Congress now had a precedent to worship."[14] It was, with regard to quarantine, a precedent that would remain largely intact for nearly a century.

Three years later (1799) the Fifth Congress revised the quarantine law of 1796, strengthening the hand of federal authority to a very small degree.[15] By that time, however, all moves to strengthen the central government had come under suspicion as the federalist era neared its end. The oppressive Aliens and Sedition Laws of the previous year[16, 17] had raised the specter of oligarchy and tyranny; and Thomas Jefferson (along with Madison) had, in cold fury, responded by secretly authoring the Kentucky Resolution (later adopted also by Virginia) with its extreme emphasis on States' Rights. Partly as a result, basic quarantine authority came to be even more firmly fixed in the hands of the states, a position that

*Lyman, born at Northampton in 1755, served in the House from 1793 to 1797. He belonged to the most radical wing of the Jeffersonian Party and was later rewarded by Jefferson with a Consulship in London. He died in England in 1811 and is interred at Gloucester Cathedral.[11]

was subsequently upheld by Chief Justice John Marshall.

The occasion was the famous *Gibbons vs Ogden* decision which was precipitated when New York State awarded a steamboat monopoly on its navigable streams to Robert Fulton and Robert Livingston. The issue was one of interstate commerce but the question of quarantine authority was brought into the argument by analogy. In his decision, Marshall denied that quarantine (inspection) laws derive from the right to regulate commerce:

That inspection laws may have a remote and considerable influence on commerce will not be denied; but that a power to regulate commerce is the source from which the right to pass them is derived, cannot be admitted. . . . They form a portion of that immense mass of legislation, which embraces everything within the territory of a State, not surrendered to the general government. . . . Inspection laws, quarantine laws, health laws of every description . . . are component parts of this mass. No direct general power over these objects is granted to Congress; and consequently they remain subject to State legislation. If the legislative power of the Union can reach them, it must be for national purposes.[18]

Although somewhat ambiguous, Marshall's opinion stood virtually unchallenged for decades. It recognized an obligation at the level of state government to protect the health of the public but made it clear that where quarantine laws ". . . might interfere with . . . the laws of the United States made for the regulation of Commerce. . . . , the Congress may control the State laws. . . ." The decision went a long way toward consolidating federal control on interstate and foreign commerce but it clearly confirmed the precedent of the 1796 quarantine law in that it assigned basic quarantine authority to the states.

But an earlier Congress had already acknowledged a degree of federal obligation in protecting the Nation's health. In an action which has been surprisingly neglected by historians, Congress had, in 1813, rejected the view that health matters belong solely in the hands of the states and acknowledged some degree of obligation at the federal level to guarantee the citizen's right to health. The law was one that required the federal government to

guarantee the efficacy of cowpox vaccine and to distribute it, free of charge, to anyone requesting it. Cowpox vaccination had been introduced into the United States by Benjamin Waterhouse, Professor of the Theory and Practice of Physick at Harvard, in 1800. Waterhouse sought the patronage of Thomas Jefferson by sending him a copy of his pamphlet on the subject later the same year and Jefferson responded, expressing great interest, in a letter written on Christmas Day.[19] Once Jefferson's interest was aroused, he pursued the problem of obtaining a potent and safe vaccine with characteristic thoroughness and was instrumental, in the first decade of the nineteenth century, in making effective vaccine available to the country's major population centers.

State government had entered the effort three years earlier when the Commonwealth of Massachusetts required "towns, districts, and plantations," to choose three or more suitable persons to superintend inoculation of Massachusetts residents.[20] But the problem of obtaining an effective vaccine was (and sometimes still is) a difficult one. Partly at Jefferson's urging, the Twelfth Congress passed a law (27 February 1813) requiring the President to appoint an agent ". . . to preserve the genuine vaccine matter, and to furnish the same [free of charge] to *any citizen* of the United States."[21] (Italics ours.) It was, in effect, a reversal of Jefferson's antifederalist stand and suggests that, where health was concerned, he was willing to modify his customary views.

The vaccination law, in principle, went a good deal further than earlier quarantine legislation and came close to demonstrating a positive across-theboard concern for the health of all American citizens up to and including the supply of the necessary biologic agent at federal expense. The law was apparently enacted with little or no opposition and remained in force for nine years. It might have remained permanently on the books had not a federal vaccine agent sent a batch of smallpox (instead of cowpox) vaccine to North Carolina with dire results. As a result, the House set up a Select Committee to inquire into the matter and the conclusion was that the 1813 law should be repealed. The Committee doubted

... that Congress can, in any instance, devise a system which will not be more liable to abuses in its operation, and less subject to a prompt and salutary control, than such as may be adopted by local authorities.[22]

Congress repealed the law of 1813 on 4 May 1822,[23] the honorable members having obviously been moved more by the outcry from North Carolina than by their concern for constitutional principles. But unlike quarantine legislation, a relatively passive exercise of police power, the 1813 act had reached out to the individual citizen by offering him guaranteed vaccine if he applied for it. In this sense, it was a precedent of considerable importance. And although the vaccination law was finally repealed on the ground that it constituted federal intrusion on the states' prerogatives, it was never actually challenged on that ground.

Subsequent decades saw a decline in federal interest in health legislation except for measures that were concerned with special groups including the military and various wards of the government. The quarantine system continued virtually unchanged except for a minor procedural alteration enacted in 1832 (for one year only).[24] The system was not, judging from the record, effective against yellow fever which continued to afflict the Nation's seaport areas, often in epidemic proportions, almost every year.[25]

But the health of the Nation was, by existing standards, undoubtedly good. As its territory expanded (it doubled between 1790 and 1840), and as the center of population shifted from just east of Baltimore (in 1790) to the vicinity of Clarksburg, West Virginia (1840), food supply and distribution improved rapidly.[26] Except in a few large cities, overcrowding was no problem. Under the circumstances government, both federal and state, felt little need to consider health legislation.

Organized Medicine and Government, 1846 to 1910

The medical profession to this time, having no national organization, found itself at a disadvantage where health matters of national significance were concerned. The impetus for a national medical organization came from the New York State Medical Society which organized a convention of delegates from medical societies and schools primarily to discuss means of improving medical education. The convention met in New York in 1846 and laid the groundwork for the formal founding of the American Medical Association the next year in Philadelphia.[27] The founding resolution listed the Asosciation's purposes as "... cultivating and advancing medical knowledge ..., elevating the standard of medical education, ..., promoting the usefulness, honour, and interests of the Medical Profession ... [etc.]."[28, 29] Speaking at the Association's first annual meeting, held in Baltimore in 1848, its first president introduced another theme. The profession, said Nathaniel Chapman of Philadelphia, had fallen to a low state and should, through the Association, cleanse itself. But, he added, "we do not want, nor will condescend to accept of any extraneous assistance."[30] Chapman's emphasis on the profession's territorial rights struck a responsive chord; the emphasis remains to this day, although the boundaries of the profession's exclusive territory have been repeatedly redefined.

The new organization devoted its attention at first to medical ethics, education and scientific matters; but, in its first year, it urged Congress to pass a law concerning adultered drugs and medicines[31] Congress quickly obliged.[32] In 1849, however, the Association set up numerous committees (Hygiene and Sanitation, Vital Statistics, and others), and also sought to protect the public, within the limits of its power, from quacks and nostrums. Its concern for the public good became apparent very early through these and other actions; but it as yet lacked the strength and status to influence legislation very effectively. As late as 1901, the AMA had, in the words of its president for that year (Charles Reed) "... exerted relatively little influence on legislation, either state or national ..." during its first fifty years.[33]

In the first decade of its life, the new association seems to have attracted relatively little attention in the press. The New York Times first mentioned it on 6 May 1858 and next day, poked fun at it ("a little business and a large row") because of a ruckus at its annual meeting over the seating of a delegate.[34, 35]

The Times continued thereafter to report its meetings more or less favorably but on 9 June 1882 a Times editorial writer delivered a blast against the Association. The occasion was the ejection of the New York State Medical Society for not conforming to the AMA's ban on consulting with homeopaths. The AMA, said the Times, had in this action "... displayed ... an amount of bigotry and stupidity which is to the last degree discreditable to them. ..."[36] The Times was also critical of the poor quality of the papers read at AMA meetings (only 20 per cent worthwhile) but, in general, press comment was either noncommittal or favorable.

The Association quite early recognized the need for a federal department of health and for federal legislation in support of adequate vital statistics. In the seventies and eighties, it was pressing at the state level for adequate licensure laws and, in the last quarter of the century, for the establishment of state boards of health. In this noble endeavor, the Association was, in effect, stressing the obligation, as well as the power, of local and state government to guarantee the implied right of all citizens to protection from public health hazards. But the policy was still thoroughly in accord with Congressman Lyman's eighteenth century concept of the right to health.

The first suggestion that the Association should be better informed about federal actions in health affairs came in 1867 when one of the founders, Dr. Nathan Smith Davis, moved that the annual meeting be held on alternate years in Washington.[37] The motion passed and the 1870 session was held in the capital; but meetings on alternate years proved to be impracticable. A section on State Medicine and Hygiene was created in 1872 and a definition of state medicine was composed for the first time. It ran:

... State Medicine consists in the application of medical knowledge and skill to the benefit of communities, which is obviously a very different thing from their application to the benefit of individuals in private or curative medicine.[38]

A similar view was put forward in 1878 by the Association's in-coming president, Dr. T. G. Richardson of New Orleans, who told the members that public hygiene was the "... prevention or arrest of all diseases which are not in their nature strictly limited to the individual . . . but which have a tendency to spread throughout . . . communities and which cannot otherwise be controlled. . . ."[39]

These semi-official definitions may be taken as the beginning of conflict between the AMA and government; but at the time they were put forward, the AMA was actually ahead of the national government in its attitude toward the right to health. Yet in defining public and private health as they did, the Association's leaders were drawing a very fine line, one which was even then rapidly becoming blurred.

At the state level, Massachusetts had (in 1850) taken a significant action when it set up a Sanitary Commission to inquire into conditions affecting the public's health in the Bay State. The result was a memorable report written largely by Lemuel Shattuck, a statistician.[40] In the report, Shattuck firmly points to the need for control of the public's health by "public authority and public administration." He thought the state should protect the citizen ". . . from injury from any influences connected with his locality, his dwelling house, his occupation, or those of his associates or neighbors; or from any other social causes." His emphasis was obviously on the prevention of disease rather than on curative medicine (". . . measures for prevention will affect infinitely more, than remedies for the cure of disease."). But there is an unmistakable inference in his comments that the individual citizen has the *right* to be protected by government from identifiable health hazards.

Shattuck's recommendations led to the establishment of the Massachusetts Board of Health (1869) but apparently had little immediate effect on Federal legislation. Congress did, however, move a year later to give the Marine Hospital Service coherent structure. To that time, the Service had been concerned solely with the health of merchant seamen and was badly organized even for that limited purpose. It now began to take shape as a health unit of more general purpose. The Act of 29 June, 1870 put the Servce under the Treasury Department and authorized the appointment of a Supervising Surgeon at $2,000 a year.[41] Viewed at the

time as a necessary but routine administrative action, it was to assume much greater significance after the turn of the century.

The National Board of Health

Eighteen seventy-eight was a major turning point in federal attitudes toward the government's obligation to protect the health of the Nation and, once again, it was a massive epidemic of yellow fever that produced the change. An epidemic of the disease had been reported in Rio de Janeiro in April[42] and by mid-summer had reached New Orleans. By late August the city was paralyzed and the disease had made its appearance in cities well upriver from New Orleans. Credence was given in retrospect to an earlier prediction by a black voodoo sorcerer that a plague would strike New Orleans in the summer of 1878 and that it would not begin to subside until the daily death toll equalled the degrees of the thermometer.[43] He turned out to be approximately, if not exactly, correct. By December, the epidemic had taken an estimated total of 30,000 lives in the Mississippi Valley and, well before it had run its course, the country was in an uproar. While the disease was still localized in the New Orleans area, Congress passed an inoffensive quarantine measure requiring U.S. Consuls at foreign posts to report epidemics of contagious disease to the Marine Hospital Service on a regular basis. The new law also authorized the Service to make new rules and regulations on quarantine as appropriate provided that ". . . such rules and regulations shall not conflict with or impair any sanitary or quarantine laws or regulations of any State or municipal authority. . . ."[44]

The action was much too weak to influence the catastrophe that was so soon to break and events during the epidemic showed with abundant clarity that local quarantine laws were inadequate in time of crisis.[25] The epidemic ran its natural course largely uninfluenced by quarantine measures, local or federal.

The subsidence of the epidemic in November 1878 brought with it vigorous debate conerning the best means of excluding the disease from the United States. The American Public Health Association, meeting in Richmond, Va., called for effective

quarantine measures and assigned responsibility for it to the "General Government."[45] The AMA had earlier passed several resolutions to the same effect.[46] In December, 1878, both houses of Congress set up special committees to investigate ways and means of controlling epidemics of all types of contagious disease and the Senate's Select Committee, reporting on 7 February 1879, made a number of recommendations mostly aimed at centralization of quarantine authority; one proposal was the creation of a National Board of Health.[47]

There ensued several weeks of contest and conflict within the federal government,[48] the net effect of which was the hasty passage of a law on 3 March setting up a National Board which was charged, among other things, with ". . . *obtaining information upon all matters affecting the public health.* . . ."[49]

The Board was organized on 2 April and included in its membership some of the most able medical men in the country; John Shaw Billings, Henry I. Bowditch, and Samuel Bemiss were among them. The Board was reluctant to accept responsibility for administering national quarantine laws until it had the benefit of epidemiologic research on yellow fever, but despite this, Congress gave it rather vaguely defined authority over quarantine in a law passed on 2 June.[50] It was hotly debated in the House.[51] Representative Jonas H. McGowan of Michigan (who had introduced the Bill setting up the National Board) derived federal authority over quarantine squarely from the Commerce clause of the constitution, a view that was contested by many other members. Representative Van H. Manning of Mississippi sought to settle the conflict by resort to semantics: he noted that the word commerce meant much more than exchange of merchandise and must include other types of interstate and international relations as well. Most southerners, however, opposed the proposal on the grounds of states' rights and Representative Omar D. Conger of Michigan finally lost patience:

Show me a southern States-rights democrat on this floor . . . and I will show you the man whose conscience has been relieved from all obligations as a States-rights man if he had a harbor to build within his district, or a river to deepen and improve.[51]

But the bill, which was to run for four years, passed despite the foes of centralization. The Nation thus, in time of crisis, acquired its first national health authority which, although badly designed and in difficulty from the start, was the closest Congress has ever come to sanctioning a Ministry of Health. The Board was charged with redesigning and implementing the Nation's quarantine system and, ostensibly, it had the legal authority to do so. But in Billings' words, "the only powers possessed by the National Board lay . . . in the character and reputation of its members and the probability that their advice would be received with respect by local organizations." [52] Its authority to initiate a research program was, however, much clearer. It was authorized to spend $500,000 as grants-in-aid for the purpose and it allocated a portion of the sum to nonfederal scientists working in private laboratories.

It was, in fact, the federal government's first move to support biomedical research *pro bono publico* and, as it turned out, the Board's sponsorship of extramural research was its most successful activity.* It funded a large number of epidemiologic and laboratory studies, some of them quite sophisticated for the time, during the four years of its existence. [48] Among its grantees were Ira Remsen of Johns Hopkins, P. C. Chandler of Columbia, James Low of Cornell, and George Sternberg of the U.S. Army.

The Board's chief problems arose in connection with the charge to design and implement a new national quarantine system. The effort to do so quickly brought it into conflict with the state health authorities (especially in Louisiana), officials of the Marine Hospital Service, and the Treasury Department. Probably its most implacable enemy was the Marine Hospital Service which saw itself being displaced by the National Board. The Board was commended for its sponsorship of research by the National Academy of Science but by 1882 its demise was a foregone

conclusion. [53] It ceased to meet in 1884 when the law that created it expired.

The National Board episode was an important but unsuccessful step toward consolidation of quarantine authority in federal hands. Probably a good deal more important was its demonstration to Congress of the value of research in the public interest. But the consensus in later years was that it was well ahead of its time and too hastily conceived to be viable.

Objections to a national quarantine authority were, however, unmistakably subsiding and an effective national quarantine law, giving appropriate authority to the Marine Hospital Service, was finally passed in 1893. [54] A Supreme Court decision handed down six years earlier had virtually invited the action. The Court at that time had said:

> But it may be conceded that whenever Congress shall undertake to provide for the commercial cities of the United States a general system of quarantine, or shall confide the execution . . . of such a system to a national board of health . . . all state laws on the subject will be abrogated, at least so far as the two are inconsistent. [55]

It was, in Faulkner's words, the beginning of the decline of *laissez-faire,* a process which he dates to the Interstate Commerce Act of 1887. [56] But, in fact, the process may be viewed as having begun much earlier when Congress made its first timid moves to establish national authority over quarantine, attempting unsuccessfully to separate the right to protection from epidemic disease from the right to free enterprise in economic affairs.

In later years, the U.S. Public Health Service, successor to the Marine Hospital Service, became the federal government's health arm, but in health matters other than quarantine, it was forced by weak federal legislation to carry on its work more by diplomacy and tact than by legal authority. The precedent of the 1796 quarantine law, backed up by the Supreme Court decision of 1824, still applied in many respects at the turn of the century.

The American Medical Association had, unofficially but effectively, gone further. It had distinguished between the public's health and private health; government at all levels could only be concerned with the public's health—

the health of the millions—and not with private health—the health of the individual. The distinction also involved another line of cleavage: preventive versus curative medicine. Preventive medicine was public; curative medicine was private with few exceptions.

The turn of the century saw the passing, for the most part, of huge epidemics of infectious disease. A federal health research arm was reestablished in 1887 with the founding of the Hygienic Laboratory within the Marine Hospital Service, and funds for a building were appropriated in 1901. [57] On 14 August 1912 an act of Congress completed the conversion of the Marine Hospital Service to the U.S. Public Health Service and specified that the Service should ". . . *study and investigate* the diseases of man and conditions influencing the propagation and spread thereof. . . ." [58] (Italics ours.) As in the case of the National Board Act of 1879, the research provision of the action taken in 1912 was clearly a pragmatic one in the minds of federal legislators: research was one means— and a politically inert one at that—by which the national government could guarantee the citizen's right to protection from disease.

Reform and Reorganization
The Age of Reform, by Hofstadter's definition [59] ran from 1890 to 1920, his reference being primarily to reform in economic affairs. It brought federal action limiting *laissez-faire* and monopolistic practices in business, the individual income tax, and other legislation all of which had the effect of strengthening the central government. But federal action in the health field was unimpressive. There was continued agitation for a National Department of Health which came to naught despite the recommendations of several presidents and the continuing support of the AMA. The Pure Food and Drugs law [60] was finally passed in 1906 owing, in considerable measure, to active support by the AMA. The Association continued the battle when the 1906 law proved to be inadequate and was instrumental in inducing Congress to pass the Sherley Amendment in 1912. [61]

But for some time prior to the turn of the century, AMA leaders had realized

---

*The practice of awarding research grants to private individuals working in nonfederal institutions was reinstated briefly during World War I. In 1937 it was incorporated in the National Cancer Act and, from 1948 onward, formed a major feature of the vastly expanded activities of the National Institutes of Health.

that the structure of the organization was too loose and clumsy to permit it to act effectively in the formation of policy. Under its old general assembly system, it was difficult to reach convincing agreement, especially on controversial matters, and concerted political action was well-nigh impossible. A few years after its founding it had disclaimed unofficial statements of AMA views,[62] but it lacked an efficient mechanism for creating or proclaiming official policy. In 1901, a new system was adopted which vested policy-making authority in an all-powerful House of Delegates whose members were chosen by the governing bodies of constituent state medical societies, instead of by direct popular vote.[63] In adopting the procedure, the AMA may well have been following the constitutional precedent of placing the selection of U.S. Senators in the hands of state legislatures, a practice that was abolished in 1913 when the seventeenth amendment was ratified. And by this means, the AMA converted itself into a less representative but much more cohesive and politically effective organization. Under the old system, said an editorial at the time, ". . . prolonged discussion almost always meant defeat or postponement."[64] Under the new, power could be channeled and concentrated for specific purposes. The Association retains the House of Delegates' structure today. Delegates are, not unnaturally, chosen from the relatively small group of physicians, usually conservative, who have shown a sustained and active interest in medical politics.

The power structure in the AMA came, in succeeding decades, to be misunderstood within and without the Association. In practice, editorials in the *Journal of the AMA* and statements by its officers are usually in line with official policy but no policy is binding unless it has been approved by the House of Delegates. At times, editorials and widely publicized comments by AMA officers seem to have been used as straws in the wind, like many so-called leaks within the federal government, that can be disowned if the response is unfavorable. But the one thing the Association cannot disown is an action of the House of Delegates.

Even the Board of Trustees, where policy is concerned, is subordinate; it is chosen by—and responsible to—the House of Delegates.

By 1910 the Association had sought to increase its influence on health legislation by the creation of special committees, bureaus, and councils to deal with the topic. Beginning much earlier, it had undertaken to improve and standardize medical education. Probably its most effective move in this direction was the creation of a permanent Council on Medical Education (1904). The Council laid the groundwork and set the stage for a joint effort with the Carnegie Foundation, beginning in 1908. The result was the Flexner Report of 1910; but the basic work, without which the Flexner Report would have had little or no effect, was done by the AMA's Council.

With so much good work to its credit, the Association acquired an unchallengeable reputation in the minds of laymen and legislators alike. It seldom came under public attack, except from dissident health groups; and in the public eye, more prominently than the federal government, it was the primary protector of the public's health.

Health Insurance and the Genesis of Conflict, 1908–1932

On the national scene, economic reform and federal legislation designed to check monopolistic practices, along with demands for better conditions for the worker, were becoming daily news items. Emerging labor unions very early turned their attention to industrial safety and to compensation insurance, and in this climate, European social and health insurance schemes began to come under national scrutiny.

Except for active interest in the prevention of industrial accidents, the AMA at first showed little interest in such matters. But between 1902 and 1914, eighteen states passed workmen's compensation laws. In 1908, the Russell Sage Foundation financed a study of European social and health insurance systems and the resulting report, published in 1910,[65] aroused the interest of a great many liberal groups in this country. The *Journal of the AMA*, at the time, published no original comments on health insurance, but from 1905 on it abstracted many articles from foreign journals on the topic.

It was the passage of the National Health Insurance Act in Britain toward the end of 1911* that stimulated the *Journal*'s first editorial on health insurance. The editorial said, in part:

. . . this law marks the beginning of the end of the old system of the individual practice of medicine, and of the old relationship between patient and physician. . . ."[66]

The developments in Britain were reported sketchily in the American press but the medical profession received detailed coverage in the *Journal of the AMA* beginning in early 1911.† The British Medical Association (BMA) had, by mid-1911, begun a campaign that was sometimes in total opposition, sometimes in favor of modifications that seemed to be designed basically to protect the physician's income and autonomy. Ultimately, the controversy split British physicians into two camps, both in effect opposed to the national health insurance bill as it had been introduced. A threat by the BMA to refuse service under the new law could not, in the end, be enforced, and after obtaining certain concessions from the government, the BMA reluctantly went along. The final result was damage to public confidence in the BMA itself, and a legislative compromise providing inadequate coverage to wage-earners and excluding their families altogether.

In the United States, the right to health concept was unquestionably coming to be defined more broadly. One of the most vocal proponents of the concept was the American Section of the International Association for Labor Legislation, organized in 1906, which espoused the health insurance cause about 1910.‡ In 1911 Louis Brandeis echoed the views of the country's Progressives§ when he told the Conference on Charities and Corrections that a comprehensive system of workingman's insurance was an "incentive to justice," and that govern-

*It went into force on 1 July 1912.
†In the form of *London Letters,* written by a correspondent. The first to deal with the British health insurance proposal appeared on 3 June 1911. There were about 30 of them over the next eighteen months.
‡The American Association held its first meeting in Madison, Wisconsin 30–31 December 1907 and was disbanded in 1942.
§Members of a political movement which was later to become Theodore Roosevelt's "Bull Moose" third party.

ment should not permit the existence of conditions that made large classes of citizens financially dependent. If it does, he continued, it should ". . . assume the burden incident to its own shortcoming."[67] The next year, the same organization called for insurance against accident, sickness, old age, and unemployment. And in the same year, Teddy Roosevelt's Progressive Party pledged itself to work increasingly for a ". . . system of social insurance [including health insurance] adapted to American use."[68]

Undoubtedly influenced by Brandeis, Woodrow Wilson lent impetus to the agitation for social legislation in his first inaugural address. Anticipating presidential health messages of the sixties, Wilson said:

There can be no equality of opportunity if men and women and children be not shielded in their lives, in their very vitality, from the consequences of great industrial and social processes which they cannot alter, control, or singly cope with. . . . The first duty of law is to keep sound the society it serves. Sanitary laws, pure food laws, and laws determining conditions of labor which individuals are powerless to determine for themselves are intimate parts of the very business of justice and legal efficiency. *We have not . . . studied and perfected the means safeguarding the health of the Nation, the health of its men and women and its children, as well as their rights in the struggle for existence.*[69] (Italics ours.)

Wilson seems, in all probability, to have had in mind a considerable expansion of the right to health concept and not to have been bound in his outlook by the rigid distinction between the public's health and private health. But his administration, so soon to be preoccupied by other matters, never followed the health issue up.

Health Insurance Viewed with Interest
The AMA seems to have taken no official notice of Wilson's reference to health, but in 1914 the *Journal* published an article favorable to health insurance by Dr. James P. Warbasse of Brooklyn, a surgeon and medical sociologist. Warbasse condemned commercialization in medicine and emphasized the need for preventive health care. "The socialization of medicine is coming," Warbasse declared, "and medical practice withholds itself from the field of science as long as it continues [to be] a competi-

tive business."[70] And less than six months later, the *Journal* carried an authoritative article on compulsory health insurance by Isaac Max Rubinow, M.D., then the Nation's leading authority on the subject, urging American physicians to react constructively to the matter (as British physicians had conspicuously failed to do in 1911).[71]

Two years earlier, the American Association for Labor Legislation had set up a Committee on Social Insurance (December, 1912) which included Rubinow in its membership. Within a few months two other physicians were added to the committee, one of whom was Dr. Alexander Lambert of New York.[72]

Rubinow and Lambert were later to join forces in temporarily converting the AMA to a position which, on balance, favored compulsory health insurance. Rubinow, born in Russia of Jewish parentage, had emigrated to the United States in 1893 at the age of 18. Within a remarkably short time he obtained the M.D. degree at New York University and was practicing in New York. An early interest in economics and social insurance grew to such proportions that he abandoned practice after a few years, and by 1913 he had published an authoritative book on social insurance.[73] In 1914 he received a Ph.D. degree from Columbia, and until he died in 1936, he worked actively in the fields of social insurance and health economics.

Lambert's background was in striking contrast to Rubinow's. Born in comfortable circumstances in New York, he graduated from Yale in 1884 and from the College of Physicians and Surgeons (Columbia) in 1888. A cardiologist by inclination, he was Professor of Clinical Medicine at Cornell for thirty-three years, and was Teddy Roosevelt's personal physician, hunting companion, and confidant. He was also very active in AMA politics, serving (between 1904 and 1920) in some of its most important offices including the presidency. Lambert, a staunch Progressive politically,* became interested in health insurance early in his career and in late 1916 delivered an address entitled

*The leadership of the Progressive Party, as studied by Chandler,[74] was upper middle class. Most had earlier been Republicans and most were businessmen, lawyers, editors, or university professors, in that order. Very few were physicians.

Medical Organization Under Health Insurance before a joint session of the American Sociologic Society, the American Association for Labor Legislation, and other liberal groups. The address left no doubt as to where he stood on the health insurance issue, and in comments on the presentation Dr. Frank Billings of Chicago unmistakably identified himself as a supporter of Lambert's views.[75] Billings, having served as President of the AMA in 1903, was one of the most prominent physicians and medical academicians of the day. His reputation was unassailable, and his support was very meaningful especially within the ranks of the AMA membership. But his comments got him into an embarrassing position within the AMA a few years later.

In mid-1916 the Committee on Social Insurance of the Association for Labor Legislation, with Lambert and Rubinow participating, had produced a Model Health Insurance Bill, an activity to which the AMA lent its counsel.[76]

In its opening sentence, the model bill rejected the term "sickness insurance" in favor of *health insurance*, ". . . because it calls attention to the main object of the act, the conservation of health. . . ." The bill proposed that the cost of insurance be distributed on a sliding scale between employer, employee, and the state, with special provision for employees in unusually low income brackets. Benefits included medical and nursing care (in- and out-patient), medical and surgical supplies for a limited time, cash payments during illness for up to 26 weeks, maternity benefits, and burial coverage. Participation was compulsory with certain exceptions. Carriers were to be mutual associations supervised by the state. No federal involvement was proposed.*[77]

*The signal importance of the model bill seems to have been largely forgotten in our own time. Drafted with great care, it avoided some of the defects of European systems and has influenced planners, directly or indirectly, ever since. Neither federal nor state government was involved in its preparation. It was introduced into the New York legislature with Governor Al Smith's endorsement; it passed the Senate but was defeated in the House. Commissions to study the proposal were set up in California, Illinois, New Jersey, Ohio, Pennsylvania, Wisconsin and others. Some reports were favorable but no legislation resulted.

The AMA's Progressive Era

To 1915, the AMA had, through its *Journal,* shown only modest interest in the changing social and political climate. But in that year, Alexander Lambert, then chairman of the Association's powerful Judicial Council, addressed the House of Delegates on the subject of health insurance. His report was a detailed account of European health insurance systems, setting them out in a very favorable light; and the House was sufficiently impressed to direct, through a reference committee, that the report be brought by state medical societies to the attention of the rank and file.[78]

A few months later, the *Journal* took favorable notice of the Model Health Insurance Bill of the American Association for Labor Legislation. All American physicians should study the bill carefully, said the *Journal,* its inference being that better health insurance legislation might result if they did so.[79] Early in 1916, a *Journal* editorial, noting the introduction of the model bill into the Massachusetts and New York legislatures, said that the move ". . . marks the inauguration of a great movement which ought to result in an improvement in the health of the industrial population and improve the conditions for medical service among the wage earners."[80]

It is difficult today to believe that such sentiments could ever have appeared in the *Journal of the AMA,* long noted for its ultraconservative views in support of *laissez-faire* medical care. But in late 1915 and early 1916, the *Journal* undoubtedly was reflecting the views of the AMA's leadership. To this point, however, the Association had, except for participating in construction of the model bill, taken no action. It now moved, partly at the suggestion of the Association for Labor Legislation but also at Lambert's urging, to set up its own Committee on Social Insurance. The AMA Board of Trustees, which approved the Committee in February 1916, instructed it ". . . to do everything in [its] power to secure such constructions of the proposed laws [on health insurance] as will work the most harmonious adjustment of the new sociologic relations between physicians and laymen which will necessarily result therefrom. . . ."[81] All of which leaves little doubt that the AMA leadership was convinced that some form of

compulsory health insurance, backed by government, was in the offing and could be made to serve a useful social purpose.

Lambert, asked to serve as chairman of the new committee, lost no time in taking action. By mid-1916 the Committee had set up offices in New York, conveniently near to those of the American Association for Labor Legislation, and had employed Rubinow as executive secretary. Rubinow energetically set to work writing, speaking, and travelling in support of health insurance. In April, 1916, he found time to testify in support of a health insurance proposal introduced into Congress by Meyer London,* Socialist representative from New York's east side.[83] In hearings before the House Labor Committee, Rubinow said that he was appearing at the request of the Socialist Party of America to which, he affirmed, he had belonged for twenty years. Later in the hearings he and Samuel Gompers traded verbal blows at some length. Toward the end of the exchange, Rubinow said ". . . most emphatically that in my official position as executive secretary of the social insurance committee of the American Medical Association I am authorized to state that [the AMA] is heartily in support of Mr. London's resolution, and . . . is committed to the general principle of social sickness insurance in this country."[84]

He was, in fact, too emphatic. His authorization most likely came from Lambert, and possibly from other AMA leaders. But it was not a position that had been approved by the House of Delegates. London's resolution was never officially backed or opposed by the AMA. Its defeat, which came in 1917, was due largely to opposition from the insurance industry and from organized labor. The vote was 189 yea, 138 nay, and 106 abstentions; but it needed a two-thirds majority to pass.[85] The affirmative vote was not negligible but the defeat of the resolution was a turning point of sorts. And about this time Ernst Freund, Professor of Law at Chicago, implied that the proponents of

*London, like Rubinow, was born in Russia (1871). He came to the United States in 1891 and served in the 64th, 65th and 66th Congresses representing the 12th New York District. Also like Rubinow, he was an active supporter of the American Association for Labor Legislation.[82]

health insurance might be pushing a bit too hard. He said that use of public funds to improve health was probably justified ". . . upon any reasonably liberal view of constitutional power," but that compulsory contributions by employers were vulnerable to attack in the courts. "Let the advocates of health insurance agree upon a minimum program and urge the adoption of that. The well-known expansive tendency of relief legislation may be relied upon to take care of the future."[86]

In May, 1917, Lambert and Rubinow produced a massive report for the House of Delegates spelling out the details of German experience with compulsory health insurance, and describing the transition in other countries from voluntary health insurance to schemes that were partly subsidized by the state and to compulsory insurance. It also condemned "blind opposition, indignant repudiation [and] bitter denunciation of [compulsory health insurance] laws." The House of Delegates, its mood now more cautious, instructed Lambert's Committee to continue its study and to make certain stipulations concerning the protection of the profession's interest.[87]

Counterreaction from the Rank and File

But the political mood of the country, now on the verge of declaring war on Germany, was rapidly moving counter to earlier progressive trends. And within the AMA, Lambert and Rubinow had reckoned without the grass roots. It seemed to have gone unnoticed that the medical profession, once a remarkably unified organization, had begun to develop two important factions. On one side stood men like Billings and Lambert whose education had gone beyond the minimal requirements for the M.D. degree, who had moved from general to specialty practice, and who were prominent in academic medicine and research. It was to such men that, prior to World War I, the leadership of the AMA was frequently entrusted. On the other side was the great body of general practitioners, men whose formal education was often limited, who usually had no connection with academic medicine, and whose long hours of exacting service, day in and day out, kept them relatively isolated from currents of social and professional change. The health insurance issue, combined with the rising tide of political reaction, brought them out of isolation.

Letters critical of Lambert and his committee, mostly moderate in tone, began to appear in the *Journal of the AMA* and in state medical journals early in 1917. But it was Eden V. Delphey, a New York general practitioner, who more than any other, converted moderate criticism to a holy war, and initiated a sharp and permanent swing to the right within organized medicine.*

In March 1917, Delphey wrote that the model health insurance bill, then before the New York legislature (and endorsed by the State Medical Society), would convert physicians into mere cogs in a huge political machine. In May, he addressed a letter to the editor of the *Journal of the AMA* condemning compulsory health insurance

. . . Because it is un-American. Americanism means that the individual amounts to something; paternalism, that the individual is nonimportant but that the state is all important. Even a beneficent paternalism is harmful because it destroys individualism and discourages thrift.

He went on to say that very few Americans were without adequate medical care, and that surveys indicating the contrary were worthless because they had been done by "medically unqualified and therefore incompetent persons." [88]

As it turned out, Delphey was obviously saying what a good many of the nation's physicians wanted to hear. Many of them, in retrospect, may have read or heard Lambert's reports in silence, possibly owing to the stature of the man who had produced them. But Delphey's move opened the floodgates of opposition.

From that point on, Lambert and colleagues fought a losing battle. Lambert himself went off to war, and by the time he returned health insurance of all kinds was discredited within the AMA. At its annual meeting in 1919, the House of Delegates heard a final plea for adequate and informed consideration of the health insurance issue, deliv-

*Eden Vinson Delphey (1858–1925) graduated from the Medical Department of Columbia College in 1889 and practiced at 171 W. 71st Street for many years.

ered by one of Lambert's colleagues. Lambert himself, now president-elect of the Association but still in Europe, sent a strong statement attacking his opposition and urging continuing study of compulsory health insurance. But it was to no avail; the receptive spirit of 1915 and 1916 was a thing of the past, and the House now created a stalemate in Lambert's small committee by adding outspoken conservatives to it. [89]

Even this was not enough for the conservative faction of the AMA. Thoroughly alarmed at any prospect of health insurance and determined to close the issue once and for all, conservatives contributed a steady stream of outspoken cricitism of Lambert's Committee to medical publications. Rubinow was singled out for increasingly vituperative attack. The Association for Labor Legislation, with which the AMA had maintained cordial rapport a scant four years earlier, was now characterized as a Bolshevist organization in disguise, and it was claimed that Rubinow had all along been acting secretly as an agent for the Labor Legislation group. [90] On this ground, in the midst of the postwar spy scare and anti-Bolshevist hysteria, Rubinow was summarily fired, the Committee's reports discredited and suppressed, and the Committee itself allowed to die. Its last report to the House of Delegates, given by Victor Vaughan in 1920, was brief and defensive. [91] Rubinow, undaunted, continued to battle for health insurance and exerted a considerable influence on the planners of New Deal social legislation. But the AMA never forgave him. It was in its Progressive Era when it hired him in 1916; it had taken the opposite tack by the time it fired him in 1919.*

Repudiation and Backlash

Meantime Delphey was still in full pursuit of the health insurance demon. Acting as Chairman of the New York

*Rubinow, chairing a session on health insurance at the Seventh National Conference on Social Security in 1934 said:

. . . I feel that I am called upon to give a word of caution, which may partly be explained by my own age. I don't look forward to waiting another thirty or forty years before these various research programs . . . culminate in a system. I can't help feeling a little bit depressed . . . by the fact that so much that has been said here this morning has been said . . . some twenty years ago. . . . [92]

Rubinow died in September, 1936.

State Medical Society's Committee on Compulsory Health Insurance, he wrote all state medical societies early in 1920, asking if they had instructed their delegates to the national House of Delegates on the health insurance issue. Subsequently he wrote all the delegates themselves, warning them against ". . . propaganda for a scheme which could but have a serious and destructive effect upon the most altruistic profession on earth. . . ." [93]

His efforts and those of the *Journal*, which published a series of articles by the new member of Lambert's committee condemning health insurance, bore fruit. By a series of maneuvers in the House of Delegates, opponents of health insurance obtained approval of the following in May, 1920:

Resolved: that the American Medical Association declares its opposition to the institution of any plan embodying the system of compulsory contributory insurance against illness, or any other plan of compulsory insurance against illness which provides for medical service to be rendered contributors or their dependents provided, controlled, or regulated by the federal government. [94]

The action, in effect, closed the door to any possibility of cooperation between organized medicine and the federal government where compulsory health insurance was concerned but made no specific mention of voluntary insurance. Involvement of local government was not specifically excluded, an omission that was soon to be set right.

The 1920 resolution against federally-sponsored health insurance was the basic dogma on which all future action in the field of health insurance was built. But the backlash within the AMA had not yet run its full course. The national climate that developed after World War I was producing some extraordinary social and political results. Congress passed a sequel to the Espionage Act of 1917, permitting wholesale deportation of aliens and forbidding reentry of many already deported. [95] New York State launched an investigation on "revolutionary radicalism" which culminated in the Lusk Report of 1920, recommending Americanization through education. [96] "Within a year after the armistice," said W. J. Ghent, in *The Reds Bring Reaction*, "we were in the midst of a tide of reaction which threatened to sweep away every social achievement gained during . . . the two previous decades. By that time or a bit later the whole fabric of social control had been rent and raveled."[97]

Delphey by now had able associates in carrying forward the repudiation of compulsory health insurance and anything else that threatened to bring medical practice under any sort of regulation. Prominent among them was E. H. Ochsner, a Chicago surgeon, who directed his attacks at health insurance, health centers, and Frank Billings. In 1919 Ochsner was among the many who attacked Lambert's committee and in 1920, writing in the Illinois Medical Journal, he had said:

The mental processes of some of our ultra highbrows are beyond comprehension. . . . Compulsory health insurance is but the entering wedge. If this gets by, the next will be old age pensions and the next unemployment pensions and finally . . . the last act in the tragedy of errors will be revolution, anarchy, and chaos. . . .[98]

A few months later, writing in the same journal, Ochsner disposed of health centers ("the same old baby with a new name and its feet cut off . . ."). Quoting Billings' published comments in favor of health insurance and health centers, he turned to the personal attack:

I wonder, gentlemen, whether we have not a right to conclude that this gentleman [Billings] is no longer a safe adviser for the American medical profession on matters of medical economics?[99]

He then went on to a number of other themes that were then new to professional debate. "When I was on the farm," he wrote, "we had occasionally to deal with skunks and rattlesnakes. . . . There is just one way to deal with a skunk or a rattlesnake and that is a good, dependable, reliable double-barrelled shotgun. I would no more temporize or compromise with any of the schemes so far proposed than I would . . . with a rattlesnake, a skunk, or a hyena. I would hit, shoot or kill them while they are still in embryo. . . ."

Ochsner seems to have carried his antipathy for Billings one step further. At the seventy-fourth annual meeting of the AMA, convened in Boston in 1921, an unsigned circular attacking Billings and quoting his earlier comments in favor of compulsory health insurance

was distributed to the members of the House of Delegates. Billings was required to defend himself and he did so by recanting.

I have declared [Billings said] in published articles that compulsory health insurance was not applicable to the United States and that I am opposed to it. . . .

The House, apparently somewhat embarrassed by it all, accepted Billings' defense and affirmed its confidence in him.[100] It also made a weak but unsuccessful effort to discover the perpetrator of the attacks on Billings. According to Morris Fishbein, editor of the Journal, it was probably Ochsner.[101]

In any event, nothing quite like the incident had ever been seen in the House and, although Billings survived the attack, its chief purpose was achieved: no one was likely to bring up health insurance again, except to condemn it, before the House. Lambert, who had served as President of the AMA in 1919–20, had already bowed out of the controversy; his presidential address dealt with various nonpolitical aspects of war medicine.[102]

The Final Action: State Medicine Again
The conservative wing of the AMA was now firmly in the saddle. And while the House of Delegates seems to have been unwilling to censure so eminent a person as Billings, the language and methods used by men like Ochsner and Delphey came to be acceptable provided they were directed against compulsory health insurance. The leadership was, in fact, still preoccupied with the threat of government intervention in health. The Shepherd-Towner Act (providing funds for maternal and child health) had become law[103] despite the Association's disapproval.[104] New legislation providing hospital benefits to veterans at government expense was being discussed. As a consequence, the official policy opposing federally backed health insurance that had been adopted in 1920 was viewed as inadequate to cover all possibilities. The question of state medicine again arose* and the old un-

*It had come up at the 1921 annual session. Delphey had introduced a resolution defining state medicine as ". . . the practice of medicine by the state by physicians on a salary to the exclusion of all other and individual practice of medicine."[105] His resolution, and several other similar ones, were buried in various committees.

official definition, describing State Medicine as public hygiene was, by action of 25 May 1922, superseded by the following:

The American Medical Association hereby declares its opposition to all forms of "state medicine" because of the ultimate harm that would come to the public weal through such form of medical practice.

"State Medicine" is . . . any form of medical treatment provided, conducted, controlled or subsidized by the federal or any state government, or municipality. . . .

The definition excepted the services provided by the Army, Navy, or Public Health Service and those needed in coping with communicable disease, mental illness, and the health of indigents. It also included a loophole in the form of reference to "such other services" as may be under the control of county medical societies provided that the appropriate state society did not disapprove.[106]

The action represented a curious inversion of the unofficial definition of 1871. At that time, state medicine had to do, in the eyes of the Association, mainly with control of communicable disease and the AMA approved of it. But in 1922, state medicine became medical treatment of nonindigent citizens provided by government at any level.

The official actions of 1920 and 1922, both in some sense historical accidents, were the foundation on which the organization built the image it still possesses today. The transformation of the AMA from a more or less flexible professional organization to a strongly partisan one, functioning as a cross between a medieval guild and a modern labor union, was completed within a remarkably short time. The Association largely ignored a chorus of external attacks as well as words of caution from a few of its own leaders. In 1923, incoming president Ray Lyman Wilbur* attempted to moderate the organiza-

*Ray Lyman Wilbur (1875–1949) was one of the most distinguished men of his time. He was an accomplished physician, President of Stanford from 1916 to 1943, Secretary of the Interior in Hoover's cabinet (1929–1933), President of the AMA in 1923–24 and President of the Association of American Medical Colleges in 1924.

tion's rigid new dogma in his inaugural address:

The social relationships of medicine are so intimate and imperative that they are bound to multiply and continue. We cannot stop them by calling them Bolshevik or socialistic or pro-German but we can guide them if we get away from the brake and begin to steer.[107]

But the members were by that time in no mood to listen to leaders with the instincts of statesmen. They subsequently sought and found leaders who were not afflicted with doubts as to the wisdom of the policies of the twenties and who followed them to the letter.

Social Security and After

Actions of the AMA since the twenties have had the effect of obscuring its record during its Progressive Era, and the events that led up to it. The tenacity with which AMA leaders have adhered to the policies of the twenties, despite criticism from without and within, has been remarkable indeed.

Even the Great Depression failed to shake the organization's faith in its post-war policies. Any form of interference from outside the profession—but especially from government—was to be condemned. Along these lines, W. G. Morgan, president of the AMA in 1930, lectured the members on paternalism: trade unions represented a sort of group paternalism, voluntary health insurance had its paternalistic aspects, and compulsory health insurance would allow the "paternalistic hand of the government" to throttle and degrade medical practice as it had in Germany and Britain. He also warned against nongovernmental paternalistic tendencies such as the mental hygiene movement.[108] In a similar vein was the AMA's official condemnation in 1932 of the majority report submitted by the Committee on the Costs of Medical Care, a prestigious body chaired by ex-president Wilbur and supported by eight major foundations.* The majority of the Committee's 48 members solidly supported the group practice concept and urged that ". . . the costs of medical care be placed on a group payment

*The Carnegie Corporation, the Josiah Macy, Jr. Foundation, the Milbank Memorial Fund, the New York Foundation, the Rockefeller Foundation, the Julius Rosenwald Fund, the Russell Sage Foundation, and the Twentieth Century Fund.

basis, through the use of insurance, through the use of taxation, or through the use of both these methods."[109] A powerful minority, which included a number of AMA conservatives, disagreed. Its report put the emphasis on "medical care furnished by the individual physician with the general practitioner in a central place," and on insurance schemes only when they can be kept under professional control. It opposed the ". . . adoption by medicine of the technique of big business, that is, mass production." Its first recommendation, drawing its substance from the policy of 1922, urged the discontinuance of government competition in the practice of medicine except in the special instances contained in the policy.

The AMA officially endorsed the minority view and a *Journal* editorial said that the majority was made up of "the forces representing the great foundations, public health officialdom, social theory—even socialism and communism—inciting to revolution."[110] The long-term effect of the decision and, of lesser importance, of the *Journal's* extravagant language is a matter of conjecture. But the decision, at the time and in retrospect, indicated clearly that AMA policy-makers found their policies so binding that they could not accept the conclusions of the nation's most able authorities in the health field.*

Things were no different when the federal government began to look into matters of health. When Franklin Roosevelt set up the Committee on Economic Security in 1934, the AMA thought that the Committee's Medical Advisory Subcommittee was not representative.[111] Even broadening the membership of the Subcommittee

*The Committee (17 practicing physicians and dentists, six public health authorities, six social scientists, ten representatives of health institutions, and nine members representing the public) could hardly have been more carefully chosen. Eight of the 15 practicing physicians, and one Ph.D., wrote the minority report. The two dentists also submitted a minority report. One social scientist submitted a critical personal statement and Edgar Sydenstricker (public health) declined to sign the final report because, in his view, it dealt inadequately with "the fundamental economic question which the Committee was formed . . . to consider." The majority report was supported by 35 of the 48 members.

failed to appease the Association although it moderated its critical tone as a result. But the possibility that the federal government might bring health insurance under study was enough to persuade AMA leaders that an emergency meeting of the House of Delegates was needed. The House convened in February 1935 and it found cause for alarm on several counts.[112] Most menacing was the content of the Wagner-Doughton Economic Security Bill which had been introduced on 17 January. Title IV of the bill called for a Social Insurance Board and one of its duties was to study and make recommendations as to ". . . legislation and matters of administrative policy concerning old-age insurance . . . , health insurance, and related subjects."[113]

That was bad enough. Only slightly less acceptable was the drafting of a second Model Bill by the American Association for Social Security. The proposal, made public on 5 January 1935, was a state measure and was to be introduced simultaneously into 43 state legislatures (it reached the New York Legislature on 25 January). It called for compulsory health insurance to be paid for by employers, employees, and state government. The employee's contribution varied from one to 3 per cent, according to the level of his income. The employer's payment went from 3½ per cent for employees making $20 or less a week, to 1½ per cent for those receiving $40 or more. The state was to put in 1½ per cent.[114] There was a suggestion that the federal government should put up 38 cents for each insured employee but the program was still to be administered by the individual states. To the House of Delegates, the Epstein Bill, named after the executive director of the organization that composed it, was unmitigated evil. The House of Delegates condemned it and reaffirmed its old stand against health insurance backed by government; but it yielded a little with regard to voluntary health insurance.

AMA opposition to Title IV of the Economic Security Bill following the special session of the House of Delegates was, under the circumstances, sufficient to dispose of it. A redraft of the proposal, submitted by Congressman Doughton in April, changed the name and purpose of the Board: it now became the Social Security Board and had no charge relating to health insurance.[115] The new draft passed the House with 372 yeas and 33 nays on 19 April.[116] It was signed into law on 14 August, 1935.[117]

The deletion represented a victory for the AMA* but the passage of the law led to a Supreme Court decision that politically and socially was more important than the law itself. When the law came under attack in 1937, Benjamin Cardozo, speaking for the Court in *Steward Machine Company vs. Davis,* quoted the general welfare clause of the Constitution† as the basis for upholding the law.[119] In a companion decision delivered the same day (*Helvering vs. Davis*), Cardozo, again speaking for the Court, said that the Federal Old Age Benefits provision (Title II) of the Social Security Law does not contravene the Tenth Amendment‡ and that Congress may spend money in aid of the general welfare. "Nor," said the Court, "is the concept of the general welfare static. What is critical or urgent changes with time. . . . When money is spent to promote the general welfare, the concept of welfare or the opposite is shaped by Congress, not the states."[120] The decision made no mention of health as such, but the inference with regard to it was clear: Congress might, whenever it was persuaded that the state of the country's general welfare required it, pass legislation guaranteeing the right to health and it might, also by inference, use federal tax funds for the purpose.

Meantime, the AMA was moving largely by improvisation as the occasion seemed to demand but always with the policies of the twenties in mind. In 1920 it had not actually condemned voluntary health insurance but its action left the impression that it might be undesirable. In a special session of the House of Delegates in 1938, the AMA dealt again with voluntary insurance

but said that it should be confined ". . . to provision of hospital facilities and should not include any type of medical care." Cash indemnity insurance for such purposes was, however, accepted. Under such policies, the insurance organization pays the patient according to rates specified in the policy; the patient, in turn, pays the physician who sets his own rates. No third party should come between the patient and his physician in the view of the House. Opposition to compulsory health insurance was reaffirmed.[121]

The AMA's intransigent stands had, meantime, not gone unnoticed in some segments of the nation's press. The *New York Times* had taken a dim view of its opposition to the Shepherd-Towner Act[122] and in 1929, a writer in *Forum* said the Association's primary interest was in the financial status of the physician.[123] In the thirties, Michael Rorty, among others, pounded away at the AMA's conservatism in traditionally liberal journals.[124,125] But in 1938, even *Fortune* found the AMA's stands too strong to stomach:

. . . Between the elders [Trustees and Delegates], and Dr. Fishbein the AMA has worked against its own purposes by clinging to ideas that rightly or wrongly have been discredited and it finds itself within hailing distance of its own downfall.[126]

By this time, few indeed remembered the Association's good work in the nineteenth century or its brief Progressive Era. A revolt in the ranks led by Dr. [James] Howard Means of Boston in 1938 came to very little,[127] but in September of the same year Attorney General Thurmond Arnold served notice that the AMA had gone too far.

Organized medicine [said Arnold] should not be allowed to extend its necessary and proper control over [professional] standards . . . , to include control over methods of payment for services involving the economic freedom and welfare for consumers and the legal rights of individual doctors.[128]

A short time later, the AMA was indicted by a federal grand jury charging violation of the Sherman Anti-Trust Act. The AMA and the Medical Society of the District of Columbia were subsequently convicted and nominal fines were imposed.[129] But the most significant result of the sequence was an opinion, handed down by the U.S.

Court of Appeals for the District of Columbia, which held that, under the circumstances of the indictment, the medical profession was unmistakably conducting itself as a trade and not as a profession.[130] And while the message got through to some members of the profession,[131] AMA leaders altered their tactics but not their policies.

Compulsory Health Insurance: Modern Times

The introduction by Senator Robert Wagner* of an amendment to the social security law in February, 1939 marked the beginning of a long and bitter battle between the AMA and the Senator. The amendment, called the National Health Act of 1939, was a relatively mild one and contained no provision for compulsory health insurance.[132] But the AMA opposed it on the ground that it would lead ultimately to complete federal control of medicine. The bill was a principal topic at the meeting of the House of Delegates in May, 1939 and a negative report by a reference committee was, in the words of the *Journal,* "adopted . . . without a dissenting vote and even without any attempt at discussion by individual members."[133]

But when Senators Murray and Wagner, and Congressman Dingell, introduced the first of their proposals to create a system for federal compulsory health insurance and federal support of medical education in June, 1943,[134] the *Journal's* language became pugnacious and abusive. "It would," said a *Journal* editorial, "make the Surgeon General of the Public Health Service . . . a virtual Gauleiter of American medicine."[135] Subsequent editorials rhetorically inquired "does the United States need a medical revolution? Does medical education need to be revolutionized?"[136,137] The answers were predictably negative on the grounds that the American health care system was the best in the world and that federal grants to medical schools would install bureaucratic control and destroy

---

*Interaction between the AMA and the Committee on Economic Security is described in detail in a memoir by Edwin Witte, Executive Director of the Committee.[118]

†Article I, Section 8, (1): The Congress shall have the power to lay and collect taxes . . . , to pay the debts and provide for the common defense and general welfare of the United States. . . .

‡"The powers not delegated to the United States by the Constitution, nor prohibited by it to the States, are reserved to the States respectively, or to the people."

*Robert Ferdinand Wagner (1877–1953) was born in Germany and came to the United States at an early age. He and Franklin Roosevelt were elected to the New York State Senate about the same time (1910). Wagner served in the U.S. Senate from 1927 to 1949 and was one of the New Deal's staunchest supporters.

standards of excellence. The first Murray-Wagner-Dingell bill came to nothing but Roosevelt's State of the Union message, delivered in January 1944 affirmed "the right to adequate medical care and the opportunity to achieve and enjoy good health."[138] Over a year later, the Murray-Wagner-Dingell bill was introduced anew (24 May 1945)[139] and the *Journal of the AMA* promptly took note in a hostile editorial attacking the bill and professional groups which supported it. These, said the *Journal,* were "inclined toward communism."[140] A letter from Senator Wagner, pleading for careful study of the bill and constructive suggestions from physicians[141] was published in June and a duel between the Senator and AMA officials ensued. Wagner noted that the AMA ". . . has condemned every proposal which had a chance to deal with our large national needs on an adequate basis." He went on to mention specific criticisms brought by the AMA and hoped that ". . . instead of pursuing a negative policy you will join with those of us who are trying to find constructive solutions to one of America's basic problems."[142]

Senator Wagner's efforts were largely wasted. Commenting at length on his letter, the Secretary of the AMA, Dr. Olin West, made it clear that the chief bone of contention was still the matter of compulsory health insurance. "They (the Senator and the Social Security Board) refuse to listen to any other proposals. . . ."[143] But he offered no evidence that the AMA was willing to listen to proposals for any but voluntary insurance proposals under control of the profession. At best, it was a matter of the pot calling the kettle black; the polarization with regard to federal health insurance was absolute.

It was otherwise with regard to the use of federal grants-in-aid, via the states, for hospital construction. The proposal had been considered during the New Deal era and had not been opposed by the AMA. Toward the end of the war it was introduced as S.191 (10 January 1945) by Senators Lister Hill of Alabama and Harold H. Burton of Ohio.[144] The House of Delegates accepted the proposal in December but, at the same time, reaffirmed its opposition to compulsory health insurance.[145]

The Hill-Burton Bill, somewhat amended, became law on 13 August 1946.[146]

The Murray-Wagner-Dingell proposal never actually came to a vote but was reintroduced several times. In 1945 it was first introduced as an amendment to the Social Security act, then was introduced as the National Health Act after Truman's health message to Congress.[147] The AMA continued its resolute opposition throughout. The *Journal* carried verbatim accounts of various hearings and, in an editorial in 1946, outdid itself in the Delphey-Ochsner tradition. Commenting on the hearings that began in April, 1946, it referred to ". . . the propaganda of Pepper, the diatribe of Dingell, the weasel words of Wagner, and the modulations of Murray. . . ."[148] The proposal was, in every sense, a "taking over of medicine by the state" that would abolish free choice of physicians and that would inevitably lead to "political degradation of medical practice."[149] At no time was there serious consideration of the possibility that government and the profession might come together to evolve a workable solution to a pressing national problem, something the existence of which the AMA denied altogether.

The climax of the battle came in 1947 and 1948. Senator Murray (joined by Senators Pepper, Chavez, Taylor, McGrath and Humphrey) reintroduced the bill on 20 May 1947.[150] Shortly thereafter, Secretary Ewing announced his ten year plan, calling for more health manpower, 600,000 new hospital beds, and compulsory health insurance.[151] In late 1948, the House of Delegates authorized the Board of Trustees to levy a $25 assessment on all members of the AMA and to employ professional public relations counsel to put down the menace of compulsory health insurance.[152] Under the direction of Whitaker and Baxter, a California firm, the campaign turned out to be one of the most expensive lobbying activities the country had ever seen. "The voluntary way is the American way" became the slogan, the threat was creeping socialism, and the American doctor could, Leone Baxter told the House of Delegates, save and preserve the American Way of Life by defeating compulsory health insurance.[153] The House of Delegates, adhering to the letter of the policies of the twenties,

said that "compulsory sickness insurance . . . is a variety of socialized medicine or state medicine. . . . It is contrary to the American tradition."[154]

Committee hearings on the Murray-Wagner-Dingell proposal began for the final time on 23 May 1949, the bill having been reintroduced in January,[155] and in April.[156] But by July the *Journal* stopped publishing transcripts of hearings because ". . . both legislators and the medical profession seem to have lost much of their interest."[157,158]* For one reason or another, the battle was beginning to subside despite which the AMA's campaign continued for another two years. Not all physicians approved of the assessment or of the Whitaker-Baxter campaign; but their contract was renewed through 1951. Looking back on it all, the AMA's president (Dr. Louis Bauer) said in 1952:

I realize that some members may have disapproved of the employment of Whitaker and Baxter and . . . have disapproved of some of [their] activities.

But without them, Dr. Bauer went on, ". . . we should in all probability now be operating under a government-controlled medical care plan."[160]

The Association breathed somewhat easier in late 1952 when Eisenhower won the presidency and announced his opposition to compulsory health insurance. Dingell's reintroduction of the national health insurance bill in 1953[161] caused no great alarm in the ranks of the AMA. But the new administration was unable to ignore the health problem altogether. In late 1954, Oveta Culp Hobby, HEW Secretary, proposed a system of spreading health insurance risks, using federal reinsurance funds, as a means of expanding the coverage of those who already had some form of health insurance.[162] It was to no avail. The AMA and some portions of the insurance industry joined in opposing the proposal despite the fact that it had no compulsory feature. The *Journal* for 18 December 1954 listed 14 bills on national

---

*It was at this juncture that the faithful and indefatigable Dr. Morris Fishbein, for years editor of the *Journal* and a major spokesman for the AMA was fired. "For thirty-seven years he had been crying 'wolf,'" said Milton Mayer. "Now," Mayer continued, "he was blamed for bringing on the wolves and was thrown to them."[159]

health program, including the reinsurance proposal, that were then pending in Congress. The AMA was actively opposed to 12 of them and took no action on the other two, one of which recommended nothing more startling than a study of health and accident insurance.[163]*

The AMA thus made it clear that it would not willingly lend its support to any federal health proposal of consequence and that its policies of 1920 and 1922 were still very much intact. However federal planners might define right to health, the AMA still doggedly pursued the view that the individual's right to curative medicine should not be guaranteed by government unless he was indigent. But a new cloud was on the horizon.

Climax: Medicare

The word *Medicare* first came into view when the Medicare Act of 7 June 1956 was passed, relating solely to the dependents of members of the Armed Forces.[165] Even so, it was thought by the *Journal* to carry with it "... some danger to the private practice of medicine."[166]

By this time, the focus was on the plight of the aged and in 1957 Congressman Forand (D., Rhode Island) introduced a bill providing hospital and medical care for the aged through Social Security.[167] Other bills were produced and one of them (the Kerr-Mills bill), which did not employ the social security mechanism for financing, was unopposed by the AMA. It became law in 1960.[168] But the matter would not rest. The Kerr-Mills law required that those over 65 who were not indigent should pay $24 annually for health insurance and that the whole program should be administered by the states. This was acceptable to the AMA; but the King-Anderson bill, introduced in early 1961 was unacceptable because it, like the Forand bill, called for financing through the social security mechanism.[169] In any case, AMA leaders considered the situation threatening enough to justify resort to a political

action technique it had used once before. In December, 1961, it created the American Medical Political Action Committee (AMPAC) to "... stimulate physicians and others to take a more active part in government ... and to help ... in organizing for more effective political action."[170] The AMA's own Board of Trustees appointed the nine members of AMPAC's Board of Directors of which Gunnar Gundersen, a former AMA president, was chairman. In practice, AMPAC's chief function was to solicit funds for the support of candidates for national office who accepted the AMA's views on federal health legislation.

The fight over the King-Anderson bill reached a peak when, on 20 May 1962, President Kennedy addressed an overflow crowd, many of them elderly, at Madison Square Garden urging public support for the measure. The AMA responded dramatically the next evening. At a cost estimated at $100,000 it staged its own TV show, taped in the empty auditorium shortly after Kennedy's audience had left. "This is the inside of that same arena," said an announcer, "just a few hours after yesterday's spectacle had ended. ... The clean-up crews will arrive shortly." Then Dr. Leonard Larson, president of the AMA, took over and introduced the prime speaker, Dr. Edward R. Annis. The line Annis took was basically the theme of the twenties, artfully framed and delivered. "England's nationalized medical program is what they have in mind for us eventually," he maintained. The King-Anderson bill was "a cruel hoax and a delusion," of limited benefits, inordinate cost, and the "forerunner of a different system of medicine for all Americans." His admonition was to go slow by defeating the bill.[171]

It was an expensive but probably effective antic. In July, the King-Anderson bill went down to defeat, although it never came, as such, to a vote.[172] But two years later a similar proposal was passed by the Senate as part of an amendment (the Gore Amendment) to the Social Security law.[173, 174] The House declined to go along and efforts at resolving House and Senate differences failed.

Meantime the AMA produced a proposal to which it attached the title *Eldercare* and which it persuaded

Senator Tower of Texas to introduce.[175] It was the first time the AMA had produced a countermeasure of its own design instead of reacting negatively to health bills from other sources. The Eldercare proposal was a relatively comprehensive one but still excluded the social security financing feature. The final result was the present Medicare law, passed in mid-1965, which adopted Eldercare's comprehensiveness in large measure but settled solidly on the social security method of financing.[176] Participation on the part of the elderly was, however, voluntary and in this regard the AMA won a pyrrhic victory. But federally backed health insurance was, despite decades of AMA opposition, finally on the books for an important group of American citizens not all of whom are indigent.

The AMA's hope of defeating the Medicare proposal had suffered a severe blow when, in December 1964, Wilbur Mills reversed his earlier opposition to it.* Hope had almost been abandoned by the time of the annual meeting in June, 1965. Various explanations of the Association's failure to block the legislation were offered. Outgoing President Donovan Ward said that on the evening of 21 November 1963, after AMA spokesmen had testified against the Medicare proposal, "... we were on our way to the most resounding legislative victory in our history as an organization." But by early afternoon the next day, President John F. Kennedy had been assassinated and a new Chief Executive, beholden (according to Ward) to labor and liberal forces, was in office.[178] The incoming President, Dr. James Z. Appel said that the AMA's political fortunes were on the wane because "... many members of Congress—acting as political sheep—are not being responsive to the people in this issue." But he counselled against boycott, if the law should pass;[179] and in this he was subsequently supported by the Board of Trustees.[180]

The passage of Medicare and other

---

*Several years earlier, an exasperated Congressman, Andrew Biemiller of Wisconsin, had said for the record: "Apparently the only kind of medical aid bill the AMA would approve is a measure which would place unlimited public funds in the hands of the AMA itself, to dispense as it sees fit after paying its lobbying and propaganda expenses. ..."[164]

---

*Mills' reasoning, and the means by which the successful Medicare proposal was put together, are described in detail by Harold B. Meyers.[177] The compromise is said to have crystallized in a conference between Mills and Secretary Wilbur Cohen of HEW in March, 1965.

health legislation thus left the Association's leaders disgruntled and bewildered but not openly rebellious. And in 1968, another incoming president inquired in his inaugural address:

Will we learn the lessons of our experience, particularly those that led to the laws affecting health that were passed by the 89th Congress?

He followed his question by a plea for enlightened guidance by the Association of the federal health planning process; steering rather than braking.[181] It was basically the same plea that had been made, and ignored, 45 years earlier by Ray Lyman Wilbur; and it was his son, Dwight L. Wilbur, who eloquently restated it in 1968. . . .

Since 1965, new proposals for major federal health legislation have been noticeably lacking. The succession of health and health-related laws enacted by the 89th Congress in 1965 left the country gasping. Implementation of the new laws has been difficult, partly owing to the shortage of administrative personnel and trained professionals.

But the hiatus is approaching its end.

Summary and Prospects for the Seventies

Neither the federal government nor the AMA is irreversibly committed to its precedents; nor is either likely to be uninfluenced by them. Since the first quarantine law was enacted in 1796, the federal definition of the right to health has been steadily broadened. But except for the short-lived vaccination law of 1813, federal health legislation did not begin to approach a guarantee of adequate health services to individual American citizens until comparatively modern times. With the passage of the Social Security Law in 1935, and the Cardozo decision two years later, a new climate was created. The several health bills introduced by Senator Robert Wagner and colleagues beginning in 1939 followed in due course. The passage of the Medicare-Medicaid Law and other health legislation in 1965 brought the process to its present state.

Since its founding in 1848, the AMA has played a key role in the development and passage of health legislation. Prior to the passage of Social Security, the federal government and the AMA, for the most part, saw comfortably eye-to-eye. As long as the definition of the right to health was a conservative

one—encompassing the health of the millions but not curative medicine for the individual—the AMA was, in fact, ahead of government, federal and state. The Model Health Insurance Bill of 1916, which the AMA helped to draft, was the real beginning of conflict. It embodied compulsory health insurance, financed by tripartite contributions: employee, employer, and state (but not federal) government. The Association's policies of 1920 and 1922 declared the proposal, and most others in which government control and financing are involved, to be anathema. The stage was then set for the battles over Social Security, the various Wagner bills, and those having to do with health care for the elderly. In the course of the long struggle, the AMA has ceded very little. The Kerr-Mills Law, which the Association approved, focussed on the states, held the federal government more or less at arm's length, and did no great violence to the AMA's view that only the indigent should receive personal health services at taxpayer's expense. But the Forand Bill and its successors put the federal government in the central position and extended benefits to all eligibles, regardless of economic status. In this sense Medicare was a watershed; it breached the AMA's 1922 definition of state medicine solidly and definitely. The extension of the Medicare system to virtually all citizens (and the revision or elimination of the state-oriented Medicaid provision), or possibly a new law having the same effect, is the prospect of the seventies.

Few organizations in American history have been so thoroughly dissected and criticized as the AMA. Some of the analyses are scholarly and relatively dispassionate;[182-185] others are strident and doctrinaire. Many have predicted that unless the AMA changes its ways, it is headed for oblivion. But the Association has ignored them all and has doggedly gone its conservative way. It is a remarkably durable institution; dire prophecies of oblivion, some dating back many decades, show little sign of becoming fact. But the Association's tactics have changed remarkably. Gone are the editorial polemics against the federal government in the *Journal,* and so are full extracts of the Minutes of the House of Delegates. The Association's *American Medical News* and

Today's Health both reflect its political and social point of view; but reports are likely to be more reportorial and less overtly propagandistic than formerly. Nor is there any suggestion that the spectacular Madison Square Garden countermeasure of 1962 will be repeated in the foreseeable future. Yet the Delphey-Ochsner style has not completely disappeared. It cropped up recently in a letter to the editor of the *American Medical News* when an AMA constituent described the *News* as a "blatant organ of the left-wing conspiracy."[186]

It is hardly that. But in the face of mounting pressure for national health insurance, the AMA has put forward its own plan to which it applies the title *Medicredit.*[187,188] The proposal is based on a scale of federal income tax credit to encourage the voluntary purchase of health insurance from existing organizations, private and semi-public. It would not alter the existing fee-for-service system nor does it contain specific inducements for physicians to locate in low-income or rural areas. It is basically a voluntary financing measure, not one that is designed to create a new health care system. At the opposite pole is a proposal backed by the Committee for National Health Insurance. It calls for compulsory health insurance for everyone and embodies the tripartite (employer, employee, and government) financing system put forward by the Model Bill of 1916.* It would virtually abolish fee-for-service practice and private health insurance plans. It would provide "financial and other" incentives to physicians willing to form medical care groups and to those who move into various low-income areas. It would assign highest priority in payment of funds collected by the system to salaried physicians in institutions, to those working in group practice prepayment units, and to physicians who agree to "accept capitation payments for the care of a defined population."[189]

It is difficult to see how more features that have traditionally been repugnant to the AMA could be incorporated into a single health insurance proposal. The Association's strenuous

*Forty per cent would come from federal tax revenues, 35 per cent from a tax on employer payrolls, and 25 per cent from a tax on individual adjusted gross income.

opposition to some features of the Committee's proposal is a certainty. It is not likely, however, to go back to the tactics of the forties, fifties and early sixties. For one thing, the Association's approach to the public is more sophisticated than it was then. For another, the AMA's political arm (AM-PAC) is said to exert more direct influence on the White House than was the case in earlier administrations.[190] But nothing that took place at the 1970 AMA Convention suggests that the AMA is as yet ready to reconsider all the present implications of its policies of the twenties.[191]

The dilemma the AMA faces in the early seventies is, in many respects, more stringent than that faced by the present Administration in Washington. The latter is as yet committed to nothing, beyond the recognition by the President of a health crisis. It can move in many directions, according to its sense of public opinion and the mood of Congress. But the AMA still labors under the self-imposed strictures of the twenties and the disadvantages under which it must now work are formidable. It must, on the one hand, continue to represent the interests of its members; and it must, on the other hand, participate in the creation of a system that will finally guarantee the right to health of all American citizens. The Association is not wrong in pointing out the dangers inherent in a health care system that is controlled absolutely by government; it could as well point out the obvious dangers of complete control by the consumer. But it cannot continue to confuse professional control of health care standards with professional control of the system itself.

To play its vital role in the guarantee of the right to health in the seventies, the AMA needs to reconsider its own precedents. Those of 1920 and 1922, developed in time of great political stress, stand today in sharp contrast to the enlightened and relevant precedents of earlier times. The policies of the twenties, more than anything else, have brought the Association to its present dilemma.

Its future may well depend on how convincingly it can rewrite—or expunge—those policies and on whether or not the House of Delegates' resolution of 1969 really means what it seems to say:

It is the basic right of every citizen to have available to him adequate health care.

References

1. Rouse, Milford O., Inaugural Address: To Whom Much Has Been Given. *JAMA* 201:169–171, 17 July 1967.

2. AMA Convention news. *New York Times.* 18 July 1969, p. 21.

3. Capen, Edward Warren, *The Historical Development of the Poor Law of Connecticut.* New York: Columbia University Press, 1905.

4. *Records of the Governor and Company of the Massachusetts Bay in New England, 1642–1649* 2:237, March 1647–8. Boston: William White, 1853.

5. Gordon, Maurice Bear, *Aesculapius Comes to the Colonies.* Ventnor, N.J.: Ventnor Publishers, Inc., 1949.

6. *Gazette of the United States.* 11 September 1793, p. 535.

7. Washington, George, Letter to the Attorney General; Mt. Vernon, 30 September 1793. In: *Writings of Washington* 33:107–109. Washington: U.S. Govt. Printing Office, 1940.

8. *Gazette of the United States.* 2 April 1794, pp. 2–3.

9. An Act to Authorize the President of the United States in Certain Cases to Alter the Place for Holding a Session of Congress. Third Cong., 1st Sess. *Pub. Stat. at Large U.S.* 1:353, 3 April 1794.

10. *Gazette of the United States.* 29 April 1796, p. 2.

11. Dexter, Franklin B., *Biographical Sketches of the Graduates of Yale College* 3:619–620, 1903. New York: H. Holt and Company, 1885–1913.

12. Lyman, William, Comment in House of Representatives. Fourth Cong., 1st Sess. Cong. Rec. (Ann. Cong.), 11 May 1796, p. 1348.

13. An Act Relative to Quarantine. Fourth Cong., 1st Sess. *Pub. Stat. at Large U.S.* 1:474, 27 May 1796.

14. Allen, William H., The Rise of the National Board of Health. *Ann. Amer. Acad. Polit. and Soc. Sci.* 15:51–68, January–May, 1900.

15. An Act Respecting Quarantine and Health Laws. Fifth Cong., 3rd Sess. *Pub. Stat. at Large U.S.* 1:619, 25 February 1799.

16. An Act Concerning Aliens. Fifth Cong., 2nd Sess. *Pub. Stat. at Large U.S.* 1:570–572, 25 June 1798.

17. An Act in Addition to the Act, Entitled "An Act for the Punishment of Certain Crimes Against the United States." Fifth Cong., 2nd Sess. *Pub. Stat. at Large U.S.* 1:596–597, 14 July 1798.

18. Gibbons *vs.* Ogden. *Reports of Cases Argued and Adjudged by the Supreme Court of the United States* (Wheaton); February term 9:1–222, 1824, p. 203.

19. Martin, Henry A., Jefferson as a Vaccinator. *North Carolina Med. J.* 7:1–34, January, 1881.

20. An Act to Diffuse the Benefits of Inoculation for the Cow Pox. *Laws of the Commonwealth of Massachusetts From February 28, 1807 to February 28, 1814.* 1(n.s.):167, 6 March 1810.

21. An Act to Encourage Vaccination. Twelfth Cong., 2nd Sess. *Pub. Stat. at Large U.S.* 2:806–807, 27 February 1813.

22. Report of the Select Committee . . . to Inquire Into the Propriety of Repealing the Act of 1813, to Encourage Vaccination, Accompanied With a Bill to Repeal the Act, Entitled "An Act to Encourage Vaccination." Seventeenth Cong., 1st Sess. *House Report* No. 93, 13 April 1822.

23. An Act to Repeal the Act Entitled "An Act to Encourage Vaccination." Seventeenth Cong., 1st Sess. *Pub. Stat. at Large U.S.* 3:677, 4 May 1822.

24. An Act to Enforce Quarantine Regulations. Twenty-second Cong., 1st Sess. *Pub. Stat. at Large U.S.* 4:577–578, 13 July 1832.

25. Keating, J. M., *A History of the Yellow Fever. The Yellow Fever Epidemic of 1878 in Memphis, Tenn.* Memphis: The Howard Association, 1879, pp. 327–443.

26. *The 1970 World Almanac and Book of Facts.* New York: Newspaper Enterprise Asso., Inc., 1969, p. 254.

27. *Evening Post* (New York). 6 May 1846, p. 2.

28. *Proceedings of the National Medical Conventions Held in New York, May, 1846, and in Philadelphia, May, 1847.* Philadelphia: T. K. and P. G. Collins, Printers, 1847.

29. Davis, N. S., *History of the American Medical Association From Its Organization up to January, 1855.* Philadelphia: Lippincott, Grambo, and Co., 1855.

30. Chapman, Nathaniel, President's Address. *Trans. Amer. Med. Asso.* 1:7–9, 1848.

31. Memorial to Congress on Adulterated Drugs and Medicines. *Trans. Amer. Asso. Med.* 1:335, 4 May 1848.

32. An Act to Prevent the Importation of Adulterated and Spurious Drugs and Medicine. Thirtieth Cong., 1st Sess. *Pub. Stat. at Large U.S.* 9:237–239, 26 June 1848.

33. Reed, Charles, President's Address. *JAMA* 36:1599–1606, 8 June 1901.

34. Editorial: The Medical Association. *New York Times,* 6 May 1858, p. 1.

35. Editorial: American Medical Association. A Little Business and a Large Row. *New York Times,* 7 May 1858, p. 1.

36. Editorial: Medical Ethics. *New York Times,* 9 June 1882, p. 4.

37. Davis, Nathan Smith, Resolution at the Eighteenth Annual Meeting. *Trans. Amer. Med. Asso.* 18:33–34, 1867.

38. Logan, Thomas M., Report of the Committee on a National Health Council. *Trans. Amer. Med. Asso.* 23:46–51, 9 May 1872.

39. Richardson, T. G., Presidential Address, Twenty-Ninth Annual Meeting. *Trans. Amer. Med. Asso.* 29:93–111, 1878, p. 111.

40. Commissioners of the Sanitary Survey, *Report of a General Plan for the Promotion of Public and Personal Health . . .* [Lemuel Shattuck]. Boston: Dutton and Wentworth, 1850, p. 10.

41. An Act to Reorganize the Marine Hospital Service and to Provide for the Relief of Sick and Disabled Seamen. Forty-first Cong., 2nd Sess. *Pub. Stat. at Large U.S.* 16:169–170, 29 June 1870.

42. Yellow Fever at Rio de Janeiro. *New York Times,* 17 April 1878, p. 8.

43. Desolation in the South. *New York Times,* 5 September 1878, p. 1.

44. An Act to Prevent the Introduction of Contagious or Infectious Diseases Into the United States. Forty-fifth Cong., 2nd Sess. *Pub. Stat. at Large U.S.* 20:37–38, 29 April 1878.

45. American Public Health Association. Reports and Resolutions Relating to Sanitary Legislation. Presented at Its Meeting in Richmond, Va., November 19–22, 1878. *Rep. Amer. Pub. Health Asso.* 5:101, 1879.

46. Resolution Calling for More Stringent Quarantine Laws to Be Enacted by Congress. *Trans. Amer. Med. Asso.* 8:37–38, 2 May 1855.

47. *Senate Report* No. 734; to Accompany S.1784. Forty-fifth Cong., 3rd Sess. 7 February 1879.

48. Cabell, J. L., A Review of the Operations of the National Board of Health. *Rep. Amer. Pub. Health Asso.* 8:71–101, 1883.

49. An Act to Prevent the Introduction of Infectious or Contagious Diseases Into the United States, and to Establish a National Board of Health. Forty-fifth Cong., 3rd Sess. *Pub. Stat. at Large U.S.* 20:484–485, 3 March 1879.

50. An Act to Prevent the Introduction of Contagious or Infectious Diseases Into the United States. Forty-sixth Cong., 1st Sess. *Pub. Stat. at Large U.S.* 21:5–7, 2 June 1879.

51. Debate on Quarantine Act of 2 June 1879. Forty-sixth Cong., 1st Sess. *Cong. Rec.* 9(2):1637–1650, 27 May 1879.

52. Billings, John Shaw, Reports and Resolutions Relating to Sanitary Legislation. *Amer. J. Med. Sci.* 78:471–479, October, 1879.

53. Editorial: The National Board of Health and the American Public Health Association. *Boston Med. and Surg. J.* 107:450–451, 9 November 1882.

54. An Act Granting Additional Quarantine Powers and Imposing Additional Duties Upon the Marine-Hospital Service. Fifty-second Cong., 2nd Sess. *Pub. Stat. at Large U.S.* 27:449–452, 15 February 1893.

55. Morgan's Louisiana and Texas Railroad and Steamship Company *vs.* Board of Health of the State of Louisiana and the State of Louisiana. *U.S. Supreme Court Reps.* (Lawyers Edition) 30:237–243, 10 May 1886.

56. Faulkner, Harold U., *The Decline of Laissez-faire, 1897–1917.* New York: Harper and Row, 1951.

57. An Act Making Appropriations for Sundry Civil Expenses of the Government for the Fiscal Year Ending June Thirtieth, 1902, and for Other Purposes. Fifty-sixth Cong., 2nd Sess. *Pub. Stat. at Large U.S.* 31:1137, 3 March 1901.

58. An Act to Change the Name of the Public Health and Marine Hospital Service to the Public Health Service, to Increase the Pay of Officers of Said Service, and for Other Purposes. Sixty-second Cong., 2nd Sess. *Pub. Stat. at Large U.S.* 37(1):309, 14 August 1912.

59. Hofstadter, Richard, *The Age of Reform: From Bryan to F.D.R.* New York: Alfred Knopf, 1955, 328 pp.

60. An Act for Preventing the Manufacture, Sale, or Transportation of Adulterated or Misbranded or Poisonous or Deleterious Food, Drugs, Medicines, and Liquors, and for Regulating Traffic Therein, and for Other Purposes. Fifty-ninth Cong., 1st Sess. *Pub. Stat. at Large U.S.* 34(1):768–772, 30 June 1906.

61. An Act to Amend Section Eight of the Food and Drugs Act Approved June Thirtieth, Nineteen Hundred and Six. Sixty-second Cong., 2nd Sess. *Pub. Stat. at Large U.S.* 37(1):416–417, 23 August 1912.

62. Resolution on Official Policy of the Association. *Trans. Amer. Med. Asso.* 4:39, 9 May 1851.

63. Official Minutes of the General Sessions, Report of the Transactions of the Reorganization Committee on Revision of Constitution and By-laws. *JAMA* 36:1643–1648, 8 June 1901.

64. Editorial: The House of Delegates. *American Medicine* 3:1030, 21 June 1902.

65. Frankel, Lee K., and Dawson, Miles M., *Workman's Insurance in Europe.* New York: Charities Publication Committee, 1910.

66. Editorial: Socializing the British Medical Profession. *JAMA* 59:1890–1891, 23 November 1912.

67. Brandeis, Louis D., Workingman's Insurance—The Road to Social Efficiency. *Proc. Conf. of Charities and Corrections,* 38th Annual Session, 8 June 1911, pp. 156–162.

68. *A Contract With the People.* Platform of the Progressive Party Adopted at Its First National Convention. Chicago, 7 August 1912. New York: Progressive National Committee, 1912.

69. Wilson, Woodrow, First Inaugural Address as President of the United States, 4 March 1913. *The Public Papers of Woodrow Wilson. The New Democracy, vol. 1.* New York: Harper and Brothers, 1926.

70. Warbasse, James P., The Socialization of Medicine. *JAMA* 63:264–266, 18 July 1914.

71. Rubinow, Isaac M., Social Insurance and the Medical Profession. *JAMA* 64:381–386, 30 January 1915.

72. American Association for Labor Legislation. Annual Business Meeting, December 1912. *Amer. Labor Legislation Rev.* 3:121, 1913.

73. Rubinow, I. M., *Social Insurance, With Special Reference to American Conditions.* New York: Henry Holt and Company, 1913.

74. Chandler, Alfred D., The Origins of Progressive Leadership. In *The Letters of Theodore Roosevelt.* Vol. 8, Elting Morrison, ed. Cambridge: Harvard University Press, 1954, pp. 1462–1465.

75. Lambert, Alexander, Medical Organization Under Health Insurance. *Amer. Labor Legislation Rev.* 7:36–50, March, 1917.

76. Editorial: Industrial Insurance. *JAMA* 66:433, 5 February 1916.

77. Health Insurance: Tentative Draft of an Act. *Amer. Labor Legislation Rev.* 6:239–268, June, 1916.

78. Minutes of House of Delegates: Report of the Judicial Council of the House of Delegates [21 June]. *JAMA* 65:73–92, 3 July 1915.

79. Current Comment: A Model Bill for Health Insurance. *JAMA* 65:1824, 20 November 1915.

80. Editorial: Cooperation in Social Insurance Investigation. *JAMA* 66:1469–1470, 6 May 1916.

81. Minutes of House of Delegates: Report of Committee on Social Insurance. *JAMA* 66:1951–1985, 17 June 1916.

82. Rogoff, Hillel, *An East Side Epic; the Life and Work of Meyer London.* New York: Vanguard Press, 1930.

83. House Joint Resolution 159: For the Appointment of a Commission to Prepare and Recommend a Plan for the Establishment of a National Insurance Fund, and for the Mitigation of the Evil of Unemployment. Sixty-fourth Cong., 1st Sess. *Cong. Rec.* 53:2856, 19 February 1916.

84. *Hearings Before the Committee on Labor (HR),* Commission to Study Social Insurance and Unemployment. April 6 and 11, 1916. Sixty-fourth Cong., 1st Sess. Washington: U.S. Govt. Printing Office, 1916.

85. Debate on National Insurance. Sixty-fourth Cong., 2nd Sess. *Cong. Rec.* 54(3):2650–2654, 5 February 1917.

86. Freund, Ernst, Constitutional and Legal Aspects of Health Insurance. *Nat. Conf. Social Work* 1917:553–558.

87. Minutes of House of Delegates, Reports of Committee on Social Insurance Regarding Invalidity, Old Age, and Unemployment Insurance, and a General Summary Concerning Social Insurance. *JAMA* 68:1721–1755, 9 June 1917.

88. Delphey, Eden V., Arguments Against the "Standard Bill" for Compulsory Health Insurance. *JAMA* 68:1500–1501, 19 May 1917.

89. Minutes of House of Delegates, Report of the Council on Health and Public Instruction. *JAMA* 72:1750–1751, 14 June 1919.

90. Fishbein, Morris, *History of the American Medical Association*. Philadelphia: W. B. Saunders Company, 1947, p. 318.

91. Minutes of House of Delegates, Report of Committee on Social Insurance. *JAMA* 74:1241–1242, 1 May 1920.

92. Wanted—A Health Insurance Program. In *Social Security in the United States*, 1934, p. 112. New York: American Association for Social Security, 1934.

93. Delphey, Eden V., Report of the Committee on Compulsory Health and Workmen's Compensation Insurance of the Medical Society of the County of New York. *New York State J. Med.* 20:394–396, December, 1920.

94. Minutes of House of Delegates, Report of Reference Committee on Hygiene and Public Health (27 April). *JAMA* 74:1319, 8 May 1920.

95. An Act to Deport Certain Undesirable Aliens and to Deny Readmission to Those Deported. Sixty-sixth Cong., 2nd Sess. *Pub. Stat. at Large U.S.* 41(1):593–594, 10 May 1920.

96. Lusk, Clayton R. (Chairman), *Revolutionary Radicalism. . . . Report of the Joint Legislative Committee* [Lusk Report], 4 vols. Albany: J. B. Lyon Co., 1920.

97. Ghent, W. J., *The Reds Bring Reaction*. Princeton: Princeton University Press, 1923.

98. Ochsner, Edward H., Compulsory Health Insurance, a Modern Fallacy. *Illinois Med. J.* 38:77–80, August, 1920.

99. Ochsner, Edward H.: Some Medical Economics Problems. *Illinois Med. J.* 39:406–413, May, 1921.

100. Minutes of House of Delegates for 9 June 1921. *JAMA* 76:1757–1758, 18 June 1921.

101. Fishbein, Morris, *History of the American Medical Association*. Philadelphia: W. B. Saunders Company, 1947, pp. 324–325.

102. Lambert, Alexander, Medicine, a Determining Factor in War. Presidential Address. *JAMA* 72:1713–1721, 14 June 1919.

103. An Act for the Promotion of the Welfare and Hygiene of Maternity and Infancy, and for Other Purposes (P.L.67–97). Sixty-seventh Cong., 1st Sess. *Pub. Stat. at Large U.S.* 42(1):224–226, 23 November 1921.

104. Editorial: Federal Care of Maternity and Infancy. The Shepherd-Towner Bill. *JAMA* 76:383, 5 February 1921.

105. Minutes of House of Delegates: Various Resolutions. *JAMA* 76:1756–1757, 18 June 1921.

106. Minutes of House of Delegates 25 May 1922. Supplementary Report of Reference Committee on Legislation and Public Relations. *JAMA* 78:1715, 3 June 1922.

107. Wilbur, Ray Lyman, Human Welfare and Modern Medicine. Inaugural Address. *JAMA* 80:1889–1893, 30 June 1923.

108. Morgan, William G., The Medical Profession and the Paternalistic Tendencies of the Times. President's Address. *JAMA* 94:2035–2042, 28 June 1930.

109. Committee on the Costs of Medical Care, *Medical Care for the American People: The Final Report*. Chicago: University of Chicago Press, 1932 (Publication No. 28).

110. Editorial: The Committee on the Costs of Medical Care. *JAMA* 99:1950–1952, 3 December 1932.

111. Editorial: The Conference on Economic Security. *JAMA* 103:1624–1625, 24 November 1934.

112. Minutes of the Special Session of the House of Delegates of the American Medical Association, Chicago, 15–16 February 1935. *JAMA* 104:747–753, 2 March 1935.

113. The Economic Security Act (S.1130). Seventy-fourth Cong., 1st Sess. *Cong. Rec.* 79(1):549–556, 17 January 1935.

114. Model Bill Maps Health Insurance. *New York Times*, 6 January 1935, Sec. 2, p. 2.

115. A Bill (H.R. 7260) to Provide for the General Welfare by Establishing a System of Federal Old-Age Benefits, . . . to Establish a Social Security Board; etc. Seventy-fourth Cong., 1st Sess. *Cong. Rec.* 79(5):5079, 4 April 1935.

116. Debate on Social Security Act. Seventy-fourth Cong., 1st Sess. *Cong. Rec.* 79(6):6069–6070, 19 April 1935.

117. An Act to Provide for the General Welfare by Establishing a System of Federal Old-Age Benefits . . . ; to Establish a Social Security Board; etc. Seventy-fourth Cong., 1st Sess. *Pub. Stat. at Large U.S.* 49(1): 620–648, 14 August 1935.

118. Witte, Edwin E., *Development of Social Security Act*. Madison: University of Wisconsin Press, 1962.

119. Steward Machine Co. vs. Davis, Collector of Internal Revenue. *United States Reports* 301:548–618, 24 May 1937.

120. Helvering, Commissioner of Internal Revenue, et al. vs. Davis. *United States Reports* 301:619–646, 24 May 1937.

121. Minutes of House of Delegates: Report of Reference Committee on Consideration of the National Health Program. *JAMA* 111:1215–1217, 24 September 1938.

122. Editorial: Evidently Change Is Needed. *New York Times*, 7 February 1921, p. 10.

123. Harding, T. Swann, How Scientific Are Our Doctors? *Forum* 81:345–351, June, 1929.

124. Rorty, James, Whose Medicine? *Nation* 143:42–44, 11 July 1936.

125. Rorty, James, Medicine's Misalliance. *Nation* 146:666–669, 11 June 1938.

126. The American Medical Association. *Fortune* 18:88–92, 150, 152, 156, 160, 162, 164, 166, 168, November, 1938.

127. Stephenson, H., Revolt in the AMA. *Current History* 48:24–26, June, 1938.

128. Arnold, T., Department of Justice: Statement About Group Health Insurance Case. *Current History* 49:49–50, September, 1938.

129. Minutes of House of Delegates: Report of Board of Trustees. *JAMA* 116:2791–2792, 21 June 1941.

130. United States vs. American Medical Assn., et al., U.S. Court of Appeals for the District of Columbia. No. 7488. *Federal Reporter*, Series 2 110:703–716, 4 March 1940.

131. Morgan, Hugh J., *Professio. Ann. Int. Med.* 28:887–891, May, 1948.

132. National Health Act of 1939 (S.1620). Seventy-sixth Cong., 1st Sess. *Cong. Rec.* 84(2):1976–1982, 28 February 1939.

133. Minutes of House of Delegates: Report of Reference Committee on Consideration of Wagner National Health Bill [17 May]. *JAMA* 112:2295–2297, 3 June 1939.

134. Social Security Act Amendment of 1943. Unified National Social Insurance (S.1161). Seventy-eighth Cong., 1st Sess. *Cong. Rec.* 89(4):5260–5262, 3 June 1943.

135. Editorial: Wagner-Murray-Dingell Bill for Social Security. *JAMA* 122:600–601, 26 June 1943.

136. Editorial: Does the United States Need a Medical Revolution? *JAMA* 123:418, 16 October 1943.

137. Editorial: Does Medical Education Need to Be Revolutionized? *JAMA* 123:484, 23 October 1943.

138. Roosevelt, Franklin D., Message From the President of the United States on the State of the Union. Seventy-eighth Cong., 2nd Sess. *Cong. Rec.* 90(1):55–57, 11 January 1944, p. 57.

139. Social Security Amendments of 1945 (S.1050). Seventy-ninth Cong., 1st Sess. *Cong. Rec.* 91(4):4920–4927, 24 May 1945.

140. Editorial: The Wagner-Murray-Dingell Bill (S. 1050) of 1945. *JAMA* 128:364–365, 2 June 1945.

141. Wagner, Robert F., The Wagner-Murray-Dingell Bill [Letter to the Editor]. *JAMA* 128:461, 9 June 1945.

142. The Wagner-Murray-Dingell Bill. Senator Wagner Comments on the Journal Editorial. . . . *JAMA* 128:672–673, 30 June 1945.

143. Editorial: Senator Wagner's Comments. *JAMA* 128:667–668, 30 June 1945.

144. A Bill . . . to Authorize Grants to the States for Surveying Their Hospitals . . . and for Planning Construction of Additional Facilities, and to Authorize Grants to Assist in Such Construction . . . (S.191). Seventy-ninth Cong., 1st Sess. *Cong. Rec.* 91 (1):158, 10 January 1945.

145. Minutes of House of Delegates, Report of Reference Committee on Legislation and Public Relations. *JAMA* 129:1200–1201, 22 December 1945.

146. An Act to Amend the Public Health Service Act to Authorize Grants to the States for Surveying Their Hospitals . . . and for Planning Construction of Additional Facilities, and to Authorize Grants to Assist in Such Construction (P.L.79–725). Seventy-ninth Cong., 2nd Sess. *Pub. Stat. at Large U.S.* 60(1):1040–1049, 13 August 1946.

147. National Health Act of 1945 (S.1606). Seventy-ninth Cong., 1st Sess. *Cong. Rec.* 91(8):10793–10795, 19 November 1945.

148. Editorial: Senate Hearings on the National Health Program. *JAMA* 130:1016, 13 April 1946.

149. Editorial: The Hearings on the Wagner-Murray-Dingell Bill. *JAMA* 131:1424, 24 August 1946.

150. National Health Insurance and Public Health Act (S.1320). Eightieth Cong., 1st Sess. *Cong. Rec.* 93(4):5516–5522, 20 May 1947.

151. Editorial: Mr. Ewing's Ten Year Health Program. *JAMA* 138:297–298, 25 September 1947.

152. Minutes of House of Delegates: Report of Reference Committee on Legislation and Public Relations [1 December 1948]. *JAMA* 138:1241, 25 December 1948.

153. Baxter, Leone: Address to House of Delegates. *JAMA* 140:694–696, 25 June 1949.

154. Minutes of House of Delegates: Statement of Policy of American Medical Association. *JAMA* 138:1171, 18 December 1948.

155. A Bill to Provide a National Health Insurance and Public Health Program (S.5). Eighty-first Cong., 1st Sess. *Cong. Rec.* 95(1):38, 5 January 1949.

156. A Bill to Provide a Program of National Health Insurance and Public Health and to Assist in Increasing the Number of Adequately Trained Professional and Other Health Personnel (S. 1679). Eighty-first Cong., 1st Sess. *Cong. Rec.* 95(4):4946, 4959–4962, 25 April 1949.

157. Washington Letter: Compulsory Insurance Chief Issue as Hearings Open. *JAMA* 140:481–482, 4 June 1949.

158. Editorial: Hearings on Health Legislation. *JAMA* 140:962, 16 July 1949.

159. Mayer, Milton, The Rise and Fall of Dr. Fishbein. *Harper's Magazine* 199:76–85, November, 1949.

160. The President's Page [Louis H. Bauer], The Chicago Meeting. *JAMA* 149:843, 28 June 1952.

161. A Bill to Provide a Program of National Health Insurance and Public Health, etc. (H.R.1817). Eighty-third Cong., 1st Sess. *Cong. Rec.* 99(1):434, 16 January 1953.

162. Hobby, Oveta Culp, Address of HEW Secretary Before House of Delegates, AMA. *JAMA* 156:1506–1508, 18 December 1954.

163. Organization Section: Legislative Review. *JAMA* 156:1514, 18 December 1954.

164. American Medical Association Opposes All Progressive Legislation. New Rival for NAM. Eighty-first Cong., 2nd Sess. *Cong. Rec.* 96(10):13904–13918, 30 August 1950.

165. An Act to Provide Medical Care for Dependents of Members of the Uniformed Services, and for Other Purposes (P.L.84–569). Eighty-fourth Cong., 2nd Sess. *Pub. Stat. at Large U.S.* 70:250–254, 7 June 1956.

166. Editorial: Morale and Medicine. *JAMA* 163:119, 12 January 1957.

167. A Bill to Amend the Social Security Act . . . so as to Increase the Benefits Payable Under the Federal Old-Age, Survivors, and Disability Insurance Program, to Provide Insurance Against the Costs of Hospital, Nursing Home, and Surgical Services, etc. (H.R.9467). Eighty-fifth Cong., 1st Sess. *Cong. Rec.* 103(12):16173, 27 August 1957.

168. An Act to Extend and Improve Coverage under the Federal Old-Age, Survivors and Disability Insurance System . . . ; to Provide Grants to the States for Medical Care for Aged Individuals of Low Income; . . . etc. (P.L.86–778). Eighty-sixth Cong., 2nd Sess. *Pub. Stat. at Large U.S.* 74:924–997, 13 September 1960.

169. A Bill to Provide for Payment for Hospital Services, Skilled Nursing Home Services, and Home Health Services Furnished to Aged Beneficiaries Under the Old-Age Survivors and Disability Insurance Program (H.R.4222). Eighty-seventh Cong., 1st Sess. *Cong. Rec.* 107(2):2136, 13 February 1961.

170. Medical News: Delegates Endorse Kerr-Mills and AMPAC, Criticize "Public Airing of Disagreements," *JAMA* 178(11):31, 16 December 1961.

171. Kihss, Peter, AMA Rebuttal to Kennedy Sees Aged Care Hoax. *New York Times,* 22 May 1962, p. 1.

172. Public Welfare Amendments of 1962 (H.R.10606). Eighty-seventh Cong., 2nd Sess. *Cong. Rec.* 108(10):13848–13873, 17 July 1962.

173. Social Security Amendments of 1964. Gore Amendment (No. 1256). Eighty-eighth Cong., 2nd Sess. *Cong. Rec.* 110 (16):21113–21122, 31 August 1964.

174. Social Security Amendments of 1964 (H.R.11865). Eighty-eighth Cong., 2nd Sess. *Cong. Rec.* 110(16):21351–21354, 2 September 1964.

175. A Bill to Amend Titles I and XVI of the Social Security Act to . . . [Authorize] Any State to Provide Medical Assistance for the Aged . . . Under Voluntary Private Health Insurance Plans and to Amend the Internal Revenue Code of 1954 to Provide Tax Incentives to Encourage Prepayment Health Insurance for the Aged . . . (S.820). Eighty-ninth Cong., 1st Sess. *Cong. Rec.* 111(2):1461, 28 January 1965.

176. An Act to Provide a Hospital Insurance Program for the Aged Under the Social Security Act With a Supplementary Benefits Program and an Expanded Program of Medical Assistance . . . etc. Eighty-ninth Cong., 1st Sess. *Pub. Stat. at Large U.S.* 79:286–423, 30 July 1965.

177. Meyers, Harold B., Mr. Mills' Elder-medi-better Care. *Fortune* 71:166–168, 196, June, 1965.

178. Ward, Donovan F., Remarks of the President [20 June 1965]. *JAMA* 193:23–25, 5 July 1965.

179. Appel, James Z., Inaugural Address. We the People of the United States—Are We Sheep? [20 June 1965]. *JAMA* 193:26–30, 5 July 1965.

180. Special Announcement: Board of Trustees Action. *JAMA* 193:689, 23 August 1965.

181. Wilbur, Dwight L., Emphasize Steering Instead of the Brake. Inaugural Address. *JAMA* 205:89–91, 8 July 1968.

182. Hyde, David R., Wolff, Payson, Gross, Anne, and Hoffman, Elliott Lee, The American Medical Association: Power, Purpose, and Politics in Organized Medicine. *Yale Law J.* 63:937–1022, May, 1954.

183. Garceau, Oliver, *The Political Life of the American Medical Association.* Cambridge: Harvard University Press, 1941.

184. Burrow, James G., *AMA. Voice of American Medicine.* Baltimore: Johns Hopkins Press, 1963.

185. Rayack, Elton, *Professional Power and American Medicine: The Economics of the American Medical Association.* Cleveland: World Publishing Company, 1967.

186. Greely, Horace, Jr., M.D., Letter to the Editor. *Amer. Med. News* 12:5, 3 November 1969.

187. National Health Care—The Gathering Storm. *Amer. Med. News* 12:1; 8–9, 27 October 1969.

188. Watt, Linda, NHI Is Nigh. *Today's Health* 48:26–29; 71, July, 1970.

189. Committee for National Health Insurance: Press Release. Washington, D.C., 7 July 1970.

190. Washington Rounds. *Med. World News* 11:10f, 19 June 1970.

191. AMA, 70. *Med. World News* 11:19–21, 10 July 1970.

91

Robert M. Sade

Medical Care as a Right: A Refutation

Reprinted with permission of the publisher from the *New England Journal of Medicine*, vol. 285, 1971, pp. 1288–1292.

The current debate on health care in the United States is of the first order of importance to the health professions, and of no less importance to the political future of the nation, for precedents are now being set that will be applied to the rest of American society in the future. In the enormous volume of verbiage that has poured forth, certain fundamental issues have been so often misrepresented that they have now become commonly accepted fallacies. This paper will be concerned with the most important of these misconceptions, that health care is a right, as well as a brief consideration of some of its corollary fallacies.

Rights—Morality and Politics

The concept of rights has its roots in the moral nature of man and its practical expression in the political system that he creates. Both morality and politics must be discussed before the relation between political rights and health care can be appreciated.

A "right" defines a freedom of action. For instance, a right to a material object is the uncoerced choice of the use to which that object will be put; a right to a specific action, such as free speech, is the freedom to engage in that activity without forceful repression. The moral foundation of the rights of man begins with the fact that he is a living creature: he has the right to his own life. All other rights are corollaries of this primary one; without the right to life, there can be no others, and the concept of rights itself becomes meaningless.

The freedom to live, however, does not automatically ensure life. For man, a specific course of action is required to sustain his life, a course of action that must be guided by reason and reality and has as its goal the creation or acquisition of material values, such as food and clothing, and intellectual values, such as self-esteem and integrity. His moral system is the means by which he is able to select the values that will support his life and achieve his happiness.

Man must maintain a rather delicate homeostasis in a highly demanding and threatening environment, but has at his disposal a unique and efficient mechanism for dealing with it: his mind. His mind is able to perceive, to identify percepts, to integrate them into concepts, and to use those concepts in choosing actions suitable to the maintenance of his life. The rational function of mind is volitional, however; a man must *choose* to think, to be aware, to evaluate, to make conscious decisions. The extent to which he is able to achieve his goals will be directly proportional to his commitment to reason in seeking them.

The right to life implies three corollaries: the right to select the values that one deems necessary to sustain one's own life; the right to exercise one's own judgment of the best course of action to achieve the chosen values; and the right to dispose of those values, once gained, in any way one chooses, without coercion by other men. The denial of any one of these corollaries severely compromises or destroys the right to life itself. A man who is not allowed to choose his own goals, is prevented from setting his own course in achieving those goals and is not free to dispose of the values he has earned is no less than a slave to those who usurp those rights. The right to private property, therefore, is essential and indispensable to maintaining free men in a free society.

Thus, it is the nature of man as a living, thinking being that determines his rights—his "natural rights." The concept of natural rights was slow in dawning on human civilization. The first political expression of that concept had its beginnings in 17th and 18th century England through such exponents as John Locke and Edmund Burke, but came to its brilliant debut as a form of government after the American Revolution. Under the leadership of such men as Thomas Paine and Thomas Jefferson, the concept of man as a being sovereign unto himself, rather than a subdivision of the sovereignty of a king, emperor or state, was incorporated into the formal structure of government for the first time. Protection of the lives and property of individual citizens was the salient characteristic of the Constitution of 1787. Ayn Rand has pointed out that the principle of protection of the individual against the coercive force of government made the United States the first moral society in history.[1]

In a free society, man exercises his right to sustain his own life by producing economic values in the form of goods and services that he is, or should be, free to exchange with other men who are similarly free to trade with him or not. The economic values produced, however, are not given as gifts by nature, but exist only by virtue of the thought and effort of individual men. Goods and services are thus owned as a consequence of the right to sustain life by one's own physical and mental effort.

If the chain of natural rights is interrupted, and the right to a loaf of bread, for example, is proclaimed as primary (avoiding the necessity of earning it), every man owns a loaf of bread, regardless of who produced it. Since ownership is the power of disposal,[2] every man may take his loaf from the baker and dispose of it as he wishes with or without the baker's permission. Another element has thus been introduced into the relation between men: the use of force. It is crucial to observe who has initiated the use of force: it is the man who demands unearned bread as a right, not the man who produced it. At the level of an unstructured society it is clear who is moral and who immoral. The man who acted rationally by producing food to support his own life is moral. The man who expropriated the bread by force is immoral.

To protect this basic right to provide for the support of one's own life, men band together for their mutual protection and form governments. This is the only proper function of government: to provide for the defense of individuals against those who would take their lives or property by force. The state is the repository for retaliatory force in a just society wherein the only actions prohibited to individuals are those of physical harm or the threat of physical harm to other men. The closest that man has ever come to achieving this ideal of government was in this country after its War of Independence.

When a government ignores the progression of natural rights arising from the right to life, and agrees with a man, a group of men, or even a majority of its citizens, that every man has a right to a loaf of bread, it must protect that right by the passage of laws ensuring that everyone gets his loaf—in the process depriving the baker of the freedom to dispose of his own product. If the baker disobeys the law, asserting the priority of his right to support himself by his own rational disposition of the fruits of his mental and physical

labor, he will be taken to court by force or threat of force where he will have more property forcibly taken from him (by fine) or have his liberty taken away (by incarceration). Now the initiator of violence is the government itself. The degree to which a government exercises its monopoly on the retaliatory use of force by asserting a claim to the lives and property of its citizens is the degree to which it has eroded its own legitimacy. It is a frequently overlooked fact that behind every law is a policeman's gun or a soldier's bayonet. When that gun and bayonet are used to initiate violence, to take property or to restrict liberty by force, there are no longer any rights, for the lives of the citizens belong to the state. In a just society with a moral government, it is clear that the only "right" to the bread belongs to the baker, and that a claim by any other man to that right is unjustified and can be enforced only by violence or the threat of violence.

Rights—Politics and Medicine

The concept of medical care as the patient's right is immoral because it denies the most fundamental of all rights, that of a man to his own life and the freedom of action to support it. Medical care is neither a right nor a privilege: it is a service that is provided by doctors and others to people who wish to purchase it. It is the provision of this service that a doctor depends upon for his livelihood, and is his means of supporting his own life. If the right to health care belongs to the patient, he starts out owning the services of a doctor without the necessity of either earning them or receiving them as a gift from the only man who has the right to give them: the doctor himself. In the narrative above substitute "doctor" for "baker" and "medical service" for "bread." American medicine is now at the point in the story where the state has proclaimed the non-existent "right" to medical care as a fact of public policy, and has begun to pass the laws to enforce it. The doctor finds himself less and less his own master and more and more controlled by forces outside of his own judgment.

For instance, under the proposed Kennedy-Griffiths bill,[3] there will be a "Health Security Board," which will be responsible for administering the new

controls to be imposed on doctors, hospitals and other "providers" of health care (Sec. 121). Specialized services, such as major surgery, will be done by "qualified specialists" [Sec. 22(b)(2)], such qualifications being determined by the Board (Sec. 42). Furthermore, the patient can no longer exercise his own initiative in finding a specialist to do his operation, since he must be referred to the specialist by a nonspecialist—i.e., a general practitioner or family doctor [Sec. 22(b)]. Licensure by his own state will not be enough to be a qualified practitioner; physicians will also be subject to a second set of standards, those established by the Board [Sec. 42(a)]. Doctors will no longer be considered competent to determine their own needs for continuing education, but must meet requirements established by the Board [Sec. 42(c)]. The professional staff of a hospital will no longer be able to determine which of its members are qualified to perform which kinds of major surgery; specialty-board certification or eligibility will be required, with certain exceptions that include meeting standards established by the Board [Sec. 42(d)].

Control of doctors through control of the hospitals in which they practice will also be exercised by the Board by way of a list of requirements, the last of which is a "sleeper" that will by its vagueness allow the Board almost any regulation of the hospital: the hospital must meet "such other requirements as the Board finds necessary in the interest of quality of care and the safety of patients in the institution" [Sec. 43(i)]. Hospitals will also not be allowed to undertake construction without higher approval by a state agency or by the Board (Sec. 52).

In the name of better organization and co-ordination of services, hospitals, nursing homes and other providers will be further controlled through the Board's power to issue directives forcing the provider to furnish services selected by the Board [Sec. 131 (a)(1),(2)] at a place selected by the Board [Sec. 131(a)(3)]. The Board can also direct these providers to form associations with one another of various sorts, including "making available to one provider the professional and technical skills of another" [Sec.

131(a)(B)], and such other linkages as the Board thinks best [Sec. 131 (a)(4)(C)].

These are only a few of the bill's controls of the health-care industry. It is difficult to believe that such patent subjugation of an entire profession could ever be considered a fit topic for discussion in any but the darkest corner of a country founded on the principles of life and liberty. Yet the Kennedy-Griffiths bill is being seriously debated today in the Congress of the United States.

The irony of this bill is that, on the basis of the philosophic premises of its authors, it does provide a rationally organized system for attempting to fulfill its goals, such as "making health services available to all residents of the United States." If the government is to spend tens of billions of dollars on health services, it must assure in some way that the money is not being wasted. Every bill currently before the national legislature does, should, and must provide some such controls. The Kennedy-Griffiths bill is the closest we have yet come to the logical conclusion and inevitable consequence of two fundamental fallacies: that health care is a right, and that doctors and other health workers will function as efficiently serving as chattels of the state as they will living as sovereign human beings. It is not, and they will not.

Any act of force is anti-mind. It is a confession of the failure of persuasion, the failure of reason. When politicians say that the health system must be forced into a mold of their own design, they are admitting their inability to persuade doctors and patients to use the plan voluntarily; they are proclaiming the supremacy of the state's logic over the judgments of the individual minds of all concerned with health care. Statists throughout history have never learned that compulsion and reason are contradictory, that a forced mind cannot think effectively and, by extension, that a regimented profession will eventually choke and stagnate from its own lack of freedom. A persuasive example of this is the moribund condition of medicine as a profession in Sweden, a country that has enjoyed socialized medicine since 1955. Werkö, a

Swedish physician, has stated: "The details and the complicated working schedule have not yet been determined in all hospitals and districts, but the general feeling of belonging to a free profession, free to decide—at least in principle—how to organize its work has been lost. Many hospital-based physicians regard their work now with an apathy previously unknown."[4] One wonders how American legislators will like having their myocardial infarctions treated by apathetic internists, their mitral valves replaced by apathetic surgeons, their wives' tumors removed by apathetic gynecologists. They will find it very difficult to legislate self-esteem, integrity and competence into the doctors whose minds and judgments they have throttled.

If anyone doubts that health legislation involves the use of force, a dramatic demonstration of the practical political meaning of the "right to health care" was acted out in Quebec in the closing months of 1970.[5] In that unprecedented threat of violence by a modern Western government against a group of its citizens, the doctors of Quebec were literally imprisoned in the province by Bill 41, possibly the most repressive piece of legislation ever enacted against the medical profession, and far more worthy of the Soviet Union or Red China than a western democracy. Doctors objecting to a new Medicare law were forced to continue working under penalty of jail sentence and fines of up to $500 a day away from their practices. Those who spoke out publicly against the bill were subject to jail sentences of up to a year and fines of up to $50,000 a day. The facts that the doctors did return to work and that no one was therefore jailed or fined do not mitigate the nature or implications of the passage of Bill 41. Although the dispute between the Quebec physicians and their government was not one of principle but of the details of compensation, the reaction of the state to resistance against coercive professional regulation was a classic example of the naked force that lies behind every act of social legislation.

Any doctor who is forced by law to join a group or a hospital he does not choose, or is prevented by law from prescribing a drug he thinks is best for his patient, or is compelled by law to

make any decision he would not otherwise have made, is being forced to act against his own mind, which means forced to act against his own life. He is also being forced to violate his most fundamental professional commitment, that of using his own best judgment at all times for the greatest benefit of his patient. It is remarkable that this principle has never been identified by a public voice in the medical profession, and that the vast majority of doctors in this country are being led down the path to civil servitude, never knowing that their feelings of uneasy foreboding have a profoundly moral origin, and never recognizing that the main issues at stake are not those being formulated in Washington, but are their own honor, integrity and freedom, and their own survival as sovereign human beings.

Some Corollaries

The basic fallacy that health care is a right has led to several corollary fallacies, among them the following:

That health is primarily a community or social rather than an individual concern.[6] A simple calculation from American mortality statistics[7] quickly corrects that false concept: 67 per cent of deaths in 1967 were due to diseases known to be caused or exacerbated by alcohol, tobacco smoking or overeating, or were due to accidents. Each of those factors is either largely or wholly correctable by individual action. Although no statistics are available, it is likely that morbidity, with the exception of common respiratory infections, has a relation like that of mortality to personal habits and excesses.

That state medicine has worked better in other countries than free enterprise has worked here. There is no evidence to support that contention, other than anecdotal testimonials and the spurious citation of infant mortality and longevity statistics. There is, on the other hand, a good deal of evidence to the contrary.[8,9]

That the provision of medical care somehow lies outside the laws of supply and demand, and that government-controlled health care will be free care. In fact, no service or commodity lies outside the economic laws. Regarding health care, market demand, individual want, and medical need are entirely different things, and have a very complex relation with the cost and the total supply of available care, as recently discussed and clarified by Jeffers et al.[10] They point out that "'health is purchaseable,' meaning that somebody has to pay for it, individually or collectively, at the expense of foregoing the current or future consumption of other things." The question is whether the decision of how to allocate the consumer's dollar should belong to the consumer or to the state. It has already been shown that the choice of how a doctor's services should be rendered belongs only to the doctor: in the same way the choice of whether to buy a doctor's service rather than some other commodity or service belongs to the consumer as a logical consequence of the right to his own life.

That opposition to national health legislation is tantamount to opposition to progress in health care. Progress is made by the free interaction of free minds developing new ideas in an atmosphere conducive to experimentation and trial. If group practice really is better than solo, we will find out because the success of groups will result in more groups (which has, in fact, been happening); if prepaid comprehensive care really is the best form of practice, it will succeed and the health industry will swell with new Kaiser-Permanente plans. But let one of these or any other form of practice become the law, and the system is in a straitjacket that will stifle progress. Progress requires freedom of action, and that is precisely what national health legislation aims at restricting.

That doctors should help design the legislation for a national health system, since they must live with and within whatever legislation is enacted. To accept this concept is to concede to the opposition its philosophic premises, and thus to lose the battle. The means by which nonproducers and hangers-on throughout history have been able to expropriate material and intellectual values from the producers has been identified only relatively recently: the sanction of the victim.[11] Historically, few people have lost their freedom and

their rights without some degree of complicity in the plunder. If the American medical profession accepts the concept of health care as the right of the patient, it will have earned the Kennedy-Griffiths bill by default. The alternative for any health professional is to withhold his sanction and make clear who is being victimized. Any physician can say to those who would shackle his judgment and control his profession: I do not recognize your right to my life and my mind, which belong to me and me alone; I will not participate in any legislated solution to any health problem.

In the face of the raw power that lies behind government programs, nonparticipation is the only way in which personal values can be maintained. And it is only with the attainment of the highest of those values—integrity, honesty and self-esteem—that the physician can achieve his most important professional value, the absolute priority of the welfare of his patients.

The preceding discussion should not be interpreted as proposing that there are no problems in the delivery of medical care. Problems such as high cost, few doctors, low quantity of available care in economically depressed areas may be real, but it is naïve to believe that governmental solutions through coercive legislation can be anything but shortsighted and formulated on the basis of political expediency. The only long-range plan that can hope to provide for the day after tomorrow is a "nonsystem"—that is, a system that proscribes the imposition by force (legislation) of any one group's conception of the best forms of medical care. We must identify our problems and seek to solve them by experimentation and trial in an atmosphere of freedom from compulsion. Our sanction of anything less will mean the loss of our personal values, the death of our profession, and a heavy blow to political liberty.

References

1. Rand, A., *Man's Rights, Capitalism: The Unknown Ideal.* New York: New American Library, Inc., 1967, pp. 320–329.

2. Von Mises, L., *Socialism: An Economic and Sociological Analysis.* New Haven: Yale University Press, 1951, pp. 37–55.

3. Kennedy, E. M., Introduction of the Health Security Act. *Congressional Record* 116:S 14338–S 14361, 1970.

4. Werkö, L. Swedish medical care in transition. *N. Engl. J. Med.* 284:360–366, 1971.

5. *Quebec Medicare and Medical Services Withdrawal.* Toronto: Canadian Medical Association, October 19, 1970.

6. Millis, J. S., Wisdom? Health? Can society guarantee them? *N. Engl. J. Med.* 283:260–261, 1970.

7. Department of Health, Education, and Welfare, Public Health Service, *Vital Statistics of the United States 1967.* Vol. II, *Mortality,* Part A. Washington, D.C.: Government Printing Office, 1969, pp. 1–7.

8. *Financing Medical Care: An Appraisal of Foreign Programs.* Edited by H. Shoeck. Caldwell, Idaho: Caxton Printers, Inc., 1962.

9. Lynch, M. J., Raphael, S. S., *Medicine and the State.* Springfield, Ill.: Charles C Thomas, 1963.

10. Jeffers, J. R., Bognanno, M. F., Bartlett, J. C., On the demand versus need for medical services and the concept of "shortage." *Am. J. Publ. Health.* 61:46–63, 1971.

11. Rand, A., *Atlas Shrugged.* New York: Random House, 1957, p. 1066.

92

Letters to the Editor in Response to Sade's Essay

Reprinted with permission of the publisher from the *New England Journal of Medicine*, vol. 286, 1972, pp. 488–493.

Medical Care as a Right

To the Editor: To anyone concerned with this society's headlong rush into the New Dark Age, the essay by Dr. Sade is a thoughtful, concise statement of the most important issue of our time: the abrogation of individual rights. The society that fosters the notion that its members have a right to health care, or to the minds and services of any person or group, will have no compunctions about forcing individuals or groups to provide those services. The final inversion will be for government to assume control over professional education. Those with certain aptitudes, as established and judged by the state, will be given the "free choice" of entering designated "needy professions of low personnel density" or receiving no higher education at all. Specialist training and physician placement will be determined by a population-profession ratio determined by some bureaucratic "boffin" (scientific or technical expert) whose main concern is control of his peers rather than care of people. The wishes and aspirations of the individual will be dismissed as irrelevant—as indeed they are in a controlled society. As the quality of medical care declines, those in authority will place the blame upon their victims, the practicing doctors. The laymen will be told that avarice and greed and lack of altruistic motivation on the part of doctors are responsible for the slow disintegration of medicine. Governments are not interested in quality, for excellence cannot be controlled. The goal is a standard level of mediocrity. Only doctors who regard themselves as chattels of society can find any comfort in these certainties. There will be little or no protest from the other professions, or from anyone else. People whose minds have been numbed by those modern comprachicos, the educators, who believe that moral values are relative and negotiable, that the state has a valid claim to the lives of its citizens, that government by extortion is justified, that the "rights of society" are in some indefinable manner greater than the rights of an individual, will not balk at the total subjugation of the medical profession. A society that has meekly acquiesced in the military draft, compulsory arbitration, compulsory unionism and wage and price controls,

and has accepted the notion that any demand, no matter how whimsical or irrational, that is put forward under the egis of "social action" constitutes a right, is philosophically bankrupt. The psychologic cripples in medicine and government who seek control of our or any other profession can succeed only by achieving control over individuals. Once the right of a single man to his own life and the product of his own mind is abrogated, all men shortly find themselves pawns of the state to be manipulated or sacrificed as the exigencies of the moment demand. Every Utopia is built of the bricks of "controlled freedom" held together by the blood of free men, and is dedicated to the obscenity: "from each according to his ability, to each according to his need."

If anyone thinks the foregoing is simplistic alarmism, let him contemplate the recent activities of the governments of British Columbia and Quebec. In the former province, an attempt is being made to seize control of hospital accreditation committees with the express purpose of deciding who can go where and do what. Dr. Sade has described what happened in Quebec. He did not mention the "regionalization boards," committees of anyone at all preferably containing no practicing doctors, that purport to define the medical needs of a given area, and to direct the placement of suitable "personnel."

It is time for responsible and honest men in and out of medicine to wake up and appreciate the extent of the assault being directed at our professional and personal freedom.

A. L. Amacher, M.D., F.R.C.S. (C)
Victoria Hospital
London, Ontario, Canada

To the Editor: I read with interest Dr. Sade's recent article entitled "Medical Care as a Right: A refutation." At a time when many aspects of our lives seem to be controlled by large, impersonal forces beyond our influence, I am certainly sympathetic and agree with Dr. Sade's deep concern for the freedom of the individual to direct his life as he chooses. However, we live in complex times. It is no longer possible—if it in fact ever was—to pursue one set of rights or interest to their logical conclusions while disregarding the consequences that this may have for those who are affected by our actions.

Today's physician, regardless of his form of practice, is not a rugged individualist who has "made it" on his own. On the contrary, society has provided a helping hand every step of the way. No medical student or physician during his period of postgraduate training completely supports his own educational process. Public funds are utilized in the support of his education either as direct subsidies or as part of grants from government, foundations and voluntary health agencies. Public monies also fund the research that improves the state of the physician's art, helps to build the hospital where he works and as often as not pays the fees of his patients.

Our society has come to consider health care more a matter of public interest and safety than a straightforward marketing of services. Clearly, the consumers of health care are no longer prepared to step aside and allow the physician to continue to act as an individual entrepreneur with no regard for the effects of his actions on the society around him. The consumers' perceived right to health and to life itself are no less strongly held than the perceived right of the physician to regulate his delivery of services.

This is not a win-or-lose situation. The consumer will not accept a "public-be-damned attitude," and the physician will not and should not work on demand. As an intelligent community of professionals we must work with those who represent the public interest to develop new methods of attaining a relation between the physician and the consumer that maximizes the rights and interests of all concerned.

Stanley S. Bergen, Jr., M.D.
College of Medicine and
Dentistry of New Jersey
Newark, N.J.

To the Editor: The article by Dr. Robert Sade, "Medical Care as a Right: A refutation" itself deserves to be refuted. Dr. Sade considers the concept of medical care as a right to be immoral because it requires governmental involvement in medical-care provision. In his view, medical care is properly a matter of self-determined action by free individuals; the seeking of services by patients; the providing of services by physicians. Governmental involvement is coercive and violates the free society of physicians and patients.

The trouble with this libertarian concept of medical-care provision is that it is almost totally unreal. Medical care may have been purely a matter of freely contracting individuals in the days of Locke and Burke, to whom Dr. Sade refers. It is certainly no longer that today. A variety of corporate bodies play major parts on the medical-care scene—hospital boards, hospital staffs, medical societies, specialty boards, accrediting bodies, insurance companies, labor unions, businesses, health and welfare funds, citizens' organizations. Can anyone pretend that medical care in the United States is not powerfully influenced by organizations like these? Do physicians and patients really function solely as autonomous individuals?

At the clinical level, transactions between physician and patient are still, and should remain, a matter of individual determination. However, the organizational and financial framework in which they take place are determined by a host of groups—groups that are mostly nongovernmental but impose major constraints on individuals nevertheless. This private structure of medical care has failed to serve satisfactorily an increasing number of citizens. That is why government involvement has grown. Dr. Sade may believe that government's only proper function is to provide people with physical security. For many of us, however, government is much more: it is the mechanism through which people may deal collectively with their problems in the most just and equitable manner.

David Savitz, M.D.
Reynolds Memorial Hospital
Winston-Salem, N.C.

To the Editor: I was surprised and dismayed to read the special article "Medical Care as a Right: A refutation" by Dr. Robert M. Sade in the Journal.

The article reveals clearly that Dr. Sade is fighting valiantly in a war that his side lost a long time ago. He says, "The only proper function of government: to provide for the defense of individuals against those who would take their lives or property by force." Should public schools, including most of our medical schools be closed? Should health departments, government-owned utilities and highways be abandoned? Or does he think all government functions except the police and armed forces should be turned over to private enterprise?

Whether an individual is a baker or a physician, the product or service provided by his labor is not his to do with as he pleases. Whether we like it or not there must be restrictions if we are to have a stable just society.

Dr. Sade states that medicine as a profession is moribund in Sweden and uses a quotation from Dr. Werkö's article to support this allegation. Dr. Werkö's article gave a very good description of the Swedish medical system and its problems, particularly from the point of view of the hospital-based specialist, but it did not even suggest that the Swedish medical profession was moribund.

My own observation of the Swedish medical system showed that all Swedish citizens have access to good medical care without severe financial strain. I dislike much in their system, but they have accomplished this and we have not. The medical facilities and the medicine practiced in Sweden are excellent.

Dr. Sade says that we should not help design a national health system. If we want to practice good medicine in the future, we had better help design it. Swedish physicians have said that if they had participated fully in the development of their national medical-care system from the first, instead of resisting it, the physicians there would now have things more to their liking.

The South continued to fight the Civil War long after it lost, with resulting bitterness and slowed progress that has not yet been completely overcome. Will the medical profession continue to battle against a co-ordinated comprehensive health-care system now that the question is decided? The "reconstruction period" will be rough if we are victims instead of participants.

James H. Sanders, Jr., M.D.
Brevard, N.C.

To the Editor: If I understand Dr. Sade, his logic goes something like this: a doctor's ability to earn a living is defined solely by his own "thought and effort"; furthermore, doctors must be allowed to earn this living at all cost, therefore, doctors must be allowed to earn this living in any way they choose, without "outside" interference from well meaning but morally myopic patients and politicians.

Terrific! Now I can forget about all the dumb people who paid millions in taxes to help build my medical school and finance my education: now I can forget about poor city and farm folk whom I need not worry about serving any more, and now I can forget about peers and professors "immorally" persecuting me with obnoxious reviews and re-examinations. Best of all, I can forget about the non-dollar "relationship" part of the doctor-patient relationship. After all, anyone bothering me on the telephone about warts or worries when I could be seeing another paying patient is wasting my time and his.

Yet I sometimes do feel the prick of an obligation toward those who put me in the position of maximizing the gains of my "thought and effort." Sometimes, I do believe that not everyone is in the position of being able to put dollars down for my professional services, let alone being in a posh enough suburban location to get them. Sometimes, I do think that we doctors and future doctors are going to use our "thought and effort" to earn a living by manipulating our patients' market demand for medical services far more than we like to admit.[1] Sometimes, I do regard our medical profession's history of building a "rigid, self-perpetuating mystique about its knowledge, its jurisdiction, its practices, its prerogatives, and its mission"[2] as introducing an inequality into Dr. Sade's moral equations. Worst of all, sometimes I get the uncomfortable feeling that those I will serve should have some say so about how I serve them.

Silly thoughts, I know. Immoral, even. So let us put them aside and instead take up the heroic struggle of Quebec's courageous defenders of professional integrity. Let us unite and fight the repressive, evil patient-

bureaucrat-politician complex until we have shed our last green drop.

Jeff Brown, M.P.H.
Stanford Medical School
Stanford, Cal.

1. Brown, J., Diagnosing and Rehabilitating the Medical Marketplace. Bennett essay on the business and politics of medical care in America. Berkeley, University of California Archives, May, 1971.

2. Freidson, E., *Profession of Medicine: A Study of the Sociology of Applied Knowledge.* New York: Dodd, Mead, and Company, 1970, p. 374.

To the Editor: Dr. Sade's defense of a racist and discriminatory American health system is but a natural consequence of his support for the American economic system. He asserts that "The right to private property . . . is essential and indispensable to maintaining free men in a free society." The "freedoms" and "rights" to which he refers are bourgeois freedoms and rights—they are reserved principally for America's ruling class. That such a ruling class exists is easily demonstrable. From the Wall Street Journal we learn that the 200 largest corporations in America own 40 per cent of this country. From the FCC we learn that 90 per cent of all campaign funds come from approximately 1 per cent of the people. American imperialism abroad is but a logical extension of domestic imperialism; the ruling class in America owns 40 per cent of the world's natural resources.

Dr. Sade is under the illusion that the American worker has control over his or her life. In reality, the American worker (assuming that he or she is fortunate enough to be able to find a job) has little control over where, when or how he or she works and has no influence at all over what is produced, why it is produced, for whom it is produced, or what is done with the products of labor. Rather, it is the capitalist class and its various appendages that makes these crucial decisions owing to the fact that this class owns and controls the means of production and, consequently, the working class.

"Free enterprise," then, means the freedom for the ruling class freely to oppress and exploit the working class with relative impunity. Profit motive, and the demands of the market place predominate: human needs are important only so far as they may contribute

to the maintenance of the status quo. It is upon the economic base of corporate capitalism that the various suprastructures are built, the medical-care system included. It should therefore come as no surprise that medical care in America is reserved primarily for those who have enough money to pay its exorbitant costs.

Thus, it is no coincidence that in the richest country in the world, over 60 million people live in poverty or deprivation (as defined by the United States Government). It is no coincidence that America ranks 15th in the world infant mortality rates, and that four times as many black women die at childbirth as white women.

Dr. Sade's defense of the present American medical system is a defense of racism, inequality and oppression. The end of such a system will come with the end of corporate capitalism, and only then will the full potential of man and womankind, as well as the full potential of medicine as a liberating and creative force, be realized.

Mark Nelson
Case Western Reserve University
Medical School
Cleveland, O.

Sade on the Right: A Refutation

To the Editor:

Bread is life. And the price is right—
   for the Baker King. What's more, he bakes
the kind he likes — and bids the rest
   eat cake.

The hungry line outside his door
   can wait. "No help needed, Mr. Kennedy,"
Too many bakers spoil . . .
   the spoils.

It's late. And while the leavened coffers rise,
   with a golden glow that fills his eyes,
he does not see those hungry guys
   turn toward a different bakery.

J. Dennis Mull, M.D.
Cohasset, Mass.

The above letters were referred to the author of the article in question, who offers the following reply:

To the Editor: Because of limited rebuttal space, I include a few general references that provide detailed refutation of those objections to my argument that are not discussed here.[1-3] I urge the objectors who have obviously not done so to read the references appended to my original article.

Wishful thinking and a conciliatory attitude cannot change the fact that all legislation is ultimately dependent upon the threat of physical violence. Initiation of the use of force in the name of the public good, social welfare, the state, the king and so forth is the great destroyer of civilized society. The consequence of the destruction of the free interaction of physicians with their patients and society as a whole will be the disintegration of quality in American medical care. Nonparticipation remains the most effective and moral method to avoid professional self-immolation.

An open marketplace is not "demeaning," and can be threatening only to one who has something to hide in the quality of his product or service. There is no higher mark of respect for one's fellow than to trade with him openly and freely, value for value. For physicians, the value received need not always be money: American physicians traditionally have often accepted as fair exchange for their services the intangible value of their patient's appreciative "Thank you." But when the relation between men is altered by the intrusion of a legislative gun, benevolence disappears, and fear becomes the currency of exchange. One wonders who really projects a "calloused disregard for human interaction based upon trust and compassion," the man who wishes to trade voluntarily with others to their mutual benefit with mutual respect, or the man who thinks it necessary and proper to deal with other men in terms of whose legislative power is greater.

It is certainly true that there are many "groups that are nongovernmental but impose major constraints on individuals nonetheless." However, one cannot fail to recognize the elementary difference between those groups and the government: the first cannot use force to settle a disagreement; the second can and does. Hospital boards, medical societies, insurance companies and the rest have a very important role in the care of patients and in the professional lives of physicians, but they cannot *force* either patients or physicians to do anything, except by voluntary contract.

By the same token, the patient does indeed have just as much a right to his own life as the physician has to his, but both rights end where the other's physical integrity begins. The "right" of a patient or his agent to force a physician to take care of his medical needs has the same moral basis as the "right" of Nazi physicians to force concentration-camp "patients" to lie down on their operating tables. Those "rights" are exactly reciprocal and equally nonexistent.

The argument that society has paid part of the educational costs of the physician and therefore has the right to force him to practice on the terms that it dictates reveals a totalitarian mentality. Nearly everyone in the country has had at least some of his education subsidized by the state; therefore, the argument logically concludes, the state has the right to direct the lives of all its citizens. A very neat package, indeed.

Finally, it cannot be emphasized enough that in the attempt to solve medical-care problems by legislative fiat, American political freedom is being sacrificed to a system that has failed to achieve its own goals wherever it has been tried.[4]

Robert M. Sade, M.D.
Boston, Mass.

1. Rand, A., *Capitalism: The Unknown Ideal*. New York: New American Library, Inc., 1967.

2. Von Mises, L., *Socialism: An Economic and Sociological Analysis*. New Haven: Yale University Press, 1951.

3. Rand, A., *Atlas Shrugged*. New York: Random House, 1957.

4. Lynch, M. J., Raphael, S. S., *Medicine and the State*. Springfield, Ill.: Charles C Thomas, 1963.

93

Charles Fried
From "Equality and Rights in Medical Care"

Reprinted with deletions by permission of the author. Copyright ©1976 by Charles Fried. Originally published in *Hastings Center Report,* vol. 6, no. 1, February 1976, pp. 30–32.

... A right is more than just an interest that an individual might have, a state of affairs or a state of being which an individual might prefer. A claim of right invokes entitlements; and when we speak of entitlements, we mean not those things which it would be nice for people to have, or which they would prefer to have, but which they must have, and which if they do not have they may demand, whether we like it or not. Although I would not want to say that a right is something we must recognize "no matter what," nevertheless a right is something we must accord unless _____ and what we put in to fill in the unless clause should be tightly confined and specific.

This notion of rights has interesting and not altogether obvious relations to the concept of equality, and confusions about those relations are very likely to lead to confused arguments about the very area before us—rights to health care and equality in respect to health care.

First, it should be noted that equality itself may be considered a right. Thus, a person can argue that he is not necessarily entitled to any particular thing—whether it be income, or housing, or education, or health care—but that he is entitled to equality in respect to that thing, so that whatever anyone gets he should get, too. And this is a nice example of my previous proposition about the notion of rights generally. For to recognize a right to equality may very well be—I suppose it often is—contrary to many other policies that we may have, and particularly contrary to attempts to attain some kind of efficiency. Yet, by the very notion of rights, if there is a right to equality, then granting equality cannot depend on whether or not it is efficient to do so.

Second, there is the relation between rights and equality which runs the other way, too: to say that a class of persons, or all persons, have a certain right implies that they all have that right equally. If it is said that all persons within the jurisdiction of the United States have a constitutionally protected right to freedom of speech, whatever that may mean, one thing seems clear: that this right should not depend on what it is one wants to say,

who one is, and the like. Indeed, if the government against whom this right is protected were to make such distinctions, for instance, subjecting to constraints the speech of "irresponsible persons," that would be the exact concept of denial of freedom of speech to those persons.

These relations between the notion of right and of equality suggest the great importance of being very clear and precise about how a particular right is conceived: confusions in this regard are rampant in respect to health, and are the source of much pointless controversy. But because the point is quite general, let me first take an example from another area. If we were sloppy in our thinking about what the right of freedom of speech is—and many people are as sloppy about that as they are about their definition of the rights in the area which is our immediate concern—if we were sloppy about that definition, we might, for instance, consider that there has been a denial of right because some people have access to radio or television in getting their ideas across, while others have only the street-corner soapbox to broadcast their views. Indeed, there are those who might find it unjust that even on the soapbox the timid or inarticulate are much less effective than the bold or eloquent. All of these disparities, of course, may or may not be regrettable but they have nothing to do with freedom of speech as a right, given the premise that there is a right to free speech and that this right must be an equal right. It seems clear to me that it is very different from the right to be heard, believed, admired, and applauded. The right to speak freely is just that: a right to be free of constraints and impositions on whatever speaking one might wish to do, should you be able to find someone to listen.

Now this analogy is offered as more than a distant irrelevance. Is it not very similar to many things that are said in the area of health? For analogous to the claim that the right to freedom of speech really implies a right to be heard by the multitude, is the notion that whatever rights might exist in respect to health care are rights to health, rather than to health *care*. And of course the claim is equally absurd in both instances. We may sensibly guarantee that all will be equally free of constraints on the speaking they

wish to do, but we should not guarantee that all will be equally effective in getting their views across. Similarly, we may or may not choose to guarantee all equality of access to health care, but we cannot possibly guarantee to all equality of health. . . .

Equality and Rights: Analytical Distinctions

. . . Our present dilemma comes from the fact that there are very many expensive things that medicine can do which might possibly help. And if we commit ourselves to the notion that there is a right to whatever health care might be available, we do indeed get ourselves into a difficult situation where overall national expenditure on health must reach absurd proportions—absurd in the sense that far more is devoted to health at the expense of other important social goals than the population in general wants. Indeed, more is devoted to health than the population wants relative not only to important social goals—for example, education or housing—but relative to all the other things which people would like to have money left over to pay for. And if we recognize that it would be absurd to commit our society to devote more than a certain proportion of our national income to health, while at the same time recognizing a "right to health care," we might then be caught on the other horn of the dilemma. For we might then be required to say that because a right to health care implies a right to equality of health care, then we must limit, we must lower the quality of the health care that might be purchased by some lest our commitment to equality require us to provide such care to all and thus carry us over a reasonable budget limit.

Consider the case of the artificial heart. It seems to me not too fanciful an assumption that such a device is technically feasible within a reasonable time, and likely to be hugely expensive both in terms of its actual implantation and in terms of the subsequent care required by those benefiting from the device. Now if the right to health care is taken to mean the right to whatever health care is available to anybody, and if this entails that it is a right to an equal enjoyment of whatever care anyone else enjoys, then what are we to do with respect to the artificial heart?

Might we decide not to develop such a device? Though the development and experimental use of it involves an entirely tolerable burden, the general provision of the artificial heart would be an intolerable burden, and since if we provide it to any we must provide it to all, therefore perhaps we should provide it to none.

This solution seems to me to be both uncomfortable and unstable. For surely there is something odd, if not perverse, about foregoing research on such devices, not because the research might fail, but because it might succeed. Might not this research then go on under some kinds of private auspices if such a governmental decision were made? Would we then go further and forbid even private research, rather than simply refusing to fund it? I can well imagine the next step, where artificial heart research and implantation would become like abortion or sex change operations in the old days: something one went to Sweden or Denmark for. Nor is a lottery device for distributing a limited number of artificial hearts likely to be more stable or satisfactory. For there, too, would we forbid people to go outside the lottery? Would it be a crime to cross national boundaries with the intent of obtaining an artificial heart? The example makes a general point about instituting an all-inclusive "right to health care," with the necessary concomitant of an equal right to whatever health care is available. For if we really instituted such a right and limited the provision of health care to a reasonable level, we would have to institute as well a degree of stringent state control, which it is both unlikely we can achieve and undesirable for us even to try to achieve. There is something that goes very deeply against the grain about any scheme which prohibits scientists from making discoveries which no one claims are harmful as such, but which will cause trouble because we can't give them to everybody. There is something which goes against the grain in a system which might forbid individual doctors to render a service, not because it is harmful, but because its benefits are not available to all.

Or take a much less dramatic case—dental care. It is said that ordinary basic prophylactic care is so lacking for tens of millions of our citizens that quite unnecessarily they do not have their own teeth while still in their prime. I take it that to provide the kind of elaborate dental care deployed on affluent suburban families to rural populations, and to all even poorer urban dwellers, would be a prodigiously expensive undertaking, one that would cost each of us quite heavily. But if we followed the slogan, "The best available made available to all," that is what is meant. My guess is the American people would not want to bear this burden and that as a form of transfer payment the poor would prefer just to have the money to spend on other things. But this shows the dangerousness of slogans, for perhaps the greatest part of the dental damage could be remedied at far less cost by fluoridation and by relatively routine care provided by a type of modestly trained person who is only now beginning to exist. Care of this sort can be afforded and should be provided. But this would mean abandoning the concept of equality and accepting the fact that the poor would be getting less elaborate care than those who are not poor.

Now it might be said that I am exaggerating. The case put forward is the British National Health Service, which is alleged to provide a model of high level care at reasonable costs with equality for all. But I would caution planners and enthusiasts from drawing too much from this example. The situation in Great Britain is very different in many ways. The country is smaller and more homogeneous. Moreover, even in Great Britain there are disparities between the care available between urban and rural areas; there are long waits for so-called elective procedures; and there is a small but significant and distinguished private sector outside of National Health which is the focus of great controversy and rancor. Finally, Great Britain is a country where a substantial portion of the citizenry is committed to the socialist ideal of equalizing incomes and nationalizing the provisions of all vital services. Surely this is a very different situation from that in the United States. Indeed, it may be that the cry for equality of access to health care bears to a general yearning for social equality much the same relation that the opposition to fetal research bears to the opposition to abortion. In each case it is a very large ideological tail wagging a relatively small and confused dog.

My point is analytical. My point is that apart from a rather general commitment to equality and, indeed, to state control of the allocation and distribution of resources, to insist on the right to health care, where that right means a right to equal access, is an anomaly. For as long as our society considers that inequalities of wealth and income are morally acceptable—acceptable in the sense that the system that produces these inequalities is in itself not morally suspect—it is anomalous to carve out a sector like health care and say that *there* equality must reign.

Towards a Better Definition of the Rights Involved

After all, is health care so special? Is it different from education, housing, food, legal assistance? In respect to all of these things, we recognize in our society a right, whose enjoyment may not be made wholly dependent upon the ability to pay. But just as surely in respect to all these things, we do not believe that this right entails equality of enjoyment, so that whatever diet one person or class of persons enjoys must be enjoyed by all. The argument, put forward for instance by some members of the Labor Party in Great Britain, that the independent schools in that country should be abolished because they offer a level of education better than that available in state schools, is an argument which would be found strange and repellent in the United States. Rather, in all of these areas—education, housing, food, legal assistance—there obtains a notion of a decent, fair standard, such that when this standard is satisfied all that exists in the way of *rights* has been accorded. And it is necessarily so; were we to insist on equality all the way up, that is, past this minimum, we would have committed ourselves to a political philosophy which I take it is not the dominant one in our society.

Is health care different? Everything that can be said about health care is true of food and is at least by analogy true of education, housing, and legal assistance. The real task before us is not, therefore, I think, to explain why there must be complete equality in medicine, but the more subtle and perilous task of determining the decent minimum in respect to health which accords with sound ethical judgments, while maintaining the virtues of freedom, variety, and flexibility which are thought to flow from a mixed system such as ours. The decent minimum should reflect some conception of what constitutes tolerable life prospects in general. It should speak quite strongly to things like maternal health and child health, which set the terms under which individuals will compete and develop. On the other hand, techniques which will offer some remote relief from conditions that rarely strike in the prime of life, and which strike late in life because something must, might be thought of as too esoteric to be part of the concept of minimum decent care.

On the other hand, the notion of a decent minimum should include humane and, I would say, worthy surroundings of care for those whom we know we are not going to be able to treat. Here, it seems to me, the emphasis on technology and the attention of highly trained specialists is seriously mistaken. Not only is it unrealistic to imagine that such fancy services can be provided for everyone "as a right," but there is serious doubt whether these kinds of services are what most people really want or can benefit from.

In the end, I will concede very readily that the notion of minimum health care, which it does make sense for our society to recognize as a right, is itself an unstable and changing notion. . . . [T]he concept of a decent minimum is always relative to what is available over all, and what the best which is available might be. I suppose (to revert to my parable of the artificial heart) that if we allowed an artificial heart to be developed under private auspices and to be available only to those who could pay for it, or who could obtain it from specialized eleemosynary institutions, then the time might well come when it would have been so perfected that it would be a reasonable component of what one would consider minimum decent care. And the process of arriving at this new situation would be a process imbued with struggle and political controversy. But since I do not believe in utopias or final solutions, a resolution of the problem of the right to health care having these kinds of tensions within it neither worries me nor leads me to suspect that I am on the wrong track. To my mind, the right track consists in identifying what it is that health care can and cannot provide, in identifying also the cost of health care, and then in deciding how much of this health care, what level of health care, we are ready to underwrite as a floor for our citizenry.

94

Gene Outka
Social Justice and Equal Access to Health Care

Reprinted with permission of author and editor from the *Journal of Religious Ethics*, vol. 2/1, 1974, pp. 11–32.

I want to consider the following question. Is it possible to understand and to justify morally a societal goal which increasing numbers of people, including Americans, accept as normative? The goal is: the assurance of comprehensive health services for every person irrespective of income or geographic location. Indeed, the goal now has almost the status of a platitude. Currently in the United States politicians in various camps give it at least verbal endorsement (see, e.g., Nixon, 1972:1; Kennedy, 1972:234–252). I do not propose to examine the possible sociological determinants in this emergent consensus. I hope to show that whatever these determinants are, one may offer a plausible case in defense of the goal on reasonable grounds. To demonstrate why appeals to the goal get so successfully under our skins, I shall have recourse to a set of conceptions of social justice. Some of the standard conceptions, found in a number of writings on justice, will do (these writings include Bedau, 1971; Hospers, 1961:416–468; Lucas, 1972; Perelman, 1963; Rescher, 1966; Ryan, 1916; Vlastos, 1962). By reflecting on them it seems to me a prima facie case can be established, namely, that every person in the entire resident population should have equal access to health care delivery.

The case is prima facie only. I wish to set aside as far as possible a related question which comes readily enough to mind. In the world of "suboptimal alternatives," with the constraints for example which impinge on the government as it makes decisions about resource allocation, what is one to say? What criteria should be employed? Paul Ramsey, in *The Patient as Person* (1970:240), thinks that the large question of how to choose between medical and other societal priorities is "almost, if not altogether, incorrigible to moral reasoning." Whether it is or not is a matter which must be ignored for the present. One may simply observe in passing that choices are unavoidable nonetheless, as Ramsey acknowledges, even where the government allows them to be made by default, so that in some instances they are determined largely by which private pressure groups prove to be dominant. In any event, there is virtue in taking up one complicated question at a time and we need to get the thrust of the case for

equal access before us. It is enough to observe now that Americans attach an obviously high priority to organized health care. National health expenditures for the fiscal year 1972 were $83.4 billion (Hicks, 1973:52). Even if such an enormous sum is not entirely adequate, we may still ask: how are we to justify spending whatever we do in accordance as far as possible with the goal of equal access? The answer I propose involves distinguishing various conceptions of social justice and trying to show which of these apply or fail to apply to health care considerations. Only toward the end of the paper will some institutional implications be given more than passing attention, and then in a strictly programmatic way.

Another sort of query should be noted as we begin. What stake does someone in religious ethics have in this discussion? For the reasonable case envisaged is offered after all in the public forum. If the issue is how to justify morally the societal goal which seems so obvious to so many, whether or not they are religious believers, does the religious ethicist then simply participate qua citizen? Here I think we should be wary of simplifying formulae. Why for example should a Jew or a Christian not welcome wide support for a societal goal which he or she can affirm and reaffirm, or reflect only on instances where such support is not forthcoming? If a number of ethical schemes, both religious and humanist, converge in their acceptance of the goal of equal access to health care, so be it. Secularists can join forces with believers, at least at some levels or points, without implying there must be unanimity on every moral issue. Yet it also seems too simple if one claims to wear only the citizen's hat when making the case in question. At least I should admit that a commitment to the basic normative principle which in Christian writings is often called *agape* may influence the account to follow in ways large and small (see Outka, 1972). For example, someone with such a commitment will quite naturally take a special interest in appeals to the generic characteristics all persons share rather than the idiosyncratic attainments which distinguish persons from one another, and in the playing down of desert considerations. As I shall try to show, such appeals are centrally relevant to the case for equal access. And they are nicely in line with the normative pressures agapeic considerations typically exert.

One issue of theoretical importance in religious ethics also emerges in connection with this last point. The approach in this paper may throw a little indirect light on the traditional question, especially prominent in Christian ethics, of how love and justice are related. To distinguish different conceptions of social justice will put us in a better position, I think, to recognize that often it is ambiguous to ask about "*the* relation." There may be different relations to different conceptions. For the conceptions themselves may sometimes produce discordant indications, or turn out to be incommensurable, or reflect, when different ones are seized upon, rival moral points of view. I shall note several of these relations as we proceed.

Which then among the standard conceptions of social justice appear to be particularly relevant or irrelevant? Let us consider the following five:
1. To each according to his merit or desert.
2. To each according to his societal contribution.
3. To each according to his contribution in satisfying whatever is freely desired by others in the open marketplace of supply and demand.
4. To each according to his needs.
5. Similar treatment for similar cases.
In general I shall argue that the first three of these are less relevant because of certain distinctive features which health crises possess. I shall focus on crises here not because I think preventive care is unimportant (the opposite is true), but because the crisis situation shows most clearly the special significance we attach to medical treatment as an institutionalized activity or social practice, and the basic purpose we suppose it to have.

I

To each according to his merit or desert. Meritarian conceptions, above all perhaps, are grading ones: advantages are allocated in accordance with amounts of energy expended or kinds of results achieved. What is judged is particular conduct which distinguishes persons from one another and not only

the fact that all the parties are human beings. Sometimes a competitive aspect looms large.

In certain contexts it is illuminating to distinguish between efforts and achievements. In the case of efforts one characteristically focuses on the individual: rewards are based on the pains one takes. Some have supposed, for example, that entry into the kingdom of heaven is linked more directly to energy displayed and fidelity shown than to successful results attained.

To assess achievements is to weigh actual performance and productive contributions. The academic prize is awarded to the student with the highest grade-point average, regardless of the amount of midnight oil he or she burned in preparing for the examinations. Sometimes we may exclaim, "it's just not fair," when person X writes a brilliant paper with little effort while we are forced to devote more time with less impressive results. But then our complaint may be directed against differences in innate ability and talent which no expenditure of effort altogether removes.

After the difference between effort and achievement, and related distinctions, have been acknowledged, what should be stressed I think is the general importance of meritarian or desert criteria in the thinking of most people about justice. These criteria may serve to illuminate a number of disputes about the justice of various practices and institutional arrangements in our society. It may help to explain, for instance, the resentment among the working class against the welfare system. However wrongheaded or self-deceptive the resentment often is, particularly when directed toward those who want to work but for various reasons beyond their control cannot, at its better moments it involves in effect an appeal to desert considerations. "Something for nothing" is repudiated as unjust; benefits should be proportional (or at least related) to costs; those who can make an effort should do so, whatever the degree of their training or significance of their contribution to society; and so on. So, too, persons deserve to have what they have labored for; unless they infringe on the works of others their efforts and achievements are justly theirs.

Occasionally the appeal to desert extends to a wholesale rejection of other considerations as grounds for just claims. The most conspicuous target is need. Consider this statement by Ayn Rand.

A morality that holds *need* as a claim, holds emptiness—nonexistence—as its standard of value; it rewards an absence, a defect: weakness, inability, incompetence, suffering, disease, disaster, the lack, the fault, the flaw—the *zero*.
Who provides the account to pay these claims? Those who are cursed for being non-zeros, each to the extent of his distance from that ideal. Since all values are the product of virtues, the degree of your virtue is used as the measure of your penalty; the degree of your faults is used as the measure of your gain. Your code declares that the rational man must sacrifice himself to the irrational, the independent man to parasites, the honest man to the dishonest, the man of justice to the unjust, the productive man to thieving loafers, the man of integrity to compromising knaves, the man of self-esteem to sniveling neurotics. Do you wonder at the meanness of soul in those you see around you? The man who achieves these virtues will not accept your moral code; the man who accepts your moral code will not achieve these virtues. (1957:958)

I have noted elsewhere (1972:89–90, 165–167) that *agape*, while it characteristically plays down, need not formally disallow attention to considerations falling under merit or desert; for in the case of merit as well as need it may be possible, the quotation above notwithstanding, to reason solely from egalitarian premises. A major reason such attention is warranted concerns what was called there the differential exercise of an equal liberty. That is, one may fittingly revere another's moral capacities and thus the efforts he makes as well as the ends he seeks. Such reverence may lead one to weigh expenditure of energy and specific achievements. I would simply hold now (1) that the idea of justice is not exhaustively characterized by the notion of desert, even if one agrees that the latter plays an important role; and (2) that the notion of desert is especially ill-suited to play an important role in the determination of policies which should govern a system of health care.

Why is it so ill-suited? Here we encounter some of the distinctive features which it seems to me health crises possess. Let me put it in this way. Health crises seem non-meritarian because they occur so often for reasons beyond our control or power to predict. They frequently fall without discrimination on the (according-to-merit) just and unjust, i.e., the virtuous and the wicked, the industrious and the slothful alike.

While we may believe that virtues and vices cannot depend upon natural contingencies, we are bound to admit, it seems, that many health crises do. It makes sense therefore to say that we are equal in being randomly susceptible to these crises. Even those who ascribe a prominent role to desert acknowledge that justice has also properly to do with pleas of "But I could not help it" (Lucas, 1972:321). One seeks to distinguish such cases from those acknowledged to be praiseworthy or blameworthy. Then it seems unfair as well as unkind to discriminate among those who suffer health crises on the basis of their personal deserts. For it would be odd to maintain that a newborn child deserves his hemophilia or the tumor afflicting her spine.

These considerations help to explain why the following rough distinction is often made. Bernard Williams, for example, in his discussion of "equality in unequal circumstances," identifies two different sorts of inequality, inequality of merit and inequality of need, and two corresponding goods, those earned by effort and those demanded by need (1971:126–137). Medical treatment in the event of illness is located under the umbrella of need. He concludes: "Leaving aside preventive medicine, the proper ground of distribution of medical care is ill health: this is a necessary truth" (1971:127). An irrational state of affairs is held to obtain if those whose needs are the same are treated unequally, when needs are the ground of the treatment. One might put the point this way. When people are equal in the relevant respects—in this case when their needs are the same and occur in a context of random, undeserved susceptibility—that by itself is a good reason for treating them equally (see also Nagel, 1973:354).

In many societies, however, a second necessary condition for the receipt of medical treatment exists de facto: the possession of money. This is not the place to consider the general question of when inequalities in wealth may be regarded as just. It is enough to note that one can plausibly appeal to all of the conceptions of justice we are embarked in sorting out. A person may be thought to be entitled to a higher income when he works more, contributes more, risks more, and not simply when he needs more. We may think it fair that the industrious should have more money than the slothful and the surgeon more than the tobacconist. The difficulty comes in the misfit between the reasons for differential incomes and the reasons for receiving medical treatment. The former may include a pluralistic set of claims in which different notions of justice must be meshed. The latter are more monistically focused on needs, and the other notions not accorded a similar relevance. Yet money may nonetheless remain as a causally necessary condition for receiving medical treatment. It may be the power to secure what one needs. The senses in which health crises are distinctive may then be insufficiently determinative for the policies which govern the actual availability of treatment. The nearly automatic links between income, prestige, and the receipt of comparatively higher quality medical treatment should then be subjected to critical scrutiny. For unequal treatment of the rich ill and the poor ill is unjust if, again, needs rather than differential income constitute the ground of such treatment.

Suppose one agrees that it is important to recognize the misfit between the reasons for differential incomes and the reasons for receiving medical treatment, and that therefore income as such should not govern the actual availability of treatment. One may still ask whether the case so far relies excessively on "pure" instances where desert considerations are admittedly out of place. That there are such pure instances, tumors afflicting the spine, hemophilia, and so on, is not denied. Yet it is an exaggeration if we go on and regard all health crises as utterly unconnected with desert. Note for example that Williams leaves aside preventive medicine. And if in a cool hour we examine the statistics, we find that a vast number of deaths occur each year due to causes not always beyond our control, e.g., automobile accidents, drugs, alcohol, tobacco, obesity, and so on. In some final reckoning it seems that many persons (though crucially, not all) have an effect on, and arguably a responsibility for, their own medical needs. Consider the following bidders for emergency care: (1) a person with a heart attack who is seriously overweight; (2) a football hero who has suffered a concussion; (3) a man with lung cancer who has smoked cigarettes for forty years; (4) a 60-year-old man who has always taken excellent care of himself and is suddenly stricken with leukemia; (5) a three-year-old girl who has swallowed poison left out carelessly by her parents; (6) a 14-year-old boy who has been beaten without provocation by a gang and suffers brain damage and recurrent attacks of uncontrollable terror; (7) a college student who has slashed his wrists (and not for the first time) from a psychological need for attention; (8) a woman raised in the ghetto who is found unconscious due to an overdose of heroin.

These cases help to show why the whole subject of medical treatment is so crucial and so perplexing. They attest to some melancholy elements in human experience. People suffer in varying ratios the effects of their natural and undeserved vulnerabilities, the irresponsibility and brutality of others, and their own desires and weaknesses. In some final reckoning then desert considerations seem not irrelevant to many health crises. The practical applicability of this admission, however, in the instance of health care delivery, appears limited. We may agree that it underscores the importance of preventive health care by stressing the influence we sometimes have over our medical needs. But if we try to foster such care by increasing the penalties for neglect, we normally confine ourselves to calculations about incentives. At the risk of being denounced in some quarters as censorious and puritanical, perhaps we should for example levy far higher taxes on alcohol and tobacco and pump the dollars directly into health care programs rather than (say) into highway building. Yet these steps would by no means lead necessarily to a demand that we correlate in some strict way a demonstrated effort to be temperate with the receipt of privileged medical treatment as a reward. Would it be feasible to allocate the additional

587 Equal Access to Health Care

tax monies to the man with leukemia before the overweight man suffering a heart attack on the ground of a difference in desert? At the point of emergency care at least, it seems impracticable for the doctor to discriminate between these cases, to make meritarian judgments at the point of catastrophe. And the number of persons who are in need of medical treatment for reasons utterly beyond their control remains a datum with tenacious relevance. There are those who suffer the ravages of a tornado, are handicapped by a genetic defect, beaten without provocation, etc. A commitment to the basic purpose of medical care and to the institutions for achieving it involves the recognition of this persistent state of affairs.

II

To each according to his societal contribution. This conception gives moral primacy to notions such as the public interest, the common good, the welfare of the community, or the greatest good of the greatest number. Here one judges the social consequences of particular conduct. The formula can be construed in at least two ways (Rescher, 1966:79–80). It may refer to the interest of the social group considered collectively, where the group has some independent life all its own. The group's welfare is the decisive criterion for determining what constitutes any member's proper share. Or the common good may refer only to an aggregation of distinct individuals and considered distributively.

Either version accords such a primacy to what is socially advantageous as to be unacceptable not only to defenders of need, but also, it would seem, of desert. For the criteria of effort and achievement are often conceived along rather individualistic lines. The pains an agent takes or the results he brings about deserve recompense, whether or not the public interest is directly served. No automatic harmony then is necessarily assumed between his just share as individually earned and his proper share from the vantage point of the common good. Moreover, the test of social advantage *simpliciter* obviously threatens the agapeic concern with some minimal consideration

due each person which is never to be disregarded for the sake of long-range social benefits. No one should be considered as *merely* a means or instrument.

The relevance of the canon of social productiveness to health crises may accordingly also be challenged. Indeed, such crises may cut against it in that they occur more frequently to those whose comparative contribution to the general welfare is less, e.g., the aged, the disabled, children.

Consider for example Paul Ramsey's persuasive critique of social and economic criteria for the allocation of a single scarce medical resource. He begins by recounting the imponderables which faced the widely discussed "public committee" at the Swedish Hospital in Seattle when it deliberated in the early 1960's. The sparse resource in this case was the kidney machine. The committee was charged with the responsibility of selecting among patients suffering chronic renal failure those who were to receive dialysis. Its criteria were broadly social and economic. Considerations weighed included age, sex, marital status, number of dependents, income, net worth, educational background, occupation, past performance and future potential. The application of such criteria proved to be exceedingly problematic. Should someone with six children always have priority over an artist or composer? Were those who arranged matters so that their families would not burden society to be penalized in effect for being provident? And so on. Two critics of the committee found "a disturbing picture of the bourgeoisie sparing the bourgeoisie" and observed that "the Pacific Northwest is no place for a Henry David Thoreau with bad kidneys" (quoted in Ramsey, 1970:248).

The mistake, Ramsey believes, is to introduce criteria of social worthiness in the first place. In those situations of choice where not all can be saved and yet all need not die, "the equal right of every human being to live, and not relative personal or social worth, should be the ruling principle" (1970:256). The principle leads to a criterion of "random choice among equals" expressed by a lottery scheme or a practice of "first-come, first-served." Several reasons stand behind Ramsey's defense of the criterion of random choice. First, a religious belief in the equality

of persons before God leads intelligibly to a refusal to choose between those who are dying in any way other than random patient selection. Otherwise their equal value as human beings is threatened. Second, a moral primacy is ascribed to survival over other (perhaps superior) interests persons may have, in that it is the condition of everything else. ". . . Life is a value incommensurate with all others, and so not negotiable by bartering one man's worth against another's" (1970:256). Third, the entire enterprise of estimating a person's social worth is viewed with final skepticism. ". . . We have no way of knowing how really and truly to estimate a man's societal worth or his worth to others or to himself in unfocused social situations in the ordinary lives of men in their communities" (1970:256). This statement, incidentally, appears to allow something other than randomness in *focused* social situations; when, say, a President or Prime Minister and the owner of the local bar rush for the last place in the bomb shelter, and the knowledge of the former can save many lives. In any event, I have been concerned with a restricted point to which Ramsey's discussion brings illustrative support. The canon of social productiveness is notoriously difficult to apply as a workable criterion for distributing medical services to those who need them.

One may go further. A system of health care delivery which treats people on the basis of the medical care required may often go against (at least narrowly conceived) calculations of societal advantage. For example, the health care needs of people tend to rise during that period of their lives, signaled by retirement, when their incomes and social productivity are declining. More generally:

Some 40 to 50 per cent of the American people—the aged, children, the dependent poor, and those with some significant chronic disability are in categories requiring relatively large amounts of medical care but with inadequate resources to purchase such care. (Somers, 1971a:20)

If one agrees, for whatever reasons, with the agapeic judgment that each person should be regarded as irreducibly valuable, then one cannot succumb to a social productiveness criterion of human worth. Interests are to be equally considered even when people have ceased to be, or are not yet, or perhaps never will be, public assets.

III

To each according to his contribution in satisfying whatever is freely desired by others in the open marketplace of supply and demand. Here we have a test which, though similar to the preceding one, concentrates on what is desired de facto by certain segments of the community rather than the community as a whole, and on the relative scarcity of the service rendered. It is tantamount to the canon of supply and demand as espoused by various laissez-faire theoreticians (cf. Rescher, 1966:80–81). Rewards should be given to those who by virtue of special skill, prescience, risk-taking, and the like discern what is desired and are able to take the requisite steps to bring satisfaction. A surgeon, it may be argued, contributes more than a nurse because of the greater training and skill required, burdens borne, and effective care provided, and should be compensated accordingly. So too perhaps, a star quarterback on a pro-football team should be remunerated even more highly because of the rare athletic prowess needed, hazards involved, and widespread demand to watch him play.

This formula does not then call for the weighing of the value of various contributions, and tends to conflate needs and wants under a notion of desires. It also assumes that a prominent part is assigned to consumer free-choice. The consumer should be at liberty to express his preferences, and to select from a variety of competing goods and services. Those who resist many changes currently proposed in the organization and financing of health care delivery in the U.S.A.—such as national health insurance—often do so by appealing to some variant of this formula.

Yet it seems health crises are often of overriding importance when they occur. They appear therefore not satisfactorily accommodated to the context of a free marketplace where consumers may freely choose among alternative goods and services.

To clarify what is at stake in the above contention, let us examine an opposing case. Robert M. Sade, M.D., published an article in *The New England Journal of Medicine* entitled "Medical Care as a Right: A Refutation" (1971) [Chapter 91, this volume]. He attacks programs of national health insurance in the name of a person's right to select one's own values, determine how they may be realized, and dispose of them if one chooses without coercion from other men. The values in question are construed as economic ones in the context of supply and demand. So we read:

In a free society, man exercises his right to sustain his own life by producing economic values in the form of goods and services that he is, or should be, free to exchange with other men who are similarly free to trade with him or not. The economic values produced, however, are not given as gifts by nature, but exist only by virtue of the thought and effort of individual men. Goods and services are thus owned as a consequence of the right to sustain life by one's own physical and mental effort. (1971:1289)

Sade compares the situation of the physician to that of the baker. The one who produces a loaf of bread should as owner have the power to dispose of his own product. It is immoral simply to expropriate the bread without the baker's permission. Similarly, "medical care is neither a right nor a privilege: it is a service that is provided by doctors and others to people who wish to purchase it" (1971:1289). Any coercive regulation of professional practices by the society at large is held to be analogous to taking the bread from the baker without his consent. Such regulation violates the freedom of the physician over his own services and will lead inevitably to provider-apathy.

The analogy surely misleads. To assume that doctors autonomously produce goods and services in a fashion closely akin to a baker is grossly oversimplified. The baker may himself rely on the agricultural produce of others, yet there is a crucial difference in the degree of dependence. Modern physicians depend on the achievements of medical technology and the entire scientific base underlying it, all of which is made possible by a host of persons whose salaries are often notably less. Moreover, the amount of taxpayer support for medical research and education is too enormous to make any such unqualified case for provider-autonomy plausible.

However conceptually clouded Sade's article may be, its stress on a free exchange of goods and services reflects one historically influential rationale for much American medical practice. And he applies it not only to physicians but also to patients or "consumers."

The question is whether the decision of how to allocate the consumer's dollar should belong to the consumer or to the state. It has already been shown that the choice of how a doctor's services should be rendered belongs only to the doctor: in the same way the choice of whether to buy a doctor's service rather than some other commodity or service belongs to the consumer as a logical consequence of the right to his own life. (1971:1291)

This account is misguided, I think, because it ignores the overriding importance which is so often attached to health crises. When lumps appear on someone's neck, it usually makes little sense to talk of choosing whether to buy a doctor's service rather than a color television set. References to just trade-offs suddenly seem out of place. No compensation suffices, since the penalties may differ so much.

There is even a further restriction on consumer choice. One's knowledge in these circumstances is comparatively so limited. The physician makes most of the decisions: about diagnosis, treatment, hospitalization, number of return visits, and so on. In brief:

The consumer knows very little about the medical services he is buying—probably less than about any other service he purchases. . . . While [he] can still play a role in policing the market, that role is much more limited in the field of health care than in almost any other area of private economic activity. (Schultze, 1972:214–215)

For much of the way, then, an appeal to supply and demand and consumer choice is not quite fitting. It neglects the issue of the value of various contributions. And it fails to allow for the recognition that medical treatments may be overridingly desired. In contexts of catastrophe at any rate, when life itself is threatened, most persons (other than those who are apathetic or seek to escape from the terrifying prospects) cannot take medical care to be merely one option among others.

IV

To each according to his needs. The concept of needs is sometimes taken to apply to an entire range of interests which concern a person's "psychophysical existence" (Outka, 1972:esp. 264–265). On this wide usage, to attribute a need to someone is to say that the person lacks what is thought to conduce to his or her "welfare"—understood in both a physiological sense (e.g., for food, drink, shelter, and health) and a psychological one (e.g., for continuous human affection and support).

Yet even in the case of such a wide usage, what the person lacks is typically assumed to be basic. Attention is restricted to recurrent considerations rather than to every possible individual whim or frivolous pursuit. So one is not surprised to meet with the contention that a preferable rendering of this formula would be: "to each according to his essential needs" (Perelman, 1963:22). This contention seems to me well taken. It implies, for one thing, that basic needs are distinguishable from felt needs or wants. For the latter may encompass expressions of personal preference unrelated to considerations of survival or subsistence, and sometimes artificially generated by circumstances of rising affluence in the society at large.

Essential needs are also typically assumed to be given rather than acquired. They are not constituted by any action for which the person is responsible by virtue of his or her distinctively greater effort. It is almost as if the designation "innocent" may be linked illuminatingly to need, as retribution, punishment, and so on, are to desert, and in complex ways, to freedom. Thus essential needs are likewise distinguishable from deserts. Where needs are unequal, one thinks of them as fortuitously distributed; as part, perhaps, of a kind of "natural lottery" (see Rawls, 1971: e.g., 104). So very often the advantages of health and the burdens of illness, for example, strike one as arbitrary effects of the lottery. It seems wrong to say that a newborn child deserves as a reward all of his faculties when he has done nothing in particular which distinguishes him from another newborn who comes into the world deprived of one or more of them. Similarly, though crudely, many religious believers do not look on

natural events as personal deserts. They are not inclined to pronounce sentences such as, "That evil person with incurable cancer got what he deserved." They are disposed instead to search for some distinction between what they may call the conditions of finitude on the one hand and sin and moral evil on the other. If the distinction is "ultimately" invalid, in this life it seems inscrutably so. Here and now it may be usefully drawn. Inequalities in the need for medical treatment are taken, it appears, to reflect the conditions of finitude more than anything else.

One can even go on to argue that among our basic or essential needs, the case of medical treatment is conspicuous in the following sense. While food and shelter are not matters about which we are at liberty to please ourselves, they are at least predictable. We can plan, for instance, to store up food and fuel for the winter. It may be held that responsibility increases along with the power to predict. If so, then many health crises seem peculiarly random and uncontrollable. Cancer, given the present state of knowledge at any rate, is a contingent disaster, whereas hunger is a steady threat. Who will need serious medical care, and when, is then perhaps a classic example of uncertainty.

Finally, and more theoretically, it is often observed that a need-conception of justice comes closest to charity or *agape* (e.g., Perelman, 1963:23). I think there are indeed crucial overlaps (see Outka, 1972:91–92, 309–312). To cite several of them: the equal consideration *agape* enjoins has to do in the first instance with those generic endowments which people share, the characteristics of a person qua human existent. Needs, as we have seen, likewise concern those things essential to the life and welfare of men considered simply as men (see also Honoré, 1968). They are not based on particular conduct alone, on those idiosyncratic attainments which contribute to someone's being such-and-such a kind of person. Yet a certain sort of inequality is recognized, for needs differ in divergent circumstances and so treatments must if benefits are to be equalized. *Agape* too allows for a distinction between equal consideration and identi-

cal treatment. The aim of equalizing benefits is implied by the injunction to consider the interests of each party equally. This may require differential treatments of differing interests.

Overlaps such as these will doubtless strike some as so extensive that it may be asked whether *agape* and a need-conception of justice are virtually equivalent. I think not. One contrast was pointed out before. The differential treatment enjoined by *agape* is more complex and goes deeper. In the case of *agape*, attention may be appropriately given to varying *efforts* as well as to unequal *needs*. More generally one may say that agapeic considerations extend to all of the psychological nuances and contextual details of individual persons and their circumstances. Imaginative concern is enjoined for concrete human beings: for what someone is uniquely, for what he or she—as a matter of personal history and distinctive identity—wants, feels, thinks, celebrates, and endures. The attempt to establish and enhance mutual affection between individual persons is taken likewise to be fitting. Conceptions of social justice, including "to each according to his essential needs," tend to be more restrictive; they call attention to considerations which obtain for a number of persons, to impersonally specified criteria for assessing collective policies and practices. *Agape* involves more, even if one supposes never less.

Other differences could be noted. What is important now however is the recognition that, in matters of health care in particular, *agape* and a need-conception of justice are conjoined in a number of relevant respects. At least this is so for those who think that, again, justice has properly to do with pleas of "But I could not help it." It seeks to distinguish such cases from those acknowledged to be praiseworthy or blameworthy. The formula "to each according to his needs" is one cogent way of identifying the moral relevance of these pleas. To ignore them may be thought to be unfair as well as unkind when they arise from the deprivation of some essential need. The move to confine the notion of justice wholly to desert considerations is thereby resisted as well. Hence we may say that sometimes "questions of social justice arise just because people are unequal in ways they can do very little to change and . . . only by attending to these inequalities can one be said to be giving their interests equal consideration'' (Benn, 1971:164).

V

Similar treatment for similar cases. This conception is perhaps the most familiar of all. Certainly it is the most formal and inclusive one. It is frequently taken as an elementary appeal to consistency and linked to the universalizability test. One should not make an arbitrary exception on one's own behalf, but rather should apply impartially whatever standards one accepts. The conception can be fruitfully applied to health care questions and I shall assume its relevance. Yet as literally interpreted, it is necessary but not sufficient. For rightly or not, it is often held to be as compatible with no positive treatment whatever as with active promotion of other peoples' interests, as long as all are equally and impartially included. Its exponents sometimes assume such active promotion without demonstrating clearly how this is built into the conception itself. Moreover, it may obscure a distinction which we have seen agapists and others make: between equal consideration and identical treatment. Needs may differ and so treatments must, if benefits are to be equalized.

I have placed this conception at the end of the list partly because it moves us, despite its formality, toward practice. Let me suggest briefly how it does so. Suppose first of all one agrees with the case so far offered. Suppose, that is, it has been shown convincingly that a need-conception of justice applies with greater relevance than the earlier three when one reflects about the basic purpose of medical care. To treat one class of people differently from another because of income or geographic location should therefore be ruled out, because such reasons are irrelevant. (The irrelevance is conceptual, rather than always, unfortunately, causal.) In short, all persons should have equal access, ''as needed, without financial, geographic, or other barriers, to the whole spectrum of health services'' (Somers and Somers, 1972a:122).

Suppose however, secondly, that the goal of equal access collides on some occasions with the realities of finite medical resources and needs which prove to be insatiable. That such collisions occur in fact it would be idle to deny. And it is here that the practical bearing of the formula of similar treatment for similar cases should be noticed. Let us recall Williams' conclusion: ''the proper ground of distribution of medical care is ill health: this is a necessary truth.'' While I agree with the essentials of his argument—for all the reasons above—I would prefer, for practical purposes, a slightly more modest formulation. Illness is the proper ground for the *receipt* of medical care. However, the *distribution* of medical care in less-than-optimal circumstances requires us to face the collisions. I would argue that in such circumstances the formula of similar treatment for similar cases may be construed so as to guide actual choices in the way most compatible with the goal of equal access. The formula's allowance of no positive treatment whatever may justify exclusion of entire classes of cases from a priority list. Yet it forbids doing so for irrelevant or arbitrary reasons. So (1) if we accept the case for equal access, but (2) if we simply cannot, physically cannot, treat all who are in need, it seems more just to discriminate by virtue of categories of illness, for example, rather than between the rich ill and poor ill. All persons with a certain rare, noncommunicable disease would not receive priority, let us say, where the costs were inordinate, the prospects for rehabilitation remote, and for the sake of equalized benefits to many more. Or with Ramsey we may urge a policy of random patient selection when one must decide between claimants for a medical treatment unavailable to all. Or we may acknowledge that any notion of ''comprehensive benefits'' to which persons should have equal access is subject to practical restrictions which will vary from society to society depending on resources at a given time. Even in a country as affluent as the United States there will surely always be items excluded, e.g., perhaps over-the-counter drugs, some teenage orthodontia, cosmetic surgery, and the like (Somers and Somers, 1972b:182). Here too the formula of similar treatment for similar cases may serve to modify the application of a need-conception of justice in order to address the insatiability-problem and limit

frivolous use. In all of the foregoing instances of restriction, however, the relevant feature remains the illness, discomfort, etc. itself. The goal of equal access then retains its prima facie authoritativeness. It is imperfectly realized rather than disregarded.

VI

These latter comments lead on to the question of institutional implications. I cannot aim here of course for the specificity rightly sought by policy-makers. My endeavor has been conceptual elucidation. While the ethicist needs to be apprised about the facts, he or she does not, qua ethicist, don the mantle of·the policy-expert. In any case, only rarely does anyone do both things equally well. Yet cross-fertilization is extremely desirable. For experts should not be isolated from the wider assumptions their recommendations may reflect. I shall merely list some of the topics which would have to be discussed at length if we were to get clear about the implications. Examples will be limited to the current situation in the United States.

Anyone who accepts the case for equal access will naturally be concerned about de facto disparities in the availability of medical treatment. Let us consider two relevant indictments of current American practice. They appear in the writings not only of those who attack indiscriminately a system seen to be governed only by the appetite for profit and power, but also of those who denounce in less sweeping terms and espouse more cautiously reformist positions. The first shortcoming has to do with the maldistribution of supply. Per capita ratios of physicians to populations served vary, sometimes notoriously, between affluent suburbs and rural and inner city areas. This problem is exacerbated by the distressing data concerning the greater health needs of the poor. Chronic disease, frequency and duration of hospitalization, psychiatric disorders, infant death rates, etc.—these occur in significantly larger proportions to lower income members of American society (Appel, 1970; Hubbard, 1970). A further complication is that ''the distribution of health insurance coverage is badly skewed. Practically all the rich have insurance.

But among the poor, about two-thirds have none. As a result, among people aged 25 to 64 who die, some 45 to 50 per cent have neither hospital nor surgical coverage" (Somers, 1971a:46). This last point connects with a second shortcoming frequently cited. Even those who are otherwise economically independent may be shattered by the high cost of a "catastrophic illness" (see some eloquent examples in Kennedy, 1972).

Proposals for institutional reforms designed to overcome such disparities are bound to be taken seriously by any defender of equal access. What he or she will be disposed to press for, of course, is the removal of any double standard or "two class" system of care. The viable procedures for bringing this about are not obvious, and comparisons with certain other societies (for relevant alternative models) are drawn now with perhaps less confidence (see Anderson, 1973). One set of commonly discussed proposals includes (1) incentive subsidies to physicians, hospitals, and medical centers to provide services in regions of poverty (to overcome in part the unwillingness—to which no unique culpability need be ascribed—of many providers and their spouses to work and live in grim surroundings); (2) licensure controls to avoid comparatively excessive concentrations of physicians in regions of affluence; (3) a period of time (say, two years) in an underserved area as a requirement for licensing; (4) redistribution facilities which allow for population shifts.

A second set of proposals is linked with health insurance itself. While I cannot venture into the intricacies of medical economics or comment on the various bills for national health insurance presently inundating Congress, it may be instructive to take brief note of one proposal in which, once more, the defender of equal access is bound to take an interest (even if he or she finally rejects it on certain practical grounds). The precise details of the proposal are unimportant for our purposes (for one much-discussed version, see Feldstein, 1971). Consider this crude sketch. Each citizen is (in effect) issued a card by the government. Whenever "legitimate" medical expenses (however determined for a given society) exceed, say, 10 per cent of his or her annual taxable income, the card may be presented so that

additional costs incurred will be paid for out of general tax revenues. The reasons urged on behalf of this sort of arrangement include the following. In the case of medical care there is warrant for proportionately equalizing what is spent from anyone's total taxable income. This warrant reflects the conditions, discussed earlier, of the natural lottery. Insofar as the advantages of health and the burdens of illness are random and undeserved, we may find it in our common interest to share risks. A fixed percentage of income attests to the misfit, also mentioned previously, between the reasons for differential total income and the reasons for receiving medical treatment. If money remains a causally necessary condition for receiving medical treatment, then a way must be found to place it in the hands of those who need it. The card is one such means. It is designed effectively to equalize purchasing power. In this way it seems to accord nicely with the goal of equal access. On the other side, the requirement of initial out-of-pocket expenses—sufficiently large in comparison to average family expenditures on health care—is designed to discourage frivolous use and foster awareness that medical care is a benefit not to be simply taken as a matter of course. It also safeguards against an excessively large tax burden while providing universal protection against the often disastrous costs of serious illnesses. Whether 10 per cent is too great a chunk for the very poor to pay, and whether by itself the proposal will feed price inflation and neglect of preventive medicine are questions which would have to be answered.

Another kind of possible institutional reform will also greatly interest the defender of equal access. This has to do with the "design of health care systems" or "care settings." The prevalent setting in American society has always been "fee-for-service." It is left up to each person to obtain the requisite care and to pay for it as he or she goes along. Because costs for medical treatment have accelerated at such an alarming rate, and because the sheer diffusion of energy and effort so characteristic of American medical practice leaves more and more people

dissatisfied, alternatives to fee-for-service have been considered of late with unprecedented seriousness. The alternative care setting most widely discussed is prepaid practice, and specifically the "health maintenance organization" (HMO). Here one finds "an organized system of care which accepts the responsibility to provide or otherwise assure comprehensive care to a defined population for a fixed periodic payment per person or per family . . ." (Somers, 1972b:v). The best-known HMO is the Kaiser-Permanente Medical Care Program (see also Garfield, 1971). Does the HMO serve to realize the goal of equal access more fully? One line of argument in its favor is this. It is plausible to think that equal access will be fostered by the more economical care setting. HMO's are held to be less costly per capita in at least two respects: hospitalization rates are much below the national average; and less often noted, physician manpower·is as well. To be sure, one should be sensitive to the corruptions in each type of setting. While fee-for-service has resulted in a suspiciously high number of surgeries (twice as many per capita in the United States as in Great Britain), the HMO physician may more frequently permit the patient's needs to be overridden by the organization's pressure to economize. It may also be more difficult in an HMO setting to provide for close personal relations between a particular physician and a particular patient (something commended, of course, on all sides). After such corruptions are allowed for, the data seem encouraging to such an extent that a defender of equal access will certainly support the repeal of any law which limits the development of prepaid practice, to approve of "front-aid" subsidies for HMO's to increase their number overall and achieve a more equitable distribution throughout the country, and so on. At a minimum, each care setting should be available in every region. If we assume a common freedom to choose between them, each may help to guard against the peculiar temptations to which the other is exposed.

To assess in any serious way proposals for institutional reform such as the above is beyond the scope of this paper. We would eventually be led, for example, into the question of whether it is consistent for the rich to pay more than the poor for the same treatment when, again, needs rather than income constitute the ground of the treatment (Ward, 1973), and from there into the tangled subject of the "ethics of redistribution" in general (see, e.g., Benn and Peters, 1965:155–178; de Jouvenal, 1952). Other complex issues deserve to be considered as well, e.g., the criteria for allocation of limited resources,[1] and how conceptions of justice apply to the providers of health care.[2]

Those committed to self-conscious moral and religious reflection about subjects in medicine have concentrated, perhaps unduly, on issues about care of individual patients (as death approaches, for instance). These issues plainly warrant the most careful consideration. One would like to see in addition, however, more attention paid to social questions in medical ethics. To attend to them is not necessarily to leave behind all of the matters which reach deeply into the human condition. Any detailed case for institutional reforms, for example, will be enriched if the proponent asks soberly whether certain conflicts and certain perplexities allow for more than partial improvements and provisional resolutions. Can public and private interests ever be made fully to coincide by legislative and administrative means? Will the commitment of a physician to an individual patient and the commitment of the legislator to the "common good" ever be harmonized in every case? Our anxiety may be too intractable. Our fear of illness and of dying may be so pronounced and immediate that we will seize the nearly automatic connections between privilege, wealth, and power if we can. We will do everything possible to have our kidney machines even if the charts make it clear that many more would benefit from mandatory immunization at a fraction of the cost. And our capacity for taking in rival points of view may be too limited. Once we have witnessed tangible suffering, we cannot just return with ease to public policies aimed at statistical patients. Those who believe that justice is the pre-eminent virtue of institutions and that a case

can be convincingly made on behalf of justice for equal access to health care would do well to ponder such conflicts and perplexities. Our reforms might then seem, to ourselves and to others, less abstract and jargon-filled in formulation and less sanguine and piecemeal in substance. They would reflect a greater awareness of what we have to confront.

Notes

1. The issue of priorities is at least threefold: (1) between improved medical care and other social needs, e.g., to restrain auto accidents and pollution; (2) between different sorts of medical treatments for different illnesses, e.g., prevention vs. crisis intervention and exotic treatments; (3) between persons all of whom need a single scarce resource and not all can have it, e.g., Ramsey's discussion of how to decide among those who are to receive dialysis. Moreover, (1) can be subdivided between (a) improved medical care and other social needs which affect health directly, e.g., drug addiction, auto accidents, and pollution; (b) improved medical care and other social needs which serve the overall aim of community-survival, e.g., a common defense. In the case of (2), one would like to see far more careful discussion of some general criteria which might be employed, e.g., numbers affected, degree of contagion, prospects for rehabilitation, and so on.

2. What sorts of appeals to justice might be cogently made to warrant, for instance, the differentially high income physicians receive? Here are three possibilities: (1) the greater skill and responsibility involved should be rewarded proportionately, i.e., one should attend to considerations of *desert*; (2) there should be *compensation* for the money invested for education and facilities in order to restore circumstances of approximate equality (this argument, while a common one in medical circles, would need to consider that medical education is received in part at public expense and that the modern physician is the highest paid professional in the country); (3) the difference should benefit the least advantaged more than an alternative arrangement where disparities are less. We prefer a society where the medical profession flourishes and everyone has a longer life expectancy to one where everyone is poverty-stricken with a shorter life expectancy ("splendidly equalized destitution"). Yet how are we to ascertain the minimum degree of differential income required for the least advantaged members of the society to be better off? Discussions of "justice and the interests of providers" are, I think, badly needed. Physicians in the United States have suffered a decline in prestige for various reasons, e.g., the way many used Medicare to support and increase their own incomes. Yet one should endeavor to assess their interests fairly. A concern for professional autonomy is clearly important, though one may ask whether adequate attention has been paid to

the distinction between the imposition of cost-controls from outside and interference with professional medical judgments. One may affirm the former, it seems, and still reject—energetically—the latter.

References

Anderson, Odin, *Health Care: Can There Be Equity? The United States, Sweden and England.* New York: Wiley, 1973.

Appel, James Z., "Health Care Delivery." Pp. 141–166 in Boisfeuillet Jones (ed.), *The Health of Americans.* Englewood Cliffs, N.J.: Prentice-Hall, Inc., 1970.

Bedau, Hugo A., "Radical Egalitarianism." Pp. 168–180 in Hugo A. Bedau (ed.), *Justice and Equality.* Englewood Cliffs, N.J.: Prentice-Hall, Inc., 1971.

Benn, Stanley I., "Egalitarianism and the Equal Consideration of Interests." Pp. 152–167 in Hugo A. Bedau (ed.), *Justice and Equality.* Englewood Cliffs, N.J.: Prentice-Hall, Inc., 1971.

Benn, Stanley I., and Richard S. Peters, *The Principles of Political Thought.* New York: The Free Press, 1965.

de Jouvenel, Bertrand, *The Ethics of Redistribution.* Cambridge: University Press, 1952.

Feldstein, Martin S., "A New Approach to National Health Insurance." *The Public Interest* 23 (Spring 1971): 93–105.

Garfield, Sidney R., "Prevention of Dissipation of Health Services Resources." *American Journal of Public Health* 61: 1499–1506 (1971).

Hicks, Nancy, "Nation's Doctors Move to Police Medical Care." Pp. 1, 52 in *New York Times,* Sunday, October 28, 1973.

Honoré, A. M., "Social Justice." Pp. 61–94 in Robert S. Summers (ed.), *Essays in Legal Philosophy.* Oxford: Basil Blackwell, 1968.

Hospers, John, *Human Conduct.* New York: Harcourt, Brace and World, Inc., 1961.

Hubbard, William N., "Health Knowledge." Pp. 93–120 in Boisfeuillet Jones (ed.), *The Health of Americans.* Englewood Cliffs, N.J.: Prentice-Hall, Inc., 1970.

Kennedy, Edward M., *In Critical Condition: The Crisis in America's Health Care.* New York: Simon and Schuster, 1972.

Lucas, J. R., "Justice." *Philosophy* 47, No. 181 (July 1972): 229–248.

Nagel, Thomas, "Equal Treatment and Compensatory Discrimination." *Philosophy and Public Affairs* 2, No. 4 (Summer 1973): 348–363.

Nixon, Richard M., "President's Message on Health Care System." Document No. 92–261 (March 2). House of Representatives, Washington, D.C., 1972.

Outka, Gene, *Agape: An Ethical Analysis.* New Haven and London: Yale University Press, 1972.

Perelman, Ch., *The Ideal of Justice and the Problem of Argument.* Trans. John Petrie. London: Routledge and Kegan Paul, 1963.

Ramsey, Paul, *The Patient as Person.* New Haven and London: Yale University Press, 1970.

Rand, Ayn, *Atlas Shrugged.* New York: Signet, 1957.

Rawls, John, *A Theory of Justice.* Cambridge, Mass.: Harvard University Press, 1971.

Rescher, Nicholas, *Distributive Justice.* Indianapolis: Bobbs-Merrill, 1966.

Ryan, John A., *Distributive Justice.* New York: Macmillan, 1916.

Sade, Robert M., "Medical Care as a Right: A Refutation." *The New England Journal of Medicine* 285 (December 1971): 1288–1292. [Reprinted as Chapter 91 of this volume.]

Schultze, Charles L., Edward R. Fried, Alice M. Rivlin, and Nancy H. Teeters, *Setting National Priorities: The 1973 Budget.* Washington, D.C.: The Brookings Institution, 1972.

Somers, Anne R., *Health Care in Transition: Directions for the Future.* Chicago: Hospital Research and Educational Trust, 1971a.

——— (ed.), *The Kaiser-Permanente Medical Care Program.* New York: The Commonwealth Fund, 1971b.

Somers, Anne R., and Herman M. Somers, "The Organization and Financing of Health Care: Issues and Directions for the Future." *American Journal of Orthopsychiatry* 42 (January 1972a), 119–136.

———, "Major Issues in National Health Insurance." *Milbank Memorial Fund Quarterly* 50, No. 2, Part 1 (April 1972b): 177–210.

Vlastos, Gregory, "Justice and Equality." Pp. 31–72 in Richard B. Brandt (ed.), *Social Justice.* Englewood Cliffs, N.J.: Prentice-Hall, 1962.

Ward, Andrew, "The Idea of Equality Reconsidered." *Philosophy* 48 (January 1973): 85–90.

Williams, Bernard A. O., "The Idea of Equality." Pp. 116–137 in Hugo A. Bedau (ed.), *Justice and Equality.* Englewood Cliffs, N.J.: Prentice-Hall, 1971.

95

The Honorable David L. Bazelon

The Right to Treatment: The Court's Role

Reprinted with permission of author and publisher from *Hospital and Community Psychiatry*, vol. 20, 1969, pp. 129–135.

A little more than two years ago, I wrote in an opinion for the District of Columbia Court of Appeals that a young man committed to St. Elizabeths Hospital following an acquittal for insanity had the right to adequate treatment, failing which the hospital might have to release him. That opinion (*Rouse* v. *Cameron*) attracted mixed reviews. It sounded like a good thing. After all, why should anyone be in a mental hospital if he is not being treated? But some people wondered whether a court was the proper institution to announce such a right. And their doubts about whether mere judges should announce the right to treatment were dwarfed by their conviction that courts should certainly not aspire to administer the right.

The American Psychiatric Association leaped to the ramparts with an official position statement, saying in part that "The definition of treatment and the appraisal of its adequacy are matters for medical determination."[1] Even student lawyers, who above all should be, but rarely are, deferential to their professional elders, muttered uneasily about the prospect of courts enforcing the right to treatment. The editors of the *Harvard Law Review* admonished me, "the difficulty of formulating standards of adequacy seems very great." The future lawyers of Yale, a supposed bastion of judicial activism, fretted at length about "the difficult problems courts will face in administering a right to treatment."

The argument that physicians, who alone are qualified to provide treatment, should also define and appraise treatment is temptingly simple and clear-cut. The corollary, that courts should stay well clear of such complicated questions, is equally enticing. But both propositions ignore two factors. The first is that when important rights, such as the right to treatment, are at stake, courts must become involved, whether they are ill-informed or well-informed. The second is that courts have a long history of participating in disputes of the most technical and esoteric sort. Sometimes that participation has resulted in the unalloyed disaster that is predicted for courts administering a right to treatment, but often it has not.

Before I talk about the physicians' role and the courts' role in protecting the right to treatment, I should explain some reasons why courts are and must be involved with the right to treatment. I well recognize that the courts' action poses problems for the medical director of a public hospital. He and his staff are working with only minimal support. They are making the best possible use of their limited budgets and using all the volunteer help they can muster. They are doing those things despite the knowledge that they could lead more comfortable professional lives in private practice, because they feel a social responsiblity to bring as many of the benefits of modern psychiatry as they possibly can to a group of underprivileged patients.

If now the courts in effect tell them that their efforts are inadequate because they cannot provide for their patients the level of care that the middle-class citizen can buy with his health insurance, they fear that a veritable Pandora's Box may be opened. Further, they may wonder whether other patients in the hospital who are getting no better treatment than the committed patient might institute malpractice suits for having received only the best treatment available within the hospital's limited resources, rather than adequate treatment by private-hospital standards.

All those are reasons why publichospital directors may greet the concept of court-enforced right to treatment with glacial coolness. But I hope they will not. For there are even stronger reasons why a court-enforced right must exist. The rationale is syllogistic in its simplicity: if society confines an individual for the professed benevolent purpose of helping him—"for his own good," in the standard phrase—then its right to so withhold his freedom depends entirely on whether help is in fact provided. If there is no treatment, the justification for commitment to a hospital disappears, and the individual should be released.

This argument has such force that few would dispute it. The rub lies in the fact that hospital commitments frequently have a dual justification: an individual is confined both because he needs help and because he is dangerous. If both requirements were carefully observed, the individual would be doubly protected. Unfortunately, in practice, the presence of two criteria has tended not to double the difficulty

of commitment, but to make it far easier. In criminal law, we imprison men only with the most scrupulous attention to substantive standards and procedures. The state must prove beyond a reasonable doubt that the defendant committed the specific act charged, and the Bill of Rights places strict limitations upon the tactics it may use in doing so. But in committing a mental patient, there has long been a tendency to almost ignore, both substantively and procedurally, the requirement that he be dangerous; after all, he is going to a hospital, not to a prison, and we are helping him, not punishing him. Unfortunately, if the hospital has woefully few psychiatrists and pathetically inadequate facilities, we then justify his confinement with the apology "Well, that's too bad, but you're dangerous." That sort of shell game is intolerable. Courts cannot force legislatures to provide adequate resources for treatment. But neither should they allow legislatures to justify commitment by a false promise of treatment.

In speaking of legislatures, I place the blame squarely where I believe it belongs. There may be cases where an admirably equipped mental hospital fails to make a bona fide effort to provide treatment. But those are exceptional cases, and the problem is usually not what the hospital deliberately fails to do, but what it cannot do. In view of this, I confess to some surprise at the hostility many mental hospital administrators display toward the concept of a right to treatment. The fact that courts will release committed patients unless treatment can be provided for them seems to offer a compelling argument for a larger appropriation from the legislature. Of course, it might be argued that legislatures may simply eliminate the promise of treatment and rely solely upon dangerousness to justify commitment. Such a development, however distressing, would at least eliminate much of the present hypocrisy. But a legislature wishing to take such a step would face the stiff constitutional requirements that hedge the criminal law.

Realizing that the state must fulfill its promise of treatment for involuntarily committed mental patients is merely

one aspect of a broader development in the law. The power of parens patriae has been invoked in other areas to justify interferences with individual freedom, and the benevolent purposes of those actions have equally often been unfulfilled. The Supreme Court has acknowledged that failure by setting new standards for our juvenile courts. Lax procedures and unexamined promises of rehabilitation were long tolerated on the ground that young offenders would not be punished, but rather helped. Two recent Supreme Court cases have dramatically demonstrated that, as Mr. Justice Fortas phrased it, "The condition of being a boy does not justify a kangaroo court." Those cases dealt with procedural matters. My own Court of Appeals, in dealing with the juvenile courts, has concluded that a young offender is entitled not only to a fair trial to determine his involvement, but also to appropriate treatment if he is confined as mentally disturbed.

Similarly, we have found that the statute in the District of Columbia recognizing alcoholism as a disease and promising treatment to those afflicted prevents the government from punishing alcoholics as criminals. Other examples are readily at hand. New York State allows a narcotic addict to accept an indeterminate commitment for treatment as an alternative to punishment as a criminal. If an addict has elected commitment, and after several years has received no treatment or rehabilitation, it seems doubtful that his continued commitment can be justified—certainly not after the maximum prison sentence he might have received would have expired.

Right to treatment will, of course, differ in each of those contexts, as will the techniques for enforcing the right. Indeed, perhaps the greatest common denominator is the ignorance of courts, which extends equally to the causes and cure of alcoholism, the nature of drug addiction, the proper therapy for a mental patient, and the best form of rehabilitation for a juvenile delinquent. Because of that ignorance, you may well ask why courts should attempt to enforce the right. Even if there must be the right, and even if courts are the proper institution to declare its existence, why is continued meddling necessary? Doctors are honorable men. Once told that the patient has a right to treatment, why can't they be trusted to protect it?

In large measure they can and must be so trusted. But at some stage, in some cases, a referee will be needed. The hospital administrator is poorly situated to take a fully dispassionate view of the adequacy of treatment. In the first place, the very sincerity of his wish to help and of his conviction that the person needs help interferes with his ability to hold the scale true between the patient's interest in his liberty and the state's interest in treating him.

Second, there is the problem that many patients, rightly or wrongly, have been labeled dangerous. The hospital entrusted with their care has a natural reluctance to release them while the faintest doubt about their mental health persists. Sometimes this reluctance may represent oversensitivity to criticism if a released patient hurts someone; more often it may be the product of a responsibility felt toward society. But in either case the scales are weighted against release.

The courts are needed, in short, to ensure that moral as well as medical values enter into the decision about whether treatment is adequate to justify commitment. In an important sense the definition of treatment is a matter for medical expertise. But courts too have their special expertise. From long experience in dealing with legislative enactments reviewing administrative decisions, and interpreting constitutional provisions, the courts in our society are pre-eminently accustomed to fashioning tolerable accommodations between competing values. To do so, they must appreciate the considerations at stake. When something so complex and controversial as the appropriate treatment for a mentally ill person is involved, the task is formidable. But it is not impossible. As a responsible jurist, I would not argue for a right to treatment unless I believed that courts can and will cope with the task of appraising adequacy of treatment. Our success will, however, depend to a large extent upon hospital administrators.

The process of delineating and implementing a right to treatment stretches from the legislatures to our

mental hospitals and, ultimately, to the courts. The role of hospital administrators as the middlemen in the process is particularly vital. In playing their part, they must look to the legislature, developing whatever broad standards it provides into workable rules and procedures, and to the courts, providing reliable records of what they have done and why. Only thus can the legislatures give enlightened responses when further statutes are needed and can the courts review administrators' medical judgment with awareness of the issues involved.

Hospital administrators have a task not unlike that of the administrative agencies that play a growing role in our government; their activities provide a useful model for developing the right to treatment. The granddaddy of the federal agencies was the Interstate Commerce Commission, created in 1887 to deal with the complicated problems of regulating railroad rates and services. Since then the jurisdiction of the ICC has been broadened to encompass other modes of surface transportation, and a host of other agencies have been created—the Federal Trade Commission, the National Labor Relations Board, the Federal Communications Commission, the Civil Aeronautics Board, the Federal Power Commission, and others too numerous to mention. Each of those agencies is charged with enforcing a broad regulatory statute or statutes.

In launching those programs, Congress has spelled out its goals with varying degrees of specificity, and it has entrusted the agencies with varying authority and responsibilities. The members of each agency, building from the expertise they bring to their positions or acquire while there, must administer programs that are in quite literal terms vast. They formulate rules, conduct enforcement proceedings, and attend to a variety of other regulatory tasks. Some of these agencies have performed with distinction; others have fared less well. Their successes and failures are a product of many factors, not the least of which is the enthusiasm displayed by legislatures and courts to assume their responsibilities.

In the field of the right to treatment, as in the area of administrative agencies, the most important task of the legislature is to outline the standards to be enforced, or at least the goals it

wishes pursued. A recurrent source of chaos in administrative law is nebulous statutes that direct the agency "to promote the public interest," leaving the agency to wallow in uncharted seas and the reviewing court with no map by which to judge the chosen course. At the other extreme, the legislature may prematurely lay down too-detailed standards that leave the agency no leeway to exercise its expertise in seeking solutions for problems unforeseen or incompletely analyzed by the legislature.

Whether we regard the right to treatment as arising from the Constitution or from statutes promising treatment to those involuntarily committed, there is no question that legislators have failed to grapple with the problem of standards. That is unfortunate, because if a legislature could avoid the rock of being prematurely specific and the whirlpool of being too vague, it could provide a valuable start toward a definition of adequate treatment. For unlike a court, a legislature has the resources to examine a complicated, technical problem in depth. And unlike an administrative agency, as a democratically elected body it can represent the community values in its actions.

Because I am no more a legislator than I am a psychiatrist, I cannot presume to spell out what such a definition of treatment should be. But a few suggestions may be useful as a framework for discussion. The concept of treatment has two levels. The first might be termed, prosaically, treatment in general: the degree to which a mental hospital possesses the staff and resources to help all its patients. A recent bill proposed in the Pennsylvania legislature thus provided for a mental treatment standards committee to compile a manual of minimum treatment standards covering such matters as the number of professional and nonprofessional staff, the minimum number of consultations and the number of hours of individual consultations to be provided for each patient over a given period, and the frequency of physical examinations.

An adumbration of such general standards for treatment is valuable, for obviously a hospital cannot provide adequate treatment for a given individual if it provides no treatment for any patient. But the mere fact that a hospital can provide generally adequate treatment for all patients should not, as some courts have been content to conclude, satisfy the requirement of adequate treatment for a specific patient. The most important aspect of the right to treatment is not that the hospital does something for everyone, but that it does the right thing for the right patient. Because individual patients, particularly mental patients, vary so much in their needs, considerable attention must be paid to each patient as an individual.

Any legislative definition of adequate treatment should therefore ensure not only that the hospital provide adequate treatment in general, but that it tailor the treatment offered to the specific patient. One possible beginning would be the sort of standards set up by the Social Security Administration in defining "active treatment" for the purpose of reimbursing hospitals for services given to medicare patients. The guidelines proposed by SSA provide, in summary, that for services in a psychiatric hospital to be designated as active treatment, they must be (a) provided under an individualized treatment or diagnostic plan, (b) reasonably expected to improve the patient's condition or for the purpose of diagnosis, and (c) supervised and evaluated by a physician.

The need for an individualized treatment plan cannot be overemphasized. Without such a plan, there can be no evidence that the patient has been singled out from the general population of the hospital for treatment as an individual with his own unique problems. And unless the plan is refined and improved on the basis of experience with the patient, there can be no guarantee that the promise of treatment has taken root in reality.

Legislative standards, however desirable, can provide no more than a beginning. The very fact that treatment must be an individual thing means that the legislature can at best specify substantive guidelines and procedures to assure the implementation of standards. The actual treatment is and must be the responsibility of the hospital.

In saying that there must be a treatment plan, I have of course been vague. Professionals of long experience may snicker at my judicial naiveté. More likely, they may think that I am simply asking them to sacrifice part of their already scant time available for

patient consultations to do more paperwork, paperwork that they may consider unrealistic. I have heard the argument in court that a treatment plan "can't be developed overnight." I do not dispute that, and I hope that any legislation directing the preparation of a treatment plan for each patient would leave the hospital adequate flexibility to decide just when the plan should be prepared. Unquestionably some time is needed for initial evaluation of the patient. And perhaps some tentative treatment may be necessary before a meaningful plan is possible.

Questions of timing are thus for the experts. But I am wary of the next argument that inevitably crops up, that *no* written treatment plan is necessary because such paperwork merely burdens the busy doctor who knows what he wants to do for his own good and professional reasons. I share that distaste for paperwork. Unrealistic requirements for voluminous records are the bane of the administrative process. But several strong reasons support the demand for a written individual treatment plan. The patient, his family or lawyer, and perhaps eventually a reviewing agency or court are entitled to know what therapy is contemplated and why. The doctor can only assure himself that he has given the patient the individual consideration to which he is entitled by setting forth on paper his evaluation of the patient and his plan for treatment. And finally, it is only by the process of planning and providing for feedback and re-evaluation that experience with present patients can contribute to better treatment of future ones.

The administration of treatment is only one aspect of the hospital's role as a *de facto* administrative agency, however. Equally important is its responsibility to settle disputes that arise concerning the adequacy of treatment. I suggested in *Rouse* v. *Cameron* that St. Elizabeths Hospital might establish internal procedures to review patients' claims that they were receiving inadequate treatment. To the best of my knowledge, no such procedures have been created. The bill proposed in Pennsylvania, to which I alluded earlier, wisely provided for a patient-treatment review board. Such internal

review has several purposes. Even if nothing else is accomplished, it provides an outlet for patient frustrations. That cathartic function is not unimportant. Some patients, and particularly involuntary patients, will be dissatisfied with their lot. Their discontent is at best a hindrance to treatment, and at worst may disrupt hospital routine. Some fairly formal way is needed for them to present their complaints and receive meaningful answers.

But the more forceful arguments for internal review rest on the hope that it will do more than merely provide a safety valve for patient frustrations. In even the best-administered hospitals, some patients will have justifiable complaints. With the present inadequate resources of most public hospitals, some patients may simply be warehoused in the back wards. In other cases, friction between doctor and patient may require an outside mediator. For whatever reason treatment is inadequate, internal review promises the quickest and best remedy. The current treatment, or lack of it, can be scrutinized by professionals, and the necessary changes can be made expeditiously.

Internal review may take a number of forms. In time, legislation may provide for such review by bodies partly or wholly divorced from the hospital administration. Whether such a separation of functions is desirable, I cannot presume to say. In the courts, of course, this country has always insisted upon a rigid separation between the roles of prosecutor and judge. Our administrative agencies have tended to blur the lines, although there are still wide differences between them. In some agencies, such as the National Labor Relations Board, there is a sharp segregation of those responsible for basic administration, those responsible for initiating enforcement proceedings, and those responsible for adjudicating disputes. The more typical pattern, perhaps, is a more unified approach, with some internal bulkheads—which may be more or less porous—between the groups responsible for different functions.

Until legislatures consider the problem, however, the hospital administration must be all things. But its dual role in both administering treatment and reviewing its adequacy requires certain precautions. The reviewing body should certainly be independent from the psychiatrist or psychiatrists responsible for treating the patient involved. Some provision should be made to give the patient an advocate to present his position. Indeed, because patients may be unaware of the review procedure or too timorous to invoke it, there should be some internal watchdog to initiate proceedings in appropriate cases.

In advocating the establishment of internal procedures to review claims of inadequate treatment, I do not wish to imply that such ad hoc proceedings can eliminate the need for periodic review of each patient's condition. Even aside from the right to treatment, legislatures have increasingly recognized that the burden of inertia should favor release rather than continued commitment. That condition can be achieved only by obligating the hospital to justify continued commitment at regular intervals.

Nor do I wish to imply that internal review can wholly eliminate the need for court review of patient claims concerning the treatment they are receiving. Internal review is more aptly regarded as a screen that disposes of egregious cases, and in others provides an initial decision while preparing a record that will permit intelligent review by the courts. Some familiarity with legal standards is required. But in applying the law, administrators, although important participants, are ultimately supporting actors. Their task is to translate legislative pronouncements into practice. To do so, or to implement court opinions in the absence of statutory standards, some interpretative skill is required. But the final responsibility for interpreting the law belongs to the courts. And as a fair *quid pro quo* for judges' recognition that they are not doctors, doctors should recognize that they are not judges. If the interaction between courts and hospital administrators is to be constructive, administrators must accept in good faith the law as announced by courts and legislatures.

In other fields, administrative agencies occasionally display too much initiative. The temptation is all too strong for their members to believe, rightly or wrongly, that they know the proper policies better than the legislature or the court. With the purest of intentions the agency may try, sometimes subtly

and sometimes obviously, to ignore the statutory mandate and to hoodwink the reviewing court. Because the agency members often know more about the field regulated than the court or legislature, such administrative runaways may be difficult to detect and bridle. The same may sometimes be the case in the mental health field. I have been told that some doctors, believing that a patient needs medical treatment, regard the statutory requirement that he be dangerous as mere surplusage, an irrelevancy to be ignored because they know better.

While in some cases those agencies or those doctors may do good, at best they have usurped a role rightfully entrusted to others. And at worst, which is frequently, they conceal a problem behind a facade of administrative ritual that prevents courts and legislators from recognizing the difficulty and working toward a better, more visible solution.

In short, the success with which courts deal with the right to treatment will depend critically on the thoroughness with which other institutions fulfill their functions. That is shown time and again by administrative law. Judges, after all, know fully as little about aviation, telecommunications, or atomic energy as about medicine. Yet the courts have for many years scrutinized the work of the Civil Aeronautics Board, the Federal Communications Commission, and the Atomic Energy Commission. When the legislature has provided some yardsticks against which administrative performance may be judged, and when the administrative agency has conscientiously examined the problem and explained its actions, the reviewing courts have coped quite competently with issues fully as technical as medical treatment. The issues requiring professional expertise are clearly set forth in the record, and judges can assess whether the agency has carried out its responsibility. If the statute has been misconstrued, or an important public policy slighted, the agency can be called to task. If, on the other hand, the agency has acted wisely, the court can provide its authoritative imprimatur.

The court's role in reviewing the action of an administrative agency is

quite different from its role in a normal trial. Recognizing the greater familiarity of the agency members with the technical issues calling for special expertise, the court need not attempt to assess whether the agency decision is "right" or "wrong" in the sense of whether the court itself would have reached the same result had it faced the issue without the benefit of the agency's deliberations. Instead, the court scrutinizes the administrative decisions, the reasoning advanced by the agency to support them, and the record of whatever proceedings were conducted by the agency, to determine whether the result is supported by "substantial evidence."

And what precisely is "substantial evidence"? That question has troubled courts for decades. Several formulations have enjoyed their vogue. However the test is phrased, "substantial evidence" is something of a matter of feel. It's less than a "preponderance of the evidence," and certainly less than "proof beyond a reasonable doubt." On the other hand, it's more than "a mere scintilla" of evidence. Perhaps a good loose-lipped definition is "enough evidence to convince the court that the agency knows what it's doing, and did its work thoroughly, but not necessarily enough evidence to convince the courts that this is the best of all possible decisions."

If that standard is to be workable, the court must be informed of what the agency did, and why. Indeed, because judges must often place a fair amount of trust in the substantive results achieved by agencies, the courts have tended to focus with particular zeal on the procedures followed. Thus in many circumstances agencies must make specific findings of fact, in writing, and discuss in some detail their reasons for a decision. If that has been done, the reviewing court can satisfy itself that the path has been trodden with care, if perhaps not with perfect wisdom.

The story will be far different if the court must face an issue calling for expertise beyond its capability without the aid of legislation or a record compiled by professionals. The untutored judge will flounder, his results will be erratic, and the parties will be predictably disgusted with the whole process. In saying this, I do not claim that there are no poor judges, nor any judges who meddle where they should not.

Some courts misfire with even the best assistance. But many examples of judicial misfeasance are the products of judges attempting to struggle with problems quite beyond their competence. President Truman's famous desk motto, "The buck stops here," applies to courts as well. Faced with an important issue, such as the right to treatment, the court must do the best it can, even if those more qualified are unwilling to grapple with the problem.

Courts will enforce the right to treatment. Whether the legislatures will help is beyond the control of all of us. But in the interim and in the long run, the willingness hospital administrators show to develop and protect that right will set the horizons for our success. I do not by any means suggest that, even with good faith and good will each for the other, the path will be strewn with petals. The recognition of the right to treatment will be attended by problems of the most subtle sort. To deny the right or to resist its vigorous enforcement because of a reluctance to face and resolve those problems would be tragic. I trust that the courts will not flinch; I am equally confident that psychiatry will not.

Note

1. "Position Statement on the Question of Adequacy of Treatment," *American Journal of Psychiatry*, Vol. 123, May 1967, pp. 1458–1460.

96

Thomas S. Szasz
The Right to Health

Reprinted with permission of the publisher from *Georgetown Law Journal*, vol. 57, 1969, pp. 734–751.

When Is Inequality Inequity?

In every society—whether it be tribal or industrial, theologic or secular, capitalist or communist—goods and services are distributed unequally. This is, in fact, what words such as "rich" and "poor" really mean; it is their operational definition: The rich "have," and the poor "have not." The "haves" eat more nutritious food, dwell in more comfortable and spacious homes, and travel by means of more luxurious transportation than do the "have nots." Similar differences exist between the same persons and groups with respect to medical care. When the rich man falls ill, he occupies a hospital bed in a single room or private suite and receives treatment from the best—or, at least, the most expensive—physicians in town. When the poor man falls ill, he occupies a bed in the charity ward (though it may no longer be called that) and receives treatment from young men who, though called "doctors," are only medical students. In short, while it is not a disgrace to be poor, it is not a great honor either.

Although it is self-evident that the poor will always have more needs than the rich, and the rich more satisfactions than the poor, this fact is now repeatedly rediscovered and denounced by psychiatric epidemiologists. For example, Ernest Gruenberg has stated that there is in our society "a pattern in which the prevalence of illness is an inverse function of family income, while the volume of medical care received is a direct function of family income."[1] In plain English, this means that poverty begets sickness, while affluence begets medical attention. The same statement, of course, could be made about every other important human need and satisfaction. An example of this would be: To earn a living, a poor man has a greater need for transportation than does a rich man, who could stay at home and live off his investments; yet the former must do with the inferior public transportation system provided by the community, whereas the latter enjoys a fleet of private cars, boats, and airplanes. Such considerations do not deter Gruenberg and the many other physicians addressing themselves to this subject from observing plaintively and, I think, rather naively that "one may doubt . . . [that] efforts to redistribute medical care have eliminated the paradox."[2] But there is no paradox, except, that is, in the eyes of the utopian social reformer who views all social differences as contagious diseases waiting to be wiped out by his therapeutic efforts.

The concept that medical treatment is a right rather than a privilege has gained increasing acceptance during the past decade.[3] Its advocates are no doubt motivated by good intentions; they wish to correct certain inequalities existent in the distribution of health services in American society. That such inequalities exist is not in dispute. What is in dispute, however, is how to distinguish between inequalities and inequities,[4] and how to determine which governmental policies are best suited to the securing of good medical care for the maximum number of persons.

The desire to improve the lot of less fortunate people is laudable; indeed, I share this desire. Still, unless all inequalities are considered inequities—a view clearly incompatible with social organization and human life as we now know it—two important questions remain. First, which inequalities should be considered inequities? Second, what are the most appropriate means for minimizing or abolishing the inequalities we deem "unjust"? Appeals to good intentions are of no help in answering these questions.

There are two groups of people whose conditions with respect to medical care the advocates of a right to treatment regard as especially unfair or unjust, and whose situations they seek to ameliorate. One is the poor, who need ordinary medical care; the other group is composed of the inmates of public mental hospitals, presumably in need of psychiatric care. The proposition, however, that poor people ought to have access to more, better, or less expensive medical care than they now do and that people in public mental hospitals ought to receive better psychiatric care than they now do pose two quite different problems. I shall, therefore, deal with each separately.

The availability of medical services for a particular person, or group of persons, in a particular society depends principally upon the supply of the services desired and the prospective user's power to command these services. No government or organization—whether it be the United States Government, the American Medical Association, or the Communist Party of the Soviet Union—can provide medical care, except to the degree it has the power to control the education of physicians, their right to practice medicine, and the manner in which they dispose of their time and energies. In other words, only individuals can provide medical treatment for the sick; institutions, such as the Church and the State, can promote, permit, or prohibit certain therapeutic activities but cannot by themselves provide medical services.

Social groups wielding power are notoriously prone, of course, to prohibit the free exercise of certain human skills and the availability of certain drugs and devices. For example, during the declining Middle Ages and the early Renaissance Period, the Church repeatedly prohibited Jewish physicians from practicing medicine and non-Jewish patients from seeking the former's services. The same prohibition was imposed by the Government of Nazi Germany. In the modern democracies of the free West, the State continues to exercise its prerogative to prohibit individuals from engaging in certain kinds of therapeutic activities. This prohibition is, to be sure, not on religious grounds, but rather because they are untrained or inadequately trained as physicians. This situation is an inevitable consequence of the fact that the State's licensing powers fulfill two unrelated and mutually incompatible functions: (1) to protect the public, i.e., the actual or potential patients, from incompetent medical practitioners by ensuring an adequate level of training and competence on the part of all physicians; and (2) to protect the members of a special vested interest group, the physicians, from competition from an excessive number of similarly trained practitioners and from healers of different persuasions and skills who might prove more useful to their would-be clients than those officially approved.[5] The result is a complex and powerful alliance—first between the Church and medicine, and subsequently, between the State and medicine—with physicians playing double roles, both as medical healers and as agents of social control. This restrictive function of the State with respect to medical practice has been, and continues to be, especially significant in the United States.

Without delving further into the intricacies of this large and complex subject, it should suffice to note that our present system of medical training and practice is far removed from that of laissez-faire capitalism for which many, especially its opponents, mistake it. In actuality, the American Medical Association is not only an immensely powerful lobby of medical-vested interests—a force that liberal socialists generally oppose—but it is also a state-protected monopoly, in effect, a covert arm of the government—a force that the same reformers ardently support.[6] The result of this alliance between organized medicine and the American Government has been the creation of a system of education and licensure with strict controls over the production and distribution of health care, which leads to an artificially created chronic shortage of medical personnel. This result has been achieved by limiting the number of students to be trained in medicine through the regulation of medical education and by limiting the number of practitioners through the regulation of medical licensure.

A basic economic precept is that when the supply of a given service is smaller than the demand for it, we have a seller's market. This is obviously beneficial for the sellers—in this case, the medical profession. Conversely, when the supply is greater than the demand, we have a buyer's market. This is beneficial for the buyers—in this case the potential patients. One way—and, according to the supporters of a free market economy, the best way—to help buyers get more of what they want at the lowest possible price is to increase the supply of the needed product or service. This would suggest that instead of government grants for special Neighborhood Health Centers and Community Mental Health Centers, the medical needs of the less affluent members of American society could be better served simply by repealing laws governing medical licensure. As logical as this may seem, in medical and liberal circles this suggestion is regarded as "hairbrained," or worse.[7]

Since medical care in the United States is in short supply, its availability to the poor may be improved by redistributing the existing supply, by increasing the supply, or by both. Many individuals and groups clamoring for an improvement in our medical care system fail to scrutinize this artificially created shortage of medical personnel and to look to a free market economy for restoration of the balance between demand and supply. Instead, they seek to remedy the imbalance by redistributing the existing supply—in effect, robbing Peter to pay Paul. This proposal is in the tradition of other modern liberal social reforms, such as the redistribution of wealth by progressive taxation and a system of compulsory social security. No doubt, a political and economic system more socialistic in character than the one we now have could promote an equalization in the quality of the health care received by rich and poor. Whether this would result in the quality of the medical care of the poor approximating that of the rich, or vice versa, would remain to be seen. Experience suggests the latter. For over a century, we have had our version of state-supported psychiatric care for all who need it: the state mental hospitals system. The results of this effort are available for all to see.

Ironically, it is precisely this inadequacy of care in public mental institutions that has inspired the concept of a "right to treatment." In two landmark decisions the U.S. Court of Appeals for the District of Columbia Circuit, under the impetus of Chief Judge David Bazelon, affirmed the concept of a right to treatment for persons confined in public mental hospitals. In *Rouse* v. *Cameron*,[8] Chief Judge Bazelon, speaking for the majority, declared: "The purpose of involuntary hospitalization is treatment, not punishment."[9] Since "Congress [had] established a *statutory* 'right to treatment' in the 1964 Hospitalization of the Mentally Ill Act,"[10] he concluded: "The patient's right to treatment is clear."[11]

On the day the *Rouse* decision was handed down, the same court reiterated and extended its views on the right to treatment in *Millard* v. *Cameron*.[12] Millard had been charged with indecent exposure in June 1962, pleaded guilty to this charge, and was subsequently committed to Saint

Elizabeths Hospital as a "sexual psychopath." His appeal in this case was based on his allegation that he was receiving no treatment. Judge Bazelon, again speaking for the court, stated: "In *Rouse* v. *Cameron* . . . [we] held that the petitioner was entitled to relief upon showing that he was not receiving reasonably suitable and adequate treatment. Lack of such treatment, we said, could not be justified by lack of staff or facilities. We think the same principles apply to a person involuntarily committed to a public hospital as a sexual psychopath."[13]

In neither *Rouse* nor *Millard,* however, did Chief Judge Bazelon define what "adequate treatment" was, or say what, in the court's opinion, would constitute clearly *inadequate* treatment. Let us, therefore, examine what the concept of a right to medical, or psychiatric, treatment does in fact both entail and imply.

The Right to Psychiatric Treatment: Rhetoric and Reality

Most people in public mental hospitals do not receive what one would ordinarily consider treatment.[14] With this as his starting point, Birnbaum has advocated "the recognition and enforcement of the legal right of a mentally ill inmate of a public mental institution to adequate medical treatment for his mental illness."[15] Although it defined neither "mental illness" nor "adequate medical treatment," this proposal was received with enthusiasm in both legal and medical circles.[16] Why? Because it supported the myth that mental illness is a medical problem that can be best solved by medical means.

The idea of a "right" to mental treatment is both naive and dangerous. It is naive because it considers the problem of the publicly hospitalized mental patient as a medical one, ignoring its educational, economic, moral, religious, and social aspects. It is dangerous because its proposed remedy creates another problem—compulsory mental treatment—for in a context of involuntary confinement the treatment too shall have to be compulsory.

Hailing the right to treatment as "A New Right," the editor of *The American Bar Association Journal* compared psychiatric treatment for patients in

public mental hospitals with monetary compensation for the unemployed.[17] In both cases, we are told, the principle is to help "the victims of unfortunate circumstances."[18]

But things are not so simple. We know what unemployment is, but are not so clear regarding the definition of mental illness. Moreover, a person without a job does not usually object to receiving money; and if he does, no one compels him to take it. The situation of the so-called "mental patient" is quite different. Usually he does not want psychiatric treatment. Yet, the more he objects to it, the more firmly society insists that he must have it.

Of course, if we *define* psychiatric treatment as "help" for the "victims of unfortunate circumstances," how can anyone object to it? But the real question is twofold: What is meant by psychiatric help and what should the helpers do if a victim refuses to be helped?

From a legal and sociologic point of view, the only way to define mental illness is to enumerate the types of behavior psychiatrists consider to be indicative of such illness. Similarly, we may define psychiatric treatment by listing the procedures which psychiatrists regard as instances of such therapy. A brief illustration should suffice.

Levine lists 40 methods of psychotherapy.[19] Among these, he includes: physical treatment, medicinal treatment, reassurance, authoritative firmness, hospitalization, ignoring of certain symptoms and attitudes, satisfaction of neurotic needs, and bibliotherapy. In addition, there are physical methods of psychiatric therapy, such as the prescription of sedatives and tranquilizers, the induction of convulsions by drugs or electricity, and brain surgery.[20] Obviously, the term "psychiatric treatment" covers everything that may be done to a person under medical auspices—and more.

If mental treatment is all the things Levine and others tell us it is, how are we to determine whether or not patients in mental hospitals receive adequate amounts of it? Surely, many of them are already being treated with large doses of "authoritative firmness," with "ignoring of symptoms," and, certainly, with "satisfaction of neurotic needs." This last therapeutic agent has particularly sinister possibilities for offenders. Psychoanalysts have long maintained that many criminals commit antisocial acts out of a sense of guilt. What they "neurotically" crave is punishment. By this reasoning, indefinite incarceration might itself be regarded as psychiatric treatment.

At present, our publicly operated psychiatric institutions perform their services based on the premise that it is morally legitimate to treat so-called "mentally sick" persons against their will. Illustrative is a document prepared by the Advisory Committee on the Recodification of the New York State Mental Hygiene Law.[21] It begins with the declaration: "It is axiomatic that the entire Mental Hygiene Law is concerned with patients' rights, especially rights to *adequate care and treatment.*[22]

In my opinion, this assertion is a brazen falsehood. The primary concern of any mental hygiene law is to empower physicians to imprison innocent citizens, under the rubic of "civil commitment," and to justify torturing them by means of a variety of violent acts called "psychiatric treatments." As one might expect, among the members of the above-mentioned committee were the Commissioner and two Assistant Commissioners of the New York State Department of Mental Hygiene. Conspicuous by their absence from the committee were either the inmates or former inmates of public mental hospitals or the experts selected by these "patients" to represent them.

In relation to psychiatric treatment, then, the most fundamental and vexing problem becomes: How can a treatment which is compulsory also be a right? As I have shown elsewhere,[23] the problem posed by the neglect and mistreatment of the publicly hospitalized mentally ill is not derived from any insufficiency in the treatment they receive, but rather from the basic conceptual fallacy inherent in the notion of mental illness and the moral evil inherent in the practice of involuntary mental hospitalization. Preserving the concept of mental illness and the social practices it has justified and papering over its glaring cognitive and ethical defects by means of a superimposed "right to mental treatment" only aggravates an already tragically inhuman situation.

The problem posed by the "warehousing" of vast numbers of unwanted, helpless, and stigmatized people in huge state mental hospitals may be better resolved—better, that is, for the victimized "patients," though not necessarily for the society that is victimizing them or the professionals who profit from this arrangement—by asking: What do involuntarily hospitalized mental patients need more—a right to receive treatments they do not wish or a right to refuse such interventions? The answer should come from the imprisoned patients, not from the institutional psychiatrists.

Fallacies of the Concept "Right to Treatment"

As my foregoing remarks indicate, I see two fundamental defects in the concept of a right to treatment. The first is scientific and medical, stemming from unclarified issues concerning what constitutes an illness or treatment and who qualifies as a patient or physician. The other is political and moral, stemming from unclarified issues concerning the differences between rights and claims.

In the present state of medical practice and popular opinion, definitions of the terms "illness," "treatment," "physician," and "patient" are so imprecise that a concept of a right to treatment can only serve to further muddy an already very confused situation. One example will illustrate what I mean.

One can "treat," in the medical sense of this term, only a disease, or, more precisely, only a person, now called a "patient," suffering from a disease. But what is a disease? Certainly, cancer, stroke, and heart disease are. But is obesity a disease? How about smoking cigarettes? Using heroin or marijuana? Malingering to avoid the draft or collect insurance compensation? Homosexuality? Kleptomania? Grief? Each one of these conditions has been declared a disease by medical and psychiatric authorities who hold impeccable institutional credentials. Furthermore, innumerable other conditions, varying from bachelorhood and divorce to political and religious prejudices, have been so termed.

Similarly, what is treatment? Certainly, the surgical removal of a cancerous breast is. But is an organ transplant treatment? If it is, and if such treatment is a right, how can those charged with guaranteeing people the protection of their right to treatment discharge their duties without having access to the requisite number of transplantable organs? On a simpler level, if ordinary obesity, due to eating too much, is a disease, how can a doctor treat it when its treatment depends on the patient eating less? What does it mean, then, that a patient has a right to be treated for obesity? I have already alluded to the facility with which this kind of right becomes equated with a societal and medical obligation to deprive the patient of his freedom—to eat, to drink, to take drugs, and so forth.

Who is a patient? Is he one who has a demonstrable bodily illness or injury, such as cancer or a fracture? A person who complains of bodily symptoms, but has no demonstrable illness, like the so-called "hypochondriac"? The person who feels perfectly well but is said to be ill by others, for example, the paranoid schizophrenic? Or is he a person, such as Senator Barry Goldwater, who professes political views differing from those of the psychiatrist who brands him insane?

Finally, who is a physician? Is he a person licensed to practice medicine? One certified to have completed a specified educational curriculum? One possessing certain medical skills as demonstrated by public performance? Or is he one claiming to possess such skills?

It seems to me that improvement in the health care of poor people and those now said to be mentally ill depends less on declarations about their rights to treatment and more on certain reforms in the language and conduct of those professing a desire to help them. In particular, such reforms must entail refinements in the use of medical concepts, such as illness and treatment, and a recognition of the basic differences between medical intervention as a service, which the individual is free to seek or reject, and medical intervention as a method of social control, which is imposed on him by force or fraud.

I can perhaps best illustrate this unsolved dilemma by citing some actual cases. As recently as 1965, a Connecticut statute made it a crime for any person to artifically prevent conception.[24] Accordingly, a mother of ten requesting contraceptive help from a physician in a public hospital in Connecticut would have been refused this assistance. Did what she seek constitute "treatment"? Not according to the legislators who defined the prescription of birth control devices as immoral and illegal acts, rather than as interventions aimed at preserving health.[25]

Today, a similar situation exists with respect to a woman's unwanted pregnancy and her wish for an abortion. Is being pregnant, when one does not want to be, an illness? Is an abortion a treatment? Or is it murder of the fetus? If it is murder, why is no "abortionist" ever prosecuted for murder? How can the preservation of a pregnant woman's mental health justify such murder, now called "therapeutic abortion"?[26]

On the other hand, should a wholly secular, utilitarian point of view prevail, and the use of birth control devices and abortion be considered treatments, what would it mean for a woman to have a right to such interventions? Clearly, it would result in her having unhampered access to physicians willing to both prescribe birth control devices and perform abortions. Where would such a medico-legal posture leave a Roman Catholic obstetrician? By refusing to abort a woman wishing a termination of her pregnancy, he would be interfering with her right to treatment in a way that might be analogized to a white barber's refusing to cut the hair of a black customer, or vice versa, thus, interfering with his customer's civil rights.

As still another example, consider the situation of an unhappily married couple. Are they sick? If they define themselves as having a "neurotic marriage" and consult a psychiatrist, they would be considered sick and their insurance coverage might even pay for their treatment. But if they seek the solution of the problem in divorce and consult an attorney, they would not be considered sick. Thus, although unhappily married people are often considered "ill," divorce is never considered a treatment. If it were, it too would have to be a right. Where would that leave our present divorce laws?

One could go on and on. I shall cite, however, only one more instance—the practice of involuntary mental hospitalization—to show how deeply confused and confusing is our present situation with respect to the concept of treatment; and hence how very mischievous any extension of this concept, as a right secured by the government, is bound to be.

In most jurisdictions, persons said to be mentally ill and dangerous to themselves or others may be committed to a mental hospital. Such incarceration in a building called a "hospital" is considered a form of psychiatric, and hence medical, treatment. But who, in fact, is the patient? Who is being treated? Ostensibly, the person treated is the one who is incarcerated. But since he did not seek medical assistance, whereas those who secured his confinement did, one might argue that involuntary mental hospitalization is treatment for those who seek commitment, rather than for those who are committed. This would be analogous to arguing that a "therapeutic abortion" is a treatment for the pregnant woman, not for the aborted fetus—an assertion few would deny. If this argument is accepted, then, in any conflict, an injury to one party could be defined as a treatment to his opponent. The following recent statement on the psychiatric treatment of "acting-out adolescents" is illustrative: "The move toward 'freedom, love, peace' has encouraged anti-social acting out, including the increasing use of marijuana and psychedelic drugs. Consequently, emotionally disturbed young men who are acting in a way that directly conflicts with their parents' standards are being hospitalized in increasing numbers."[27] In this sort of situation, whose right to treatment do the advocates of this concept wish to guarantee—that of the parent to commit his rebellious son as mentally ill or that of the child to defy his parents without being subjected to quasi-medical penalties?

The Distinction between "Rights" and "Claims"

The second difficulty which the concept of a right to treatment poses is of a political and moral nature. It stems from confusing "rights" with "claims," and protection from injuries with provision for goods or services.

For a definition of right, I can do no better than to quote John Stuart Mill: "I have treated the idea of a right as *residing in the injured person and violated by the injury.*... When we call anything a person's right, we mean that he has a valid claim on society to protect him in the possession of it, either by force of law, or by that of education and opinion.... To have a right, then, is, I conceive, to have something which *society ought to defend me in the possession of.*"[28]

This helps us distinguish rights from claims. Rights, Mill says, are "possessions"; they are things people have by nature, like liberty; acquire by dint of hard work, like property; create by inventiveness, like a new machine; or inherit, like money. Characteristically, possessions are what a person *has,* and of which others, including the State, can therefore deprive him. Mill's point is the classic libertarian one: The State should protect the individual in his rights. This is what the Declaration of Independence means when it refers to the inalienable rights to life, liberty and the pursuit of happiness. It is important to note that, in political theory, no less than in everyday practice, this requires that the State be strong and resolute enough to protect the rights of the individual from infringement by others and that it be decentralized and restrained enough, typically through federalism and a constitution, to insure that it will not itself violate the rights of its people.

In the sense specified above, then, there can be no such thing as a right to treatment. Conceiving of a person's body as his possession—like his automobile or watch (though, no doubt, more valuable)—it is just as nonsensical to speak of his right to have his body repaired as it would be to speak of his right to have his automobile or watch repaired.

It is thus evident that in its current usage and especially in the phrase "right to treatment" the term "right" actually means claim. More specifically, "right" here means the recognition of the claims of one party, considered to be *in the right,* and the repudiation of the claims of another, opposing party, considered to be *in the wrong*—

the "rightful" party having allied himself with the interests of the community and having enlisted the coercive powers of the State on his behalf. Let us analyze this situation in the case of medical treatment for an ordinary bodily disease. The patient, having lost some of his health, tries to regain it by means of medical attention and drugs. The medical attention he needs is, however, the property of his physician, and the drug he needs is the property of the manufacturer who produced it. The patient's right to treatment thus conflicts with the physician's right to liberty, *i.e.*, to sell his services freely, and the pharmaceutical manufacturer's rights in his own property, *i.e.*, to sell his products as he chooses. The advocates of a right to treatment for the patient are less than candid regarding their proposals for reconciling this proposed right with the right of the physician to liberty and that of the pharmaceutical manufacturer to property.[29]

Nor is it clear how the right to treatment concept can be reconciled with the traditional Western concept of the patient's right to choose his physician. If the patient has a right to choose the doctor by whom he wishes to be treated, and if he *also* has a right to treatment, then, in effect, the doctor is the patient's slave. Obviously, the patient's right to choose his physician cannot be wrenched from its context and survive; its corollary is the physician's right to accept or reject a patient, except for rare cases of emergency treatment. No one, of course, envisions the absurdity of physicians being at the personal beck and call of individual patients, becoming literally their medical slaves, as some had been in ancient Greece and Rome.

The concept of a right to treatment has a different, much less absurd but far more ominous, implication. For just as the corollary of the individual's freedom to choose his physician is the physician's freedom to refuse to treat any particular patient, so the corollary of the individual's right to treatment is the denial of the physician's right to reject, as a patient, anyone officially so designated. This transformation removes, in one fell swoop, the individual's right to define himself as sick and to seek medical care as he sees fit, and the physician's right to define whom he considers sick and wishes to treat; it

places these decisions instead in the hands of the State's medical bureaucracy. To see how this works in the United States on a less-than-total scale and coexisting with a flourishing system of private medical practice, one need only to look at our state mental hospitals. Every patient admitted to such a hospital has a right to treatment, and every physician serving in this hospital system has an obligation to treat each patient assigned to him by his superiors or committed to his care by the courts. Missing from this system, and similar systems, are the patient's traditional economic and legal controls over the medical relationship and the physician's traditional economic dependence on, and legal obligations to, the individual he has accepted for treatment.

As a result, bureaucratic care, as contrasted with its entrepreneurial counterpart, ceases to be a system of healing the sick and instead becomes a system of controlling the deviant. Although this outcome seems to be inevitable in the case of psychiatry (in view of the fact that ascription of the label "mental illness" so often functions as a quasi-medical rhetoric concealing social conflicts), it need not be inevitable for nonpsychiatric medical services. However, in every situation where medical care is provided bureaucratically, as in communist societies, the physician's role as agent of the sick patient is necessarily alloyed with, and often seriously compromised by, his role as agent of the State. Thus, the doctor becomes a kind of medical policeman—at times helping the individual, and at times harming him.

Returning to Mill's definition of a "right," one could say, further, that just as a man has a right to life and liberty, so, too, has he a right to health and, hence, a claim on the State to protect his health. It is important to note here that the right to health differs from the right to treatment in the same way as the right to property differs from the right to theft. Recognition of a right to health would obligate the State to prevent individuals from depriving each other of their health, just as recognition of the two other rights now prevents each individual from depriving every other individual of liberty and property. It would also obligate the State to respect the health of the individual and

to deprive him of that asset only in accordance with due process of law, just as it now respects the individual's liberty and property and deprives him of them only in accordance with due process of law.

As matters now stand, the State not only fails to protect the individual's health, but it actually hinders him in his efforts to safeguard his own health, as in the case of its permitting industries to befoul the waters we drink and the air we breathe. The State similarly prohibits individuals from obtaining medical care from certain, officially "unqualified," experts and from buying and ingesting certain, officially "dangerous," drugs. Sometimes, the State even deliberately deprives the individual of treatment under the very guise of providing treatment.[30]

To be sure, there are good reasons, in an age in which the powerful, centralized State is idolized as the source of all benefits, why the concept of a right to treatment is considered progressive and is popular, and why the concept of a right to health has, so far as I know, never even been articulated, much less recognized by legislators and the courts. On the one hand, recognition of a right to health, rather than to treatment, would impose greater obligations on the State to insure domestic peace, especially the protection of an individual's health as a type of private property; on the other hand, it would impose greater restraints on its own powers vis-à-vis the citizen, especially on its jurisdiction over the licensure of physicians and the dispensing of drugs. These would require a government to shoulder greater responsibilities for its duties as policeman, while limiting its alleged responsibilities for dispensing services—in short, the very antithesis of the type of State which modern liberal social reformers consider desirable and necessary for the attainment of their goals. Instead of fostering the independent judgment of the individual, such reformers encourage his submission to an ostensibly competent and benevolent authority; hence, they project the image of the medical therapist unto the State, while casting the citizen in the complementary role of sick patient. This, of course, places the individual in precisely that inferior and submissive role vis-à-vis the government from which the founding fathers sought, by means of the Constitution, to rescue him. Politically, the right to treatment is thus simply the right to submit to authority—a right which has always been dear both to those in power and those incapable of managing their own lives.

Conclusion

The State can protect and promote the interests of its sick, or potentially sick, citizens in one of only two ways: either by coercing physicians, and other medical and paramedical personnel, to serve patients—as State-owned slaves in the last analysis[31]—or by creating economic, moral, and political circumstances favorable to a plentiful supply of competent physicians and effective drugs.

The former solution corresponds to and reflects efforts to solve human problems by recourse to the all-powerful State. The rights promised by such a state—exemplified by the right to treatment—are not opportunities for uncoerced choices by individuals, but rather are powers vested in the State for the subjection of the interests of one group to those of another.

The latter solution corresponds to, and reflects efforts to, solve human problems by recourse to individual initiative and voluntary associations without interference by the State. The rights exacted from such a State—exemplified by the right to life, liberty, and health—are limitations on its own powers and sphere of action and provide the conditions necessary for, but of course do not insure the proper exercise of, free and responsible individual choices.

In these two solutions we recognize the fundamental polarities of the great ideological conflict of our age, perhaps of all ages and of the human condition itself, namely, individualism and capitalism on the one side, collectivism and communism on the other. *Tertium non datur*: There is no other choice.

Notes

1. Gruenberg, Book Review, 161 *Science* 347 (1968).

2. *Id.*

3. "Concisely stated, the standard [of law as public policy] is that every individual has a right to treatment, a right to good treatment, a right to the best treatment." Brown, Psychiatric Practice and Public Policy, 125 *Am. J. Psychiatry* 141, 142–43 (1968).

4. Since the French Revolution, and increasingly during the past century, virtually all Western governments have fostered the belief that not only great inequalities of wealth, but also inequalities of all kinds—ambition, talent, and, of course, health—are inequities. The result has been described with unmatched irony by C. S. Lewis: "Men are not angered by mere misfortune but by misfortune conceived as injury. And the sense of injury depends on the feeling that a legitimate claim has been denied. The more claims on life, therefore, that your patient can be induced to make, the more often he will feel injured and, as a result, ill-tempered." C. S. Lewis, *The Screwtape Letters & Screwtape Proposes a Toast* 106 (1961).

5. The overprotection granted the latter group prompted S. Jerome Bronson, the Oakland (Michigan) County prosecutor, to state publicly: "When the state medical licensing board is more interested in protecting the doctor than the public, the whole question of licensing procedures needs review." *Med. World News*, Aug. 2, 1968, at 25.

The proposition that medical licensing procedures serve the purpose of protecting the public rather than the profession is largely rhetoric. *See* note 7 *infra*.

6. Joseph S. Clark, Jr., the then Mayor of Philadelphia, defined a "liberal" as: "[O]ne who believes in utilizing the full force of government for the advancement of social, political, and economic justice at the municipal, state, national, and international levels." Clark, Can the Liberals Rally?, *The Atlantic Monthly*, July 1953, at 27.

7. For an excellent discussion of the deleterious effects of professional licensure requirements, see M. Friedman, *Capitalism and Freedom* 137–60 (1962). Friedman correctly recognizes that the justification for enacting special licensure provisions, especially for regulating medical practice, "is always said to be the necessity of protecting the public interest. However, the pressure on the legislature to license an occupation rarely comes from the members of the public. . . . On the contrary, the pressure invariably comes from members of the occupation itself." *Id.* at 140.

Unless one believes in the unique altruism of physicians, for which, it may be noted, there is no evidence, the conclusion is inescapable that the actual aim of restrictive licensure laws—as compared to the certification of a special competence of persons, such as mathematicians or physicists, which carries no implication of legal restraints on others not so certified—is the very opposite of their ostensible or professed aim. Under the pretense of protecting the public from incompetent practitioners, licensing laws protect the medical profes-

sion from the competition of other vendors of desired services and from the scrutiny of the enlightened public.

8. 125 U.S. App. D.C. 366, 373 F.2d 451 (1966).

9. *Id.* at 367, 373 F.2d at 452. Individuals imprisoned in mental institutions against their will, however, consider their confinement punishment, not treatment. Also, in ordinary English usage, involuntary confinement is synonymous with imprisonment. "Imprisonment" has been defined as "constraint of a person either by force or by such other coercion as restrains him within limits against his will." 2 *Webster's New International Dictionary* 1252 (2d ed. unabridged 1958). Our use of language is crucial in this connection. If we accept, as Chief Judge Bazelon does, that mental hospitalization is treatment, we adopt an idiom designed to justify psychiatric violence as "therapy." See generally Szasz, Science and Public Policy: The Crime of Involuntary Mental Hospitalization, 4 *Med. Op. & Rev.*, May 1968, at 24.

10. 125 U.S. App. D.C. at 368, 373 F.2d at 453. The Act provides: "A person hospitalized in a public hospital for a mental illness shall, during his hospitalization, be entitled to medical and psychiatric care and treatment." *D.C. Code Ann.* § 21–562 (1967).

11. 125 U.S. App. D.C. at 371, 373 F.2d at 456. Rouse, it is interesting to note, had been involuntarily committed to Saint Elizabeths Hospital in Nov. 1962, after having been found not guilty by reason of insanity to the charge of carrying a dangerous weapon. Had Rouse been found guilty of this offense, the maximum sentence would have been one year in prison. Having been acquitted, he had already been confined for four years in Saint Elizabeths Hospital at the time of his appeal. Moreover, Rouse contended that he had never been mentally ill, was presently not mentally ill, and that he never needed psychiatric treatment—all arguments which Judge Bazelon simply ignored.

12. 125 U.S App. D.C. 383, 373 F.2d 468 (1966).

13. *Id.* at 387, 373 F.2d at 472.

14. This section of the article is adapted, with minor modifications and additions, from one of my books: T. S. Szasz, *Law, Liberty, and Psychiatry* 214–16 (1963). My objections to the concept of a right to mental treatment, formulated in 1962, seem to me as valid today as they were then.

15. Birnbaum, The Right to Treatment, 46 *A.B.A.J.* 499 (1960).

16. *See, e.g.*, Editorial, A New Right, 46 *A.B.A.J.* 516 (1960); *N.Y. Times*, Dec. 15, 1967, at 21, col. 1.

17. Editorial, A New Right, *supra* note 16, at 516.

18. *Id.*

19. M. Levine, *Psychotherapy in Medical Practice* 17–19 (1942).

20. The following is a curious, though by no means rare, example of the kind of thing that passes nowadays for mental treatment. In Sydney, Australia, "a former tax inspector on trial for murdering his sleeping family was found not guilty on the grounds of mental illness. . . . A psychiatrist told the court yesterday that Sharp . . . had apparently cured his mental illness when he shot himself in the head." *N.Y. Herald-Tribune* (Paris), July 5, 1968, at 5, col. 8. Murder is here considered an "illness," and a brain injury a "treatment" and indeed a "cure" for it. In the "Brave New World" where treatment is a right, will every murderer have the right to a brain injury—if not by means of a gun, then perhaps by that of a leucotome?

21. Institute of Public Administration, *A New Mental Hygiene Law for New York State* art. 37 (Feb. 1968 Draft).

22. *Id.* at 31 (emphasis added). This statement is true in the same sense and in the same way as would have been the claim of a 16th century Spanish inquisitor that: "It is axiomatic that the entire Inquisition is concerned with the rights of the faithful, especially rights to true belief and salvation."

23. *See* T. S. Szasz, *Psychiatric Justice* (1965); T. S. Szasz, *supra* note 14; T. S. Szasz, *The Myth of Mental Illness* (1961).

24. *Conn. Gen. Stat. Rev.* § 53–32 (Supp. 1965), ruled invalid in *Griswold* v. *Connecticut,* 381 U.S. 479 (1965). In *Griswold* the anticontraceptive statute was declared unconstitutional by the Supreme Court on the ground that it violated the right of marital privacy, a right the Court considered within the penumbra of the specific guarantees of the Bill of Rights.

The significance of this case lies in its offering an instance in which a state's duly appointed legislators denied a certain medical assistance to their constituents while a majority of the Supreme Court deemed such assistance to be a "right."

Justice White's concurring opinion represents what was, in all likelihood, the real reason for the Court's overturning of the statute before it: "[T]he clear effect of these statutes, as enforced, is to deny disadvantaged citizens of Connecticut, those without either adequate knowledge or resources to obtain private counseling, access to medical assistance and up-to-date information in respect to proper methods of birth control." 381 U.S. at 503.

25. There exist endless variations on this theme. For example, recently a group of Negro women in Pittsburgh sought the return of a birth control clinic which had left their neighborhood "after a militant black leader had accused it of committing 'black genocide.'" *N.Y. Times*, Aug. 11, 1968, at 44, col. 1. Again, the issue revolved around the definition of birth control, as "medical help" or as "genocide"; and, more specifically, around who has the *power* of definition and the power to impose his definition by threat or law on his fellows.

For another pertinent example, consider the recent ruling of Louis J. Lefkowitz, the New York State Attorney General, that medicaid does not cover surgical sterilization for strictly contraceptive purposes, but does include surgical sterilization for medical reasons. *AMA News,* Aug. 26, 1968, at 13, col. 1.

26. *See* Szasz, The Ethics of Abortion, 26 *The Humanist* 147 (1966); Szasz, The Ethics of Birth Control, 20 *The Humanist* 332 (1960).

27. Krinsky & Jennings, The Management and Treatment of Acting-Out Adolescents in a Separate Unit, 19 *Hosp. & Community Psychiatry* 72 (1968).

28. J. S. Mill, *Utilitarianism* 78–79 (1863) (emphasis added).

29. The proposition that sick people have a special claim to the protection of the State—in other words, that they be allowed to use the coercive apparatus of the State to expropriate the fruits of the labor of others—is a part of a much larger theme, namely, the inevitable tendency in a society for each special interest group to enlist the powers of the State on its own behalf. In this connection, R. A. Childs has recently written:

Economically, the state uses its monopoly on expropriation of wealth to create political castes, or "classes." . . . Thus, today, we see the state being supported by businessmen who are being benefited by defense contracts and other state patronage, tariffs, subsidies, and special tax "loopholes"; unions which are benefited by labor laws; farmers benefited by price supports, and other groups benefited by other state-granted privileges. . . . Of course, almost every group is harmed more by the benefits heaped on other groups than it is helped by its own special privileges, but since the state has gotten people to believe that the only valid approach to problems is to increase, rather than to decrease, state powers, no one mentions the possibility of benefiting each group by removing the special privileges of all other groups. Instead, each group supports the state, to benefit itself at the expense of all other groups.

Childs, Autarchy and the Statist Abyss. 4 *Rampart J.* 1, 4–5 (1968).

Long ago de Tocqueville had perceived this phenomenon and warned of its dangerous consequences for individual liberty: "The government having stepped into the place of Divine Providence in France it was but natural that everyone, when in difficulties, invoked its aid." A. de Tocqueville, *The Old Regime and the French Revolution* 70 (1856).

30. The following is an illustrative example. In June 1968, the Santa Monica Synanon center was raided by agents of the California Narcotic Authority. Two of the residents were removed for tests to determine if they were "clean." This interference with their voluntary effort to break the narcotic habit in accordance with the Synanon principles was lawful inasmuch as the persons arrested were parolees from California's Narcotic

Rehabilitation Center at Corona, and as such, subject to periodic surprise testing by state authorities. On the advice of Synanon lawyers, the defendants refused to take the test. Their paroles were thereupon revoked, and they were recommitted to the Corona facility to serve out the full terms of their "psychiatric sentence." *Time,* July 12, 1968, at 74.

The relapse rate of addicts treated at rehabilitation centers such as Corona is approximately 90%, whereas for those treated at Synanon, it is 20%. It can hardly be said, then, that the two patients, over whose abstinence from narcotics the State of California appears to have shown such touching solicitude, were being guaranteed their right to treatment at Corona, though such no doubt would be the official interpretation of their fate. In a larger sense, this is also an instance of the bureaucratic perversion of language which Orwell so eloquently described. To his lexicon of Newspeak, in which "war" means "peace" and "slavery" means "freedom," we may add "punishment" to mean "treatment." G. Orwell, *1984,* at 6 (1949).

31. The position of the physician in Czechoslovakia is illustrative. "The constitution [of Czechoslovakia] declares that health care is a right of the people and that it is the duty of the state to satisfy that right." In practice, this "right" is assured through "the assignment [by the Communist State] of a low economic (productive) status to the health services. . . . A skilled factory worker may earn much more than a doctor through premium pay. Even a taxi driver may earn more than a doctor. . . . Almost universal was the comment: 'We are not attracting the best people into medicine.'" Cooper, Czechoslovakia Reflects Regional Plan Problems, *Hospital Tribune,* Sept. 9, 1968, at 1, col. 1.

Allocation of Scarce Medical Resources

97

David Sanders and Jesse Dukeminier, Jr.

From "Medical Advance and Legal Lag: Hemodialysis and Kidney Transplantation"

Reprinted with permission of the publisher from *UCLA Law Review,* vol. 15, February 1968, pp. 366–380.

Patient Selection[1]

The number of persons who seek hemodialysis is far greater than the number who can be served. In the United States there are now approximately 800 persons on hemodialysis in 121 centers; less than 100 of these are on home hemodialysis.[2] Dr. Scribner and his associates estimate that from 5,000 to 10,000 *new* patients each year in the United States need hemodialysis,[3] which would require at least 20,000 hemodialysis machines.[4] Dr. Kolff estimates that "there are between 60,000 and 90,000 persons with chronic renal failure in the United States who need treatment with the artificial kidney."[5] Regardless of which estimate is correct, it is obvious that rigid selection of patients is currently taking place and is likely to continue in the foreseeable future.

The selection of patients for hemodialysis raises an ethical question of great perplexity. The issue is sharply posed: selection means a chance for life; rejection means death.[6] How should selection be made? Any useful answer can be reached only after untangling many matters, including, first, how selection is currently made.

In all hemodialysis centers a medical evaluation is made by physicians. In some, psychiatric, social worth, and financial evaluations are also made, either by a medical committee or a lay committee or both. Here is a cryptic description of the selection process at Los Angeles County General Hospital and San Francisco General Hospital:

Only physicians licensed to practice medicine in California are authorized to refer patients. The initial contact is with the medical director, who advises the physician concerning the course of action he considers indicated.

If the patient is to be evaluated at the center, referral forms are provided and a date of evaluation set. Transportation costs to the center and costs for evaluation are borne by the patient, his family or by third party payments. Patients found medically suitable for chronic hemodialysis, on original evaluation, are then referred to a Patient Selection Committee composed of physicians, social workers, rehabilitation workers and other specialists as indicated.

The committee then considers the patient from an overall standpoint as to the feasibility of accepting him for the program. Upon selection, a plan of payment for services is arranged and chronic hemodialysis is initiated.[7]

To see the moral and legal questions hidden in this short passage requires a fuller description of the selection procedures.

Medical Evaluation

The medical evaluation of a candidate includes an analysis of the candidate's general health. If the candidate has cardiac disease, diabetes, or systemic diseases of various kinds, his life expectancy is not as great as one with kidney disease alone. The candidate with kidney disease alone, uncomplicated with other illnesses, is preferred on the theory that if the kidney's function is replaced by the artificial kidney, he will be relatively well. The healthier the candidate generally, the better chance he has for selection.

At most hospitals the age of the candidate is also important. Most hemodialysis centers are unwilling to begin dialyzing persons over 50 years of age (and some set the limit much younger).[8] At the other end of the age scale, children under 13 are rejected for chronic hemodialysis both because they lack the extreme self-discipline required by the dialysis regime and because puberty is unlikely to develop if hemodialysis is begun before adolescence.

Psychiatric Evaluation

Physicians are now aware of the psychiatric problems attending the actual physical process of hemodialysis[9] and of the psychiatric problems involved in a new way of life where the patient is dependent upon the machine.[10] Some hemodialysis units have therefore set up a series of psychiatric examinations to screen candidates. These include an interview by a psychiatrist and standard intelligence and personality tests.

A patient on hemodialysis must have the emotional and intellectual ability to cooperate with the treatment regime. Dr. Scribner and his associates in Seattle have found cooperation to be the most essential factor in successful chronic hemodialysis: "It now appears that picking the cooperative patient is a far more important criterion of selection for chronic dialysis than the other needlessly rigid criteria originally proposed by our group."[11]

What is cooperation? Following is a list of characteristics that are considered to be minimal for success in the treatment regime of hemodialysis. (1) The ability to learn to take care of the cannulas, to keep them clean and free from infection. (2) The ability to adhere to a diet. Perhaps in no other medical condition is adherence to a strictly controlled diet as important in avoiding complications, or indeed in preserving life, as in hemodialysis. The diet is bland and limiting, the intake of salt and water must be kept to a minimum. (3) The ability to tolerate complications. Experience has taught the hospital staff at most hemodialysis centers that in the normal course of hemodialysis complications will develop. The ability to tolerate these, to be cooperative, to go along with the medical regime without getting too depressed or discouraged is an essential ingredient in "cooperation." (4) The psychological ability to tolerate the stress of being "saved twice a week." (5) The ability to live with uncertainty. Although a patient may be stabilized on hemodialysis for long periods of time, there is no way to predict when a complication, either mild or serious, may occur. The quality of personality that is important is the ability to live with this uncertainty without its unduly interfering with outside functioning. (6) The ability to tolerate dependence. Patients on hemodialysis are dependent upon a mechanical device for their life. They are dependent on continued medical care as long as they are on the hemodialysis program. They cannot change doctors or change institutions. Personality difficulties may develop between the patient and the staff. These have to be dealt with and worked through, and this is much easier if the patient has the ability to view his conduct with some detachment. (7) Rehabilitation potential. This can be defined as the ability and desire to continue in active life, despite the constant fluctuations of bodily state. Hemodialysis often requires a change in occupations.

A person on chronic hemodialysis must develop a life style that includes dependence on the machine and the personnel providing medical care. It is not easy for psychiatrists and social workers to predict who has or will develop the qualities that a person must have to adjust to life with a machine.[12]

At Cedars-Sinai Medical Center in Los Angeles some patients regarded at the beginning as poor risks have shown surprising strength and ability to deal with the life-threatening continual crises of hemodialysis—crises which may be remarkably different from what psychiatrists could normally predict. When the candidate is being evaluated for the hemodialysis program, he is sick, has been in chronic renal failure for some time, and personality changes, usually irritability and depression, accompany the uremic syndrome. When his uremia is ameliorated by hemodialysis, his depression may lift and the personality initially presented the psychiatrist may change.

Moreover, psychiatric evaluation is difficult because it is not just the patient who must be evaluated. The success of a patient in adjusting to a life of hemodialysis depends not on himself alone, but also upon the support he receives from his family, from the hospital staff, and from others of the group on the hemodialysis program. The patient will be interacting with all these other persons. One of the most common psychiatric problems occurring with hemodialysis patients is depression. The degree and manifestations of depression vary, depending on the patient's previous personality type and the dynamic structure and defense mechanisms of the patient. A common manifestation of depression is relaxation of self-care and diet control. When depression occurs the reactions of those around the patient will affect the patient's ability to cope further.

Hemodialysis is a family affair. The emotional and economic burdens put on the family by this procedure are enormous. When the prospect of hemodialysis comes up, most families respond positively to it, but when they find that their relatives are being saved twice a week and the burdens continue or increase, many hidden resentments develop. The relatives may even go through a premature mourning process causing psychological isolation of the patient. As in any illness that may require role reversals, the psychological equilibrium that has developed between husband and wife is upset, and this can cause psychological problems of great intensity. Families often need to deny their anger and frustration with the patient because of the seriousness of the illness. It is as crucial to work with the families as it is to work with the patients.[13]

The close and continuing relationships that develop between the staff and patients on hemodialysis can cause difficulty for staff members and for patients. Patients' transference reactions or depressions that manifest themselves by disturbed behavior in relation to the staff can evoke strong feelings in and from the staff. These patients sometimes are then labeled uncooperative, causing stress in the whole hemodialysis situation. When a patient does poorly or dies the staff—and the whole dialysis unit including the other patients—may be precipitated into crisis. How the unit interacts in crisis affects the success of the program. At Cedars-Sinai Medical Center it has been found useful to have weekly meetings to discuss patient problems and staff reactions to these problems, similar to the kinds of regular meetings that are held in mental hospitals and chronic disease hospitals.

Social Worth Evaluation

The pioneering Seattle Artificial Kidney Center at the University of Washington bases its decisions upon an evaluation by an anonymous committee of the social worth of the candidate.[14] No moral or ethical guidelines are given the committee. The members are guided by their individual consciences. The deliberations of this committee were described several years ago in an article in Life[15] and more recently in an article in Redbook:

Dr. Scribner supports—he feels from necessity—the system of weeding out applicants by a civilian board that obtains in Seattle, Washington. He says, "The purpose is to represent the community and to assure that choices are made objectively, without outside pressure."

All candidates for treatment must be under 40 years of age. They must be self-supporting and residents of the state of Washington. A first panel, composed of physicians, eliminates the medically unfit. These include heart patients, diabetics . . . and those with other chronic illnesses.

The second panel consists of seven persons. At present they are a clergyman, a housewife, a banker, a labor leader and two physicians. This group makes the final decision, and they remain anonymous in order to be protected from public pressures. "And of course," as one of them admits, "the

importunate pressures of those who are on their way to die."

This civilian group bases its decisions on social and economic criteria. Other factors equal, the group chooses those with dependents. It favors patients who are stable in their behavior and appear to be emotionally mature. To have a record of public service is a help—scout leader, Sunday-school teacher, Red Cross volunteer. They frown on those who have a record of skipping appointments.[16]

Other hemodialysis centers may have a lay committee or a hospital staff committee evaluate social worth, or they may not attempt such an evaluation. In some centers an evaluation of social worth may be hidden in obscurantist language such as that used in the mimeographed procedure for selection of patients at the San Francisco General Hospital. The general criteria are given first:

Two primary, interrelated and equally weighted general criteria will apply in determining acceptance. These are medical data indicating that the patient is suitable to this treatment and vocational data indicating that the patient can be effectively rehabilitated with the treatment. Other social values must not influence the decision.[17]

When the directive gets down to business, however, it does not take a very firm grip on specifics. The specific criteria weighed in the selection process include:

1. Vocational history suggesting rehabilitation is feasible on chronic hemodialysis.
2. Medical data indicating that the patient's present disability will be significantly helped by chronic hemodialysis therapy.
3. Medical data indicating that the patient is emotionally and intellectually capable of managing chronic hemodialysis therapy.
4. Medical data indicating that there are no disabling irreversible complications of renal failure.
5. Medical data indicating that there are no associated diseases likely to (1) prove fatal or disabling over the next 5 years or (2) significantly complicate effective rehabilitation through chronic hemodialysis therapy.
6. Data regarding the feasibility of transplant.
7. Data indicating the feasibility of home dialysis therapy.
8. Data indicating the feasibility of center dialysis therapy.[18]

How is the selection made between two patients with equally good medical histories and equally good rehabilitation potential? What undisclosed preferences and prejudices, as well as objective criteria, may be contained in such a large, roomy word as "feasibility"?

Should Social Worth Evaluations Be Made?

Selection procedures using evaluations of social worth need to be re-examined carefully. Who should be saved? Should we save Jones because of his past achievements or Smith because of his great potential as a brilliant chemist or Allen because by dying with four children he imposes a greater burden on society? Should we save the poor rather than the rich, because the families of the rich will be well provided for and not burden society?[19] Should we save a woman with six children or a great composer? Obviously selection for hemodialysis raises moral questions of immense perplexity.[20] When this decision is made by publicly owned hospitals[21] or by hospitals with enough government contacts to make them instruments of the state,[22] or possibly by any hospital,[23] constitutional problems of due process and equal protection of the law are also presented.

It is not necessary here to go into the meaning of the constitutional command of equal protection,[24] nor into the meaning of equality, which in recent years has been emerging as the primary force in constitutional law.[25] It suffices to point out that selection procedures that permit men to evaluate and compare the social worth of human beings and, on that basis, to spare the life of some and doom others may well not meet that command. Judicial notions of morality and fair play, which finally determine the limits of the equal protection clause of the Constitution, may require a more impersonal method of selecting who is to be saved from among the dying.

The precise issue raised by selection for hemodialysis seems not to be discussed in the legal literature. The well-known shipwreck cases[26] present the closest analogy. In those cases some of the persons apparently doomed to die in an overcrowded lifeboat made the decision as to which passengers would be killed; they were convicted of homicide.[27] Selection by the doomed was also a feature of Professor Lon Fuller's celebrated *Case of the Speluncean Explorers*,[28] a hypothetical case where four men, trapped in a cave, killed and dined on one of their fellows to stay alive. In selection for hemodialysis, however, the decision is made by persons not doomed. Selection for hemodialysis is analogous to a situation where there are thirty persons in a sinking boat and a second boat, with room for five persons, comes by. A committee on land is to decide and advise by radio which five persons will be transferred to the second boat. The issue is not one of jettison of men by those imperiled; the issue is who shall be rescued from the dying.[29]

Although selection for hemodialysis involves human rescue rather than human jettison, one of the principles underlying the rule of equality of all men applied in the shipwreck cases should be applicable to selection for hemodialysis. If the rule of the shipwreck cases is based solely on a desire to prevent A from killing B in order to save A's own life, the rule is not applicable since the selection committee for hemodialysis is not motivated by self-preservation. There is, however, another principle underlying the rule of equality in the shipwreck cases, a principle applicable to human rescue as well as jettison. In his Gay Lecture to the Harvard Medical School, Professor Paul Freund said, in illustrating how protective is the law of human life:

If a human life is deliberately taken it is, moreover, no mitigation of the crime that the victim was, by worldly standards, someone of little merit, or someone having little time left to live. The governing principle is not the merit or need or value of the victim but equality of worth as a human being. The governing principle, it might be said, is that man shall not play God with human lives.[30]

This principle—that man shall not play God with human lives—which bases the rule of equality in the shipwreck cases ought to be applicable to committees allocating life-saving resources as well as to private individuals taking life. This principle would, in our judgment, proscribe selection for hemodialysis on the basis of ad hoc comparisons of the social worth of

candidates. The essence of playing God is to look at A and to look at B, assay them, declare B is worth more than A, and save B. The principle that man shall not play God with human lives would not, however, necessarily proscribe selection by criteria announced in advance of the appearance of any candidate, provided the criteria can be supported rationally and are not unconstitutionally discriminatory.

It can be argued that there is precedent for selecting who lives on the basis of social worth both in the different sentences meted out by judge or jury to persons convicted of the same crime and in the commutation power of the governor. A person convicted of the crime of murder may be given a death sentence or some lesser penalty, and if given a death sentence it may be commuted by the governor to some lesser penalty. In determining the penalty, under criminal law procedures, doubtless some kind of evaluation of "social worth" of the convicted criminal affects the decision as to the penalty.[31] However, there is an essential distinction between the penalty procedures of criminal law and the selection of patients for hemodialysis. In criminal law the convicted murderer may escape death by reason of an evaluation of *his* social worth alone.[32] His social worth is not directly compared to the social worth of any other individual, and a choice made between them, as in hemodialysis selection. All convicted murderers might escape the electric chair because each—assessed individually—deserved to escape. But of persons with uremia, some must be left to die.

The selection of persons for hemodialysis raises problems of procedural due process as well as equal protection. The committee may be a secret committee, or there may be no articulated standards or procedures. Although it has been suggested that it is possible to establish usable criteria for measuring social worth,[33] the task is not an easy one. The complexities are such that it is difficult to get agreement on criteria in the specificity required to make the criteria meaningful. A simple rule, "women are preferred to men," would be clear enough, but once one begins to add qualifications such as

"parents are preferred to persons without children" and "the younger are preferred to the older" difficulties rapidly mount. When the faculty of Christ Church College at Oxford was of many opinions concerning the design of a new belfry, even the mathematical genius of Charles Dodgson (better known as Lewis Carroll) could not devise a voting method that could resolve their differences.[34] Opinions of social worth are infinitely more diverse than opinions concerning the design of a belfry. If no understandable criteria of social worth can be agreed upon, committees measuring social worth must decide upon an ad hoc basis. Ad hockery is not the stuff from which the constitutional guaranties of equal protection and due process are made.[35]

The ethical muddle of selection committees comparing human worth is well illustrated by the operations of the selection committee at the Seattle Artificial Kidney Center. The descriptions of how this committee makes its decisions, published in *Life*[36] and *Redbook*,[37] are numbing accounts of how close to the surface lie the prejudices and mindless clichés that pollute the committee's deliberations. The committee of seven, appointed by the King County Medical Society, is said to be anonymous. It has from time to time consisted of a lawyer, minister, banker, housewife, labor leader, official of the state government, and physicians. In the published accounts of their deliberations they have considered such factors as "age and sex of patient; marital status and number of dependents; income; net worth; emotional stability, with particular regard to the patient's capacity to accept the treatment; educational background; nature of occupation, past performance and future potential; and names of people who could serve as references."[38] How these factors are weighted, or how they relate to social worth, is undisclosed. One member thought the surviving spouse's chances of remarriage should be considered. Another member (not the minister) thought people of good character should be saved, and good character was indicated by active church work. "To have a record of public service is a help—scout leader, Sunday-school teacher, Red Cross volunteer."[39] What is meant by "public service," a phrase so difficult to define in a pluralistic society? Were the persons who got themselves jailed in the South while working for civil rights doing a "public service"? What about working for the Antivivisection League? Why should a Sunday-school teacher be saved rather than Madalyn Murray? The magazines paint a disturbing picture of the bourgeoisie sparing the bourgeoisie, of the Seattle committee measuring persons in accordance with its own middle-class suburban value system: scouts, Sunday school, Red Cross.[40] This rules out creative nonconformists, who rub the bourgeoisie the wrong way but who historically have contributed so much to the making of America. The Pacific Northwest is no place for a Henry David Thoreau with bad kidneys.

The Seattle selection system was begun when chronic hemodialysis for renal failure was truly an experimental program. If a project is experimental, the use of broad discretion in selecting candidates who can demonstrate the validity of the project is not objectionable. Once a procedure proves its merit and passes from the experimental to the standard, however, as has happened with chronic hemodialysis, justice requires that selection be made by a fairer method than the unbridled consciences, the built-in biases, and the fantasies of omnipotence of a secret committee. Selection by a secret committee operating without explicit criteria is a grotesque conceit worthy of Franz Kafka.[41]

If selection of patients by ad hoc comparisons of social worth is objectionable, comparisons by a committee composed of physicians, hospital personnel, and social workers rather than by a lay committee is no less objectionable.[42] Medical men are no more qualified to play God—to look at two persons and say one is worth more than the other—than ordinary mortals. Moreover, it may be even more objectionable for the decision to be made by physicians. The physician owes to his patient a high degree of fidelity and care for his welfare. Disciplined by this duty, the medical profession has built up an enormous reservoir of public trust. When physicians select who is to live and who is to die without reference to any medical criteria, this trust

may dissipate.[43] It is in the best interests of medicine to keep it as free as possible of comparisons of social worth.

On the other hand it may be argued that the internists and nurses who take care of inpatients over a long period of time should have a hand in their selection. Several internists involved in hemodialysis programs have said in private conversations that they have to like the patient and get some psychological satisfaction from the patient. Though the internists and nurses deserve gratitude and, when they have an uncooperative patient, sympathy and a psychiatrist's aid, life and death judgments cannot ethically be decided by whether the medical staff likes the patient.

Physicians, in making medical and psychiatric evaluations, are not applying discrete criteria. Social worth considerations, as well as unconscious biases, can secrete themselves within a medical or psychiatric evaluation. Hence selection procedures ought to be devised which keep these judgments as free as possible from such considerations. When the stake is life itself, procedures respecting equality of persons must be stringently observed.

Psychiatric assessments of a candidate's ability to cope with life on a machine are admittedly useful to selection committees in determining whether the patient can adjust to life on hemodialysis. Nonetheless, we are troubled if these assessments are used for more than weeding out candidates with psychoses or gross personality disorders that would make them incapable of cooperation. Psychiatric and psychological tests predicting cooperation do not have enough empirical support to justify conclusive assertions about their effectiveness. Moreover, the future personality problems of the patient depend so much on interactions with other persons as to make any prediction questionable. Psychiatric and psychological assessments can also reflect unconscious prejudices. Not even psychiatrists can rid themselves of all their predilections. We think psychiatrists, psychologists, and social workers can be more useful in providing crisis therapy during hemodialysis—crisis therapy for the patient and his family and the hospital staff—than in selecting out candidates through tests of highly uncertain efficacy.

How Should Patients Be Selected?

One can know what is a bad method without knowing what is the best method. As Professor Fuller has said, "We can . . . know what is plainly unjust without committing ourselves to declare with finality what perfect justice would be like.[44] Once the judgment has been made by physicians that Smith and Jones are equally good medical risks, the choice between them should be made by some method that does not require or permit ad hoc comparisons of their social worth. There are a number of possible methods: e.g., (1) ability to pay; (2) first-come, first served; (3) lottery or random selection; (4) rules announced in advance that are not unconstitutionally discriminatory.[45] None of these methods is perfect; each has its defects. But any of these methods is preferable to selection by ad hoc comparative judgments of social worth.

Notes

1. Gorney, The New Biology and the Future of Man, and Grad, Legislative Responses to the New Biology: Limits and Possibilities. 15 UCLA Law Review 267 (1968).

2. Personal communication to the authors from Dr. Alfred Katz, School of Public Health, University of California, Los Angeles, Dec. 1967.

3. Scribner, Fergus, Boen, and Thomas, Some Therapeutic Approaches to Chronic Renal Insufficiency, 16 Annual Review of Medicine 298 (1965).

4. Robbins and Robbins, The Rest Are Simply Left to Die, Redbook, Nov. 1967, p. 1133.

5. Kolff, To Live without Heart and Kidneys, 1 Proceedings European Dialysis and Transplant Association 97, 99 (1964).

6. "In the past three years, 120 suitable patients have been considered for chronic haemodialysis [by the Royal Free Hospital in London], but only 21 patients have been treated because of limitations of space and equipment. The 21 patients are all alive, whereas of the remaining 99, only 1 is surviving and he was rejected only a month ago." Shaldon, Comty & Baillod, Letters to the Editor, 2 Lancet 1182, 1183 (1965).

7. Breslow, Public Health Report, Calif. Med. 360 (1967).

8. In Proceedings of the Conference on Dialysis as a Practical Workshop, New York, June 26–28, 1966, at 5, it is noted that a few patients up to 70 years of age have been accepted in some centers and have responded to hemodialysis.

9. For discussion of some of the psychological reactions before, during, and after the

physical process of hemodialysis see Shea, Bogden, Freeman, and Schreiner, Hemodialysis for Chronic Renal Failure: IV. Psychological Considerations, 62 *Annals Internal Med.* 558 (1965).

10. Kemph, Renal Failure, Artificial Kidney and Kidney Transplants, 122 *Am. J. Psychiatry* 1270 (1966); Wright, Sand, and Livingston, Psychological Stress During Hemodialysis for Chronic Renal Failure, 64 *Annals Internal Med.* 611 (1966).

11. Scribner, Fergus, Boen, and Thomas, *supra* note 3, at 291. They add: "What to do with the deserving but uncooperative patient remains a most difficult medical, moral, and economic problem." *Id.*

12. Psychological requirements for successful adaptation to the chronic hemodialysis regime are discussed in Sand, Livingston, and Wright, Psychological Assessment of Candidates for a Hemodialysis Program, 64 *Annals Internal Med.* 602 (1966). The authors, who worked with the Seattle Artificial Kidney Center, used psychiatric interviews and standard intelligence and personality tests for screening. They are rather more sanguine than we are about the general reliability of psychiatric predictions. See also Gombos, Lee, Harton, and Cummings, One Year's Experience with an Intermittent Dialysis Program, 61 *Annals Internal Med.* 462 (1964).

13. In a description of the dialysis program at the Georgetown University Hospital appear three poignant lines about two patients who chose death: "Two of these voluntarily withdrew from the program. One thought that he was dying slowly, without dignity, and leaving an unpleasant memory for his teen-age children as well as intemperate demands on their sympathy, attention, and devotion. The other patient felt discouraged at the realities of the program and did not desire a prolongation of what he considered ill-health." Schreiner and Maher, Hemodialysis for Chronic Renal Failure: III. Medical, Moral and Ethical, and Socioeconomic Problems, 62 *Annals Internal Med.* 551, 554 (1965).

14. Murray, Albers, Burnell, and Scribner, A Community Hemodialysis Center for the Treatment of Chronic Uremia, 8 *Transactions Am. Soc'y Artificial Internal Organs* 315 (1962). "Another purpose of this committee is to protect those in charge of the Center from pressure to take a given patient." *Id.* at 316.

15. Alexander, They Decide Who Lives, Who Dies, *Life,* Nov. 9, 1962, at 102.

16. Robbins and Robbins, *supra* note 4, at 132–33.

17. *Northern California Chronic Hemodialysis Center, Procedure for Selection of Patients for Chronic Hemodialysis Therapy* 2 (mimeographed 1967).

The legislation establishing the hemodialysis centers in Los Angeles and San Francisco provided:

The dialysis centers shall be designed primarily to provide lifesaving dialysis services to approximately 30 patients in each

center. Funds shall be provided for developing home dialysis treatment services for approximately 20 patients in each center and the necessary specialized personnel and equipment to operate each center.
Cal. Health and Safety Code § 417.1 (West Supp. 1966). The act did not provide how the patients at each center were to be selected.

The Los Angeles center uses a selection procedure different from the procedure used in San Francisco. It selects by lot among candidates with equally good medical conditions:

"The patient's medical, psychiatric and sociologic history will be reviewed and the patient will be judged to be either an optimum or alternate candidate largely on the basis of medical findings.

"An optimum candidate is a patient who is disabled because of chronic renal insufficiency and who does not have any other disabling illness or significant organ involvement. Patients who have cerebrovascular accidents with paralyses, severe coronary artery disease and heart failure, another disabling systemic disease or who show unwillingness to cooperate with the prescribed hemodialysis program are examples of alternate candidates. Each time an opening occurs on the program, all referrals will be classified into one or the other category. The group of optimum candidates will be pooled and one of them will be selected by lot for therapy. If there are no optimum candidates, then the alternate pool will be used to draw the patient for treatment." Barbour, Meihaus, Berne, and Orellana, *Los Angeles County General Hospital Renal-Dialysis Center, Operational Plans I,* at 3 (mimeographed 1967).

18. *Northern California Chronic Hemodialysis Center, Procedure for Selection of Patients for Chronic Hemodialysis Therapy* 5 (mimeographed 1967).

19. "More recently the Admissions and Policy Committee [in the Seattle Center] had to select one of 4 candidates on the basis of sociological factors. . . . They selected a 33-year-old electrician whose 7 dependents almost certainly would become dependent upon state aid if he were unable to work." Murray, Albers, Burnell, and Scribner, *supra* note 14, at 316.

20. For discussions in medical journals of the ethical aspects of the issue, see Colloquium, The Changing Mores of Biomedical Research, 67 *Annals Internal Med.* Supp. 7 (Sept. 1967); Elkinton, Moral Problems in the Use of Borrowed Organs, 60 *Annals Internal Med.* 309 (1964); Robin, Rapid Scientific Advances Bring New Ethical Questions, 189 *J.A.M.A.* 624 (1964); Schreiner and Maher, *supra* note 13; Scribner, Ethical Problems of Using Artificial Organs to Sustain Human Life, 10 *Transactions Am. Soc'y Artificial Internal Organs* 209 (1964), Stumpf, Some Moral Dimensions of Medicine, 64 *Annals Internal Med.* 460 (1966).

21. The question may be asked: What is meant by "hospital"? In Darling v. Charleston Community Memorial Hosp., 33 Ill. 2d

326, 211 N.E.2d 253 (1965), *cert. denied,* 383 U.S. 946 (1966), the court held a "hospital" liable for negligence, apparently including both the hospital administration and the medical staff. See Chayet, Hospital Responsibility for Medical Care, 274 *N. Eng. J. Med.* 507 (1966).

22. *See* Lewis, The Meaning of State Action, 60 *Colum. L. Rev.* 1083, 1099–1108 (1960); Van Alstyne and Karst, State Action, 14 *Stan. L. Rev.* 3, 52–57 (1961). In Simkins v. Moses H. Cone Memorial Hosp., 323 F.2d 959 (4th Cir. 1963), *cert. denied,* 376 U.S. 938 (1964), the court held that a private nonprofit hospital, which received federal construction grants under the Hill-Burton Act, could not deny admission to patients on grounds of race.

23. "In the hospital case [Simkins v. Moses H. Cone Memorial Hosp., 323 F.2d 959 (4th Cir. 1963)], there was injury of great magnitude to the discriminatees: denial to the patients of admission to a facility essential to the preservation of their lives. . . . In view of the magnitude of injury to the discriminatees in the hospital case it would appear sound to conclude that state law could not constitutionally permit the discrimination even though a hospital was not included in an overall 'state plan' and did not receive public funds to meet a substantial part of the costs of construction." Horowitz, Fourteenth Amendment Aspects of Racial Discrimination in "Private" Housing, 52 *Calif. L. Rev. 1,* 21 (1964). Professor Horowitz's position that all hospitals, public and private, should be subject to the fourteenth amendment is espoused in the Brief of the American Civil Liberties Union as Amicus Curiae in the Simkins case. See also Horowitz, The Misleading Search for "State Action" Under the Fourteenth Amendment, 30 *S. Cal. L. Rev.* 208 (1957).

24. For recent discussions of the meaning of equal protection, see Black, Foreword: "State Action," Equal Protection, and California's Proposition 14, 81 *Harv. L. Rev.* 69 (1967); Harvith, Federal Equal Protection and Welfare Assistance, 31 *Albany L. Rev.* 210, 223–26 (1967); Karst and Horowitz, Reitman v. Mulkey: A Telophase of Substantive Equal Protection, 1967 *Sup. Ct. Rev.* 39.

25. See Kellett, The Expansion of Equality, 37 *S. Cal. L. Rev.* 400 (1964); Roche, Equality in America: The Expansion of a Concept, 43 *N.C.L. Rev.* 249 (1965).

26. United States v. Holmes, 26 F. Cas. 360 (No. 15,383) (C.C.E.D. Pa. 1842); Regina v. Dudley, 14 Q.B.D. 273 (1884).

27. The American court suggested the selection of who is to be killed might be made by a lottery. The English court rejected a lottery as "grotesque"; under its view, all must wait and die or be rescued together. "Who shall know," Cardozo asked, in approving the English view, "when masts and sails of rescue may emerge out of the fog?" B. Cardozo, What Medicine Can Do for Law, in *Selected Writings of Benjamin Nathan Cardozo* 371, 390 (1947). For discussion of the shipwreck cases, see E. Cahn, *The Moral Decision* 61–71 (1955) (concluding all must

die together); J. Hall, *General Principles of Criminal Law* 427–36 (2d ed. 1960) (not disapproving a lottery); R. Perkins, *Criminal Law* 847–51 (1957) (remarking that a lottery has "much to commend it").

28. 62 *Harv. L. Rev.* 616 (1949).

29. A similar issue arises in abortion cases, when a choice is presented of saving either the mother or the child. See G. Williams, *The Sanctity of Life and the Criminal Law* 146–247 (1957). Abortion differs in so many ways from selection for hemodialysis, however, that little seems to be gained by way of analogy.

30. Freund, Ethical Problems in Human Experimentation, 273 *N. Eng. J. Med.* 687 (1965).

31. See Proceedings of the 1967 California Sentencing Institute for Superior Court Judges, 62 *Cal. Rptr. App.* 11–36 (1967); Proceedings of the Institute on Sentencing, 42 *F.R.D.* 175–233 (1966); Proceedings of First Philadelphia Sentencing Institute, 40 *F.R.D.* 399–477 (1965).

32. Even a non-comparative evaluation of social worth in sentencing has recently come in for some sharp criticism. Baab and Furgeson, Texas Sentencing Practices, 45 *Texas L. Rev.* 471 (1967); Rubin, Disparity and Equality of Sentences, 40 *F.R.D.* 55 (1966); Comment, A Review of Sentencing in Missouri, 11 *St. Louis U.L.J.* 69 (1966).

33. Shatin, Medical Care and the Social Worth of Man, 36 *Am. J. Orthopsychiatry* 96 (1966), proposes to allocate medical care according to the social value of the individual. His determinants of value, listed without rank, are made up of such vague words that they would impose no practical control on the decision maker.

34. D. Black, *The Theory of Committees and Elections* 189–213 (1958).

35. Compare L. Fuller, *The Morality of Law* 31 (1964): "Wherever distinctions are granted or deprivations imposed it is natural to select some umpire or committee to make the decision, and, no matter whether the issue be that of penalty or award, the deciding agency is expected to act with intelligence and impartiality. Nevertheless there is a great difference in the procedures generally established for meting out penalties as contrasted with those which grant awards. When penalties or deprivations are involved we surround the decision with procedural guaranties of due process, often elaborate ones, and we are likely to impose an obligation of public accountability. Where awards and honors are granted we are content with more informal, less scrutinized methods of decision." Is selection for hemodialysis an "award"? Or is rejection a "deprivation"?

36. Alexander, *supra* note 15, at 102.

37. Robbins and Robbins, *supra* note 4, at 132–33.

38. Alexander, *supra* note 15, at 106.

39. Robbins and Robbins, *supra* note 4, at 133. The Seattle committee evaluates scout leaders somewhat differently than did one of the most eminent American psychiatrists, Harry Stack Sullivan. Wrote he: "The interviewer also inquires whether his patient, before he became a father—or before she became a mother—showed any particular interest in leading boys' or girls' clubs, in being a 'big brother' or a 'big sister,' for a period of years. If he did, I think it is a fairly important clue to deficiencies in his preadolescent experience." H. Sullivan, *The Psychiatric Interview* 158 (1954).

40. "[A] rather difficult philosophical position arises should there be any change in the status of the patient. If you really believe in the right of society to make decisions on medical availability on these criteria you should be logical and say that when a man stops going to church or is divorced or loses his job, he ought to be removed from the programme and somebody else who fulfills these criteria substituted. Obviously no-one faces up to this logical consequence." Schreiner, Problems of Ethics in Relation to Haemodialysis and Transplantation, in *Ethics in Medical Progress*, (ed. G. Wolstenholin, 1966), at 126, 128.

41. The phrase is borrowed from Professor Fuller, who used it in speaking of a system of law composed exclusively of retrospective rules. L. Fuller, *supra* note 35, at 74.

42. Dr. Kolff, inventor of the artificial kidney for human use, has consistently opposed selection by committees of any kind. "Lay committees tend to legalize and give a pretext of respectability to a deficiency that should not be condoned. Committees should be formed not to exclude certain patients from treatment, but to establish possibilities for more treatment. Do we really subscribe to the principle that social standing should determine selection? Do we allow patients to be treated with dialysis only when they are married, go to church, have children, have a job, a good income and give to the Community Chest? . . .

"As far as the selection by a medical committee is concerned, very high on the list is whether or not the patient is an emotionally mature adult. To have seen a psychiatrist once in one's life jeopardizes one's employment with many companies. Are we from now on also going to exclude the same people from the treatment of uremia? I refuse to believe that this is the kind of society we want to build up in the United States." Kolff, Letters and Comments, 61 *Annals Internal Med.* 359, 360 (1964).

43. Compare the vast public distrust of zoning variance administrators, which has arisen largely because they often allocate valuable resources without resort to any discoverable criteria except their own personal value systems. Anderson, The Board of Zoning Appeals—Villain or Victim?, 13 *Syracuse L. Rev.* 353 (1962); Dukeminier and Stapleton, The Zoning Board of Adjustment: A Case Study in Misrule, 50 *Ky. L.J.* 273 (1962).

44. L. Fuller, *supra* note 35, at 12.

45. A somewhat analogous problem, with less drastic consequences from the selection, arises respecting the draft of men to fight wars. A random selection method was recommended by the President's *National Advisory Commission on Selective Service, In Pursuit of Equity* 37–40 (1967). Random selection was rejected in the *Civilian Advisory Panel on Military Manpower Procurement, Report to the Committee on Armed Services, U.S. House of Representatives* 18–20 (1967). In the 1967 act extending selective service, the random selection method was forbidden. Military Selective Service Act of 1967, 50 App. U.S.C.A. § 455(a)(2) (Supp. 1967). The draft act prescribes some arbitrary criteria announced in advance, but draft boards have considerable discretion in classifying men.

98

Nicholas Rescher

The Allocation of Exotic Medical Lifesaving Therapy

Reprinted with permission of the publisher from *Ethics,* vol. 79, 1969, pp. 173–186.

The Problem

Technological progress has in recent years transformed the limits of the possible in medical therapy. However, the elevated state of sophistication of modern medical technology has brought the economists' classic problem of scarcity in its wake as an unfortunate side product. The enormously sophisticated and complex equipment and the highly trained teams of experts requisite for its utilization are scarce resources in relation to potential demand. The administrators of the great medical institutions that preside over these scarce resources thus come to be faced increasingly with the awesome choice: *Whose life to save?*

A (somewhat hypothetical) paradigm example of this problem may be sketched within the following set of definitive assumptions: We suppose that persons in some particular medically morbid condition are "mortally afflicted": It is virtually certain that they will die within a short time period (say ninety days). We assume that some very complex course of treatment (e.g., a heart transplant) represents a substantial probability of life prolongation for persons in this mortally afflicted condition. We assume that the facilities available in terms of human resources, mechanical instrumentalities, and requisite materials (e.g., hearts in the case of a heart transplant) make it possible to give a certain treatment—this "exotic (medical) lifesaving therapy," or ELT for short—to a certain, relatively small number of people. And finally we assume that a substantially greater pool of people in the mortally afflicted condition is at hand. The problem then may be formulated as follows: How is one to select within the pool of afflicted patients the ones to be given the ELT treatment in question; how to select those "whose lives are to be saved"? Faced with many candidates for an ELT process that can be made available to only a few, doctors and medical administrators confront the decision of who is to be given a chance at survival and who is, in effect, to be condemned to die.

As has already been implied, the "heroic" variety of spare-part surgery can pretty well be assimilated to this paradigm. One can foresee the time when heart transplantation, for example, will have become pretty much a routine medical procedure, albeit on a very limited basis, since a cardiac surgeon with the technical competence to transplant hearts can operate at best a rather small number of times each week and the elaborate facilities for such operations will most probably exist on a modest scale. Moreover, in "spare-part" surgery there is always the problem of availability of the "spare parts" themselves. A report in one British newspaper gives the following picture: "Of the 150,000 who die of heart disease each year [in the U.K.], Mr. Donald Longmore, research surgeon at the National Heart Hospital [in London] estimates that 22,000 might be eligible for heart surgery. Another 30,000 would need heart and lung transplants. But there are probably only between 7,000 and 14,000 potential donors a year."[1] Envisaging this situation in which at the very most something like one in four heart-malfunction victims can be saved, we clearly confront a problem in ELT allocation.

A perhaps even more drastic case in point is afforded by long-term haemodialysis, an ongoing process by which a complex device—an "artificial kidney machine"—is used periodically in cases of chronic renal failure to substitute for a non-functional kidney in "cleaning" potential poisons from the blood. Only a few major institutions have chronic haemodialysis units, whose complex operation is an extremely expensive proposition. For the present and the foreseeable future the situation is that "the number of places available for chronic haemodialysis is hopelessly inadequate."[2]

The traditional medical ethos has insulated the physician against facing the very existence of this problem. When swearing the Hippocratic Oath, he commits himself to work for the benefit of the sick in "whatsoever house I enter."[3] In taking this stance, the physician substantially renounces the explicit choice of saving certain lives rather than others. Of course, doctors have always in fact had to face such choices on the battlefield or in times of disaster, but there the issue had to be resolved hurriedly, under pressure, and in circumstances in which the very nature of the case effectively precluded calm deliberation by the decision maker as well as criticism by others. In sharp contrast, however, cases of the type we have postulated in the present discussion arise predictably, and represent choices to be made deliberately and "in cold blood."

It is, to begin with, appropriate to remark that this problem is not fundamentally a medical problem. For when there are sufficiently many afflicted candidates for ELT then—so we may assume—there will also be more than enough for whom the purely medical grounds for ELT allocation are decisively strong in any individual case, and just about equally strong throughout the group. But in this circumstance a selection of some afflicted patients over and against others cannot ex hypothesi be made on the basis of purely medical considerations.

The selection problem, as we have said, is in substantial measure not a medical one. It is a problem for medical men, which must somehow be solved by them, but that does not make it a medical issue—any more than the problem of hospital building is a medical issue. As a problem it belongs to the category of philosophical problems—specifically a problem of moral philosophy or ethics. Structurally, it bears a substantial kinship with those issues in this field that revolve about the notorious whom-to-save-on-the-lifeboat and whom-to-throw-to-the-wolves-pursuing-the-sled questions. But whereas questions of this just-indicated sort are artificial, hypothetical, and far-fetched, the ELT issue poses a genuine policy question for the responsible administrators in medical institutions, indeed a question that threatens to become commonplace in the foreseeable future.

Now what the medical administrator needs to have, and what the philosopher is presumably ex officio in a position to help in providing, is a body of rational guidelines for making choices in these literally life-or-death situations. This is an issue in which many interested parties have a substantial stake, including the responsible decision maker who wants to satisfy his conscience that he is acting in a reasonable way. Moreover, the family and associates of the man who is turned away—to say nothing of the man himself—have the right to an acceptable explanation. And indeed even the general public wants to know that what

is being done is fitting and proper. All of these interested parties are entitled to insist that a reasonable code of operating principles provides a defensible rationale for making the life-and-death choices involved in ELT.

The Two Types of Criteria

Two distinguishable types of criteria are bound up in the issue of making ELT choices. We shall call these Criteria of Inclusion and Criteria of Comparison, respectively. The distinction at issue here requires some explanation. We can think of the selection as being made by a two-stage process: (1) the selection from among all possible candidates (by a suitable screening process) of a group to be taken under serious consideration as candidates for therapy, and then (2) the actual singling out, within this group, of the particular individuals to whom therapy is to be given. Thus the first process narrows down the range of comparative choice by eliminating en bloc whole categories of potential candidates. The second process calls for a more refined, case-by-case comparison of those candidates that remain. By means of the first set of criteria one forms a selection group; by means of the second set, an actual selection is made within this group.

Thus what we shall call a "selection system" for the choice of patients to receive therapy of the ELT type will consist of criteria of these two kinds. Such a system will be acceptable only when the reasonableness of its component criteria can be established.

Essential Features of an Acceptable ELT Selection System

To qualify as reasonable, an ELT selection must meet two important "regulative" requirements: it must be simple enough to be readily intelligible, and it must be plausible, that is, patently reasonable in a way that can be apprehended easily and without involving ramified subtleties. Those medical administrators responsible for ELT choices must follow a modus operandi that virtually all the people involved can readily understand to be acceptable (at a reasonable level of generality, at any rate). Appearances are critically important here. It is not enough that the

choice be made in a justifiable way; it must be possible for people—plain people—to "see" (i.e., understand without elaborate teaching or indoctrination) that it is justified, insofar as any mode of procedure can be justified in cases of this sort.

One "constitutive" requirement is obviously an essential feature of a reasonable selection system: all of its component criteria—those of inclusion and those of comparison alike—must be reasonable in the sense of being rationally defensible. The ramifications of this requirement call for detailed consideration. But one of its aspects should be noted without further ado: it must be fair—it must treat relevantly like cases alike, leaving no room for "influence" or favoritism, etc.

The Basic Screening Stage: Criteria of Inclusion (and Exclusion)

Three sorts of considerations are prominent among the plausible criteria of inclusion/exclusion at the basic screening stage: the constituency factor, the progress-of-science factor, and the prospect-of-success factor.

The Constituency Factor

It is a "fact of life" that ELT can be available only in the institutional setting of a hospital or medical institute or the like. Such institutions generally have normal clientele boundaries. A veterans' hospital will not concern itself primarily with treating nonveterans, a children's hospital cannot be expected to accommodate the "senior citizen," an army hospital can regard college professors as outside its sphere. Sometimes the boundaries are geographic—a state hospital may admit only residents of a certain state. (There are, of course, indefensible constituency principles—say race or religion, party membership, or ability to pay; and there are cases of borderline legitimacy, e.g., sex.[4]) A medical institution is justified in considering for ELT only persons within its own constituency, provided this constituency is constituted upon a defensible basis. Thus the haemodialysis selection committee in Seattle "agreed to consider only those applications who were residents of the state of Washington. . . . They justified this stand on the grounds that since the basic research

... had been done at ... a state-supported institution—the people whose taxes had paid for the research should be its first beneficiaries."[5]

While thus insisting that constituency considerations represent a valid and legitimate factor in ELT selection, I do feel there is much to be said for minimizing their role in life-or-death cases. Indeed a refusal to recognize them at all is a significant part of medical tradition, going back to the very oath of Hippocrates. They represent a departure from the ideal arising with the institutionalization of medicine, moving it away from its original status as an art practiced by an individual practitioner.

The Progress-of-Science Factor

The needs of medical research can provide a second valid principle of inclusion. The research interests of the medical staff in relation to the specific nature of the cases at issue is a significant consideration. It may be important for the progress of medical science—and thus of potential benefit to many persons in the future—to determine how effective the ELT at issue is with diabetics or persons over sixty or with a negative RH factor. Considerations of this sort represent another type of legitimate factor in ELT selection.

A very definitely *borderline* case under this head would revolve around the question of a patient's willingness to pay, not in monetary terms, but in offering himself as an experimental subject, say by contracting to return at designated times for a series of tests substantially unrelated to his own health, but yielding data of importance to medical knowledge in general.

The Prospect-of-Success Factor

It may be that while the ELT at issue is not without *some* effectiveness in general, it has been established to be highly effective only with patients in certain specific categories (e.g., females under forty of a specific blood type). This difference in effectiveness—in the absolute or in the probability of success—is (we assume) so marked as to constitute virtually a difference in kind rather than in degree. In this case, it would be perfectly legitimate to adopt the general rule of making the

ELT at issue available only or primarily to persons in this substantial-promise-of-success category. (It is on grounds of this sort that young children and persons over fifty are generally ruled out as candidates for haemodialysis.)

We have maintained that the three factors of constituency, progress of science, and prospect of success represent legitimate criteria of inclusion for ELT selection. But it remains to examine the considerations which legitimate them. The legitimating factors are in the final analysis practical or pragmatic in nature. From the practical angle it is advantageous—indeed to some extent necessary—that the arrangements governing medical institutions should embody certain constituency principles. It makes good pragmatic and utilitarian sense that progress-of-science considerations should be operative here. And, finally, the practical aspect is reinforced by a whole host of other considerations—including moral ones—in supporting the prospect-of-success criterion. The workings of each of these factors are of course conditioned by the ever-present element of limited availability. They are operative only in this context, that is, prospect of success is a legitimate consideration at all only because we are dealing with a situation of scarcity.

The Final Selection Stage: Criteria of Selection

Five sorts of elements must, as we see it, figure primarily among the plausible criteria of selection that are to be brought to bear in further screening the group constituted after application of the criteria of inclusion: the relative-likelihood-of-success factor, the life-expectancy factor, the family role factor, the potential-contributions factor, and the services-rendered factor. The first two represent the *biomedical* aspect, the second three the *social* aspect.

The Relative-Likelihood-of-Success Factor

It is clear that the relative likelihood of success is a legitimate and appropriate factor in making a selection within the group of qualified patients that are to receive ELT. This is obviously one of the considerations that must count very significantly in a reasonable selection procedure.

The present criterion is of course closely related to [the third] item of the preceding section. There we were concerned with prospect-of-success considerations categorically and *en bloc*. Here at present they come into play in a particularized case-by-case comparison among individuals. If the therapy at issue is not a once-and-for-all proposition and requires ongoing treatment, cognate considerations must be brought in. Thus, for example, in the case of a chronic ELT procedure such as haemodialysis it would clearly make sense to give priority to patients with a potentially reversible condition (who would thus need treatment for only a fraction of their remaining lives).

The Life-Expectancy Factor

Even if the ELT is "successful" in the patient's case he may, considering his age and/or other aspects of his general medical condition, look forward to only a very short probable future life. This is obviously another factor that must be taken into account.

The Family Role Factor

A person's life is a thing of importance not only to himself but to others—friends, associates, neighbors, colleagues, etc. But his (or her) relationship to his immediate family is a thing of unique intimacy and significance. The nature of his relationship to his wife, children, and parents, and the issue of their financial and psychological dependence upon him, are obviously matters that deserve to be given weight in the ELT selection process. Other things being anything like equal, the mother of minor children must take priority over the middle-aged bachelor.

The Potential-Future-Contributions Factor (Prospective Service)

In "choosing to save" one life rather than another, "the society," through the mediation of the particular medical institution in question—which should certainly look upon itself as a trustee for the social interest—is clearly warranted in considering the likely pattern of future *services to be rendered* by the patient (adequate recovery assumed), considering his age, talent, training, and past record of performance. In its allocations of ELT, society "invests" a scarce resource in one person as against another and is thus entitled to look to the probable prospective "return" on its investment.

It may well be that a thoroughly egalitarian society is reluctant to put someone's social contribution into the scale in situations of the sort at issue. One popular article states that "the most difficult standard would be the candidate's value to society," and goes on to quote someone who said: "You can't just pick a brilliant painter over a laborer. The average citizen would be quickly eliminated."[6] But what if it were not a brilliant painter but a brilliant surgeon or medical researcher that was at issue? One wonders if the author of the *obiter dictum* that one "can't just pick" would still feel equally sure of his ground. In any case, the fact that the standard is difficult to apply is certainly no reason for not attempting to apply it. The problem of ELT selection is inevitably burdened with difficult standards.

Some might feel that in assessing a patient's value to society one should ask not only who if permitted to continue living can make the greatest contribution to society in some creative or constructive way, but also who by dying would leave behind the greatest burden on society in assuming the discharge of their residual responsibilities.[7] Certainly the philosophical utilitarian would give equal weight to both these considerations. Just here is where I would part ways with orthodox utilitarianism. For—though this is not the place to do so—I should be prepared to argue that a civilized society has an obligation to promote the furtherance of positive achievements in cultural and related areas even if this means the assumption of certain added burdens.[8]

The Past-Services-Rendered Factor (Retrospective Service)

A person's services to another person or group have always been taken to constitute a valid basis for a claim upon this person or group—of course a moral and not necessarily a legal claim. Society's obligation for the recognition and reward of services rendered—an obligation whose discharge is also very possibly conducive to self-interest in the long run—is thus another factor to be taken into account.

This should be viewed as a morally necessary correlative of the previously considered factor of *prospective* service. It would be morally indefensible of society in effect to say: "Never mind about services you rendered yesterday—it is only the services to be rendered tomorrow that will count with us today." We live in very future-oriented times, constantly preoccupied in a distinctly utilitarian way with future satisfactions. And this disinclines us to give much recognition to past services. But parity considerations of the sort just adduced indicate that such recognition should be given *on grounds of equity*. No doubt a justification for giving weight to services rendered can also be attempted along utilitarian lines. ("The reward of past services rendered spurs people on to greater future efforts and is thus socially advantageous in the long-run future.") In saying that past services should be counted "on grounds of equity"—rather than "on grounds of utility"—I take the view that even if this utilitarian defense could somehow be shown to be fallacious, I should still be prepared to maintain the propriety of taking services rendered into account. The position does not rest on a utilitarian basis and so would not collapse with the removal of such a basis.[9]

As we have said, these five factors fall into three groups: the biomedical factors, the familial factor, and the social factors. With [the first two] items the need for a detailed analysis of the medical considerations comes to the fore. The age of the patient, his medical history, his physical and psychological condition, his specific disease, etc., will all need to be taken into exact account. These biomedical factors represent technical issues: they call for the physicians' expert judgment and the medical statisticians' hard data. And they are ethically uncontroversial factors—their legitimacy and appropriateness are evident from the very nature of the case.

Greater problems arise with the familial and social factors. They involve intangibles that are difficult to judge. How is one to develop subcriteria for weighing the relative social contributions of (say) an architect or a librarian or a mother of young children? And they involve highly problematic issues.

(For example, should good moral character be rated a plus and bad a minus in judging services rendered?) And there is something strikingly unpleasant in grappling with issues of this sort for people brought up in times greatly inclined towards maxims of the type "Judge not!" and "Live and let live!" All the same, in the situation that concerns us here such distasteful problems must be faced, since a failure to choose to save some is tantamount to sentencing all. Unpleasant choices are intrinsic to the problem of ELT selection; they are of the very essence of the matter.[10]

But is reference to all these factors indeed inevitable? The justification for taking acount of the medical factors is pretty obvious. But why should the social aspect of services rendered and to be rendered be taken into account at all? The answer is that they must be taken into account not from the *medical* but from the *ethical* point of view. Despite disagreement on many fundamental issues, moral philosophers of the present day are pretty well in consensus that the justification of human actions is to be sought largely and primarily—if not exclusively—in the principles of utility and of justice.[11] But utility requires reference of services to be rendered and justice calls for a recognition of services that have been rendered. Moral considerations would thus demand recognition of these two factors. (This, of course, still leaves open the question of whether the point of view provides a valid basis of action: Why base one's actions upon moral principles?—or, to put it bluntly—Why be moral? The present paper is, however, hardly the place to grapple with so fundamental an issue, which has been canvassed in the literature of philosophical ethics since Plato.)

More Than Medical Issues Is Involved

An active controversy has of late sprung up in medical circles over the question of whether non-physician laymen should be given a role in ELT selection (in the specific context of chronic haemodialysis). One physician writes: "I think that the assessment of the candidates should be made by a senior doctor on the [dialysis] unit, but

I am sure that it would be helpful to him—both in sharing responsibility and in avoiding personal pressure—if a small unnamed group of people [presumably including laymen] officially made the final decision. I visualize the doctor bringing the data to the group, explaining the points in relation to each case, and obtaining their approval of his order of priority.[12]

Essentially this procedure of a selection committee of laymen has for some years been in use in one of the most publicized chronic dialysis units, that of the Swedish Hospital of Seattle, Washington.[13] Many physicians are apparently reluctant to see the choice of allocation of medical therapy pass out of strictly medical hands. Thus in a recent symposium on the "Selection of Patients for Haemodialysis,[14] Dr. Ralph Shakman writes: "Who is to implement the selection? In my opinion it must ultimately be the responsibility of the consultants in charge of the renal units . . . I can see no reason for delegating this responsibility to lay persons. Surely the latter would be better employed if they could be persuaded to devote their time and energy to raise more and more money for us to spend on our patients."[15] Other contributors to this symposium strike much the same note. Dr. F. M. Parsons writes: "In an attempt to overcome . . . difficulties in selection some have advocated introducing certain specified lay people into the discussions. Is it wise? I doubt whether a committee of this type can adjudicate as satisfactorily as two medical colleagues, particularly as successful therapy involves close cooperation between doctor and patient."[16] And Dr. M. A. Wilson writes in the same symposium: "The suggestion has been made that lay panels should select individuals for dialysis from among a group who are medically suitable. Though this would relieve the doctor-in-charge of a heavy load of responsibility, it would place the burden on those who have no personal knowledge and have to base their judgments on medical or social reports. I do not believe this would result in better decisions for the group or improve the doctor-patient relationship in individual cases."[17]

But no amount of flag waving about the doctor's facing up to his responsibility—or prostrations before the idol of the doctor-patient relationship and reluctance to admit laymen into the sacred precincts of the conference chambers of medical consultations—can obscure the essential fact that ELT selection is not a wholly medical problem. When there are more than enough places in an ELT program to accommodate all who need it, then it will clearly be a medical question to decide who does have the need and which among these would successfully respond. But when an admitted gross insufficiency of places exists, when there are ten or fifty or one hundred highly eligible candidates for each place in the program, then it is unrealistic to take the view that purely medical criteria can furnish a sufficient basis for selection. The question of ELT selection becomes serious as a phenomenon of scale—because, as more candidates present themselves, strictly medical factors are increasingly less adequate as a selection criterion precisely because by numerical category-crowding there will be more and more cases whose "status is much the same" so far as purely medical considerations go.

The ELT selection problem clearly poses issues that transcend the medical sphere because—in the nature of the case—many residual issues remain to be dealt with once all of the medical questions have been faced. Because of this there is good reason why laymen as well as physicians should be involved in the selection process. Once the medical considerations have been brought to bear, fundamental social issues remain to be resolved. The instrumentalities of ELT have been created through the social investment of scarce resources, and the interests of the society deserve to play a role in their utilization. As representatives of their social interests, lay opinions should function to complement and supplement medical views once the proper arena of medical considerations is left behind.[18] Those physicians who have urged the presence of lay members on selection panels can, from this point of view, be recognized as having seen the issue in proper perspective.

One physician has argued against lay representation on selection panels for haemodialysis as follows: "If the doctor advises dialysis and the lay panel refuses, the patient will regard this as a death sentence passed by an anonymous court from which he has no right of appeal."[19] But this drawback is not specific to the use of a lay panel. Rather, it is a feature inherent in every *selection* procedure, regardless of whether the selection is done by the head doctor of the unit, by a panel of physicians, etc. No matter who does the selecting among patients recommended for dialysis, the feelings of the patient who has been rejected (and knows it) can be expected to be much the same, provided that he recognizes the actual nature of the choice (and is not deceived by the possibly convenient but ultimately poisonous fiction that because the selection was made by physicians it was made entirely on medical grounds).

In summary, then, the question of ELT selection would appear to be one that is in its very nature heavily laden with issues of medical research, practice, and administration. But it will not be a question that can be resolved on solely medical grounds. Strictly social issues of justice and utility will invariably arise in this area—questions going outside the medical area in whose resolution medical laymen can and should play a substantial role.

The Inherent Imperfection (Nonoptimality) of Any Selection System

Our discussion to this point of the design of a selection system for ELT has left a gap that is a very fundamental and serious omission. We have argued that five factors must be taken into substantial and explicit account:

A. *Relative likelihood of success.*—Is the chance of the treatment's being "successful" to be rated as high, good, average, etc.?[20]

B. *Expectancy of future life.*—Assuming the "success" of the treatment, how much longer does the patient stand a good chance (75 per cent or better) of living—considering his age and general condition?

C. *Family role.*—To what extent does the patient have responsibilities to others in his immediate family?

D. *Social contributions rendered.*—Are the patient's past services to his society outstanding, substantial, average, etc.?

E. *Social contributions to be rendered.*—Considering his age, talents, training, and past record of performance, is there a substantial probability that the patient will—*adequate recovery being assumed*—render in the future services to his society that can be characterized as outstanding, substantial, average, etc.?

This list is clearly insufficient for the construction of a reasonable selection system, since that would require not only *that these factors be taken into account* (somehow or other), but—going beyond this—would specify *a specific set of procedures for taking account of them.* The specific procedures that would constitute such a system would have to take account of the interrelationship of these factors (e.g., B and E), and to set out exact guidelines as to the relevant weight that is to be given to each of them. This is something our discussion has not as yet considered.

In fact, I should want to maintain that there is no such thing here as a single rationally superior selection system. The position of affairs seems to me to be something like this: (1) It is necessary (for reasons already canvassed) to *have* a system, and to have a system that is rationally defensible, and (2) to be rationally defensible, this system must take the factors A–E into substantial and explicit account. But (3) the exact manner in which a rationally defensible system takes account of these factors cannot be fixed in any one specific way on the basis of general considerations. Any of the variety of ways that give A–E "their due" will be acceptable and viable. One cannot hope to find within this range of workable systems some one that is *optimal* in relation to the alternatives. There is no one system that does "the (uniquely) best"—only a variety of systems that do "as well as one can expect to do" in cases of this sort.

The situation is structurally very much akin to that of rules of partition of an estate among the relations of a decedent. It is important *that there be* such rules. And it is reasonable that spouse, children, parents, siblings, etc., be taken account of in rules. But the question of the exact method of division—say that when the decedent has neither living spouse nor living

children then his estate is to be divided, dividing 60 per cent between parents, 40 per cent between siblings versus dividing 90 per cent between parents, 10 per cent between siblings—cannot be settled on the basis of any general abstract considerations of reasonableness. Within broad limits, a *variety* of resolutions are all perfectly acceptable—so that no one procedure can justifiably be regarded as "the (uniquely) best" because it is superior to all others.[21]

A Possible Basis for a Reasonable Selection System

Having said that there is no such thing as *the optimal* selection system for ELT, I want now to sketch out the broad features of what I would regard as *one acceptable* system.

The basis for the system would be a point rating. The scoring here at issue would give roughly equal weight to the medical considerations (A and B) in comparison with the extramedical considerations (C = family role, D = services rendered, and E = services to be rendered), also giving roughly equal weight to the three items involved here (C, D, and E). The result of such a scoring procedure would provide the essential *starting point* of our ELT selection mechanism. I deliberately say "starting point" because it seems to me that one should not follow the results of this scoring in an *automatic* way. I would propose that the actual selection should only be guided but not actually be dictated by this scoring procedure, along lines now to be explained.

The Desirability of Introducing an Element of Chance

The detailed procedure I would propose—not of course as optimal (for reasons we have seen), but as eminently acceptable—would combine the scoring procedure just discussed with an element of chance. The resulting selection system would function as follows:

1. First the criteria of inclusion of [the fourth] section above would be applied to constitute a *first phase selection group*—which (we shall suppose) is substantially larger than the number *n* of persons who can actually be accommodated with ELT.

2. Next the criteria of selection of [the fifth] section are brought to bear

via a scoring procedure of the type described in [the last] section. On this basis a *second phase selection group* is constituted which is only *somewhat* larger—say by a third or a half—than the critical number *n* at issue.

3. If this second phase selection group is relatively homogeneous as regards rating by the scoring procedure—that is, if there are no really major disparities within this group (as would be likely if the initial group was significantly larger than *n*)—then the final selection is made by *random selection* of *n* persons from within this group.

This introduction of the element of chance—in what could be dramatized as a "lottery of life and death"—must be justified. The fact is that such a procedure would bring with it three substantial advantages.

First, as we have argued above, any acceptable selection system is inherently nonoptimal. The introduction of the element of chance prevents the results that life-and-death choices are made by the automatic application of an admittedly imperfect selection method.

Second, a recourse to chance would doubtless make matters easier for the rejected patient and those who have a specific interest in him. It would surely be quite hard for them to accept his exclusion by relatively mechanical application of objective criteria in whose implementation subjective judgment is involved. But the circumstances of life have conditioned us to accept the workings of chance and to tolerate the element of luck (good or bad): human life is an inherently contingent process. Nobody, after all, has an absolute right to ELT—but most of us would feel that we have "every bit as much right" to it as anyone else in significantly similar circumstances. The introduction of the element of chance assures a like handling of like cases over the widest possible area that seems reasonable in the circumstances.

Third (and perhaps least), such a recourse to random selection does much to relieve the administrators of the selection system of the awesome burden of ultimate and absolute responsibility.

These three considerations would seem to build up a substantial case for introducing the element of chance into the mechanism of the system for ELT selection in a way limited and circumscribed by other weightier considerations, along some such lines as those set forth above.[22]

It should be recognized that this injection of *man-made* chance supplements the element of *natural* chance that is present inevitably and in any case (apart from the role of chance in singling out certain persons as victims for the affliction at issue). As F. M. Parsons has observed: "any vacancies [in an ELT program—specifically haemodialysis] will be filled immediately by the first suitable patients, even though their claims for therapy may subsequently prove less than those of other patients refused later."[23] Life is a chancy business and even the most rational of human arrangements can cover this over to a very limited extent at best.

Bibliography[24]

S. Alexander, "They Decide Who Lives, Who Dies," *Life,* LIII (November 9, 1962), 102–25.

C. Doyle, "Spare-Part Heart Surgeons Worried by Their Success," *Observer* (London), May 12, 1968.

J. Fletcher, *Morals and Medicine.* London, 1955.

S. Gorovitz, "Ethics and the Allocation of Medical Resources," *Medical Research Engineering,* V (1966), 5–7.

L. Lader, "Who Has the Right To Live?" *Good Housekeeping* (January, 1968), pp. 85 and 144–50.

J. D. N. Nabarro, F. M. Parsons, R. Shakman, and M. A. Wilson, "Selection of Patients for Haemodialysis," *British Medical Journal* (March 11, 1967), pp. 622–24.

H. M. Schmeck, Jr., "Panel Holds Life-or-Death Vote in Allotting of Artificial Kidney," *New York Times,* May 6, 1962, pp. 1, 83.

G. E. W. Wolstenholme and M. O'Connor (eds.), *Ethics in Medical Progress.* London, 1969.

Notes

1. Christine Doyle, "Spare-Part Heart Surgeons Worried by Their Success," *Observer,* May 12, 1968.

2. J. D. N. Nabarro, "Selection of Patients for Haemodialysis," *British Medical Journal* (March 11, 1967), p. 623. Although several thousand patients die in the U.K. each year from renal failure—there are about thirty new cases per million of population—only 10 per cent of these can for the foreseeable future be accommodated with chronic haemodialysis. Kidney transplantation—itself a very tricky procedure—cannot make a more than minor contribution here. As this article goes to press, I learn that patients can be maintained in home dialysis at an operating cost about half that of maintaining them in a hospital dialysis unit (roughly an $8,000 minimum). In the United States, around 7,000 patients with terminal uremia who could benefit from haemodialysis evolve yearly. As of mid-1968, some 1,000 of these can be accommodated in existing hospital units. By June 1967, a world-wide total of some 120 patients were in treatment by home dialysis. (Data from a forthcoming paper, "Home Dialysis," by C. M. Conty and H. V. Murdaugh. See also R. A. Baillod et al., "Overnight Haemodialysis in the Home," *Proceedings of the European Dialysis and Transplant Association,* VI [1965], 99 ff.).

3. For the Hippocratic Oath see *Hippocrates: Works* (Loeb ed.; London, 1959), I, p. 298. [Reprinted in Chapter 1 of this volume.]

4. Another example of borderline legitimacy is posed by an endowment "with strings attached," e.g., "In accepting this legacy the hospital agrees to admit and provide all needed treatment for any direct descendant of myself, its founder."

5. Shana Alexander, "They Decide Who Lives, Who Dies," *Life,* LIII (November 9, 1962), 102–25 (see p. 107).

6. Lawrence Lader, "Who Has the Right To Live?" *Good Housekeeping* (January 1968), p. 144.

7. This approach could thus be continued to embrace the previous factor, that of family role, the preceding item.

8. Moreover a doctrinaire utilitarian would presumably be willing to withdraw a continuing mode of ELT such as haemodialysis from a patient to make room for a more promising candidate who came to view at a later stage and who could not otherwise be accommodated. I should be unwilling to adopt this course, partly on grounds of utility (with a view to the demoralization of insecurity), partly on the non-utilitarian ground that a "moral commitment" has been made and must be honored.

9. Of course the difficult question remains of the relative weight that should be given to prospective and retrospective service in cases where these factors conflict. There is good reason to treat them on a par.

10. This in the symposium on "Selection of Patients for Haemodialysis," *British Medical Journal* (March 11, 1967), pp. 622–24. F. M. Parsons writes: "But other forms of selecting patients [distinct from first come, first served] are suspect in my view if they imply evaluation of man by man. What criteria could be used? Who could justify a claim that the life of a mayor would be more valuable than that of the humblest citizen of his borough? Whatever we may think as individuals none of us is indispensable." But having just set out this hard-line view he immediately backs away from it: "On the other hand, to assume that there was little to choose between Alexander Fleming and Adolf Hitler . . . would be nonsense, and we should be naive if we were to pretend that we could not be influenced by their achievements and characters if we had to choose between the two of them. Whether we like it or not we cannot escape the fact that this kind of selection for long-term haemodialysis will be required until very large sums of money become available for equipment and services [so that *everyone* who needs treatment can be accommodated]."

11. The relative fundamentality of these principles is, however, a substantially disputed issue.

12. J. D. N. Nabarro, *op. cit.,* p. 622.

13. See Shana Alexander, *op. cit.*

14. *British Medical Journal* (March 11, 1967), pp. 622–24.

15. *Ibid.,* p. 624. Another contributor writes in the same symposium, "The selection of the few [to receive haemodialysis] is proving very difficult—a true 'Doctor's Dilemma'—for almost everybody would agree that this must be a medical decision, preferably reached by consultation among colleagues" (Dr. F. M. Parsons, *ibid.,* p. 623).

16. "The Selection of Patients for Haemodialysis," *op. cit.* (n. 10 above), p. 623.

17. Dr. Wilson's article concludes with the perplexing suggestion—wildly beside the point given the structure of the situation at issue—that "the final decision will be made by the patient." But this contention is only marginally more ludicrous than Parson's contention that in selecting patients for haemodialysis "gainful employment in a well chosen occupation is necessary to achieve the best results" since "only the minority wish to live on charity" (*ibid.*).

18. To say this is of course not to deny that such questions of applied medical ethics will invariably involve a host of medical considerations—it is only to insist that extramedical considerations will also invariably be at issue.

19. M. A. Wilson, "Selection of Patients for Haemodialysis," *op. cit.,* p. 624.

20. In the case of an ongoing treatment involving complex procedure and dietary and other mode-of-life restrictions—and chronic haemodialysis definitely falls into this category—the patient's psychological makeup, his willpower to "stick with it" in the face of substantial discouragements—will obviously also be a substantial factor here. The man who gives up, takes not his life alone, but (figuratively speaking) also that of the person he replaced in the treatment schedule.

21. To say that acceptable solutions can range over broad limits is *not* to say that there are no limits at all. It is an obviously intriguing and fundamental problem to raise the question of the factors that set these limits. This complex issue cannot be dealt

with adequately here. Suffice it to say that considerations regarding precedent and people's expectations, factors of social utility, and matters of fairness and sense of justice all come into play.

22. One writer has mooted the suggestion that: "Perhaps the right thing to do, difficult as it may be to accept, is to select [for haemodialysis] from among the medical and psychologically qualified patients on a strictly random basis" (S. Gorovitz, "Ethics and the Allocation of Medical Resources," *Medical Research Engineering,* V [1966], p. 7). Outright random selection would, however, seem indefensible because of its refusal to give weight to considerations which, under the circumstances, *deserve* to be given weight. The proposed procedure of superimposing a certain degree of randomness upon the rational-choice criteria would seem to combine the advantages of the two without importing the worst defects of either.

23. "Selection of Patients for Haemodialysis," *op. cit.,* p. 623. The question of whether a patient for chronic treatment should ever be terminated from the program (say if he contracts cancer) poses a variety of difficult ethical problems with which we need not at present concern ourselves. But it does seem plausible to take the (somewhat anti-utilitarian) view that a patient should not be terminated simply because a "better qualified" patient comes along later on. It would seem that a quasi-contractual relationship has been created through established expectations and reciprocal understandings, and that the situation is in this regard akin to that of the man who, having undertaken to sell his house to one buyer, cannot afterward unilaterally undo this arrangement to sell it to a higher bidder who "needs it worse" (thus maximizing the over-all utility).

24. I acknowledge with thanks the help of Miss Hazel Johnson, Reference Librarian at the University of Pittsburgh Library, in connection with the bibliography.

99

James F. Childress
Who Shall Live When Not All Can Live?

Reprinted with permission of the editor from *Soundings,* vol. 53, 1970, pp. 339–355.

Who shall live when not all can live? Although this question has been urgently forced upon us by the dramatic use of artificial internal organs and organ transplantations, it is hardly new. George Bernard Shaw dealt with it in "The Doctor's Dilemma":

Sir Patrick. Well, Mr. Savior of Lives: which is it to be? that honest decent man Blenkinsop, or that rotten blackguard of an artist, eh?

Ridgeon. It's not an easy case to judge, is it? Blenkinsop's an honest decent man; but is he any use? Dubedat's a rotten blackguard; but he's a genuine source of pretty and pleasant and good things.

Sir Patrick. What will he be a source of for that poor innocent wife of his, when she finds him out?

Ridgeon. That's true. Her life will be a hell.

Sir Patrick. And tell me this. Suppose you had this choice put before you: either to go through life and find all the pictures bad but all the men and women good, or go through life and find all the pictures good and all the men and women rotten. Which would you choose?[1]

A significant example of the distribution of scarce medical resources is seen in the use of penicillin shortly after its discovery. Military officers had to determine which soldiers would be treated—those with venereal disease or those wounded in combat.[2] In many respects such decisions have become routine in medical circles. Day after day physicians and others make judgments and decisions "about allocations of medical care to various segments of our population, to various types of hospitalized patients, and to specific individuals,"[3] for example, whether mental illness or cancer will receive the higher proportion of available funds. Nevertheless, the dramatic forms of "Scarce Life-Saving Medical Resources" (hereafter abbreviated as SLMR) such as hemodialysis and kidney and heart transplants have compelled us to examine the moral questions that have been concealed in many routine decisions. I do not attempt in this paper to show how a resolution of SLMR cases can help us in the more routine ones which do not involve a conflict of life with life. Rather I develop an argument for a particular method of determining who shall live when not all can live. No conclusions are implied about criteria and procedures for determining who shall receive medical resources that are not directly related to the preservation of life (e.g. corneal transplants) or about standards for allocating money and time for studying and treating certain diseases.

Just as current SLMR decisions are not totally discontinuous with other medical decisions, so we must ask whether some other cases might, at least by analogy, help us develop the needed criteria and procedures. Some have looked at the principles at work in our responses to abortion, euthanasia, and artificial insemination.[4] Usually they have concluded that these cases do not cast light on the selection of patients for artificial and transplanted organs. The reason is evident: in abortion, euthanasia, and artificial insemination, there is no conflict of life with life for limited but indispensable resources (with the possible exception of therapeutic abortion). In current SLMR decisions, such a conflict is inescapable, and it makes them so morally perplexing and fascinating. If analogous cases are to be found, I think that we shall locate them in moral conflict situations.

Analogous Conflict Situations

An especially interesting and pertinent one is *U.S. v. Holmes*.[5] In 1841 an American ship, the *William Brown*, which was near Newfoundland on a trip from Liverpool to Philadelphia, struck an iceberg. The crew and half the passengers were able to escape in the two available vessels. One of these, a longboat, carrying too many passengers and leaking seriously, began to founder in the turbulent sea after about twenty-four hours. In a desperate attempt to keep it from sinking, the crew threw overboard fourteen men. Two sisters of one of the men either jumped overboard to join their brother in death or instructed the crew to throw them over. The criteria for determining who should live were "not to part man and wife, and not to throw over any women." Several hours later the others were rescued. Returning to Philadelphia, most of the crew disappeared, but one, Holmes, who had acted upon orders from the mate, was indicted, tried, and convicted on the charge of "unlawful homicide."

We are interested in this case from a moral rather than a legal standpoint,

and there are several possible responses to and judgments about it. Without attempting to be exhaustive I shall sketch a few of these. The judge contended that lots should have been cast, for in such conflict situations, there is no other procedure "so consonant both to humanity and to justice." Counsel for Holmes, on the other hand, maintained that the "sailors adopted the only principle of selection which was possible in an emergency like theirs,—a principle more humane than lots."

Another version of selection might extend and systematize the maxims of the sailors in the direction of "utility"; those are saved who will contribute to the greatest good for the greatest number. Yet another possible option is defended by Edmond Cahn in *The Moral Decision*. He argues that in this case we encounter the "morals of the last days." By this phrase he indicates that an apocalyptic crisis renders totally irrelevant the normal differences between individuals. He continues,

In a strait of this extremity, all men are reduced—or raised, as one may choose to denominate it—to members of the genus, mere congeners and nothing else. Truly and literally, all were "in the same boat," and thus none could be saved separately from the others. I am driven to conclude that otherwise—that is, if none sacrifice themselves of free will to spare the others—they must all wait and die together. For where all have become congeners, pure and simple, no one can save himself by killing another.[6]

Cahn's answer to the question "who shall live when not all can live" is "none" unless the voluntary sacrifice by some persons permits it.

Few would deny the importance of Cahn's approach although many, including this writer, would suggest that it is relevant mainly as an affirmation of an elevated and, indeed, heroic or saintly morality which one hopes would find expression in the voluntary actions of many persons trapped in "borderline" situations involving a conflict of life with life. It is a maximal demand which some moral principles impose on the individual in the recognition that self-preservation is not a good which is to be defended at all costs. The absence of this saintly or heroic morality should not mean, however, that everyone perishes. Without making survival an absolute value and without justifying all means to achieve

it, we can maintain that simply letting everyone die is irresponsible. This charge can be supported from several different standpoints, including society at large as well as the individuals involved. Among a group of self-interested individuals, none of whom volunteers to relinquish his life, there may be better and worse ways of determining who shall survive. One task of social ethics, whether religious or philosophical, is to propose relatively just institutional arrangements within which self-interested and biased men can live. The question then becomes: which set of arrangements—which criteria and procedures of selection—is most satisfactory in view of the human condition (man's limited altruism and inclination to seek his own good) and the conflicting values that are to be realized?

There are several significant differences between the *Holmes* and SLMR cases, a major one being that the former involves *direct* killing of another person, while the latter involve only *permitting* a person to die when it is not possible to save all. Furthermore, in extreme situations such as *Holmes*, the restraints of civilization have been stripped away, and something approximating a state of nature prevails, in which life is "solitary, poor, nasty, brutish and short." The state of nature does not mean that moral standards are irrelevant and that might should prevail, but it does suggest that much of the matrix which normally supports morality has been removed. Also, the necessary but unfortunate decisions about who shall live and die are made by men who are existentially and personally involved in the outcome. Their survival too is at stake. Even though the institutional role of sailors seems to require greater sacrificial actions, there is obviously no assurance that they will adequately assess the number of sailors required to man the vessel or that they will impartially and objectively weigh the common good at stake. As the judge insisted in his defense of casting lots in the *Holmes* case: "In no other than this [casting lots] or some like way are those having equal rights put upon an equal footing, and in no other way is it possible to guard against partiality and oppression, violence, and conflict.'' This difference should not be exaggerated since self-interest, professional pride, and the like obviously affect the outcome of many medical decisions. Nor do the remaining differences cancel *Holmes'* instructiveness.

Criteria of Selection for SLMR

Which set of arrangements should be adopted for SLMR? Two questions are involved: Which standards and criteria should be used? and, Who should make the decision? The first question is basic, since the debate about implementation, e.g., whether by a lay committee or physician, makes little progress until the criteria are determined.

We need two sets of criteria which will be applied at two different stages in the selection of recipients of SLMR. First, medical criteria should be used to exclude those who are not ''medically acceptable.'' Second, from this group of ''medically acceptable'' applicants, the final selection can be made. Occasionally in current American medical practice, the first stage is omitted, but such an omission is unwarranted. Ethical and social responsibility would seem to require distributing these SLMR only to those who have some reasonable prospect of responding to the treatment. Furthermore, in transplants such medical tests as tissue and blood typing are necessary, although they are hardly fully developed.

''Medical acceptability'' is not as easily determined as many non-physicians assume since there is considerable debate in medical circles about the relevant factors (e.g., age and complicating diseases). Although ethicists can contribute little or nothing to this debate, two proposals may be in order. First, ''medical acceptability'' should be used only to determine the group from which the final selection will be made, and the attempt to establish fine degrees of prospective response to treatment should be avoided. Medical criteria, then, would exclude some applicants but would not serve as a basis of comparison between those who pass the first stage. For example, if two applicants for dialysis were medically acceptable, the physicians would *not* choose the one with the *better* medical prospects. Final selection

would be made on other grounds. Second, psychological and environmental factors should be kept to an absolute minimum and should be considered only when they are without doubt critically related to medical acceptability (e.g., the inability to cope with the requirements of dialysis which might lead to suicide).[7]

The most significant moral questions emerge when we turn to the final selection. Once the pool of medically acceptable applicants has been defined and still the number is larger than the resources, what other criteria should be used? How should the final selection be made? First, I shall examine some of the difficulties that stem from efforts to make the final selection in terms of social value; these difficulties raise serious doubts about the feasibility and justifiability of the utilitarian approach. Then I shall consider the possible justification for random selection or chance.

Occasionally criteria of social worth focus on past contributions but most often they are primarily future-oriented. The patient's potential and probable contribution to the society is stressed, although this obviously cannot be abstracted from his present web of relationships (e.g., dependents) and occupational activities (e.g., nuclear physicist). Indeed, the magnitude of his contribution to society (as an abstraction) is measured in terms of these social roles, relations, and functions. Enough has already been said to suggest the tremendous range of factors that affect social value or worth.[8] Here we encounter the first major difficulty of this approach: How do we determine the relevant criteria of social value?

The difficulties of quantifying various social needs are only too obvious. How does one quantify and compare the needs of the spirit (e.g., education, art, religion), political life, economic activity, technological development? Joseph Fletcher suggests that ''some day we may learn how to 'quantify' or 'mathematicate' or 'computerize' the value problem in selection, in the same careful and thorough way that diagnosis has been.''[9] I am not convinced that we can ever quantify values, or that we should attempt to do so. But even if the various social and human needs, in principle, could be quantified, how do we determine how much weight we will give to each one?

Which will have priority in case of conflict? Or even more basically, in the light of which values and principles do we recognize social ''needs''?

One possible way of determining the values which should be emphasized in selection has been proposed by Leo Shatin.[10] He insists that our medical decisions about allocating resources are already based on an unconscious scale of values (usually dominated by material worth). Since there is really no way of escaping this, we should be self-conscious and critical about it. How should we proceed? He recommends that we discover the values that most people in our society hold and then use them as criteria for distributing SLMR. These values can be discovered by attitude or opinion surveys. Presumably if fifty-one percent in this testing period put a greater premium on military needs than technological development, military men would have a greater claim on our SLMR than experimental researchers. But valuations of what is significant change, and the student revolutionary who was denied SLMR in 1970 might be celebrated in 1990 as the greatest American hero since George Washington.

Shatin presumably is seeking criteria that could be applied nationally, but at the present, regional and local as well as individual prejudices tincture the criteria of social value that are used in selection. Nowhere is this more evident than in the deliberations and decisions of the anonymous selection committee of the Seattle Artificial Kidney Center where such factors as church membership and Scout leadership have been deemed significant for determining who shall live.[11] As two critics conclude after examining these criteria and procedures, they rule out ''creative nonconformists, who rub the bourgeoisie the wrong way but who historically have contributed so much to the making of America. The Pacific Northwest is no place for a Henry David Thoreau with bad kidneys.''[12]

Closely connected to this first problem of determining social values is a second one. Not only is it difficult if not impossible to reach agreement on social values, but it is also rarely easy to predict what our needs will be in a few years and what the consequences of present actions will be. Furthermore it is difficult to predict which persons will fulfill their potential function in society. Admissions committees in colleges and universities experience the frustrations of predicting realization of potential. For these reasons, as someone has indicated, God might be a utilitarian, but we cannot be. We simply lack the capacity to predict very accurately the consequences which we then must evaluate. Our incapacity is never more evident than when we think in societal terms.

Other difficulties make us even less confident that such an approach to SLMR is advisable. Many critics raise the spectre of abuse, but this should not be overemphasized. The fundamental difficulty appears on another level: the utilitarian approach would in effect reduce the person to his social role, relations, and functions. Ultimately it dulls and perhaps even eliminates the sense of the person's transcendence, his dignity as a person which cannot be reduced to his past or future contribution to society. It is not at all clear that we are willing to live with these implications of utilitarian selection. Wilhelm Kolff, who invented the artificial kidney, has asked: "Do we really subscribe to the principle that social standing should determine selection? Do we allow patients to be treated with dialysis only when they are married, go to church, have children, have a job, a good income and give to the Community Chest?"[13]

The German theologian Helmut Thielicke contends that any search for "objective criteria" for selection is already a capitulation to the utilitarian point of view which violates man's dignity.[14] The solution is not to let all die, but to recognize that SLMR cases are "borderline situations" which inevitably involve guilt. The agent, however, can have courage and freedom (which, for Thielicke, come from justification by faith) and can

go ahead anyway and seek for criteria for deciding the question of life or death in the matter of the artificial kidney. Since these criteria are . . . questionable, necessarily alien to the meaning of human existence, the decision to which they lead can be little more than that arrived at by casting lots.[15]

The resulting criteria, he suggests, will probably be very similar to those already employed in American medical practice.

He is most concerned to preserve a certain *attitude* or *disposition* in SLMR—the sense of guilt which arises when man's dignity is violated. With this sense of guilt, the agent remains "sound and healthy where it really counts."[16] Thielicke uses man's dignity only as a judgmental, critical, and negative standard. It only tells us how all selection criteria and procedures (and even the refusal to act) implicate us in the ambiguity of the human condition and its metaphysical guilt. This approach is consistent with his view of the task of theological ethics: "to teach us how to understand and endure—not 'solve'—the borderline situation."[17] But ethics, I would contend, can help us discern the factors and norms in whose light relative, discriminate judgments can be made. Even if all actions in SLMR should involve guilt, some may preserve human dignity to a greater extent than others. Thielicke recognizes that a decision based on any criteria is "little more than that arrived at by casting lots." But perhaps selection by chance would come the closest to embodying the moral and nonmoral values that we are trying to maintain (including a sense of man's dignity).

The Values of Random Selection

My proposal is that we use some form of randomness or chance (either natural, such as "first come, first served," or artificial, such as a lottery) to determine who shall be saved. Many reject randomness as a surrender to non-rationality when responsible and rational judgments can and must be made. Edmond Cahn criticizes "Holmes' judge" who recommended the casting of lots because, as Cahn puts it, "the crisis involves stakes too high for gambling and responsibilities too deep for destiny."[18] Similarly, other critics see randomness as a surrender to "non-human" forces which necessarily vitiates human values. Sometimes these values are identified with the process of decision-making (e.g., it is important to have persons rather than impersonal forces determining who shall live). Sometimes they are identified with the outcome of the process (e.g., the features such as creativity and fullness of being which make human life what it is are to be considered and respected in the decision). Regarding the former, it must be admitted that the

use of chance seems cold and impersonal. But presumably the defenders of utilitarian criteria in SLMR want to make their application as objective and impersonal as possible so that subjective bias does not determine who shall live.

Such criticisms, however, ignore the moral and nonmoral values which might be supported by selection by randomness or chance. A more important criticism is that the procedure that I develop draws the relevant moral context too narrowly. That context, so the argument might run, includes the society and its future and not merely the individual with his illness and claim upon SLMR. But my contention is that the values and principles at work in the narrower context may well take precedence over those operative in the broader context both because of their weight and significance and because of the weaknesses of selection in terms of social worth. As Paul Freund rightly insists, "The more nearly total is the estimate to be made of an individual, and the more nearly the consequence determines life and death, the more unfit the judgment becomes for human reckoning. . . . Randomness as a moral principle deserves serious study."[19] Serious study would, I think, point toward its implementation in certain conflict situations, primarily because it preserves a significant degree of *personal dignity* by providing *equality* of opportunity. Thus it cannot be dismissed as a "non-rational" and "non-human" procedure without an inquiry into the reasons, including human values, which might justify it. Paul Ramsey stresses this point about the *Holmes* case:

Instead of fixing our attention upon "gambling" as the solution—with all the frivolous and often corrupt associations the word raises in our minds—we should think rather of *equality* of opportunity as the ethical substance of the relations of those individuals to one another that might have been guarded and expressed by casting lots.[20]

The individual's personal and transcendent dignity, which on the utilitarian approach would be submerged in his social role and function, can be protected and witnessed to by a recognition of his equal right to be saved. Such a right is best preserved by procedures which establish equality of opportunity. Thus selection by chance more closely approximates the requirements established by human dignity than does utilitarian calculation. It is not infallibly just, but it is preferable to the alternatives of letting all die or saving only those who have the greatest social responsibilities and potential contribution.

This argument can be extended by examining values other than individual dignity and equality of opportunity. Another basic value in the medical sphere is the relationship of trust between physician and patient. Which selection criteria are most in accord with this relationship of trust? Which will maintain, extend, and deepen it? My contention is that selection by randomness or chance is preferable from this standpoint too.

Trust, which is inextricably bound to respect for human dignity, is an attitude of expectation about another. It is not simply the expectation that another will perform a particular act, but more specifically that another will act toward him in certain ways—which will respect him as a person. As Charles Fried writes:

Although trust has to do with reliance on a disposition of another person, it is reliance on a disposition of a special sort: the disposition to act morally, to deal fairly with others, to live up to one's undertakings, and so on. Thus to trust another is first of all to expect him to accept the principle of morality in his dealings with you, to respect your status as a person, your personality.[21]

This trust cannot be preserved in life-and-death situations when a person expects decisions about him to be made in terms of his social worth, for such decisions violate his status as a person. An applicant rejected on grounds of inadequacy in social value or virtue would have reason for feeling that his "trust" had been betrayed. Indeed, the sense that one is being viewed not as an end in himself but as a means in medical progress or the achievement of a greater social good is incompatible with attitudes and relationships of trust. We recognize this in the billboard which was erected after the first heart transplants: "Drive Carefully. Christiaan Barnard Is Watching You." The relationship of trust between the physician and patient is not only an instrumental value in the sense of

being an important factor in the patient's treatment. It is also to be endorsed because of its intrinsic worth as a relationship.

Thus the related values of individual dignity and trust are best maintained in selection by chance. But other factors also buttress the argument for this approach. Which criteria and procedures would men agree upon? We have to suppose a hypothetical situation in which several men are going to determine for themselves and their families the criteria and procedures by which they would want to be admitted to and excluded from SLMR if the need arose.[22] We need to assume two restrictions and then ask which set of criteria and procedures would be chosen as the most rational and, indeed, the fairest. The restrictions are these: (1) The men are self-interested. They are interested in their own welfare (and that of members of their families), and this, of course, includes survival. Basically, they are not motivated by altruism. (2) Furthermore, they are ignorant of their own talents, abilities, potential, and probable contribution to the social good. They do not know how they would fare in a competitive situation, e.g., the competition for SLMR in terms of social contribution. Under these conditions which institution would be chosen—letting all die, utilitarian selection, or the use of chance? Which would seem the most rational? the fairest? By which set of criteria would they want to be included in or excluded from the list of those who will be saved? The rational choice in this setting (assuming self-interest and ignorance of one's competitive success) would be random selection or chance since this alone provides equality of opportunity. A possible response is that one would prefer to take a "risk" and therefore choose the utilitarian approach. But I think not, especially since I added that the participants in this hypothetical situation are choosing for their children as well as for themselves; random selection or chance could be more easily justified to the children. It would make more sense for men who are self-interested but uncertain about their relative contribution to society to elect a set of criteria which would build in equality of opportunity. They would consider selection by chance as relatively just and fair.[23]

An important psychological point supplements earlier arguments for using chance or random selection. The psychological stress and strain among those who are rejected would be greater if the rejection is based on insufficient social worth than if it is based on chance. Obviously stress and strain cannot be eliminated in these borderline situations, but they would almost certainly be increased by the opprobrium of being judged relatively "unfit" by society's agents using society's values. Nicholas Rescher makes this point very effectively:

a recourse to chance would doubtless make matters easier for the rejected patient and those who have a specific interest in him. It would surely be quite hard for them to accept his exclusion by relatively mechanical application of objective criteria in whose implementation subjective judgment is involved. But the circumstances of life have conditioned us to accept the workings of chance and to tolerate the element of luck (good or bad): human life is an inherently contingent process. Nobody, after all, has an absolute right to ELT [Exotic Lifesaving Therapy]—but most of us would feel that we have "every bit as much right" to it as anyone else in significantly similar circumstances.[24]

Although it is seldom recognized as such, selection by chance is already in operation in practically every dialysis unit. I am not aware of any unit which removes some of its patients from kidney machines in order to make room for later applicants who are better qualified in terms of social worth. Furthermore, very few people would recommend it. Indeed, few would even consider removing a person from a kidney machine on the grounds that a person better qualified medically had just applied. In a discussion of the treatment of chronic renal failure by dialysis at the University of Virginia Hospital Renal Unit from November 15, 1965 to November 15, 1966, Dr. Harry Abram writes: "Thirteen patients sought treatment but were not considered because the program had reached its limit of nine patients."[25] Thus, in practice and theory, natural chance is accepted at least within certain limits.

My proposal is that we extend this principle (first come, first served) to determine who among the medically acceptable patients shall live or that we utilize artificial chance such as a lottery or randomness. "First come, first served" would be more feasible than a lottery since the applicants make their claims over a period of time rather than as a group at one time. This procedure would be in accord with at least one principle in our present practices and with our sense of individual dignity, trust, and fairness. Its significance in relation to these values can be underlined by asking how the decision can be justified to the rejected applicant. Of course, one easy way of avoiding this task is to maintain the traditional cloak of secrecy, which works to a great extent because patients are often not aware that they are being considered for SLMR in addition to the usual treatment. But whether public justification is instituted or not is not the significant question; it is rather what reasons for rejection would be most acceptable to the unsuccessful patient. My contention is that rejection can be accepted more readily if equality of opportunity, fairness, and trust are preserved, and that they are best preserved by selection by randomness or chance.

This proposal has yet another advantage since it would eliminate the need for a committee to examine applicants in terms of their social value. This onerous responsibility can be avoided.

Finally, there is a possible indirect consequence of widespread use of random selection which is interesting to ponder, although I do *not* adduce it as a good reason for adopting random selection. It can be argued, as Professor Mason Willrich of the University of Virginia Law School has suggested, that SLMR cases would practically disappear if these scarce resources were distributed randomly rather than on social worth grounds. Scarcity would no longer be a problem because the holders of economic and political power would make certain that they would not be excluded by a random selection procedure; hence they would help to redirect public priorities or establish private funding so that life-saving medical treatment would be widely and perhaps universally available.

In the framework that I have delineated, are the decrees of chance to be taken without exception? If we recognize exceptions, would we not open Pandora's box again just after we had succeeded in getting it closed? The direction of my argument has been

against any exceptions, and I would defend this as the proper way to go. But let me indicate one possible way of admitting exceptions while at the same time circumscribing them so narrowly that they would be very rare indeed.

An obvious advantage of the utilitarian approach is that occasionally circumstances arise which make it necessary to say that one man is practically indispensable for a society in view of a particular set of problems it faces (e.g., the President when the nation is waging a war for survival). Certainly the argument to this point has stressed that the burden of proof would fall on those who think that the social danger in this instance is so great that they simply cannot abide by the outcome of a lottery or a first come, first served policy. Also, the reason must be negative rather than positive; that is, we depart from chance in this instance not because we want to take advantage of this person's potential contribution to the improvement of our society, but because his immediate loss would possibly (even probably) be disastrous (again, the President in a grave national emergency). Finally, social value (in the negative sense) should be used as a standard of exception in dialysis, for example, only if it would provide a reason strong enough to warrant removing another person from a kidney machine if all machines were taken. Assuming this strong reluctance to remove anyone once the commitment has been made for him, we would be willing to put this patient ahead of another applicant for a vacant machine only if we would be willing (in circumstances in which all machines are being used) to vacate a machine by removing someone from it. These restrictions would make an exception almost impossible.

While I do not recommend this procedure of recognizing exceptions, I think that one can defend it while accepting my general thesis about selection by randomness or chance. If it is used, a lay committee (perhaps advisory, perhaps even stronger) would be called upon to deal with the alleged exceptions since the doctors or others would in effect be appealing the outcome of chance (either natural or artificial). This lay committee would determine whether this patient was so indispensable at this time and place that he had to be saved even by sacrificing

the values preserved by random selection. It would make it quite clear that exception is warranted, if at all, only as the "lesser of two evils." Such a defense would be recognized only rarely, if ever, primarily because chance and randomness preserve so many important moral and nonmoral values in SLMR cases.[26]

Notes

1. George Bernard Shaw, *The Doctor's Dilemma* (New York, 1941), pp. 132–133.

2. Henry K. Beecher, "Scarce Resources and Medical Advancement," *Daedalus* (Spring 1969), pp. 279–280.

3. Leo Shatin, "Medical Care and the Social Worth of a Man," *American Journal of Orthopsychiatry*, 36 (1967), 97.

4. Harry S. Abram and Walter Wadlington, "Selection of Patients for Artificial and Transplanted Organs," *Annals of Internal Medicine*, 69 (September 1968), 615–620.

5. *United States v. Holmes* 26 Fed. Cas. 360 (C.C.E.D. Pa. 1842). All references are to the text of the trial as reprinted in Philip E. Davis, ed., *Moral Duty and Legal Responsibility: A Philosophical-Legal Casebook* (New York, 1966), pp. 102–118.

6. *The Moral Decision* (Bloomington, Ind., 1955), p. 71.

7. For a discussion of the higher suicide rate among dialysis patients than among the general population and an interpretation of some of the factors at work, see H. S. Abram, G. L. Moore, and F. B. Westervelt, "Suicidal Behavior in Chronic Dialysis Patients," *American Journal of Psychiatry* (in press). This study shows that even "if one does not include death through not following the regimen the incidence of suicide is still more than 100 times the normal population."

8. I am excluding from consideration the question of the ability to pay because most of the people involved have to secure funds from other sources, public or private, anyway.

9. Joseph Fletcher, "Donor Nephrectomies and Moral Responsibility," *Journal of the American Medical Women's Association*, 23 (Dec. 1968), p. 1090.

10. Leo Shatin, op. cit., pp. 96–101.

11. For a discussion of the Seattle selection committee, see Shana Alexander, "They Decide Who Lives, Who Dies," *Life*, 53 (Nov. 9, 1962), 102. For an examination of general selection practices in dialysis see "Scarce Medical Resources," *Columbia Law Review*, 69:620 (1969) and Harry S. Abram and Walter Wadlington, op cit.

12. David Sanders and Jesse Dukeminier, Jr., "Medical Advance and Legal Lag: Hemodialysis and Kidney Transplantation," *UCLA Law Review* 15:367 (1968) 378. [Reprinted in part as Chapter 97 of this volume.]

13. "Letters and Comments," *Annals of Internal Medicine,* 61 (Aug. 1964), 360. Dr. G. E. Schreiner contends that "if you really believe in the right of society to make decisions on medical availability on these criteria you should be logical and say that when a man stops going to church or is divorced or loses his job, he ought to be removed from the programme and somebody else who fulfills these criteria substituted. Obviously no one faces up to this logical consequence" (G.E.W. Wolstenholme and Maeve O'Connor, eds. *Ethics in Medical Progress: With Special Reference to Transplantation,* A Ciba Foundation Symposium [Boston, 1966], p. 127).

14. Helmut Thielicke, "The Doctor as Judge of Who Shall Live and Who Shall Die," *Who Shall Live?* ed. by Kenneth Vaux (Philadelphia, 1970), p. 172.

15. Ibid., pp. 173–174.

16. Ibid., p. 173

17. Thielicke, *Theological Ethics,* Vol. I, *Foundations* (Philadelphia, 1966), p. 602.

18. Cahn, op. cit., p. 71.

19. Paul Freund, "Introduction," *Daedalus* (Spring 1969), xiii.

20. Paul Ramsey, *Nine Modern Moralists* (Englewood Cliffs, N.J., 1962), p. 245.

21. Charles Fried, "Privacy," In *Law, Reason, and Justice,* ed. by Graham Hughes (New York, 1969), p. 52.

22. My argument is greatly dependent on John Rawls's version of justice as fairness, which is a reinterpretation of social contract theory. Rawls, however, would probably not apply his ideas to "borderline situations." See "Distributive Justice: Some Addenda," *Natural Law Forum,* 13 (1968), 53. For Rawls's general theory, see "Justice as Fairness," *Philosophy, Politics and Society* (Second Series), ed. by Peter Laslett and W. G. Runciman (Oxford, 1962), pp. 132–157 and his other essays on aspects of this topic.

23. Occasionally someone contends that random selection may reward vice. Leo Shatin (op. cit., p. 100) insists that random selection "would reward socially disvalued qualities by giving their bearers the same special medical care opportunities as those received by the bearers of socially valued qualities. Personally I do not favor such a method." Obviously society must engender certain qualities in its members, but not all of its institutions must be devoted to that purpose. Furthermore, there are strong reasons, I have contended, for exempting SLMR from that sort of function.

24. Nicholas Rescher, "The Allocation of Exotic Medical Lifesaving Therapy," *Ethics,* 79 (April 1969), 184 [reprinted as Chapter 98 of this volume]. He defends random selection's use only after utilitarian and other judgments have been made. If there are no "major disparities" in terms of utility, etc., in the second stage of selection, then final selection could be made randomly. He fails to give attention to the moral values that random selection might preserve.

25. Harry S. Abram, M.D., "The Psychiatrist, the Treatment of Chronic Renal Failure, and the Prolongation of Life: II" *American Journal of Psychiatry* 126:157–167 (1969), 158.

26. I read a draft of this paper in a seminar on "Social Implications of Advances in Biomedical Science and Technology: Artificial and Transplanted Internal Organs," sponsored by the Center for the Study of Science, Technology, and Public Policy of the University of Virginia, Spring 1970. I am indebted to the participants in that seminar, and especially to its leaders, Mason Willrich, Professor of Law, and Dr. Harry Abram, Associate Professor of Psychiatry, for criticisms which helped me to sharpen these ideas. Good discussions of the legal questions raised by selection (e.g., equal protection of the law and due process) which I have not considered can be found in "Scarce Medical Resources," *Columbia Law Review,* 69:620 (1969); "Patient Selection for Artificial and Transplanted Organs," *Harvard Law Review,* 82:1322 (1969); and Sanders and Dukeminier, op. cit.

100

Ralph B. Potter

Labeling the Mentally Retarded: The Just Allocation of Therapy

Reprinted with permission of the author and delivered at "Choices of our Conscience," International Symposium on Human Rights, Retardation and Research, sponsored by the Joseph P. Kennedy, Jr. Foundation, Washington, D.C., October 16, 1971.

Labels serve as convenient means for ordering experience and determining appropriate reactions. Labels create roles and define relations. They may be applied formally or informally, officially or unofficially. The official use of labels such as "retarded," "handicapped," "culturally deprived," or "exceptional" raises questions of public policy. The application of such labels may have significant effects upon the life chances of those to whom they are applied. When the welfare of any neighbor is at stake, citizens must scrutinize public practice to assess the purpose and precision of labels, the procedural fairness and reliability in their application, the suitability and effectiveness of consequent treatment, and the impact of such intervention upon immediate subjects, families, institutions, communities and the ethos of the entire society.

The use of a label such as "mentally retarded" is a highly risky and ambiguous moral enterprise. On the one hand, resort to some distinctive label may bring benefit to those in need of special aid. Application of a label is necessary to establish eligibility for special treatment shaped in the hope of enhancing the fulfillment of human potential. On the other hand, the same act of labeling may bring harm by assigning one to a social category or role that is disfavored.

The presumed weakness or need of the mentally retarded creates a claim for ameliorative aid from society at large. But the particular type of weakness that qualifies the mentally retarded for special assistance tends, paradoxically, on the basis of some patterns of moral reasoning, to disqualify or attenuate their claim upon the scarce resources that any society must parcel out in competition with other possible worthy claims. Errol E. Harris, in an essay entitled "Respect for Persons," sketches the context of social philosophy which generates an ambiguous attitude toward the needs of the mentally retarded.

The ultimate aim of the whole social way of life is the fullest possible development of the capacities of the individuals who make up the society concerned, giving the fullest possible satisfaction of the complete personality. This complete development and satisfaction of the individual as an integrated personality is the ultimate criterion of all human value. . . . In sum,

the full and satisfactory realization of human personality is attainable only in a complete way of life, led with knowledge and insight into the principles, moral, philosophical and religious, which govern its satisfactory character. It was this, or something like it, that Aristotle had in mind when he defined the good for man as "an activity of the soul in accordance with excellence, in a complete life."[1]

The state exists in order to facilitate the attainment of the good life by its members. But the good life is held to be contingent upon the exercise of the distinctively human powers of reason reflected in a high degree of self-consciousness and awareness: it must be "led with knowledge and insight into the principles, moral, philosophical and religious, which govern its satisfactory character." The community bears a responsibility to facilitate each person in the realization of his potential for self-conscious fulfillment of his powers. But, given the scarcity of many forms of resources, questions of justice can arise in the allocation of opportunities. As Harris notes, "Some human individuals appear incapable of intellectual or moral development and so of the realization of value. Should such people be respected at the expense of others who have definite potentialities?"[2] In suggesting that "the consideration and treatment to which any person is entitled should be commensurate with his potentiality,"[3] Harris renders the mentally retarded vulnerable to crude utilitarian arguments that might be invoked to justify neglecting their needs to reap a greater social good by investing resources in the nurture of those held to have "greater potential." A dilemma is created by espousal of a simple maxim such as, "It is wrong to condone the waste of human potential." Such dimensions of human potential will surely be wasted if the mentally retarded are not provided with special aid. But other dimensions of human potential will be neglected if the costs of aiding the mentally retarded make it impossible to nurture fully the powers of those believed to be endowed with greater gifts. . . .

Our purpose is to dramatize the point that the practice of assigning labels such as "mentally retarded" is not to be taken lightly or performed carelessly. In applying such a label, an

official assigns an individual to a highly vulnerable role which has a tenuous hold upon the sympathy and support of the populace. Officials who must preside over the apportionment of opportunities cannot abstain from labeling. To do so would be to deprive those in need of access to the special care to which they are entitled. Injustice may be done through excessively naive or sentimental scrupulosity. Labels must, on due occasions, be assigned. But the labels must be precisely and relevantly defined. They must be accurately applied. And they must lead to treatment that serves the welfare of those that are labeled. Prospects for achieving justice in the right use of labels may be enhanced by consideration of the forms of injustice that stem from the misuse of the power of labeling.

Injustice in the Definition of Labels

The administrative function of the type of label we are concerned with is to establish eligibility for special treatment by public agencies on the basis of an identifiable need. Receipt of the label qualifies one for a presumed benefit. The situation is complicated, however, by a concomitant fact of social life: the same labeling process assigns one to membership in a disfavored group bearing a stigma that may reduce life chances. The status of "mentally retarded" tends to be a "master status" within which all subordinate statuses and characteristics are submerged.[4] Those who bear the label of mentally retarded are set apart and marked as different. Whereas they are different specifically in relation to activities demanding the exercise of high mental powers, the impact of their differentness is commonly allowed to spread into a wide range of endeavors. A specific weakness is taken as the grounds for a general discrimination diminishing the opportunity for full participation in activities not directly effected by their mental retardation. A concern for justice in the definition of labels requires that this contagion of statuses be controlled.

Social justice is grounded upon the presumption that all are to be treated equally unless some relevant difference can be brought forward to vindicate an unequal distribution of benefits or burdens. There are many valid purposes that can justify the creation of special categories for the distribution of benefits and burdens. Membership within these categories can be determined on the basis of an indefinite number of different attributes. But the recurring question of justice is, "Which attributes are relevant for membership in a category bearing a claim to a specific benefit or a liability to a particular burden?" Should good looks be taken as the basis of eligibility for military conscription? Or should the color of hair qualify one for a pension? The boundaries of the "domains of relevance"[5] must be carefully drawn. Men differ in their judgments concerning what attributes should qualify or disqualify one for particular benefits and burdens. Aristotle noted that it is plain "that awards should be 'according to merit'; for all men agree that what is just in distribution must be according to merit in some sense, though they do not all specify the same sort of merit, but democrats identify it with the status of free man, supporters of oligarchy with wealth (or with noble birth), and supporters of aristocracy with excellence."[6]

Among the diverse, pluralistic subcultures of the United States there is little consensus concerning what constitutes merit and hence little agreement concerning the bases for the distribution of benefits and burdens. The democratic, egalitarian heritage has discredited reliance upon indices such as race, creed, national origin, social class, sex, or clan. The rise of the meritocracy has brought a widely welcomed emphasis upon "individual ability" as the proper qualification for reward and advancement. In a highly mobile society in which individual acquaintance can seldom be the basis for assessment of relative ability, certification by public schools has served as a primary credential. The public schools have been the great sorting bins in which future members of the work force are prepared, assessed and labeled in relation to their predicted efficacy as members of the community.

Within the schools, there has been the temptation to allow performance upon standardized intelligence tests to serve as a general index of merit. The effect has been to collapse consideration of a great range of independent and incommensurable human qualities into a single measure yielding a scale upon which persons with highly diverse constellations of admirable and less admirable characteristics can be placed in rank order. Intelligence tests purport to measure the most fundamental abilities that are inborn, constant and indispensable for successful performance of the widest range of activities. The results of the tests are quantifiable, permitting easy comparison, ranking and grouping. They are taken to provide an index of "trainability" and can be used, or misused, as predictors of future capacity to contribute to the public good and even for estimates of the ability to enjoy assorted experiences of life. Exaggerated emphasis upon the import of intelligence test scores can greatly ease the philosophical discomfort of utilitarians by making the hedonic calculus required to determine which mix or distribution of pleasures would insure "the greatest happiness for the greatest number" more plausible. By maximizing the significance of the measurable characteristic of intelligence it seems possible to reduce perplexities concerning the assessment of merit in the process of apportioning opportunities. Incommensurable qualities are reduced to commensurable status when intelligence is taken as a general measure of "human potential." Then the rule suggested by Harris, that "the consideration and treatment to which any person is entitled should be commensurate with his potentiality," can be invoked to aid in the apportionment of benefits and burdens.

Questions of the validity and reliability of intelligence tests come thus to be of central moral significance when heavy weight is placed upon them as determinants of social stratification through the allotment of opportunities. Psychologists and others possessed of technical training must be pressed to provide ever more clear accounts of what it is that intelligence tests measure, how constant results are likely to be, and what factors may lead to variation in performance. But what difference differences in performance will make in the allotment of benefits and burdens is a matter of public policy to be decided by the community at large. The question of justice in the definition of labels is, "What benefits and burdens are properly to be linked to estimates of intelligence?" What realms of activity and participation should be effected by a presumed weakness of intelligence? The domain of relevance should be circumscribed as narrowly as possible in order to enable those who are mentally retarded to have fullest opportunity to realize the widest range of human capacities in the most extensive interaction of which they are capable within a community sensitive enough to create labels with care and caution and confine their effects to relevant domains. The justification of assuming the risk of creating and applying a label must be to open a wider future for those who need special forms of assistance. It is contradictory to allow the irrelevant extension or unsuitable retention of a label to foreclose future opportunities.

To avoid injustice in the definition of a label, the criteria for the official application of every label must be specific, clear, precise, open to public understanding and review, relevant to anticipated treatment, and able to be fairly applied for stated purposes.

Injustice in the Application of Labels

The risk entailed in the definition and application of the types of labels we are concerned with can be justified only by the prospect of benefiting those in need of special care. It follows that those having some lack must be correctly identified and their exact need accurately diagnosed and relieved by discriminating intervention if those who apply potentially embarrassing labels are not to be held guilty of compounding rather than relieving the difficulties of the mentally retarded by drawing attention to the undesired differentness which makes them unintentional nonconformists vulnerable to stigmatization even though they are blameless of any moral fault through purposeful wrongdoing. Those who apply labels must be held accountable for the accuracy and fairness of the process of labeling.

But how can labels be verified or falsified? What is the appropriate test of the accuracy of a label and the veracity of a labeler? An attempt to answer such questions reveals the manifold ambiguity of labels. They can be taken to refer either to some characteristic of the subject or to the response of labelers themselves. If a label is understood to refer to a capacity of a subject it may be seen either as a report of past performance or as a prediction of future capacity. A label held to be nothing more than a report upon past performance might gain a measure of reliability and definiteness, but it would do so at the cost of losing interest. It is as a predictor of future capacity and behavior that a label has significance for those who must orient their action in response to the presumed characteristics of one who bears a label. There is always a gap between past observation and future prediction, a gap filled with the uncertain effects of an indeterminant number of variables influencing the future. Sociologists who emphasize that labels may be taken to refer most clearly to the reactions of those doing the labeling rather than to any fixed and "objective" characteristic of the one who is labeled, point to an important source of contingency within the gap between past observation and future performance. Labeling always takes place in an interactive framework in which the application of the label is itself a determinant of the future. Many have observed the working of "self-fulfilling prophecies" and have drawn attention to the inclination of the one labeled to take on the self-image and the patterns of conduct suggested by the expectations of others made manifest in the labeling. It is also to be noted that those who do the labeling, in the very process of affixing the label, develop a vested interest in vindicating their veracity. Once they have assigned a label, they can be proved right and competent only if future capacities and conduct conform to that which is indicated by the label. Thus, once a child is labeled as "mentally retarded," the only way the veracity of those applying the label can be verified is to have the child continue indefinitely to manifest the attributes of the mentally retarded. Such a circumstance seems unlikely to stimulate vigorous remedial action that would contradict the diagnosis.

The greater the role of environmental factors in determining the degree of observed retardation the greater is the possibility that future performance will contradict the diagnosis. New constellations of factors may elicit new patterns of performance. In cases of very gross mental deficiency involving extensive malfunctioning of the central nervous system the likelihood of the falsification of diagnosis through the action of new constellations of variables is much less than it is in the case of school children whose marginal retardation may reasonably be expected to be significantly influenced by linguistic, racial, economic, social, familial, or cultural disadvantages. There is a wide range in the degree of permanence or biological fixedness of the factors that may produce the symptoms taken as grounds for the application of the label "mentally retarded." The use of a single label to cover both conditions that are biologically grounded and virtually irreparable and also conditions stemming from different causes which are open to change through variation of individual social circumstance wrongfully obscures possibilities for successful intervention. The assimilation of one category to the other has a conservative effect by lending credence to the assumption that little can be done for any of those who are labeled "mentally retarded." The belief that little can be done serves to diminish awareness of moral responsibility and erode a sense of urgency in bringing about new conditions in which those whose retardation may be traced to factors directly or indirectly under human control may be enabled to flourish. That which can be done to release hidden potential ought to be done. But it is in cases in which much could be repaired through the reformation of environmental factors that those who make diagnoses are most menaced by the threat of contradiction and, ironically, develop the highest stake in maintaining the status quo for the sake of their veracity.

The verification of a label must have reference to the future. But the future is always uncertain and the action of those who apply and act in accordance with labels is itself a significant determinant of the future. An accurate label must always express the contingency of the future. It should be no more fixed and static in its quality than the imperfectly predictable outcome of the complex patterns of interaction that shape lives. It is not simply a euphemism, but rather, a recognition of modesty fully appropriate in light of the current state of the art of predicting, to suggest that, in many cases, "mentally retarded" should be replaced with a term such as "of seemingly limited potential for intellectual development." As long as there is the well-grounded suspicion that intelligence tests do not enable even the best trained evaluator to assess accurately the level and quality of problem-solving behavior outside of the testing situation, as long as it can be supposed that intelligence tests give an incomplete accounting of abilities necessary for adaptation and successful functioning in a future world in which the value to be assigned to intellectual capacities is uncertain, so long is it necessary to impose restraint upon the tendency to employ the increasing ability to test, track, and file in a manner that forecloses the future options of those who were meant to be benefited rather than harmed by the diagnosis of their need.

Justice in the application of labels requires close attention to the question of the validity of the tests that provide the evidence offered to justify specific applications of labels. It requires also procedural fairness and interpretive frameworks that are not flagrantly culture-bound. Those who misuse their professional training to perpetuate the institutionalized Anglocentrism documented in the researches of Jane Mercer need to be exposed as violators of the canons of veracity who hide social injustice behind the mask of biological inevitability. They commit crimes against truth insofar as they misconstrue the etiology of educational retardation by implying that its causes are to be found in innate characteristics of individuals rather than in the nexus of social factors shaping behavior in particular settings. Injury is thereby done not only to those who are slandered by inaccurately applied labels but also to conscientious fellow citizens who, being desirous of doing justice to their neighbors, are led to be in default of their obligations to change those elements of their own practice that in fact have the overlooked effect of reducing the opportunity of those labeled as retarded to realize to the fullest possible extent all the dimensions of humanity that are common to us all. A test that is culturally unfair and leads to a diagnosis that misplaces the causes of retarded development is a source of deception and injustice in the application of labels.

Injustice in the Treatment of the Mentally Retarded

The treatment of the mentally retarded should be aimed at expanding as far as possible their participation in the common life of the community. Two limits that could be acknowledged in assessing the prospects for fuller participation are considerations of cost and the possibility of danger to other members of the community. The task of balancing costs has been delegated to other panels. The possibility that the presence of the mentally retarded in the everyday round of communal activities may increase dangers for other citizens raises interesting questions concerning the determinants of behavior and the propriety of segregation. If it were true that failure to identify the mentally retarded might somehow increase the hazards of life for other persons, a second justification of the practice of labeling would be available which would be grounded not in the obligation to facilitate the self-realization of the mentally retarded but, rather, in the obligation to protect the innocent from possible harm.

It is possible to combine a series of assumptions to create a fear that the mentally retarded constitute a serious menace to society. For instance, if the report that a significant portion of the "undesirable classes" of criminals, prostitutes, paupers, narcotic addicts and other deviants are of very low intelligence is combined with the assumption that intelligence is a factor determined fully by heredity and both these ideas are joined to the belief that these segments of the population are especially prolific, a scare can be engendered. A vision of the persistent degradation of the community can be conjured up to support proposals to segregate, sterilize, or otherwise prevent the reproduction of the bearers of an inferior genetic heritage. It becomes possible to portray the mentally retarded as a danger to the species, to the society, and to individual members of the community.

But even if intelligence were conceded to be an attribute determined strictly by heredity, it cannot be claimed that possession of an inherited level of intelligence disposes or determines one to pursue dangerous or deviant courses of conduct. Mental retardation cannot "explain" particular forms of behavior. Behavior is shaped by manifold influences within specific settings formed by sets of expectations, opportunities, institutions, and patterns that are variable from society to society and from time to time. The encompassing context that influences behavior is always open to change. The mentally retarded may possess a reduced capacity for judgment in certain situations. But the scope of activities within which judgment must be exercised in the course of daily life is itself open to modification. It is possible to reorder institutions and relations in a manner that can expand the scope of participation for the mentally retarded by thoughtful creation of roles and situations in which the capacity they lack is not a constant requisite. Mental retardation does not predispose one to deviant and dangerous patterns of behavior. Constant failure and frustration within a society that takes little care to provide suitable opportunities for satisfying participation for those who are slower to learn may very well force victims of such thoughtlessness into marginal careers of high risk to themselves and others. Any dangerous tendencies that might be feared flow not from the existence of those who may be labeled "mentally retarded" but from tensions generated in the efforts of some to cope with a particular constellation of social institutions and attitudes that are always open to modification.

In considering arguments for the segregation of the mentally retarded or for other forms of restriction upon their participation in the common life of the community, the concept of "danger" to the wider populace must not be confused with their "discomfort." The most likely danger that the "normal" community suffers is that they will be deprived of a realistic understanding of the nature of the world they live in if the mentally retarded and other less perfectly endowed elements of the population are segregated and removed from public consciousness and view. If family life and school experience is designed to prepare children for life in "the real world" it is a fraud to force them to grow up in a setting in which

the handicapped are absent. A distorted, naive, pollyanna view of the world is likely to evolve that will prove to be brittle when children must eventually confront the unexpurgated version of their world.

To avoid injustice in the treatment of the mentally retarded it is necessary, first of all, to treat them as persons, as persons with a very specific weakness, possession of which should not prejudice expectations concerning the presence of a wide range of other valuable human qualities. Which of these qualities will be drawn forth to shape character and conduct throughout a lifetime depends upon the presently unfathomable complexities of human interaction. The outcome of this interactive process escapes prediction. Respect for the contingency of the future, the unpredictability of the career of a mentally retarded child who is allowed to interact to the fullest possible degree with fellow human beings, should guide public policy concerning labeling, testing, tracking, and filing. No label should be indelible. None should be attached for a span of time longer than reach of the predictive accuracy of fallible men forced to cope with intricacies of human formation beyond present comprehension. The purpose of the ambiguous activity of labeling is to establish the eligibility of those with specific needs for special assistance designed to expand their opportunities to participate in the processes of interaction within which personality is formed and enriched. Any use of labels that contracts rather than expands such opportunities constitutes a reprehensible misuse of public power.

Notes

1. Errol E. Harris, "Respect for Persons," in *Ethics and Society*, ed. Richard T. De George (Garden City, New York: Doubleday Anchor Books, 1966), pp. 111–132, at pp. 118ff.

2. Ibid., p. 125.

3. Ibid., p. 128.

4. Howard S. Becker, *Outsiders: Studies in the Sociology of Divorce* (New York: The Free Press, 1963), pp. 33ff.

5. Alfred Schutz, "Equality and the Meaning Structure of the Social World," in *Aspects of Human Equality*, ed. Lyman Bryson, Clarence H. Faust, Louis Finkelstein, and R. M. MacIver (New York: Harper and Brothers, 1956), pp. 33–78.

6. *Nicomachean Ethics*, V, 3 (1131ª27).

101

Stanley Hauerwas

Having and Learning How to Care for Retarded Children: Some Reflections

Reprinted by permission from *Catholic Mind*, April 1976, pp. 24–33.

Why Do We Have Retarded Children?

A recent letter to the "Wise Man's Corner" of the *St. Anthony Messenger* asked a question I suspect we have all asked, but supressed for fear of the answer that we might give to it. It read: "How does one believe in God, Who is supposedly good, when there is so much unhappiness in the world? I have a mentally retarded sister who is in a state institution. On every visiting day it tears me apart to see such ugliness. I know I will never understand God's purpose in allowing these poor human beings to exist with the resulting heartbreak it causes their families every day of their lives. I do very much want to believe in God, but I guess my sister's existence has caused me to resent Him. How do I believe?" (June, 1975, p. 44)

There is much that is theologically naive about this letter. For example, it mistakenly assumes that God is to be held directly responsible for every unfortunate event that occurs in the world. But this kind of theological point fails to come to grips with the agony that gives birth to such letters. For we want to know why, or how, we can learn to welcome retarded children into our lives without self-pity or false courage. The "Wise Man" attempted to answer this letter by suggesting that the writer contemplate Job and consider the many accounts of people who have had retarded children and the richness they often add to family life.

Yet, while no one can deny that many families have come to see retarded children as a blessing, this response fails to be sufficient. For every case that one can quote that has been morally and spiritually rewarding, you can find a case that has been destructive for all the participants. In other words, I am suggesting that our attitudes about retarded children cannot be based on whether or not they enliven certain families. Rather we must ask what kind of families and communities we should be so that we could welcome retarded children into our midst regardless of the happy or unhappy consequences they may bring.

Of course, some may feel that the question of why and how we should learn to accept retarded children is, morally and practically, a bad faith question. For, morally, it seems to be prejudicial against those who have made tremendous sacrifices in order to raise and care for retarded children. In other words, it seems to make a matter of doubt what they have taken to be a matter of moral necessity. Thus, even to raise the question is to change the moral parameters of the case for them.

However, as I hope to show, unless we can give an answer to the question of why such children are to be welcomed in the world, we will have no satisfactory moral stance that can give our care of such children moral direction. For, as those who work with the retarded soon discover, caring for such children means more than simply providing them with the latest means of therapy or subjecting them to the current forms of educational or behavior-modification theory. For care is not simply "doing" things for these children, even when such "doing" involves our best technologies, but it means knowing how to be with and regard these children with the respect they demand. Thus, the forms of care with which we approach these children must be guided by our basic beliefs about why we have them at all.

Practically, the question of why we have these children may seem to be nonsense because it is obvious that we cannot avoid them. But, in fact, this is no longer true. For techniques have been developed, e.g., amniocentesis, that will allow for the early diagnosis and abortion of many children who are suffering from various forms of retardation. Moreover, we are increasingly confronting cases today where parents are refusing life saving surgery because the child happens to have been born retarded. Or, less dramatically, we know we have often avoided the reality of these children by unnecessary institutionalization.

It, of course, may be thought that these developments are not particularly important for Christians because our attitudes toward abortion preclude the use of amniocentesis for such purposes. Yet I want us to bracket these kinds of concerns about abortion, for I think we will learn more about ourselves, and in particular why abortion is abhorrent to Christians, if we do. For I want to try to show that even if abortion were permissible for Christians, we would still have no special or overriding reason to abort a child simply because he or she is destined to be born retarded.

This is the case because the reasons we have these children give essential clues for why we have any children. Moreover, I shall try to suggest that the presence of these retarded children provides us with important skills from which we learn how to care for and raise children not retarded. For contrary to our normal assumptions, the having of children is not just a natural event, but rather one of the most highly charged moral events of our lives. The difficulty many feel at the prospect of raising a retarded child is but an indication that we have lost the substantive stories that should inform and give direction to why we have children at all. It is my purpose therefore to try to remind us what it is we do when we have children and why the presence of retarded children is so important for helping us understand that story.

Choosing Our Children

It is a common presumption that we choose or do not choose to have children. Not only do we choose to have children, but since having children has been freed from the necessity of the past, we feel we *should* make having or not having children a matter of choice. Even Catholics who refuse to use contraception still feel that they must describe having children as something they choose to do. For we are people who feel it is important that we have control of our lives, that we not be subject to fate, and one of the ways that we have such control is by choosing to have, or not to have, children.

Moreover, this seems to be in accordance with our basic responsibilities as parents for biology does not make us parents. Rather parenting is a role that requires that we be concerned about the conditions into which our children are born and the kind of moral and material care that we can provide them with. Thus the church talks about the importance of "responsible parenthood" indicating that the mere production of children is not a good in itself but having children in a context in which they can receive appropriate forms of care.

Yet it is unclear how responsible we must be before we can choose to have children. Does it mean that we must own a good house, have a secure job, and be able to send our children to college? Moreover, what moral prerequisites are required for the having of children and are moral conditions more important than material conditions? The phrase "responsible parenthood" does little to help us negotiate these kinds of questions.

The ambiguity surrounding the questions has placed a heavy burden on parenting today. For the strong assumption that we choose our children has made us claim unwarranted responsibility for their well being. Some even go so far as to blame themselves when their children do not get the proper genes to prevent certain aesthetic problems (baldness); or some worry about when their children should be conceived in order that their children be formed by the best sperm and ova. Mothers worry if they are giving their children just the right amount of love or attention. This kind of list, cataloging the extraordinary commitments that some parents are willing to accept in order to justify the choice of having children, can almost be extended indefinitely. For when there is no reason to have children beyond our individual choice, then it seems that we must claim full responsibility or none at all. Against such a background it is clear why more and more people are deciding that they would rather not have children—it is too great a moral burden.

Even though we think we have and should exercise the physical and moral freedom to have children, we have no reason, no story, which says why we should exercise this freedom to decide to have children. We thus have children because they are "fun" or because we want to continue the family name; or because our parents or society expect us to have children; or because it just seems to be something that people ought to do. But none of these, or other reasons that are often given for having children, are sufficient to provide us with adequate skills for knowing what we should do with children once we have had them. We thus seem trapped to live and raise our children as if the only object is to secure for them a better basis for the acquisition of goods than we had, e.g., so that they can go to a better college than we did, have a better job, home, boat, etc. In such a context, however, children end by hating the sacrifices parents have made for their welfare since they perceive the goal was not worth the sacrifice.

For the sacrifice, what we do for our children, becomes a way of claiming our children as our own. They are made our property by our choice to have them and by what we do for them—they are our product. As our product they have no independent existence except as they are able to wrench it from us through psychological and finally physical power.

But, ironically, just to the extent that we must choose our children we feel that we must also place a demand on them—namely that they be perfect. They must be physically and psychologically perfect in order to justify all the energy, all the sacrifices that have gone into our choice to have and raise children. After all, who wants to go to all the trouble that children represent for an inferior product.

Moreover, it is the sense that children are our total responsibility that makes some parents feel so defeated when their children do something wrong. For if the children are ours, then the natural question, when they do something wrong, is: "Where did we go wrong?" But it is important to notice that such a question, though appearing to be a willingness to assume guilt, is an extraordinary assertion of parental power over the lives of our children. For there is no better way to control another than to claim responsibility for them.

Now I think it is exactly the notion that we choose our children, and the demand that they be perfect, that has created the difficulty of explaining why we have retarded children and has, moreover, corrupted our child-rearing practices for normal children. I want to suggest that it is an extremely odd idea that we *choose* our children. In fact, we know from our having and rearing children, we do not so much choose them, as discover them as gifts that are not of our making. Indeed, the notion of choosing our children is as misleading as the assumption that we decide to get married.

Thus, I will try to show that, if the language of choice is to be used at all in describing our willingness to have children, it must be qualified and controlled by the more fundamental metaphor of gift. For, only when we understand that our children are gifts, can we have an intelligible story that makes clear our duties to them and the form that our care, and in particular the care of our children born retarded, should take.

The Christian Obligation to Have Children

As Christians, we do not choose to have our children; nor do we have them because we cannot avoid them. This was true before and after contraception became a widespread practice. (In fact, the condemnation of contraception was an attempt to take the having of children out of the realm of necessity and make it part of the moral order.) Rather Christians (and Jews) have children because it is our duty—we are commanded to do so.

Many may find this terrible, as it seems to rob us of our freedom to decide to have or not to have children. But such a criticism misses the point of why we are obligated to have children —namely that we wish to continue and people the world created by a gracious God. For our having children draws on our deepest convictions that God is the Lord of this world—that in spite of all the evidence of misery in this world, it is a world and an existence that we can affirm as good as long as we have the assurance that He is its creator and redeemer. Even though we know that this is an existence racked with sin and disobedience, our Lord has provided us with skills to deal with sin, in ourselves and others, in a manner that will not destroy us or them. Children are, thus, our promissory note, our sign to present and future generations, that we Christians trust the Lord who has called us together to be His people. (This is the basis of our conviction about abortion, not that life is sacred, but that this is the way we should regard children.)

The having of the children is hard to make intelligible, unless we are members of a people. But we are not just any people, we are a people who are charged to carry the story of God who gives us the basis for our existence as His people. Thus, we do not have our children because we have some obligation to keep the species intact or because we wish to furnish our country with a population large enough to secure worldly power but because we are pledged to exist as a Christian community.

The character of that community is, therefore, crucial for answering the questions of why and how we learn to rear our children. The Christian community is formed by the conviction that the power of this world is not the determining sway of our existence, but rather it is the power we find in the cross of Jesus Christ. Thus, our willingness to have children, our obligation to have children, is one of the ways we serve the community formed by such a story—namely, children witness to our determination to exist as a people formed by the Cross even though the world wishes to deny that a people can exist without the power protected and acquired through the sword.

To many, such a stance will appear foolish or, perhaps, even immoral. For there is much that could be done that might be considered more important than having children. Children take time and energy, psychologically and physically, that prevents us from being better scholars, important businessmen, serving the poor, or attacking the structures of injustice. But it is the Christian claim that God's kingdom is not to be built by us that gives us the patience, in a world of injustice, to insist that nothing is more important than the having and rearing of children. We do this, not because we assume our children will somehow be better than we are, but because we hope our children will choose to be the next generation of those that carry the story of God in the world. We must remember that our hope is not in our children but in the God who gives us and them grounds of hope.

Of course, this does not mean that everyone who identifies with the Christian faith is called to have children or that each of us should have as many children as we can. Rather it is to remind us that, for Christians, having children is a vocation—it is one of the highest callings that we can have in such a community. Some among us (and not just women) will see it as their special vocation to gain the particular skills of learning how to care for and educate children. But all of us who find ourselves members of this people called Christians recognize that this vocation is basic, however we view our own particular calling.

Moreover, this makes clear that as parents we act on the behest of our community as we raise our children. In other words, we do not raise our children to conform just to what we, the child's particular parents, think right. Rather, parents are agents of communities' commitments to which both child and parents are, or should be, loyal. Indeed, such commitments are the necessary condition for giving the child independence from the parents, for the child, as well as the parents, can appeal to the community for the limits of each one's responsibilities.

That is one of the reasons why the church becomes so important, if families are not to be left to their own devices. For, unless the child has a community that also provides him or her with symbols of significance beyond the family, then in fact the child is at the mercy of his parents. The church, by insisting that the child is not just the parents' but that the parents have authority insofar as they are agents of the communities' values, gives the necessary moral and physical space for children to gain independence from their parents. (Indeed one of the reasons that our children today seem so much at the mercy of their peer group is the attempt of the subculture of youth to gain an institution, in the absence of the church, for protection from the good and bad will of their parents. It is the attempt to find a space not dominated by their parents but, unfortunately, the teen culture is not a substantive enough institution to prevent the worst forms of manipulation.)

The Gift of Children

Once the having of children is put in the context of this story and the people formed by it, we can see how inappropriate the language of choice is to describe our parenting. For children are not beings created by our wills—we do not choose them, but, rather, they are called into the world as beings separate and independent from us. They are not ours, for they, like each of us, have a Father who wills them as His own prior to our choice of them.

Thus, children must be seen as a gift for they are possible exactly because we do not determine their right to exist or not to exist. Now it is important to notice that the language of gift involves an extremely interesting grammar. For gifts come to us as a given—they are not under our control. Moreover, they are not always what we want or expect and thus they necessarily have an independence from us.

Insofar as gifts are independent, they do not always bring joy and surprise, but they may equally bring pain and suffering. But just such pain and suffering is the condition for their being genuine gifts. Gifts that are genuine do not just supply needs or wants. If they did, they would then be subject to our limitations. Rather, genuine gifts create needs, that is, they teach us what wants we should have, as they remind us how limited we were without them.

Now children are the basic and, perhaps, the most essential gifts we have because they teach us how to be. That is, they create in us the proper need to want to love and regard another. For love born of need is always manipulative love unless it is based on the regard of the other as an entity who is not in my control but who is all the more valuable because I do not control him. Children are gifts exactly because they draw our love to themselves while refusing to be as we wish them to be.

But, to the extent that we realize that our children are a duty, we can also be freed from the excessive concern and claims of responsibility associated with our decision to have children. For, contrary to contemporary assumptions, duties bring freedom by helping us learn to accept the proper moral limitations of being human. We destroy ourselves and our children just to the extent that we act as if there are no such limits.

The Retarded as Gifts

Thus, we must learn to accept the retarded into our lives as providing a peculiar and intense instance of the way we should regard all children. They are not, to be sure, the kind of children we would choose to have, for we would wish on no one any unnecessary suffering or pain. But they are not different than other children insofar as any child is not of our choice.

It is, of course, true that retarded children destroy our plans and fantasies about what we wish our children to be. They thus call us to reality quicker than most children for they remind us that the plans we have for our children may not be commensurate with the purposes of having children at all. Thus, these retarded children are particularly special gifts reminding us that we have children, not that they be a success, nor for what they may be able to do for the good and betterment of mankind, but because we are members of a people who are gathered around the table of Christ.

I want to be very clear about this. I am not suggesting that Christians should rejoice that their children are born retarded rather than normal. Rather, I am suggesting that as Christians the story that informs and directs our having children at all, provides us with the skill to know how to welcome these particular children into our existence without telling ourselves self-deceiving stories about our heroism for doing so. For such heroic stories can also serve to subject the retarded child to forms of care that he should not be forced to undergo.

For example, such heroic stories can lead us to forms of sentimental care and protection that rob these children of the demands to grow as they are able. For the love of the retarded, like any love, must be hard if we are not to stifle the other in overprotective care. To care for these children as if they are somehow specially innocent—that is "children of God"—is to rob them of the right to be the kind of selfish, grasping, and manipulative children other children have the right to be. Retarded children are not to be cared for because they are especially loving, though some of them may be, but because they are children. We forget that there is no more disparaging way to treat others than to assume that they can do nothing wrong.

But, just as the retarded child is a gift like any other child, he also requires special skills if we are to care for him appropriately. What is important is not that we Christians have retarded children, but that we know why and to what end we have them. To have them in order to witness to what nice people we are is only another subtle way of using them. We have them because they are children—no special reason beyond that needs to be given—but as children they present special needs that we must know how to meet responsibly. We must know how to care for them in ways that respect their independence from us for their existence, as well as our own, is grounded in the fact that we are each called to service in God's kingdom.

The Care of the Retarded

How one cares for the retarded child will of course differ in terms of the kind of retardation and from child to child—no two Down's syndrome children are alike just as no two normal children, are the same. Moreover, I have no competency to try to suggest what kind of care or training is better than another. However, I think it is important and necessary to try to articulate some general guidelines that should govern our care of retarded children irrespective of the kind of retardation and the best techniques for dealing with it.

The great temptation in caring for the retarded, as for any child, is to make them conform to what we think they should want to be—namely, that they should wish to be "normal." We thus often care for the retarded on the assumption that our task is to make them as much like the rest of us as we can. But, as I have suggested, the very way we learn to accept these children into our lives requires us to learn to see and love them as gifts that are not at our disposal.

We must, therefore, be very careful that we do not impose on them a form of life born from our frustration because they are not and cannot be like us. For example, the so-called "principle of normalization" is a valuable check against the sentimental and often cruel care of the retarded that tries to spare them the pain of learning basic skills of living. But, as an ideology, it tends to suggest that our aim is to make the retarded "normal." This, of course, ignores entirely the fact that we have no clear idea of what it means to be "normal." Thus, in the name of "normalcy," we stand the risk of making the retarded conform to convention because they lack the power to resist.

As Milton Mayeroff reminds us, to care for another person, in the most

significant sense, is to help him grow and actualize himself. [*On Caring* (New York: Harper and Row, 1971), p. 1.] That is, to care for another is to help him establish an independent existence from us—so as not to be under our power. "To help another person grow is at least to help him to care for something or someone apart from himself, and it involves encouraging and assisting him to find and create areas of his own in which he is able to care. Also, it is to help that other person to come to care for himself, and by becoming responsive to his own need to care to become responsible for his own life" (Mayeroff, *op. cit.*, pp.10–11). The retarded must be cared for in a way, therefore, that will develop their ability to care for others as we care for them.

To so care, requires the supporting virtues of patience, for we must learn to wait, even when the other fails; honesty, for we must learn how to tell the truth to the other even when it is unpleasant; trust, so as to let the other take the risk of the unknown; and humor, so that the other knows that no mistake is a decisive defeat. Therefore, learning to live with the retarded requires a substantive story that will give us the patience, honesty, trust, and humor to provide those children with the space they need to acquire such virtues themselves.

Such virtues and such a story are required for all child rearing, but it may be that they are especially intensified in learning how to care for the retarded. For to know how to care for the retarded, requires the special skill not to be overprotective. Such a skill is possible when we have the confidence that the destiny of retarded children is not finally in our hands—that they and we are both sustained by a power beyond our capacity. In the presence of such a power we have the grounds for taking the risk of caring for the retarded exactly because their existence and ours is called forth by the God we have come to know in the history of Israel and the cross of Christ. For we have learned that this power refuses to sustain our existence as though existence were an end in itself. Rather we are sustained by service to a God who asks nothing more from us than to be His people who continue to have time, in the business of this world, to have children, even if they are retarded.

**The Economics of
Resource Allocation**

102

Rashi Fein

On Measuring Economic Benefits of Health Programmes

Reprinted with permission of the publisher and editors from Gordon McLachlan and Thomas McKeown, eds., *Medical History and Medical Care: A Symposium of Perspectives* (London: Oxford University Press, 1971), pp. 181–217.

Early History

When the sentimentalist and the moralist fails, he will have as a last resource to call in the aid of the economist, who has in some instances proved the power of his art to draw iron tears from the cheeks of a city Plutus (1).

Economic data and analysis have long been used in efforts to influence programme and expenditure decisions in the public sector. Those who have favoured particular policies have sought allies and supporting arguments for their positions. Particularly appealing have been the arguments that were cast in economic terms, and this has, perhaps, been especially the case in areas involving programmes with clear, visible, and direct impact on people. This appeal would appear to have been based on two factors. The general attractiveness of economic arguments has, at least in part, derived from the belief that economics is value-free, neutral, and objective. Thus, economic arguments relying on the hard criteria of the market, on "profit" and on "loss," carried a special weight (a weight that was, perhaps, increased by the fact that economists use data, jargon, and methodology that are somewhat mysterious to the uninitiated). The specific attractiveness of economic arguments in social areas (for example in the case of programmes that deal directly with people) is increased by the fact that these fields generally lack rigorous monetary guidelines for decision-making. In Chadwick's terms, these are the areas favoured by "the sentimentalist and moralist." Therefore, to find that economic criteria were not at variance with humanitarian considerations seemed to be especially useful. Chadwick was correct when he suggested that the economist could prove a useful ally.

The power of the economic argument that the proponents of social programmes found useful was not derived from the literary quality with which the arguments were offered, or from the elegance of the economist's prose. Nor, as will become clear, did it result from the fact that the analytical methodology was so refined and the data so exact that disagreement with the conclusions was impossible. Rather it was because the economic argument embodied an appealing pattern of thought and a way of looking at a problem: the economic rationale for various social programmes was presented in investment terms. Ill-health, ignorance, disability, and death caused by war were costly to an economy. Investment in medical care, public health, education, and in the pursuit of peace, brought significant economic rewards in increasing the value of human capital. Such investment concepts were looked upon with favour at a time when economic progress was seen as deriving from capital growth brought about by investment.

Thus, the early literature of economics as well as articles in applied areas of public policy, contains references to the economic value of an education, of acquired skills, of better health, and to the economic costs and gains of war, emigration, and immigration. These subjects were examined at irregular intervals by persons concerned with practical policy matters. Unfortunately none of these contributions developed a general theory and methodology concerning the economic value of a human being. They were not integrated into the main body of the economic literature, remaining on, if not beyond, the fringe. Furthermore, because they were derived from a specific interest in a particular applied problem, there was little attempt to generalize or to show the usefulness of the approach to other problems. Those writing on the economic value of an immigrant seemed unaware that a similar type of problem was examined by persons concerned with the economic value of an education; those writing on the economic loss suffered through emigration seemed unaware that other scholars were concerned with the economic loss caused by disease or by casualties in war.

This situation, I might note, makes the examination of early references to human capital a fascinating but time-consuming task. Some years ago, in undertaking just such an examination, I found that in order to locate useful examples of the quantitative application of the concept of human capital, one had to consider the various fields in which such a concept might be used and then search for articles, bibliographies, and references in these applied

fields. General indexes were hardly useful since they contained no classification heading called human resources or human capital. Even titles of articles could be, and were, misleading.

Perhaps the first estimates of the money value of a person were offered by Sir William Petty writing in the latter decades of the seventeenth century. At various times Petty offered estimates of the value of a person residing in England. These estimates ranged between £60 and £90. In his *Political Arithmetick,* for example, Petty calculates the value by deriving the productive contributions of labour (£26 million), multiplying by 20 ("The Mass of Mankind being worth Twenty Years purchase . . .") and by dividing by 6 million (the population of England). Thus ". . . makes about £80. Sterling, to be valued of each Head of Man Woman and Child . . . : from whence we may learn to compute the loss we have sustained by the Plague, by the Slaughter of Men in War, and by the sending them abroad into the Service of Foreign Princes" (2). Petty then used estimates of the value of human capital to derive a number of policy implications. He asked: "From whence it follows, that 100,000 persons dying of the Plague, above the ordinary number is near 7 Millions loss to the Kingdom [this was based upon an estimate that each person was worth £69]; and consequently how well might £70,000 have been bestowed in preventing this Centuple loss?" (3). In another work he asked: "The value of 140^m people at £90. per head is 12 millions 600^m pounds; soe as the Question seems to be what sum of money, and Meanes ought to be prudently ventured for the probable cutting off 3 fifths of this Calamity" (4). In Petty's plan, dated 7 October 1667, "Of Lesening ye Plagues of London," he attempted to provide an answer to the question. He estimated that, given the value of an individual and the cost of transporting people outside of London and caring for them for three months, thus increasing the probability of survival, every pound expended would yield a return of £84 (5). Here, then, was an economic argument, cast in monetary terms, in favour of a course of action to prevent deaths and thus to increase the value of the nation's human resources.

Petty also used the concept of human capital in advocating lying-in hospitals for illegitimate children. He calculated that the cost of thirty days in child-bed would only be 30s. Since the value of mankind was some £70 "a new born Child, bread up to fair and hard work for 25 yeares, will be very well worth 3 times 30 Shillings, as may be seen in the price of Negros Children in the American plantations" (4). It is not without interest to note that Petty advocated lying-in hospitals in order to increase the population. Perhaps, however, to insure that the government receive a direct return on its investment, he also advocated that the child should be the servant of government for twenty-five years. Today, with the growth of income taxation, the argument is often made in terms of the direct returns to government resulting from the increase in tax revenue.

Some twenty-one years earlier, in 1676, in a lecture on anatomy, Petty noted that the state should intervene to assure better medicine. The value of better medicine, he felt, was that it could save 200,000 subjects a year. Even valued at only £20, the lowest price of slaves, this was a large sum and better medicine, therefore represented a sensible state expenditure. "Wherefore it is not in the Interest of the State to leave Phisitians and Patients (as now) to their own shifts" (6). Almost three hundred years later, the same arguments are presented (though the data are more refined) to advocate similar policies.

It is also of interest to note that not only was Petty the precurser of present discussions of investment in health activities, but he also presented arguments analogous to those used today in discussions concerning migration and economic development policies. Petty argued that an individual in England was worth £90, but that in Ireland only £70. This differential value led to the conclusion that transplantation would be economically wise (4).

Over a century passes before the economic value of man concept reappears again in a major way in the literature. Edwin Chadwick, in his *Sanitary Report* for 1842, estimated that the loss due to excessive sickness and premature disability and death, including the loss of productive power equalled £14 million (7). In 1844 he argued that bad sanitation increased the proportion of dependent hands to workers and that sanitation could be viewed "as an economical question of production" (8). He also suggested that it could be shown "how much, by expenditure in well-executed measures, directed by engineering science, they may gain in the reduction of existing pecuniary burdens alone, that are entailed by an excessive mortality" (10). Chadwick, of course, was particularly interested in sanitation, and a number of his many articles contain references to the economic value of sanitation and to the costs that society bears in ". . . excessive sickness, excessive death-rates and funerals, and premature disablement and lost labour . . ." due to poor sanitation (9).

In 1862, Chadwick argued, ". . . as the artist for his purpose views the human being as a subject for the cultivation of the beautiful—as the physiologist for the cultivation of his art views him solely as a material organism, so the economist for the advancement of his science may well treat the human being simply as an investment of capital, in productive force" (1). He then presented detailed estimates of the value of a person based on the cost of rearing a child, taking account of the factor of death before becoming productive (at age 11!) and the number of productive years. He used these estimates to derive the costs associated with poor housing and sanitation, and offered additional comments related to the value of human capital. Suggesting that economists should strive to unite personal and pecuniary motives, he defended education on economic grounds and, in words which remain applicable today, argued: ". . . it is well to subscribe to reformatories as to hospitals for the treatment of the sick, but giving exclusive attention to them is like giving exclusive attention to the foundation and maintenance of hospitals for the alleviation of marsh and foul air diseases, without regard to the drainage of the marshes, or to the removal of the sources of the foul air whence the diseases arise" (1).

Lemuel Shattuck in the Report of a General Plan for the Promotion of Public and Personal Health, presented in 1850, also viewed public health measures from an economic perspective. In arguing for preventive sanitary measures to lessen epidemics, he wrote: "In this case economy is on the side of humanity, and the most expensive of all things is—to do nothing" (10). The expenses and losses caused by the neglect of sanitary measures included "A loss sustained by the state, in consequence of the diminished physical power and general liability to disease" (10). Shattuck estimated that the failure of the State of Massachusetts to adopt an efficient sanitary system resulted in 6,000 unnecessary deaths and that the average individual might have been productive for an additional eighteen years. Thus, society lost 108,000 years of labour at $50 per year, equalling $5.4 million. When this was added to the lost labour of the sick, the cost of sickness and of supporting widows and orphans, Shattuck estimated that the cost to the state was $7.5 million. Interestingly, he felt that this cost could be eliminated by an expenditure of only $3,000 (largely in planning and, what we would call today "technical assistance") (10). Shattuck thus argued:

According to the estimate above presented, the State suffers, from its imperfect sanitary condition, an unnecessary annual loss of more than 7½ millions of dollars! and this arises, partly at least, from the non-adoption of a measure which will cost but about $3,000. If saved, it would add that amount to the wealth of the State, besides the indefinite amount of increased happiness which would accompany it! Should any one consider this an extravagant estimate, let him reduce it to 3 millions, more than one half, and then the relation of expenditure to the savings, or to the income, will be as one dollar to one thousand dollars! And even if nine tenths of this latter sum be deducted, it will be like paying out one dollar, and receiving back again ten, as the return profit! What more wise expenditure of money can be desired? (10).

In the latter half of the nineteenth century others were writing in much the same vein as Chadwick and applying the same concepts to a number of different fields. They would have accepted the statement by the Revd. J. E. Thorold Rogers: "It seems to me wholly un-philosophical to ignore capital in the person of a labourer, and to recognize it in a machine" (11). One writer, however, stands out above all others because of the method by which he calculated what he termed the "money value of a man" and because he applied the concept to general taxation problems as well as to social programmes. William Farr, in a paper presented in 1853 discussing income and property taxes, used a method that is surprisingly close to the methods used today since he did not base values on the costs of rearing the child (producing the machine) but rather on the wages that will be earned, on the future income stream (12). In his volume Vital Statistics, Farr stated:

Life has a pecuniary value. In its production and education a certain amount of capital is sunk for a longer or shorter time, and that capital, with its interest, as a general rule, reappears in the wages of the labourer, the pay of the officer, and the income of the professional man. At first it is all expenditure, and a certain necessary expenditure goes on to the end to keep life in being, even when its economic results are negative (13).

The sum of future earnings and the cost of future maintenance determines the value. Thus Farr estimates the following values for a Norfolk agricultural labourer: at birth £5; age 5, £56; age 10, £117; age 15, £192; age 20, £234; age 25, £246; age 30, £241 declining to £138 at age 55, and £1 at age 70, following which the values become negative (maintenance exceeds income) and, thus, at age 80 the value is −£41. Farr uses these data to justify particular concern with those events that destroy lives at their prime—"fever, consumption, cholera, violence in all its forms, and childbirth" (13).

The estimates provided by Farr in his Vital Statistics that a human life was worth $770 a head were used by Gary Calkins in estimating that sanitation saved 856,804 lives with a value of $650 million from 1880 to 1890. This saving, he noted, exceeded the cost of sanitary improvements between 1875 and 1890, since the latter totalled $583.5 million (14).

If Petty was the first to examine the concept of human capital and Chadwick the first to present detailed estimates and apply these quite carefully and extensively to justify various public expenditures, Farr deserves recognition as the first to analyse value in terms of future income streams and to do this in relation to the general question of taxation rather than in a specific context of health (or other) expenditures.

In the period 1870–1920, the concept of human capital continued to be applied in a number of specific areas. The economic value of man entered into discussions on the cost of war (perhaps with the hope that war would be eliminated if it were recognized that when the loss in human capital was included in the "profit and loss statement" even the victor could be found to have made a poor investment). Detailed studies on the cost of the Franco-Prussian War of 1870 were undertaken (chiefly by Sir Robert Giffen). Additional studies on the South African War and the First World War included estimates of the production foregone during the war (because men were in the armed forces) as well as losses due to deaths and injuries (15–18).

A second group of economists applied the concept of human capital to problems of emigration and immigration. British writers tended to focus on the loss that Britain was suffering because of emigration. Migration, it was felt, represented the loss of a capital asset (though the value of the asset was not always measured in terms of future income, but on occasion in terms of the cost of "creating" the asset, for example, the cost of upbringing and education). Archibald Hamilton, writing in 1877, noted that the value of an immigrant to the community has been estimated in the United States at £166. 13s. 4d. and "they have been computed to be worth £200 in New Zealand" (11). In response, Dr Guy suggested that the value of an immigrant was £400 "and when it was remembered that an emigrant . . . married and became the father of children who . . . had families, it was difficult to say what the true value of an emigrant was" (20). There was general agreement, however, that the value of an immigrant depended upon the demand for labour in the place to which he emigrated. Thus Farr noted that the ex-Prime Minister of New Zealand, Sir Julius Vogel, had done "An admirable work . . . to remove some of the agricultural labourers from a place where they were worth very little, to a place where they were worth a great deal" (20).

A third area of economic inquiry that utilized a capital concept of man dealt with health and with the costs associated with specific diseases. Among the diseases studied were tuberculosis and typhoid fever (21–22). These studies did not break new methodological ground, nor did they lead the general economist to a greater interest in the field of health. Just as the profession neglected the field of human resources in general, so too, it neglected the area of health.

It is not clear why there was relatively little discussion of the economic value of human resources, except by scholars interested in applied specific problem areas. Economists, after all, have long referred to land, labour, and capital inputs and resources. They have devoted considerable analysis to the consequences derived from the observed fact that land is not homogeneous and from the observation that capital equipment differs in its productivity. Yet, to a considerable extent, much of economics has been written as if labour were all the same. Even when cognizance was taken of the obvious and observable differences in labour quality, there seemed to be little concern with analysis of the factors that brought about these differences, almost as if it were felt that the factors could not be controlled or were not amenable to change. It is significant, perhaps, that to the extent that human capital was considered (even by those in applied areas), greatest attention was paid to problems of mortality, total incapacity, or migration—issues involving the addition or subtraction of total productivity rather than an increase in productivity resulting from the individual's becoming more effective in his work.

We can only speculate why human capital was largely ignored by the main body of economics. In part it may be due to the fact that during the period of rapid economic growth (the period of rapid industrial growth and the period when economics was developing as an organized discipline), striking and rapid changes were taking place in the amount of capital equipment available to the society and at the disposal of the worker. The capital/labour ratio was increasing. It is, therefore, to be expected that capital equipment occupied

the centre of the stage and was the chief focus of interest. Higher standards of living were seen as the result of the process of industrialization. Industrialization, in turn, was seen as the consequence (synonomous with) investment in addition to the stock of capital equipment. Changes in the quality of human resources were not as obvious, certainly not as easy to measure or as dramatic, not as apparently the result of deliberate policies. Thus, they were given small parts in the chorus along with other actors called custom, organization, entrepreneurship, and so forth.

Secondly, capital and differences in capital could easily be measured in economic terms. Capital is traded in the market and no conversion to economic or monetary terms is required. The common denominator that expresses the value of capital equipment is there for all to see. One-time investments in capital yield future income streams. Labour, however, is not bought and sold. Only labour services are. In general (with exceptions in discussions of insurance), one did not think in terms of income streams when discussing labour.

Thirdly, labour plays a dual role in the economic system: as input and as final consumer. Many of the things that increase the value and contribution of the worker as input (things that could be termed investments) are considered as part of consumption. They involve expenditures on goods and services that, in many cases, would be purchased even if they did nothing to improve the skill levels and productivity of the working force. Thus, the costs of recreation are classified as consumption expenditures even if they might be considered as part of the necessary costs required to maintain productivity. So, too, with health expenditures and with education expenditures. Surely people want health and education, and would purchase some of these two commodities, even in the absence of any impact on productivity and earning power? Surely, however, health and education do have such impacts and are not, therefore, entirely consumption expenditures? Some portion can be viewed (and in recent years this has been the case) as investment.

Fourth, the early orientation of economics failed to take account of the importance of "externalities." Expenditures on health and education that increased the productivity of the worker were viewed as private matters since they increased the individual's income. It was not fully appreciated that all of us are the beneficiaries when some of us are more productive. Nor was it recognized that certain expenditures might make sound economic sense for society as a whole even though they did not do so for the individual. If externalities are ignored much of the rationale for public intervention disappears—much, but not all—and with a weaker rationale there was a lesser interest in such, clearly, private matters.

Fifth, economists, as others, failed to examine some expenditures as investments and failed to view human capital as capital, at least in part because the terminology was felt repellent when applied to man. Man is not a machine. How then could one use such terms as "human capital" or "investment in human beings." The notion of man as something that can be assigned some dollar value reminds one of slavery. It seems to violate the concept of the sacredness of life. The notion is rejected as repugnant. Even when the ideas are explored and man is assigned an economic value, writers often felt it necessary to make disclaimers that man is much more than a robot merely embodying some set of skills. The fact that the writer felt that he might be misunderstood in the absence of such disclaimers is in itself significant.

In recent years, however, there has been a significant change in the place that human resources occupy in the literature of economics. The 1950s saw rekindled interest in health economics and the economics of education. This was built upon in the decade of the 1960s as economists turned their attention to a variety of issues relating to investment in human capital. No longer were these considered fringe areas. Today there is a field known as the economics of human resources. There are economists, courses, workshops, seminars, conferences, and a journal —perhaps the final evidence that a field exists—devoted to this area of inquiry. In little more than a decade the situation has changed from the case where individuals, who had not yet

succeeded in defining a field or having it accepted by their professional colleagues, were working in relative isolation on problems that today would be defined as part of the "economics of human resources." In the course of this change, there has been an altered orientation to the questions that have been studied. It is to this altered orientation, particularly as it applies to questions in the health areas, that we now turn.

Recent Developments

We recall that many of the early contributions already referred to were designed to promote specific policies by demonstrating that funds expended for various social programmes would bring economic returns. Economists or their analytical techniques were called upon "when the sentimentalist and the moralist" needed additional support. In this heavily investment-oriented approach one discovers little reference to programmes that do not yield a high return. Nor do we find suggestions that expenditures for certain activities should be cut. This may be because economists chose not to address problems that might yield "negative" answers, because they chose not to publish "negative" results, or because there are few, if any, general social programmes that have very low yields. While there may have been an element of the first two reasons—most of the articles, after all, were written by persons actively working in and dedicated to action in the particular applied field— the last reason is, perhaps, of even greater importance. The absence of low rates of return is particularly true if the analysis is cast in general and broad dimension rather than as an examination of a specific programme, designed to accomplish a narrow and specific purpose in which the outcome can be measured. What was being evaluated was whether better health or more education had a substantial payoff, not whether this particular educational technique raised reading levels to a degree commensurate with the resources required to implement the technique or whether a particular health programme in a particular location and designed to help a

particular population group had a substantial payoff. Most of the literature spoke of health in general, education in general. Most of the literature did not describe the particular programme that would be designed to alter the existing situation and surely did not examine the likelihood that the programme would accomplish its goals. The analysis was based on "average" data for large population groups and did not concern itself with whether or not the population groups to be served by the expenditures which were being advocated would, in fact, exhibit an average response to the new programme. Given the broad nature of the questions being addressed, it is not surprising that the returns were found to be high.

To be sure, part of the reason that one would expect to find high rates of return also relates to the methodology that was used to calculate the yields (the absence of discounting, for example). This, however, is not the critical element for even today when a more refined methodology (much of which works to lower the calculated rate of return) is utilized, rates remain high when one speaks of education in general (as contrasted with a particular programme for particular students). Similarly, with health.

Even during the 1950s, the decade in which the revival of interest in the economics of human resources began, elements of the older tradition were maintained. Much of the new work undertaken, related to the economic rates of return to various levels of education and the economic costs of various disease—not to the rate of return to specific education or health programmes. The analysis did, of course, demonstrate that education had a high yield and that disease was costly. It did not ask, however, what specific programmes could—in the real world— lower the incidence of disease and by how much. It did not ask what the rates of return would be for those programmes. Similarly, it did not ask how learning could be increased and what the returns to new educational programmes were likely to be. Yet, even the work that was done, limited as it was, was extremely important both in introducing economists to various applied fields in the social programme areas and in introducing an economic dimension to the discussion of these kinds of activities.

The reasons for the revival of interest in the economics of health and education in the 1950s are many. Concern about rapidly increasing budgets for education (and to a smaller degree for health) led to attempts to "justify" those budgets by examination of the economic benefits of education and health activities. Concern about under-developed economies brought us face to face with the question of skills and productivity, with the costs to production that result from lack of adequate education and health. It was clear that plant, equipment, roads, and electric power were not enough to insure development, and that quality of the labour force also made a difference. In the United States, concern about Soviet scientific advances and the growth in Soviet Gross National Product led to attempts to put empirical content into the statements that a nation's richest resource was its skilled manpower and that its wealth included its stock of engineers and scientists. Attempts to examine problems of economic growth in developed economies led to intensive examination of the sources of growth. United States Gross National Product, it is clear, has grown more rapidly than can be accounted for by increases in land, labour, and capital. There have, therefore, been attempts to provide more precise measurements and explanations of the part not accounted for, the residual element in growth. While primary emphasis has often been given to research and technology, a spill-over effect has directed considerable attention to capital invested in men. Finally, economists have directed more and more attention not only to income differences between nations but also to differences between groups in the same nation, to the reasons for these differences and to socio-economic policies that might narrow the differences. In the United States, the economic problems of Negroes has been an important focus of interest for economists (and others), and many have attributed much of the income part of the problem to the underinvestment in education and health for this part of our population.

During the 1960s, however, the nature of much of the empirical effort in the economics of health (and of education) began to change. Increasingly,

many felt that the work of economists on rates of return was interesting and illuminating, but not very helpful in guiding public policy and in choosing between public programmes. High rates of return are encouraging to the practitioner in a given field and they make for fine banquet address material, but they do not answer two questions that government budgeteers raise: (1) are the specific programmes for which support is sought "good" investments, i.e., what are the rates of return for the various proposals that come before the decision-maker; (2) which particular programmes should be favoured over other programmes, i.e., how does the rate of return for each programme compare with rates of return for alternatives? In the government sector these are the kinds of questions that are asked and, particularly, in the mid 1960s, the kinds of questions that United States government departments began asking of economists.

It should be remembered that there was a flavour, a "climate of opinion" in the early 1960s. Ideology was "dead," and the problems were, to a considerable measure, viewed as technical ones which required "technical" solutions. The analyst was not only necessary but sufficient. Those were the days of "the whizz kids" in the Pentagon, those were the days when it was felt that hard intellectual effort, the power of logic, and rationality would provide the answers to the society. In such an atmosphere, the importance of economists in government grew considerably. Thus, economists were among those asking (and answering) the questions of allocation of budget resources.

The issue confronting the budget officer and other decision-makers, after all, is not whether there is or is not (which in terms of the analysis often means "has or has not been") a high rate of return (an economic payoff) to health activities in general. Government budgets do not allocate funds to health in general but to specific programmes and activities. The question, therefore, is and should be how specific programmes and activities measure up and how they will do *in the future* since the future may differ from the past (if only because the population

groups to be served may become successively harder to reach). This is true whether one is conducting an economic analysis or any other type of evaluative effort. Furthermore, the decision-maker does not have free resources. He is subject to a budget constraint. He must *choose* between a large number of alternative programmes. It is, therefore, necessary to compare the likely gains and costs of the various possible courses of action that are open to him. He needs to ask how a particular programme compares with other programmes, how an *incremental* expenditure in one area compares with others.

Thus, in the mid 1960s we witnessed a conscious attempt to utilize the economist's tools in behalf of the decision-maker. Economists, called upon to examine specific programmes, had to shift their attention from the aggregative and macro aspects to the micro level. They were asked to compare programmes and rank them in terms of the relationship between costs and benefits. These economists (and the data for analysis) were most often found in government rather than outside. They were at work for and at the behest of the decision-maker himself, not for persons in an applied area who were trying to influence the decisions in their favour.

It can be noted that the intervention of economists in the process was not without difficulties. There was some controversy whether the analytical effort could best proceed at the highest level, say in the Bureau of the Budget (i.e., the President's staff), in the office of the Secretary of a Department, or in the individual operating agencies. The problem of where to carry forward such work to insure that the analyst has access to data and to the experience of persons intimately acquainted with programme operations and yet does not become a special pleader for the operating agency is important. Though we shall not discuss this at further length, we must note that success or failure in analysis and in influencing the decision-making process may hinge on the locational decision.

We speak of the economist's role in helping conduct *ex-ante* analysis of the consequences of decisions. This attempt often involved the application of quantitative methods to the analysis of the various alternatives open to the decision-maker. If it is granted that the essential characteristic of decision-making is that of choice as between alternatives (including, of course, the option of postponing the decision), then the process of choice involves some kind of a comparison of the likely gains and the likely costs of the various courses of action or inaction. This pattern of thought—though not necessarily in quantitative terms—is applicable to all facets of rational decision-making. Certainly it existed before 1965. What was new was the attempted quantification of costs and benefits, the attention to economic benefits, the involvement of economists, and the attempt to compare programmes in an explicit way. It should be clear, however, that gains and costs need not be limited to or expressed in monetary terms. They must include any number of other considerations which are relevant to the problem or decision at hand: gains or costs in prestige, political fortune, satisfaction, goodwill, effort, energy, and so forth. What is important is that in the evaluation, the comparisons be made explicit. It is also helpful if they be made in units which are commensurable.*

That economists were heavily involved thus does not mean that the only benefits that were or need to be considered are economic benefits, though, of course, there is the danger that a particular profession may tend to overlook the importance of things that lie outside its area of professional competence. Economists were involved for many reasons. They had developed a reputation in subjecting public decisions (particularly in the areas of water resources and defence) to analysis and in forcing the consideration of alternatives. They were used to empirical methods and to the pattern of thought that explicitly attempts to compare benefits and costs. They were conversant with the language of the men who

prepare budgets. Finally, they were viewed as "objective," i.e., not special pleaders for a particular programme or area.

Perhaps most important, economists had been most concerned with economic growth policies and with measures to increase the rate of growth. Many of the programmes that were to be analysed were examined from the perspective of growth. Furthermore, economists were concerned with the constraint of limited resources and the necessity for choice. The analysis was to involve the comparison of alternatives.

I do not propose to examine the details of the effort begun in the 1960s to bring the new type of analysis to bear on the governmental policy decision-making process. This is not the place to review that history. To do so would require that we move well beyond the area of our specific interests since the analytical effort was tied in with a number of other new activities in the planning and budgeting process, all of them designed collectively to make for better decisions and for wider range of choice. Our purposes are better served by examination of some of the conceptual difficulties that are involved in the effort to assess costs and benefits of programmes for people, particularly programmes which are viewed as human investment programmes. Let us, therefore, examine some of the issues that arise and that are involved in the quantitative analysis of benefits and costs.

Conceptual Issues

Basic to all considerations of programmes is the need to specify the objectives of the programme in question and to develop techniques and reporting systems that enable one to assess the degree to which the objectives are being met. It is clear that these are first and important steps. It is also clear that, in many cases, these steps entail great difficulty. The difficulties arise in part because the final objectives of many government programmes are to produce outputs which, at least at the present time, cannot be measured directly. The difficulties also arise because, often, we know relatively little

about the production process whereby these final outputs are created. I do not ignore the difficulties involved in creating data and reporting systems to measure the achievement of limited and well-defined goals (e.g., reduction in incidence of a particular disease). In no small measure our relative ignorance about many health matters relates to the fact that our data systems are underdeveloped and—in terms of funds and personnel—undernourished. Far too often we simply do not have the data we need for analytical purposes. These difficulties, however, are surmountable, and better reporting and data systems can be created. I refer instead to the even greater problems associated with the measurement of outputs which are amorphous in concept, outputs such as "higher levels of health" and which are contributed to by many factors (e.g., housing, income, nutrition, environment, medical care of all kinds), factors whose relative contribution may differ for different persons and whose relative contribution is largely unknown.

The difficulty of measuring the achievement of goals which lie on a continuum is apparent. We do not do as well in measuring pain, concern, or functional ability, as we do in measuring states which are discontinuous, such as life and death. Two consequences arise as a result of the problem of measurement and of understanding how various states of health are or can be produced. First, our lack of understanding of the production process and our inability to measure outputs leads programme administrators to define their goals in resource input terms: the goal is more hospital beds, more physicians, more patient visits, more examinations, more research, above all more money. It is an article of faith that good things are accomplished by more resources and that things will be even better if even more resources are utilized. This may indeed be the case, but it is not the issue for the question must be, "how much better." It is analogous to saying that a health programme is effective because it produces a positive change. The argument that we present says that that is not a sufficient guideline to the policy-maker since he must choose between different programmes and, therefore, must be concerned with levels of

*When the argument is cast in its broadest and most general terms it loses some of its operational significance since it can presumably be argued that when comparisons are not made (and decisions are arrived at on bases that, to some, may appear irrational) that the individual making the decision felt that the benefits of undertaking more refined comparisons and of reaching decisions in a more deliberate and explicit manner were outweighed by the costs involved.

effectiveness. His concern cannot be with whether a form of treatment or a government programme is likely to do some good, but rather with the amount of good accomplished per unit of resource input. He cannot be satisfied with a goal of more inputs, unless he understands how inputs relate to outputs, in which case he might as well speak in output terms.

There exists a second important consequence of our difficulty in measuring outputs. This arises most often in the development of new programme alternatives. The pressure to quantify, to measure, to be able to assess whether the goal is being achieved and in what degree, creates a bias in favour of developing those programmes that have output goals that can be measured, where data can be gathered, where the achievement of limited (but specified) goals can be documented. These, however, are not necessarily the most desirable, needed, or highest yield programmes. They may be, but they need not be.

The problem of measurement of output is a real one and the consequences are real as well. There is no reason, however, to be totally pessimistic about their solution. First, we must recognize that except for the bias in selection of programmes (a bias which I believe can be guarded against) these problems leave us no worse off than we are in the absence of the evaluation effort. It is not the attempt to calculate cost-benefit ratios that leaves us at sea, that makes us ignorant of production functions and forces us to speak of inputs rather than of outputs. These problems are with us all the time. Indeed the cost-benefit analysis leads to a greater level of understanding of the deficiencies in our measurement techniques, of the vagueness of some of our goals. It does not make us ignorant but makes us aware of our ignorance. It forces us to question the "conventional wisdom"—a discreet phrase that often really means well-accepted, but not fully documented, professional judgements. In the long run—and because of the recognition of the inadequate state of our knowledge—many of the problems will be partially solved. Some of them, I believe, are not fully solvable since they involve interpersonal comparisons and changing standards of need and adequacy, and thus changing measurements of the

benefits derived from various programmes. In the short run (and the short run may be a very long time indeed), we will be forced to find proxy measures for the outputs that are our ultimate interests. Thus, even if we are unable to develop a satisfactory index of health, there would be agreement that the absence of illness—while not a fully satisfactory measure of health—might serve as one of a number of proxy measures. It is necessary, of course, to be careful not to subvert the real aims of a programme by adjusting it to serve the proxy measure—a programme designed to improve the health of children with the consequence that they have fewer days of absence from school (the proxy measure) is different from a programme that focuses so heavily on the proxy that its attempt to achieve success leads sick children to be sent to school, perhaps contributing to even more illness. The danger that new (and measurable) aims are substituted for the real ones can, however, be guarded against.

Let us assume that, alert to the difficulties and biases and the dangers that they entail, the goals of the programmes have been specified and measures of the outputs have been developed. The difficulties are not yet over. Since the interest lies in the comparison of programmes, there develops a need to find a common denominator for the different outputs, a way of translating different things into a common unit of measure, a way, for example, of comparing the value of a life saved with a case of blindness prevented, of the life of a 10-year-old with the life of a 50-year-old, and so forth.

As has already been pointed out, these kinds of questions (e.g., the value of human life) are often found to be distasteful. None the less, whether formulated explicitly or implicitly, they are being asked—and are being answered—all the time. Often, however, because they are not formulated explicitly, one may find that governments pursue expenditure policies that imply that some lives are worth much more than others (e.g., aeroplane passengers as contrasted with coal miners). Thus, distasteful as it may be to articulate these types of questions, it is better that we do so than that we reach

policy decisions without being explicitly aware of their value implications.

The search for a common unit of measurement is, however, fraught with danger. We are unable to measure units of satisfaction or of happiness generated by various government activities. Nor are we able to compare A's satisfaction with B's. None the less, the climate of opinion places a premium on measurement. Since the evaluation of alternative programmes is carried forward by economists who are responding to budget and treasury officials, themselves sensitive to data that are presented in financial terms, and since the evaluation of programmes is being undertaken in an atmosphere that is investment and economic growth-oriented (while in the United States this atmosphere may be changing—one hopes that is the case—cost-benefit and programme analysis is still too young to have outgrown its early and very recent history), the common denominator that is most often sought is a monetary unit and the benefits most often measured are monetary ones. The fact that the monetary benefits are measured does not imply that economists are less concerned about other benefits than are historians, philosophers, or the general public. It simply means that economists (as others) tend to measure that which is measurable and tend first to address their attention to those things that they are familiar with: dollar costs and dollar benefits. Thus, as with the writings of economists and others in an earlier period, benefits are often translated into dollars (more correctly, the benefits that are measured are those that can be cast in dollar terms). This is the case even though it is total benefits of all kinds that we are interested in. Monetary benefits are—at best—only a proxy for total benefits. They are only part (perhaps only a small part) of all benefits and do not represent a stable or constant fraction of all benefits. The problems that may, therefore, arise are many.

In measuring the economic benefits of programmes it has become traditional to assess the increase in earning power of the individual that results from the improved health brought about by the programme under review. The increase in earning power is a measure of the gain to the economy since the contribution to production is measured by wages and salary income. This is not different from the evaluation made by those whose writings we examined above. It will be recalled that in those writings the value of a human being was assessed in different ways at different times: sometimes in terms of the cost of rearing (of producing the "machine") but later—and as is still done today—in terms of future earnings, a measure of expected future productive contribution. Using this measure entails some decisions about conceptual problems: what value should be placed on productive contribution and work effort that does not receive monetary rewards through the market system, a problem not confined to but often found in the case of women; what adjustments, if any, should be made to the gross earnings figure to take account of the individual's consumption; should adjustment be made for the additional investments that the individual or that society might make in the future in order to increase the individual's skills and his productive contribution and his earning power; what account should be taken of unemployment at the national level and at the regional level (what assumptions are reasonable as regards mobility and migration); should the future earnings figures be adjusted when there is evidence that because of market imperfections the individual is being rewarded at too low a rate?* These and numerous other issues arise and require a measure of agreement. Important as these issues are, we can only note them. Our discussion moves on to two matters that, it seems to me, are particularly troublesome.

The first issue, not unlike some of the difficulties that we have discussed earlier, relates to the problems and biases that may result from the inability to specify or measure the outputs that

are sought. If only some of the outputs are measured, however eloquent the words concerning other outputs, a budget or treasury official may tend to focus on those outputs which have numbers (economic values) attached to them. Further, because of the investment orientation of the analysis, often reflecting the investment orientation of the policy-maker, we may come to overvalue programmes that have an impact on future productivity and undervalue programmes that relieve pain, distress, concern, and suffering but have little or no impact (or measurable impact) on productivity. It may, indeed, be that programmes addressed to disabling conditions and to diseases involving mortality rather than to conditions that do not remove the person from economic activity should be favoured. That conclusion, however, should not be reached primarily because some things can be measured while others cannot. The analyst may discount the nature of the difficulty and the likelihood that this might occur, believing that his description of the items (particularly, benefits) that cannot be measured will suffice to alert the decision-maker to the inadequacy of the numbers. I suggest, however, that the analyst may underestimate the problem. He would do well to consider how compelling numbers are to finance officials and how high a rate of discount is applied to words, however well turned the phrases may be. There are those who feel that this danger is surmounted because all programmes are likely to have non-measurable by-products. They, therefore, believe that there is value in assessing the part of the iceberg that is visible (even if one cannot do the same for that part that lies below the surface of the waters). It is argued that it is, after all, better to know something than to know nothing (knowledge thus being equated with measurement and the inability to quantify equated with ignorance). Yet, there is little reason to believe that the ratio of measured to nonmeasured is the same in all programmes. If in some icebergs a higher proportion is visible than is the case in others, how do we assess which icebergs are larger in total and which are smaller? It is better to know something than to know nothing, but we dare not minimize the danger that in knowing something we may behave as if we know everything.

In reference to quantification and its dangers, one cannot help but be impressed by the words of Charles Henry Hull who, in his introduction to *The Economic Writings of Sir William Petty*, published in 1899, noted that Petty was sometimes careless in his calculations. He indicated that Petty was aware of the conjectural character of his numbers and that Petty had written: "I hope that no man takes what I say about the living and dyeing of men for a mathematical demonstration." Hull continued:

But in the ardour of argument he was himself more than once mislead into fancying that his conclusions were accurate because their form was definite. His mistake is not without its modern analogies. Mathematical presentations of industrial facts, both symbolic and graphic, have by their definiteness, encouraged many as investigator in the false conceit that he now knew what he sought, whereas he had at most but a neat name for what he sought to know. Nevertheless the substitution of symbols for Petty's "terms of number" is an improvement in this, that calculations made in symbols must be consciously translated into the terms of actual life before any practical use—or misuse—can be made of them, whereas calculations in figures of number, weight, and measure are already concrete and appear to tell something intelligible even to a common man (24).

The danger that Hull recognized is our concern. Almost three-quarters of a century have passed since Hull, but the problem has not been solved.

The second problem that arises when we concentrate our measurement on earnings is even more basic. The previous discussion addressed itself to difficulties that can, perhaps, be solved by acquainting the decision-maker with the inadequacy of the methodology, by requiring that all analysts be humble and all decision-makers be wise (requirements that are not easy to achieve). They can be solved by recognizing that *quantification is not a substitute for judgement* but a contributor to it. The problem to which we now turn is, I believe, even more severe for it asks the basic question whether programmes are to be evaluated primarily on the basis of "investment criteria"? Does the measurement of a person's worth in terms of his productive contribution really represent our social values?

*Market imperfections arise in many areas. As early as 1861, it was suggested that ". . . the value of compulsory servitude in the Army . . . (should include) . . . the value between the market price of labour and the price paid for it by government . . ." (23). This issue has, once again, arisen in the debates in the United States concerning the comparison of the cost of a volunteer and of a conscripted army.

I believe that it does not do so. In particular, it fails adequately to take account of equity and distributional considerations (which many believe to be one of the major functions of government). Note that the theory says that in instituting a programme and measuring the benefits we ask what impact the programme would have on the earning power of the individual. Because we cannot count *the* individual we tend, in our measurements, to deal with groups of individuals and with averages. Always, however, the theory would have us include as many characteristics of individuals as are relevant to the projection of future income and as are available to us: the sex and age of the people affected, their urban-rural and racial characteristics, their income and education levels, and so forth. A programme directed at women would use the average income of women as a measure of benefit. A programme directed at a specific age-group should (and does) use the discounted value of future earnings of that age-group (yielding different answers for persons in the age-group 45–55 than for persons in the age-group 25–35). Yet, taking account of the individual's characteristics (or classifying the individual as a member of a group that has certain average behaviour patterns) could lead us to direct our health activities towards those with the highest potential incomes and away from those whose earning capacity would be low: away from those with less education and skills, from the poor (whose increase in potential income may also be low), from those in low productivity sectors such as agriculture, and so forth. It would also mean that programmes directed at females would compete unfavourably with programmes for males, that the old would compete unfavourably with the young. The latter two biases are offset because income is often imputed to women since the difficulty with using an earned income test is obvious and because in the case of the young the discount rate that is applied to future earnings has a very powerful effect in reducing the present value of future earnings. None the less, the problem is clear and particularly so for the present poor since their potential increase in earnings, however large in percentage terms, may be small in absolute terms, and it is the absolute that is measured.

It is apparent that the theory and the results that would be obtained were the theory followed, stand in conflict with our value system. The victims, in many cases, of past discrimination would be discriminated against again because, as a result of past discrimination, they are "worth less" in economic terms—and all this at a time when many feel that past discrimination justifies and necessitates compensation. In fact, the conflict does not arise because practice departs from theory. The analysis does not include all the information that it might. We are sufficiently sensitive to the problem of distributional equity that we do not include all the characteristics of the population to be affected in the projection of future income and thus in the benefit-cost calculation. In general, we ignore differences in education, in present income (at given ages), in occupation, and in other variables that might affect future earnings of different groups. The issue, therefore, is not raised because we are "getting the wrong answers" but, rather, in order to alert us to the fact that the conceptual and philosophical problems at issue have not been adequately addressed or resolved. These may not have been problems in earlier days when the arguments presented were cast in general terms and were in support of health, education, and other general programmes. It is an issue when the analysis and arguments are addressed to problems of choice as between alternative programmes *for alternative population groups*. Often the analytical issues are viewed as technical matters relating to how economists measure value. We must recognize that measurement is more than a matter of technical procedures but that it carries with it an implicit value system and orientation. To suppose that economics is value free and that measurement is neutral is incorrect. Explicit discussion of the value system would be valuable for the debate would illuminate matters which now are buried within jargon, regression equations, and technical considerations that few decision-makers are totally familiar with. Cost-benefit analysis is too important to be left to analysts or economists. It is more than regrettable that philosophers, historians, students of intellectual thought,

and others have neglected this area of inquiry.

That the calculation of benefit-cost ratios entails other difficulties is well known. Many of these difficulties bear discussion. I propose, however, to address one remaining question, not technical in nature. It relates to the impact of the kind of analysis that we are reviewing. While much of the analytical effort stems from an attempt at rational decision-making and involves a pressure to depart from incremental budget-making, I would suggest that the (benefit-cost) analytical effort is likely to result in the development of small, innovative, experimental programmes (all this is desirable) but likely to favour a "conservative" response towards bold, new, and large departures from existing policies, programmes, and patterns of organization and funding. In my view this is undesirable. There are times when large changes are needed.

Social revolutions, bold new departures in social policy, massive changes in the prevailing patterns of health financing or organization can probably not be subjected to rigorous benefit-cost analysis. Nor is it likely that when analysis could be undertaken, it could withstand the critics of the benefit-cost ratios that might offer support for such changes and departures. At the present time we do not know how much good is created by a physician visit, what benefits more medical care brings, what the contribution of other factors is to the level of health. If policies must be justified with quantitative arguments and economic data, we are likely to find that those who would delay the institution of new programmes could argue that more experimental effort is required, that we are not quite ready, that the programme is "good" but that it may not be the "best." I rather doubt Britain would have a National Health Service had the decision involved the kind of analysis I describe. This is not because the analysis would have suggested that the NHS was undesirable (though since benefit-cost analysis would likely not have taken adequate account of one of the important objectives of the programme, distributional equity, benefits would have been understated) but rather because the analysis would have revealed many "unknowns" and would thus have favoured the point of view of those who believed in more small experiments. The analytical effort is likely to reveal that there is much we do not know and thus will favour marginal change in the *status quo* "until we know more." But there will always be more to know, more programmes to analyse.

I do not argue that every revolution is good (though that may often be the case with social programmes involving distributional equity). I simply argue that it is difficult to justify most revolutions on an *ex-ante* basis in the face of critics who are trying to avoid risks. In the analytical effort, after all, there is a climate of opinion which says that the programme can be justified only when we are certain that there is no other programme that is better. As I look at the social legislation enacted in the United States in recent years, I am forced to conclude that we have been well served by decision-makers who were willing to reach decisions and move on to new paths, battling for the answers given them by their ideological convictions. The programmes might, of course, have been better constructed. Not all of them have been successes, and some of them have left much to be desired. It is not clear, however, that had the analyst been listened to that the programmes would have been better. They might simply not have existed ("let's wait and do more research").

The reader will note that these comments are not based on the additional possibility that the benefit-cost ratio for a programme that is massive in scope might differ greatly from the ratio for the small experiment. If this is the case then no experiment (other than one involving the massive change) can give us the right answer. This may well be the case with social programmes that involve behavioural characteristics that are influenced by the fact that one is involved in an experiment, discontinuities, or long periods of time before their impacts can be fully assessed. The argument presented here is a more limited one, however. Here the issue is the flavour of the exercise, what I believe, is a bias against big changes. Perhaps benefit-cost analysis has a non-incremental impact on the budget for existing programmes and an incremental impact

on experimentation. One may, therefore, favour it. It should be recognized, none the less, that incremental experiments are different from programme changes, particularly major ones.

It should also be clear that I am not suggesting that all analysis is without value and that major changes in programmes should be supported by statements of faith. Our discussion relates to benefit-cost analysis, not to analysis in general. That economists (and others) can conduct useful analysis of the distributional impact of cash transfer programmes, for example, should be evident. Their efforts at constructing more equitable and more efficient transfer programmes—some of them, indeed, representing major new departures—should not go unrecognized. Our discussion is not meant to detract from this type of analytical work. The ability to provide economic analysis of programmes where the objective is simply distributional does not mean that there exists an equal ability to provide analysis of the ultimate benefits of programmes whose aim is not solely distributional or whose aim involves levels of performance via redistribution of services rather than money.

It is also useful to note one specific contribution to decision-making that can be derived from cost-effectiveness analysis, a mode of analysis close to, but not identical with, cost-benefit analysis. Let us assume that, in one way or another—perhaps through the political process responsive to and leading the electorate—a decision is reached to accomplish a certain purpose, to achieve a goal, to reach an objective, say in health. Whether it is the most worthwhile purpose, goal, or objective in terms of maximizing total satisfaction is no longer the issue. The particular output sought can usually be achieved in a variety of different ways, that is, with different combinations of resource inputs. In cost-effectiveness analysis we seek the optimal, economically efficient combination of these inputs so that resources are not wasted and so that they might, therefore, be available for other purposes. The object is to minimize cost per unit of output (or one may put it as maximizing output per unit cost). Because of the problems engendered by multiple outputs, each with different values and, thus, requiring some comparison of the values of the outputs (of

the benefits), cost-effectiveness analysis does tend, at times, to move closer and closer to benefit-cost analysis. None the less, the purpose to be served by the cost-effectiveness inquiry is different.

Cost-effectiveness analysis raises questions concerning trade-offs (of inputs if not of inputs and outputs). Though more limited than benefit-cost analysis, it is valuable and reinforces our need to know more about the production function. It reminds us to consider quality considerations. Above all else, perhaps, it forces the professional to respond to the question whether the fact that things have been done in a particular way in the past means that that is the best way to do them in the future. Such questions, of course, are questions that the professional should be asking himself all the time, but the fact is that oftentimes it is the outsider who can question tradition more readily than the practitioner. There are many rewards to be derived in a wide variety of government programmes from good cost-effectiveness analysis: rewards in the saving of resources in some instances and in accomplishing much more good for people in other instances. Cost-effectiveness analysis, to some, seems to involve less exciting issues than is the case in benefit-cost analysis. None the less, the benefit-cost ratio of this kind of work is likely to be extremely high. Major government stimulus of this kind of analysis is justified.

Conclusions

I have raised a number (though by no means all) of the problems that relate to the evaluation of the economic benefits of health (and other social) programmes. Yet, earlier, I indicated the need for evaluation, for the kind of thinking that is involved in the comparison of programmes, and for doing so in an explicit manner in order to improve decision-making. Where does that leave us? What contribution can the successors to Petty, Chadwick, and others make?

It should, I think, be clear that in my view we have not arrived at a stage where benefit-cost analysis can be as helpful as some (but not all) of its proponents believe to be the case in the allocation of scarce resources in public policy decisions. We are a long way (and will always remain a long way) from being able to allocate the total government budget as between competing priorities on the basis of this kind of analysis. Even more limited objectives are beyond our attainment. In the United States, major elements of the Federal budget for health, education, and welfare fall within one department, the Department of Health, Education, and Welfare. Yet, competing claims between the three major activities in that one department cannot be significantly illuminated and even partially resolved by benefit-cost analysis. Indeed, I rather doubt that, given the state of our data systems and the conceptual problems yet to be solved, the analytical effort can be more than only somewhat helpful in allocating scarce dollars within a single broad line of activity, say within the health arena. Helpful, yes, because it will force explicit statements about our ignorance, because it will help us to implement data and reporting systems, because it will provoke debate leading to questions and, in some cases, answers. The degree of usefulness will, however, depend on how wise the decision-maker is, how sceptical he is of measurement techniques even as he supports, encourages, and assists in their development.

Thus we are not called upon to declare a moratorium on this type of analysis. To do so would, in my view, be an error. That we will find fewer answers than we seek is clear, but we will learn much in the formulation of the questions and in the seeking of the answers. Economists have until recently been underrepresented in departments and agencies concerned with social programmes and all of us, I believe, have paid a price for this underrepresentation. The economist's point of view, his questions, his perspective, are useful in forcing persons to examine a problem that they are professionally familiar with from another point of view. It leads, therefore, to a more intelligent debate concerning programmes, issues, and goals. Since many of the programmes referred to are concerned with human behaviour

and response, departments should also increase the number of behavioural and social scientists involved from disciplines other than economics. By focusing on the economist, I in no sense mean to ignore the potential contribution of the sociologist, anthropologist, psychologist, social psychologist, and others. My own background does permit me, however, to speak with more knowledge about the role that economic analysis and the thought process of the economist can play.

In my view the contribution of economists and analysts can be important. The scepticism that I have concerning some of the answers provided by cost-benefit analysis in no way detracts from my view about the potential contribution derived from the thought process, from the way of thinking about problems. Furthermore, Chadwick was correct when he stated that economists had a contribution to make. The contribution does not depend on the ability to measure whether removing persons from London during a plague yields a return of £84, or of £72, or of £129 per pound expended. This will not often enable us to answer whether this or some other programme is a "better" investment. But policy-makers and others need to be reminded that there are economic returns to health programmes, that good health can be supported on investment grounds, that there are high costs (for the issue is total costs, both direct budget outlays and indirect costs associated with loss of production) as a consequence of poor health and inadequate education. Economics can help point up these issues. It can—and should—serve the protagonist (not only the decision-maker). The discipline is not debased by such analysis nor is the public decision process harmed for far too often health and education appropriations are insufficient not because other programmes yield a higher rate of return, but because it is assumed that health and education appropriations are simply money down the drain, yielding no economic benefit. In a world oriented to economic benefits, this assumption becomes a difficult obstacle to surmount. Too many economists—perhaps afraid of being accused of being part sentimentalist and moralist and because of their desire to assume the stance of "objec-

tivity"—have been on the defensive too long. Too often we have said that health and education are valuable but that society must choose the most valuable programme, and we cannot be certain which of the many possible activities are the most valuable. While this is true and important, we must recognize that in the political world those who would compete with health and education for funds often are far less objective and analytical. To subject health activities to analysis while, for example, leaving the military budget to emotional arguments is hardly to fight for scarce dollars on even terms. Surely I am not arguing for the end of the analytical effort, but rather for a greater willingness to do what Petty and Chadwick did: to bring supporting evidence for their point of view without that self-consciousness that some of us often have because we have not examined every alternative; to be willing to say that this is good even if we cannot yet say that this is best.

Earlier I noted that a major function of many government programmes is to achieve a more equitable distribution of goods and services. The early history of economic analysis in the health field did not rest its case for an increased effort on the part of government on these grounds nor, as has been indicated, does the present effort take due account of such considerations. Clearly, however, distributional equity does provide an important rationale for many health programmes. To that extent, the task of the analyst and of the data and reporting system is made easier. If the objective of the legislature is to equalize services, to make available to certain population groups services which they would otherwise not be able to purchase in the market, services which people believe to be important (even if, in fact, they are less important or beneficial than is imagined), then the evaluation effort is much simpler. At present, in the United States, beset as we are by divisions and by tensions, distributional considerations lie at the heart of many of our problems. The healing of social wounds (not an unimportant objective even if its benefits cannot be quantified in monetary terms) may, today, be more readily accomplished by providing the services that people believe to be important than by providing that which the analyst has tentatively determined is most beneficial. The healing of social wounds is, at this moment, I believe more vital than the healing of disease. Though there is surely a relationship between the two efforts, and they need not be in conflict, there may well be a trade-off between them. In that case, social harmony would, I suggest, be the overriding goal. It may, for example, be that certain medical procedures cannot be justified on economic grounds and, in fact, contribute very little to better health. If, however, they are available to many in the population and are utilized (even if this means that individuals are "wasting their money"), if the population believes them to be important, society may be compelled to make them available to all. This, though in many ways a more limited objective, is not a trivial one at all. We are a long way from its attainment and would do well to pursue it with vigour and commitment.

That distributional equity in the delivery of services is a limited goal should, none the less, be clear. An enlightened society will attempt to achieve a greater equity in outcomes rather than in inputs. In the United States, in the field of education there was a time when equality meant that children should attend schools with equal inputs. Difficult as it may be to achieve such goals, the formulas required for their attainment are easy to construct and require little knowledge of the educational process. Evaluation in such a context requires simple data. Today, however, equality of educational opportunity has come to mean that we should offer opportunities such that regardless of the circumstances of the child when he enters school and the environmental problems he faces while he attends school, the child should have equal opportunity to achieve a given level of education. Thus, the resources going to schools with a high proportion of poor children should be greater than the resources going to schools with more affluent children. The problem in evaluation when we are interested in unequal resource inputs and unequal provision of services so that we might have more equal outcomes is, of course, immensely more difficult since it requires

an understanding of the relationship between inputs and outputs and an understanding of the production process. Thus, an enlightened society can hardly avoid many of the analytical efforts we have discussed in this chapter. We cannot find an easy way out of the analytical difficulties.

We shall have to continue the kind of explorations begun by Petty and by others. We shall have to remember Chadwick's words. We shall, however, have to carry on this work with a certain modesty, remembering the words of Sir Arthur Newsholme: "There remains a further problem which must at least be mentioned. Is it possible in every instance to measure by means of statistics, influence and procedures benefiting the public health or improving social welfare?" (25).

References

1. Chadwick, E. (1862). "Opening address as President of Section F (Economic Sciences and Statistics) of the British Association for the Advancement of Science," *Jl. Statist. Soc. Lond.* 25, 504, 509, 522.

2. Petty, Sir William (1690), *Political Arithmetick,* in Hull, C. H. (1899), *The Economic Writings of Sir William Petty* (Cambridge University Press), p. 267.

3. —— (1691). *Verbum Sapienti,* in Hull, C. H., ibid., p. 109.

4. —— (n.d.). "Magnalia Regni" in Lansdowne, Marquis of (1927), *The Petty Papers, Some Unpublished Writings of Sir William Petty, edited from the Bowood Papers* (London: Constable & Co. Ltd.), pp. 265–7, 274.

5. —— (1667). "Of Lesening yᵉ Plagues of London," in Hull, C. H. (1899), *The Economic Writings of Sir William Petty* (Cambridge University Press), p. 109.

6. —— (1676). "Anatomy Lecture" in Lansdowne, Marquis of (1927), *The Petty Papers, Some Unpublished Writings of Sir William Petty, edited from the Bowood Papers* (London: Constable & Co. Ltd.), p. 176.

7. Chadwick, E. (1842). *Sanitary Report,* cited by the Right Honorable the Earl Fortescue (1877), "Extracts from the Address of the President of Section F (Economic Sciences and Statistics) of the British Association for the Advancement of Science," *Jl. Statist. Soc. Lond.* 25, 558.

8. —— (1844). "On the best modes of representing accurately, by statistical returns, the duration of life, and the pressure and progress of the causes of mortality amongst different classes of the community, and amongst the populations of different districts and countries," ibid. 7, 25, 30.

9. —— (1859). "Results of different principles of legislation and administration in Europe; of competition for the field, as compared with competition within the field, of service," ibid. 22, 405.

10. Shattuck, L. (1850). *Report of the Sanitary Commission of Massachusetts,* Facsimile Edition, 1948 (Cambridge: Harvard University Press), pp. 254, 257, 258–60.

11. Rogers, the Revd. J. E. T. (1865). "On the statistical and fiscal definitions of the word "income," *Jl. Statist. Soc. Lond.* 28, 243.

12. Farr, W. (1853). "The income and property tax," ibid. 16, 1–44.

13. —— (1885). *Vital Statistics,* ed. Humphreys, N. A. (London: Offices of the Sanitary Institute), pp. 313, 314.

14. Calkins, G. N. (1891). "Some results of sanitary legislation in England since 1875," *Am. Statist. Ass.* 2, 297–303.

15. Bogart, E. L. (1919). *Direct and Indirect Costs of the Great World War* (New York: Oxford University Press).

16. Giffen, Sir Robert (1900). "Some economic aspects of the war," *Econ. J.* 10, 194–207.

17. —— (1904). *Economic Inquiries and Studies* (London: George Bell & Sons), pp. 1–74.

18. Guillebaud, C. W. (1927). "The cost of the war in Germany," *Econ. J.* 27, 270–7.

19. Hamilton, A. (1877). "On the recent economic progress of New Zealand," *Jl. Statist. Soc. Lond.* 40, 111.

20. Guy, Dr. (1877). "Discussion on Mr. Hamilton's paper," ibid. 40, 127, 129.

21. Dublin, L. I., and Whitney, J. (1920). "On the cost of tuberculosis," *Am. Statist. Ass.* 17, 441–50.

22. Mendenhall, W. O., and Castle, E. W. (1911). "Vital and monetary losses in the United States due to typhoid fever," ibid. 12, 519–43.

23. —— (1861). "The British and French armies, comparative statements, 1860–61," *Jl. Statist. Soc. Lond.* 24, 241.

24. Hull, C. H. (1899). *The Economic Writings of Sir William Petty* (Cambridge University Press), p. lxviii.

25. Newsholme, Sir Arthur (1923). "The measurement of progress in public health," *Economica,* 3, 201.

103

Robert N. Grosse
Analysis in Health Planning

Reprinted from A. W. Drake, R. L. Keeney, and P. M. Morse, eds., *Analysis of Public Systems,* by permission of the MIT Press, Cambridge, Massachusetts. Copyright © 1972 by the Massachusetts Institute of Technology.

Systems Analysis: From DOD to HEW

This chapter discusses the application of analytical approaches to budgetary and legislative decisions in health policy at the federal level. My personal experience included some years in analysis of national security problems followed by work on domestic social policies. The initiation of such activities in domestic agencies attempted to introduce approaches that had found some success in the Department of Defense (DOD). I thought it might be useful to begin with some points of contrast between the two settings. Discussions of health analyses in this chapter include allocations among disease programs, allocations within one disease problem area, and maternal and child health program comparisons. Rather than abstracting the technical structure of our methods and procedures, I shall go directly into the types of questions we considered and the nature of the results obtained. However oversimplified they may be, many of the studies discussed here constituted the first attempts at program analysis in their respective fields.

When the Secretary of Defense in 1961 desired to institutionalize the applications of operations research and systems analysis to decision making, a major problem identified was that planning and budgeting activities were being carried out independently of each other. They were independent in the sense of the people and of the time-frame in which they looked at the problems. The planners were usually spinning their dreams 5, 10, and 20 years into the future; the budgeteers were concerned with next year. They also dealt in different dimensions. Planners looked at the missions: tactical, strategic, logistical; areas such as the central plains of Germany, the Mediterranean, or the Far East; and weapon systems and organizations, such as bombers and missile systems, naval task forces, army divisions. The budget side of the process dealt in dimensions of input, purchases of equipment, construction of facilities, maintenance and operations activities, hiring and paying of personnel.

Decisions made in each area were weaker than they might have been had planning and budgeting been integrated. Planners rarely took into explicit consideration in their designs the financial and resource implications of alternative courses of action. They did, of course, screen the total plan for economic feasibility. But this was like designing your ideal house and discovering, after you have laid out the plans, that it will cost $350,000 but that you have only something in the order of $35,000. This usually led to a hasty cutting down of plans as though one looked at the plans of the $350,000 house and eliminated nine-tenths of the items, rather than redesigning the building to optimize what one could procure for $35,000. As a consequence, much of the mid-range and long-range planning activity conducted by the Pentagon had little relevance when budget decisions were made with regard to research and development, procurement of equipment, and force structure.

The budget side of management, while in some sense more practical and obviously influencing the course of events, had little understanding of the military effects of budgetary decisions, as there was no mechanism available for determining what in the way of missions accomplishment or organization or force structure was implied by short-run purchases of inputs.

A major management objective of the early McNamara period became the construction of a link between planning and budget activities, permitting an understanding of the implications of the items and personnel procured in terms of military effectiveness and, in turn, an understanding of the resource considerations of alternative courses of actions for weapon systems and for organizational decisions made in the planning process. This bridging or translating device was given the name of "programming" or "program budgeting." Later, in nondefense applications, it was called the planning, programming and budgeting system (PPB). Four years later, President Johnson, searching for methods of improving management and decision making in the domestic side of government, ordered his cabinet to institute similar procedures and the planning, programming, budgeting system began to spread throughout the whole of the federal government.

In joining the Department of Health, Education, and Welfare (HEW), to help develop the system, I naïvely assumed that again the problem would be to link the planning and budgeting processes so that operations or systems analysis could be utilized in the planning process, and in turn affect the budgeting decisions. There were a number of significant differences, however, between the Defense Department and a department such as that of Health, Education, and Welfare.

One was that, while there were many people operating in the budget area, nobody at HEW engaged in any form of systematic planning. There were, of course, people scheming to get more money for particular programs. The problem was not one simply of linking a plan to a budgeting process but rather it also required the development almost from scratch of a planning capability and planning procedures.

A second difference was the extent of responsibility of the federal government in the areas to be studied. In defense or national security matters, the Department of Defense is responsible for most of the actions taken. There are, of course, the actions of the State Department, the Atomic Energy Commission, and, externally, those of our allies. But, by and large, what is recommended in the defense area is directed and controlled by one department. In matters such as health and education, this is not the case. The primary actors in health in the United States are private physicians, voluntary county and municipal hospitals, state and mental hospitals, state and local departments of health and welfare, and universities that train professionals and conduct research.

Further complicating the situation is the nature by which the federal government supports its activities. It does this largely through grants-in-aid. This means that the federal government transfers funds to state governments, local governments, universities, and hospitals which then organize the programs which use nonfederal funds as well. About 94 percent of the general funds of the Department of Health, Education, and Welfare is spent on grants-in-aid and an additional 1 percent or so on the administration of such grants. There are relatively few

programs run directly by the federal government. There are some intramural research activities at the National Institutes of Health, and there are Public Health Service hospitals for the merchant mariners (soon to be eliminated) and health activities run on Indian reservations by the Division of Indian Health.

So we have a situation of only partial funding by the federal government, and essentially what is done is through nonfederal agencies. This complicates understanding the systems and how government programs affect them. Designing models and developing coefficients is indeed difficult.

I would add to the problems of model building the pervasive ignorance of social production functions. There has been very little work done on determining relationships between expenditures and results in social areas. We do not know the impact of different kinds of educational programs on people's capacities, nor the effects of social service on adjustment, nor health services on the status of health. Most social problems of any consequence are not rectified by any single program. The reduction of tuberculosis is related to housing conditions, diet, immunization, isolation of affected individuals, and therapy. Diet and housing are in turn related to income and employment levels. Income and employment levels are related to educational level, skill training, racial discrimination, health, the state of business, the labor market, income supplements, job training, job creation, job placement, fiscal policy, education, legal services, community power, and more can be added to this list.

The well-known weakness or absence of our social indicators makes it difficult to say what has happened, let alone why it happened. A summary of some difficulties in program evaluation would indicate that, with few exceptions:

We lack agreement on the objectives of programs.
We lack agreement on measures of achievement of objectives.
We find it hard to estimate measures when we agree on them.
We cannot sort out cause and effect relationships because of the multiplicity of inputs and the multidimensionality of outputs.

We have little longitudinal information about programs whose effects come about over long periods of time. Usually we don't even know where we are.

A further problem was the philosophy and attitude of most of the program managers and bureau chiefs. They could hardly be described as sympathetic to the philosophy of analysis and operations research where one tries to define objectives, identify and price alternatives, trace the consequences of these alternatives, and through some test of preferredness relate costs and effectiveness to determine the preferred alternative. In most cases, program managers felt that there was a large gap between the needs of the society and what we were doing. Their preferred alternative was to spend money on expanding processes that they were already engaged in. "Desirable for what purpose," or "for what accomplishment," or "concerns about alternative methods of achievement of these accomplishments," were rare in the vocabulary or thinking processes. It was presumed that more hospitals, more nurses, more doctors, more research, and more services were what the society needed and that the only problem was to secure these on an ever increasing scale.

Finally, perhaps the most significant difference between military and domestic government is the much greater significance in the domestic area of political interests—those of the serving professions, such as medicine and education, and those of the communities and peoples to be served. The reconciling of such interests into a consensus or coalition and deciding whom you will fight and to whom you will make concessions is an important ingredient—perhaps the most important in the decision process.

Within the context described, we attempted in 1966 to develop an analytical process in the department of HEW. A small number of analysts, mostly economists, were formed into the office of the assistant secretary for Program Coordination (later called Planning and Evaluation). Despite pressure from the Bureau of the Budget to "analyze" all programs, it was obvious that only a few could be addressed. For these, program analysis teams were formed, consisting of staff from the secretary's office and the operating programs, and consultants. The time allotted to the studies was usually designed to bring results in about the time of budget formulation. This meant studies beginning in March or April were to have usable results by August or September. I shall try to sketch some examples of our initial efforts.

Disease Control Programs

One of the first applications of cost-benefit analysis was to disease control programs. Considerable work has been done during the last 10 years in estimating the economic costs of particular diseases. It was not surprising, then, that, when systematic quantitative analysis of government programs and policies began to spread from defense to civilian applications, one of the first analytical studies was a study of disease control programs.

The basic concept of the study was a simple one. The Department of Health, Education, and Welfare supports (or could support) a number of categorical disease control programs, whose objectives are to save lives or to prevent disability by controlling specific diseases. The study was an attempt to answer the question: If additional money were to be allocated to disease control programs, which programs would show the highest payoff in terms of lives saved and disability prevented per dollar spent?

I'm talking here not about research, but where a technology exists and the problem is whether to put the same or more or less federal funding behind these control programs to support activities in hospitals, states, and communities. We addressed the question of the allocation of available resources for disease control. The Department of Health, Education, and Welfare studied five programs: cancer, arthritis, tuberculosis, syphilis, and motor vehicle injury. After discussing some studies concerned with allocations among disease programs, I will describe a later study addressed to the proper mix of approaches within a single program (kidney disease).

Factors Influencing Control Programs

The effectiveness of the department's disease control programs is influenced by a number of factors. Of most significance are the abilities of medical technology to provide the scientific knowledge to prevent the disease, to diagnose disease early enough so that the impact on health can be minimized, and to treat the disease to cure the patient. In order to determine the relative emphasis on the department's disease control programs, we addressed such questions as:
Does the knowledge exist for disease prevention?
How can the knowledge be applied?
Does the knowledge exist for disease diagnosis and treatment?
What are the more productive methods for applying this knowledge?
What are the costs involved in applying the knowledge?
What benefits in terms of lives saved, disability prevented, and other economic and social losses averted can be achieved?

For each of the diseases discussed in this chapter, medical knowledge exists for some measure of disease control. However, for such diseases as head and neck cancer and colon-rectum cancer, techniques of diagnosis have not yet been developed to make it economical to screen a necessarily large number of people in order to identify even a relatively small number of these cancers. Although primitive technology exists, the cost of a control program may be too high measured by benefits forgone in programs with higher potential for saving of lives and decreasing the impact of illness.

The Federal Role

The particular federal interest in disease control programs stems from two concerns:
1. Those diseases that may be communicated across state boundaries.
2. Those diseases where people are not getting adequate medical care because either personnel, knowledge, or facilities may not be available, or because the people cannot afford health care.

Tuberculosis and syphilis control have been of concern to the Public Health Service for many years. The national spread of these communicable diseases through personal contact has been a key reason for the federal role

in these programs. In addition, the technology (drugs and diagnostic procedures) for effective control of these diseases has been in existence for many years; penicillin and blood tests for syphilis, isoniazid and x ray for tuberculosis.

Technology for effective control of the selected cancer sites has only recently become available and in most cases is still under development. Although the Papanicolaou test for uterine cervix cancer disease dates back to 1928, its general acceptance dates to 1943; as late as 1960 fewer than 5 million tests were reported by national laboratories. With Public Health Service support for case finding and demonstration projects, including the training of technologists, utilization of this technique reached almost 15 million tests by 1965.

Arthritis includes a number of specific diseases where knowledge does not exist to permit prevention, control, or even effective amelioration of crippling and/or disabling symptoms in a large number of patients. The limited knowledge that is available is not widely disseminated, and only a small portion of the estimated 10 to 13 million people suffering from arthritis have access to good quality diagnosis and care. The federal concern here is to assure that more people receive better care. The method of approach is similar to that applied to the cancer programs—demonstration projects that have as a major component the training of physicians and technicians and developing and testing diagnostic and treatment methods.

Public Health Service programs in motor vehicle injury prevention are in their initial stages. The magnitude of this problem would indicate a major interest for all health agencies.

Selected Disease Alternative Analysis

The Department of Health, Education, and Welfare task groups were established to develop detailed analyses of the individual selected disease control programs. Each of these studied and analyzed a number of alternative programs. Program cost and anticipated benefits were compared for the alternatives within each of the programs.

Two principal criteria were used as a basis for recommending funding allocation among the programs within each

Table 103-1
Cancer Control Program: 1968–1972

	Uterine Cervix	Breast	Head and Neck	Colon-Rectum
Grant costs ($000)	97,750	17,750	13,250	13,300
Number of examinations (000)	9,363	2,280	609	662
Cost per examination	$10.44	$7.79	$21.76	$20.10
Examinations per case found	87.5	167.3	620.2	496.0
Cancer cases found	107,045	13,628	982	1,334
Cost per case found	$913	$1,302	$13,493	$9,970
Cancer deaths averted	44,084	2,936	303	288
Cost per death averted	$2,217	$6,046	$43,729	$46,181

Source: "Program Analysis: Cancer," Office of the Assistant Secretary for Program Coordination, U.S. Department of Health, Education, and Welfare, Washington, D.C., October 1966.

disease category as well as among the different diseases analyzed. These criteria were the cost per death averted and the benefit cost ratio.

Cost per Death Averted

The "cost per death averted" is the 5-year program cost, divided by the deaths averted owing to the programs. These costs range from an estimated $87 per death averted for a seat belt use program to over $40,000 for such programs as head and neck cancer control, increasing driver skills, and emergency medical services.

The cost per death averted for each of the programs is an average cost figure. It would be expected that some of the costs would actually be many times the average cost. For example, a uterine cervix program recommended has an average cost per death averted of $3,470. However, of the 34,000 lives expected to be saved owing to the programs through 1972, 30,000 have an average cost of about $2,000; 2,300 have an average cost of over $3,500, and 400 have an average cost of over $7,000. While it may sometime be possible to add additional lives saved at the lower figure, any significant investment of funds in this program would probably be oriented toward the more expensive cases averaging over $7,000.

The Benefit Cost Ratio

There are at least two problems with cost per death averted as a sole criterion for evaluating program effectiveness.
1. There is no distinction made regarding the age at which the death is averted, and

2. There is no way to rank those diseases that are not primarily killers. The benefit cost ratio includes both morbidity and mortality implications of the disease. The benefit cost ratio, simply stated, is the amount of dollars invested divided into the amount of dollars saved.

The economic savings for disease are composed of direct savings of dollars that would have been spent on medical care cost including physician's fees, hospital services, drugs, and so on, and indirect savings such as the earnings saved because the patient did not die or was not incapacitated due to illness or injury. The average lifetime earnings for different age groups is related to the age at which death occurs and a calculation of the present value of lost lifetime earnings. For example, if a 27-year-old man died this year of one of the diseases, his aggregate earnings would have been estimated at $245,000 had he lived a full life. However, discounting this at 4 percent to the current year, the economic loss is actually closer to $125,000. Included in this analysis are economic losses based on future earnings discounted to present value.

For the purposes of estimating benefits among diseases, it is recognized that economic loss or even death do not completely state the damage and harm caused by disease. Pain and the impact on family relationships are among the more obvious additional items. We do not know how to bring such items into this kind of analysis as yet, but it seems likely that these additional considerations argue in the same direction as the other benefits. We have no reason at this moment to

believe that such considerations would have changed the relative preferences among programs.

Some of the programs are designed to have an effect beyond the directly supported federal operations. For example, the uterine cervix program and the proposed arthritis program have major demonstration and training objectives. The training of specialists who will take the newly learned or developed technology outside the public sector is a major benefit of these programs. This analysis does not credit these programs with such benefits since data are not currently available.

Costs Other Than Health, Education, and Welfare

The costs attributed to the programs are primarily the direct Health, Education, and Welfare program costs. In the syphilis and uterine cervix programs there are additional direct costs; serological screening costs for the syphilis program and early treatment cost of the uterine cervix program. These costs are directly related to the federal decision about the size and scope of the programs. There are other expenses, costs, and benefits that may be indirectly attributed to the other programs, but since there is not a direct link between the federal decision and these costs, they have not been charged to the program. For example, the seat belt use educational program will probably cause an increased consumption of these devices. However, the program attempts to encourage people to use the belts that are already

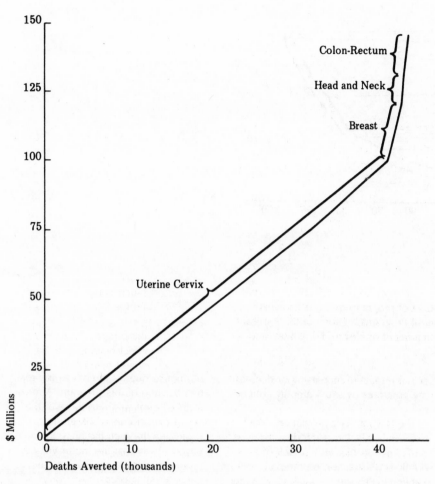

Figure 103-1
Programs for control of cancer. (Source: "Program Analysis: Cancer," Office of the Assistant Secretary for Program Coordination, U.S. Department of Health, Education, and Welfare, Washington, D.C., October 1966.)

installed in the vehicle. The cost of the belts is not attributed to this program. The benefits of a successful injury prevention program could result in lower auto insurance rates; these are not credited to the programs in this analysis.

Examples of the Results
Table 103-1 illustrates the costs of various control programs for cancer. We estimated cost per examination and the number of examinations that would be required before a case would probably be found. From this was derived the number of cases that would be found, and estimates of the cost per case found. An estimate was made of the number of deaths that could be averted by the treatment following the detection of the cancers and then we calculated the cost per death averted which

ranged from about $2,200 in the case of cervical cancer up to $40,000 to $45,000 in the case of head and neck and colon-rectum cancer.

On the vertical axis of Figure 103-1 we have plotted the program costs; including the cost of treatment in addition to the federal detection program. On the horizontal axis estimates of death averted are ordered by increase in cost per death averted in each program. Segments of the curve identified to each disease cover the extent of the program which it was estimated could be mounted in the years 1968–1972 before running into sharply increasing costs. In concept, the cervical cancer curve is cut off where costs become higher than the breast cancer program, and so on. From this analysis one might say that if there is only available $50 million, cervical cancer should get all the funds. If we have $115 million, then breast cancer control programs

look quite competitive. Head and neck and colon-rectum cancer detection programs as major control programs did not look attractive when viewed in this context. The analysts recommended that they concentrate on research and development.

The same kind of analysis for each of the five programs studied is illustrated in Figure 103-2. There seemed to be a very high potential payoff for certain educational programs in motor vehicle injury prevention (that is, trying to persuade people that "the lump you're sitting on is a seat belt, use it; don't walk in front of a car," and so on). Again, as we move up this curve, ordered by cost of averting death, we begin adding other efforts. This particular criterion, deaths averted, was not completely satisfactory. The number of fatalities attributed to arthritis, for instance, is not

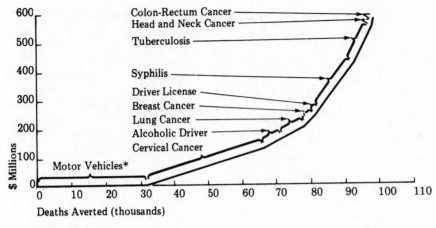

Deaths Averted (thousands)

*Seat Belt Restraint
Pedestrian Injury

Figure 103-2
Analysis of programs for selected diseases: Cost of programs and deaths averted,
1968–1972. (Source: "Selected Disease Control Programs," Office of the Assistant
Secretary for Program Coordination, U.S. Department of Health, Education, and
Welfare, Washington, D.C., September 1966.)

very impressive. Secondly, we had returned to the question: Did it matter
who died? Did it matter whether it was
a 30-year-old mother or a 40-year-old
father of a family or a 75-year-old
grandfather? On Figure 103-3 I have
used dollar savings, counting the
avoidance of death, the use of lower
cost treatment, and a crude estimate of
the average (discounted) lifetime earnings saved, as a criterion in place of
deaths averted. You will notice two
changes in results: cervical cancer and
syphilis change places in priority order,
and we are able to justify arthritis programs.

The way we developed programs
from such analyses was to use information such as this and the preceding
charts as another insight to give us an
additional feel for what were relatively
high- and low-priority programs, and
then to feed these insights into the
decision-making process, which also
considers other viewpoints, the existing
commitments, political situation, rate of
spending, and the ability to get people
moving on programs, and so on.

Some Criticisms
These studies were not greeted with
universal acclaim. Criticisms focused
on a number of problems. First, with
almost no exception, the conclusions
were based on average and approximate relationships. That is, the total
benefits were divided by the total costs.
There was little evidence of what the

actual impact of increasing or decreasing programs by small amounts might
be.

The lack of marginal data resulted
from both a lack of such data for most
programs together with a lack of economic sophistication on the part of the
Public Health Service analysts who performed the studies. As in all modeling
efforts, some common sense was required in applying the results.

Practical obstacles of existing commitments made it almost impossible to
recommend *reductions* in any program.
So the actual policy decisions dealt
with the allocation of modest incre-
ments.

In the case of oral and colon-rectum
cancers, the average cost per death
averted seemed so high that the department recommended emphasis on research and development rather than a
control program to demonstrate and extend current technology.

In cervical cancer, investigation indicated a sizable number of hospitals in
low socioeconomic areas without detection programs that would establish
these if supported by federal funds. The
unit costs for increasing the number of
hospitals seemed to be the same as for
those already in the program. Shifting
the approach to reach out for additional women in the community
would increase costs per examination

but not so high as to change the relative position of this program. At most,
it raised costs to about those of the
breast cancer control program.

Despite the seeming high potential
payoff of some of the motor vehicle
programs, there was far more uncertainty about success. As a consequence, recommendations were for
small programs with a large emphasis
on evaluation for use in future decisions. The same philosophy was
applied to the arthritis program.

What resulted then was a setting of
priorities for additional funding, based
on the analytical results, judgment
about their reliability, and other practical considerations.

A second type of criticism was concerned with the criteria, especially the
calculation of benefits. [11, 13, 14]
These were considered inadequate in
that they paid attention to economic
productivity alone and omitted other
considerations. In particular, they were
thought to discriminate against the old
who might be past employment years
and women whose earnings were relatively low. It was also feared that the
logic, if vigorously pursued, would
penalize not only health programs for
the aged, such as the newly launched
Medicare, but also programs aimed at
assisting the poor whose relative earning power is low by definition.

In actual practice, for the particular
programs studied, these concerns were

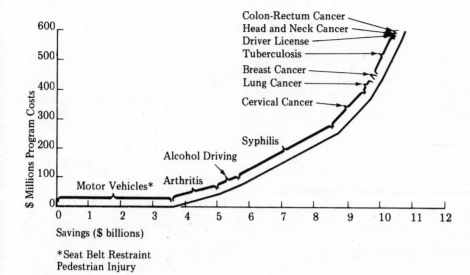

Figure 103-3
Cost of benefit: Selected diseases, 1968–1972. (Source: "Selected Disease Control Programs," Office of the Assistant Secretary for Program Coordination, U.S. Department of Health, Education, and Welfare, Washington, D.C., September 1966.)

not critical. The programs for cervical and breast cancer looked to be good despite their being for women. As for the poor, most of the programs considered, especially cervical cancer, syphilis, and tuberculosis, were aimed primarily at them, and projects were usually located to serve low-income residents.

Another type of objection was raised not against the technique of analysis but against its being done at all. Choices among diseases to be controlled and concern with costs of saving lives can be viewed as contrary to physicians' attitudes in the care of an individual patient. Prior decisions on allocations to various health problems (and such decisions are *always* made, with or without analysis) rested upon a combination of perception of the magnitude of the problem and the political strength organized to secure funding, for example the National Tuberculosis Association.

The disease control cost-benefit analyses suggest that additional considerations are very relevant. Given scarce resources (if they are not scarce, there is no allocation problem), one ought to estimate the costs of achieving improvements in health. If we can save more lives by applying resources to a small (in numbers affected) rather than a large problem, we ought to consider doing so.

A somewhat separate issue is that of the disease control approach to personal health. This is too large an issue to deal with here, but it may make more sense to develop programs of delivering comprehensive health care, including preventive services, than to maintain categorical disease programs. But that is another cost-benefit analysis.

Analysis of Kidney Disease Programs

The following year a number of additional disease control studies were performed. One of the most interesting and important was on kidney diseases [12]. This analysis was launched at a time when the public was becoming conscious of a new technique, the artificial kidney (chronic dialysis), which could preserve the life and productivity of individuals who would otherwise die of end-stage kidney disease. About 50,000 persons a year do so die. It is estimated that about 7,500 of these were "suited" by criteria of age, temperament, and the absence of other damaging illnesses for dialysis treatment. The national capacity could handle only about 900, who would remain on intermittent dialysis the rest of their lives. About 90 percent would survive from one year to the next. The operating cost of dialysis treatment in hospitals was estimated at about $15,000 per patient per year. A home

treatment approach might reduce this to about $5,000 per year.

The federal government was under great pressure to expand the national capacity, which was limited not only by the large money costs but also by shortages of trained personnel and supplies of blood. Indeed, at the same time as this analysis was being performed, an advisory group to the U.S. Bureau of the Budget was studying the problem of end-stage kidney disease. This group came in with recommendations for a massive national dialysis program.*

The HEW program analysis was somewhat more broadly charged and took a more systems-oriented approach. It concerned itself not only about the 7,500 annual candidates for dialysis but also about the other 40,000 or so who would suffer the end-stage disease but were unsuited to dialysis. If

*The Bureau of the Budget convened an expert Committee on Chronic Kidney Disease. See [6]. Klarman, Francis, and Rosenthal [10] analyzed the committee's data to explore what is the best mix of center dialysis, home dialysis, and kidney transplantations. The authors restricted their beneficiaries to those in end-stage kidney disease and concluded that transplantation is economically the most effective way to increase life expectancy of persons with chronic kidney disease, although they recognize the factors that constrain the expansion of transplantation capability.

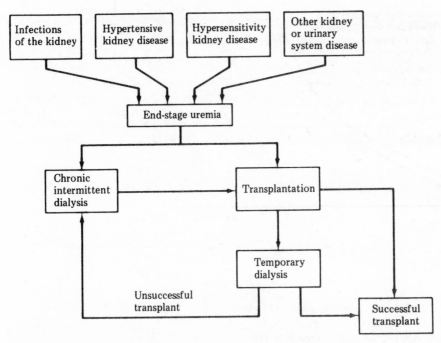

Figure 103-4
Schematic of transplant and dialysis patients. (Source: "Kidney Disease Program Analysis: A Report to the Surgeon General," Public Health Service, U.S. Department of Health, Education, and Welfare, Bethesda, Maryland, 1967.)

some way could be found to reduce the numbers falling into the pool of end-stage patients, perhaps a larger number of people could be helped. Figure 103-4 presents the classes of kidney diseases leading to end-stage disease. If these could be better prevented or treated we might keep down the number of patients requiring dialysis or transplantation.

The analysis group, therefore, examined a number of mechanisms or program components. Among these were:
1. Expanded use of existing preventive techniques.
2. Expanded use of existing diagnostic techniques.
3. Expanded use of existing treatments, including chronic dialysis, kidney transplantation and conservative management (drugs, diets, and so on).
4. Laboratory and clinical research to produce new preventive, diagnostic, therapeutic, and rehabilitative methods.
5. Increased specialized scientific medical and paramedical training to provide the manpower needed for the research and treatment attack on the kidney disease problem. This also includes continued postgraduate education to train practicing physicians in the use of the latest diagnostic and treatment modalities.

6. Increased public education to alert potential victims of kidney disease to seek medical help at the earliest possible emergence of warning signs.
7. Provision of specialized facilities not currently in existence that are essential for the execution of any of the above programs.

It must be understood that in most cases these program components are interdependent. For example, preventive techniques exist that need further research to make them maximally effective for broad application. New treatment methods are useless even if existing diagnostic techniques are not being applied in medical practice. Because of the present inadequacies of existing treatments, be they dialysis, transplantation, or conservative management, a considerable research effort is called for to increase their efficacy and economy to make them more broadly useful.

A detailed description of the analysis cannot be presented here. Costs were estimated for relevant public and private expenditures for the nationwide treatment of kidney disease. The latter includes cost of physician care, hospital care, nursing home care, and other

professional services for diagnosis and therapy of kidney diseases, as well as the cost of drugs and net insurance costs. In addition, the cost was estimated for ongoing research efforts, for demonstration, screening and detection programs, for education and training efforts and for that portion of the cost of construction of hospital and medical facilities which can be prorated to the use of patients with kidney disease.

Based on the substantive information obtained and statistical and economic data collected, estimates were made of the benefits to be gained by different approaches to the solution or amelioration of the overall national kidney disease problem at different expenditure levels of HEW funds.

Several different funding levels were assumed, and estimates were made assuming both the current state of the art and an expected advanced state of the art in 1975.

Each program consisted of a hypothetical situation where a specific level of HEW program funding was divided among a rational mix of program components (screening, diagnosis and treatment, research, training, and so on) based on the particular characteristics of the specific disease group involved, and was applied to specifically involved or particularly vulnerable groups or, as the case may be, to the entire population. The benefits accruable from these programs were then estimated and stated in terms of overall reduction of mortality, prevalence, and morbidity due to kidney disease.

Benefit indices were quantified in terms of the reduction in annual mortality, the reduction in annual morbidity (number of sick days per year) and in terms of the disease prevalence in the total population due to the specific type of kidney disorder analyzed, which would accrue because of the impact of the various program components—such as research advances, disease prevention, and improved treatment.

The analysis group originally chose to avoid estimates of the impact on economic productivity in their results, although such calculations have been made independently [7,8].

The HEW study concluded that concentration in future programs merely on the treatment of end-stage kidney disease is not likely to solve the problem of annual deaths due to irreversible uremia unless nearly unlimited funds are available for an indefinite continuation of such a program. Thus, steps must be taken to decrease the number of people who enter the irreversible fatal stage each year by a systematic prevention or treatment of the primary kidney diseases which initiate their progressive downhill course. It is obvious from the analyses in the three major kidney disease groups— infectious, hypersensitive, and hypertensive—that the otherwise inevitable annual reservoir of patients with irreversible kidney failure can be diminished considerably through vigorous programs activated to deal with each of these groups. The application of relatively minor funds in the group of infectious kidney diseases to stimulate systematic screening of high-risk groups followed by diagnosis and treatment, even within the current state of the art and without awaiting additional advances due to ongoing or future research, can bring about a significant future reduction in the number of end-stage patients. Continued and expanded research activities will be necessary to increase the percentage of

patients ultimately benefited by this approach.

In the area of hypersensitivity diseases involving the kidney there appears to be no promising mode of attack in sight except for the launching of a systematic research effort intended to increase our knowledge of the disease mechanisms involved. The promise for benefits to be derived from this type of research effort is believed to be such that it should not be postponed— particularly since any new effective treatment or prevention modality would produce major benefits in the entire field of hypersensitivity diseases, such as rheumatic heart disease, rheumatoid arthritis, and others.

In the group of hypertensive diseases of the kidney an immediate start, within the current state of the art, of screening, diagnosis, and treatment can begin to diminish the number of patients who will eventually require end-stage treatment because of their progressive renal involvement. Simultaneous research efforts are likely to make this particular portion of the overall program more effective as time goes by, in the same fashion in which the new antihypertensive drugs developed during the last ten years have succeeded in decreasing by about 50 percent the mortality due to malignant hypertension.

Thus, a meaningful federal program to reduce the annual mortality due to kidney disease and aimed at a general reduction of the prevalence of the various kidney diseases must perforce be a multifactorial one that brings into play all of the program components— research, prevention, treatment, and education. An optimally proportioned mix of these program components should be present to yield maximum benefits in overall number of lives saved. This last concept includes not only deaths avoided today but deaths to be prevented in the years to come. Needless to say, such a total program, to be effective and productive, must be aimed at all three major primary kidney diseases, as well as at end-stage kidney failure.

Figure 103-5 shows a hypothetical program mix that might come from such conclusions. Note the early emphasis on research to offset the state of the art and the growth in allocations to

the prevention and treatment of primary kidney diseases as relative allocations to dialysis are diminished.

To illustrate some of the cost and benefit calculations developed in the study, Table 103-2 summarizes the federal HEW costs. A similar tabulation was developed for all costs. As another illustration, Table 103-3 estimates the impacts of these programs on deaths, numbers of cases of each disease, and days of illness.

Maternal and Child Health Programs

HEW also did a rather different type of analysis in the field of health: a study of alternative ways of improving the health of children. The president had focused public attention on the problem of child health and expressed a desire to introduce new legislation in this field. The HEW study was an attempt to assess the state of health of the nation's children (to what extent the children have correctable health problems and in what groups in the population the problems were concentrated), and to estimate the cost and effectiveness of various kinds of programs to improve the health of children.

The study proved more difficult than anticipated. Hard information on the state of health of children is hard to come by. Surprisingly, estimates of improvement in general health attributable to medical care are almost nonexistent. It is not easy to demonstrate statistically that children who see doctors regularly are healthier than children who do not.

In regard to maternal and child care programs the stated goal was to make needed maternal and child health services available and accessible to all, in particular to all expectant mothers and children in health depressed areas. Health depressed areas could be characterized as areas with excessive infant mortality rates. There is no universal index of good or bad health among children. Two measurable areas were selected—mortality and the prevalence of chronic handicapping conditions. Over a dozen possible programs aimed at reducing these were examined. In

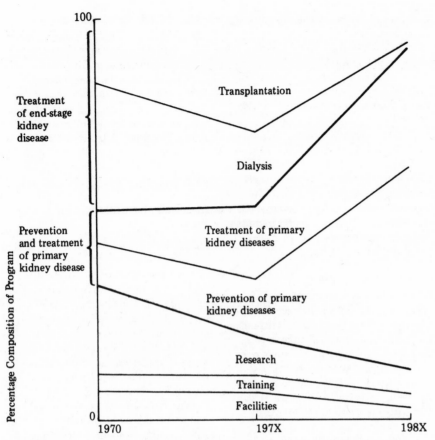

Figure 103-5
Effect of advancing state of the art on future program composition. (Percentages are wholly arbitrary and merely serve to illustrate shifting trends.) (Source: "Kidney Disease Program Analysis: A Report to the Surgeon General," Public Health Service, U.S. Department of Health, Education, and Welfare, Bethesda, Maryland, 1967.)

Table 103-4, three selected programs addressed to the problem of coverage of maternal and child health are illustrated, two of them comprehensive programs of care to expectant mothers and children. This table shows the estimated annual effects of spending the same amount of money, $10 million a year, in different ways. The analysts examined comprehensive care programs covering up to age 18 and up to age 5 with estimates based on the best assumptions derived from the literature and advisers on the probabilities of prevention of maternal deaths, premature deaths, infant deaths, and mental retardation, and handicapping conditions prevented or corrected by age 18. They also looked at a program of early case finding and assured treatment which focused on children at ages four days and again every other year until they were nine. Expending the same amounts, changing where one puts the

money yields different results. With respect to reduction of infant mortality, several other programs had higher payoffs than these. For example, a program of intensive care units for high-risk newborns was estimated annually to eliminate 367 deaths if we put all our money in that basket—it would cost about $27,000 per infant death prevented. The programs shown cost about four times that, but they do other good things too.

The HEW analysts also looked at programs with a given amount of money (Table 103-5) aimed at reducing the number of children who will have decayed and unfilled teeth by age 18. Fluoridation programs in communities which do not possess this, will, for the same amount of money, give us close to 300,000 fewer children in this condition, compared to 18 or 44 thousand fewer in other programs noted. Fluoridation looks like a very attractive program. It was so attractive that one can

assume that a program as cheap as this is not being inhibited by lack of financial support by the federal government; there are other factors at work.

One other program, additional funds on family planning, looked like a very good way not only to reduce the number of infant deaths but also the rate of infant mortality in high-risk communities.

Despite the information difficulties, several conclusions emerged clearly from the study. Two of these conclusions resulted in new legislation being requested from Congress. First, it seemed clear that a program of early case findings and treatment of handicapping conditions would have considerable payoff. It was also clear that if the large number of children who do not now have access to good medical care were to be provided with conventional pediatric services, an acute shortage of doctors would be precipitated.

Table 103-2

HEW Cost Summary ($1,000)

| Program Level | Kidney Disease Categories | | | | Total | |
	Infectious	Hypersensitivity	Hypertensive§	End-Stage	Cost	Percent
Current Expending Level*						
Diagnosis, Prevention, Treatment						
Prevention (including education & administration)	3,803	1,500	4,000	—	9,303	19.92
Diagnosis and Treatment	—	—	—	7,240	7,240	15.50
Subtotal	3,803	1,500	4,000	7,240	16,543	35.42
Research	4,000	5,250	3,800	12,100	25,150	53.85
Training	400	560	380	1,000	2,340	5.01
Facilities	1,000	170	1,000	500	2,670	5.72
Total	9,203	7,480	9,180	20,840	46,703	100.00
Intermediate Expenditure Level*						
Diagnosis, Prevention, Treatment						
Prevention (including education & administration)	5,929	3,000	8,057	—	16,986	14.47
Diagnosis and Treatment	—	—	—	30,000	30,000	25.56
Subtotal	5,929	3,000	8,057	30,000	46,986	40.03
Research	5,500	8,250	4,650	18,000	36,400	31.01
Training	750	750	500	5,500	7,500	6.39
Facilities	8,000	8,000	8,000	2,500	26,500	22.57
Total	20,179	20,000	21,207	56,000	117,386	100.00
Accelerated Expenditure Level*						
Diagnosis, Prevention, Treatment						
Prevention (including education & administration)	9,919	3,000	10,114	—	23,033	7.94
Diagnosis and Treatment	—	—	—	171,000	171,000	58.98
Subtotal	9,919	3,000	10,114	171,000	194,033	66.92
Research	6,500	10,125	5,500	24,000	46,125	15.91
Training	975	750	1,425	10,000	13,150	4.54
Facilities	10,000	10,000	11,600	5,000	36,600	12.63
Total	27,394	23,875	28,639	210,000	289,908	100.00
Accelerated Expenditure Level—1975†						
Diagnosis, Prevention, Treatment						
Prevention (including education & administration)	11,308	{ 43,000 Vaccine { 13,000	11,732	—	76,040	25.94
Diagnosis and Treatment	—	—	—	132,225	132,225	45.11
Subtotal	11,308	56,000	11,732	132,225	208,265	71.05
Research	7,410	12,450	9,500	1,500	30,860	10.53
Training	1,110	1,870	3,000	5,000	10,980	3.75
Facilities	11,400	10,000	11,600	10,000	43,000	14.67
Total	31,228	77,320	35,832	148,725	293,105	100.00

*Current state of the art
†Advanced state of the art
§Attributable to renal disease associated with hypertension.
Source: "Kidney Disease Program Analysis: A Report to the Surgeon General," Public Health Service, U.S. Department of Health, Education, and Welfare, Bethesda, Maryland, 1967.

Table 103-3
Program Benefits

Program Level	Kidney Disease Categories				
	Infectious	Hypersensitivity	Hypertensive§	End-Stage	Total
Current Expenditure Level*					
Short-Term Benefit-Reductions:					
Mortality	70 Deaths	610 Deaths	2,190 Deaths	690 Deaths	3,560 Deaths
Prevalence	3,231,260 Cases	—	27,000 Cases	—	3,258,260 Cases
Morbid Days	15,962,420 Days	—	1,802,000 Days	—	17,764,420 Days
Long-Term Benefit-Reductions:					
Annual	1,750 Deaths	—	4,330 Deaths	—	6,080 Deaths
Cumulative	25,850 Deaths	—	86,560 Deaths	—	112,410 Deaths
Intermediate Expenditure Level*					
Short-Term Benefit-Reductions:					
Mortality	70 Deaths	610 Deaths	2,270 Deaths	1,560 Deaths	4,520 Deaths
Prevalence	3,243,860 Cases	—	34,880 Cases	—	3,278,740 Cases
Morbid Days	16,273,640 Days	—	2,056,820 Days	—	18,330,460 Days
Long-Term Benefit-Reductions:					
Annual	1,770 Deaths	—	4,820 Deaths	—	6,590 Deaths
Cumulative	26,190 Deaths	—	96,300 Deaths	—	122,490 Deaths
Accelerated Expenditure Level*					
Short-Term Benefit-Reductions:					
Mortality	70 Deaths	610 Deaths	2,380 Deaths	7,675 Deaths	10,735 Deaths
Prevalence	3,292,860 Cases	—	42,750 Cases	—	3,335,610 Cases
Morbid Days	17,483,880 Days	—	2,311,340 Days	—	19,795,220 Days
Long-Term Benefit-Reductions:					
Annual	1,870 Deaths	—	4,820 Deaths	—	6,690 Deaths
Cumulative	27,480 Deaths	—	96,300 Deaths	—	123,780 Deaths
Accelerated Expenditure Level—					
Short-Term Benefit-Reductions:					
Mortality	80 Deaths	770 Deaths	9,300 Deaths	27,399 Deaths	37,549 Deaths
Prevalence	5,630,780 Cases	62,250 Cases	289,690 Cases	—	5,991,723 Cases
Morbid Days	26,064,430 Days	2,610,000 Days	5,578,860 Days	—	34,253,290 Days
Long-Term Benefit-Reductions:					
Annual	4,125 Deaths	8,610 Deaths	9,480 Deaths	—	21,090 Deaths
Cumulative	76,500 Deaths	320,000 Deaths	189,660 Deaths	—	586,160 Deaths

*Current state of the art
†Advanced state of the art
§Renal disease associated with hypertension.
Short-term benefits, reduction in *annual* mortality, and so on, when program is fully operative.
Long-term annual benefits, eventual *annual* reduction in number of cases reaching end-stage kidney disease.
Long-term cumulative benefits, sum total of long-term annual benefits.
Source: "Kidney Disease Program Analysis: A Report to the Surgeon General," Public Health Service, U.S. Department of Health, Education, and Welfare, Bethesda, Maryland, 1967.

Table 103-4

Yearly Effects per $10,000,000 Expended in Health Depressed Areas

	Comprehensive programs to age		Case finding of treatment
	18	5	0, 1, 3, 5, 7, 9
Maternal deaths prevented	1.6	3	
Premature births prevented	100–250	200–485	
Infant deaths prevented	40–60	85–120	
Mental retardation prevented	5–7	7–14	
Handicaps prevented or corrected by age 18:			
Vision problems:	350	195	3470
all amblyopia	60	119	1140
Hearing loss:	90	70	7290
all binaural	7	5	60
Other physical handicaps	200	63	1470

Source: "Maternal Child Health Care Programs," Office of the Assistant Secretary for Program Coordination, U.S. Department of Health, Education, and Welfare, Washington, D.C., 1966.

Table 103-5

Reduction in Number of 18-Year-Olds with Decayed and Unfilled Teeth per $10,000,000 Expended in Health Depressed Areas

Fluoridation	294,000
Comprehensive dental care without fluoridation	18,000
Comprehensive dental care with fluoridation	44,000

Source: "Maternal Child Health Care Programs," Office of the Assistant Secretary for Program Coordination, U.S. Department of Health, Education, and Welfare, Washington, D.C., October 1966.

Ways have to be found to use medical manpower more efficiently. The Social Security Amendments of 1967 include provision for programs of early case finding and treatment of defects and chronic conditions in children and for research and demonstration programs in the training and use of physician assistants.

Afterword

The health analyses sampled here were done in 1966 and 1967. On what has taken place since that time, I have little evidence. The only analysis published since that time was the tardy release of a cost-effectiveness analysis of family planning program components.
1968 was a year of reorganizations in the Public Health Service, and many studies aborted because staffs were shifted, and because attention was given to organizational survival, elections, transition, and defense against budget cutting. Despite the Bureau of the Budget's zeal in promoting analytical activities, their own staff's approach was to hold to incremental budgeting and cut down any new programs in the interest of fighting inflation and the Vietnam War.

The Nixon administration in its first years placed little emphasis on systematic analysis, although the planning and evaluation office was much more a center of power than it had been. Little addition was made to the analytical staff, even to replace attrition. Thus far, little has been published. This phase appears to be changing. A new assistant secretary for planning and evaluation has been appointed who is a professor of business administration with experience in systems analysis in national security. His projected deputy for health planning and evaluation is an economist with analytical experience in defense and health. The shift back to economists from lawyers should bring new efforts to carry on analytical work in greater scale and depth.

References

1. Cheit, E. F., *Injury and Recovery in the Course of Employment*, John Wiley & Sons, New York, 1961.

2. Cohen, J., "Routine Morbidity Statistics as a Tool for Defining Public Health Priorities," *Israel Journal of Medical Sciences*, May 1965, pp. 457–460.

3. Conley, R., M. Cromwell, and M. Arrill, "An Approach to Measuring the Cost of Mental Illness," *American Journal of Psychiatry*, 12416, December 1967, pp. 63–70.

4. Dublin, L. I., and A. J. Latka, *The Money Value of a Man*, The Ronald Press Company, New York, 1930.

5. Fein, R., *Economics of Mental Illness*, Basic Books, Inc., Publishers, New York, 1958.

6. Gottschalk, C. W., *Report on the Committee on Chronic Kidney Disease*, Chairman, Bureau of the Budget, Washington, D.C., September 1967.

7. Hallan, J. B., and B. S. H. Harris, III, "The Economic Cost of End-Stage Uremia," *Inquiry,* Vol. V, No. 4, December 1968, pp. 20–25.

8. Hallan, J. B., B. S. H. Harris, III, and A. V. Alhadeff, *The Economic Costs of Kidney Disease,* Research Triangle Institute, North Carolina, 1967.

9. Klarman, H. E., "Syphilis Control Programs," *Measuring Benefits of Government Investments,* edited by Robert Dorfman, The Brookings Institution, Washington, D.C., 1956, pp. 367–410.

10. Klarman, H. E., J. O'S. Francis, and G. D. Rosenthal, "Cost Effectiveness Analysis Applied to the Treatment of Chronic Renal Disease," *Medical Care,* Vol. VI, No. 1, Jan.–Feb. 1968, pp. 48–54.

11. Pan American Health Organization, *Health Planning: Problems of Concept and Method,* Scientific Publication No. 111, April 1965, see especially pp. 4–5.

12. Rice, D. P., *Estimating the Cost of Illness,* Public Health Service Publication 947-6, Washington, D.C., May 1966.

13. Rice, D. P., "Measurement and Application of Illness Costs," *Public Health Reports,* February 1969, pp. 95–101.

14. Schelling, T. C., "The Life You Save May Be Your Own," *Problems in Public Expenditure Analysis,* edited by Samuel B. Chase, Jr., The Brookings Institution, Washington, D.C., 1968, pp. 127–176.

15. U.S. Department of Health, Education, and Welfare, Office of Assistant Secretary for Program Coordination, *Motor Vehicle Injury Prevention Program,* August 1966.

16. U.S. Department of Health, Education, and Welfare, Office of Assistant Secretary for Program Coordination, *Arthritis,* September 1966.

17. U.S. Department of Health, Education, and Welfare, Office of Assistant Secretary for Program Coordination, *Selected Disease Control Programs,* September 1966.

18. U.S. Department of Health, Education, and Welfare, Office of Assistant Secretary for Program Coordination, *Cancer,* October 1966.

19. U.S. Department of Health, Education, and Welfare, Office of the Assistant Secretary for Planning and Evaluation, *Kidney Disease,* December 1967.

20. U.S. Department of Health, Education, and Welfare, *Economic Costs of Cardiovascular Diseases and Cancer, 1962,* Public Health Service Publication 947–5, Washington, D.C., May 1965.

21. Weisbrod, B. A., *Economics of Public Health: Measuring the Economic Impact of Diseases,* University of Pennsylvania Press, Philadelphia, 1961.

22. Winslow, C. E. A., *The Cost of Sickness and the Price of Health,* World Health Organization, Geneva, Switzerland, 1951.

Illustrative Cases

As chairman of a committee on health care of the U.S. Congress, you are responsible for drafting a bill to provide health services to the population. Some of your constituents are urging you to write a bill that entitles all Americans to receive any benefit that medical art and science can confer on them. Others ask you to draft a bill that gives a "limited package" of health-care benefits to all citizens. Still other constituents urge that you make this "limited package" of benefits available only to groups in the population whose members generally cannot afford to adequately insure themselves against illness, such as the aged, unemployed, and low-income families or individuals. And a fourth block of constituents are against any direct government subsidy for health care and insist that you press the Congress to allow the free marketplace and charitable institutions to provide the means to solve the nation's health-care problems.

1. Which of these positions would you favor, and what are the moral grounds on which you base your judgment?
2. If you choose either of the two "limited-package" approaches, how would you define the boundaries of the health-care services you would make available?
3. Can you identify other public policy positions that offer a more satisfactory moral solution to the distribution of health services?

The private yacht *Mignonette* sailed from Southampton on May 19, 1884, bound for Sydney, Australia, where it was to be delivered to its owner. There were four persons aboard, all members of the crew: Dudley, the captain; Stephens, mate; Brooks, seaman; and Parker, a 17-year-old cabin boy and apprentice seaman. The yacht went down in the South Atlantic and all put off in a 13-foot lifeboat. After twenty days in the boat, during which they had no fresh water except rainwater and during the last eight of which they had no food, Dudley, with Stephens' assent, killed the boy. Brooks objected. Thereafter all three fed on the body of the boy for four days. On the fifth day they were rescued. According to the jury's verdict, there was no likelihood that any of them would have survived unless one were killed and eaten, and it so appeared to the men.

1. Consider the different alternatives of picking out one member, as was done; all risking death together; or drawing lots to decide who should be sacrificed.
2. In the last alternative, should all have been forced to participate, even though one or two might not wish to?
3. Would the case be different if one member had navigational experience indispensable to the group?

A 5-year-old boy has an IQ below 40. He also has, among other defects, a heart condition that causes excessive blood flow into the lungs. The increased pressure produced by this flow damages the blood vessels in the lungs and diminishes the intake of oxygen into the blood. These circumstances carry a poor prognosis and frequently cause early death. Without surgery this boy would survive less than a year. Open-heart surgery at this early age is extremely dangerous, but a procedure known as pulmonary artery banding is feasible: it reduces the blood flow to the lungs and prevents vessel damage. This operation is effective for approximately five to ten years, allowing time for a child to develop to an age when open-heart surgery can take place. However, in the case of this child, the other defects he has make it unlikely that he would survive more than a few years even after such surgery.

In your opinion, would the decision of whether to proceed with pulmonary artery banding be affected by the following factors?

1. Scarce medical resources.
2. The fact that the child's IQ is extremely low.
3. The fact that he is not likely to live to his teens.
4. The cost to society and to his family of maintaining him.

At an infant intensive-care unit, the conclusion has been reached that a particular child, John, will in all likelihood die in the next few days. Although prognosis is sometimes difficult to establish with infants less than a year old, the physician in charge and his team are virtually certain that John's massive brain hemorrhage will be fatal. At this very time, an urgent call has come to the intensive care unit to admit another infant as soon as possible. The physician in charge of John and of the whole infant intensive-care unit would like to take John off the respirator, now needed for someone else. But John's parents would like every effort to be made to save their son. The hospital where this infant intensive-care unit is located is known to have the best care for infants available within the area they serve.

1. What moral issues are raised for the physician in charge of the infant judged to be dying?
2. What alternatives do you see for this physician in this particular case and for the policy of the infant intensive-care unit as a whole?
3. What do you think the physician in charge should do and what policy should be adopted by the intensive-care unit?

Appendix

California Natural Death Act

Approved by Governor September 30, 1976. Filed with Secretary of State September 30, 1976.

The people of the State of California do enact as follows:

Section 1

Chapter 3.9 (commencing with Section 7185) is added to Part 1 of Division 7 of the Health and Safety Code, to read:

7185. This act shall be known and may be cited as the Natural Death Act.

7186. The Legislature finds that adult persons have the fundamental right to control the decisions relating to the rendering of their own medical care, including the decision to have life-sustaining procedures withheld or withdrawn in instances of a terminal condition.

The Legislature further finds that modern medical technology has made possible the artificial prolongation of human life beyond natural limits.

The Legislature further finds that, in the interest of protecting individual autonomy, such prolongation of life for persons with a terminal condition may cause loss of patient dignity and unnecessary pain and suffering, while providing nothing medically necessary or beneficial to the patient.

The Legislature further finds that there exists considerable uncertainty in the medical and legal professions as to the legality of terminating the use or application of life-sustaining procedures where the patient has voluntarily and in sound mind evidenced a desire that such procedures be withheld or withdrawn.

In recognition of the dignity and privacy which patients have a right to expect, the Legislature hereby declares that the laws of the State of California shall recognize the right of an adult person to make a written directive instructing his physician to withhold or withdraw life-sustaining procedures in the event of a terminal condition.

7187. The following definitions shall govern the construction of this chapter:

(a) "Attending physician" means the physician selected by, or assigned to, the patient who has primary responsibility for the treatment and care of the patient.

(b) "Directive" means a written document voluntarily executed by the declarant in accordance with the requirements of Section 7188. The directive, or a copy of the directive, shall be made part of the patient's medical records.

(c) "Life-sustaining procedure" means any medical procedure or intervention which utilizes mechanical or other artificial means to sustain, restore, or supplant a vital function, which, when applied to a qualified patient, would serve only to artificially prolong the moment of death and where, in the judgment of the attending physician, death is imminent whether or not such procedures are utilized. "Life-sustaining procedure" shall not include the administration of medication or the performance of any medical procedure deemed necessary to alleviate pain.

(d) "Physician" means a physician and surgeon licensed by the Board of Medical Quality Assurance or the Board of Osteopathic Examiners.

(e) "Qualified patient" means a patient diagnosed and certified in writing to be afflicted with a terminal condition by two physicians, one of whom shall be the attending physician, who have personally examined the patient.

(f) "Terminal condition" means an incurable condition caused by injury, disease, or illness, which, regardless of the application of life-sustaining procedures, would, within reasonable medical judgment, produce death, and where the application of life-sustaining procedures serve only to postpone the moment of death of the patient.

7188. Any adult person may execute a directive directing the withholding or withdrawal of life-sustaining procedures in a terminal condition. The directive shall be signed by the declarant in the presence of two witnesses not related to the declarant by blood or marriage and who would not be entitled to any portion of the estate of the declarant upon his decease under any will of the declarant or codicil thereto then existing or, at the time of the directive, by operation of law then existing. In addition, a witness to a directive shall not be the attending physician, an employee of the attending physician or a health facility in which the declarant is a patient, or any person who has a claim against any portion of the estate of the declarant upon his decease at the time of the execution of the directive. The directive shall be in the following form:

Directive to Physicians

Directive made this _____ day of _____ (month, year).

I _____, being of sound mind, willfully, and voluntarily make known my desire that my life shall not be artificially prolonged under the circumstances set forth below, do hereby declare:

1. If at any time I should have an incurable injury, disease, or illness certified to be a terminal condition by two physicians, and where the application of life-sustaining procedures would serve only to artificially prolong the moment of my death and where my physician determines that my death is imminent whether or not life sustaining procedures are utilized, I direct that such procedures be withheld or withdrawn, and that I be permitted to die naturally.

2. In the absence of my ability to give directions regarding the use of such life-sustaining procedures, it is my intention that this directive shall be honored by my family and physician(s) as the final expression of my legal right to refuse medical or surgical treatment and accept the consequences from such refusal.

3. If I have been diagnosed as pregnant and that diagnosis is known to my physician, this directive shall have no force or effect during the course of my pregnancy.

4. I have been diagnosed and notified at least 14 days ago as having a terminal condition by _____, M.D., whose address is _____, and whose telephone number is _____. I understand that if I have not filled in the physician's name and address, it shall be presumed that I did not have a terminal condition when I made out this directive.

5. This directive shall have no force or effect five years from the date filled in above.

6. I understand the full import of this directive and I am emotionally and mentally competent to make this directive.

Signed:
City, County and State of Residence:

The declarant has been personally known to me and I believe him or her to be of sound mind.

Witness:
Witness:

7188.5. A directive shall have no force or effect if the declarant is a patient in a skilled nursing facility as defined in subdivision (c) of Section 1250

at the time the directive is executed unless one of the two witnesses to the directive is a patient advocate or ombudsman as may be designated by the State Department of Aging for this purpose pursuant to any other applicable provision of law. The patient advocate or ombudsman shall have the same qualifications as a witness under Section 7188.

The intent of this section is to recognize that some patients in skilled nursing facilities may be so insulated from a voluntary decisionmaking role, by virtue of the custodial nature of their care, as to require special assurance that they are capable of willfully and voluntarily executing a directive.

7189. (a) A directive may be revoked at any time by the declarant, without regard to his mental state or competency, by any of the following methods:

(1) By being canceled, defaced, obliterated, or burnt, torn, or otherwise destroyed by the declarant or by some person in his presence and by his direction.

(2) By a written revocation of the declarant expressing his intent to revoke, signed and dated by the declarant. Such revocation shall become effective only upon communication to the attending physician by the declarant or by a person acting on behalf of the declarant. The attending physician shall record in the patient's medical record the time and date when he received notification of the written revocation.

(3) By a verbal expression by the declarant of his intent to revoke the directive. Such revocation shall become effective only upon communication to the attending physician by the declarant or by a person acting on behalf of the declarant. The attending physician shall record in the patient's medical record the time, date, and place of the revocation and the time, date, and place, if different, of when he received notification of the revocation.

(b) There shall be no criminal or civil liability on the part of any person for failure to act upon a revocation made pursuant to this section unless that person has actual knowledge of the revocation.

7189.5. A directive shall be effective for five years from the date of execution thereof unless sooner revoked in a manner prescribed in Section 7189.

Nothing in this chapter shall be construed to prevent a declarant from reexecuting a directive at any time in accordance with the formalities of Section 7188, including reexecution subsequent to a diagnosis of a terminal condition. If the declarant has executed more than one directive, such time shall be determined from the date of execution of the last directive known to the attending physician. If the declarant becomes comatose or is rendered incapable of communicating with the attending physician, the directive shall remain in effect for the duration of the comatose condition or until such time as the declarant's condition renders him or her able to communicate with the attending physician.

7190. No physician or health facility which, acting in accordance with the requirements of this chapter, causes the withholding or withdrawal of life-sustaining procedures from a qualified patient, shall be subject to civil liability therefrom. No licensed health professional, acting under the direction of a physician, who participates in the withholding or withdrawal of life-sustaining procedures in accordance with the provisions of this chapter shall be subject to any civil liability. No physician, or licensed health professional acting under the direction of a physician, who participates in the withholding or withdrawal of life-sustaining procedures in accordance with the provisions of this chapter shall be guilty of any criminal act or of unprofessional conduct.

7191. (a) Prior to effecting a withholding or withdrawal of life-sustaining procedures from a qualified patient pursuant to the directive, the attending physician shall determine that the directive complies with Section 7188, and, if the patient is mentally competent, that the directive and all steps proposed by the attending physician to be undertaken are in accord with the desires of the qualified patient.

(b) If the declarant was a qualified patient at least 14 days prior to executing or reexecuting the directive, the directive shall be conclusively presumed, unless revoked, to be the directions of the patient regarding the withholding or withdrawal of life-sustaining procedures. No physician, and no licensed health professional acting under the direction of a physician, shall be criminally or civilly liable for failing to effectuate the directive of the qualified patient pursuant to this subdivision. A failure by a physician to effectuate the directive of a qualified patient pursuant to this division shall constitute unprofessional conduct if the physician refuses to make the necessary arrangements, or fails to take the necessary steps, to effect the transfer of the qualified patient to another physician who will effectuate the directive of the qualified patient.

(c) If the declarant becomes a qualified patient subsequent to executing the directive, and has not subsequently reexecuted the directive, the attending physician may give weight to the directive as evidence of the patient's directions regarding the withholding or withdrawal of life-sustaining procedures and may consider other factors, such as information from the affected family or the nature of the patient's illness, injury, or disease, in determining whether the totality of circumstances known to the attending physician justify effectuating the directive. No physician, and no licensed health professional acting under the direction of a physician, shall be criminally or civilly liable for failing to effectuate the directive of the qualified patient pursuant to this subdivision.

7192. (a) The withholding or withdrawal of life-sustaining procedures from a qualified patient in accordance with the provisions of this chapter shall not, for any purpose, constitute a suicide.

(b) The making of a directive pursuant to Section 7188 shall not restrict, inhibit, or impair in any manner the sale, procurement, or issuance of any policy of life insurance, nor shall it be deemed to modify the terms of an existing policy of life insurance. No policy of life insurance shall be legally impaired or invalidated in any manner by the withholding or withdrawal of life-sustaining procedures from an insured qualified patient, notwithstanding any term of the policy to the contrary.

(c) No physician, health facility, or other health provider, and no health care service plan, insurer issuing disability insurance, self-insured employee welfare benefit plan, or nonprofit hospital service plan, shall require any person to execute a directive as a condition for being insured for, or receiving, health care services.

7193. Nothing in this chapter shall impair or supersede any legal right or legal responsibility which any person may have to effect the withholding or withdrawal of life-sustaining procedures in any lawful manner. In such respect the provisions of this chapter are cumulative.

7194. Any person who willfully conceals, cancels, defaces, obliterates, or damages the directive of another without such declarant's consent shall be guilty of a misdemeanor. Any person who, except where justified or excused by law, falsifies or forges the directive of another, or willfully conceals or withholds personal knowledge of a revocation as provided in Section 7189, with the intent to cause a withholding or withdrawal of life-sustaining procedures contrary to the wishes of the declarant, and thereby, because of any such act, directly causes life-sustaining procedures to be withheld or withdrawn and death to thereby be hastened, shall be subject to prosecution for unlawful homicide as provided in Chapter 1 (commencing with Section 187) of Title 8 of Part 1 of the Penal Code.

7195. Nothing in this chapter shall be construed to condone, authorize, or approve mercy killing, or to permit any affirmative or deliberate act or omission to end life other than to permit the natural process of dying as provided in this chapter.

Section 2

If any provision of this act or the application thereof to any person or circumstances is held invalid, such invalidity shall not affect other provisions or applications of the act which can be given effect without the invalid provisions or application, and to this end the provisions of this act are severable.

Section 3

Notwithstanding Section 2231 of the Revenue and Taxation Code, there shall be no reimbursement pursuant to this section nor shall there by any appropriation made by this act because the Legislature recognizes that during any legislative session a variety of changes to laws relating to crimes and infractions may cause both increased and decreased costs to local government entities and school districts which, in the aggregate, do not result in significant identifiable cost changes.

Bibliographical Note

Each year, the Institute of Society, Ethics, and the Life Sciences at Hastings-on-Hudson, New York, publishes a medical ethics bibliography that is partially annotated. Also valuable is the *Bibliography of Bioethics*, edited by LeRoy Walters, published yearly under the auspices of the Kennedy Center for Bioethics at Georgetown University, Washington, D.C.

Some journals are directly concerned with medical ethics: *Hastings Center Report*, *Journal of Medicine and Philosophy*, *Journal of Medical Ethics*, *Man and Medicine: The Journal of Values and Ethics in Health Care*, and the *Linacre Quarterly*. Articles on medical ethics may often be found in *Philosophy and Public Affairs*, the *New England Journal of Medicine*, the *Journal of Religious Ethics*, and the *American Journal of Law and Medicine*.

An *Encyclopedia of Bioethics* is forthcoming from the Kennedy Center for Bioethics at Georgetown University.

Index